WR 175 RIE   £28.99

Fisher's CONTACT DERMATITIS 6

Robert L. Rietschel, MD

Professor of Clinical Medicine
University of Arizona College of Medicine
Chief, Dermatology Service
Southern Arizona VA Health Care System
Tucson, Arizona

Joseph F. Fowler, Jr, MD

Clinical Professor of Dermatology
Director of Occupational Dermatology
University of Louisville School of Medicine
Louisville, Kentucky

2008
BC Decker Inc
Hamilton

BC Decker Inc
P.O. Box 620, L.C.D. 1
Hamilton, Ontario L8N 3K7
Tel: 905-522-7017; 800-568-7281
Fax: 905-522-7839; 888-311-4987
E-mail: info@bcdecker.com
www.bcdecker.com

ISBN 978-1-55009-378-0
Printed in India by Ajanta Offset & Packaging Ltd.
Production Editor: Margaret Holmes
Typesetter: Integra
Cover Design: Alex Wheldon

Sales & Distribution

United States
BC Decker Inc
P.O. Box 785
Lewiston, NY 14092-0785
Tel: 905-522-7017; 800-568-7281
Fax: 905-522-7839; 888-311-4987
E-mail: info@bcdecker.com
www.bcdecker.com

Canada
McGraw-Hill Ryerson Education
Customer Care
300 Water Street
Whitby, Ontario, L1N 9B6
Tel: 1-800-565-5758
Fax: 1-800-463-5885

Foreign Rights
John Scott & Company
International Publishers' Agency
P.O. Box 878
Kimberton, PA 19442
Tel: 610-827-1640
Fax: 610-827-1671
E-mail: jsco@voicenet.com

Japan
United Publishers Services Limited
1-32-5 Higashi-Shinagawa
Shinagawa-Ku, Tokyo 140-0002
Tel: 03 5479 7251
Fax: 03 5479 7307

UK, Europe, Middle East
McGraw-Hill Education
Shoppenhangers Road
Maidenhead
Berkshire, England SL6 2QL
Tel: 44-0-1628-502500
Fax: 44-0-1628-635895
www.mcgraw-hill.co.uk

*Singapore, Malaysia, Thailand,
Philippines, Indonesia, Vietnam,
Pacific Rim, Korea*
McGraw-Hill Education
60 Tuas Basin Link
Singapore 638775
Tel: 65-6863-1580
Fax: 65-6862-3354

Australia, New Zealand
McGraw-Hill Australia
Pty Ltd Level 2, 82 Waterloo Road
North Ryde, NSW, 2113 Australia
Customer Service Australia
Phone: +61 (2) 9900 1800
Fax: +61 (2) 9900 1980
Email: cservice_sydney@mcgraw-hill.com

Customer Service New Zealand
Tel (Free): +64 (0) 800 449 312
Fax (Free): +64 (0) 800 449 318
Email: cservice@mcgraw-hill.co.nz

Mexico and Central America
ETM SA de CV
Calle de Tula 59
Colonia Condesa
06140 Mexico DF, Mexico
Tel: 52-5-5553-6657
Fax: 52-5-5211-8468
E-mail: editoresdetextosmex@prodigy.net.mx

Brazil
Tecmedd Importadora E Distribuidora De
Livros Ltda.
Avenida Maurílio Biagi, 2850
City Ribeirão, Ribeirão Preto – SP – Brasil
CEP: 14021-000
Tel: 0800 992236
Fax: (16) 3993-9000
E-mail: tecmedd@tecmedd.com.br

India, Bangladesh, Pakistan, Sri Lanka
CBS Publishers & Distributors
4596/1A-11, Darya Ganj
New Delhi-2, India
Tel: 232 71632
Fax: 232 76712
E-mail: cbspubs@vsnl.com

To Alex and his inspiration, Lillian.
You are both missed.
Alex, your wit and wisdom live on in the work you created.

To Connie, Eric, and Penny, a wonderful supportive family.

To Lynn, for all her love, friendship and support.

CONTENTS

Preface

PREFACE

This is the first revision of Alexander Fisher's book that the original author will not see. We mourn Dr. Fisher's passing and in this sixth edition we hope to honor his memory. When we took over this task with the production of the fourth edition, Dr. Fisher remarked that we had taken a classic and turned it into a masterpiece. While his very kind words might have been something of an overstatement, his description of this book as a classic remains appropriate and we have endeavored to maintain that tradition. Much of the history of contact dermatitis remains in these pages, and we have changed Dr. Fisher's original wording as little as possible.

The organization of the book has been slightly modified in this edition. We have removed the Aquatic Dermatoses chapter (since it was less an account of contact dermatitis than a reflection of one of Dr. Fisher's personal interests), and some chapters have been combined in an effort to eliminate redundancy. A substantial amount of new information has been added and is to be found in the body of the text rather than in tables. The "boxes" that were part of the first five editions have been replaced by executive summaries to the chapters, since we felt that the boxes were redundant to the text and not as complete. In addition, a mini-atlas has been added to highlight some of the principles noted in various chapters.

It is inevitable that a computer search will turn up items that we have failed to include. However, a computer search will not provide the context that this classic attempts to provide. Most of what is "out there" has found a place "in here." We hope you will find this edition a useful alternative to spending valuable hours at your computer in search of relevant information on contact dermatitis.

Robert L. Rietschel, MD
Joseph F. Fowler, Jr, MD

GLOSSARY OF COMMONLY USED ABBREVIATIONS

ACD	allergic contact dermatitis
acet	acetone
alc	alcohol
aq	aqueous
as is	undiluted
BP	balsam of Peru (now called *Myroxylon pereirae*)
chlor	chloroform
co	castor oil
eth	ethanol
FDA	Food and Drug Administration
ICD	irritant contact dermatitis
ICU	immunologic contact urticaria
MP	*Myroxylon pereirae*
pdr	powder
NACDG	North American Contact Dermatitis Group
oo	olive oil
pet	petrolatum
PPDA	paraphenylediamine
RAST	radioallergosorbent test
sat	saturated
ROAT	repeated open application test

CHAPTER 1

PATHOGENESIS OF ALLERGIC CONTACT HYPERSENSITIVITY

EXECUTIVE SUMMARY

Allergic contact dermatitis is a T cell-driven process that begins when haptens come into contact with Langerhans cells in the epidermis. When properly stimulated, Langerhans cells migrate to regional lymph nodes. Here, antigen is processed by T lymphocytes, which become specifically reactive to the presented allergen. The T cells that respond when the individual is re-exposed to the allergen are now known as CD8+T cells and are under the control of subsets of CD4+ T cells. A role has also been proposed for B cell participation in allergic contact dermatitis, and an animal model devoid of T and B cells has been found to demonstrate allergic contact dermatitis using natural killer cells.

Neurologic factors have also been found to play an important role in allergic contact dermatitis. Destroying the nerve fibers to draining lymph nodes can abolish the reaction. Neuropeptides Substance P, neurokinin A, and calcitonin gene-related peptide and their receptors all play regulatory roles. T regulatory cells play a critical role in downregulating the contact sensitivity reaction. IL-10 production by these cells is one of the mechanisms. A cell-to-cell, contact-dependent, cytokine-independent mechanism is also found. Skin memory of contact dermatitis may be due to a chemokine (CCL27) that causes retention of a specific type of T cell in the skin site where the allergen was encountered.

Jadassohn,[1] who described contact allergy to mercury in 1895, can be considered the "father" of contact dermatitis. Prior to this time, and indeed for some years thereafter, contact hypersensitivity was essentially unknown except by a few workers in dermatology.[2–5] In 1927, Landsteiner[6] published studies regarding antigens containing "simple chemical compounds." Sulzberger,[7] in 1929, published one of the earliest American works on the subject.

Another important development was the recognition that a close similarity existed between contact allergy and delayed-type hypersensitivity to microbial antigens, after Landsteiner and Chase published their findings that both contact allergy to small molecular allergens and delayed-type hypersensitivity to microbial antigens could be passively transferred with lymphocytes in guinea pigs.[8,9] As a matter of fact, this finding precipitated an era in which many investigators considered contact allergy and microbial allergy to be based on identical mechanisms. Despite many important fundamental similarities, however, certain differences were always evident between these forms of allergy.[10,11]

Teleologically, one assumes that cell-mediated hypersensitivity serves the purpose of defending the body against foreign antigens, like those derived from bacteria, fungi, viruses, and foreign tissues, and against autologous tumor antigens and other undesirable autologous antigens. However, although cell-mediated hypersensitivity to these antigens in general helps to preserve the body's integrity, allergic-contact hypersensitivity to small molecular allergens (which, in fact, is hypersensitivity to autologous proteins made "foreign" by complexing with small molecular compounds) is damaging to the skin. In a sense, therefore, contact allergy can be considered a deviant form of cell-mediated hypersensitivity.

Overview

Contact allergens almost invariably are small-molecule substances of less than 500 daltons (Da).[12] Because of their small size, they penetrate the skin barrier, which is relatively impermeable under normal circumstances to large molecules, and reach the living layers of the skin. In order to induce contact allergy, these substances must be presented by antigen-presenting cells, principally epidermal

Langerhans cells (LCs), and other dendritic cells, to T lymphocytes in an immunologically effective "processed" form. The effector cells, which mediate allergic contact hypersensitivity, are descendants of these T lymphocytes.

In order to interact with antigen presented by the LCs in the course of both induction of hypersensitivity and elicitation of a reaction, the T lymphocytes must possess surface receptors ("idiotypes") that are complementary to the physicochemical features of that antigen. Furthermore, the antigen-presenting cells must bear immune response–associated antigens for which the T lymphocytes possess receptors. The T lymphocytes must also be activated by interleukin-1 (IL-1), which is released from LCs and keratinocytes.

Under ordinary conditions, exposure to contact allergens sets in motion two competing mechanisms, the one mediated by effector T lymphocytes and leading to a state of hypersensitivity that becomes clinically manifest as an eczematous skin reaction. The other is mediated by suppressor cells and leads to relative or complete tolerance of the allergen. The state of reactivity of the skin at any particular time and site is principally the result of the existing balance between the effector and the suppressor cells present.

Contact Allergens

Normally, only small molecular compounds (<500 Da) can penetrate through the horny layer into the living layers of the epidermis. Yet, in order to induce and elicit contact allergy, an antigen with a molecular weight of at least 5,000 Da is required. Antigenicity is accomplished by the conjugation of small molecules with autologous proteins present in the skin. Other requirements for antigenicity are the appropriate number of antigenic determinants and the appropriate tertiary structural features in the resulting molecule. Activation of the innate immune response is also part of this process. Sensitization is more easily induced when the skin barrier is compromised by dermatitis or ulceration.

It was originally thought that such conjugates were formed with the fibrous proteins of prokeratins, keratins, procollagens and collagens, epidermal cell membranes, or soluble tissue, and serum proteins. Although a role for these conjugates cannot be dismissed, it now appears that conjugation takes place mainly with cell membrane proteins in the course of "processing" by the antigen-presenting LCs.

Linkage to the protein moiety is frequently covalent; for example, the epsilon-amino group of lysine and the sulfhydryl groups of cystine and cysteine have been suggested as binding sites for certain allergens. In many instances, however, it is difficult to predict the sensitizing capacity of a substance on the basis of its chemical structure. In the past it has not been adequately emphasized that some of the most common contact allergens, like nickel, chromates, and other metal salts, do not form covalent bonds with proteins; the fact that they can combine in some form with components of LCs provides a reasonable explanation for their allergenicity.[13] Current research suggests that a "successful" contact allergen causes an increase in the size of LCs along with an increase of Ia (major histocompatibility complex) molecules on the LC surfaces. In addition, the allergen may induce LC migration to lymph nodes.[14] Langerhans cells migrate out of the epidermis not only when exposed to allergens, but also when exposed to toxic concentrations of irritants.[15]

GENETIC FACTORS

Susceptibility to the development of contact sensitivity is genetically controlled. The mode of inheritance in guinea pigs is autosomal and irregularly dominant.[16] Different strains of guinea pigs can make an immune response to different contact allergens. For example, one strain responds to potassium dichromate and beryllium fluoride, but not to mercuric chloride, whereas another strain makes a response to mercuric chloride but responds poorly to potassium dichromate and beryllium fluoride.[17] These differences apparently relate to different hapten–amino acid linkages.

Other studies have shown that ultraviolet-B (UVB) exposure inhibits contact sensitivity in certain strains of mice, but not in other genetically distinct strains.[18,19] It has been postulated that tumor necrosis factor-a (TNF-a) may be an important mediator of these effects.[20]

Studies of the mode of inheritance in humans are still inadequate, but the very limited available data suggest that here also genetic factors control susceptibility to sensitization to particular allergens.[21] A number of European studies have compared the frequency of human leucocyte antigens (HLA) antigens in patients with allergic contact dermatitis (ACD), usually to nickel, with local controls.[22–24] Several studies have purported to show increased occurrence of one or two HLA types in patients, but for reasons that are obscure, no two studies have found the same HLA antigen to be increased in a statistically significant fashion. Among the antigens reported to be increased to some degree are HLA-B7, -B21, -B12, -Bw22, -B35, -B40, -DR4, and -DRw6. Because the expression of the HLA antigen system is essential for the development of ACD, it is tempting to search for HLA-ACD associations.

Gene products of the TAP-1 and TAP-2 genes (transporter associated with antigen processing) are involved in antigen processing. A Finnish study showed that nickel-allergic persons were much more likely to possess the TAP-2B gene allele and much less likely to be TAP-2C positive than nonallergic subjects.[25] This study further supports the likelihood of inborn genetic factors regulating one's ability to develop contact allergy.

In a search for a genetic basis for susceptibility to contact allergy, a study was done looking at polymorphisms in cytokine genes. Individuals with multiple contact allergens were compared to individuals without eczema or contact allergy. Carriers of TNFA-308*1/2(*GA) and TNFA-308*2.2(*A/A), which are tumor necrosis factor alpha genes, were more likely to be polysensitized.[26] Another role for genetic polymorphism in contact dermatitis in humans has been identified. Susceptibility to *p*-phenylenediamine sensitization was related to genotype coding for rapid acetylation in 52.9% of patients with contact dermatitis and 37% of control subjects. The frequency of the NAT2*4 allele and NAT2*4/*4 genotype, which code for rapid acetylation, was significantly higher in the patients with contact dermatitis (p= 0.003).[27]

ANTIGEN PRESENTATION

It is not possible for T lymphocytes to interact directly with the contact antigen even when they possess the appropriate surface receptors for that antigen. The antigen must first be "processed," and then must be presented in suitable form on the surface of LCs[28] that bear immune response–associated surface antigens (HLA-DR in humans; called Ia in mice) for which the T lymphocytes have the specific receptors. To induce contact allergy, the allergen is displayed in close association with these antigens or perhaps becomes conjugated with them.[29,30] Random T lymphocytes circulating through the epidermis, dermis, dermal lymphatics, and regional lymph nodes can become apposed to the LCs, but only T lymphocytes, which have the complementary receptors for the contact antigen that is being presented, can become irreversibly apposed.

LANGERHANS CELLS

Epidermal LCs have properties that make them particularly well suited to serve the function of presenting contact allergens. They have a pronounced capacity to bind small molecular compounds, among them well-recognized contact allergens, to their surface.[13] Their capacity to do this binding is greater than that of peripheral blood macrophages.[31] Similar antigen-presenting cells are found in the spleen and lymph nodes. These and LCs are all derived from bone marrow precursors.
Antigen-processing capacity of LCs involves, first, plasma membrane changes with endocytosis of the antigen and digestion of proteins to active peptides in acidic organelles.[32,33] Birbeck granule expression increases at this

time, apparently in relation to antigen processing. As processing continues, LC morphology changes to a more dendritic cell type, which is associated with enhanced antigen-presenting capacity.

Experimental proof of the antigen-presenting functions of LCs derives from studies in inbred guinea pigs and mice and from the demonstration in mice that antigen presentation cannot take place in the absence of adequate numbers of functionally intact LCs at sites of exposure to the allergen.[34]

Irradiation with UVB or application of a topical corticosteroid reduces the density of LCs in skin and inhibits induction of contact sensitization.[14] In vitro cyclosporine A inhibits the antigen-presenting capability of LCs, apparently without affecting cell surface expression of Ia molecules.[35]

Induction of Contact Allergy

Shortly after contact with an allergen, various cytokines are released that enhance the development of contact sensitivity.[36] Interleukin-1B (IL-1B) increases the level of intercellular adhesive molecule (ICAM-1). Other molecules are then expressed on the LC surface, which facilitates interaction with CD4+ T cells.

Within 24 hours of antigen application, LCs migrate to regional lymph nodes. There they present the antigen to compatible T lymphocytes. The T lymphocytes must bear receptors for complementary major histocompatibility complex protein as well as receptors for the contact allergen. Ultrastructural observations indicate that the contact allergens reside on the surfaces of LCs as well as in the intracytoplasmic Birbeck granules.[37] In the lymph nodes, certain T lymphocytes become physically apposed to the LCs facilitating transfer of antigen. These T cells are CD4+ and CD45RA+ and may be referred to as Th-0 cells.[38] Other cytokines are important at this stage of sensitization, including IL-6, TGF-B, and IL-12. Lack of IL-12 can prevent development of Th-1 cells, which cause ACD, and therefore may allow development of tolerance to the particular allergen.[39] Through clonal proliferation, a subset of T lymphocytes is produced that will be capable of responding to the particular antigen when future exposure occurs. It will be 7 to 10 days before there are sufficient numbers of these specific T lymphocytes to cause contact dermatitis. After that time, elicitation of contact dermatitis, by patch test or routine exposure, is possible.

EFFECTOR AND SUPPRESSOR CELLS

As noted previously, exposure of individuals who are genetically susceptible to sensitization to a specific contact allergen sets in motion two competing mechanisms, namely, allergic sensitization mediated by effector cells and specific immunologic tolerance mediated by suppressor cells. In an unsensitized individual, oral or parenteral administration of an antigen can lead to reduced immune reactivity, whereas the same allergen may cause contact sensitization when applied topically.[40] The key role played by lymphocytes as the source and carriers of the hypersensitivity in contact allergy was demonstrated by Landsteiner and Chase[9] 60 years ago in experiments on guinea pigs. Peritoneal exudate cells, predominantly lymphocytes, from contact-allergic donor animals, injected intraperitoneally or intravenously into recipient animals that had not previously been sensitized, passively transferred the hypersensitivity. In humans, however, such passive transfer experiments have yielded contradictory results. Both failure and success have been reported with intracutaneous and intravenous passive transfer of sensitized cells.[41–45] The immunologic changes, which ensue during the early days following sensitizing exposure, usually have a lasting impact on the outcome of the competition between effector and suppressor lymphocytes. The state of specific allergic hypersensitivity may last indefinitely. Once established, it cannot be deliberately altered, except for transient hyposensitization. Contact hypersensitivity is thought to often wane spontaneously in elderly people. In some patients, this hypersensitivity wanes spontaneously at a much earlier age (at times within a few years) despite continued exposure to the specific contact allergen. As yet, no explanation for this finding has been discovered. Contact allergy can develop from earliest infancy to old age, but it is most common in the intermediate age groups.

The spleen plays an important role in generating suppressor cells.[46] Tolerance, once established, apparently persists indefinitely in humans. In laboratory animals, tolerance can be broken deliberately with cyclophosphamide.[47]

The induction of contact allergy is sometimes referred to as the afferent phase and elicitation as the efferent phase. Vocanson and colleagues reviewed the role of various factors involved in the study of contact dermatitis in mouse models. To summarize some of their observations, most mouse work is done with strong sensitizers, such as 2,4-dinitrochlorobenzene (DNCB) and oxazolone. However, weak haptens such as dyes, preservatives, perfumes, metal ions, and drugs are the common haptens in human medicine. In the afferent phase CD8+ T cells in draining lymph nodes are primed. The efferent phase results in the recruitment of these cells to the site of hapten challenge. The authors of this study, showed that CD8+ T cells were the effector cells in weak allergens when studied in mice. The cells that downregulate contact dermatitis to strong haptens in animal models include various CD4+ T cell subsets. Th2 cells, IL-10-producing Tr1 cells, and natural CD4+CD25+ T cells have been implicated in down regulation. Vocanson and colleagues further found that CD4+CD25+ T cells both natural and hapten-induced regulate the CD8+ T cell response to a weak hapten (such as fragrances). They found that the sensitizing potential of haptens correlated to their proinflammatory properties. This provided the activation of the skin-innate immunity required for differentiation and mobilization of dendritic cells from skin to lymph node and the priming of CD8+ T cell precursors. Since factors in the control of the development of allergic contact dermatitis include frequency, dose, duration and route of administration of hapten, genetic polymorphisms of xenobiotic-metabolizing enzymes, and environmental factors such as psychological stress,[48] CD8+ cytotoxic lymphocytes are now implicated in the elicitation of contact dermatitis. CD4+ T cells perform regulatory functions, but CD8+ T cells can mediate contact hypersensitivity, even in the absence of the CD4+ cells. Skin biopsies taken 3 days after patch testing show that Interleukin-12 (IL-12) is present in the cytoplasm of dermal dendritic cells such as macrophages and Langerhans cells. IL-12 can also be found in keratinocytes where there is exocytosis of cells and spongiosis. It is thought that IL-12 enhances the activation of cytotoxic lymphocytes and plays an important role in contact dermatitis.[49]

The focus of immunologists on T cell and B cell factors in contact hypersensitivity was questioned by O'Leary and colleagues, who demonstrated substantial contact hypersensitivity to 2,4-dinitroflurobenzene and oxazolone in mice devoid of T and B cells. Natural killer cells were believed to account for this phenomenon.[50] The role of B cells has been clarified in mouse models. A role for IL-5 in activating eosinophils and B-1 cells was recently described. The B-1 cell-derived antigen-specific immunoglobulin M antibodies recruit effector T cells into skin. Infiltration of antigen-nonspecific mononuclear cells and polymorphonuclear cells then follows.[51]

GENERALIZATION OF CONTACT SENSITIVITY

Antigen presentation by LCs to T lymphocytes has been thought to take place primarily in the lymph nodes. Whether antigen presentation occurs in the skin also is uncertain.[52] In laboratory animals, enlargement of the regional lymph nodes is observed during this period of proliferation. There they undergo further proliferation, which accounts for the production of large numbers of specifically sensitized effector cells and T memory cells. Their descendants enter the collecting sinus of the lymph node and from there are transferred to the blood, which then circulates them to other parts of the lymphoid system.[53] This finding explains why all areas of the body's surface almost invariably become hypersensitive to the contact allergen.

LOCALIZED DIFFERENCES IN SENSITIVITY

Contact sensitivity usually involves the entire integument, but it is not unusual to find differences in degree of sensitivity at different skin sites. For example, a greater degree of sensitivity is often present at the site of originally induced sensitization and at other sites of previous exposure to the particular allergen, such as sites at which patch tests had been done.[54] The mechanism for this has not yet been elucidated, but one theory is that clones of sensitized cells have established themselves in the dermis during a previous encounter with the allergen. Re-exposure to the allergen may then trigger interaction with and proliferation of the clones of specifically sensitized cells at these particular sites, thus creating the increased capability to react.

Elicitation of Reactions

After sensitization has taken place, re-exposure to the specific allergen leads to a series of events that eventually result in the inflammatory response clinically recognized as an eczematous dermatitis. It is characterized histologically by spongiosis and lymphocytes in the epidermis and by lymphocytes, histiocytes, and varying numbers of eosinophils and basophils in the papillary dermis (see Chapter 4). The spongiosis, at least in part, could be due to the destructive effects of hapten-specific cytotoxic effector cells on keratinocytes and LCs.[55] The presence of eosinophils and basophils points to the participation of IgE antibodies and of cutaneous basophil hypersensitivity in the production of contact allergic reactions.[56,57] Basophils are sources of transforming growth factor (TGF-b) and therefore may play a role in downregulating expression of ACD.

Elicitation of ACD in a sensitized individual starts with antigen uptake and presentation by LCs. T lymphocytes specifically reactive to the allergen in question accumulate at the site of exposure. It is uncertain whether this accumulation is due to localized retention or proliferation of the specific T cells once they have arrived at the site, or to preferential migration to the site.[58] Kalish,[14] however, feels that migration of T lymphocytes is random, and therefore on-site retention or proliferation is likely. Antigen-specific T cells make up only 1% or less of the total T-cell population of the site, but this is still 10 to 100 times more than are present in the circulation.

Both antigen-specific and nonspecific T cells produce a number of inflammatory mediators once they arrive on-site. Tumor necrosis factor b (TNF-b) has direct cytotoxic effects on epidermal cells. In addition, it induces ICAM-1 on keratinocytes, which aids binding of lymphocytes. g-Interferon also induces ICAM-1 as well as HLA-DR antigen expression on keratinocytes. This, too, facilitates attachment by lymphocytes. Various interleukins stimulate growth and activation of T lymphocytes and attract neutrophils. Granulocyte-monocyte colony-stimulating factor (GM-CSF) activates monocytes and neutrophils.[59–61]

Mast Cells and Basophils

Mast cells and basophils are routinely found at sites of ACD and are usually confined to the upper dermis. They release histamine, serotonin, and leukotrienes.[62] Pruritus and vascular dilation leading to tissue edema may result. Leukotrienes act to attract both neutrophils and lymphocytes. Mast cells and basophils are not essential for the development of ACD, however, as demonstrated by the development of ACD in most cell-deficient mice.[63]

Keratinocytes

Keratinocytes are not passive bystanders in the process of ACD. Multiple cytokines are produced and/or released by damaged or "activated" keratinocytes. These include interleukin and GM-CSF, with the function noted above. In addition, ICAM-1 is expressed in damaged but not normal keratinocytes and aids T-cell attachment. Furthermore, involved keratinocytes produce HLA-DR antigens in the cell surface, which allows attachment of autoreactive T lymphocytes.

IL-1, which was one of the first cytokines identified from keratinocytes, enhances the activation of accessory dendritic cells, which in turn activates resting T lymphocytes.[64] IL-5, also expressed by keratinocytes, further stimulates T-cell proliferation. IL-8 is another keratinocyte product that has a strong chemotactic effect on T cells. Nozaki and colleagues[65] have prepared an excellent review of currently understood cytokine effects.

Neurologic Factors

Neuropeptides may influence ACD development, because nerve fibers of skin are in direct contact with LCs.[66] Unmyelinated sensory neurons release cutaneous neuropeptide in response to epicutaneously applied allergens. These include Substance P, neurokinin A, and calcitonin gene-related peptide (CGRP). Substance P may increase ACD by increasing levels of TNF-a and IL-2. Substance P stimulates its principal receptor, neurokinin 1R. Substance P is also known as neurokinin 1 (NK1). The result includes the release of IL 1 and the immunologic cascade (previously discussed). A second receptor exists, known as neurokinin 2R (NK-2R). Allergic contact dermatitis is augmented when NK 2R is blocked and decreased when NK-2R is stimulated. Conversely, blocking NK-1R decreases allergic contact dermatitis and stimulating NK-1R increases it. Neurokinin A seems to work with NK-2R, and Substance P works with NK-1R. Both Substance P and NKA are released when allergen is applied. Consequently, it has been shown in mice that capsaicin-mediated depletion of neuropeptides in skin abolishes DNCB contact sensitivity. In additional, destroying the nerve fibers to draining lymph nodes can abolish the DNCB reaction.[66] Another neuropeptide, calcitonin gene-related peptide, may decrease ACD by stimulating IL-10 production.[67,68]

The interplay between the immune system and cutaneous nerves was explored by injecting calcitonin gene-related peptide (CGRP) and a CGRP-antagonist into human skin prior to challenge with an immediate reaction, a delayed reaction, and irritant inducing substances. At low doses, inhibition of CGRP resulted in inhibition of delayed but not of immediate or irritant reactions; at high doses, the opposite effect was seen on delayed reactions. This implies a role for CGRP in delayed immunologic reactions.[69]

INHIBITION OF CONTACT SENSITIVITY

Adequate antigen presentation cannot take place when exposure to the contact allergen occurs at a skin site that has an insufficient number of functionally intact LCs. Under such circumstances, the development of specific immunologic tolerance (unresponsiveness) is favored because production of effector T lymphocytes is greatly decreased or absent. Another consequence is that more of the allergen then reaches the central parts of the lymphoid system and induces the production of specific suppressor cells there. However, even when first exposure takes place by contact, a tolerogenic effect is exerted by that fraction of the allergen that bypasses the epidermal LCs and reaches the dermis, the dermal lymphatics, and the regional lymph nodes.[70] The ultraviolet radiation–resistant antigen-presenting cell described by Granstein and colleagues[71] must also be mentioned in this connection.

Under what circumstances can one expect inadequate antigen presentation and consequently suppressor cell predominance to occur? Certain skin sites in laboratory animals have contained a relatively small number of LCs (e.g., the tail skin of mice, which has approximately one-third the number of LCs present in most other areas). Although variations in the number of LCs have been observed in different areas of skin in humans, none has been described to date that is so deprived of these cells that it interferes with adequate antigen presentation.[72]

A decrease in the number or functional ability of LCs or a dysfunction of the T-lymphocyte systems can lead to diminished contact sensitivity. Ultraviolet radiation (UVR) decreases the functional capability of LCs and may impair lymphocyte function.[14,73] The actual numbers of LCs are not greatly reduced by UVR. Topical corticosteroid usage also results in functional impairment of LCs and suppression of patch test reactions.[74] Systemic corticosteroid intake may compromise T-lymphocyte function, as well as LC capability.[75] Cyclosporine A impairs LC function in vitro without cytotoxic effects on the LCs or T lymphocytes.[76] LC function may be compromised in acquired immunodeficiency syndrome.[77] The failure of LCs to stain positively for membrane Ia antigens and adenosine triphosphatase (ATPase) has demonstrated this functional impairment. It should be pointed out that, although the number of LCs, demonstrable by electron microscopy at such sites, is either unchanged or only slightly reduced, many of them are functionally impaired. The number of LCs is temporarily reduced immediately following a contact allergic reaction, but whether this reduction is sufficient to interfere with antigen presentation is not known. Recovery from functional impairment caused by glucocorticosteroids and UVR usually takes 1 to 2 weeks.

Antihistamines, although they inhibit mast cell and basophil function, do not appreciably alter contact hypersensitivity. Likewise, immunosuppressives such as methotrexate do not seem to impair contact sensitivity, as measured by patch testing.

It is safe to assume that other, as yet undiscovered factors and diseases must exist that can also interfere with antigen presentation by LCs.

DOWNREGULATION OF CONTACT SENSITIVITY BY REGULATORY T CELLS

Control of contact sensitization is mediated by two types of T cells. One type releases IL-10, which impairs the normal release of IL-12 from mature dendritic cells that are responding to an antigen. This lack of IL-12 inhibits activation of effector T cells. This type of control is under the direction of IL-10-producing regulatory T cell or Tr1. The other cell that exerts inhibitory activity on the contact sensitization reaction is the CD4+CD25+Treg cell. A cell-to-cell, contact-dependent, cytokine-independent mechanism is involved, although under certain circumstances these cells may produce IL-10 also. The Treg cell is anergic to antigen but can suppress contact sensitization in normal and naïve individuals and partially suppress the expression of allergy in the sensitized individual.[78]

IN-VITRO TESTS

The interaction between antigen-bearing LCs and sensitized lymphocytes can be demonstrated in vitro. When sensitized T lymphocytes are cultured together with syngeneic Langerhans cell–enriched epidermal cell suspensions in the presence of the specific allergen, they undergo an antigen-specific proliferative response.[79,80] Preceding treatment of the epidermal cell suspension with antibodies against Ia antigens abolishes this in-vitro response and demonstrates the important role played by the immune response–associated surface antigens in this interaction.

Several in-vitro reactions, like the lymphocyte transformation test and the macrophage migration inhibition test, often parallel clinical contact sensitivity. The results of these in-vitro procedures, however, do not yet correlate with sufficient regularity with the results of in vivo exposures to justify their regular clinical use. Also, adequate test techniques have been worked out for only a few contact allergens.

SYSTEMIC ADMINISTRATION OF CONTACT ALLERGENS

Exposure to contact allergens takes place frequently by the "systemic" route, either by ingestion or by injection and on less frequent occasions by insertion into the body (as in operative procedures and intrauterine devices). As has been discussed earlier, first exposure to contact allergens by the systemic route usually favors the development of partial or complete specific tolerance. In some instances, however, allergic contact sensitization rather than tolerance occurs after such a first exposure. The explanation presumably is that some of the allergen has reached the skin through the blood circulation and has then been taken up by antigen-presenting epidermal or lymph node LCs.

A completely different effect is exerted by contact allergens that are "systemically" administered after specific sensitization has already occurred. Under such circumstances, a clinical reaction may ensue, probably because of take-up of the blood-borne contact allergen by antigen-presenting epidermal cells and subsequent interaction with specifically sensitized lymphocytes.

A MECHANISM FOR AUTOECZEMATIZATION

In a mouse model of contact dermatitis, the induction of sensitivity to a specific hapten resulted in T cell clones that not only recognized the hapten but also recognized keratinocyte antigens. This phenomenon, which resulted in a broader degree of reactivity than expected, was seen as a possible mechanism for autoeczematization in humans.[81]

HYPOSENSITIZATION

Hyposensitization, a state of decreased sensitivity, occurs in previously sensitized subjects and can sometimes be induced by intravenous administration of the allergen and by prolonged oral administration.[82] The allergen then bypasses the epidermal Langerhans cell system and exerts a direct action on effector T lymphocytes. The suppression of hypersensitivity is antigen specific and is not mediated by suppressor cells, but its exact mechanism is unknown. The possibility of a receptor blockade has been suggested.[83] Hyposensitization usually has a short-lived effect, in contrast to specific immunologic tolerance, which is mediated by suppressor cells and tends to be long-lasting.

SKIN MEMORY

Application of patch tests to the back of a patient can recall or cause a flare-up of dermatitis on other body surfaces that previously were exposed to the allergen and part of the patient's clinical contact dermatitis. If a patch test site is re-exposed to the same allergen within 2 to 3 weeks, a reaction occurs in 4 to 6 hours rather than 2 to 4 days. This phenomenon is allergen specific, and the retest technique has been suggested as a way to evaluate whether true crossreactivity exists or whether co-reactivity is occurring.[84] It has been suggested that the mechanism for site-specific allergen skin memory is related to a chemokine (CCL27) that causes retention of CCR10+CD4+ T cells perivascularly in the dermis at the site of patch testing.[85] These cells are found at least 3 weeks after resolution of the patch-test reaction and are believed to be responsible for the rapid reactions seen on rechallenge with the same or true crossreacting allergens.

References

1. Jadassohn, J. Zur Kenntnis der medikamentösen Dermatosen. Verh Dtsch Derm Gesellschaft V Kongress 1895;103.

2. Low RC. Skin-sensitiveness to non-bacterial proteins and toxins. Br J Dermatol 1924;36:292.

3. Wedroff ES, Dolgoff AP. Über die spezifische Sensibilität der Haut einfachen chemische Stoffen gegenüber. Arch Dermatol Syphilol 1935;171:647.

4. Frei W. Über willkürliche Sensibilisierung gegen chemisch definierte Substanzen. I. Untersuchungen mit Neosalvarsan am Menschen. Klin Wochenschr 1928;7:539.

5. Mayer RL. Die Überempfindlichkeit gegen Körper von Chinonstruktur. Arch Dermatol Syphilol 1928;156:331.

6. Landsteiner K. Über komplexe Antigene. Klin Wochenschr 1927;6:103.

7. Sulzberger MB. Hypersensitiveness to arsphenamine in guinea pigs. I. Experiments in prevention and in desensitization. Arch Dermatol Syphilol 1929;20:669.

8. Chase MW. The cellular transfer of cutaneous hypersensitivity to tuberculin. Proc Soc Exp Biol Med 1945;59:134.

9. Landsteiner K, Chase MW. Experiments on transfer of cutaneous sensitivity to simple compounds. Proc Soc Exp Biol Med 1942;49:688.

10. Baer RL. Allergic eczematous sensitization in man 1936 and 1964. J Invest Dermatol 1964;43:223.

11. Storck H, Schwarz-Speck M. Different response to experimental sensitization by epicutaneous and intracutaneous application of bacterial antigens. Monogr Allergy 1974;8:79.

12. Eisen HN, Orris L, Belman S. Elicitation of delayed skin reactions with haptens: the dependence of elicitation on hapten combination with protein. J Exp Med 1952;95:473.

13. Shelley WB, Juhlin L. Langerhans cells form a reticuloepithelial trap for external contact allergens. Nature 1976;261:46.

14. Kalish RS. Recent developments in the pathogenesis of allergic contact dermatitis. Arch Dermatol 1991;127:1558.

15. Jacobs JJ, Lehé CL, Hasegawa H, et al. Skin irritants and contact sensitizers induce Langerhans cell migration and maturation at irritant concentration. Exp Dermatol 2006; 15:432.

16. Levine B, Ojeda A, Benacerraf B. Studies on artificial antigen. III. The genetic control of the immune response to hapten-poly-L-lysine conjugates in guinea pigs. J Exp Med 1963;118:953.

17. Polak L, Barnes JM, Turk JL. The genetic control of contact sensitization to inorganic metal compounds in guinea pigs. Immunology 1968;14:707.

18. Satoh T, et al. Effect of the H-2 and Igh complexes on the susceptibility to ultraviolet B–induced immunosuppression in murine contact sensitivity and contact photosensitivity. Photodermatol Photoimmunol Photomed 1990;7:73.

19. Streilein JW, Bergstresser PR. Genetic basis of ultraviolet-B effects on contact hypersensitivity. Immunogenetics 1988;27:252.

20. Yoshikawa T, Streilein JW. Tumor necrosis factor—alpha and ultraviolet B light have similar effects on contact hypersensitivity in mice. Regional Immunol 1990;3:139.

21. Walker FB, Smith PD, Maibach HI. Genetic factors in human allergic contact dermatitis. Int Arch Allergy Appl Immunol 1967;32:453.

22. Karvonen J, Silvennoinen-Kassinen S, Ilonen J, et al. HLA antigens in nickel allergy. Ann Clin Res 1984;16:211.

23. Mozzanica N, Rizzolo L, Veneroni G, et al. HLA-A, B, C, and DR antigens in nickel contact sensitivity. Br J Dermatol 1990;122:309.

24. Bergstresser PR. Contact dermatitis: old problems and new techniques. Arch Dermatol 1989;125:276.

25. Silvennoinen-Kassinen S, Ikaheimo I, Tiilikainen A. TAP1 and TAP2 genes in nickel allergy. Int Arch Allergy Immunol 1997;114:94.

26. Westphal GA, Schnuch A, Moessner R, et al. Cytokine gene polymorphisms in allergic contact dermatitis. Contact Dermatitis 2003; 48:93.

27. Baer RL, Flotte TJ, Gigli I, Thorbecke GJ. Langerhans cells—the skin-associated antigen-presenting cells. In: Daynes RA, Spikes JD, eds. Experimental and clinical photoimmunology. Boca Raton, FL: CRC Press, 1983;1:139.

28. Nacak M, Erbagci Z, Aynacioglu AS. Human arylamine N-acetyltransferase 2 polymorphism and susceptibility to allergic contact dermatitis. Int J Dermatol 2006;45:323.

29. Benacerraf B. Interrelationships between products of the major histocompatibility complex and their relevance to disease. In: Katz DH, Benacerraf B, eds. The role of products of the histocompatibility gene complex in immune response. New York: Academic Press, 1976.

30. Nalefski E, Rao A. Nature of the ligand recognized by a hapten- and carrier-specific MHC restricted T-cell receptor. J Immunol 1993;150:3806.

31. Braathen LR, Thorsby E. Human epidermal Langerhans cells are more potent than blood monocytes in inducing some antigen-specific T-cell responses. Br J Dermatol 1983;108:139.

32. Heufler C, Koch F, Schuler G. Granulocyte-macrophage colony-stimulating factor and interleukin-1 mediate the maturation of murine epidermal Langerhans cells into potent immunostimulatory dendritic cells. J Exp Med 1988;167:700.

33. Aiba S, Katz S. Phenotypic and functional characteristics of in vitro activated Langerhans cells. J Immunol 1990;145:2791.

34. Toews GB, Bergstresser PR, Streilein JW. Langerhans cells: sentinels of skin-associated lymphoid tissue. J Invest Dermatol 1980;75:78.

35. Teunissen MB, De Jager MH, Kapsenberg ML, Bos JD. Inhibitory effect of cyclosporin A on antigen and alloantigen presenting capacity of human epidermal Langerhans cells. Br J Dermatol 1991;125:309.

36. Enk A, Katz S. Early molecular events in the induction phase of contact sensitivity. Proc Natl Acad Sci USA 1992;89:1398.

37. Gawkrodger DJ, Haftek M, Botham PA, et al. The hapten in contact hypersensitivity to dinitrochlorobenzene: immunoelectron microscopic and immunofluorescent studies. Dermatologica 1989;178:126.

38. Dearman R, Basketter D, Coleman J, et al. The cellular and molecular basis for divergent allergic responses to chemicals. Chem Biol Interactions 1992;84:1.

39. Riemann H, Schwarz A, Grabbe S, et al. Neutralization of IL-12 in vivo prevents induction of contact hypersensitivity and induces hapten specific tolerance. J Immunol 1996;156:1799.

40. Gautam SC, Battisto JR. Orally induced tolerance generates an efferently acting suppressor T-cell and an acceptor T-cell that together down-regulate contact sensitivity. J Immunol 1985;135:2975.

41. Baer RL, Sulzberger MB. Attempts at passive transfer of allergic eczematous sensitivity in man. J Invest Dermatol 1952;18:53.

42. Harber LC, Baer RL. Attempts to transfer eczematous contact-type allergy with whole blood transfusions. J Invest Dermatol 1961;36:55.

43. Epstein WL, Kligman AM. Transfer of allergic contact–type delayed hypersensitivity in man. J Invest Dermatol 1957;28:291.

44. Good RA, Zak SJ, Jensen DR, Pappenheimer AM, Jr. Delayed allergy and agammaglobulinemia. J Clin Invest 1957;36:894.

45. Baer RL, Turk JL. Delayed skin reactions. In: Goldsmith LA, ed. Biochemistry and physiology of the skin. Oxford: Oxford University Press, 1982.

46. Sommer G, Parker D, Turk JL. Epicutaneous induction of hyporeactivity in contact sensitization: demonstration of suppressor cells induced by contact with 2:4 dinitrothiocyanatebenzene. Immunology 1975;29:517.

47. Polak L, Turk JL. Reversal of immunological tolerance by cyclophosphamide through inhibition of suppressor cell activity. Nature 1974;249:654.

48. Vocanson M, Hennino A, Cluzel-Tailhardat M, et al. CD8+ T cells are effector cells of contact dermatitis to common skin allergens in mice. J Invest Dermatol 2006;126:815.

49. Yawalkar N, Egli F, Brand CU, et al. Antigen-presenting cells and keratinocytes express interleukin-12 in allergic contact dermatitis. Contact Dermatitis 2000;42:50.

50. O'Leary JG, Goodarzi M, Drayton DK, et al. T cell- and B cell-independent adaptive immunity mediated by natural killer cells. Nat Immunol 2006;7:507.

51. Itakura A, Kikuchi Y, Kouro T, et al. Interleukin 5 plays an essential role in elicitation of contact sensitivity through dual effects on eosinophils and B-1 cells. Int Arch Allergy Immunol 2006;140:8.

52. Silberberg-Sinakin I, Thotbecke G, Baer R, et al. Antigen-bearing Langerhans cells in skin, dermal lymphatics and lymph nodes. Cell Immunol 1976;25:137.

53. Gowans JL. Life-span, recirculation and transformation of lymphocytes. Int Rev Exp Pathol 1966;5:1.

54. Sulzberger MB, Baer RL, Kanof A, Lowenberg C. Skin sensitization to vesicant agents of chemical warfare. J Invest Dermatol 1947;8:365.

55. Tamaki K, Fujiwara H. Levy RB, et al. Hapten-specific TNP reactive cytotoxic effector cells using epidermal cells as targets. J Invest Dermatol 1981;77:225.

56. Ray MC, Tharp MD, Sullivan TJ, Tigelaar RE. Contact hypersensitivity reaction to DNFB mediated by monoclonal IgE-DNP antibodies. J Immunol 1983;131:1096.

57. Dvorak HF, Mihm MC Jr, Dvorak A. Morphology of delayed-type hypersensitivity in man. J Invest Dermatol 1976;67:391.

58. Sterry W, Bruhn S, Künne N, et al. Dominance of memory over naive T cells in contact dermatitis is due to differential tissue immigration. Br J Dermatol 1990;123:59.

59. Brasch J, Sterry W. Expression of adhesion molecules in early allergic patch test reactions. Dermatology 1992;185:12.

60. Lewis R, Buchsbaum M, Whitaker D, Murphy GF. Intercellular adhesion molecule expression in the evolving human cutaneous delayed hypersensitivity reaction. J Invest Dermatol 1989;93:672.

61. Heufler C, Koch F, Schuler G. Granulocyte/macrophage colony stimulating factor and interleukin 1 mediate the maturation of murine epidermal Langerhans cells into potent immunostimulatory dendritic cells. J Exp Med 1988;167:700.

62. Kerdel F, Belsito D, Scotto-Chinnici R, et al. Mast cell participation during the elicitation of murine allergic contact hypersensitivity. J Invest Dermatol 1987;88:686.

63. Thestrup-Pedersen K, Larsen CG, Ronnevig J. The immunology of contact dermatitis: a review with special references to the pathophysiology of eczema. Contact Dermatitis 1989;20:81.

64. Austyn JA, et al. Dendritic cells initiate a two stage mechanism for T lymphocyte proliferation. J Exp Med 1983;157:1101.

65. Nozaki S, Feliciani C, Sauder D. Keratinocyte cytokines. In: Advances in dermatology. St. Louis: Mosby-Year Book, 1991:7.

66. Hosoi J, et al. Regulation of Langerhans cell function by nerves containing calcitonin gene–related peptide. Nature 1993;363:159.

67. Shepherd AJ, Beresford LJ, Bell EB, et al. Mobilisation of specific T cells from lymph nodes in contact sensitivity requires substance P. J Neuroimmunol 2005;164:115.

68. Calvo C, Chavanel G, Senik A. Substance P enhances IL-2 expression in activated human T-cells. J Immunol 1992;148:3498.

69. Fox F, Kubin M, Cassin M, et al. Calcitonin gene–related peptide inhibits proliferation and antigen presentation by human peripheral blood mononuclear cells. J Invest Dermatol 1997;108:43.

70. Wallengren J. Dual effects of CGRP-antagonist on allergic contact dermatitis in human skin. Contact Dermatitis 2000;43:137.

71. Macher E, Chase MW. Studies on the sensitization of animals with simple chemical compounds. XII. The influence of excision of allergenic depots on onset of delayed hypersensitivity and tolerance. J Exp Med 1969;129:103.

72. Granstein RD, Lowy A, Greene MI. Epidermal antigen presenting cells in activation of suppression: identification of a new functional type of ultraviolet radiation–resistant epidermal cell. J Immunol 1984;132:563.

73. Bergstresser PR, Toews GB, Gilliam JN, Streilein JW. Unusual numbers and distributions of Langerhans cells in skin with unique immunologic properties. J Invest Dermatol 1980;74:312.

74. Aberer W, Schuler G, Stingl G, et al. Ultraviolet light depletes surface markers of Langerhans cells. J Invest Dermatol 1981;76:202.

75. Rietschel RL. Irritant and allergic responses as influenced by Triamcinolone in patch test materials. Arch Dermatol 1985;121:68.

76. Belsito DV, Flotte TJ, Lim HW, et al. Effect of glucocorticosteroids on epidermal Langerhans cells. J Exp Med 1982;155:291.

77. Belsito D, Epstein S, Schulz J, et al. Enhancement by various cytokines or 2-B-mercaptoethanol of Ia antigen expression on Langerhans cells in skin from normal aged and young mice: effect of cyclosporine A. J Immunol 1989;143:1530.

78. Belsito DV, Sanchez MR, Baer RL, et al. Reduced Langerhans cell Ia antigen and ATPase activity in patients with acquired immune deficiency syndrome. N Engl J Med 1984;310:1279.

79. Moed H, von Blomberg BME, Bruynzeel DP, et al. Regulation of nickel-induced T-cell responsiveness by CD4+CD25+ cells in contact allergic patients and healthy individuals. Contact Dermatitis 2005;53:71.

80. Stingl G, Katz SI, Shevach EM, et al. Analogous functions of macrophages and Langerhans cells in the initiation of the immune response. J Invest Dermatol 1978;71:59.

81. Fehr BS, Takashima A, Bergstresser PR, et al. T cells reactive to keratinocyte antigens are generated during induction of contact hypersensitivity in mice. A model for autoeczematization in human? Am J Contact Dermat 2000;11:145.

82. Van Scott E, Kalmanson JD. Complete remissions of mycosis fungoides lymphoma induced by topical nitrogen mustard. Cancer 1973;32:18.

83. Polak L, Rinck C. Mechanism of desensitization in DNCB-contact sensitivity guinea pigs. J Invest Dermatol 1978;20:98.

84. Rustemeyer T, de Groot J, von Blomberg BM, et al. Assessment of contact allergen cross-reactivity by retesting. Exp Dermatol 2002;11:257.

85. Moed H, Boorsma DM, Tensen CP, et al. Increased CCL27-CCR10 expression in allergic contact dermatitis: implications for local skin memory. J Pathol 2004;204:39.

PRACTICAL ASPECTS OF PATCH TESTING

EXECUTIVE SUMMARY

The patch test is a bioassay that, when properly performed, approximates the rigorous approach required by the Henle-Kock postulates in the field of microbiology. Steps must be taken to avoid irritant reactions, but weak reactions continue to challenge the physician in terms of interpretation. Clinical relevance has been reported to weak or doubtful patch test reactions, but this low level of reactivity can also represent a false positive reaction. A positive patch test may provoke reactivation of dormant dermatitis, thus confirming the relevance of the test. Undesired reactions to patch tests include prolonged persistent patch test responses, alterations of pigmentation, anaphylactoid reactions, pustular reaction, infections, and scarring.

The inability to confirm a patch test reaction, which occurs in the setting of multiple positive tests, led to the concept of an "angry back." This concept envisioned a spillover effect modifying nearby tests, leading to false or unverifiable reactions when the allergens were individually retested. However, more recent studies have found the same degree of non-reproducibility when tests are applied simultaneously or sequentially. Furthermore, the reactive threshold is now known to vary by as much as 250 fold when allergens are retested. This has led to the term "twinkling back" to reflect the biologic fluctuations inherent in patch testing.

Traditionally, groups of allergens that investigate similar environmental hazards are referred to as "trays" or "series." A basic screening series is commonly supplemented by these more specialized trays. The size of the basic screening series has increased as our knowledge of environmental sources of dermatitis and the complexity of our environment have evolved. Currently, the North American Contact Dermatitis Group screening series comprises 65 items. The current sources of patch test materials are included in this chapter.

Basic Assumptions

The patch test is generally required to identify the cause of allergic contact dermatitis. When performed and interpreted properly, it is a scientific method of investigation with definite rules, regulations, and fundamentals. The achievement of valid results from the patch test—a test that seems simple to apply and read—is in fact a complicated procedure, and this test should not be undertaken without sufficient experience under the supervision of trained personnel. Modification of the standard methods may lead to confusion and misinterpretation and should not be undertaken lightly.

The patch test is artificial and does not necessarily duplicate clinical exposure, in which sweating, maceration, and multiple applications may play roles in producing dermatitis. The real-life exposure of skin to allergen will have variable contact time for the transfer of allergen to skin, whereas the patch test is applied for a fixed, standardized time. The concentration of allergen in a real-life exposure is seldom known, whereas the patch test exposure is defined and adjusted to minimize the chance for an irritant reaction. Patch testing, however, is a better method of finding an offending contactant than clinical "trial and error." A history of reactions to cheap jewelry, zippers, snaps, or metal buttons might be clinically equated with nickel allergy. This assumption would be incorrect over 53% of the time and would miss true nickel allergy in an additional 35% of those surveyed.[1] History simply cannot replace the more complete information obtained by patch testing.

Because the patch test exposes only a small skin area and may be performed on covered parts of the body, even strongly positive reactions need not be disabling or disfiguring. Patch-test reactions properly obtained and interpreted are acceptable as "scientific proof" of a state of allergic sensitization. If this allergic state can be correlated with known exposures, positive use tests, or improvement by avoidance of substances containing the allergen identified by patch testing, then the validity of the patch test is said to be relevant and may be medicolegally important.

Dermatologists who regularly use the patch test realize that the discovery of a specific chemical responsible for dermatitis is fundamentally important to prevent recurrence. That this knowledge is attainable only through intelligent and careful patch testing has been demonstrated time and again, as a review of the medical literature of the past 60 years confirms. Education in the technique of patch testing is as essential to physicians in training as the learning of most surgical procedures.

The four reasons for dermatologists' reluctance to use patch testing are (a) the amount of time required of the physician, (b) the number of visits required of the patient, (c) the unavailability of suitable test materials, and (d) the risk of complications. In general, these beliefs are not supported by the facts: (a) The confirmatory value of patch testing enables the physician to proceed with confidence; (b) patients usually appreciate efforts to investigate their case (the default rate in a dermatology clinic that performs patch tests is lower than that in most other clinics); (c) guidelines have been published on the relative risk of complications and the means to avoid them; and (d) after more than two visits for contact dermatitis, patch testing becomes clearly cost-effective.[2] Rajagopalan and colleagues[3] demonstrated that patch-tested patients have a better outcome than patients who were not patch tested, as evidenced by a decrease in disease severity index and percentage of disease activity. They further demonstrated that dermatitis lasting from 2 months to 1 year was the most cost-effective group for evaluation by patch tests.

The patch test is not perfect, but as a bioassay it approximates the rigors required in the field of microbiology by the Henle-Koch postulates. These postulates require that a specific microorganism be found in every case in question and account for the pathologic changes and clinical course of the disease, that the organism not occur as a nonpathogen in other clinical disease settings, and that the organism could be grown in pure culture and reintroduced to produce the disease.[4] A proper patch test uses a specific substance that produces the disease, contact dermatitis, in miniature; it is the purified etiologic agent reproducing the clinical disease in a susceptible host and causing no disease outside the proper clinical setting (ie, no reaction in a nonsensitized host). It is a very complete bioassay. To achieve maximum accuracy, the principles in Table 2.1 should be used.

PROVOCATIVE USE TEST OR OPEN USE TEST

The provocative use test is valuable in confirming positive reactions to nonirritating substances, such as cosmetics, in which at least one of the ingredients was previously found positive by conventional closed testing. The suspected material is rubbed directly onto normal skin in the antecubital fossa, twice daily for 1 week, over an area approximately 3 cm in diameter. If no reaction occurs, the test may be considered negative. False-negative reactions are common

Table 2-1 Principles of Patch Testing
1. Test only with known substances in "standard" concentrations. If in doubt, do open or "use" tests with controls. Do not test with industrial substances of unknown concentration.
2. Do not test if the dermatitis is acute. The test site must be *completely* free of dermatitis.
3. Instruct the patient to leave the patches on for 48 hours. If any patch burns and itches severely, the patient should remove that patch carefully without disturbing the others.
4. Instruct the patient not to shower, get the back wet, or engage in sports while the patches are in place. Certain types of heavy work are contraindicated as well, especially if the patient sweats considerably.
5. Patch tests can be read initially at 48 hours after allowing the tape reaction to subside, but an additional reading should be taken between 72 and 120 hours using the interpretation key of the North American Contact Dermatitis Group (see Table 2.5).[16]
6. Irritant and allergic reactions may be difficult to distinguish. As a rule, allergic reactions tend to itch more than irritant reactions. Certain patch test substances commonly produce weak irritant reactions, especially on highly sensitive skin or on skin of subjects who have several strong allergic reactions simultaneously.

with this method of testing. The "open use" or "provocative use" test may sometimes distinguish an allergic from an irritant response because open testing is far less likely than closed testing to produce an irritant reaction.

In the detection of contact urticaria, the test may be read 15 to 30 minutes following application, but otherwise the reading is the same as with the open patch test. Cosmetics, such as perfumes, hair sprays, conditioners, aftershave lotions, and plant oleoresins, are tested frequently in this manner. The recommended sites for testing are the retroauricular area, or the outer aspect of the arm immediately above the elbow.

The open or provocative use test is administered (a) before closed patch testing if no safe concentration for closed patch testing is known, (b) to confirm suspected contact urticaria within 15 to 30 minutes by applying the suspect material close to skin that is normally dermatitic and observing for whealing, or (c) to confirm that a substance at its normal "use" concentration in a finished product is capable of inducing contact dermatitis.

Causes of Irritant Patch Test Reactions

Irritant patch test responses are due to either hyperirritability of the skin or the application of an irritating concentration of a test substance (Figure 2-1). Often a combination of both factors is present. Hyperirritable skin has been attributed to strong allergic responses (the "angry back" or "excited skin state"). However, this is an oversimplification. Memon and Friedmann[5] tried to reproduce a hyperirritable state by patch testing standard allergens adjacent to and various distances from strong allergic and irritant reactions. They could not demonstrate a reproducible effect on the standard substance. Although the ability of positive patch tests in close proximity to influence the responsiveness of each other has been questioned, the ability of distant dermatitis to influence the threshold of reactivity is well established. Patients with active hand eczema are more reactive to irritants applied to the back as compared with similarly tested normal individuals, and patients with healed hand eczema react to such irritants the same as normal subjects.[6] The phenomenon of conditioned hyperirritability has been reviewed and an animal model for the production of hyperirritable skin demonstrated.[7] "Spillover" is the term used to indicate that one positive patch test has influenced another test to appear positive when it would not have done so in the absence of the former positive test. When the influence of strongly positive nickel tests was evaluated on chromate patch tests at a distance of 1, 3, or 7 cm from the nickel site, no evidence of spillover was found. Rather, the exact opposite was observed, namely, a significant attenuation of chromate reactions when the chromate was closer to the positive nickel test.[8]

If hyperirritable skin is suspected as the cause of false-positive irritant tests, the test can be repeated in a month or two when the patient's skin may be less irritable. Only clinically normal skin should be tested, and the previously active dermatitis should be allowed to disappear completely. When confronted with a possible irritant test from an industrial or other environmental agent, one must determine the irritancy of the material by patch testing volunteers. This method is not entirely without risk, as one may induce sensitization or produce a severe primary irritant reaction. The concentration that is nonirritating in a few normal test subjects should not be used for patch testing patients. Because patients more frequently have hyperirritable skin than normal volunteers as noted above, one-half or one-third of the concentration that is "safe" in a normal subject will probably prove nonirritating when tested on the patient.

AVOIDING IRRITANT TESTS

Because irritant tests can closely mimic allergic patch test responses, it is important to avoid producing irritant tests. Four cardinal rules should be followed:

1. Test only skin that appears completely normal.
2. Avoid concentrations of patch test materials that are irritating.
3. Do not prepare the skin by cleansing it with soaps or solvents.
4. Avoid patch testing with materials other than the standard series to minimize irritant reactions. *Seek consultation for testing with nonstandard substances.*

It is usually stated that one should not patch test patients who are in status eczematicus or who have widespread dermatoses because of the frequent occurrence of irritable skin. Unfortunately, matters are not so simple in practice. Patients who have widespread dermatitis may have normally reacting skin, whereas other patients who have only hand dermatitis or other limited processes may have markedly irritable skin. The requirement of normal skin for the patch test site is absolute. Failure to limit patch testing to normal skin may result in false-positive test results, which are worse than useless because they are misleading. Skin to be tested (usually on the back) should be examined with good sidelighting to ensure that not even a minimal trace of dermatitis is present. Unless an area of skin can be cleared completely of dermatitis, reliable patch testing is difficult. Patch testing is best done 2 weeks after a patient is completely clear of dermatitis.

The second requirement, that of not testing with irritant materials, is more difficult. Many allergens, such as formalin, chrome, and nickel, are potent irritants. Obtaining a completely nonirritating concentration of these compounds is impossible, as such a concentration would be so diluted it would produce false-negative reactions. It has been the usual practice to determine "safe" or "nonirritating" concentrations by patch testing normal subjects. Even such "safe" concentrations, however, may produce false-positive irritant reactions because the clinician does not test a normal person but a patient whose skin may be more sensitive to irritants than a normal subject.

It should be understood that the term "irritant" as applied to standard commercially available screening allergens is a misnomer or wastebasket term. The test concentration is not one that produces a glazed or scalded patch test reaction typical of what would be generally accepted as an irritant reaction. The false-positive test seen with standard screening allergens more commonly is an erythematous, slightly edematous reaction that would be morphologically a 1+ "allergic" reaction. However, this mild reaction is either unconfirmable on repeated testing or highly suspect because of other circumstances. An example would be an isolated positive patch test to carba mix with a negative reaction to thiuram mix in an individual who was tested while active dermatitis was present elsewhere on the body. Common usage has permitted a broad concept of "irritant" to include these reactions. The patch test is a bioassay that does not by itself distinguish mechanisms. The patch test can result in weak allergic reactions of little or no clinical relevance, mild reactions that do not require specifically sensitized T cells and cannot be morphologically distinguished from reactions that do, or mild reactions that are relevant but may be undervalued by the physician conducting the test. This imprecise terminology has prompted one of us (Robert L. Rietschel) to propose that those nonpapulovesicular patch test reactions consisting of slightly palpable erythema and edema be called Janus reactions. These are reactions that are at or very near the threshold of reactivity. The mythological figure Janus was a symbol found on gates or doorways and looked in both directions simultaneously (double-faced). This would recognize the possibility that this mild reaction may or may not be relevant and only further correlation can establish that (see Table 2.2). The evaluation of macular erythema as a patch-test reading presents the challenge of determining whether the reaction represents weak allergy or some other inflammatory process that is not relevant. A Mayo Clinic study of 2,833 patients found 7,274 reactions and 3,082 (42.4%) were macular erythema. Of the macular erythema responses 2,430 (78.8%) were considered relevant.[9]

Use testing of mild reactions of this type with cosmetic chemicals showed that 44% of "doubtful" patch test reactions were actually relevant.[10] However, weak reactions have also been found to be less likely to have relevance. Fischer and Rystedt[11] found that doubtful reactions to metal salts were relevant 1% to 5% of the time, 1+ reactions were relevant about 20% of the time, 2+ were relevant 80% to 90% of the time, and 3+ reactions were relevant 95% to 100% of the time. Stronger reactions were also associated with greater relevance based on use tests results. Hannuksela and Salo[10] found 1+ and 2+ reactions relevant 80% of the time, in contrast to the 44% relevance of doubtful reactions. The 2+ and 3+ reactions require the presence of papulovesicles. This morphologic criterion more than any other militates against irritation and in favor of an allergic reaction. However, no firm criteria have yet been established that can reliably make this distinction on the basis of one finding. The similarity between irritant and allergic contact dermatitis extends into the immunologic mechanisms that participate in these inflammatory reactions. Virtually all of the events thought to be unique to allergy have also been found in irritant reactions.[12]

A technique known as the RNase protection assay (RPA), which allows for the measurement of small quantities of RNA obtained from tape stripping of human skin, has been found to be extremely sensitive. In a pilot study, when the RPA was used to analyze tape strippings from patch test reactions, the RPA was able to discriminate between irritant and allergic patch test reactions. Interleukin-4 was found to be increased in allergic but not irritant reactions.[13] If this technique is verified in larger trials, then a determination of the true nature of Janus reactions could be readily made.

Interpreting Patch Test Reactions

RELEVANCE (EXPLAINED OR NOT EXPLAINED)

The clinician's task is not ended once the allergic state of the patient has been established. The fact that certain allergens have been demonstrated reliably by careful patch testing does not prove that such allergens were responsible for the dermatitis. The clinician must determine whether or not the allergy is relevant to the dermatitis, either as a primary cause or as an aggravating factor.

In analyzing the question of relevance, it may be helpful to consider the possibilities as follows:

1. relevance to present dermatitis

   A. primary cause
   B. aggravating factor

2. relevance to a preceding bout of dermatitis

   A. primary cause
   B. aggravating factor

3. not relevant

It is impossible to provide absolute rules for the determining relevance, because it depends on that blend of knowledge and experience known as clinical judgment. Frequently, the clinician must decide among the roles of endogenous factors (atopic eczema, psoriasis) and external factors (irritants, contact allergens). A careful examination of the entire skin and a thorough history are helpful in yielding clues to endogenous dermatitis. The judgment of "not relevant" with regard to a positive patch test often reflects our ignorance about possible exposures rather than a patch test that is actually irrelevant.

Relevance can be considered possible, probable, or certain. If a substance produces an allergic patch test reaction and the patient is exposed to circumstances in which skin contact with materials known to contain the allergen is likely to occur, relevance can be said to be *possible*. For example, when a positive reaction to black rubber mix is found in an auto mechanic who works with black rubber hoses and fan belts, relevance is at least

Table 2-2 Criteria for a Janus Reaction
Erythema with or without edema
No vesicles
No necrosis, pustules, or epidermal glazing
The significance of these reactions can only be determined over time, based on patient outcomes.
Morphologic criteria alone are insufficient at this level of reaction to be a reliable correlate of allergy.

possible. If a chemical component of the black rubber mix can be verified to be present in hoses or fan belts with which the patient comes in contact, relevance is *probable*. If a use test with a black rubber hose rubbed over an area of normal skin produces contact dermatitis, the concentration of allergen in the item is sufficient to elicit dermatitis and relevance is *certain*. The rigor with which relevance evaluation is pursued depends on the clinical circumstances and the impact on lifestyle or job modifications required by the patch test findings.

The absence of positive patch tests does not prove the absence of allergy. "Screening" or battery patch testing is often performed on patients who have eczematous dermatoses of unknown cause as a fishing expedition to help establish etiologic factors. Negative patch tests establish only that the patient is not allergic to the relatively more common and well-established sensitizers included in such patch test batteries. The ability of a screening series to detect contact allergy has been evaluated. In a study of 732 patients referred for possible contact dermatitis, only 15.7% were found to be evaluated adequately by a screening series of 20 allergens.[14] In a separate study of 554 patients who were patch tested, a correlation was found between the size of the screening series and the amount of useful information gathered. The 20-allergen screening series detected only 55% of the information obtained by the 50-allergen North American Contact Dermatitis Group (NACDG) series. The 23 allergens of the T.R.U.E. test series identified 65% of the information found by the larger series. The use of additional supplemental series beyond the 50 allergens of the NACDG series found another 103 reactions, of which 59 were relevant.[15]

NEGATIVE PATCH TEST REACTIONS

Just as a positive reaction does not always mean that the cause of the presenting dermatitis has been found, a negative result does not mean that contact dermatitis has been excluded. Standard screening series include only statistically common allergens; we must be constantly alert to the possibility of rare, exotic, or new sensitizers.

REASONS FOR FALSE-NEGATIVE REACTIONS

False-negative reactions have various causes:

1. Insufficient reproduction by the test of the conditions that produced the dermatitis, such as sweating, friction, pressure, and the presence of damaged, ulcerated, or eczematous skin.
2. A concentration of test substance that is too low. The concentration of test substances is critical and should be "standard" because the threshold of reactivity is a narrow margin and, at even slightly higher concentrations, many substances become irritants.
3. Failure to perform delayed readings.[16] When patch tests are read only at 48 hours, some positive reactions are missed. This finding is especially true of substances such as neomycin, but delayed reactivity may occur with many allergens.
4. Wet or loosened patches.
5. Inappropriate vehicle. For example, testing with nickel suspended in petrolatum as a vehicle may produce negative results, whereas testing with nickel in an aqueous solution may produce positive results.
6. Duration of contact that is too brief. A duration of 24 to 48 hours is probably the minimum for occlusion in the closed patch test; earlier removal may prevent development of some positive reactions.
7. Failure to perform photo patch testing. Testing with a photosensitizing substance may cause a negative result if the test site is completely occluded by opaque material. Sometimes, however, sufficient light penetrates to elicit a definite reaction.
8. Influence of corticosteroids. The application of potent topical steroids to the test site for several days before testing may diminish or even obliterate weak positive results.
9. A fluctuation in the threshold of reactivity that resulted in the level of sensitivity being lower than the patch test concentration at the time chosen for testing. This variable is not under the control of the clinician and can result in mild allergens being missed at one time and found on repeated testing.

Sukanto and associates[17] found that the topical application of corticosteroids had a suppressive effect on both the intensity and the size of epicutaneous reactions; no marked difference in the suppressive effect of the four corticosteroids could be observed. However, intermediate-strength corticosteroids (triamcinolone ointment 0.1%) applied three times per day for a week prior to diagnostic patch testing did not have a significant effect.[18] The inclusion of triamcinolone ointment 0.1% directly into a patch test substance such as thimerosal was found to ablate both irritant and allergic reactions.[19] Systemic steroids in doses of 20 mg daily or less probably do not inhibit a "significant" patch test. The effect of 20 mg of prednisone daily for 1 week on nickel patch test reactivity showed that fewer extreme reactions occur on prednisone, that a greater number of weak or doubtful reactions can be expected, and a small number of truly positive cases may test negative. In this study 7 of 15 patients were unchanged in their reaction intensity, but 8 were diminished and 3 others became negative (Figure 2-2).[20]

WHAT TO TELL THE PATIENT ABOUT THE RESULTS OF THE PATCH TEST

When a clinically significant patch test reaction is obtained, the patient should be given the following information, in writing, concerning the sensitizing substance:

1. the various names and guises of the sensitizer
2. immunochemical relatives that might produce cross-reactions with the sensitizer
3. methods of avoiding clinical exposure to the contactant
4. when available, the names of suitable nonsensitizing substitutes (the Contact Allergen Replacement Database or CARD computer program, available from the American Contact Dermatitis Society and developed by James Yiannias of Mayo Clinic Scottsdale, is an excellent tool for providing this information.)

The Safety of Patch Testing

The greatest hazard is *omission* of patch testing procedures in the management of patients who have certain dermatoses. Such omission dooms these patients to repeated attacks of avoidable contact dermatitis. Table 2.3 lists possible adverse patch test reactions.

ACTIVE SENSITIZATION FROM PATCH TESTS

A reaction that occurs 7 or more days later with no preceding reaction is a late reaction caused by the interactions of residues of the allergen with newly sensitized tissues. This type of reaction is sometimes called a spontaneous flare. Such active sensitization is detected by either a positive patch test 10 to 14 days after application (flare-up) and 2 to 4 days after being repeated, or systematic retesting of patients after an interval. An exception to this general rule is gold sodium thiosulfate. Tests that show positive up to

Table 2-3 Possible Adverse Patch Test Reactions
Active sensitization
Irritant patch test reactions
"Ectopic" flare of dermatitis
Koebner phenomenon
Persistence of a positive reaction
Anaphylactoid reactions
Hyper- and hypopigmentation at the sites of positive patch test reactions
Edge effects
Pustular patch test reactions
Pressure effects
Bacterial and viral infections
Necrosis, scarring, and keloids

3 weeks after application do not represent active sensitization, and readings beyond the first week of patch test observation are required to detect all the sensitized cases.[21]

It should be emphasized that for all the standard allergens, the correct patch test concentrations are known and lists have been published. The most frequent cause of active sensitization is the use of too high a concentration of the test substance; the amount applied and how long the patch test remains on the skin are less important. However, because the proper concentration of each standard chemical has now been determined after testing thousands of patients, sensitizing reactions are increasingly being avoided.[22] Recently, the standard test for para-phenylenediamine has been questioned as being too prone to active sensitization.[23]

Cronin[24] correctly states, "Active sensitization is a *complication* of patch testing *but is not a hazard* and it should not be used as an excuse by the *indolent* for eschewing this investigation. To reject patch testing is the greater disservice to the patient" (emphasis added).

Agrup[22] reported the results of retesting 379 patients who had hand eczema with 11 substances first applied 6 to 21 months previously. In 281 patients (74%), the results were unchanged; in 73 patients (19%), tests had become positive; in 19 patients (5%), tests had become negative; and in 6 patients (2%), some tests had become positive, whereas other tests had become negative. The allergens for which there was a statistically significant change were potassium dichromate (0.29% in water), cobalt chloride (2.4% in water), paraphenylenediamine (2.2% in ethanol), para-aminoazobenzene (0.9% in methyl ethyl ketone [MEK]), and diaminophenylmethane (2% in MEK). Among the 79 patients thought to have been sensitized by the patch tests, 20% had healed, 52% had improved, 20% were the same, and 8% were worse. Agrup concluded that the course of the hand dermatitis was the same whether or not the tests had sensitized the patients. In these patients, therefore, the clinical course was unaffected by patch testing, and they were not harmed by the investigation. At the time of this investigation, the frequency with which tests may be found positive or negative on retesting was not appreciated. The tests lost were assumed false negatives once the angry back syndrome was introduced.[25] New positives were assumed to be the result of active sensitization. Although both assumptions can be true, the issues are more complex and relate to multiple factors that will be discussed in the angry back syndrome section of this chapter.

It should be noted that even though this investigative patch test procedure exposed the patients to nonstandard vehicles, no marked adverse reactions occurred. Thus, Agrup tested paraphenylenediamine 2.2% in alcohol, although the present standard is 1% in petrolatum, a much safer concentration and vehicle. Also, Agrup employed a powerful solvent, such as MEK, as a vehicle for para-aminobenzene and diaminophenylmethane, which are now tested with the much safer petrolatum vehicle. The margin of safety is thus quite great because such unorthodox vehicles did not sensitize the patient(s).

As far as paraphenylenediamine is concerned, in the "old" days when testing was performed with various concentrations of this dye, even those as high as 8%, active sensitization occurred. At present, testing this dye in a 1% concentration is safe and reasonably free of the hazard of sensitizing the tested patient.

To study the risk of patch tests sensitizing, Meneghini and colleagues[26] repeated patch testing of 181 patients who had eczema and 100 patients who had noneczematous dermatoses. New positive patch tests were found in 31 patients who had eczema and 4 patients from the other group. These authors concluded that sensitization had been due to further environmental exposure rather than to patch test active sensitization. In a follow-up study, Meneghini and Angelini[27] emphasized that patch testing does not cause new sensitization to any significant extent provided proper techniques are used. The risk of patch tests sensitizing patients is sometimes evaluated by the occurrence of late reactions 10 to 20 days after the application of the test. By this criteria, 0.3% of 7,629 patients might have been sensitized in a Danish series. However, further investigation of these late reactions failed to identify any adverse effect from the suspected patch test sensitization, indicating that clinical contact dermatitis as a result of patch test sensitization is very rare.[28]

Adams[29] stated that active sensitization is rare with standard allergens and warns that testing with substances of unknown composition that are brought in by patients presents the greatest hazard of the patch test procedure.

Malten and colleagues[30] stated that the following nonstandard substances (if applied in sufficient concentration) undoubtedly have a sensitizing capacity: DNCB (2,4-dinitro-1-chlorobenzene), NDMA (*p*-nitrosodimethylaniline), and certain natural products of plants, for example, leaves of poison ivy and of *Primula obconica*. They emphasized that precisely because these substances are such potent sensitizers they are not used industrially, which makes their use unnecessary in patch testing to determine the cause of contact eczema.

IRRITANT PATCH TEST REACTIONS

The correct concentration of an allergen produces a moderate reaction in a sensitized person but none in a control subject. With bland chemicals, this concentration is easy to determine, but for the many allergens that also are irritants, the concentration necessary to elicit an allergic reaction may differ little from that producing an irritant response. Failure to appreciate this difference causes misinterpretation of results and is a major stumbling block in patch testing.

During testing with a nonstandard allergen, the correct concentration has to be determined for most chemicals. An initial test concentration of 0.1% to 1.0% is suitable for clinical use, but for known irritants it should be weaker. If the results are negative, the concentration can be increased. To check a positive reaction that looks allergic, this same concentration should be used to test about ten controls. Many substances used in daily life, such as cosmetics and medicaments, can be used without dilution; however, under the occluded conditions of patch testing, some are mild irritants. Testing should not be performed with undiluted solvents, gasoline, soaps, or detergents.

Serious irritation can be avoided by using standard procedures. These procedures include pretesting substances of unknown composition in several volunteers (including the investigator). Substances should be investigated toxicologically and allergologically before industrial work with them is begun. This investigation also concerns any assay of possible dermatologic toxicity.

Irritant and allergic reactions to the patch test materials and to adhesive tape were quite common formerly. With the advent of the modern aluminum patch, the Finn chamber, and nonrubber acrylate adhesives (Dermicel, Scanpor), such reactions have been greatly minimized.

"ECTOPIC" FLARE OF DERMATITIS

On rare occasions, a positive patch test reaction may be accompanied by a specific flare of an existing or pre-existing dermatitis that was caused by the test allergen. Thus, a positive patch test reaction to nickel sulfate may produce a flare of a preexisting nickel-induced dermatitis of the earlobe or wrist, or even a dyshidrotic and id-like eruption (Figure 2-3). When such a flare occurs, it has proved to be a beneficial, educational experience for both patient and physician because it emphasizes the importance of avoiding the contact allergen in sensitized patients.

KOEBNER PHENOMENON

A positive patch test reaction in a patient who has active psoriasis or lichen planus may reproduce these dermatoses at the patch test site, which is known as the Koebner phenomenon. The application of a corticosteroid preparation usually quickly clears this localized "hazard."

PERSISTENCE OF A POSITIVE PATCH TEST REACTION

The only patch test reaction that is notorious for persisting for more than a month is that due to a 0.5% aqueous solution of gold chloride in a gold-sensitive person. Allergic contact dermatitis to gold is known to persist even though the patient has not been re-exposed to gold for a long time. The persistence of the positive gold patch test reaction merely confirms the clinical phenomenon. Intralesional injections of a corticosteroid into the patch test site quickly control the persistent reaction.

ALTERATION IN PIGMENTATION

Hyperpigmentation from patch tests occurs infrequently and is most likely to occur in darkly pigmented persons. The problem usually clears over time with use of topical corticosteroids to treat the dermatitic component. Hydroquinone may produce an epidermal leukoderma overlying the dermal melanophages, further disturbing the normal appearance, and should be avoided.

Sunlight exposure immediately following removal of patches on which coal tar or fragrance materials have been tested may also result in hyperpigmentation. Severe reactions sometimes cause hyperpigmentation or total depigmentation. Irritant reactions in certain patients may result in hyperpigmentation from the inflammation.

Because patch testing is usually performed on the back, which is covered by clothing, these temporary pigmentary changes do not present serious problems. Preparations such as Covermark corrective makeup may be used until the pigmentation clears.

ANAPHYLACTOID REACTION FROM PATCH TESTING

Rarely, anaphylactoid reactions are seen within 30 minutes after topical testing with certain antibiotics, such as penicillin, neomycin, gentamicin, or bacitracin. Nitrogen mustard may also produce such a reaction (see Chapter 31). Anaphylactoid reactions from patch tests are rare. A nurse developed signs and symptoms of immediate hypersensitivity manifest by wheal-and-flare after skin contact with cefotiam hydrochloride and after continued exposure she experienced cough, nausea, abdominal pain and diarrhea. When patch tested with cefotiam hydrochloride 20% in physiological saline she developed a wheal at the patch test site and then total body whealing and abdominal pain. Intravenous antihistamine and corticosteroid resolved the symptoms and a lymphocyte stimulation test was found to be positive with a stimulation index of 315%. This is considered a case of stage 3 contact urticaria syndrome. In separate prick testing immediate hypersensitivity was confirmed without systemic complications.[31] Patch tests conducted with natural rubber latex rarely cause problems of anaphylaxis even in the latex sensitive patient, but exceptions do occur. After testing over 5,000 patients safely, Parry and Beck encountered a 26-year-old female atopic hairdresser who wore latex gloves in her workplace. Within one hour of patch test application she developed generalized pruritus, nausea, abdominal pain, and difficulty breathing. A large wheal was present at the latex patch test site and no other patches were positive at 1 hour. She responded to treatment with subcutaneous adrenaline, IV hydrocortisone, and chlorpheniramine within 15 minutes.[32]

In addition to such specific allergic reactions, ammonium persulfate, used as a "booster" of hydrogen peroxide for hair-bleaching in "platinum blondes," may rarely produce a nonspecific, idiosyncratic release of histamine that results in an anaphylactoid reaction. Routine patch testing with ammonium persulfate is not advised. If the test is performed under unusual circumstances, such as a medicolegal procedure, readily available injectable epinephrine should be on hand.

EDGE EFFECT

The "edge effect" is an irritant reaction in which the reaction is greatest at the periphery of the patch test, and there is little or no reaction at the center. The effect is probably caused by an increased concentration of an irritant liquid at the margin. The edge effect usually disappears rapidly following removal of the patch. However, the edge effect seen when patch testing corticosteroids is different. This is a sign of allergy and represents the interplay of the pharmacologic and immunologic activities of corticosteroids. Lower concentrations of corticosteroids give a more traditional positive patch test as the pharmacologic effect becomes diluted more than the immunologic effect.

PUSTULAR PATCH TEST REACTIONS

These reactions occur occasionally, especially in atopic persons, from application of metallic salts, such as nickel and copper sulfates, arsenic trioxide, and mercuric chloride. Pruritus is often absent or minimal. Pustular reactions usually disappear promptly, although they may persist for some time before they disappear completely. These reactions do not signify allergy.

PRESSURE EFFECTS

The application of a solid substance to the skin of certain persons produces an edematous area that is almost always most intense at the margins (Figure 2-4). If the test substance is sufficiently large and heavy, the reaction may cover the entire test area. Persons who have a tendency to dermographism are more likely to develop this reaction. It may even be induced by rubbing the skin while the patches are in place.

BACTERIAL AND VIRAL INFECTIONS

These complications have been described, but fortunately, we have not yet encountered them.[33] It is not unusual for patients to be patch tested with leaves or stems of plants, as commercial patch test materials for most botanical agents are not available. However, this carries risk, as was pointed out by physicians at Mayo Clinic Scottsdale. They report a patient who, after being patch tested to a snapdragon from his garden, developed a necrotizing cellulitis at the patch-test site due to a mucormycosis infection with *Apophysomyces elegans*. While this is rare, it needs to be considered as a risk of using fresh plant material.[34]

NECROSIS, SCARRING, AND KELOIDS

Foolhardy testing with strong acids, alkalis, or chemicals of unknown composition may produce adverse effects. Hypertrophic scar formation is a very rare complication of a strongly positive test reaction. This type of scarring was reported in a young woman who had strong reactions to nickel and potassium dichromate. The latter was considered an irritant reaction and the potassium dichromate patch test was the site of scarring. Intralesional triamcinolone resolved the scar.[35]

MILIA

Milia have rarely been reported as sequelae of contact dermatitis. They have not been reported at the allergen patch test site but at the site of dermatitis or positive use test, as was reported by Thormann and Andersen. Their patient had a blistering reaction to a use test with chloroatranol which is a component of oak moss.[36]

Role of Excited Skin Syndrome ("Angry Back") in Patch Testing

There has been a revival of interest in a phenomenon that Dr. Max Jessner of the old New York Skin and Cancer Unit called the "crazy back."

Mitchell[25,37,38] used the term "angry back" to describe a regional phenomenon caused by the presence of a strongly positive reaction, a state of skin hyperreactivity in which other patch test sites become reactive, especially to marginal irritants, such as formalin and potassium dichromate. Mitchell[37] believed that these concomitant "positive" reactions cannot be relied on. He tested 35 patients who showed 90 positive 1+ reactions to 28 substances at 48 hours. He then retested these patients on day 7. On day 9, 42% of the reactions were negative, suggesting that false-positive reactions were common when one

strong positive reaction occurred. Mitchell suggested that the true index of sensitivity is falsely exaggerated by concomitant testing. To confirm or deny the significance of individual reactions found on the "angry back," Mitchell recommended sequential testing later with each substance alone.

Strongly positive patch test reactions to nickel sulfate and potassium dichromate (the two "standard" patch test allergens most likely to engender nonspecific reactions in adjacent patch test materials) may be confused with allergic reactions. Whenever the clinical history of a patient suggests strongly that either one of these common allergens may produce a positive reaction, it may be placed on the patient's arm away from the other patches and thus minimize the "crazy back," or what Calnan[33] called the "status eczematicus."

Because patch tests may be performed elsewhere besides the back, Maibach and Mitchell[39,40] have broadened the term "angry back" to the "excited skin syndrome" (ESS).

Some clinical investigators have begun to think seriously about the possibility or indeed the likelihood that some 40% of the positive patch test reactions observed in routine concomitant screening patch testing are in fact false positives. Thus, in order to avoid misinformation, sequential retesting would be mandatory.

Maibach and Mitchell[39,40] have tested patients who have ESS on both arms and have found a similar response; the reproducible or nonreproducible tests could be demonstrated on the arm as well as on the back. In other words, a strong reaction on the right arm can produce a nonspecific response on the left arm. This finding suggests that, whatever the mechanism may be, it is not necessarily localized. This would account for the strong positive result and spillover from one site to adjacent sites. But it is not the sole explanation, or one would not see enhanced reactivity over such a wide area as from one arm to the contralateral arm.

Since the original description of the angry back syndrome, much has been learned about the reproducibility of patch tests. Gollhausen and colleagues[41] applied patch tests sequentially to patients and found that 40% were lost (i.e., nonreproducible). These investigators then applied the same patch tests to the left and right side of the back (simultaneously) and again found nonreproducibility of 43.8%. All of these figures are in the range reported for the so-called angry back syndrome and question the explanation of strong reactions influencing other patch test responses. Gollhausen and colleagues tested allergens from several different manufacturers and found nonreproducibility rates of 17.9% for Pharmacia AB, Uppsala, Sweden; 18.5% for Hermal, Reinback, Germany; and 29.4% for Maser, Herne, Germany.

The differences were not statistically significant.[42] Discordance of results was found to be in part dependent on the strength of the reaction. With concomitant testing, nonreproducibility of 1+ reactions occurred 36.6% of the time, but with 2+, 3+, or 4+ reactions only 21% of the time. On sequential testing the same trend was found. The 1+ nonreproducibility was 40.4%, and the stronger reactions were nonreproducible 28.4% of the time. This work requires that the explanation for Mitchell's lost reactions be seen as something more than the work of other nearby reactions. Furthermore, entirely too much emphasis was placed on tests that were lost. Retesting leads to new or "found" reactions and does so just as frequently as reactions are "lost." This was demonstrated by Meneghini and Angelini,[27] who tested 309 cases of suspected contact dermatitis and found 208 to have one or more positive tests. They used a series of 31 allergens and repeated the patch tests to all 31 from 1 to 36 months after the initial testing. They "lost" 50 cases (25%) but found 55 new cases (26.5%). Likewise, Ayala and colleagues[43] tested 174 patients with the same 30 allergens 5 years after the original testing. They found that one or more patch tests were "lost" in 18% of cases, but 29% had more positive tests on repeat testing and 53% were exactly the same. As noted earlier in this chapter, Memon and Friedmann[5] could not demonstrate an effect on patch test results based on the proximity or distance of patch tests to strong irritants or allergens. Their work does show that reactivity across the back is not uniform to the same patch test, but this lack of uniformity cannot be accounted for by the presence or absence of other test reactions.

We now have patch test reactions that vary with location, vary to a greater degree when they are weaker, and are capable of varying either up or down. It is now known that one factor influencing the reactivity of an area of the back is how recently the area was or was not dermatitic. Nickel-sensitive patients had a controlled nickel dermatitis produced on different quadrants of their backs 8, 4, and 1 months prior to patch testing with a dilution series of nickel over each of these sites and a control site.[44] A higher reactivity was found if a previous nickel dermatitis had been present, and, furthermore, a stronger reaction was observed if the antecedent dermatitis was more recent. The findings paint a different picture than that envisioned by Mitchell, although his observation was correct. It appears that the closer a patch test exposure is to the patient's threshold of reactivity, the greater the chance that the test will vary over time. Because patch test reactions can vary up or down, the back can be visualized as "twinkling" rather than angry (Figure 2-5). Because diagnostic patch testing is usually done one time and with only one concentration of an allergen rather than a dilution

series, the dynamic aspect of the immunologic variability of the skin will not be noted unless the tests are repeated or placed at varying sites. The proven value of routine testing in patient outcome attests to how well these variables have been overcome with standard screening allergens. This has been achieved by moving away from the threshold of reactivity as much as possible without inducing nonspecific inflammation (Janus-type reactions).

That the threshold of reactivity is highly variable was ably demonstrated by Hindsen and colleagues They tested 30 women with patch tests positive to nickel at a 2+ or higher level on 4 different occasions at 2-month intervals.[45] An extensive nickel dilution series was used on each occasion to define the threshold of reactivity. The minimal concentration to elicit a reaction differed on all four occasions in all of the patients and the variation was 250 fold. Two of the women tested negative to all test concentrations once.[45]

An additional variable that can amplify threshold events is neurogenic inflammation. It has been suggested that "noise" or stochastic resonance may be another factor modifying skin reactivity and that this effect is mediated by cutaneous nerves in contact with Langerhans cells.[46] The presence or absence of this neurologic static may modify the threshold response of numerous biological systems.

The concept of spillover was not found by Memon and Friedmann,[5] but this author (RLR) has observed this as envisioned originally by Mitchell. A case that I will describe illustrates the specificity of spillover that may make the phenomenon very difficult to study. At day 2 of diagnostic patch testing a young woman had a 2+ reaction to colophony. No other reactions were present. Patch tests were applied with Scanpor tape to all four quadrants of her back. At the day 4 patch test reading the 2+ colophony reaction was still present, but a tape reaction to Scanpor was now present surrounding the colophony reaction and covering all the area of Scanpor application on the left upper quadrant of her back. There were no reactions at any other sites and no Scanpor reaction at any of the other three quadrants of the back. The Scanpor reaction on the left upper quadrant surrounded all of the standard allergens of the 20-allergen screening series in common use at the time of evaluation (Figure 2-6). Not one of those tests became positive. The enhanced reactivity was confined to an area about 10 cm by 10 cm roughly surrounding the positive colophony test. This enhanced reactivity was specific to colophony interacting with Scanpor. If an attempt had been made to study the influence of a positive colophony reaction on any of the standard allergens, the conclusion would be that no such influence exists and thus spillover does not exist. Spillover appears to be more specific than envisioned by Mitchell [25,37] and not the null event envisioned by the experiments of Memon and Friedmann.[5]

THRESHOLD OF IRRITANCY

In the screening series, the parabens, potassium dichromate, formalin, and wool wax alcohol (lanolin), are notorious for their production of nonreproducible positive responses with greater frequency than other allergens. This finding means that even compounds of extremely low irritancy may produce a false-positive response in some subjects. These rules are relative rather than absolute. Categorization of such reactions requires a determination of relevance as discussed for Janus reactions.

ADHESIVE TAPE REACTIONS

Adhesive tape produces a localized dermatitis in many subjectsand has several mechanisms: irritant dermatitis, miliaria, microbial infection, pressure phenomena, allergic contact dermatitis, and others (Figure 2-7).

Magnusson and Hellgren[47] studied the effect of this dermatitis on patch test reactivity. The thrust of their observations was on the irritation and adhesive characteristics of different adhesive tapes used in Scandinavia. They recorded diagnostic patch test positivity in men and women, correlating this finding to the degree of adhesive tape reactivity.

With turpentine, potassium dichromate, p-phenylenediamine (PPD), and formalin, they noticed a striking difference in patch test positivity between subjects with and without tape dermatitis. With these four materials, the differences were statistically significant between the groups. For PPD, 17 positive responses (in a group of 26 men) were positive when a tape reaction occurred, and only 4 positive responses occurred with a tape-negative reaction. The investigators observed similar differences with irritants (detergents). Comparable results were obtained for the 26 women in the study only in regard to formalin. (This sex difference in reactivity was not researched further.) Magnusson and Hellgren interpreted the additional responses as a nonspecific increase in skin reactivity secondary to the tape dermatitis.

THE PRINCIPLES OF DEALING WITH PATIENTS WHO HAVE MORE THAN ONE POSITIVE PATCH TEST

In verifying the multiple positive responses noted in battery testing, much time and trouble are involved for both patient and physician (refer to Table 2.4). Mitchell and Maibach[40] have developed a strategy that minimizes the task of dealing with the ESS (which is actually a

Table 2-4 Battery Testing: Strategy for Dealing with the Excited Back Syndrome

When more than one positive is noted, retake the clinical history
May not be necessary to retest positives individually if:
The material is readily avoided (e.g., ammoniated mercury)
History strongly negates positive patch test results
Important to retest individually if material is ubiquitous
Preservatives (paraben mixture)
Vehicle (wool wax alcohol)
Medicament (neomycin)
Fragrance (fragrance mixture)
Rubber chemical
Formalin
Possible job change
Medicolegal situation
Regulatory situation

matter of determining relevance and is applicable to any positive patch test result):

1. If more than one positive patch test is noted, the clinical history is retaken. This by itself is often enough to solve the problem.

2. It may not be necessary to retest the positive substances individually. For example, if the material is a chemical that the patient can avoid relatively easily (such as ammoniated mercury, which is rarely used in the United States), the patient can be informed about this and questioned about previous reactions, and testing can be discontinued. If no previous history supports exposure, the impetus for delving into it deeply is diminished. Equally important, if the subject has a history that strongly negates the relevance of the positive patch test, the patient may not be interested in working through the physician's academic curiosity. It is not as important clinically to repeat that test because it presumably makes little difference to the patient even though it might make significant inroads into the diagnosis.

3. Retesting is unnecessary if the multiple reactions can be reasonably explained by a known chemical similarity or cross-reaction. If formaldehyde, quaternium-15, and imidazolidinyl urea are all positive, the release of formaldehyde by the latter two substances is a sufficient explanation. A positive patch test to benzocaine and paraphenylenediamine need not be reconfirmed because they are known to be potential cross-reactants.

4. It may be helpful to retest the patient if a positive patch test is related to a ubiquitous substance and the physician is uncertain of the validity of the result. The physician can lose credibility when the patient is told that he or she is allergic to something that is known not to cause the difficulty. Attributing the allergy to a chemical such as a preservative (the parabens), a vehicle (wool wax

alcohol or lanolin), a medicament (neomycin), a fragrance, rubber chemicals, or formalin has great import. The avoidance of these materials involves considerable effort on the part of the patient, and if it is, in fact, a false-positive response, it is a needless waste of time and causes loss of confidence in the physician.

Maibach and colleagues,[48] in a joint International Contact Dermatitis Research Group (ICDRG) study, attempted to quantify ESS. Fifty-six patients entering the study had two or more positive reactions with the basic ICDRG routine series. At approximately weekly intervals, the patients were retested one at a time with the two most clinically important positive responses. The results of this study revealed that 32 of the 56 subjects were still positive to both substances. In 16 cases, however, the patients reacted to only one of these substances, and in 8 cases, patients reacted to neither substance. This finding suggests that 24 of 56 patients (42%) may have had ESS. However, the study design did not address the number of additional allergens that would be found by retesting the initially negative results. As noted earlier in this chapter, both events occur with similar frequency. Retesting introduces new variables that were not appreciated at the time of the initial studies of excited skin syndrome. Location on the back[5] and prior dermatitis in that region can influence results[44] and the threshold of reactivity is not static.[45]

Bandmann and Agathos[49] detected a significant number of false-positive reactions by sequential testing, as did Bruynzeel and colleagues.[50]

It is prudent to place notoriously strong sensitizers at a practical distance from similarly strong allergens. Distance will be limited by the size of the patient's back, the number of allergens to be tested, and the application system employed. (Finn chambers are available in single rows of five and double rows of five, all premounted on Scanpor tape.) This provides fixed distances for allergen placement, which may require thoughtful planning when other than "standard" series of allergens are used.

Interpretation of the Mixes in the Screening Series

Mixes of closely related chemicals save valuable time and space. By using mixes containing four to five related chemicals from the same family, one can increase considerably the number of test materials.

Occasionally, a sensitive patient shows a negative reaction to a mix but a positive reaction to one of its ingredients tested separately. This finding occurs occasionally with

mercapto mix because the concentration of 2-MBT in the mix is lower than in the individual test material. Conversely, testing with tetramethylthiuram disulfide (TMTD) may sometimes be negative, whereas thiuram mix may be positive because the patient is sensitive to the monosulfide but not to the disulfide.

Mixes have assumed a valuable role, but caution must be observed in their preparation so that the concentration of each chemical is sufficient to evoke a reaction. Also, the combination must not react chemically to induce irritation or cause deactivation of one or more of its components, which results in a false-negative reaction.

Mitchell[51] states that patch testing with mixes can provide requisite information. Thus, in a patient with clinical findings strongly suggestive of rubber glove dermatitis, a positive reaction to thiuram mix leads to advice on avoidance of rubber, and further testing may be unnecessary. The multitude of allergenic rubber chemicals leads us to test them in groups because it would require too much effort to test each substance individually. The detailed analysis of reactions to rubber chemicals is only necessary in specific cases, for example, for research or legal purposes.

Phenomena of aging, maturity, balance, stability, and quenching have been studied for mixtures of aroma chemicals (fragrances and flavorings). These problems limit the utility of mixes and represent an area for further study.

NATURALLY OCCURRING MIXES

In the case of balsam of Peru, a naturally occurring mix of plant origin, patients can show positive patch tests to the balsam but to none of its known allergenic constituents, suggesting that allergens as yet unknown are present in the natural product.

A relatively high patch test concentration is required because most of the material is immunologically indifferent. The allergen(s) may be unstable.

The allergen content of turpentine initially increases and then declines during storage. During the period of increase, patch test sensitization can occur. During the period of decline, false-negative reactions have been noted.

If only a small fraction of a test mixture is allergenic, the very bulk of inert material may preclude an adequate concentration. Lanolin sensitivity is best demonstrated by patch testing with wool alcohols, which contain a concentrate of the allergens.

PARABEN MIX

The name "parabens" is applied to the alkylesters, butyl, ethyl, methyl, and propyl of *p*-hydroxybenzoic acid, which are widely used as preservatives in the pharmaceutical and cosmetic industries, as well as in certain foods. The parabens are the most commonly used preservatives in dermatologic topical medicaments, drugs, dentifrices, and suppositories.

The high incidence of cross-reactions between the esters and the frequent use of two or more esters in the same preparation makes a paraben mixture desirable for detecting hypersensitivity to any or all of them. The topical application of pharmaceuticals with high concentrations of parabens is not a prerequisite for sensitization. Repeated applications of relatively low concentrations of parabens in medicaments, proprietaries, cosmetics, and dentifrices appear to be sufficient. Sensitivity reactions to orally ingested parabens, however, have not been reported.

The following facts concerning topical medications should be taken into consideration when treating a paraben-sensitive person:

1. Some corticosteroid ointments are paraben-free.
2. Many corticosteroid creams contain parabens.
3. Many other topical preparations contain parabens.

Some paraben-sensitive patients who develop allergic contact dermatitis when parabens are applied to eczematous skin tolerate their use on normal skin (i.e., cosmetics). It has not been established whether the following medicaments, which contain paraben, are "safe" for paraben-sensitive persons: Lidocaine hydrochloride, prednisone, Solu-Medrol and penicillin, as well as Syrup of Aristocort, Achromycin Pediatric Drops, Maalox, and Terfonyl Suspensions. *Positive weak reactions to the paraben mix should be interpreted with caution because the mixture is near the irritancy threshold for many patients. Testing with the individual paraben components should help clarify these weak responses to the mix or retesting with the mix.*

Screening Patch Test Kit

The Screening Patch Test Kit, which was sold by Hermal in the United States until its discontinuation in 1997, contained the 20 clinically common agents known to cause contact dermatitis, as specified by the North American Contact Dermatitis Group (NACDG) (Table 2.5). Many studies were based on this series, and it is included here for historical purposes.

Several allergens grouped together for the purpose of patch testing are referred to as a "test series" or "battery." The series may be general, that is, a "screening" group, or specific, such as a "therapeutic," "metal," or "rubber" series (Figure 2-8). Such groupings often overlap because the screening series may contain metals, rubber chemicals, and topical therapeutic agents that are common sensitizers. Differences between physician input and regulatory restrictions have led to a slight difference between the two widely used screening series found in Table 2.5 (North American and International Contact Dermatitis Group Series) and the T.R.U.E. test system. As noted earlier in this chapter in the section "Interpreting Patch Test Reactions," larger screening series capture more relevant information. Presently, the 2007 North American Contact Dermatitis Group screening series contains 65 allergens and this series is commonly supplemented with additional allergens based on the patient's history (Table 2.6).

The Hermal screening allergens were applied on Finn chambers because allergen concentrations have been customized to this system. These shallow aluminum chambers are mounted in units of 10, 5, or single chambers on Scanpor tape. (Available from Allerderm division of SmartPractice, 3400 Mcdowell Rd., Phoenix, AZ 85008 (602) 225–9090). Petrolatum-based allergens are available today from three North American sources, all in Canada (Omniderm/Pharmascience, Dormer Laboratories, and SmartPractice Canada). Two strips of 10 patch tests are usually applied to the back of an adult patient. The T.R.U.E. test system is premounted on tape and is applied to the back, as are Finn chambers.

The allergen-petrolatum mixtures are applied directly into the Finn chambers, filling slightly more than half their volume. For the aqueous allergen mixtures, a filter paper disc (Whatman 3 MM) is placed into the chamber and saturated with the mixture. Patient patch test record sheets should be used to record the allergens tested, their position, and the test results.

During application of patch tests to the upper back, the patient should stand erect with shoulders dorsiflexed in a military "attention" posture (Figure 2-9). This allows the tape to fit tightly against the back when the patient assumes normal standing, sitting, and reclining postures. The lower portion of the test strip is adhered first; the chambers at the lower end of the tape are then fixed by pressing them from below in order to let the air escape from the chambers. Next, the top of the chambers should be pressed gently to obtain an even distribution of the allergen against the skin. The surrounding tape is then pressed against the skin. This process is repeated with each chamber, working up the back to the top of the test strip.

After the tests are affixed to the patient's back, the skin around the top and bottom of each strip is outlined by a Pilot Spotlighter pen. This fluoresces a bluish-white under a Wood's light. Upon removal of the Finn chamber, it is helpful to leave the top 0.5 cm of Scanpor tape adherent to the skin as a second marking device for taking delayed readings. The kit comes with a template that aligns with the markings or residual tape to identify patch test sites. The serrated edge of the template can be held against the top of the Finn chambers to keep a small rim of tape in place during removal of the bulk of the patches.

Table 2-5 Screening Patch Test Series

Hermal (based on North American Contact Dermatitis Group recommendations and now of historical interest only)	International Contact Dermatitis Research Group Recommended Series	T.R.U.E. Test
Benzocaine 5% in petrolatum, USP	Benzocaine 5% in petrolatum	(Not tested separately; see caine mix)
Mercaptobenzothiazole 1% in petrolatum, USP	Mercaptobenzothiazole 2% in petrolatum	Mercaptobenzothiazole 0.075 mg/cm^2
Colophony 20% in petrolatum, USP	Colophony 20% in petrolatum	Colophony 0.85 mg/cm^2
p-phenylenediamine 1% in petrolatum, USP	p-phenylenediamine base 1% in petrolatum	p-phenylenediamine 0.09 mg/cm^2
Imidazolidinyl urea 2% in water for injection	Not tested	Not tested
Cinnamic aldehyde 1% in petrolatum, USP	Not tested separately; see fragrance mix	Not tested separately; see fragrance mix
Lanolin alcohol (wool wax alcohol)30% in petrolatum, USP	Wool alcohols 30% in petrolatum	Wool alcohols 1 mg/cm^2
Carba mix 3% in petrolatum, USP1,3 diphenylguanidine 1%zinc diethyldithiocarbamate 1%zinc dibutyldithiocarbamate 1%	Not tested	Carba mix: same 3 as Hermal in equal parts Patch contains 0.25 mg/cm^2 carba mix
Neomycin sulfate 20% in petrolatum, USP	Neomycin sulfate 20% in petrolatum	Neomycin sulfate 0.23 mg/cm^2
Thiuram mix 1% in petrolatum, USP Tetramethylthiuram disulfide 0.25% Tetramethylthiuram monosulfide (0.25%) Tetramethylthiuram disulfide 0.25% Dipentamethylenethiuram disulfide 0.25%	Thiuram mix 1% in petrolatum (same)	Thiuram mix equal parts: tetramethylthiuram monosulfide, tetramethylthiuram disulfide, dipentamethylenethiuram disulfide, 0.25% mg/cm^2 of thiuram mix tetraethylthiuram disulfide,
Formaldehyde (contains methanol) 1% in water for injection	Formaldehyde 1% aqueous	N-hydroxymethyl succinimide, which forms formaldehyde in contact with skin 0.18 mg/cm^2 formaldehyde
Ethylenediamine dihydrochloride 1% in petrolatum, USP	Ethylenediamine dihydrochloride 1% in petrolatum	Ethylenediamine dihydrochloride 0.018 mg/cm^2
Epoxy resin 1% in petrolatum, USP	Epoxy resin 1% in petrolatum	Epoxy resin 0.05 mg/cm^2
Quaternium-15 [N-(3 chloroallyl)-hexaminium chloride] 2% in petrolatum USP	Quaternium-15 1% in petrolatum	Quaternium-15 0.081 mg/cm^2
p-tert-butylphenol formaldehyde resin 1% in petrolatum, USP	4-tert-butylphenol formaldehyde resin 1% in petrolatum	p-tert-butylphenol formaldehyde resin 0.32 mg/cm^2
Mercapto mix 1% in petrolatum, USP N-cyclohexyl-2-benzothiazole-sulfenamide 0.333% 2,29-benzothiazyl disulfide 0.333% Morpholinyl-2-benzothiazyl disulfide 0.333%	Mercapto mix 2% in petrolatum N-cyclohexylbenzothiazyl sulfenamide 0.5% Mercaptobenzothiazole 0.5% Dibenzothiazyl disulfide 0.5% Morphodinylmercapto-benzothiazole 0.5%	Mercapto mix; equal parts: N-cyclohexylbenzothiazyl sulphenamide, dibenzothiazyl disulfide, morpholinylmercaptobenzo- thiazole at 0.075 mg/cm^2
Black rubber-p-phenylenediamine mix 0.6% in petrolatum, USP N-phenyl-N'-cyclohexyl-p-phenylenediamine 0.25% N-isopropyl-N'-phenyl-p-phenylenediamine 0.10% N,N'-diphenyl-p-phenyl-enediamine 0.25%	Black rubber mix 0.6% in petrolatum (same)	N-isopropyl-N'-phenyl paraphenylenediamine, N-cyclohexyl-N'-phenyl paraphenylenediamine, N,N'-diphenyl paraphenylenediamine in a ratio of 2:5:5 at 0.075 mg mix/cm^2
Potassium dichromate, 0.25% in petrolatum, USP	Potassium dichromate 0.5% in petrolatum	Potassium dichromate 0.023 mg/cm^2
Balsam of Peru 25% in petrolatum, USP	Balsam of Peru 25% in petrolatum	Balsam of Peru 0.8 mg/cm^2
Nickel sulfate (anhydrous) 2.5%	Nickel sulfate (NiSo$_4$ • 6H$_2$O) 5% in petrolatum	Nickel sulfate 0.2 mg/cm^2
Not tested	Cobalt chloride (CoCl$_2$ • 6H$_2$O) 1% in petrolatum	Cobalt chloride 0.02 mg/cm^2
Not tested	Quinoline mix 6% in petrolatum and Clioquinol 3% Chlorquinaldol 3% Benzyl-4-hydroxybenzoate 3.0	Quinoline mix, clioquinol, chlorquinaldol in equal parts at 0.19 mg/cm^2 (omitted from series in 1998)
Not tested	Parabens 15% in petrolatum Methyl-4-hydroxybenzoate 3.0 Ethyl-4-hydroxybenzoate 3.0 Propyl-4-hydroxybenzoate 3.0 Butyl-4-hydroxybenzoate 3.0B enzyl-4-hydroxybenzoate 3.0	Paraben mix same as European series at 1mg/cm^2

Table 2.5 (Cont.) Screening Patch Test Series

Not tested	Fragrance mix 8% in petrolatum Cinnamic aldehyde 1% Hydroxycitronellal 1% Amylcinnamaldehyde 1% Geraniol 1% Eugenol 1% Isoeugenol 1% Oak moss absolute 1%	Fragrance mix same 8 ingredients as European series at 0.43 mg/ cm^2
Not tested	Primin 0.01% in petrolatum	Not tested
Not tested	5-chloro-2-methyl-4-isothiazolin- 3-one + 2- methyl-4-isothiazolin- 3-one (3:1 in water) 0.01% aqueous	5-chloro-2-methyl-4-isothiazolin-3-one + 2-methyl-4-isothiazolin-3-one (3:1) (Kathon CG) 0.004 mg/cm^2
Not tested	Not tested	Thimerosal 0.008 mg/cm^2
Tested as benzocaine only	Tested as benzocaine only	Caine mix: Benzocaine 0.364 mg/patch Tetracaine 0.063 mg/patch Dibucaine 0.064 mg/patch

In the United States, the Hermal Kit of 20 allergens is no longer distributed by Hermal Pharmaceutical Laboratories, Inc., Oak Hill, NY 12460. The European series is available in Canada from Pharmascience, Inc., 8400 Ch. Darnley Rd., Montreal, Quebec H4T 1M4 and in Europe from Hermal Kurt Herrmann, P.O. Box 1228, D-2057 Reinbek/Hamburg, Germany, or Chemotechnique Diagnostique AB, Ringugnsgatan 7, S-21616 Malmo, Sweden. Dormer Laboratories has begun distribution of an expanded series of allergens that includes the former 20 allergens of the Hermal series and additional allergens commonly used for screening by the North American Contact Dermatitis Group. T.R.U.E. Test is distributed by Glaxo Dermatology, Research Triangle Park, NC. The gel vehicles vary among the patches and are listed on the package insert.

ALTERNATIVE MARKING SYSTEMS

Use of a marking paint to delineate the sites of the various tests at the time of test application is an essential step in the technique of testing when several hours or days elapse between the time of test removal and test reading. There is no perfect marking paint. One-half percent gentian violet solution, Castellani's paint, and similar dyestuffs are effective marking paints but permanently smudge overlying clothing. In whites, a concentrated solution of dihydroxyacetone in a mixture of water, alcohol, and acetone provides an effective brown stain that does not discolor clothing. Occasionally this paint fails completely, and it is unsuitable in dark-skinned persons. *Whatever paint is used, it should be reapplied at the time of patch test reading, and also when delayed readings are performed, so that the sites of any delayed positive tests can be identified precisely.*

AIDS IN ADHESION

In hot weather, extra adhesion can be obtained by spraying a pressure-sensitive silicone adhesive (Hollister Medical Adhesive No. 7730, Hollister Inc., 200 Hollister Drive, Libertyville, IL 60048) to the upper and lower exposed adhesive edges of the tape. This is rarely necessary. An extra strip of 2-in.-wide Scanpor tape is more than adequate. Patch tests should not be applied to the area directly over the vertebrae because false-positive tests from mechanical trauma can result. If one allergen is specifically suspect, it should be applied as a separate test strip so that the patient can remove the patch test if marked itching occurs. The upper arm can be used in this instance to facilitate removal.

Screening Patch Test Series

Some chemicals have proved to be frequent or otherwise important causes of allergic contact dermatitis. These sensitizers may be included in a "screening" patch test series. Such screening series have been variously labeled as "diagnostic," "basic," "standard," or "battery." The term "standard" should be avoided as it implies that other test materials are nonstandard. This is not the case. The proper tests must be selected based on the patient's history. Testing with a screening group of substances has proved of great value when allergic contact dermatitis is suspected and the offending agent cannot be pinpointed by careful history.

Patch test screening only supplements, never supplants, patch testing with suspected environmental agents. No screening series could ever encompass the many allergens encountered in cosmetics, in industry, and in gardening.

Screening by a series of patch tests revealed that as many as one-half of all cases of contact dermatitis may be caused or complicated by an allergic contact sensitivity. Hence, patch testing may be a useful procedure for the investigation of any case of dermatitis. The examination is useful as a guide to substances that should be avoided to reduce the risk of a relapse.

Table 2-6 2007–2008 North American Contact Dermatitis Group Screening Series

1. Benzocaine 5.0% pet	23. Imidazolidinyl urea 2.0% pet	45. Glyceryl thioglycolate 1.0% pet
2. Mercaptobenzothiazole 1.0% pet	24. Bacitracin 20.0% pet	46. Tosylamide formaldehyde resin 10% pet
3. Rosin (colophony) 20.0% pet	25. Mixed dialkyl thioureas 1.0% pet	47. Methyl methacrylate 2.0% pet
4. P-phenylenediamine 1.0% pet	26. Methylchloroisothiazolinone/ Methylisothiazolinone 100 ppm aq	48. Cobalt chloride 1.0% pet
5. Imidazolidinyl urea 2.0% aq	27. Paraben mix 12.0% pet	49. Tixocortol-21-pivalate 1.0% pet
6. Fragrance mix II 14% pet	28. Cinnamic aldehyde 1.0% pet	50. Budesonide 0.1% pet
7. Lanolin alcohol 30.0% pet	29. Fragrance mix I 8.0%	51. Hydrocortisone-17-butyrate 1.0% alc
8. Carba mix 3.0%	30. Amidoamine 0.1%aq	52. Disperse blue 106 1.0% pet
9. Neomycin sulfate 20.0% pet	31. 2-Bromo-2-nitropropane-1, 3diol 0.5% pet	53. Propolis 10.0% pet
10. Thiuram mix 1.0%	32. Sesquiterpene lactone mix 0.1% pet	54. Lidocaine 15% pet
11. Formaldehyde 1.0% aq	33. 2-Hydroxyethyl methacrylate 2.0% pet	55. Dibucaine 2.5% pet
12. Ethylenediamine Dihydrochloride 1.0% pet	34. Propylene glycol 30% aq	56. Clobetasol-17-propionate 1.0% pet
13. Bisphenol A epoxy resin 1.0% pet	35. Benzophenone 3 3.0% pet	57. Cocamidopropyl betaine 1.0% aq
14. Quaternium 15 2.0% pet	36. Chloroxylenol (PCMX) 1.0% pet	58. Bisphenol F epoxy resin 0.25% pet
15. 4-tert-butylphenol formaldehyde Resin 1.0% pet	37. DMDM hydantoin 1.0% aq	59. Triamcinolone acetonide 1.0% pet
16. Mercapto mix 1.0% pet	38. Diazolidinyl urea 1.0% aq	60. Dimethyloldihydroxyethylene urea 4.5% pet
17. Black rubber mix 0.6% pet	39. Desoximetasone 1.0% pet	61. Cocamide DEA 0.5% pet
18. Potassium dichromate 0.25% pet	40. Methyldibromoglutaronitrile/ phenoxyethanol 2.0% pet	62. Compositae mix 5.0%
19. *Myroxylon pereirae* (Balsum of Peru) 25% pet	41. Benzyl alcohol 1.0% pet	63. Glutaral 1.0% pet
20. Nickel sulfate 2.5% pet	42. DI alpha tocopherol 100.0%	64. Tea tree oil, oxidized 5.0% pet
21. Diazolidinyl urea 1.0% pet	43. Iodopropynyl butyl carbamate 0.5% pet	65. Ylang-ylang oil 2.0% pet
22. DMDM hydantoin 1.0% pet	44. Ethyl acrylate 0.1% pet	

New sensitizing chemicals and products are introduced regularly into the environment. Hence, the selection of substances for a screening test series cannot be rigidly defined. Constant revision and additions are needed to adapt the standard series to the sensitivities currently most prevalent in the populations served by any particular clinic. The North American Contact Dermatitis Group revises its 65 allergen screening series every 2 years based on a review of the frequency of positive reactions, the relevance of the reactions, a review of the literature on newer allergens, and the collective experience of the Group.

A positive patch test reaction to one or more substances in the screening series gives the physician and the patient a lead to investigate and may help to determine in retrospect how contact could possibly have been made with the substance that produced the positive patch test reaction. It enables the physician to investigate the possibility that the dermatitis was produced by a chemical that cross-reacts with the substance that produced the reaction. Thus, a positive patch test reaction to paraphenylenediamine may not only incriminate the dye itself but also alert the physician to the possibility that a group of immunochemically related substances, such as local anesthetics and other chemicals, which have an amino group in the "para" position, may have to be investigated.

Patch Test Reading and Interpretation

READING THE TEST RESULTS

At each test reading, it is traditional to note the result as negative or positive, and grade the positive results on a quantitative scale. The International Contact Dermatitis Research Group has recommended a 1+ to 3+ scoring system, with 1+ representing erythema and edema; 2+ representing erythema, edema, and vesicles; and 3+ representing a very severe reaction (Figure 2-10). Weak and questionable reactions are recorded by a question mark. Irritant reactions are recorded as IR. When the reactions are to be computer codes, the designations are as follows: 1+ = 1; 2+ = 2; 3+ = 3; doubtful = 4; irritant = 5; and negative = 6. This convention is followed by the North American Contact Dermatitis Group and has been adopted by T.R.U.E. test also. The important point in evaluating a positive test response, however, is not how many pluses one should assign to the test response but whether it is a true positive result caused by allergy or a nonspecific irritant reaction. Irritant reactions, also known as false-positive tests, are the bane of patch testing.

Patch test reactions may have features of more than one category. A doubtful reaction is a macular erythema that may not confluently fill the area of the patch test but is sustained beyond a day 2 reading. This level of intensity may represent mild irritancy or weak allergy whether or not the response is confluent. Because the patch test is a bioassay, the point at which irritancy ends or weak allergy begins in any one individual may overlap the contrary reactions in another individual. Only by clinical correlation can the distinction be sorted out; even then, it cannot be done in all cases because there are no *absolute* criteria to morphologically distinguish macular erythema of allergic etiology from that of irritant etiology. If erythema is palpable, accompanied by edema, and covers at least 50% of the patch test site, it is scored 1+. This is considered a morphologic grade in which allergy is probable, although some irritant reactions may still encroach on this level of reactivity. A Janus reaction incorporates both doubtful and 1+ levels of reactivity and gives recognition to the uncertainty associated with this level of response. When papules (microvesicles) occupy up to 50% of the patch test surface, a 2+ reaction is appropriate; however, if greater than 50% of the surface is vesicular or bullous, the reaction is scored 3+. Spreading reactions that are not secondary to overfilling of chambers are by definition scored 3+. Irritant reactions are rare with the standard allergens, but 1+ reactions are commonly encountered and are the most difficult to interpret (Table 2.7, Figure 2-11).

While it is common to examine patch test reactions 1 or 2 days after the allergens are placed on the back, an examination done 30 minutes after allergen placement reveals that all the allergens in standard screening series can produce immediate contact urticaria (Figure 2-7). This phenomenon was observed in a study of 664 patients. Balsam of Peru produced the most such reactions.[113] Fragrance mix produced 112 reactions and paraben mix 30 reactions. There was a slight increase in the amount of delayed hypersensitivity detected in patients with immediate contact urticaria to an allergen as compared to patients who did not exhibit the phenomenon.[52]

DISTINGUISHING BETWEEN IRRITANT AND ALLERGIC PATCH TEST RESPONSES

Whereas many textbooks indicate that one can reliably decide whether a patch test response is irritant or allergic upon morphologic grounds, in actual practice the morphology of the patch test response is a poor guide to whether the response is allergic or irritant. When the patch test reaction is very strong, it is usually possible to differentiate the sharply demarcated, promptly healing, "burn-like" irritant reaction from the spreading, more slowly disappearing, eczematous reaction to an allergen. Unfortunately, whereas the criteria for distinguishing between irritant and allergic patch test responses are of some value when the patch test is strongly positive, they are of *absolutely no value* when the physician is confronted with a relatively weak reaction. *There is no morphologic way to distinguish a weak irritant patch test from a weak allergic test.*

Suppliers of Patch Testing materials

1. Screening Series Allergens
   T.R.U.E. Test
   Allerderm Division, SmartPractice
   3400 E. McDowell Rd.
   Phoenix, AZ 85008
   (602) 225-9090

   Hermal Patch Test Allergens
   Omniderm Pharma Canada Inc.
   997 Seguin
   Hudson, Quebec JOP 1HO
   (450) 458-0158
   Dormer Laboratories (supplier of Chemotechnique allergens)
   91 Kelfield, Suite 5
   Rexdale, Ontario M9W 5A3
   Canada
   (416) 242-6167

   AllergEAZE Patch Test Allergens
   SmartPractice Canada
   2175 29th Street NE, Unit 90
   Calgary, AB T1Y 7H8
   (866) 903-2671

2. Patch Testing Devices
   Finn Chambers on Scanpor
   Allerderm Division, SmartPractice
   3400 E. Mcdowell Rd.
   Phoenix, AZ 85008
   (602) 225-9090

Table 2-7 Interpretation Key	
?	*doubtful* reaction; faint macular erythema only
+	*weak* (nonvesicular) positive reaction; erythema, infiltration, possibly papules
++	*strong* (vesicular) positive reaction; erythema, infiltration, papules, vesicles
+++	*extreme* positive reaction; bullous reaction
2	*negative* reaction
IR	*irritant* reaction of different types
NT	*not tested*

*May be obtained from: OmniDerm/Pharmascience or Dormer Laboratories. (See above)

3. Patch Test Adhesive Tapes
   Scanpor Tape
   Allerderm Labs (see above)
   Blenderm
   3M Company (consult your local surgical supply)

4. Black Light Eastern Division of Spectronics
   Westbury, Long Island, New York
   Model BLF 6

5. Uni-Solve Adhesive Remover
   (Active ingredients 1,1,1, trichloroethane)
   United, Division of Howmedica, Inc.
   11775 Starkey Road
   Largo, FL 33540

6. Hollister Adhesive Remover
   No. 7731, 6-oz spray can (contains a
   fluorocarbon)
   Distributed by Hollister, Inc.
   211 East Chicago Avenue
   Chicago, IL 60611

7. Detachol
   Ferndale Laboratories
   780 West Eight Mile Road
   Ferndale, MI 48220

References

1. Kieffer M. Nickel sensitivity: relationship between history and patch test reaction. Contact Dermatitis 1979;5:398.

2. Rietschel RL. Is patch testing cost-effective? J Am Acad Dermatol 1989;21:885.

3. Rajagopalan R, Kallal JE, Fowler JF Jr, Sherertz EF. A retrospective evaluation of patch testing in patients diagnosed with allergic contact dermatitis. Cutis 1996;57:360.

4. Evans AS. Causation and disease: the Henle-Koch postulates revisited. Yale J Biol Med 1976;49:175.

5. Memon AA, Friedmann PS. 'Angry back syndrome': a non-reproducible phenomenon. Br J Dermatol 1996;135:924.

6. Bjornberg A. Increased skin reactivity to primary irritants provoked by hand eczema. Arch Dermatol Forsch 1974;249:389.

7. Roper SS, Jones HE. An animal model for altering the irritability threshold of normal skin. Contact Dermatitis 1985;13:91.

8. Brasch J, Kreilgard B, Henseler T, et al. Positive nickel patch tests do not intensify positive reactions to adjacent patch tests with dichromate. Contact Dermatitis 2000;43:144.

9. Davis MDP, Yiannias JA. Should macular erythema reactions be counted as positive allergic patch-test reactions? Dermatitis 2006;17:12.

10. Hannuksela M, Salo H. The repeated open application test (ROAT). Contact Dermatitis 1986;14:221.

11. Fischer T, Rystedt I. False-positive, follicular and irritant patch test reactions to metal salts. Contact Dermatitis 1985;12:93.

12. Rietschel RL. Mechanisms in irritant contact dermatitis. Clin Dermatol 1997;15:557.

13. Morhenn VB, Chang E-Y, Rheins LA. A noninvasive method for quantifying and distinguishing inflammatory skin reactions. J Am Acad Dermatol 1999;41:687.

14. Cohen DE, Brancaccio R, Andersen D, Belsito DV. Utility of a standard allergen series alone in the evaluation of allergic contact dermatitis: a retrospective study of 732 patients. J Am Acad Dermatol 1997;36(6 Pt 1):914.

15. Larkin A, Rietschel RL. The utility of patch tests using larger screening series of allergens. Am J Contact Dermat 1998;9:142.

16. Rietschel RL, Adams RM, Maibach HI, et al. The case for patch test readings beyond day 2. J Am Acad Dermatol 1988;18:42.

17. Sukanto H, et al. Influence of topically applied corticosteroids on patch test reactions. Contact Dermatitis 1981;7:180.

18. Clark RA, Rietschel RL. 0.1% triamcinolone acetonide ointment and patch test responses. Arch Dermatol 1982;118:163.

19. Rietschel RL. Irritant and allergic responses as influenced by triamcinolone in patch test materials. Arch Dermatol 1985;121:68.

20. Anveden I, Lindberg M, Andersen KE, et al. Oral prednisone suppresses allergic but not irritant patch test reactions in individuals hypersensitive to nickel. Contact Dermatitis 2004; 50:298.

21. Bruze M, Hedman H, Bjorkner B, Moller H. The development and course of test reactions to gold sodium thiosulfate. Contact Dermatitis 1995;33:386.

22. Agrup G. Sensitization induced by patch testing. Br J Dermatol 1968;80:631.

23. Devos SA, Van Der Valk PG. The risk of active sensitization to PPD. Contact Dermatitis 2001;44:273.

24. Cronin F. Clinical prediction of patch tests. Trans St. John's Hosp Dermatol Soc 1972;58:153.

25. Mitchell JC. The angry back syndrome: Eczema creates eczema. Contact Dermatitis 1975;1:193.

26. Meneghini CL, Rantuccio F, Lomuto M. A propos de réactions de sensibilisation active après l'execution des tests diagnostiques picutanes: observations sur 281 cas. [Active sensitization reactions after execution of diagnostic epicutaneous tests: 281 cases.] Annales de Dermatologie et de Syphiliographie 1972;99:161.

27. Meneghini CL, Angelini G. Behaviour of contact allergy and new sensitivities on subsequent patch tests. Contact Dermatitis 1977;3:138.

28. Jensen CD, Paulsen E, Andersen KE. Retrospective evaluation of the consequence of alleged patch test sensitization. Contact Dermatitis 2006;55:30.

29. Adams RM. Patch testing—a recapitulation. J Am Acad Dermatol 1981;5:637.

30. Malten KE, Nater JP, van Ketek WG. Patch testing guidelines. Nijmegen, Dekker & van de Begt, 1976.

31. Yoshiyuki C, Takahashi S, Yamakawa Y, et al. Contact urticaria syndrome caused by patch testing with cefotiam hydrochloride. Contact Dermatitis 1999;41:234.

32. Parry EJ, Beck MH. Acute anaphylaxis resulting from routine patch testing with latex. Contact Dermatitis 1999;41:236.

33. Calnan CD. The use and abuse of patch tests. In: Maibach HI, Gellin GA, eds. Occupational and Industrial Dermatology. Chicago: Year Book Medical Publishers, 1982.

34. LeSueur BW, Warschaw K, Fredrikson L. Necrotizing cellulitis caused by Apophysomyces elegans at a patch test site. Am J Contact Dermat 2002;13:140.

35. Ariffin N, Felton JR, Price ML. Hypertrophic scar following patch testing. Clin Exp Dermatol 2005;31:281.

36. Thormann H, Andersen KE. Milia as sequelae to allergic contact dermatitis. Contact Dermatitis 2005;53:239.

37. Mitchell JC. Angry back syndrome [letter]. Contact Dermatitis 1981;7:359

38. Mitchell J. Multiple concomitant positive patch test reactions. Contact Dermatitis 1977;3:315.

39. Maibach HI. The ESS-excited skin syndrome (alias the "angry back"). In: Ring J, Burg G, eds. New Trends in Allergy. Berlin: Springer-Verlag, 1981.

40. Mitchell JC, Maibach HI. The angry back syndrome—the excited skin syndrome. Semin Dermatol 1982;1:9.

41. Gollhausen R, Przybilla B, Ring J. Reproducibility of patch tests. J Am Acad Dermatol 1989;21:1196.

42. Gollhausen R, Przybilla B, Ring J. Reproducibility of patch test results: comparison of T.R.U.E. Test and Finn Chamber test results. J Am Acad Dermatol 1989;21(4 Pt 2):843.

43. Ayala F, Balato N, Lembo G, et al. Statistical evaluation of the persistence of acquired hypersensitivity by standardized patch tests. Contact Dermatitis 1996;34:354.

44. Hindsen M, Bruze M, Christensen OB. The significance of previous allergic contact dermatitis for elicitation of delayed hypersensitivity to nickel. Contact Dermatitis 1997;37:101.

45. Hindsen M, Bruze M, Christensen OB. Individual variation in nickel patch test reactivity. Am J Contact Dermat 1999;10:62.

46. Rietschel RL. Stochastic resonance and angry back syndrome: noisy skin. Am J Contact Dermat 1996;7:152.

47. Magnusson B, Hellgren L. Skin irritating and adhesive characteristics of some different tapes. Acta Derm Venereol 1962;42:463.

48. Maibach H, Fregert S, Magnusson B, et al. Quantification of the excited skin syndrome (the 'angry back'): Retesting one patch at a time. Contact Dermatitis 1982;8:78.

49. Bandmann HJ, Agathos M. New results and some remarks to the "angry back syndrome." Contact Dermatitis 1981;7:23.

50. Bruynzeel DP, van Ketel WG, von Blomberg-van der Flier BM, et al. The angry back syndrome—a retrospective study. Contact Dermatitis 1981;7:293.

51. Mitchell JC. Patch testing with mixes. Contact Dermatitis 1981;7:98.

52. Katsarou A, Armenaka, Ale I, et al. Frequency of immediate reactions to the European standard series. Contact Dermatitis 1999;1:76.

CHAPTER 3

PREDICTIVE TESTING FOR HUMAN CONTACT DERMATITIS

EXECUTIVE SUMMARY

The identification of the sensitizing capacity of individual compounds or finished products can be undertaken in human or animal systems. Some animal systems can detect weak allergens that would affect only 10 of 100,000 humans. In order to identify with confidence a sensitizer that would affect 0.1% of the population a human panel of 5,300 subjects would be needed. Most human test panels contain only 200 subjects. Agreement between test systems and different laboratories was problematic until the development of the local lymph node assay (LLNA). This in-vitro system has shown good correlation between in-vitro data and human patch test experience. Inter and intra-laboratory consistency has been another advantage. The modified Draize test and the maximization test are the human predictive tests most commonly employed. The use of patch test clinic data to make judgments about the frequency of allergy in the general population will result in an overestimate of 10 to 30-fold.

The factors that create the sensitizing potential of a chemical, such as molecular weight, charge, and electrophilic potential, are unique to that chemical. However, a structural analysis of the chemical rarely gives a clue to its sensitizing potential. This is probably because of the complex and poorly understood genetic factors required for sensitization and is related to T-lymphocyte cell surface-receptor expression of the genetic code. It has been estimated that 50% to 70% of the United States population is capable of sensitization to *Toxicodendron,* given an adequate sensitizing exposure, but about 30% are genetically incapable of responding regardless of exposure (antigen-specific tolerance).[1] Few compounds rival *Toxicodendron* for both sensitizing potential on a chemical basis and abundance of environmental exposures—much of this potential can be recognized as poison ivy, poison oak, and poison sumac. However, the quest to find a chemical structure-activity relationship has been able, at times, to produce useful information. A combination of electrophilicity and hydrophobicity was used to calculate a relative alkylation index for chemicals. For reactive hard electrophilic carbonyl compounds, a good correlation was found with the sensitization potential identified by the LLNA (local lymph node assay). This provides a physical chemical basis for the reason why some compounds sensitize while others do not.[2]

Expression of the sensitizing potential of a chemical is restricted by the circumstances of exposure. This has been studied extensively for the preservative methyl-chloroisothiazolinone/methylisothiazolinone (MCI/MI).[3] The potential of MCI/MI to sensitize at concentrations of 100 to 250 ppm from a single exposure in a closed 48-hour patch test attests to a considerable potential for sensitization. This potential is not always expressed, because this biocide is extremely effective at low concentrations (15 ppm or less); thus, the question arises whether this potential will be recognized in normal use. The answer appears to be dependent on the type of skin exposed to MCI/MI. Application to eczematous skin of products that contain no more than 12.5 ppm appears to be capable of producing sensitizing reactions.[4] Similar products applied to normal skin may also produce sensitizing reactions, but products intended for skin application that are subsequently washed off, such as shampoo and liquid soap, were found to pose virtually no problem. This was true even when patients known to be patch test sensitive to MCI/MI bathed in products preserved with 15 ppm MCI/MI.[5] This points out the importance of intended skin use, use concentration, duration of skin contact, and type of skin in the assessment of the risk of skin sensitization. These factors, as well as the human genetic variable, make the process of predicting sensitization risk difficult and complex. In-vitro predictive work with MCI/MI has found that the vehicle is also a factor in allergenicity. The LLNA found an effect of vehicle on sensitization to MCI/MI. The EC3 value, which is the concentration of chemical that produces a threefold increase in the proliferation assay, showed a significant difference between an acetone/olive oil vehicle vs. propylene glycol vehicle in terms of sensitization.[6]

The Patch Test Clinic as a Source of Epidemiologic Perspective on Sensitization

Historically, groups of dermatologists have pooled their collective data on the frequency with which positive patch tests occur in patients seeking diagnostic evaluation of persistent or new-onset dermatitis. The frequency of positive tests depends on the knowledge and skill of the clinician, as well as societal or environmental factors, referral patterns, health care systems, and other confounding variables. This type of data can be used to gather clinical insight but cannot be used for epidemiologic purposes. Ability to accurately predict what is occurring in a population requires proper epidemiologic methods.[7] When Prystowsky and colleagues[8] compared the prevalence of ethylenediamine and benzocaine sensitization in a random sample of the population to patch test clinic data, the true prevalence in the population was 10 to 30 times less than expected.

The database for patch test clinic data is historically large, whereas population-based studies are few. Efforts to define the difference between "strong" and "weak" sensitizers have used a 1% threshold from patch test clinic data as a crude guide. That is, if more than 1% of patients test positive in response to a substance, it is deemed a "strong" sensitizer.[9] What, then, becomes of materials thought to be sensitizers, which are routinely tested but found positive in less than 1% of patients tested? Are these nonsensitizers or "weak" sensitizers? Or is it the current usage pattern of a product that is increasing or decreasing and thus truly responsible for the number of patients identified in patch test clinics?

For example, in the early 1970s, parabens were found to have sensitized greater than 1% of tested patients, as evaluated by the North American Contact Dermatitis Group (NACDG) (3% of 1,200 patients tested).[10] In the 1980s, the NACDG did not include parabens in its routine screening series of allergens because it had been concluded that most paraben sensitivity occurred in the presence of stasis dermatitis.[11] Did the sensitizing poten-

tial of parabens change? It is more likely that the sample drawn from clinic-based patch test data rather than from population-based data will always show this type of variation and cannot be used to accurately gauge the sensitizing potential of a substance, even on a scale as simple as "strong" versus "weak."

The same phenomena were recently seen with patch test clinic-based reports of the prevalence of sensitivity to MCI/MI. Patients were reported to have anywhere from 1% to 16% frequency of positive reactions to MCI/MI. A critical analysis of these findings revealed an inverse linear correlation between the "prevalence" and the log size of the population tested.[12] The sample sizes used to generate the reports did not provide sufficient reliability, nor were study groups matched for age, sex, occupation, usage, or climate. Because patch test clinic data do not report on the same group of patients tested sequentially, the finding may reflect different percentages of varying occupations or similar factors in the study population. One obvious example of the importance of controlling such variables is the degree to which nickel sensitivity is found in patch test clinics. Sound epidemiologic studies have repeatedly and overwhelmingly found nickel allergy to be a female allergen (10:1).[13] Nickel allergy is found in patch test clinic "epidemiologic" reports of from 4% of 2,897 tested[14] to 16% of 4,500 patients tested.[15] Without correcting for the proportion of women (or other important variables) in the two separate trials, comparison of these figures becomes meaningless.

The importance of the use of proper epidemiologic methods is required if we are to assess the potency of a sensitizer. We cannot rely solely on data derived from patients in patch test clinics. This type of information can be used only as a guide to more carefully controlled studies that address relevant variables appropriate to the material in question. Does the population at risk have intact skin or eczematous skin? Is the duration of contact an issue? What concentrations will be encountered in actual use?

Limits of Predictive Testing

A great deal of predictive patch testing is performed on populations likely to be exposed to the products under scrutiny. Sample size immediately becomes an issue; as the mathematical calculations of Henderson and Riley[16] have shown, at the 95% confidence interval there may be no reactions detected in a sample size of 200 subjects, but up to 15 of every 1,000 in the general population might still be sensitized. If the confidence limits were increased to 99% without a change in sample size, 22 of every 1,000 could still react. If only one member of a panel of 200 is sensitized, we can state with 95% confidence that between 1 and 275 of every 10,000 subjects would be sensitized. Because panel sizes of 200 humans are commonly used in such tests as the modified Draize test, these limitations must be borne in mind when results are discussed.

Animal Testing

Although the thrust of this chapter is human testing, it is helpful to know some of the common methods used for screening and preclinical work. The United States Environmental Protection Agency (EPA) recognizes seven methods of animal testing as acceptable for use under the Toxic Substances Control Act.[17] These are the Buehler method, the open epicutaneous test, the guinea pig maximization test (GPMT), the split adjuvant technique, Freund's complete adjuvant test, the Maurer optimization test, and the footpad technique.[18] The GPMT has been adopted by the OECD Test Guideline 406 along with the local lymph-node assay (LLNA) as a screen for sensitization. This in effect has created a worldwide standard. However, to eliminate laboratory variation, the guideline stipulates that three sensitizers be used and demonstrated as positive to show proficiency in performing the tests. These three chosen standards are hexyl cinnamic aldehyde, mercaptobenzothiazole, and benzocaine. The first two of these perform well in both the GPMT and the LLNA, but widely divergent results are obtained with benzocaine. In the GPMT, 0% to 60% of animals were positive, and in the LLNA 12 tests in two laboratories only occasionally found positive results.[19] A comprehensive list of local lymph node test data on 211 individual chemicals has been published.[20] The LLNA has come to the forefront of animal allergy testing. The use of EC3 has proven reproducible in inter- and intra-laboratory testing. A relationship between potency of an allergen in the LLNA and the potency in humans based on human repeated insult patch tests was compared for 26 sensitizers. A linear relationship was found that allowed the LLNA EC3 values to predict the relative human sensitizing potency of new allergens.[21] An example of the power of the LLNA can be found in work done on Euxyl K 400. The sensitizing potential of methyldibromo glutaronitrile and the commercial preservative Euxyl K 400 that contains it was investigated by LLNA, GPMT, and the cumulative contact enhancement test (CCET). The LLNA correctly identified the sensitizing potential of the preservative and its active ingredient, while the CCET identified only the active ingredient. The need for multiple induction applications was felt to be the critical factor in successfully identifying this sensitizer.[22]

Table 3-1 Degree of Sensitization in Different Phases of Animal Testing

Percentage of animals sensitized	Sensitizer grade	Class
0–8	Weak	I
9–28	Mild	II
29–64	Moderate	III
65–80	Strong	IV
81–100	Extreme	V

The GPMT bears comment. The method uses Freund's complete adjuvant to facilitate a heightened immune response to the test substance.[23] To further augment the opportunity for sensitization, 10% sodium lauryl sulfate (SLS) is applied in conjunction with the test substance if the substance fails to produce irritation by itself on day 7 of the test. After a rest period, the animals are challenged. Usually 20 to 25 animals are used in each phase of the test, and the degree of sensitization is assessed, as shown in Table 3.1. Efforts have been made to improve on the predictive value of the GPMT by focusing on the minimum induction concentration that induces a positive response and comparing the challenge concentrations that produce a standardized reaction intensity with the highest concentration for induction. This correlated well with allergen levels in causative products in human cases of contact dermatitis.[24]

Extrapolating to Humans

Maurer[25] has equated strong sensitizing capacity with a frequency of 100 individuals sensitized per 100,000 population and weak allergy with a frequency of 10 per 100,000. He believes that adjuvant-enhanced animal models like the GPMT can detect most weak sensitizers, leaving compounds with allergenicity in the 1:10,000 range as those expected to enter the marketplace. It is generally recognized that the incidence of sensitization will never be zero. Animal tests that do not employ adjuvant are less sensitive for allergen screening. These animal tests are useful guides but still do not address the issues of concentration to be employed in finished products where skin contact is intended or inevitable; contact time; vehicle and solubility; or penetration of human stratum corneum. It is generally acknowledged that hexavalent chromium is a sensitizer and potential hazard, whereas trivalent chromium is less soluble and thus frequently behaves as a nonsensitizer, because it fails to penetrate human stratum corneum.[26] These factors are required if an evaluation of the

Table 3-2 Human Sensitizer Risk Assessment Variables

Normal versus dermatitic skin
Vehicle effects on absorption
Percutaneous absorption variables such as body site
Open or occluded use
Leave-on or rinse-off exposure
Duration of skin contact
Frequency of skin exposure
Use concentration

Table 3-3 Modified Draize and Human Maximization Tests

Substance	Human predictive test sensitized/tested	Percentage sensitized by patch test clinic data (NACDG)[b]
Formaldehyde	4.5%–7.8%/331	4
Parabens	0.3%/397	3
p-paraphenylenediamine	53%/NA	8
Balsam of Peru	28%/25[a]	3.2–4.5
Nickel	48%/25[a]	11
Chromium	48%/23	8
Ammoniated mercury	59%/74[a]	5
Neomycin	28%/25[a]	6
Thiuram	16%/25[a]	4
Benzocaine	6%/99	
	22%/23[a]	5
Ethylenediamine	8%/61	7

[a] Indicates human maximization test. All others are from modified Draize test. Summarized from Marzulli, FN, Maibach HI. Predictive testing in humans for contact allergy. In: Fisher AA, ed. Contact dermatitis. 3rd ed. Philadelphia: Lea & Febiger, 1986;30–44.
[b] NACDG, North American Contact Dermatitis Group.

sensitizing potential of a substance is to become a human risk assessment (Table 3.2).

According to Cronin and Agrup,[27], human test panels have statistical limitations. In order to ensure with a confidence limit of 99.5% that no more than 0.1% of a population would be sensitized, a human panel of 5,300 subjects would have to be tested. This would still be 10 times more people sensitized than if screening were done with adjuvant animal testing. The customary human panel consists of about 200 subjects.

The most commonly cited human predictive tests are the modified Draize test and the maximization test. In the modified Draize test, a high concentration of 0.5 mL or 0.5 g of material is suspended in petrolatum applied to the arm with occlusive bandages for 48 hours on 10 occasions. After 2 weeks' rest, a nonirritant concentration is applied to a new site for 72 hours. [28] The human maximization test usually uses 25 volunteers instead of the 200 used for the modified Draize test.[29] For the maximization test, 1 mL of 5% SLS followed by 1 mL of 25% test substance in petrolatum is applied to the arm on Webril, a type of gauze, and occluded with Blenderm tape. First, the SLS is applied for 24 hours; then the subject undergoes five successive 48-hour challenges of the SLS-treated site followed by a 10-day rest. The challenge for elicitation of sensitization is performed at a different site on the back. The skin is pretreated with 0.4 mL of 10% SLS for 1 hour, followed 24 hours later by 0.4 mL of test material at 10% concentration for 48 hours.

Some sample results of common patch test allergens evaluated by "predictive" methods, such as the modified Draize and human maximization tests, are seen in Table 3.3.[30]

Most substances commonly employed for diagnostic patch test purposes would be labeled as sensitizers by such predictive tests, but the frequency with which these materials are found in patch test clinics indicates the importance of the variables seen in Table 3.1. Sensitizers that affect 10 to 100 persons per 100,000 are generally identifiable with current methodology.

References

1. Lampe KF. Cutaneous toxicology. In: Drill VA, Lazar P, eds. New York: Raven Press, 1984.

2. Roberts DW, York M, Basketter DA. Structure-activity relationships in the murine local lymph node assay for skin sensitization: alpha, beta-diketones. Contact Dermatitis 1999; 41:14.

3. Rietschel RL, Nethercott JR, Emmett EA, et al. Methyl-chloroisothiazolinone-methylisothiazolinone reactions in patients screened for vehicle and preservative hypersensitivity. J Am Acad Dermatol 1990;22:734.

4. de Groot AC, Liem DH, Weyland JW, Kathron CG. Cosmetic allergy and patch test sensitization. Contact Dermatitis 1985;12:76.

5. Weaver JE, Cardin CW, Maibach HI. Dose-response assessments of Kathron biocide (I). Diagnostic use and diagnostic threshold patch testing with sensitized humans. Contact Dermatitis 1985;12:141.

6. Warbrick EV, Dearman RJ, Basketter DA, et al. Influence of application vehicle on skin sensitization to methyl-chloroisothiazolinone/methylisothiazolinone: an analysis using the local lymph node assay. Contact Dermatitis 1999;41:325.

7. Allen AM. Use and misuse of "epidemiology" [Letter]. Arch Dermatol 1974;110:131.

8. Prystowsky SD, Allen AM, Smith RW, et al. Allergic contact hypersensitivity to nickel, neomycin, ethylenediamine and benzocaine: relationships between age, sex, history of exposure, and reactivity to standard patch tests and use tests in a general population. Arch Dermatol 1979;115:959.

9. Meneghini CL, Rantuccio F, Lomuto A. Additives, vehicles and active drugs of topical medicaments as causes of delayed type allergic dermatitis. Dermatologica 1971;143:137.

10. North American Contact Dermatitis Group. Epidemiology of contact dermatitis in North America: 1972. Arch Dermatol 1973;108:537.

11. Nethercott JR, Holness DL, Adams RM, et al. Patch testing with a routine screening tray in North America, 1985 through 1989: frequency of response. Am J Contact Dermat 1991;2:122.

12. Shuster S. Patch-test sensitivity and reproducibility in individuals and populations. Am J Contact Dermat 1992;3:74.

13. Menné T, Christopherson J, Green A. Epidemiology of nickel dermatitis. In: Maibach HI, Menné T, eds. Nickel and the skin: immunology and toxicology. Boca Raton, FL: CRC Press, 1989.

14. Korossy S. Zur Epidemiologie der allergischen Kontakt Dermatitis in Ungarn. Dermatosen 1978;27:119.

15. Husain SL. Contact dermatitis in the west of Scotland. Contact Dermatitis 1977;3:327.

16. Henderson CR, Riley EC. Certain statistical considerations in patch testing. J Invest Dermatol 1945;6:227.

17. Health Effects Test Guidelines. EPA 560/6–82–001. Washington, DC: Office of Pesticides and Toxic Substances, U.S. Environmental Protection Agency, 1982.

18. Henningsen GM. Dermal hypersensitivity: immunologic principles and current methods of assessment. In: Hubson DW, ed. Dermal and ocular toxicology fundamentals and methods. Boca Raton, FL: CRC Press, 1991;153.

19. Basketter DA, Scholes EW, Wahlkvist H, Montelius J. An evaluation of the suitability of benzocaine as a positive control skin sensitizer. Contact Dermatitis 1995;33:28.

20. Gerberick GF, Ryan CA, Kern PS, et al. Compilation of historical local lymph node data for evaluation of skin sensitization alternative methods. Dermatitis 2005;16:157.

21. Basketter DA, Clapp C, Jefferies D, et al. Predictive identification of human skin sensitization thresholds. Contact Dermatitis 2005;53:260.

22. Wahlkvist H, Boman A, Montelius J, et al. Sensitizing potential in mice, guinea pig and man of the preservative Euxyl K 400 and its ingredient methyldibromo glutaronitrile. Contact Dermatitis 1999;41:330.

23. Magnusson B, Kligman AM. The identification of contact allergens by animal assay. The guinea pig maximization test. J Invest Dermatol 1969;52:268.

24. Nakamura A, Momma J, Sekiguchi H, et al. A new protocol and criteria for quantitative determination of sensitization potencies of chemicals by guinea pig maximization test. Contact Dermatitis 1994:31:72.

25. Maurer T. Contact and photocontact allergens: a manual of predictive test methods. New York: Marcel Dekker, 1983.

26. Burrows D. Adverse chromate reactions on the skin. In: Burrows D, ed. Chromium metabolism and toxicity. Boca Raton, FL: CRC Press, 1983:137.

27. Cronin E, Agrup G. Contact dermatitis C. Br J Dermatol 1970;82:428.

28. Marzulli FN, Maibach HI. Contact allergy: predictive testing in man. Contact Dermatitis 1976;2:1.

29. Kligman AM. The identification of contact allergens by human assay. III. The maximization test: a procedure for screening and rating contact sensitizers. J Invest Dermatol 1966;47:393.

30. Marzulli FN, Maibach HI. Predictive testing in humans for contact allergy in contact dermatitis. In: Fisher AA, ed. Contact dermatitis. 3rd ed. Philadelphia: Lea & Febiger, 1986;30.

CHAPTER 4

HISTOLOGY OF CONTACT DERMATITIS

EXECUTIVE SUMMARY

Histologic evaluation of potential contact dermatitis is useful primarily to eliminate other conditions that clinically may be confused with contact dermatitis. It is not possible on biopsy to differentiate contact dermatitis from other types of spongiotic dermatitis. From a research standpoint, very early biopsies (within 8 hours or so of induction) may show some differences between allergic contact dermatitis (ACD) and irritant contact dermatitis (ICD). Clinically, when a biopsy is usually performed at least several days after onset of disease, the changes of ICD and ACD may be virtually identical.

Contact dermatitis is normally differentiated from other types of dermatitis on the basis of clinical findings, knowledge of exposure to potential allergens or irritants, and diagnostic patch testing. The histopathology of contact dermatitis shows much overlap with that of the other forms of dermatitis and is, therefore, not usually helpful in distinguishing the various forms of dermatitis. Both irritant (ICD) and allergic contact dermatitis (ACD), however, have certain histopathologic features that may at times add weight to the evidence in favor of the diagnosis.

Histology of Allergic Contact Dermatitis

Cutaneous changes viewed by light microscopy are dependent on two factors, severity of the response to an allergen and time of biopsy after allergen exposure. Severity of the response in turn is dependent on both the potency of the allergen and the degree of immunologic sensitivity of the affected individual.

Biopsies of experimentally induced ACD (e.g., to 1% dinitrochlorobenzene [DNCB]) show changes as early as 4 to 8 hours after allergen application.[1] The earliest change noted is the appearance of a few lymphocytes perivascularly in the dermis. By 6 to 8 hours, some lymphocytes migrate into the epidermis as the dermal infiltrate increases. Also at about 6 to 8 hours, focal

spongiosis (intercellular edema) in the malpighian and basal layers occurs. Both of these findings peak at 24 to 48 hours after application. A study comparing punch biopsies from allergic patch tests (quaternium-15 or colophony) with irritant patch tests (benzalkonium chloride) demonstrated follicular spongiosis in six of seven allergic reactions but only one of seven irritant reactions.[2] Vesiculation occurs when the focal areas of spongiosis coalesce. With severe reactions, an occasional neutrophil may be seen, but this is rare in comparison to ICD. Eosinophils may be found in both the dermis and the epidermis and, if present, suggest ACD rather than another form of dermatitis. Starting at about 24 hours, and perhaps even earlier, basophils begin to appear. They may comprise up to 15% of the infiltrate by day 3, at which time tissue mast cells begin to increase in number. Whereas basophils enter the site from the blood, mast cells are formed by local replication, accounting for their delayed appearance. Other changes within the 24- to 48-hour time frame may include increased vascular permeability resulting in rare erythrocyte extravasation and dermal papillary edema, as well as fibrin deposition in the reticular dermis. After 48 to 72 hours, the activity of inflammation subsides. Rebuilding and "cleanup" processes occur with infiltration of macrophages needed for removal of keratinocyte debris.[3]

In contrast to the above experimentally derived data, biopsy of suspected contact dermatitis in the clinical setting usually occurs days or even months after onset. In this case, a pattern of subacute or chronic dermatitis may be seen, which may be impossible to distinguish from nummular dermatitis or lichen simplex chronicus.[4] The inflammatory infiltrate, again primarily lymphocytes and other mononuclear cells, is less prominent and, in fact, may be absent from the epidermis. One study has shown the presence of eosinophilic spongiosis in 28% of patints compared to controls and dendritic fibrohistiocytic cells in 44% compared to 24%.[5] In the dermis, a perivascular pattern is likely. Mild spongiosis and microvesicle formation may be seen, but these changes may be absent in long-standing dermatitis. Chronically, acanthosis with hyperkeratosis and some parakeratosis may be seen. Apparent intracellular edema may actually be due to glycogen distribution. Upper dermal fibrosis may occur as the result of thickened collagen.

Histology of Irritant Contact Dermatitis

Experimentally induced irritant contact dermatitis gives a very different histopathologic picture as compared to ACD when biopsies are taken during the first day or two following exposure. This would be expected because in ICD the epidermal damage is caused directly by the toxic agent, whereas in ACD the damage is due to the host's immune reactions. Although it varies with the strength and type of irritant, ICD generally develops much more quickly than ACD.[6] Within a few hours of exposure to a moderately strong irritant such as 10% DNCB, dermoepidermal separation begins. By 24 hours, epidermal necrosis is observed, often with subepidermal blister formation.[1] Lymphocytes are relatively rare in either the dermis or the epidermis. In contrast, the bulk of the inflammatory infiltrate is made up of neutrophils, which first appear within 6 to 8 hours of exposure. In guinea pigs, Anderson[7] has shown that basophils are much more plentiful in early allergic as opposed to irritant reactions. Although presumably all allergens induce a similar immune response, different irritants produce different histologic findings, depending on their mechanism of cell damage. For example, after 48 hours the cytotoxic agent dithranol produced a balloon degeneration of the upper dermis with disruption of mitochondria, whereas the detergent sodium lauryl sulfate induced parakeratosis and intracytoplasmic vesicles and lipid vacuoles.

Unfortunately, these differences between early ACD and ICD are rarely of clinical benefit because biopsies within the first few days of onset are usually unavailable. The histologic findings of a chronic low-grade ICD may be identical to those described above for ACD. Although by no means pathognomonic, the presence of eosinophils

might suggest ACD, whereas the absence of exocytosis of lymphocytes might suggest ICD.

Differentiating Contact Dermatitis from Other Dermatoses

At times, biopsy may shed light on a confusing clinical picture to help determine if the diagnosis is within the broad category of dermatitis as opposed to some other entity. Acute ICD or ACD, for example, may be simulated by bullous impetigo or a viral vesicular eruption such as herpes. The histologic pattern of these conditions would be readily distinguished from contact dermatitis. Contact urticaria or urticarial vasculitis can likewise be suggested by biopsy examination. Persistent or "dermal" contact dermatitis may be differentiated histologically from infiltrative processes such as rosacea, sarcoid, or cutaneous T-cell lymphoma. Generalized ACD, as sometimes seen in formaldehyde allergy, for example, can be histologically separated from erythroderma due to psoriasis, a drug reaction, or Sézary syndrome. The histopathology of these other conditions is thoroughly reviewed in texts on that subject.

Unusual Histologic Patterns of Contact Dermatitis

Occasional cases of ACD, either systemic or exogenous, may show histologic and clinical patterns simulating other diseases. These include erythema multiforme, vasculitis, and granuloma formation.[8] These rare variants are reviewed in the chapters covering the allergens involved.

Confocal Microscopy of Contact Dermatitis

Reflectance confocal microscopy (RCM) utilizes a low power laser to scan intact skin, with the resulting image of similar resolution to routine histology. Acutely, changes seen in both ACD and ICD were similar. ICD showed more disruption of the stratum corneum and parakeratosis.[9] A small study (14 subjects) showed more severe acute changes in white skin as opposed to black skin after exposure to the irritant sodium lauryl sulfate.[10] Another study of 16 subjects with positive patch tests to various allergens showed that spongiosis and exocytosis at the level of the stratum spinosum correlated highly with ACD as compared to controls.[11]

References

1. Medenica M, Rostenberg A. A comparative light and electron microscopic study of primary irritant contact dermatitis and allergic contact dermatitis. J Invest Dermatol 1971;56:259–71.

2. Vestergaard L, Clemmensen O, Sorensen F, Andersen K. Histologic distinction between early allergic and irritant patch test reactions: follicular spongiosis may be characteristic of early allergic contact dermatitis. Contact Dermatitis 1999;41:207–10.

3. Dvorak H, Mihm M, Dvorak A. Morphology of delayed-type hypersensitivity reactions in man. J Invest Dermatol 1976;67:391–401.

4. Lever WF, Schaumburg-Lever G. Histopathology of the skin, 7e. Philadelphia: WB Saunders, 1990:106–10.

5. Wildemore J, Junkins-Hopkins J, James W: Evaluation of the histologic characteristics of patch test confirmed allergic contact dermatitis. J Am Acad Dermatol 2003;49:243–8.

6. Willis C, Stephens C, Wilkinson J. Epidermal damage induced by irritants in man: a light and electron microscopic study. J Invest Dermatol 1989;5:695–9.

7. Anderson C. Dermal cell infiltrates: allergic, toxic, irritant, and type I reactions. Acta Derm Venereol Suppl (Stockh) 1988;68:24–7.

8. White C. Histopathology of exogenous and systemic contact eczema. Semin Dermatol 1990;9:226–9.

9. Swindells K, Burnett N, Rius-Diaz F, et al. Reflectance confocal microscopy may differentiate acute allergic and irritant contact dermatitis in vivo. J Am Acad Dermatol 2004;50:220–8.

10. Hicks S, Swindells K, Middlekamp-Hup M, et al. Confocal histopathology of irritant contact dermatitis in vivo and the impact of skin color. J Am Acad Dermatol 2003;48:727–34.

11. Astner S, Gonzalez E, Cheung A, et al. Pilot study on the sensitivity and specifity of in vivo reflectance confocal microscopy in the diagnosis of allergic contact dermatitis. J Am Acad Dermatol 2005;53:986–92.

CHAPTER 5

ROLE OF AGE, SEX, COLOR OF SKIN, AND ATOPIC STATUS

EXECUTIVE SUMMARY

Contact dermatitis occurs from infancy onwards. Irritant contact dermatitis in the form of diaper dermatitis is common. Disposable diapers can help in its control, but colorants and dyes used in some disposable diapers can cause allergy. Footwear is another common source of allergic contact dermatitis in children, as are metal objects, plants, and medications. Standard patch test allergens are suitable for use on children, and relevant reactions are seen in numbers similar to those in adult testing.

Elderly patients may acquire allergy to topical preparations used to treat stasis dermatitis. Allergy to hair dye, cosmetics, and fragrances is frequent.

Skin-to-skin contact can result in transfer of potential contact allergens from one sex partner to the other, resulting in consort or connubial contact dermatitis. Contact dermatitis related to sexual activity can result from lubricants, hygiene products, seminal fluid, and rubber in diaphragm and condoms. Race seems to be a minor factor in contact dermatitis. Studies point to more similarities than differences. A higher incidence of para-phenylenediamine allergy is found in blacks, along with more pigment abnormalities as a result of dermatitis in this group. Likewise, pomade acne is more prevalent among blacks.

Patch tests studies of patients with atopic dermatitis have found the tests to be of similar value to those seen in nonatopic patients. This has held true even though it can be demonstrated that it is more difficult to sensitize atopic patients when their disease is active. Individuals with atopy are prone to pustular reactions when tested with nickel. The use of aeroallergens to evaluate their role in atopic dermatitis cases has been difficult to standardize, and this has been particularly true for dust mite allergens.

Age Factors

CONTACT DERMATITIS IN CHILDHOOD

Both allergic and irritant varieties of contact dermatitis occur during childhood and infancy.[1] The skin is less reactive to potent contact sensitizers in early infancy than it is later in life. Irritant dermatitis readily takes place in persons of all ages, including newborns. Allergic dermatitis due to poison ivy oleoresin and to certain topical medications is by no means rare in early life.[2] Dermatitis due to clothing, particularly wool, and to sensitizers in shoes is frequent.

Certain topical medications that produce sensitization in adults, including mercury, benzocaine, and antihista-mines, also produce dermatitis in children. Antibiotic ointments may be prescribed in the same strength as for adults. Children are also susceptible to photosensitizing reactions from tar preparations used for topical medications and to the essential oils of perfumes.

Children may acquire severe irritant dermatitis and burns from accidental contact with a host of potentially harmful household products, including caustics.

Caustic Burns

So many caustic substances are used in the home that it is inevitable that children will suffer caustic burns. Proper treatment depends on whether the burn was caused by an acidic or an alkaline substance. The burn should be touched with the pH portion of a urine dipstick. Alkali burns may be treated with orange juice or vinegar; acid burns should be treated with bicarbonate paste or milk of magnesia.

Other household irritants include polishes, waxes, solvents, detergents, bleaching agents, disinfectants, and insecticides. Widespread dermatitis may be produced by baby oils containing antiseptics, such as 8-hydroxyquinoline sulfate (oxyquinoline sulfate). The eruptions may resemble prickly heat.

Highly perfumed oils, toilet soaps, and dusting powders may also cause infantile dermatitis. These preparations may accumulate in the folds of the skin, particularly in the axillary and inguinal folds, in which staphylococcal infections may become superimposed on the dermatitis. In general, infant skin tolerates lotions better than it does oils.

The use of nonperfumed oils, powders, and soaps free of antiseptics is recommended for infants. When the infant begins to crawl, dermatitis of the legs, knees, and elbows may be produced by floor polish, floor wax, rough fabrics used in rugs and carpets, and oily dust on furniture. The wearing of cotton coveralls prevents such dermatitis.

Dermatitis in children may result from exposure to irritants and sensitizers while participating in activities such as finger painting, shop work, and chemistry experiments. Crayons may also produce dermatitis.

Soap and Detergent Dermatitis

"Detergent hands" may occur in young girls who wash doll clothes. Honigman[3] showed that a subacute primary irritant dermatitis is brought about usually by prolonged bubble baths, bathing too frequently, using excessive amounts of bubble bath concentrate, or a combination of these factors. Children who have atopic eczema and who normally have xerotic skin are often severely affected.

Asteatosis and primary irritations are the inevitable results of overindulgence in bathing. Bubble baths assuredly can contribute to this problem.

Bubble baths are available as powders, liquids, and aerosol foams. They are often packaged in containers shaped appropriately for subsequent use as a toy when empty. The attractive container, the ease of bathing the child, and the child's preference for bubble baths account for their popularity with both parents and children.

Disposable Diapers

Disposable diapers were introduced in the United States in the early 1960s and are estimated to be used exclusively on 71% of infants; they are used along with cloth diapers in 22% of infants, and only 7% of infants now use cloth diapers.[4] There are two main types of disposable diapers: conventional cellulose-core diapers and extra-absorbent diapers containing absorbent gelling material (AGM). There is usually an inner topsheet in contact with the child's skin to decrease friction and distance the skin from the moisture in the cellulose-core diapers. The AGM is positioned in different locations in various manufacturers' products and is composed of high-molecular-weight polymers that gel on hydration. The outer covering is either polypropylene or polyethylene.

AGM-containing diapers have shown superiority over home-laundered cloth diapers in preventing diaper dermatitis, reducing wetness, and normalizing pH with the buffering capacity of sodium polyacrylate.[5] Disposable diapers are also available in a variety of colors. Alberta and colleagues reported 5 cases of diaper dermatitis due to dyes present in the diapers and all cases cleared with the use of dye free diapers. Patch test reactions in these patients who ranged in age from 9 months to 3 years included disperse red 17, disperse blue 106, disperse red 1, disperse blue 124, and disperse orange 3.[4]

Psoriasiform Diaper Dermatitis

This syndrome has been variously interpreted as an early manifestation of psoriasis, a seborrheic dermatitis, a candida infection, and a disease sui generis. Fergusson and colleagues[6] stated that treatment with antimonilial dyes in the diaper area is superior to therapy with steroid creams. The clinical appearance of the diaper eruption and the fact that all infants were hospital born were thought to support a monilial etiology.

Psoriasiform diaper dermatitis can be treated with the use of equal parts of a corticosteroid cream and Lassar's paste. This combination adheres well to the diaper area and is more efficacious than a corticosteroid cream or ointment alone.[7]

Perianal Dermatitis

Frequent soft or liquid stools and undigested food particles or their split products in feces may produce perianal dermatitis. Coating the area with zinc oxide ointment is protective and healing in such instances. Mercurial, formaldehyde, or strong detergent disinfectants on a thermometer may produce contact dermatitis in the perianal area.

Toilet seat dermatitis may be produced by strong detergents used to cleanse the seat. In addition, lacquer or paint covering the seat may cause a clearly defined pattern of dermatitis on the posterior aspect of the thighs and buttocks. Holme and colleagues reported a 3-year-old with dermatitis of the posterior thighs and buttocks due to a pine toilet seat. The coating had worn off and the child reacted to the wood shaving when patch tested and not to the painted shaving.[8]

Clothing Dermatitis

Irritant contact dermatitis in childhood is not uncommonly due to woolen clothing. Rough cuffs and collars, particularly when wet, readily irritate the skin, especially in children who have atopic dermatitis.

Residues of soap and detergent in laundered clothes can also be irritating. Highly starched garments may initiate dermatitis. Clothing dyes rarely cause dermatitis in infants. New clothing and bed linens should be washed before coming into contact with the inflamed skin of children. Clothing that has been drycleaned or contaminated with moth preventatives or insecticides should be thoroughly aired before being worn by the child.

Children's flame-retardant night clothing no longer contains TRIS (2,3-dibromopropyl) phosphate, a flame retardant that was once used frequently on acetate, acetate blends, triacetate, triacetate blends, and 100% polyester children's sleepwear.

The principal manner in which children's sleepwear has to comply with the flammability standards, however, is with the use of inherently flame-resistant fibers. Examples are modacrylic (brand names Verel, SEF, Kanecaron), modacrylic blends, matrix (brand name Cordelan), matrix blends, vinyon (brand name Leavil), vinyon blends, and polyester.

Wool, while it has the advantage of being nonflammable, cannot be tolerated by atopic persons. Cotton is not generally used in children's sleepwear at present. It has been replaced by the aforementioned synthetic fibers, which are flame resistant without further treatment (report from U.S. Consumer Products Commission, Washington, DC).

Dermatitis of the Feet

This type of dermatitis in children may be due to allergic sensitization to ingredients in shoes, particularly rubber. Frequently a nonspecific dermatitis is produced by the friction and irritation of an ill-fitting shoe. The dorsal aspect of the first toe may be involved in both allergic and irritant types of shoe dermatitis. It is not uncommon for friction of tight-fitting shoes to localize atopic dermatitis to this site. It may be necessary to perform patch tests with shoe ingredients in order to differentiate such atopic dermatitis from allergic contact dermatitis due to shoes.

Children whose feet perspire excessively and who wear socks containing synthetic fibers or sneakers, rubbers, or rubber-soled shoes for prolonged periods may suffer from sweaty-sock dermatitis, an eruption of the toes and interweb areas due to maceration by unabsorbed sweat[9]. These areas readily become eczematous and

infected. Paronychial infections and dystrophic nail changes in neglected cases are not uncommon.

This syndrome must be distinguished from tinea pedis, contact dermatitis from shoes, and atopic dermatitis. Scrapings and cultures for tinea may be necessary in the differential diagnosis. Allergic contact dermatitis to shoes usually spares the interdigital areas. Patch tests may be necessary to rule out sensitization to chemicals in footwear. Sweaty sock dermatitis is often confused with atopic dermatitis of the feet, particularly if hyperhidrosis also causes dermatitis of the antecubital fossae.

Juvenile plantar dermatosis (JPD) is probably the same condition, and the precise role of atopy in producing JPD is still not understood. A glazed and fissured plantar dermatitis is found as a morphologic marker of JPD. A personal or family history of atopic dermatitis is encountered in nearly half of children with JPD.[10,11]

Children with hyperhidrosis of the feet should wear all-cotton hose and, whenever feasible, shoes with perforated uppers or sandals. Prolonged wearing of rubbers, boots, sneakers, or other occlusive footwear should be avoided. Each morning Zea-SORB Powder (Stiefel) should be dusted onto the feet and into hose and footwear.

Contact Cheilitis and Perioral Dermatitis

In children, the lips and adjacent skin are commonly irritated. Children who have a habit of licking often have inflammation of this area. In addition, saliva trapped between the thumb and the mouth of a thumb-sucking child may produce dermatitis of the lips and cheeks. Similarly, children who salivate when teething may develop facial dermatitis. The constant chewing of bubble gum can produce dermatitis of the face and cheilitis because of the macerating effect of the moist gum and the irritation of essential oils.

Children whose eating habits permit foods such as spinach, carrots, and citrus fruit to remain on the cheeks may have dermatitis from the irritation of food juices. The facial dermatitis produced by saliva or food juices may closely resemble atopic eczema. Regurgitation of food particles may cause contact dermatitis around the mouth and on the neck and chin. Rubber-sensitive children may acquire a perioral dermatitis resembling perleche from chewing rubber pencil erasers or rubber bands.

Plant Dermatitis

Poison ivy, poison sumac, and poison oak are the most common causes of allergic eczematous contact dermatitis in children. Contact with resins of trees may also produce allergic dermatitis. Anemones and buttercups contain a blister-producing lactone that can cause vesiculation in children who crush or chew the plants.

Although allergic rhinitis due to ragweed protein is common throughout childhood, ragweed oil dermatitis is extremely rare during this period.

Vick's Vaporub contains several plant substances, including oil of turpentine, oil of eucalyptus, and oil of cedar, which may irritate or sensitize a child's skin. In addition, this nostrum contains camphor, menthol, oil of nutmeg, and thymol.

Although poison ivy dermatitis is essentially a summer disease, it may occur whenever children come into contact with the dried oleoresin on the twigs of the dormant plant. Not infrequently, pets, particularly long-haired dogs, come into contact with poison ivy plants and transmit the oleoresin to children. Ingestion of *toxicodendron* plants may produce systemic symptoms, such as vomiting, diarrhea, fever, convulsions, and stupor. Acute nephritis may accompany ingestion or marked cutaneous involvement.

There is no difficulty in sensitizing newborn infants to poison ivy oleoresin.[12] Although clinically one may see many severe cases of poison ivy dermatitis in children, experimental evidence indicates that poison ivy reactions are more intense in adults and that the reactivity does not reach its zenith for several years.

Cosmetic Dermatitis

Infants and children may acquire cosmetic dermatitis by contact with cosmetics worn by the mother and other attendants or by cosmetics in play.

The cheeks and forehead of an infant may be affected by the mother's or caregiver's perfume, face powder, lipstick, or hair spray. Dermatitis may occur if an attendant handles a child before her nail polish is dry. Berloque dermatitis in children, resulting in patchy pigmentation, may be seen from the photosensitizing effect of perfumes and toilet waters. Occasionally, children use irritating or sensitizing eye makeup.

Contact Urticaria Due to Milk in Childhood

Edwards[13] described contact urticaria that developed in an 18-month-old girl as a reaction to cow's milk. The child did not have a similar reaction after the milk was heated to 80°C for 30 seconds. This child presented with urticaria on the neck, perioral, and chest areas that developed immediately after her diet was changed from an infant formula without iron to commercial, pasteurized cow's milk. A few minutes after first drinking warm cow's milk, the child developed a red eruption on the face that disappeared after 30 minutes. No systemic manifestations of allergy were present.

Lecks[14] reported that a child developed a severe urticarial reaction of the diaper area with an anaphylactoid reaction from the use of Diaparene neonatal ointment, which contains a milk protein (casein). This case report is presented to alert pediatricians, allergists, and other practicing physicians of the hazards of using Diaparene neonatal ointment in infants and young children exquisitely sensitive to cow's milk proteins (see also Chapter 31).

Patch Testing in Childhood

Veien and colleagues[15] studied 168 children, 14 years of age or younger, who were patch tested with the Standard Series of the International Contact Dermatitis Research Group (ICDRG) over a 5-year period. Seventy-seven of the children had one or more positive reactions; relevant test results were found in 80% of them.

Eight boys and 24 girls were allergic to nickel, which proved to be the most common allergen. Five boys and 6 girls reacted to chromate, and 5 boys and 4 girls reacted to one or more of the rubber chemicals.

Although it was suggested that patch testing of children may result in nonspecific reactions, these investigators encountered no difficulty in the classification of allergic or toxic patch test results. This finding was in accord with the fact that most of the positive patch tests were relevant to the current dermatitis. Therefore, they prefer the same patch test allergens and concentrations used for adults rather than the lower concentration of allergens for children suggested by Fisher.[1]

In an evaluation of the currently available screening allergens sold by Hermal, the North American Contact Dermatitis Group[16] found that irritant reactions were not a problem for children when Finn chambers were used. This proved to be the case even though some allergens were tested at concentrations later deemed to be marginal irritants in adults: 2% cinnamic aldehyde in petrolatum, 2% formaldehyde aqueous, and 0.5% potassium dichromate in petrolatum. These three marginal irritant concentrations were later halved; nonetheless, irritant reactions were always less frequent in children than in adults, and relevant positive patch tests were found in 68% of children. A study from Scotland[17] of children tested with standard diagnostic patch test concentrations found 48% of 125 reactions to be positive and 92% to be relevant.

Five recent studies confirm the value of patch testing in children.[18–22] The frequency of positive patch tests ranged from 37% to 66%. Relevance ranged from 40% to 54%. The recurring theme of these reports is that nickel and other metals are the most commonly encountered allergens. Mercury and thimerosal are frequently found, probably due to thimerosal in immunizations. Fragrance and rubber chemical additives are also common. Roul and colleagues[18] found the peak incidence around 3 years of age, whereas Giordano-Labadie and colleagues[19] found the peak to occur after the age of 5. The relevance of nickel in children was uncommon enough to be called rare by Roul and colleagues. They believe that atopic dermatitis in children leads to frequent false-positive nickel patch tests. Whereas Roul and colleagues tested children of all types, Giordano-Labadie and colleagues focused on children with atopic dermatitis. Among the children with atopic dermatitis, metals were positive in 19.3%,[19] whereas in a German study of children (regardless of atopic status), 15.9% were sensitive to nickel.[20] The German study found a lower prevalence of atopic dermatitis among children with positive patch tests. Although there may be disagreement about the relevance of positive patch tests to metals in children, particularly atopic children, there is general agreement on the value of patch testing children with suspected contact dermatitis. A more recent German study of 285 children aged 6 to 12 and 2,175 adolescents aged 13 to18 found that contact allergy was detected in 52.6% of children and 49.7% of adolescents. The most common allergens were thimerosal, gentamicin sulfate, nickel sulfate, ammoniated mercury, cobalt chloride, fragrance mix, bufexamac, Compositae mix, propylene glycol, and turpentine.[21] In a study of children patch tested in Wales, 191 cases were identified and 41% had at least one reaction to a screening series of allergens. About 52% of the positive tests were deemed relevant. The most common allergens were nickel, fragrance, thiuram, cobalt, para-phenylenediamine, tixocortol pivalate, and *Myroxylon pereirae*. All cases were in children 16 and under.[22]

Two studies have reported on the use of the T.R.U.E test patch test system in children. A study of children in the eighth grade in Odense, Denmark, attempted to establish the prevalence of contact allergy in an unselected group of children. T.R.U.E test was used to evaluate contact allergy, and 15% of those tested had at least one positive patch test. The most commonly identified allergen was nickel (positive in 8%) and fragrance mix was the next most common at 2%.[23] However, a concern was raised in the second report. A study of infants aged from birth to 18 months was undertaken with T.R.U.E Test patches of nickel at 200, 66, and 22 $\mu g/cm^2$ and a fragrance mix at 430 $\mu g/cm^2$. While 200 $\mu g/cm^2$ is the standard test for adults in children tested at age 12 and again at age 18 months, reproducible reactions were found in 8.6% (20 girls and 6 boys) and transient reactions occurred in 111. Relevance was established in only one case, and it was suggested that a lower concentration of nickel would be needed in this age group. There were no reproducible reactions to the fragrance test.[24]

Epstein[12] stated that although allergic contact dermatitis in neonates and young infants is unusual, an occasional case may be overlooked because patch testing is rarely performed in this age group. Neonates and young infants can be sensitized. The lack of contact sensitization in this age group is a consequence of the lack of exposure to the more potent allergens in the environment.

ALLERGIC DERMATITIS DUE TO SPECIFIC SENSITIZERS IN CHILDREN

Table 5.1 lists the most common causes of allergic contact dermatitis in childhood, which are not very different from those of the general population.

Nickel Dermatitis

Sensitization to nickel in childhood is caused most frequently by the piercing of ears and insertion of nickel-plated earrings. Such sensitization has been reported in the first few weeks of life. Identification bands with a plastic strap and metal clip, zippers, metal tips of shoelaces, and coins have produced dermatitis in nickel-sensitive children. Once sensitization to nickel occurs, the child is subject to nickel dermatitis indefinitely.[25,26]

Neomycin

This antibiotic applied as a powder to circumcisions at certain hospitals has sensitized many infants.[27]

Mercaptobenzothiazole

This rubber chemical, present in many shoes and used as a rubber adhesive to cement shoe linings to shoe uppers, is one of the most common causes of allergic contact reactions in childhood, particularly in boys who have hyperhidrosis.[28]

Thimerosal (Merthiolate) and Merbromin (Mercurochrome)

These antiseptics, used frequently in infancy and childhood, may cause cases of allergic contact dermatitis.[25]

Table 5-1 Most Common Sensitizers in Childhood
Poison ivy, oak, and sumac
Mercaptobenzothiazole (in shoes)
Potassium dichromate (in shoes)
Nickel (in earrings)
Ethylenediamine hydrochloride
Topical antihistamines
Ethyl aminobenzoate (benzocaine)
Neomycin
Cosmetics
Perfumes
Balsam of Peru
Thimerosal (merthiolate)

Balsam of Peru

Several topical medications for use in the diaper area containing balsam of Peru (Balmex baby powder, emollient, lotion, and ointment, as well as Diaprox ointment) have produced allergic contact dermatitis.[29]

Ethylenediamine Hydrochloride

This stabilizer in original Mycolog cream, used on the diaper area, has sensitized many infants. Mycolog II does not contain ethylenediamine, and the original formula is available only from generic suppliers.

EFFECTS OF STRONG TOPICAL CORTICOSTEROIDS IN CHILDREN

Table 5.2 lists complications from the prolonged use of strong topical corticosteroids in children. Diffuse "wasting" of the skin on the diaper area may occur.[30] Occasionally, instead of general atrophy of the skin, atrophic striae may be formed in the inguinal area.[31] On the face, so-called perioral dermatitis or a more diffuse rosacea-like eruption may occur.[32]

LARGE GRANULOMAS IN DIAPER AREA FROM TOPICAL CORTICOSTEROIDS

In recent years, a new entity in the diaper area has been observed. Firm, angioma-like, painless swellings appear on the buttocks, inner thighs, and occasionally the lower abdomen. These large, symmetrical, round or oval nodules are oriented along the axis of the buttock folds, reaching the size of a cherry or plum, and are sharply demarcated, slightly protruding, and bluish-red or maroon in color. The infants are otherwise in good health, and the condition resolves spontaneously in several months with no treatment and without sequelae. This condition was first reported by Tappeiner and Pfleger,[33] who called it "granuloma gluteale infantum." The cause of this disorder is not entirely clear, but all reported patients have been on rather prolonged application of fluorinated corticosteroids for pre-existing diaper eruption, and all cases cleared slowly on discontinuation of treatment.[34]

Table 5-2 Complications of Strong Topical Fluorinated Corticosteroids

Diaper area
 Diffuse atrophy
 Atrophic striae
 Granulomas
Face
 Rosacea-like dermatitis

Japanese investigators reported five cases of Kaposi sarcoma–like granuloma occurring on the lesion of diaper dermatitis.[35] The common characteristic features of the clinical findings in these cases are summarized, with discussion of the similarities and differences between Kaposi sarcoma and the granulomas. In their cases, the lesions were in the genitocrural region, the thigh, and the penile region and were not observed on the gluteal region. Thus, the name "granuloma gluteale infantum" is not suitable. The investigators described their cases under the title of "Kaposi sarcoma–like granuloma on diaper dermatitis."

Georgouras and Kocsard[36] described a case of a 13-year-old boy who had a diffuse facial micropapular eruption with a granulomatous histology. The diagnosis is consistent with perioral dermatitis of the Gianotti type.[37] It is postulated that bubble gum was the cause of the condition. The most likely ingredients responsible for the problem were the essential oils in the gum, which may actually be selectively absorbed by the follicle to produce a follicular granulomatous reaction. We have added yet another cause for perioral dermatitis. Histologically, a granulomatous infiltrate with "sarcoid-like" appearance was present in some cases. Table 5.3 shows the numerous ingredients of chewing gum.

CONTACT DERMATITIS IN ELDERLY PATIENTS

If we arbitrarily define an elderly person as one who is entitled to Medicare, then the most common causes of allergic dermatitis among such persons are topical medications applied to stasis ulcers.[38,39]

Sensitizing topical agents used in the treatment of stasis ulcers produce widespread and even generalized eruptions (Table 5.4). Particularly in the elderly, "autosensitization" plays a prominent role in the development of serious eruptions from injudicious treatment of varicose ulcers and stasis eczema. A combination of sensitization to bacteria, the absorption of modified protein from inflamed or ulcerated skin, and topical medications are potential causes of autosensitization.

Sensitizing Topical Medications Applied to Stasis Ulcers

Neomycin   This antibiotic sensitizes 30% of persons when it is applied to stasis ulcers.[40] Erythromycin base in petrolatum has proved a safe, nonsensitizing antibiotic to apply to infected stasis ulcers.

Nitrofurazone   This antiseptic, a favorite of some surgeons for ulcers and burns, is a potent sensitizer. In addition, the polyethylene glycols used as a vehicle for nitrofurazone can cause allergic contact dermatitis.[41]

Table 5-3 Chewing Gum Additives[a]

BHA (butylated hydroxyanisole)

BHT (butylated hydroxyaluene) as antioxidant

Butadiene styrene rubber

Butyl rubber

Chewing gum base, which includes:

  Chicle, chicuibal, crown gum, gutta hand kang, massaranduba balata, massaranduba chocolate, nespero, rosidinba, Venezuelan chicle, jelutong leche caspi, pendara, perilla, leche devaca, niger gutta, tunu, chilte, natural rubber

Chilte

Glycerine ester of partially hydrogenated wood resin

Glycerin ester of polymerized resin

Isobutylene-isoprene capolymer

Isobutylene resin

Lanolin

Latex (butadiene styrene rubber)

Paraffin wax

Polyvinyl acetate (molecular weight 2,000 minimum)

Resin, polymerized, partially hydrogenated, and/or partially dimerized, glyceral esters

Rubber (natural), smoked sheet, and latex solids

Sodium sulfate

Sodium sulfide

Terpene resin (synthetic polymers of B-pinene and natural polymers of A-pinene)

[a]Compiled by Stephen D. Lockey, Sr., M.D., 60 North West End Avenue, Lancaster, PA 17603.

Table 5-4 Common Sensitizers in Topical Agents Applied to Stasis Ulcers

Ethylenediamine hydrochloride

Lanolin

Neomycin

Nitrofurazone

Paraben preservatives

Vitamin E creams

Vehicle Ingredients Lanolin and the parabens are rather rare sensitizers, except when applied to stasis eczema and stasis ulcers.[42]

Other Causes of Allergic Contact Dermatitis in the Elderly

As far as the older age group is concerned, Fisher felt that the common potent sensitizers, such as paraphenylenediamine, nickel, the dichromates, poison ivy, and rubber compounds produce as many instances of contact dermatitis with strongly positive patch test reactions in patients over age 65 as in younger age groups. The experience of the North American Contact Dermatitis Group showed that, indeed, a wide variety of common sensitizers is regularly identified in patients age 80 and older.[16]

Aside from dermatitis owing to topical medications and poison ivy dermatitis, the following are not infrequently encountered in elderly persons.

Hair-Dye Dermatitis Allergic eczematous contact dermatitis owing to paraphenylenediamine hair dyes is not uncommon in elderly women. In 30 persons sensitive to it, 10 were over 60 years of age.[43] Furriers, occupationally sensitized to paraphenylenediamine, show positive patch test reactions long after they have retired, even if they are no longer in contact with paraphenylenediamine.[44]

Wearing-Apparel Dermatitis A dermatitis due to the finishes and dark dyes of clothes is facilitated in menopausal women because of hyperhidrosis. "Widow's dermatitis" or "mourner's dermatitis" may be produced by allergic sensitivity to the black dyes in clothing worn for the first time when the patient is in mourning. Obesity in older age groups can be a factor in producing wearing-apparel dermatitis due to friction and sweating.

Industrial Dermatitis In industry, a severe allergic contact dermatitis can develop suddenly in older workers who have handled certain substances in their occupation for decades without difficulty. This is likely to occur in cement workers, painters, tile setters, and bakers. Even prompt retirement and the avoidance of irritants or specific allergens do not necessarily prevent the dermatitis or keep it from becoming generalized. Such widespread involvement may be due to increased nonspecific irritability of the entire skin surface, which becomes hyperreactive to many irritants and even to bland substances.[39]

Ragweed Dermatitis Ragweed dermatitis is caused by ragweed oleoresin, in contrast to ragweed rhinitis and asthma, which are caused by the protein fraction of ragweed pollen. Ragweed dermatitis is almost exclusively a male dermatitis, occurring most commonly in farmers age 40 to 75.[45] However, people in other occupations and in suburban areas frequently become sensitized to ragweed oil. Even "city folk" can acquire ragweed dermatitis because ragweed pollen contaminated with the sensitizing oleoresin can be airborne for long distances and can be confused easily with a photodermatitis.

Photodermatitis Photodermatitis, owing to aftershave lotion containing musk ambrette and actinic reticuloid, is encountered in the elderly.

Dryness of the skin in elderly persons may be aggravated through normal use of toilet soaps and detergents, predisposing the elderly to allergic contact sensitization.

To relieve the dryness, the patient may use lubricants and bath oils containing lanolin products or surfactants that may be sensitizers.

In tracking down the cause of contact dermatitis in the older age group, not only must the physician question the patient concerning new contactants, but a thorough investigation must also be made of substances to which the patient has been exposed for decades. It is surprising how frequently the older patient becomes sensitized to a contactant to which he or she has been exposed intermittently throughout life without any previous reaction.[46] Properly performed patch tests are reliable in finding the causative agents in allergic contact dermatitis in persons of this age group.

Systemic Eczematous Contact Dermatitis in the Elderly Elderly persons may take one or more drugs that are chemically related to topical sensitizers. Eczematous drug eruptions may closely resemble allergic contact dermatitis. Usually an eczematous drug eruption is more widespread and symmetrical than an "external" contact eruption.

Table 5.5 lists drugs that may produce an eczematous drug reaction in which the initial sensitization may have been induced by a topically applied medication chemically related to the drug. In such instances, patch testing may be valuable in detecting the offending drug.

Features of Contact Dermatitis in Elderly Patients In older people, the disease, even during the acute stage, may show relatively little vesiculation or inflammation. Scaling is regularly a prominent feature in all phases of dermatitis in the elderly. Thickening, hyperpigmentation, and lichenification take place readily, and itching is usually pronounced. Both allergic and irritant eruptions tend to persist and be more resistant to therapy in the aged than in younger persons.

If the older patient is managed improperly or is re-exposed to irritants or sensitizers, the eruption readily becomes widespread and intractable, particularly if intercurrent disease is present.

Finally, in all cases of intractable contact dermatitis, serious systemic disease or internal malignancy may be suspected.[47] In addition, many elderly patients have persistent eczematous dermatoses that resemble contact dermatitis clinically and histopathologically and are in reality a form of mycosis fungoides.[48]

USE OF PATCH TESTS IN DRUG ERUPTIONS

In general, aside from the use of patch tests in certain types of eczematous eruptions, skin tests have not as yet proved to be of predictable value.

Table 5-5 Topical Sensitizers and Immunochemically Related Drugs that Can Cause Eruption upon Systemic Administration
TOPICAL SENSITIZERS
Hydrazine hydrobromide
Para-amino compounds
Ethyl aminobenzoate (benzocaine)
Paraphenylenediamine
Balsam of Peru
Neomycin sulfate
Resorcinol (Resorcin)
Organic and inorganic mercurials
Metallic mercury
Cobalt
Thiamine
Ethylenediamine hydrochloride
Formaldehyde
Thiram and disulfiram
Halogenated hydroxyquinolones
Chlorobutanol
Iodine
Caladryl, diphenhydramine (Benadryl Cream)
IMMUNOCHEMICALLY RELATED DRUGS
Isoniazid, hydralazine (Apresoline), phenelzine sulfate
Para-aminobenzoic acid (PABA)
Azo dyes in foods and drugs
Dymelor, Orinase, Diabinese, sulfonamides, chlorothiazide (Diuril), hydrochlorothiazide (HydroDiuril), hydroflumethiazide (Saluron), polythiazide (Renese), para-aminosalicylic acid (PAS)
Cinnamon
Streptomycin, kanamycin
Hexylresorcinol (Crystoids, Caprokol)
Mercurial diuretics
Calomel
Vitamin B_{12}
Coenzyme B (cocarboxylase)
Aminophylline, antazoline (Antistine), tripelennamine (Pyribenzamine), thonzylamine (Neohetramine), piperazine, hydroxyzine (Atarax, Vistaril), methenamine (Urotropin), methenamine mandelate (Mandelamine), urised disulfiram (Antabuse)
Iodochlorhydroxyquin (Vioform), iodoquinol (Diodoquin)
Chloral hydrate
Iodides, iodinated organic compounds
Diphenhydramine (Benadryl)

Table 5.5 lists drugs that can produce a systemic contact-type drug eruption in patients who have been sensitized originally to the drug or to a related chemical by topical application. This type of drug reaction is usually eczematous. The patch test is valuable in confirming the identity of the offending drug.[49]

Felix and Comaish[50] emphasized that, apart from clinical challenge, there is no consistently reliable test to confirm that a drug is the cause of an adverse systemic reaction. One of their patients had an eczematous reaction to diazepam and positive patch tests, although intradermal tests were negative. Another patient had two anaphylactoid reactions to meprobamate, indicating a type-1 (immediate hypersensitivity) reaction. Skin testing in this patient, however, was more in keeping with a type-4 (delayed) reaction (positive patch test).

If patch tests are positive in a patient and negative in an adequate number of controls, this finding may be considered important whenever a clinical systemic reaction has occurred.

Korbitz[51] treated a patient with quinine-induced thrombocytopenic purpura, which proved to be caused immunochemically by an IgG quinine-dependent platelet antibody. A successful "petechial" patch test of quinine was obtained using Telfa gauze pledgets saturated with a quinine solution. Parafilm was placed over the gauze, and a gauze pad was also placed on top, resulting in petechiae at 48 hours that persisted for several days.

Aside from quinidine, a patch test with a solution of carbromal or apronalide (Sedormid) may induce a petechial reaction in patients with purpura caused by these drugs. If no purpura develops spontaneously at the test site, the arm may be congested with the sphygmomanometer cuff, and the test site inspected for hemorrhages. A positive purpuric patch test may be significant, but a negative test does not exonerate the drug.

Houwerzijl and colleagues[52] observed an epileptic patient treated with carbamazepine and phenytoin (diphenylhydantoin) who developed an extensive erythematous, maculopapular rash and generalized lymphadenopathy. Positive patch tests were obtained for 1% and 5% carbamazepine but not for the phenytoin.

Van Ketel[53] tested 247 patients with a history of drug reactions. Ninety-three of these patients had had a skin reaction to penicillin. Patch testing of the 93 patients revealed that 21 showed positive delayed patch test reactions to one or more penicillins. Except possibly in one case, no patients were sensitized by the patch test procedure.

Penvy and Schroepl[54] stated that patch tests with drugs must be read with great caution because many drugs produce irritant reactions. The authors carried out epicutaneous control tests with 44 psychopharmaceutic agents in the pure state on 40 nonallergic persons. All subjects showed at least one positive epicutaneous reaction. It was concluded that tablets, either coated or uncoated, are unsuitable for epicutaneous testing.

A study of 826 patients who received patch tests to evaluate suspected drug hypersensitivity found that 89 (10.8%) had a positive patch test. The most frequent of these drugs were beta-lactams, clindamycin, and tri-methoprim. A positive skin-prick test was found in only 10 of 935 patients (1.1%). Rechallenge with the drug identified by the positive skin test in 17 patients showed that 13 of 16 patch-test–positive patients developed an exanthema and one prick-test–positive patient developed urticaria.[55]

Cutaneous adverse drug reactions are sometimes evaluated by patch tests, prick tests, or intradermal tests. Suggested guidelines for patch-testing drugs to identify the source of the eruption have been published and include:

1. Waiting 6 weeks to 6 month after the eruption has resolved
2. Testing of commercialized drug at 30% in petrolatum and/or aqueous
3. Testing of pure drug at 10% in petrolatum or aqueous, but lower concentration if the reaction was severe
4. Taking of readings at day 1 and 7 in addition to traditional readings
5. Application of the test over the most severely affected area.[56]

In fixed drug eruption, the patch may occasionally be of some help. Thus, phenolphthalein, tested 2% powder in aqueous solution left on for several days, may sometimes reproduce a fixed drug eruption. There is a greater chance that the test will be positive if the test site was part of the initial eruption. In a recent report, a generalized eruption to the antiarrhythmia agent mexiletine hydrochloride was positive at 6.25%, 12.5%, and 25% in petrolatum *only* on previously involved skin. Patch tests and scarified patch tests of noninvolved skin were negative.[57]

Role of Sex in Contact Dermatitis

There is very little difference in susceptibility to allergic contact dermatitis due to sex. Leyden and Kligman[58] have reported that bona fide sex differences in prevalence rates of response to contact allergens reflect the intensity of past exposure. Nickel sensitivity occurs predominantly in women, as would be expected from their greater contact with jewelry. Likewise, allergy to perfumes is far more frequent in women. These disparities may change as men increasingly adopt practices that were formerly the province of women. On the other hand, men predominate in chromium allergy because of occupational exposures such as those in the cement industry.

Björnberg[59] was unable to demonstrate any difference between men and women in skin reactions to primary irritants.

CONNUBIAL AND CONSORT CONTACT DERMATITIS

Wilkinson,[60] in describing two cases of connubial contact dermatitis, stated that contact dermatitis or photodermatitis in a patient may be due to the work or household activities of the spouse or to medicaments the patient is receiving. He warns us not to neglect patients' spouses when tracking down the cause of contact dermatitis.

In this day and age, however, investigation of contact with a spouse without considering other partners sometimes fails to detect many cases of contact dermatitis. The old-fashioned term "consort," which can apply to not only a spouse but also a companion or partner, seems to fit the present situation more accurately. In consort contact dermatitis, whether or not it is connubial, the dermatitis is not necessarily produced by sexual exposure.[61]

Connubial Propylene Glycol Dermatitis (K-Y Jelly Dermatitis)

A 55-year-old man had previously experienced a severe allergic contact dermatitis after using halcinonide (Halog cream). Patch test procedures had proved that the patient was allergic to the propylene glycol in the preparation. One year later, 24 hours after having intercourse with his wife, the patient developed a severe pruritic dermatitis of the penis and scrotum with marked erythema, edema, slight scaling, and crusting.

It was ascertained subsequently that his wife had for the first time used K-Y Jelly as a vaginal lubricant prior to intercourse. After 48 hours, patch tests gave positive results to the K-Y Jelly and to 5% and 10% aqueous solutions of propylene glycol. In five controls, patch tests gave negative results to K-Y Jelly. This finding was the first reported instance of connubial K-Y Jelly dermatitis.[62,63]

Feminine Hygiene Dermatitis

A 30-year-old man stated that he believed he was allergic to one of his girlfriends' secretions because each time they had intercourse he acquired a dermatitis of his penis, scrotum, and lower abdomen. Relations with other women did not produce this dermatitis. After routine patch testing, results showed a positive patch reaction only to balsam of Peru. This finding suggested the possibility of an allergic reaction to a perfume.[64] After further questioning, it was discovered that this girlfriend used a feminine hygiene spray prior to intercourse.

Positive results were obtained when this feminine hygiene spray was patch tested. Patch tests to three other feminine sprays gave positive results to two of them and negative results to the third. The patient's girlfriend is now using a feminine hygiene spray that does not produce dermatitis, and the patient no longer acquires dermatitis after intercourse.[64]

Benzoyl Peroxide Dermatitis

A 20-year-old woman believed that she was allergic to her boyfriend because an eruption developed on her face, neck, and occasionally her arms each time they had intercourse. Examination revealed a patchy, eczematous eruption on her face and neck. Patch tests to the "screening" patch test tray and the patient's cosmetics gave negative results.

Further investigation revealed that her consort used a 5% benzoyl peroxide preparation for a facial acneiform eruption. Patch tests of the benzoyl peroxide preparation and of a 1% benzoyl peroxide in petrolatum gave positive results. After the boyfriend changed the benzoyl peroxide preparation to a topical antibiotic, the patient's eruption subsided.

This case of consort contact dermatitis is quite similar to a case of connubial dermatitis reported by Caro,[65] whose patient was a physician who developed a pruritic erythematous eruption localized on the right side of the neck and the right anterior axillary fold. The patient had recently given his wife a preparation containing 5% benzoyl peroxide for mild acne on her back. Patch tests with 1% benzoyl peroxide in petrolatum also gave positive results.

Caro ascertained that the patient slept on the left side of the bed; the right side of his neck and the interior axillary fold on the right were thus in contact with the bedding, which could be contaminated by benzoyl peroxide applied to his wife's back just before she retired.[65] The wife discontinued using the preparation, and the physician has had no further dermatitis.

Consort Sunscreen Dermatitis

A young woman developed a diffuse follicular eruption of the upper arms, anterior trunk, inner thighs, and buttocks that resembled recurrent and disseminated infundibulo-folliculitis of Hitch and Lund. This eruption cleared when her fair-skinned boyfriend left town, and reappeared some months later upon his return. The couple frequently spent their weekends at the beach, where he applied a homosalate-containing sunscreen (Coppertone Lotion), but the woman, who was olive-complexioned, used no topical products. The physical contact that occurred following their beach excursions explained the distribution of the eruption, which occurred only on the woman. She was patch test positive to both Coppertone Lotion and 2% homosalate in petrolatum.[66] The patch test produced a typical eczematous reaction, but the clinical picture resembled a folliculitis most likely due to small amounts of material transferred by skin-to-skin contact through follicular diffusion shunts.

Consort Seminal Fluid Reactions

There are several reports of severe pruritus, urticaria, and even anaphylaxis owing to reactions in women who proved to have allergic hypersensitivity to seminal fluid.[67–72] These cases, divided approximately equally between connubial and nonconnubial exposure, are exquisite examples of allergic "consort" contact reactions. Postcoital vulvar dermatitis may be due to contact allergy to seminal fluid. Guillet and Dagregorio reported two cases of vulvar dermatitis that improved when condoms were used, and in their cases no IgE antiseminal antibodies were found. Rather, they performed patch tests with the partners' semen and noted 2+ reactions at day 2, persisting for several additional days. This supports a diagnosis of allergic contact dermatitis for semen.[73]

Rubber Diaphragm Dermatitis

Rubber-sensitive women may acquire vulvitis and vaginitis from contraceptive rubber diaphragms. Male rubber-sensitive partners may similarly acquire balanitis from contact with such diaphragms.

Condom Dermatitis

Because allergic hypersensitivity to rubber condoms occurs occasionally, rubber-sensitive men and women should be informed that nonrubber condoms such as Fourex (Schmidt) and Lambskin (Youngs Rubber) made of processed sheep's intestine are available. However, a better alternative is the use of polyurethane condoms, available for both men and women.

Dermatitis Due to Sensitizers in Contraceptive Spermicides

Such sensitizers include phenylmercuric acetate, oxyquinoline sulfate, quinine hydrochloride, and hexylresorcinol.

CONNUBIAL WORK CLOTHES DERMATITIS

Fiberglass Dermatitis

A 36-year-old woman and her husband had been treated for "scabies" for 3 months without results. The husband had marked folliculitis, papular urticaria, and linear erosions in the creases. The wife had a milder, pruritic follicular eruption. It was revealed that the husband recently had become employed in a fiberglass factory and had brought home his fiberglass-contaminated work clothes,

which his wife washed together with her own clothes. Because it was believed that this might be the cause of the eruption, the husband was instructed to apply talcum powder liberally to his entire body just before he put on his work clothes, and the wife was instructed to wash her husband's work clothes separately from her own. One week after this procedure was instituted, the eruption on both husband and wife subsided completely.

Fisher and Warkentin[74] also reported a case of fiberglass dermatitis in a husband and wife who washed their fiberglass curtains in the same washing machine as their clothing.

Connubial Chloracne

A persistent follicular acneiform eruption developed on the forearms of a 40-year-old woman. She then revealed that her husband delivered fuel oil and had acquired a widespread chloracne. The patient inquired whether her husband's eruption was "contagious." She also stated that before putting her husband's oil-soaked clothing in the washing machine, her forearms often came in contact with the clothing.

The patient was instructed to place the soiled work clothes in the washing machine with a long forceps. The acneiform eruption subsided completely 3 weeks after the patient started using this procedure.

IRRITANT AND TRAUMATIC DERMATITIS

This type of dermatitis is usually characterized by redness, swelling, and a burning sensation. The history may reveal unusual "gymnastic" sexual maneuvers. Patients should also be asked whether they have cleansed the skin with strong soaps or detergents or have vigorously used rough towels.

Traumatic sexual dermatitis should be suspected when abrasions, fissures, erosions, or ulcers are present on the genitalia and perirectal area. Anal sexual eroticism is a fact of modern life, playing a major role in homosexual relationships. Skin injury from various manipulations and contact with "erotic" objects must be considered in both homosexual and heterosexual exposure.

Not infrequently, traumatic contact dermatitis is complicated by a superimposed allergic reaction due to the application of various medications. The patient should be asked, "What medicine did you apply to your skin?" The most common causes of allergic contact dermatitis superimposed on traumatic dermatitis are benzocaine, neomycin, and thimerosal (merthiolate).

Patients do not always readily admit the origin of penile ulcers caused by human bites. In addition to biting, a sexual partner may produce ulcers of the penis by scratching, by burning the penis with a lighted cigarette, or by injuring the penis with some instrument.

Marked swelling of the penis in circumcised persons may occur several hours after repeated vigorous intercourse with a passive partner. The involved area may be tender. A correct diagnosis is based on the history of a young vigorous male having intercourse with a sexually nonparticipating partner. There is absence of abrasions, ulcerations, adenopathy, or urethral discharge. There is no significant incubation period, and rapid recovery occurring after sexual abstinence is the rule without any particular therapy.

Balanoposthitis, inflammation of the membrane covering the glans penis and prepuce, occurs most frequently in uncircumcised men. The amount and type of involvement depend on the presence or absence of redundant prepuce, the degree of phimosis, and the severity of the irritation.

Irritant balanitis is usually mild, but it can progress to erosive balanitis with edema, hyperemia, and bleeding of the glans. The patient should be cautioned to avoid excessive trauma and irritation from strenuous intercourse or fellatio.[75–78]

The management of contact balanoposthitis consists of retraction of the foreskin two or three times daily for careful cleansing with soap and water. The prepuce must not be left in the retracted position because paraphimosis may result. The penis is soaked for 15 minutes three times daily in Burow's solution diluted 1 to 10 in water; 1% hydrocortisone cream or lotion is then applied.

HEMORRHAGIC CHANGES OF ORAL MUCOSA DUE TO FELLATIO

Worsaae and Wanscher[75] reported a 34-year-old white woman who presented with a circular hemorrhagic lesion located on the soft palate caused by fellatio. The lesion consisted of erythema, petechiae, dilated blood vessels, and vesicles. It healed in a few days. No evidence of the major clinical alternatives, such as thrombocytopenia, venereal disease, or candida infection, were found. Injuries due to fellatio must be considered as an etiologic factor of hemorrhagic changes of the oral mucosa; patients with a positive history can be spared other investigations.

CONTACT DERMATITIS IN HOMOSEXUAL MEN

Contact dermatitis due to self-administered medications is quite common in gay men. One type of contact dermatitis, "poppers' dermatitis," is seen occasionally in gay men.

"Poppers' Dermatitis"

This dermatitis results from the inhalation of amyl or butyl nitrite, which is popularly known as "popping," to obtain a sexual "high," a common practice among gay men. The inhalation of the nitrites produces a warm sensation, dizziness, a flushing of the skin, and a "rush" as the blood vessels dilate, the heartbeat quickens, and the blood rushes to the brain.

This use of amyl or butyl nitrite is related to several unconventional sexual practices in gay men. These nitrites, perhaps more than any other illicit drugs currently in use, have a specifically sexual function: They are inhaled immediately before sexual climax. In the homosexual community in particular, use of nitrites to intensify orgasm is widespread. A guide to homosexual lovemaking states that the use of amyl nitrite "has passed into every corner of gay love."[79]

Nature and Uses of Volatile Nitrites

Lowry[79] writes that the inhaled volatile nitrites are among the most widely used sexual "enhancers" in the United States today; moreover, their use is growing.

Two volatile nitrites are most commonly used as recreational drugs: amyl nitrite ($C_5H_{11}NO_2$) and isobutyl nitrite ($CH_3(CH_2)_3ON$). Amyl nitrite is a prescription drug approved by the Food and Drug Administration for the diagnosis and treatment of heart diseases. Isobutyl nitrite is not listed as a drug but is marketed as a "room odorizer."

Amyl nitrite is a clear, yellowish, volatile, flammable liquid with a peculiarly ethereal and fruity odor. This prescription item is available from two pharmaceutical manufacturers: as Aspirols (Lilly) and as Vapolole (Burroughs Wellcome). Amyl nitrite is supplied in fragile 0.3-mL glass containers enclosed in a gauze jacket of woven absorbent covering, which can readily be crushed between the fingers and held to the nostrils for inhalation. The noise made when the bottle is crushed gives rise to the street names, "popper" and "snapper."

Isobutyl nitrite, usually distributed in a 12-mL bottle with a screw cap, does not require a prescription and is less expensive than amyl nitrite. On the street, isobutyl nitrite is sold under various names (Table 5.6) and in

Table 5-6 Street Names for Isobutyl Nitrite	
Aroma of Men	Hi Baller
Black Jac	Krypt Tonight
Bolt	Lockaroma
Bullet	Locker Room
Cat's Meow	Mama Popperer's Olde Fashioned
Climax	Fragrance
Discorama	Oz
Dr. Bananas	Rush
The Blues	Satan's Scent
Hardware	

such places as record shops, "radical" or "erotic" boutiques, "head" shops, adult book stores, and "specialty" shops as a "personal" product, "liquid scent," or "room odorizer." One manufacturer alone is currently producing 4 million bottles a year. A conservative extrapolation would yield a nationwide annual production of 250 million recreational doses of volatile nitrites.

Use of Nitrites among Homosexuals Thirty years ago, amyl nitrite was widely used by heterosexual and homosexual persons in New York City's artistic and theatrical colony. Today, the nitrites, especially isobutyl nitrite, are most widely used among homosexuals. Perhaps this is because of visible social clustering of homosexuals at clubs, discos, and baths, whereas heterosexual users are a more diffuse group that is hard to locate, measure, or identify.[80]

Goode and Troiden[81] interviewed 150 homosexual men to determine the relationship between the use of amyl nitrite and certain aspects of homosexual practice. These investigators found that the nitrites, perhaps more than any other illicit drug currently in use, have specifically sexual functions. Thus, the volatile nitrites can be inhaled either during foreplay (producing floating sensations, increased skin perception, and loss of inhibitions) or just before orgasm. In the latter instances, users report that the climax is intensified and prolonged.

Adverse reactions from the volatile nitrites. Mild transitory headache, rapid pulse, dizziness, and flushing of the face are common among all users of nitrites. Adverse reactions that may occur in susceptible patients are nausea, vomiting, weakness, restlessness, pallor, cold sweat, involuntary passing of urine and feces, tachycardia, hypotension, syncope, and collapse. Excessively high doses of amyl nitrite may cause methemoglobinemia.

Pearlman and Adams[82] call special attention to the fact that the nitrites may also produce a transient elevation of intraocular pressure. Thus, ophthalmologists should be aware of this fact when they examine young patients who complain of pain about the eyes and intense headache and in whom increased intraocular pressure may be found. These physicians must be aware of the possibility of amyl nitrite abuse in this younger age group. Recognizing the source of their symptoms and findings can largely remove the need for a more extensive glaucoma evaluation unless the intraocular pressure remains elevated for a prolonged period. The use of nitrites, however, might also harm persons with proved glaucoma.

Effects on skin and mucosa from inhaling nitrites In persons who inhale nitrites, marked vasodilation of the blood vessels in the skin is present, particularly in the "blush" zone of the head, neck, and clavicular area. In some instances, nasotracheal irritation and sinusitis develop.[83,84]

Patch testing with nitrites The volatile nitrites are irritants under a closed patch. "Open" testing in one patient who had dermatitis revealed a marked eczematous reaction that did not occur in three control subjects. A yellowish dermatitis can be a clue to nitrites as a cause of dermatitis. Three patients had facial dermatitis characterized by crusts with a distinctive yellowish tint.[83,84] Fregert and colleagues[85] have a possible explanation for this yellowish color. They noted that certain factory workers exposed to nitric acid or nitrites acquired a yellow stain on their palms. These authors state that the yellow stain caused by nitric acid or nitrites in an acid environment is known as the xanthoprotein reaction, which is presumed to arise by nitration of the aromatic nuclei of certain amino acids incorporated into the protein chain.

Finally, because some butyl nitrite preparations contain a fragrance, the possibility that an allergic reaction may develop in addition to an irritant reaction has to be considered during examination of a perfume-sensitive person.

TRAUMATIC PENILE ULCERS
Dequalinium, a quaternary ammonium compound with antimicrobial and antifungal properties, is a recognized cause of penile ulcerations. Most cases have been recognized in Europe, but the antiseptic may be acquired by travelers abroad and brought into this country. The patients are usually uncircumcised men who have been treated with dequalinium because of pre-existing balanitis. The resultant ulcers may be deep and necrotic, with sites of predilection on the glans and prepuce.

Unexplained ulcers of the penis that do not correspond to well-defined disease may be of factitial origin. Patients have produced ulcers of the penis with lighted cigarettes, razor blades, and a range of objects that demonstrate a remarkable degree of resourcefulness.

TRAUMATIC SCLEROSING LYMPHANGITIS OF THE PENIS
Male homosexuals may exhibit a specific type of edema of the glans penis and coronal area that is doughy and plastic, appearing 24 to 48 hours after intercourse.

LYMPHOCELE
This condition may occur following excessive sexual intercourse or masturbation. The lymphatics in the coronal sulcus temporarily become blocked. Clinically, the patient has wormlike translucent masses, in contrast to

the purplish, nontranslucent lesions of sclerosing lymphangitis.

SEX AND THE RISK OF CONTACT DERMATITIS

A review of the role of sex as a possible intrinsic factor in the acquisition of contact dermatitis found that women might be at somewhat greater risk of developing the condition, not however because of a biologic factor but because of different exposure patterns.[86]

Contact Dermatitis in Black Patients

McDonald[87] compared the disease incidence in a random sampling of patients from a private dermatology practice, in which most patients were white, with the disease incidence in a random sampling of black patients from several health centers. He concluded that the occurrence of the most common dermatologic diseases, such as atopic eczema, dermatitis (including contact dermatitis), and acne, is quite similar in black and in white skin. Table 5.7 lists the common complications of contact dermatitis in black skin. A review of the literature on irritant and allergic responses among different ethnic groups was undertaken by Robinson with an eye toward how such difference might cause a consumer product manufacturer to structure safety testing. He concluded that there were few scientific reasons to do safety testing in unique ethnic groups, as the literature showed only slightly less skin reactivity in blacks as compared to Caucasians and this was due to a better skin barrier among blacks. Furthermore, he could find little difference between Asians and Caucasians in regard to skin irritation or barrier function and no difference between men and women. He did find evidence for a slight decrease in reactivity to irritants among those greater than 65 years of age. In regard to allergic sensitization, he found some data to support a slight increase in sensitization among women as compared to men.[88] A comparison of acute irritation in a panel of Japanese women and Caucasian women demonstrated a statistically significant difference in that Japanese women were more responsive to stronger acute irritation. Cumulative irritation was also studied, and with weaker irritants a similar but not significant trend was seen.[89]

Table 5-7 Complications of Contact Dermatitis in Black Skin

Acne venenata
Hyperpigmentation
Hypopigmentation
Lichenification

A study of irritation induced by 20% sodium dodecyl sulphate, 100% decanol, 100% octanoic acid, and 10% acetic acid in Asians vs. Caucasians found that there was increased reactivity among Asians. Men were more significantly more reactive than women, and older subjects (56–74 years of age) were significantly less reactive than younger subjects.[90]

Complications of Contact Dermatitis in Black Skin

HYPOPIGMENTATION

Contact vitiligo, which may be due to chemicals, such as the phenolic detergents (paratertiary butylphenol, paratertiary amylphenol, paratertiary butylcatchol), alkylphenols, and monobenzylether of hydroquinone, is distressing, particularly to patients who have dark skin.[91] Several black hospital workers who acquired severe contact vitiligo from the use of phenolic detergents were observed.[92]

HYPERPIGMENTATION

McDonald[87] stressed that, in many cases, hyperpigmentation in black patients is the end result of the most innocuous irritant. Thus, acneiform lesions, in the process of either formation or regression, can cause persistent spotty hyperpigmentation. Keratolytics and other irritants used in acne therapy often cause such deep and distressing hyperpigmentation that many black patients voluntarily terminate therapy. In many instances, unless forewarned, the patients do not return for additional care because they prefer the disease to the hazards of therapy. Tretinoin may cause transient hyper- or hypopigmentation in deeply pigmented persons. In such cases, pigmentation recedes 3 to 6 months after removal of the irritant. In these situations, it cannot be overemphasized that the patient must be warned of both the potential for and the temporary nature of this type of hyperpigmentation. Constant reassurance is necessary during the course of active therapy.

LICHENIFICATION

Black skin appears to be especially predisposed to lichenification. This clinical entity, which in its most easily recognizable form consists of thickened, indurated, hyperpigmented plaques of skin, with accentuated normal skin markings, is usually associated with pruritic diseases of the skin. In most affected persons, lichenification presents early as clusters of tiny papules in skin that has been subjected to vigorous, prolonged rubbing and scratching. These papules coalesce very readily to form the more characteristically observed plaque-like skin lesions.[93]

Apparently, the papular state of lichenification not only occurs earlier in black skin but persists late into the course of pruritic dermatoses, such as atopic eczema, contact dermatitis, and localized neurodermatitis. Frequently, lichenified papules in black skin occur singly rather than in clusters and are often confused clinically with the violaceous, polygonal papules of lichen planus.

ACNE VENENATA IN BLACK SKIN

"Pomade acne" or "Vaselinoderma" is very common in black patients because of the extensive use of such preparations as Vaseline petroleum jelly, Noxzema skin cream, Wildroot Cream Oil hair dressing, mineral oil (heavy or light), Royal Crown hair dressing, and Dixie Peach pomade.

Plewig and colleagues[94] studied a total of 735 black men who used scalp creams and oils daily. About 70% of the long-term users of pomades displayed a recognizable acneiform eruption of the forehead and temples that consisted mainly of rather uniform closed comedones with occasional papulopustules. The more elaborate formulations (Noxzema, Dixie Peach, and Wildroot) induced pomade acne more frequently and more intensively than simpler preparations, such as mineral oil and Vaseline.

Application of five pomades to black skin under continuous occlusion for 8 weeks produced microscopic signs of early comedo formation. Histologically, pomade acne was indistinguishable from acne vulgaris. Plewig and colleagues[94] further stressed that although individual lesions may mimic acne vulgaris clinically and histologically, pomade acne is a quite distinctive condition. Its features include localization to the forehead and temples, uniform and often numerous closed comedones with a few scattered papulopustules in more extensive cases, and a history of long-term daily use of greasy or oily hair grooming preparations. Finally, pomade acne is primarily a disease of black patients.

The chief ingredients of the pomades are high-melting hydrocarbons that are not chemically defined. Mineral oil itself comes in a great many grades, and probably no two samples are entirely alike, no matter how much they are refined. It seems very likely that the acnegenic components reside mainly in these hydrocarbons and not in some minor, potent acnegen that is inadvertently added or is not eliminated during processing.

Because the pomades are weak acnegens, it generally takes a year or more of daily use to produce the eruption. Moreover, the lesions rarely go beyond the closed comedo stage. This is in contrast to industrial acnegens, such as chloronaphthalenes, that produce huge open comedones and marked inflammatory lesions resembling acne conglobata.

Kaidbey and Kligman[95] compared the results of continuous occlusive application of 25% crude coal tar to the backs of young black and adult white males for 3 weeks, which regularly induced an acneiform eruption. In blacks, the eruption consisted of a monomorphous crop of comedones that were of the open variety from the very start. In whites, the first lesions were papulopustules resulting from toxic disorganization of the follicular epithelium. This inflammatory phase was followed by the development of comedones.

This study demonstrated racial differences in follicular reactivity. The follicles of white subjects responded early with rupture of the wall and an outpouring of follicular contents into the dermis. This led to an inflammatory papule and was attributed to the cytotoxicity of the tar. Later, hyperkeratosis became pronounced. In black subjects, the first response was a proliferative one with excessive production and retention of coherent horny cells. The "fragility" of follicles in white subjects supports the clinical observation that the more severe manifestations of inflammatory acne are more common in whites. Pomade acne in blacks is also principally a noninflammatory comedonal disease. In black persons, the sebaceous follicles are evidently sturdier and more likely to respond with hyperkeratosis than with disintegration.

Verhagen[96] confirmed Plewig and colleagues' finding[94] that black skin is prone to the development of pomade acne. He also confirmed the demonstration by Kaidbey and Kligman (95) that artificially induced coal tar acne in blacks differed from that in whites because it was hardly inflammatory.

Verhagen and colleagues[97] also reported that Vaselinoderma was so common in Kenya that they saw 41 cases in 2 years because of the widespread practice of treating the faces of African children with petroleum jelly (Vaseline), frequently up to twice daily. In the great majority, lesions consisted only of open comedones with minute inflammation. There were, however, a few exceptions to this rule. Almost all cases were in children between the ages of 1 and 12 years. This demonstrates the susceptibility of black skin to monomorphic comedo acne in response to acne-inducing substances. Moreover, this condition not only exists in adulthood but also can begin at an age when acne vulgaris is very rare.

Black patients readily acquire allergic contact dermatitis from such contactants as paraphenylenediamine, nickel, chromates, and mercaptobenzothiazole. Such dermatitis is often complicated by hyperpigmentation and lichenification unless it is treated early and vigorously with systemic corticosteroids. Patch testing is reliable on black skin.

Andersen and Maibach[98] concluded that a review of the literature on differences between black and white human skin emphasizes the alleged importance of factors other than the obvious, that is, skin color. Physicochemical differences and differences in susceptibility to irritants and allergens suggest that black skin is more resistant than white skin. Differences exist in the frequency with which several skin diseases occur among blacks and whites. A striking feature in this literature is the disagreement between authors. Much of this information is difficult to interpret because of socioeconomic influences and other environmental factors. Pigmentation rather than race was identified as a factor in barrier function. Men and women with type II/III skin were compared with skin type V/VI. Darkly pigmented skin was found to have a more resistant barrier and recovered more rapidly than skin of individuals with lighter pigmentation.[99] This was independent of race (white vs Asian) or gender.

INDUSTRIAL DERMATITIS IN BLACKS

Schwartz and colleagues[100] and Shelley[101] state that black persons resist chemical and ultraviolet light irritation better than light-skinned persons. Marshall and colleagues,[102] who as early as 1919 used 1% dichloroethylsulfide in mineral oil on the arms of whites and blacks to produce dermatitis, found erythema in 15% of black subjects compared to 59% of white subjects.

Weigand and Mershon[103] noted that black skin was more resistant than white skin by measuring the minimal perceptible erythema (MPE) using quantitative patch test exposures to o-chlorobenzylidene malononitrile, a lacrimator. Weigand and Gaylor[104] determined the MPE in both black and white volunteers by applying increasing amounts of dinitrochlorobenzene (DNCB) to the skin of the back. The investigators reported that white subjects tended to have MPEs at lower concentrations of DNCB than did black subjects. On stripped skin, reactivity was more homogeneous. Tests were read in a room with artificial lighting indicating that, because of constant reading conditions, the differences were not due to perceptual error in reading of erythema because a dose-response curve was made for each subject and the differences were not observed on stripped skin. The possible protective effect of melanin granules in black skin was discussed, but it was concluded that melanin could not be the main protectant because it is distributed mainly below the removed stratum corneum. Frosch and Kligman[105] found that black subjects were less susceptible to irritants than were white subjects, but no data were presented.

The use of laser Doppler velocimetry and transepidermal water loss measurements showed that black skin was more sensitive to sodium lauryl sulfate than white skin when water loss was considered. However, only minimal blood flow changes were noted in response to this irritant when black subjects were compared to white subjects, even with the laser Doppler instrument.[106]

Most studies evaluated irritancy using erythema as the endpoint in equating white versus black responses. This procedure is questionable because erythema is difficult to detect in black skin, so the differences in irritancy response between the two races might be less pronounced than reported.

SPECIFIC ALLERGENS AND RACE

A significant difference in p-phenylenediamine sensitization has been identified between black and white patients. Overall, 10.6% of black patients and 4.5% of white patients were sensitive. However, when only men were considered the difference was 21.2% of black men vs. 4.2% of white men. Black men were also more sensitive to imidazolidinyl urea 9.1% vs. 2.6%. The difference was considered due to exposure patterns or possibly to variations in N-acetylation.[107]

Contact Dermatitis in Atopic Persons

"Atopic dermatitis is (at least in some cases) characterized by a susceptibility to start to itch (and persist in itching) when omnipresent, usually harmless, substances in the stratum corneum meet and react with specific circulating antibodies, presumably IgE."[108,109]

Antigen-presenting cells of both the epidermis and dermis express IgE on their surfaces in atopic dermatitis to a significantly ($p = .001$) greater degree than patients with either irritant or allergic contact dermatitis.[110] The penetration of antigen through the stratum corneum to the epidermis would be sufficient to elicit a reaction. It is the peculiarity of atopy that ordinarily harmless antigens elicit harmful reactions in certain selected shock tissues. There is some evidence suggesting that substances from the horny layer (including its own constituents, soil, and products of microorganisms that colonize it, e.g., staphylococci) may elicit reactions in persons who have atopic skin.

Extracts of human dander produced wheal reactions in most atopic persons but did so in only a minority of persons with nonatopic skin. Thus, the human dander test can help to diagnose atopy and to divide a population roughly between the atopic reactors and the nonatopic nonreactors. These wheal reactions are based on an immunologic mechanism and can be passively transferred—that is, IgE mediates them.

It is also well known that atopic persons experience reactions to skin tests with house dust, a mixture that must contain a substantial amount of desquamated human horny material. Furthermore, urticarial skin reactions occur after prick tests or intradermal injections of feathers, wool, and substances that may well contain antigenic groups in common with human stratum corneum.

Often the first signs of atopic dermatitis in the infant are itching and rubbing of the scalp and then of the cheeks. A large amount of stratum corneum material is present in young infants, exemplified by conditions such as physiologic desquamation, cradle cap, and increased scaling of the scalp. Moreover, infant skin, as well as the skin of patients who have atopic dermatitis, allows penetration of many substances more easily than does the skin of normal adults. It is an appealing hypothesis that patients who have atopic dermatitis itch when stratum corneum antigens penetrate to the superficial vessels—the shock tissue—and that scratching and rubbing enhance this penetration.

The incidence of allergic contact dermatitis superimposed on atopic dermatitis, however, is still controversial.[111–113] Some patients who have atopic conditions, such as allergic asthma and rhinitis, never suffer from atopic dermatitis. Regardless of whether atopic dermatitis is present, however, atopic individuals may acquire a contact dermatitis, which may be either the irritant or the allergic variety, or both. Atopic eczema renders the skin vulnerable to nonspecific irritants, such as heat, humidity, perspiration, dust, strong soaps, detergents, and wool.

The literature is divided on whether or not atopic individuals have skin that is more easily irritated than normal individuals. Gallacher and Maibach[114] reviewed studies supporting both points of view. They point out that most of the epidemiological data that suggest patients with atopic dermatitis are more prone to irritant dermatitis relate to hand eczema, but studies of such cases rarely test the hands. Rather, those studies are done on the forearm, back, or thigh. Variables they identified that in part account for the different positions expressed in the literature include the definition of atopic dermatitis, the definition of normal, sex, race, age, anatomic site, whether the tests were patch tests or open tests, the nature of the irritant studied, and the method of assessment.

In a carefully controlled study of sodium lauryl sulfate irritant reactions, atopic and nonatopic patients were found to react similarly with, if anything, a slightly lesser amount of reaction among the atopic patients.[115] At the time of the study, the atopic dermatitis patients had no active eczema at the test site. Assessment was visual,

chrommetric, laser Doppler flowmetric, and by transepidermal water loss.

When controlled exposures to a new antigen are compared between atopic subjects and nonatopic subjects, fewer atopic subjects become sensitized. This proved the case with dinitrochlorobenzene (DNCB).[116] The induction phase of contact dermatitis seems more susceptible to disruption by experimental inflammation even when nonatopic individuals are studied with DNCB as the potent allergen.[117] The presence of inflammatory mediators in atopic dermatitis may inhibit the acquisition of new contact allergy or delayed hypersensitivity. This downregulating effect does not provide absolute protection against the acquisition of delayed hypersensitivity, and patch tests are useful in detecting the elicitation phase of the hypersensitivity. The elicitation phase is more difficult to affect experimentally than is the induction phase. Although several studies found patients with atopic dermatitis less likely to sensitize to strong allergens such as DNCB and poison ivy extract, several other studies have shown that contact dermatitis is prevalent in patients with atopic dermatitis and frequently related to medications used to treat the dermatitis.[118] In a study of 74 atopic dermatitis patients with persistent facial dermatitis (119), 39.2% were found to have one or more positive patch tests, and 31 of the 40 such patients were female. The female predominance has been found by other authors.[119]

PATCH TESTING

When diagnostic patch tests were investigated prospectively in atopic and nonatopic patients, positive tests were seen in 37% of atopic patients versus 57% of nonatopic patients.[120]

In a study of 410 patients with chronic eczematous dermatitis, it was found that atopic patients were just as likely as nonatopic patients to have allergic contact dermatitis and to benefit from patch testing.[121] Furthermore, patients with atopic dermatitis had significantly more positive tests (2.7 vs 2.0) when compared with patients with nonatopic dermatitis. Fifty-four percent of atopic patients had definite relevant positive patch tests. In this study, the more positive patch tests occurred, the more reactions of doubtful meaning were found. The authors refer to these as irritant reactions, but they likely represent the Janus phenomenon discussed in Chapter 2. An Italian study of atopic and nonatopic patients found that the rate of positive patch test reactions was not significantly different between the two groups. They also observed that contact sensitization in atopic dermatitis was inversely related to the clinical severity of atopic dermatitis.[122] A comparison of atopic patients who were patch tested to six allergens was made to a carefully selected control group (matched for sex, age, reason for testing, and test center) likewise tested to the same six allergens. The atopic group showed only slight tendencies that were not statistically significant. There were more doubtful or irritant reactions the day after the patch tests were removed in the atopic group, fewer reactions that steadily increased from day one to day three, and a greater number of strong reactions at day 3. These differences were seen as minor.[123] A German study of allergic contact dermatitis between atopic and nonatopic individuals showed that there was no difference in the frequency of single, double, or polyvalent sensitization between the two groups. Only bufexamac was found three times more often in atopic individuals.[124]

In a similar study of 122 English patients with atopic dermatitis, 60 (49%) were found to have one or more positive patch tests.[125] The patch test reactions were deemed relevant in 44% of the cases. These findings underscore the value of patch testing atopic dermatitis cases.

When screening patch tests were used in a study of 137 children with atopic dermatitis,[126] the value of patch testing in this group was confirmed. Contact sensitization was found in 43% of all children with atopic dermatitis tested. The most common allergen category was metals (19%), then fragrance (4%) and balsam of Peru (3%), lanolin (4%), and neomycin (3%).

REACTION INDEX

In a study of 15,553 patients patch tested by 18 dermatology departments, the reaction index was calculated from the number of allergic, questionable, and irritant reactions using 13 standard screening allergens.[127] A history of atopic dermatitis did not have a consistent influence on the reaction index.

Although atopic dermatitis does not seem to render the patient particularly susceptible to allergic contact dermatitis, a search for the presence of contactants in all instances of persistent atopic dermatitis is important in the management of atopic individuals.[111] This is especially necessary when the atopic dermatitis is not responding to therapy or when the eruption suddenly flares. In an effort to allay the itching, many individuals who have atopic dermatitis are exposed to sensitizing topical medications that produce a superimposed allergic contact dermatitis.

The prompt recognition and removal of irritating and sensitizing contactants may prevent the atopic dermatitis from becoming widespread. It is surprising how often the detection and elimination of offending contactants

markedly alleviate an otherwise intractable atopic dermatitis.

Allergic contact dermatitis superimposed on atopic eczema usually appears as an insidious aggravation of the eczema rather than as an acute, easily recognized epidermal eczematous contact dermatitis. The reason may be that many patients who have atopic eczema receive topical or systemic corticosteroid therapy, which can modify the appearance of the dermatitis. Patients whose atopic eczema is not responding well to therapy, therefore, should be investigated for the possibility of a superimposed contact dermatitis from topical applications, particularly neomycin. Children with atopic dermatitis are exposed to topical corticosteroids over prolonged periods of time. A study of 71 children with atopic dermatitis and use of topical corticosteroids for greater than 6 months in the prior 2 years found that 18 (25.3%) reported aggravation or lack of improvement in the dermatitis with such treatment. While this might suggest corticosteroid allergy, only one child proved to be sensitive on patch testing with tixocortol pivalate, hydrocortisone-17-butyrate, and Locoidon cream.[128]

Aside from being modified by corticosteroid therapy, a superimposed contact dermatitis may not appear typical in atopic individuals because the so-called dermal type of contact dermatitis is especially likely to develop in such patients. Clinically, the lesions are edematous and erythematous rather than papulovesicular and may closely resemble the papular, dry form of atopic dermatitis. The allergens reported as producing "dermal" contact sensitivity include neomycin, formaldehyde, nickel, and ragweed oleoresin.[129]

PATCH TESTING IDIOSYNCRASIES IN ATOPIC INDIVIDUALS

As in nonatopic individuals, the proof of allergic contact dermatitis often consists of obtaining a positive patch test reaction with a suspected contactant (Figure 5-1). There is usually a normal incidence of typical eczematous reactions to patch tests performed on patients who have atopic dermatitis.[109] Atopic individuals, however, may have unique patch test reactions, such as pustular reactions and specific and nonspecific patch test responses to protein substances.

Pustular Patch Test Reactions

There is a high incidence of papulopustular reactions to patch tests with nickel sulfate, the halogens, and sodium arsenate that probably represent some form of irritation. In contrast to true allergic patch test reactions, pustular eruptions rarely itch, do not spread beyond the patch test site, and usually heal within 24 hours after the patch has been removed.[130] Although pustular patch test reactions, particularly to nickel sulfate, are more common in atopic individuals, such reactions occur in the nonatopic patient and are not diagnostic evidence of the atopic state.

Nonspecific Patch Test Reactions to Protein Substances

When tested with simple chemicals, the atopic individual may show either an eczematous or a pustular reaction. In addition, atopic individuals who are patch tested with certain protein substances, such as feathers, silk, and foods, may show nonspecific reactions characterized by closely aggregated, discrete, pinpoint vesicles and occasionally pustules.[131,132] There is no exudation and no crusting. Erythema and itching are minimal and are localized to the patch test site. The reaction reaches its greatest intensity in 4 to 5 days. This response has been noted in atopic individuals with or without atopic dermatitis. If dermatitis is present, a positive reaction is not associated with a flare-up of the dermatitis, and the spontaneous flare phenomenon is absent.

Atopic individuals may also have a nonspecific reaction to the tuberculin patch test that is similar to that described for feathers, silk, and foods. A specific, positive reaction to a tuberculin patch test consists of a group of tiny vesicles and papules on a reddened, indurated area. False-positive reactions to the tuberculin test may appear as vesicles and pustules with minimal erythema and no induration.

These nonallergic patch test reactions are probably due to an irritable skin and indicate that the atopic individual may react nonspecifically to many protein substances. Such reactions must be distinguished carefully from true allergic changes, which are characterized by itching and a spread of the reaction beyond the borders of the test site.

Specific Allergic Patch Test Reactions to Protein Substances

Atopic individuals may rarely react in a specific manner to patch tests with molds, feathers, dander, and wool. Allergic patch test reactions to the defatted pollen protein of grasses and ragweed are also occasionally obtained in atopic individuals. The specific allergic reaction to these substances differs from the nonspecific atopic patch test reaction in that the former is characterized by erythema, vesiculation, exudation, and crusting. Furthermore, the reaction may spread beyond the patch test site and may be associated with a flare-up of the existing dermatitis. Such positive reactions would seem to signify that inhalation of or external contact with protein substances may cause a flare-up of

atopic dermatitis. Patch testing with protein substances is not a routine procedure, and the clinical significance of the reactions is uncertain even when they seem specific.

RELATIONSHIP OF CONTACT DERMATITIS TO EXPOSURE TO SPECIFIC PROTEIN ALLERGENS IN THE ATOPIC INDIVIDUAL

Contact dermatitis can be prolonged and aggravated by the intranasal, subcutaneous, or surface application of specific protein allergens to which an atopic individual has been shown by scratch tests to be sensitive. For example, poison ivy dermatitis in an atopic individual may be made worse by the prophylactic injection of ragweed pollen extract or intradermal testing with protein antigens. Such injections on occasion render the atopic skin more irritable, and a concentration of a chemical that is usually innocuous may produce contact dermatitis. Furthermore, in atopic individuals who have contact dermatitis, external exposure to proteins in foods, pollens, and molds can produce exacerbations.[133,134] These observations indicate that there is a mechanism by which specific antigens can produce a flare-up of an existing, etiologically unrelated contact dermatitis in certain susceptible individuals, regardless of whether the antigen reaches the skin by contact, ingestion, inhalation, or injection.

It would therefore be advisable for atopic individuals who have contact dermatitis to avoid desensitization procedures or other injections with protein substances while the dermatitis is in the acute or subacute phase.

INHALATION AND AIRBORNE CONTACTANTS IN ATOPIC DERMATITIS

Occasionally, inhalation of pollens, dusts, and animal hairs causes either a flare-up of atopic dermatitis or an apparent superimposed contact dermatitis. In some instances, these airborne allergens may produce positive patch test reactions.

Champion[135] reported five patients who had atopic dermatitis in which exacerbations were provoked both by inhalation and by direct contact with algae. These patients also reacted to lichens, which contain algae in symbiosis with fungi. All of the patients had allergic rhinitis or asthma, often very mild in relation to the severity of the skin symptoms. Three of them also had a delayed hypersensitivity contact dermatitis from lichens but not from algae.

It is important to investigate patients who have suspected sensitivities to lichens and algae both by patch testing and by prick testing, because specific desensitization may help those with immediate wheal reactions.

Mold allergens were implicated in the dermatitis experienced by a 25-year-old who had childhood atopic dermatitis.[136] Face and neck dermatitis were accompanied by cough, rhinitis, and conjunctivitis when she was in her apartment but improved in other living quarters. Her apartment had mold on the ceiling, and several species of fungi were cultured. Positive patch tests were obtained with *Fusarium, Cladosporium, Pullularia, Rhizopus,* and *Penicillium* aeroallergens. Prick tests were positive to these also. Moving to a new apartment was curative.

Airborne contact dermatitis correlated with harvest season for a 42-year-old rural worker.[137] The eruption had been seasonal for 10 years. A mite associated with grain storage facilities was found to be the source of the eruption. A positive RAST and a positive patch test to the mite *Tyrophagus putrescentiae* was found. The mite can be found in pastures, as well as in grain storage areas.

Champion[135] also stated that immediate *contact* wheal reactions may occur in atopic patients handling eggs or being licked by dogs.

The aeroallergens routinely used for prick and scratch tests have been used to complement the diagnostic armamentarium in an effort to narrow the list of potential environmental sources thought to be responsible for generalized atopic dermatitis.[138] The clinical benefits described in reports, such as those of Clark,[138] demonstrate the utility of selective use of these allergens for patch test purposes, even though standardized procedures for their use are not yet agreed upon.

DUST MITES

Patch tests can be performed with allergen extracts commonly used for prick tests. Sometimes relevant reactions occur with only patch tests, at other times only prick tests, and at times both types of tests are positive.

A 49-year-old patient with atopic dermatitis who was known to have IgE antibodies to *Dermatophagoides pteronyssinus* by RAST was patch tested to a variety of allergens, including the dust mite antigen.[139] His only reaction was to *D. pteronyssinus,* and he experienced a generalized flare of his dermatitis following this positive patch test. This would either be a coincidence or a specific immunologic event that relates to the cause of his dermatitis. He was advised to keep his home free of dust mites.

The dust mites *D. pteronyssinus* and *D. farinae* have been implicated in causing atopic dermatitis based on various patch test observations. A study was undertaken using equal amounts of purified adult bodies from the two species in a 20% concentration in petrolatum.[140]

Patch tests were performed on normal skin of the back and read on day 2 and day 3. The same tests were done on 52 control subjects. About half (47.8%) of the atopic patients, and only 15.3% of normal subjects reacted. Of the 22 atopic patients with positive patch test reactions, only 15 were also positive to a prick test with the mites.

Manzini and colleagues[141] studied 313 atopic dermatitis patients and 100 healthy controls with three different commercially prepared dust mite patch test allergens. Patch test reactions did not correlate with prick test reactions to dust mite antigens. Thirty-eight percent of atopic dermatitis cases reacted to one or more dust mite patch test material, but only 13% of normal individuals reacted. One source of patch test material produced positive reactions in 54% of atopics, another in 51%, and a third source in only 20%.

To further establish a link between dust mites and dermatitis, 23 patients with atopic dermatitis and a positive patch test to *D. pteronyssinus* were studied in vitro by incubating peripheral blood mononuclear cells with the mite antigen.[142] This led to the production of cytokines typical of delayed hypersensitivity reactions rather than immediate hypersensitivity reactions. Marked secretion of IL-2 and INF-gamma but not IL-4 was observed.

Similar studies have been conducted in children with atopic dermatitis. When aeroallergens are used as patch test material and compared with the standard use as prick test allergens, there is some agreement and disagreement between the results in atopic patients. In a group of children with well-defined atopic dermatitis, 29% had at least one positive patch test and 54% had at least one positive prick test.[143] Patch and prick test results corresponded in 8 of 17 patients. The most commonly positive aeroallergens were *D. pteronyssinus* and *D. farinae* in 27% of patients, then trees in 12%, plantain in 10%, and timothy grass, mugwort, and damp area trees at 5% each. The significance of these findings is uncertain.

ATOPY PATCH TEST

The atopy patch test (APT) involves the application of intact protein allergens in customary patch test chamber methodology with readings taken 24 to 72 hours after application.[144] Foods and aeroallergens are the common test substances employed in the APT. Traditionally, these allergens have been tested by skin-prick test or specific IgE levels. At times, the APT is positive when the traditional tests are negative.[145] One example of this can be seen in the evaluation of 85 children with reactions to egg. The APT to egg was positive in 37% while the skin-prick test was positive in 19%.[146] However, the literature on the APT has suffered from a lack of standardization in allergens and methodology used to perform the tests. A large European study attempted to address this. House dust mite, cat dander, grass, birch pollen allergen, egg white, celery, and wheat flour were evaluated. The frequency of positive APT reactions ranged from 39% with dust mite to 9% with celery. Clear-cut positive APT reactions with negative skin-prick tests and specific IgE tests occurred in 7% of patients.[147] The difficulty of standardizing testing with foods and aeroallergens has led to the publication of a position paper attempting to outline indications for testing with APT, choice of allergens, test materials, and technique. In that paper it is pointed out that the commercially available house-dust mixture is at an overly high concentration. Wheat gluten was also noted to be causing many false reactions. The paper calls for further work on optimum allergen concentrations, vehicles for the various allergens, determination of the optimum-sized Finn chamber, and demonstration that test preparations are nonirritant and nontoxic in normal subjects as well as in patients with atopic dermatitis.[148]

SUBSTANCES THAT CAN PRODUCE BOTH ALLERGIC CONTACT DERMATITIS AND ATOPIC MANIFESTATIONS

Theoretically, there is no absolute difference between agents that cause eczematous allergy and those that engender urticarial (atopic-anaphylactoid) allergy. Under actual conditions, however, some agents generally cause eczematous allergy but rarely or never cause urticarial allergy. Many other agents generally cause urticarial allergy but rarely or never cause eczematous allergy. A small group of agents may cause both forms of hypersensitivity at the same time.[149]

Some allergens alternately produce asthma and contact dermatitis. Among the drugs, penicillin, quinine, sulfonamides, mercurials, and arsenicals produce both allergic contact and atopic reactions in the same individual. These drugs can produce an eczematous contact dermatitis when applied topically and, in addition, can cause asthma, urticaria, or even anaphylactic shock when ingested or injected.[150] Fortunately, procaine (Novocain), which not infrequently produces allergic eczematous hypersensitivity, rarely produces an anaphylactic reaction in atopic individuals or even in those who have epidermal hypersensitivity to the anesthetic.[151]

Paraphenylenediamine can produce both an allergic eczematous contact dermatitis and asthma in furriers. Allergic rhinitis has been described from the inhalation of epoxy resins and the amine hardeners in a patient who also had a contact dermatitis from processing these resins.[152]

ALLERGIC CONTACT DERMATITIS IN ATOPIC INDIVIDUALS

Allergic contact dermatitis in atopic individuals may appear as an eczematous eruption. If the patient is receiving topical or systemic corticosteroid therapy for an atopic dermatitis, however, the superimposed contact dermatitis may appear as an erythematous, papular, noneczematous eruption simulating the original atopic dermatitis. An allergic contact dermatitis to a topical medication, therefore, may not be suspected.

Features of "Dermal" Type of Allergic Contact Dermatitis in Atopic Individuals

Aside from being modified by corticosteroid therapy, a superimposed contact dermatitis may appear to be atypical in atopic individuals because the so-called dermal type of contact dermatitis is most likely to develop in these patients.[153]

In Fisher's experience,[154] patch tests with sensitizing contactants in atopic individuals yield positive reactions similar to those in nonatopic patients, and it is not necessary to perform intracutaneous tests, as advocated by Epstein.[153]

Most cases of contact dermatitis in atopic individuals seem to be a combination of eczematous and dermal sensitivity. Usually one can demonstrate both a positive eczematous patch test reaction and a positive dermal intracutaneous test reaction in the atopic skin with superimposed allergic contact dermatitis. It is claimed, however, that occasionally the patch test reaction is negative, and only an intracutaneous test reveals the dermal contact reaction.[155]

Diagnostic Features of Allergic Contact Sensitivity to Neomycin

Some investigators report that most individuals investigated for allergic contact hypersensitivity to neomycin had atopic dermatitis.[156,157]

Wereide[158] states that this study does not support the view that the atopic state (as it occurs in atopic dermatitis patients) predisposes to neomycin sensitivity. Patients who had stasis dermatitis of the lower part of the leg had a significantly higher incidence of neomycin sensitivity than did any other groups with eczematous dermatitis.

Both the classic form of allergic contact dermatitis with vesiculation and eczematization and the papular, erythematous "dermal" type of sensitivity may occur in patients who have neomycin sensitivity and atopic eczema. Because neomycin is frequently prescribed in a mixture with a corticosteroid preparation, the corticosteroid may modify the appearance of the superimposed neomycin dermatitis. When an individual treated with a neomycin-containing preparation fails to improve or the eruption becomes worse, neomycin sensitivity should be suspected.[158]

In order to prove the neomycin sensitivity, the patient should be patch tested with the suspected topical neomycin preparation. In some instances in which allergic contact sensitivity is present, a typical positive patch test reaction is obtained with the preparation or only with a 20% aqueous solution of neomycin. When the reaction to a neomycin preparation is negative, it may be worthwhile to perform an intradermal skin test with a 1:1,000 solution of neomycin sulfate. A positive reaction consists of a delayed indurated papule present 48 hours after testing. Intradermal testing has rarely been necessary.

When neomycin sensitivity has been demonstrated, the patient should avoid exposure to streptomycin and kanamycin, which may cross-react with neomycin and with bacitracin, which may co-react with neomycin.

Precautions in Testing Atopic Individuals for Allergic Contact Sensitivity to Nickel

Allergic contact dermatitis due to nickel may occasionally take the "dermal" form and closely mimic atopic dermatitis. Although most cases of nickel dermatitis occur in the nonatopic population, nickel sensitivity superimposed on atopic eczema may not be readily recognized.[159]

Patch testing for nickel sensitivity in atopic individuals may also present the difficulty of properly interpreting pustular patch test reactions, which occur frequently in this group. Wahlberg and Skog[160] reported that in eczematous patients who had nickel allergy, immunoglobulin E (IgE) and the threshold of sensitivity were determined by patch testing with dilutions of nickel sulfate ($NiSO_4$). In four of the 47 patients investigated, the IgE value increased. The occurrence of atopic disease in nickel-sensitive patients was 9% and, among relatives, 38%.

Although not all investigators agree, several groups have found a higher prevalence of atopy among nickel-sensitive patients.[161] However, McDonagh and colleagues[162] did not find either increased or decreased susceptibility to nickel among atopic patients undergoing diagnostic patch testing. Instead, atopic patients reported more jewelry dermatitis but were frequently negative to notorious jewelry allergens. When atopic dermatitis has been long-standing, sensitization to contact allergens has been found more commonly.[163] The most frequently encountered allergens have been nickel, fragrance mix, balsam of Peru, and neomycin. These same investigators[163] found that a 50% dilution of test allergens did not reduce the number of irritant patch test reactions.

Relationship of Allergic Contact Ragweed Oil Sensitivity to the Atopic State

Ragweed oil dermatitis may mimic a generalized atopic eczema, particularly the seasonal type.[164] Ragweed oil dermatitis is due to an oil-soluble oleoresin, whereas ragweed rhinitis, asthma, and possibly certain cases of atopic dermatitis are due to the water-soluble protein fraction of the pollen.

In Fisher's experience,[165] most patients who had ragweed dermatitis had no atopic dermatitis or evidence of the atopic state.

Wool as an Irritant and Sensitizer in Patients who Have Atopic Dermatitis

The mechanism by which wool produces dermatitis, particularly in atopic individuals, is still controversial. Some investigators[166] feel that the inhalation of wool is an important factor. Contact with wool, including house dust, which may be largely wool fibers, may readily irritate the atopic skin.[167] Although wool is usually a weak allergen, on rare occasions the degree of sensitivity is so great that mere contact of wool with the skin can produce urticaria.

Apart from allergic sensitization, wool is irritating to many individuals, particularly those with atopy.

Atopic Dermatitis Confined to Hands or Feet

Atopic dermatitis confined to the hands may be precipitated by household or occupational irritants and sensitizers. In other instances, particularly in children, primary irritant reactions from friction, perspiration, and tight shoes are factors in a recurrent dermatitis of the feet in atopic individuals.[168] Such atopic dermatitis may resemble shoe dermatitis. Occasionally, only the dorsal aspect or the large toe is involved. A study of the hands of patients with atopic dermatitis found that 458 of 777 consecutive patients, or 58.9%, had hand involvement. Hand involvement increased with age. Morphologic clues to the etiology of hand eczema were evaluated, and when the dorsal hand surface and volar wrist were involved, atopic dermatitis was more likely to be a contributing factor.[169]

Fredriksson and Faergemann[170] found, in a retrospective survey of 1,112 patients who had atopic dermatitis, that lesions localized to the lower gluteal and posterior femoral regions reached their peak in patients age 7 to 8 years. These investigators speculate that this is due to sweat retention caused by prolonged sitting when these individuals start school.

In another study of 1,385 subjects who had hand eczema in the prior 12 months, it was learned that the most important predictive factor was childhood eczema, followed by being female. Additional factors of lesser importance were occupation, asthma, and/or hay fever.[171]

Atopic Dermatitis and Occupation

Atopy has been said to be a risk factor for occupational skin disease. However, studies in Singapore and Taiwan did not support this.[172] Rather, nonatopic individuals were found to be at highest risk of occupational skin disease. Sometimes patch testing does not identify an allergen to explain what appears to be a potential case of contact dermatitis. The term "unclassified endogenous eczema" is used by some authorities in this setting. Latent late-onset atopic dermatitis was identified in a group of patch-test patients who after testing had been categorized as unclassified endogenous eczema. An elevated IgE level of greater than 100 IU/mL was used to establish this diagnosis and 12 of 34 unclassified endogenous eczema patients fell into this group. After 2 years of follow-up, 20 of 31 of the unclassified endogenous eczema patients had improved or their condition had cleared up.[173]

JUVENILE PLANTAR DERMATOSIS AND ATOPIC CONDITION

Verbov[174–176] states that juvenile plantar dermatosis (JPD) is a characteristic dermatosis of infancy and childhood localized to the distal soles, including the toes (particularly the big toe) but sparing the toe spaces. He believes that JPD describes not only a true localized atopic dermatitis but also a frictional contact dermatitis to which those with an atopic condition are prone but which may also occur in susceptible nonatopic persons. His series, dating from 1973, has reached 72 patients, of whom 33 (46%) have had a personal or family history of atopy. The criteria for a diagnosis of atopy are a personal or family history of asthma, hay fever, perennial rhinorrhea, or typical eczema of atopic type. Using similar criteria, Jepsen[177] also found a high incidence of atopy.

ATOPICS AND BEER

Three atopic patients developed urticaria after drinking beer.[178] Prick tests to grains showed immediate hypersensitivity to malt, wheat flour, barley flour, maize flour, and rice flour. Fresh cereal preparations rather than commercial products were recommended for testing. In contrast, beer was not a problem when ingested for a malt-worker who became sensitive to barley malt.[179] Patch tests were positive to barley residues (as is and 10% in petrolatum), malt radicle, and malt residues at the same concentrations. A prick test to barley was negative.

ATOPIC CHILDREN AND GRAINS

Children with atopic dermatitis may be allergic to grains such as barley, oats, rye, and wheat. Oral provocation with these cereals can provoke dermatologic, gastrointestinal, and oropharyngeal reactions that can be either immediate or delayed. Prick tests with these grains were performed on atopic children who had positive oral challenges to the grains.[180] Prick tests, RAST, or histamine release test detected the allergen in 8 of 8 children who had immediate reactions and in 9 of 14 who had delayed reactions. Five children had allergens identifiable only with patch tests to the cereals or by lymphocyte proliferation assay. Wheat was the most common cereal allergen and antibodies to gliadin of IgE, IgA, and IgG classes were found.

ATOPIC CHILDREN AND COW'S MILK

Oral challenges with cow's milk may provoke atopic dermatitis especially in children under the age of 2 years. A study of 113 infants 2 to 24 months old found a positive oral cow's milk challenge in 54.[181] Of these 54, immediate reactions were documented in 36 and delayed reactions in 18. Prick tests were useful to detect the immediate reactions, and patch tests to cow's milk detected the delayed reactions. The detection of cow's milk allergy was possible only by patch tests 26% of the time. The authors define immediate reactions as pruritus, urticaria, and/or exanthema, and delayed reactions were eczematous.[182]

References

1. Fisher AA. Childhood allergic contact dermatitis. Cutis 1975;15:635.

2. Epstein E. Contact dermatitis in children. Pediatr Clin North Am 1971;18:839.

3. Honigman, J. Bubble bath dermatitis in children. Cutis 1966;2:406.

4. Alberta L, Sweeney SM, Wiss K. Diaper dye dermatitis. Pediatrics 2005;116:450.

5. Lane AT, Rehder PA, Helm K. Evaluations of diapers containing absorbent gelling material with conventional disposable diapers in newborn infants. Am J Dis Child 1990;144:315.

6. Fergusson AG, Fraser NG, Grant PW. Napkin dermatitis with psoriasiform "Ide": a review of fifty-two cases. Br J Dermatol 1966;78:289.

7. Andersen SL, Thomsen K. Psoriasiform napkin dermatitis. Br J Dermatol 1971;84:316.

8. Holme SA, Stone NM, Mills CM. Toilet seat contact dermatitis. Pediatr Dermatol 2005;22:344.

9. Gibson WB. Sweaty sock dermatitis. Clin Pediatr (Phila) 1963;2:175.

10. Verbov JL. Atopic dermatitis and the forefoot. Br Med J 1978;11:962.

11. Jepsen LV. Dermatitis plantaris sicca: a retrospective study of children with recurrent dermatitis of the feet. Acta Derm Venereol (Stockh) 1979;59:257.

12. Epstein WL. Contact-type delayed hypersensitivity in infants and children: induction of rhus sensitivity. Pediatrics 1960;187:1130.

13. Edwards EK. Contact urticaria to cow's milk. Cutis 1981;28:450.

14. Lecks HE. Anaphylaxis from milk protein in diaper ointment [Letter]. JAMA 1980;244:1560.

15. Veien NK, Hattel T, Justesen O, Nörholm A. Contact dermatitis in children. Contact Dermatitis 1982;8:373.

16. Rietschel RL, Rosenthal LE, the North American Contact Dermatitis Group. Standard patch test screening series used diagnostically in young and elderly patients. J Am Contact Derm Soc 1990;1:53.

17. Rademaker M, Forsyth A. Contact dermatitis in children. Contact Dermatitis 1989;20:104.

18. Roul S, Ducombs G, Taieb A. Usefulness of the European standard series for patch testing in children: a 3-year single-centre study of 337 patients. Contact Dermatitis 1999;40:232.

19. Giordano-Labadie F, Rancé F, Pellegrin F et al. Frequency of contact allergy in children with atopic dermatitis: results of a prospective study of 137 cases. Contact Dermatitis 1999;40:192.

20. Brasch J, Geier J. Patch test results in schoolchildren: results from the Information Network of Departments of Dermatology (IVDK) and the German Contact Dermatitis Research Group (DKG). Contact Dermatitis 1997;37:286.

21. Heine G, Schnuch A, Uter W, et al. Frequency of contact allergy in German children and adolescents patch tested between 1995 and 2002: results from the Information Network of Departments of Dermatology and the German Contact Dermatitis Research Group. Contact Dermatitis 2004;51:111.

22. Lewis VJ, Statham BN, Chowdhury MMU. Allergic contact dermatitis in 191 consecutively patch tested children. Contact Dermatitis 2004;51:155.

23. Mortz CG, Andersen KE. Allergic contact dermatitis in children and adolescents. Contact Dermatitis 1999;41:121.

24. Johnke H, Norberg LA, Vach W, et al. Reactivity to patch tests with nickel sulfate and fragrance mix in infants. Contact Dermatitis 2004;51:141.

25. Levy A, Hanau D, Foussereau, J. Contact dermatitis in children. Arch Dermatol 1963;87:378.

26. Peltonen L. Nickel sensitivity in the general population. Contact Dermatitis 1979;5:27.

27. Prystowsky SD, Allen AM, Smith RW, et al. Allergic contact hypersensitivity to nickel, neomycin, ethylenediamine, and benzocaine: relationship between age, sex, history of exposure, and reactivity to standard patch tests and use tests in a general population. Arch Dermatol 1979;115:959.

28. Fisher AA. Prevention of shoe dermatitis by controlling hyperhidrosis with tannic acid. Cutis 1973;12:493.

29. Hjorth N. Contact dermatitis in children. Acta Derm Venerol 1981 [suppl]; 95:36.

30. Johns AM, Bower BD. Wasting of the napkin area after repeated uses of fluorinated steroid ointment. Br Med J 1970;1:347.

31. Miara RH. Atrophic striae following topical fluocinolone therapy. Br J Dermatol 1964;76:481.

32. Savin JA, Alexander S, Marks R. A rosacea-like eruption of children. Br J Dermatol 1972;87:425.

33. Tappeiner J, Pfleger L. Granuloma glutaeale infantum. Hautarzt 1971;22:383.

34. Grupper C, Bensoussan L, Duprepaire R. Granuloma facial infantile après corticoides fluores locaux. Bull Soc Fr Derm Syph 1975;82:337.

35. Uyeda K, Nakayasu K, Takaishi Y, Sotomatsu S. Kaposi sarcoma–like granuloma on diaper dermatitis: a report of five cases. Arch Dermatol 1973;107:605.

36. Georgouras K, Kocsard E. Micropapular sarcoidal facial eruption in a child: Gianotti-type perioral dermatitis. Acta Derm Venereol 1978;58:433.

37. Gianotti F. Cutaneous benign histiocytoses in childhood. In: Pediatric dermatology: modern problems in pediatrics. Basel: Karger. 71:193.

38. Breit R. Allergen change in stasis dermatitis. Contact Dermatitis 1977;3:309.

39. Coenraads PJ, Bleumink E, Nater JP. Susceptibility to primary irritants: age dependence and relation to contact allergic reactions. Contact Dermatitis 1975;1:377.

40. Angelini G, Rantuccio F, Meneghini CL. Contact dermatitis in patients with leg ulcers. Contact Dermatitis 1975;1:81.

41. Fisher AA. Contact urticaria due to polyethylene glycol. Cutis 1977;19:409.

42. Fisher AA. The paraben paradoxes. Cutis 1977;12:830.

43. Fisher AA, Pelzig A, Kanof NB. The persistence of allergic eczematous sensitivity and the cross-sensitivity pattern to para-phenylenediamine. J Invest Dermatol 1958;30:9.

44. Reiss F, Fisher AA. Is hair dyed with paraphenylenediamine allergenic? Arch Dermatol 1974;109:22.

45. Fisher AA. Some immunologic phenomena in treatment of and patch testing for ragweed oil dermatitis. J Invest Dermatol 1952;19:271.

46. Smith JG Jr, Kiem IM. Allergic contact sensitivity in the aged. J Gerontol 1961;16:118.

47. Tindall IP, Smith JG. Skin lesions of the aged and their association with internal changes. JAMA 1963;186:1039.

48. Fisher AA. Drug eruptions in geriatric patients. Cutis 1976;18:402.

49. Fisher AA. Systemic eczematous "contact-type" dermatitis medicamentosa. Ann Allerg 1966;24:406.

50. Felix RH, Comaish JS. The value of patch and other skin tests in drug eruptions. Lancet 1974;1:1017.

51. Korbitz BC. Patch tests for quinine allergy. Arch Environ Health 1973;27:409.

52. Houwerzijl J, de Gast GC, Nater JP. Patch tests in drug eruptions. Contact Dermatitis 1975;1:100.

53. Van Ketel WG. Patch testing in penicillin allergy. Contact Dermatitis 1975;1:253.

54. Penvy ME, Schroepl F. Toxic skin reactions in patch testing with tricyclic psychotropic drugs. Hautarzt 1974;25:430.

55. Lammintausta K, Kortekangas-Savolainen O. The usefulness of skin tests to prove drug hypersensitivity. Brit J Dermatol 2005;152:968.

56. Barbaud A, Goncalo M, Bruynzeel D, et al. Guidelines for performing skin tests with drugs in the investigation of cutaneous adverse drug reactions. Contact Dermatitis 2001;45:321.

57. Kikuchi K, Tsunoda T, Tagami H. Generalized drug eruption due to mexiletine hydrochloride: topical provocation on previously involved skin. Contact Dermatitis 1991;25:70.

58. Leyden JL, Kligman AM. Allergic contact dermatitis: sex differences. Contact Dermatitis 1977;3:333.

59. Björnberg A. Skin reactions to primary irritants in men and women. Acta Derm Venereol (Stockh) 1975;55:191.

60. Wilkinson DS. Connubial photodermatitis. Contact Dermatitis 1975;1:58.

61. Fisher AA. Consort contact dermatitis. Cutis 1979;24:595.

62. Fisher AA, Brancaccio RR. Allergic contact sensitivity to propylene glycol in a lubricant jelly. Arch Dermatol 1979;115:1451.

63. Fisher AA. Propylene glycol dermatitis. Cutis 1978;21:166.

64. Fisher AA. Allergic reaction to feminine hygiene sprays. Arch Dermatol 1973;108:801.

65. Caro I. Connubial contact dermatitis to benzoyl peroxide. Contact Dermatitis 1976;2:362.

66. Rietschel RL, Lewis CW. Contact dermatitis to homo-menthyl salicylate. Arch Dermatol 1978;114:442.

67. Fisher AA. Urticarial and systemic reactions to contactants varying from hair bleach to seminal fluid. Cutis 1977;19:715.

68. Levine BB, Siraganian RP, Schenkein I. Allergy to human seminal plasma. N Engl J Med 1973;288:894.

69. Schultz KH, Schirren C, Kueppers I. Allergy to seminal fluid [Letter]. N Engl J Med 1974;290:916.

70. Levine BB. Allergy to seminal fluid [Letter]. N Engl J Med 1974;290:916.

71. Frankland AW, Parish WE. Anaphylactic sensitivity to human seminal fluid. Clin Allergy 1974;4:249.

72. Mikkelsen EJ, Henderson LL, Leiferman KM, Gleich GJ. Allergy to human seminal fluid. Ann Allergy 1975;34:239.

73. Guillet G, Dagregorio G. Seminal fluid as a missed allergen in vulvar allergic contact dermatitis. Contact Dermatitis 2004;50;318.

74. Fisher BK, Warkentin JD. Fiberglass dermatitis. Arch Dermatol 1969;99:717.

75. Worsaae N, Wanscher B. Oral injury caused by fellatio. Acta Derm Venereol (Stockh) 1978;58:187.

76. Wide H, Canby JP. Penile venereal edema. Arch Dermatol 1973;108:263.

77. Wright RA, Judson FN. Penile venereal edema. JAMA 1979;241:157.

78. Gorlick G. Chronic rash of the glans penis: a differential diagnosis. JAMA 1979;242:469.

79. Lowry TP. Nitrite inhalants for sex—the quest for the ultimate orgasm. Sex Med Today 1980(July):34.

80. Louria DB. Sexual use of amyl nitrite. Med Aspects Hum Sexuality 1970;4:89.

81. Goode E, Troiden RR. Amyl nitrite use among homosexual men. Am J Psychiatry 1979;136:1067.

82. Pearlman JT, Adams GL. Amyl nitrite inhalation fad [Letter]. JAMA 1970;212:160.

83. Fisher AA, Brancaccio RR, Jelinek JE. Facial dermatitis in men due to inhalation of butyl nitrite. Cutis 1981;271:146.

84. Fisher AA, Brancaccio RR. Popper's dermatitis from sniffing butyl nitrite. The Schoch Letter 1979;29(October):item 142.

85. Fregert S, Poulsen J, Trulsson L. Yellow stained skin from sodium nitrite in an etching agent. Contact Dermatitis 1980;6:296.

86. Modjtahedi BS, Modjtahedi SP, Maibach HI. The sex of the individual as a factor in allergic contact dermatitis. Contact Dermatitis 2004;50:53.

87. McDonald CJ. Dermatological problems in black skin. Prog Dermatol 1973;4:15.

88. Robinson MK. Population differences in skin structure and physiology and the susceptibility to irritant and allergic contact dermatitis: implications for skin safety testing and risk assessment. Contact Dermatitis 1999;41:65.

89. Foy V, Weinkauf R, Whittle E, et al. Ethnic variation in the skin irritation response. Contact Dermatitis 2001;45:346.

90. Robinson MK. Population difference in acute skin irritation responses, race, sex, age and sensitive skin and repeat subject comparisons. Contact Dermatitis 2002;46:86.

91. Kahn G. Depigmentation caused by phenolic detergent germicides. Arch Dermatol 1970;102:177.

92. Fisher AA. Vitiligo due to contactants. Cutis 1976;17:431.

93. Fisher AA. Contact dermatitis in black patients. Cutis 1977;20:303.

94. Plewig G, Fulton JE, Kligman AM. Pomade acne. Arch Dermatol 1970;101:580.

95. Kaidbey KH, Kligman AM. A human model of coal tar acne. Arch Dermatol 1974;109:212.

96. Verhagen AR. Pomade acne in black skin. Arch Dermatol 1974;110:465.

97. Verhagen AR, Koten JW, Chaddah VK, Patel RI. Skin diseases in Kenya: a clinical and histopathological study of 3,168 patients. Arch Dermatol 1968;98:577.

98. Andersen KE, Maibach HI. Black and white skin differences. J Am Acad Dermatol 1979;1:276.

99. Reed JT, Ghadially R, Elias PM. Skin type, but neither race nor gender, influence epidermal permeability barrier function. Arch Dermatol 1995;131:1134.

100. Schwartz L, Tulipan L, Birmingham DJ. Occupational diseases of the skin. 3rd ed. Philadelphia: Lea & Febiger, 1957.

101. Shelley WB. Newer understanding of ecology in dermatology. In: Rees RB, ed. Dermatoses due to environmental and physical factors. Springfield: Charles C Thomas Publisher, 1962:12.

102. Marshall EK Jr, Lynch V, Smith HW. Variations in susceptibility of the skin to dichloroethylsulfide. J Pharmacol Exp Ther 1919;12:291.

103. Weigand DA, Mershon MM. The cutaneous irritant reaction to agent o-chlorobenzylidene malononitrite (CS). I. Quantitation and racial influence in human subjects. Edgewood Arsenal Technical Report 4332. February 1970.

104. Weigand DA, Gaylor JR. Irritant reaction in Negro and Caucasian skin. South Med J 1974;67:548.

105. Frosch PJ, Kligman AM. The chamber-scarification for assessing irritancy of topically applied substances. In: Drill VA, Lazar P, eds. Cutaneous toxicity. New York: Academic Press, 1977.

106. Berardesca E, Maibach HI. Racial differences in sodium lauryl sulphate induced cutaneous irritation: black and white. Contact Dermatitis 1988;18:65.

107. Dickel H, Taylor JS, Evey P, et al. comparison of patch test results with a standard series among white and black racial groups. Am J Contact Dermat 2001;12:77.

108. Dahl MV. Forum discussion: some aspects of atopic dermatitis. Arch Dermatol 1983;119:237.

109. Sulzberger MB, Witten VH. Atopic dermatitis. In: Lowenthal LJA, ed. The enzymes. Edinburgh: E. & S. Livingstone, 1954:78.

110. Ward KA, Todd D, Thornton C, et al. A comparison of expression of surface-bound immunoglobulin E on antigen-presenting cells in cutaneous tissue between patients with allergic, irritant and atopic dermatitis. Contact Dermatitis 1991;25:115.

111. Epstein S, Mohajerin AH. Incidence of contact sensitivity in atopic dermatitis. Arch Dermatol 1964;90:284.

112. Baer R, Witten V. Editorial comment. In: Year book of dermatology and syphilography. Chicago: Year Book Medical Publishers, 1955: 414.

113. Fisher AA. Contact dermatitis superimposed on atopic eczema. Dermatol Digest 1966;5:45.

114. Gallacher G, Maibach HI. Is atopic dermatitis a predisposing factor for experimental acute irritant contact dermatitis? Contact Dermatitis 1998;38:1.

115. Basketter DA, Miettinen J, Lahti A. Acute irritant reactivity to sodium lauryl sulfate in atopics and non-atopics. Contact Dermatitis 1998;38:253.

116. Rees J, Friedmann PS, Matthews JN. Contact sensitivity to dinitrochlorobenzene is impaired in atopic subjects. Arch Dermatol 1990;126:1173.

117. Rietschel RL, Klemm J, Jones HE. Chronic irritant dermatitis interferes with induction of dinitrochlorobenzene (DNCB) sensitization. Clin Res 1982;30:915A.

118. Lever R, Forsyth A. Allergic contact dermatitis in atopic dermatitis. Acta Derm Venereol Suppl (Stockh) 1992;176:95.

119. Tada J, Toi Y, Arata J. Atopic dermatitis with severe facial lesions exacerbated by contact dermatitis from topical medicaments. Contact Dermatitis 1994;31:261.

120. de Groot AC. The frequency of contact allergy in atopic patients with dermatitis. Contact Dermatitis 1990;22:273.

121. Klas PA, Corey G, Storrs FJ, et al. Allergic and irritant patch test reactions and atopic disease. Contact Dermatitis 1996;34:121.

122. Ingordo V, D'Andria G, D'Andria C, et al. Clinical relevance of contact sensitization in atopic dermatitis. Contact Dermatitis 2001;45:239.

123. Brasch J, Schnuch A, Uter W. Patch-test reaction patterns in patients with a predisposition to atopic dermatitis. Contact Dermatitis 2004;49:197.

124. Heine G, Schnuch A, Uter W, et al. Type-IV sensitization profile of individuals with atopic eczema: results from the Information Network of Departments of Dermatology (IVDK) and the German Contact Dermatitis Research Group (DKG). Allergy 2006;61:611.

125. Lewis FM, Shah M, Gawkrodger DJ. Contact sensitivity in atopic dermatitis. Am J Contact Dermat 1995;6:150.

126. Giordano-Labadie F, Rancé F, Pellegrin F, et al. Frequency of contact allergy in children with atopic dermatitis: results of a prospective study of 137 cases. Contact Dermatitis 1999;40:192.

127. Brasch J, Geier J, Henseler T. Evaluation of patch test results by use of the reaction index: an analysis of data recorded by the Information Network of Departments of Dermatology (IVDK). Contact Dermatitis 1995;33:375.

128. Foti C, Bonifazi E, Casulli C, et al. Contact allergy to topical corticosteroids in children with atopic dermatitis. Contact Dermatitis 2005;52:162.

129. Epstein S. Contact dermatitis from neomycin due to dermal delayed (tuberculin-type) sensitivity: report of 10 cases. Dermatologica 1956;113:191.

130. Fisher AA, Chargin L, Fleischmajer R, Hyman A.. Pustular patch-test reactions. AMA Arch Dermatol 1959;80:742.

131. Fisher AA. Management of atopic dermatitis. NY J Med 1966;66:236.

132. Baer RL. Conference on infantile eczema: history, definitions, concepts. J Pediatr 1965;66:248.

133. Strauss JS, Kligman AM. The relationship of atopic allergy and dermatitis. AMA Arch Dermatol 1957;75:806.

134. Jadassohn W. Contact dermatitis versus atopic eczema. Int Arch Allergy 1957;11:20.

135. Champion RH. Atopic sensitivity to algae and lichens. Br J Dermatol 1971;85:551.

136. Kanny G, Becker S, de Hauteclocque C, Moneret-Vautrin DA. Airborne eczema due to mould allergy. Contact Dermatitis 1996;35:378.

137. Vidal C, Rial A. Airborne contact dermatitis from Tyrophagus putrescentiae. Contact Dermatitis 1998;38:181.

138. Clark RAF, Adinoff AD. Aeroallergen contact can exacerbate atopic dermatitis: patch tests as a diagnostic tool. J Am Acad Dermatol 1989;21:863.

139. Stinco G, de Francesco V, Frattasio A, Patrone P. A dermatitis flare after patch testing with Dermatophagoides pteronyssinus in an atopic patient. Contact Dermatitis 1997;37:52.

140. Gaddoni G, Baldassari L, Zucchini A. A new patch test preparation of dust mites for atopic dermatitis. Contact Dermatitis 1994;31:132.

141. Manzini BM, Motolese A, Donini M, Seidenari S. Contact allergy to Dermatophagoides in atopic dermatitis patients and healthy subjects. Contact Dermatitis 1995;33:243.

142. Kubota Y, Koga T, Imayama S, Hori Y. Mite-antigen-stimulated cytokine production by peripheral blood mononuclear cells of atopic dermatitis patients with positive mite patch tests. Contact Dermatitis 1994;31:217.

143. Cabon N, Ducombs G, Mortureux P, et al. Contact allergy to aeroallergens in children with atopic dermatitis: comparison with allergic contact dermatitis. Contact Dermatitis 1996;35:27.

144. Kerschenlohr K, Darsow U, Burgdorf WH, et al. Lessons from atopy patch testing in atopic dermatitis. Curr Allergy Asthma Rep 2004;4:285.

145. Turjanmaa K. The role of atopy patch tests in the diagnosis of allergy in atopic dermatitis. Curr Opin Allergy Clin Immunol 2005;5:425.

146. Giusti F, Seidenari S. Patch testing with egg represents a useful integration to diagnosis of egg allergy in children with atopic dermatitis. Pediatric Dermatol 2005;22:109.

147. Darsow U, Laifaoui J, Kerschenlohr K, et al. The prevalence of positive reactions in the atopy patch test with aeroallergens and food allergens in subjects with atopic eczema: a European multicenter study. Allergy 2004;59:1318.

148. Turjanmaa K, Darsow U, Niggemann B, et al. EAACI/GA2LEN position paper: present status of the atopy patch test. Allergy 2006;61:1377.

149. 149.Mayer RL. Contact dermatitis versus atopic dermatitis. Int Arch Allergy 1957;11:1.

150. Fisher AA. Recent developments in the diagnosis and management of drug eruptions. Med Clin N Am 1959;43:1.

151. Fisher AA, Sturm H. Procaine sensitivity: the relationship of the allergic eczematous contact type sensitivity to the urticarial, anaphylactoid variety. Ann Allergy 1958;16:593.

152. Morris GE. Allergic rhinitis acquired during the processing of epoxy resins. Ann Allergy 1959;17:74.

153. Epstein S. Contact-dermatitis due to nickel and chromate: observations on dermal delayed (tuberculin-type) sensitivity. Arch Dermatol 1956;73:236.

154. Fisher AA. Contact dermatitis, 3e. Philadelphia: Lea & Febiger, 1986.

155. Baer RL. Allergic eczematous sensitization in man. J Invest Dermatol 1964;43:223.

156. Jillson OF, Curwen WL, Alexander BR. Problems of contact dermatitis in the atopic individual: with reference to neomycin and ragweed oil sensitivity. Ann Allergy 1959;17:215.

157. Patrick J, Panzer JD, Derbes VL. Neomycin sensitivity in the normal (nonatopic) individual. Arch Dermatol 1970;102:532.

158. Wereide K. Neomycin sensitivity in atopic dermatitis and other eczematous conditions. Acta Derm Venereol (Stockh) 1970;50:114.

159. Fisher AA, Shapiro A. Allergic eczematous contact dermatitis due to metallic nickel. JAMA 1956;161:717.

160. Wahlberg IE, Skog E. Nickel allergy and atopy threshold of nickel sensitivity and immunoglobulin E determinations. Br J Dermatol 1971;85:97.

161. Motolese A, Truzzi M, Seidenari S. Nickel sensitization and atopy. Contact Dermatitis 1992;26:274.

162. McDonagh AJ, Wright AL, Cork MJ, Gawkrodger DJ. Nickel sensitivity: the influence of ear piercing and atopy. Br J Dermatol 1992;126:16.

163. Lammintausta K, Kalimo K, Fagerlund VL. Patch test reactions in atopic patients. Contact Dermatitis 1992;26:234.

164. Fromer IL, Burrage WS. Ragweed oil dermatitis. J Allergy 1953;24:425.

165. Fisher AA. Some immunologic phenomena in treatment of and patch testing for ragweed oil dermatitis. J Invest Dermatol 1952;19:271.

166. Osborne ED, Murray PF. Atopic dermatitis: a study of its natural course and of wool as a dominant factor. AMA Arch Dermatol Syphilol 1953;68:619.

167. Hambly EM, Levia L, Wilkinson DS. Wool intolerance in atopic subjects. Contact Dermatitis 1978;4:240.

168. Silvers SH, Glickman FS. Atopy and eczema of feet in children. Am J Dis Child 1968;116:400.

169. Simpson EL, Thompson MM, Hanifin JM. Prevalence and morphology of hand eczema in patients with atopic dermatitis. Dermatitis 2006;17:123.

170. Fredriksson T, Faergemann J. The atopic thigh: a "starting-school" symptom? Acta Derm Venereol (Stockh) 1981; 61:452.

171. Meding B, Swanbeck G. Predictive factors for hand eczema. Contact Dermatitis 1990;23:154.

172. Sun C-C, Cheng C-S. Frequency and determinants of occupational contact dermatitis in 2793 consecutively-investigated patients. Contact Dermatitis 1998;38:230.

173. MacKenzie-Wood AR, Freeman S. Unclassified endogenous eczema. Contact Dermatitis 1999;41:18.

174. Verbov JL. Atopic dermatitis and the forefoot. Br Med J 1978;11:962.

175. Verbov JL. Atopic eczema localized to the forefoot: an unrecognized entity. Practitioner 1978;220:465.

176. Verbov JL. Skin problems in childhood. Practitioner 1976;217:403.

177. Jepsen LV. Dermatitis plantaris sicca: a retrospective study of children with recurrent dermatitis of the feet. Acta Derm Venereol (Stockh) 1979;59:257.

178. Santucci B, Cristaudo A, Cannistraci C, et al. Urticaria from beer in 3 patients. Contact Dermatitis 1996;34:368.

179. Pereira F, Rafael M, Lacerda MH. Contact dermatitis from barley. Contact Dermatitis 1998;39:261.

180. Rasanen L, Lehto M, Turjanmaa K, et al. Allergy to ingested cereals in atopic children. Allergy 1994;49:871.

181. Kekki OM, Turjanmaa K, Isolauri E. Differences in skin-prick and patch-test reactivity are related to the heterogeneity of atopic eczema in infants. Allergy 1997;52:755.

182. Isolauri E, Turjanmaa K. Combined skin prick and patch testing enhances identification of food allergy in infants with atopic dermatitis. J Allergy Clin Immunol 1996;97:9.

REGIONAL CONTACT DERMATITIS

EXECUTIVE SUMMARY

Eyelid dermatitis is not simply a problem of contact dermatitis. Almost as many cases are found to be due to seborrheic dermatitis, with lesser numbers identified as atopic dermatitis, psoriasis, and nonspecific xerotitic dermatitis, depending on the investigator and the country in which the study is conducted. Sources of contact dermatitis of the eyelids include mascara, cosmetic preservatives, nail polish, hair cosmetics, eyeliner, ophthalmic medications, adhesive in false eyelashes, eyelash curlers, paper products, plants, airborne materials, dyes, and phosphorus sesquisulfide in strike-anywhere matches. Newer allergens in mascara include shellac and black iron oxide. Coconut diethanolamine and cocamidopropyl betaine in shampoos, and benzophenone as well as phthalic anhydride/trimellitic anhydride/glycols copolymer in nail products, are also newer allergen sources of eyelid dermatitis.

Facial dermatitis can include sensory changes, predominantly stinging. Metal and elastic objects are common allergens for the chest and abdomen. Genital areas experience dermatitis from hygiene products, contraceptives, condoms, and seminal fluid. Nails may show changes from physical trauma, acrylate application, hardeners, enamels, hydroquinone in bleaching creams, weed killers, and insecticides.

Eyelids

The eyelids are one of the most sensitive areas. Any substance used on the scalp, face, or hands may produce allergic eczematous contact dermatitis of the eyelids, whereas those primary sites remain unaltered. Airborne pollen and dust and all types of volatile agents may affect the eyelids first and exclusively. The absence of eyelid involvement is a strong argument against an airborne exposure to volatile substances unless this is explained by the use of protective eyewear. Contamination of the fingers with small amounts of allergen can result in transfer of sufficient material to the eyelids to produce dermatitis when little or no visible sign of difficulty is found elsewhere on the body. Marked edema of the eyelids is often a feature of poison ivy or hair dye dermatitis.

The skin of the eyelid is highly susceptible to irritants and allergens. This may be because of the thinness of the eyelid (0.55 mm, as compared to the thickness of the integument of the face, measuring about 2.0 mm) or caused by rubbing the eyelid area with the hands and fingers, which become exposed to many substances.

STUDIES OF EYELID DERMATITIS

A study of 105 cases of eyelid dermatitis found that when only the eyelids were involved, the most common cause was seborrheic dermatitis (46.3%). Contact dermatitis was the next most frequent diagnosis (35.2%). When other areas of the face were affected, allergic contact dermatitis was the most frequent cause.[1] An Italian study of eyelid dermatitis in 447 patients determined that 50.2% of cases were due to allergic contact dermatitis, 20.9% to irritant contact dermatitis, 13.5% to atopic dermatitis, 6.3% to seborrheic dermatitis, 6.5% to nonspecific xerotic dermatitis, and 2.3% to psoriasis.[2] A study of 1,053 cases of allergic periorbital dermatitis and 588 nonallergic periorbital dermatitis found that about 10.4% of the allergic cases and 60.2% of the nonallergic cases were atopics. The allergens found significantly more often in the allergic vs. the nonallergic patients were thimerosal, phenylmercuric acetate, sodium disulfite, gentamicin sulfate, phenylephrine hydrochloride and benzalkonium chloride. Among the important allergens supplied by the patients were beta-blockers, oxybuprocaine, and dexpanthenol in their ophthalmic products (Figure 6-1 and 6-2).[3] Also, in a series of 215 eyelid dermatitis cases, 165 were found to be allergic contact dermatitis, 37 were atopic dermatitis (but 33 of the 37 patients also had contact allergies), 35 patients had seborrheic dermatitis, and 35 had psoriasis. There were 9 cases of protein contact dermatitis in addition. Personal care products were responsible for 54 of the contact allergen cases; 12 individuals were allergic to cosmetic applicators, and an additional 12 reacted to a botanical cosmetic ingredient. Artificial nails and fingernail polish accounted for 18 contact allergy cases.[4]

EYELID DERMATITIS DUE TO COSMETICS

Contact dermatitis of the lids and periorbital area is caused by cosmetics applied to the hair, face, or fingernails more often than by cosmetics applied to the eye area. It is important to bear in mind that the sites to which some cosmetics are applied may not be affected. This is particularly true for hair dye and nail polish. Similarly, allergic and irritant reactions to face creams, makeup (foundation lotions and bases), and blushers may be limited to the eyelids.[5]

Two principal forms of contact dermatitis attributable to eye-area cosmetics are recognized: allergic contact dermatitis and irritant (toxic) contact dermatitis.[6] The morphologic features of these two forms are not always readily distinguishable. The degree of inflammation may be of the same order (usually mild to moderate), and the interval may be the same between the initial exposure and the onset of the dermatitis. Furthermore, potential irritants in eye-area cosmetics and in cosmetics in general are usually weak; repeated exposures are often required to induce a reaction. Nor do all exposed persons react as they do generally with strong irritants.[7]

Patch-test responses to allergens and irritants may also be indistinguishable; erythema or edema and erythema at the patch test site may be elicited by either. An eczematous vesicular reaction diagnostic of delayed allergic hypersensitivity in response to potential allergens in eye makeup is by no means the rule.

The cause of contact dermatitis of the eyelid is not always readily ascertainable. The following approach is recommended, especially when more than one cosmetic is suspect:

1. Take a detailed history of exposure, which should include inquiry about agents other than eye-area cosmetics that are known to elicit localized contact dermatitis of the eyelids, the introduction of a new product, and the renewal or refill of a previously used product. Modification or revision of formulations without a change in nomenclature or packaging is not an uncommon practice in the cosmetic industry. The method used to remove eye makeup also merits attention. Eye-area cosmetics may be removed by face creams, wet (chemically treated) facial tissues, or eye makeup removers. Use of eyelash curlers may lead to contact dermatitis from the rubber edges or nickel plating.

2. When the history is not sufficiently revealing or when more than one cosmetic is involved, the use test is often helpful in pinpointing the causative agent. The use test is often more rewarding than an open or closed patch test with the product because of the high incidence of false-positive and false-negative reactions in response to patch testing. To carry out the use test, the product is generally applied to the back of the ear or to the antecubital fossa two or three times a day for at least 4 or 5 days. Although a positive test (i.e., reproduction of the dermatitis) is significant, a negative response does not necessarily exclude the test substance as causative.

3. Patch tests with the components (open or closed, depending on the chemical nature of the ingredient) of the product(s) incriminated by the history and use test are carried out in an attempt to identify causative allergen(s). Most cosmetic companies comply with a physician's request for such materials.

COSMETIC IRRITANT EYELID AND CONJUNCTIVAL REACTIONS

Stinging and burning of the eyes and lids on application of an eye-area cosmetic are the most common complaints. These subjective symptoms are usually transitory and unaccompanied by objective signs of irritation. Evaporation of volatile components, such as mineral spirits, isoparaffins, and alcohol, and the presence of potential irritants, such as propylene glycol, sunscreens, and soap emulsifiers, in eye-area formulations are among the principal causes. In some instances, tolerance increases with subsequent applications, and the offending product does not have to be discarded.

Conjunctivitis may be elicited by physical irritants (mascara flakes, eyeshadow dust, particles of eyeliner, and mascara extenders, such as nylon or rayon fibers) and by chemical irritants (e.g., solvents and soap emulsifiers), as well as by potential allergens, such as preservatives and fragrances.

IRRITATION DUE TO MASCARA

Water-based mascara may contain several soap emulsifiers, such as sodium borate and ammonium stearate, formed by the interaction of stearic acid with ammonium hydroxide, which may be irritating to certain individuals who may tolerate an anhydrous, waterproof mascara.

A person who does not tolerate waterproof mascara or waterproof eyeliner may very well tolerate water-based counterparts. In the event that neither type of mascara or eyeliner is tolerable, a cake mascara or cake eyeliner may be tried. Maybelline Cake Mascara, Lumilane Cake Mascara

(Orlane), and Maybelline Ultra Liner Cake Eyeliner have only half the number of chemicals found currently in water-based and waterproof formulations. The potential for irritation is thus considerably reduced. This is not true for Chanel's Compact Mascara, which is highly complex. Similarly, persons who cannot use cream eyeshadow may tolerate pressed-powder eyeshadow, and vice versa.

Eyelid dermatitis can result from the use of mascara, in which shellac was found to be the responsible agent. Shellac is tested at 20% in eth. and it is also known as lacca. Shellac is the resinous secretion of an insect (*Laccifer lacca*).[8] In another report, shellac in mascara also was the cause of eyelid dermatitis. These authors found that while shellac is usually tested at 20% concentration in ethanol, it can also be tested at 5% aqueous with the addition of 5% triethanolamine.[9]

A rare cause of eyelid dermatitis is black iron oxide, which can be present in mascara. It is tested at 5% in petrolatum.[10]

PRESERVATIVES IN EYE COSMETICS

With few exceptions, parabens are common to all eye-area products. These esters of parahydroxybenzoic acid not infrequently are combined with at least one other antimicrobial, such as phenyl mercuric acetate, imidazolidinyl urea (germall-115), or quaternium-15 (Dowicel 200), to ensure adequate protection against yeasts, molds, and pseudomonads, which are widely distributed in nature. Clinique's Resistant Eyeliner and Basic Eye Emphasizer are paraben-free and contain sorbic acid as a preservative.

Paraben-sensitive persons, however, do not necessarily have to avoid paraben-containing cosmetics.[11] According to Fisher, patients sensitized to parabens may nevertheless tolerate paraben-containing cosmetics even on the thin skin of the eyelids, provided the product is applied to normal skin not subjected to a dermatitis in the past. This is the so-called paraben paradox.

Quaternium-15, imidazolidinyl urea, and DMDM hydantoin are formaldehyde donors. The latter is used less frequently than the other two compounds. Quaternium-15 has a more active formaldehyde releaser than imidazolidinyl urea.[12] Allergic reactions may be elicited by the compound per se or by the released formaldehyde.[13] Fisher maintains that imidazolidinyl urea is a much safer preservative than quaternium-15 for formaldehyde-sensitive persons.[13] Potassium sorbate is also used as a preservative in eye-area products. Sensitization to this agent has been reported.[14]

Di-isopropanolamine, used in cosmetic gloss formulations to "set up" the gel, has produced allergic contact dermatitis from an eyeshadow and a "blushing" gel.[15]

Ditertiarybutyl hydroquinone, an antioxidant in eyeshadow, produced an eyelid dermatitis.[16]

NAIL POLISH DERMATITIS

Nail polish dermatitis is an "ectopic dermatitis" because sensitized persons acquire dermatitis not on the nails or paronychial area but elsewhere, such as on the eyelids and neck. Dry nail polish becomes polymerized and is not a sensitizer.[17] The sensitizing toluene-sulfonamide formaldehyde resin in ordinary nail polish may be replaced by a "hypoallergenic" polyester resin (Clinique). Reports of airborne contact dermatitis to resins that are sticky or poorly soluble with soap and water, such as epoxy resin, may represent ectopic rather than airborne contact due to similar finger-to-eyelid transfer.

While nail polish and artificial nails are known sources, a less common source associated with ultraviolet cured nail acrylates is benzophenone. This is added as an ultraviolet absorbing agent in a variety of nail enhancements, particularly nail gels.[18] Ectopic contact dermatitis from nail polish can present as dermatitis of the eyelid and neck. While tosylamide/formaldehyde resin is well known as a cause of this presentation, another cause is phthalic anhydride/trimellitic anhydride/glycols copolymer. This is tested 1% in petrolatum. Contact urticaria and contact dermatitis to this agent have been reported from factory workers exposed to it.[19]

HAIR COSMETICS

Hair dyes, bleaching agents containing ammonium persulfate, perfumed hair sprays, hair setting lotions, and shampoos containing formaldehyde may affect the eyelids without producing scalp or forehead dermatitis. Paraphenylenediamine sensitivity and ammonium persulfate, in particular, may produce marked edema of the eyelids. Sometimes eyelid dermatitis is the only manifestation of contact dermatitis to ingredients in shampoo. Dejobert and colleagues report this presentation of contact dermatitis due to coconut diethanolamide, which was positive at 0.5% petrolatum. Changing shampoo resolved the dermatitis.[20]

CONJUNCTIVAL PIGMENTATION DUE TO EYELINER

Conjunctival pigmentation caused by eyeliner is a consequence of the application of eyeliner to the conjunctival side of the lid instead of to the exterior lid just behind the lashes. Unless the upper lid is everted to bring into view the aggregates of pigment deposited along the upper margin of the tarsal conjunctiva, this complication may be missed. Twelve cases were reported by Zuckerman,[21] and another was reported by Jervey[22] in

1969. Although some patients complain of discomfort, tearing, and itching, most are asymptomatic and do not require treatment.

EYESHADOW MIMICKING ORBITAL CALCIFICATION ON A ROENTGENOGRAM

A single case of bilateral curvilinear supraorbital shadow was found on X-ray examination of the skull of a patient complaining of increasing headaches. This shadow was interpreted as calcification. It was noted that the patient wore a large amount of eye makeup, making the possibility of an artifact likely. The curvilinear shadows disappeared after the eyeshadow was removed. A subsequent survey of 25 types of eye shadow showed that many were radiopaque because of bismuth, magnesium silicate, and iron oxides within the formulation.[23]

PRESERVATIVES IN OPHTHALMIC MEDICATIONS

Some preservatives may produce not only conjunctivitis but also eyelid dermatitis in sensitized individuals.[24] Table 6.1 lists some of the items to consider for patch testing when conjunctivitis and eyelid dermatitis coexist. Preservatives are prime suspects, especially benzalkonium chloride and thimerosal (merthiolate). Less commonly used and less frequently reported ophthalmic preservatives include chlorobutanol, chlorhexidine, phenylmercuric nitrate, and acetate. Because preservative systems may change without notice, it may be necessary to consult the package insert, label, or manufacturer to ascertain product composition.

ADHESIVES USED FOR FALSE EYELASHES

Artificial eyelashes consist of synthetic or natural fibers, including human hair, mounted on a thin fabric strip. The adhesive is a mixture of rubber latex, cellulose gums, and casein solubilized with a very mild alkali or other resins and water. The adhesive is formulated to be non-irritating and to permit easy removal of the lashes by simply peeling them off. This rubber latex rarely irritates the eyelids.

EYELASH CURLERS

Nickel-sensitive patients may acquire eyelid dermatitis from nickel-plated eyelash curlers and tweezers. Such curlers and tweezers should be replaced by the stainless-steel variety. Formerly, rubber-tipped eyelash curlers produced eyelid dermatitis in rubber-sensitive patients.

PAPER

Facial tissues containing perfume, formaldehyde, or benzalkonium chloride may produce dermatitis in sensitized persons. Newsprint and carbon paper produce eyelid dermatitis, particularly in persons sensitized to formaldehyde.

PLANTS

The *Toxicodendron* genus of plants (poison ivy, poison oak, and poison sumac) in particular may produce marked swelling of the eyelids with minimum dermatitis of the face.

AIRBORNE CONTACTANTS

Household sprays, insecticides, animal hairs, and occupational volatile chemicals can produce eyelid dermatitis.

EYELID DERMATITIS DUE TO FRUITS

The oil of lemon peel and the dyes of Florida orange skin can cause eyelid dermatitis.

MATCH DERMATITIS

The phosphorous sesquisulfide in "strike-anywhere" matches may produce marked eyelid dermatitis.[25] Affected patients should use "safety" matches or cigarette lighters. Contact urticaria of the eyelids was ascribed to the use of "strike-anywhere" matches.[26]

Match dermatitis usually affects the eyelids and face, particularly on the left side. The dermatitis may also affect the thighs and hands. Even nonsmokers who do not use matches may acquire dermatitis, if they are near

Table 6-1 Patch Test "Series"
Topical Ophthalmic Preparations, Including Contact Lens Solutions
Acetozolamide 0.1%
Benzalkonium chloride 0.01% pet
Benzethonium chloride 0.1% aq
Chlorhexidine 1% aq
Chlorobutanol 1% aq
Epifrin 1%
Epinephrine chloride 0.1% aq
Isopto carbachol 1%
Mannitol 2% in alcohol
Paraben mix 15% (3% ea. ethyl, methyl, butyl, benzyl, propyl) pet
Phenylmercuric acetate 0.05% pet
Phenylmercuric nitrate 0.05% pet
Pilocarpine chloride 0.1% aq
Propylene glycol 10% ag
Sorbic acid 5% pet
Thimerosal 0.1% pet

persons who use matches, apparently because the allergen may become airborne.[27]

EYELID DERMATITIS FROM QUINAZOLINE YELLOW DYE (D & C YELLOW NO. 11)

Calnan[28] reported that Yellow D & C No. 11 dye produced an eyelid dermatitis owing to the presence of this dye in an eye cream.

EYELID DERMATITIS DUE TO ORTHODONTIC DEVICES

Eyelid dermatitis was the sole manifestation of nickel allergy whose source was an orthodontic appliance. Removal of the appliance resulted in resolution of the dermatitis in 2 weeks. Oral administration of 2.5 mg of nickel sulfate caused the ocular lesions to appear within 24 hours. A placebo produced no reaction.[29]

SEQUELAE OF EYELID DERMATITIS

Periocular dermatitis may result in ectropion, which resolves with resolution of the dermatitis. De Groot and Poelhuis reported this phenomenon in a patient with unclassified periorbital dermatitis and pointed out that topical fluorouracil and tretinoin had previously been noted to produce this effect.[30] Contact dermatitis of the eyelids due to para-phenylenediamine in an eyelash dye was followed by the development of xanthelasma palpebrarum. This rare complication has been reported to occur following erythroderma in the presence of normal serum lipid profiles. The contact dermatitis case also had normal serum lipids.[31]

Face

Allergens can be transferred to the face not only by direct exposure but also indirectly from airborne or hand-to-face exposure. Thus, the face is the most common and often the main site of photodermatitis. Ragweed dermatitis, which occurs predominantly in men and boys, is most marked on the face. Toxicodendron dermatitis is often most prominent in the facial area.

An airborne exposure once weekly to a fish food caused a facial eczema from a combination of immediate and delayed hypersensitivity reactions to chironomids (nonbiting flies, midges) placed in an aquarium.[32]

UNILATERAL FACIAL DERMATITIS

In general, cosmetic dermatitis is bilateral, with the exception of nail polish dermatitis, which may be uni-

lateral. Connubial or consort contact dermatitis owing to hair dyes, fragrances, and topical medication used by the partner may also occur on one side of the face.

Facial dermatitis owing to an allergic reaction to phosphorous sesquisulfide (P_4S_3), the sensitizer in "strike-anywhere" matches, may be unilateral and airborne and may occur in nonsmokers.[25] Crushing match heads, soaking match heads in water, and transferring the resulting mushy material to the patch test paper is the most satisfactory method of applying the allergen. Patch testing may also be performed with 0.5% of phosphorous sesquisulfide in petrolatum.

"STATUS COSMETICUS" DUE TO "STINGING" COMPOUNDS IN COSMETICS

Many currently available cosmetics are free of compounds that produce most allergic hypersensitivity. However, nonspecific irritation from cosmetics still occurs. Thus, some persons appear to be in a condition of "status cosmeticus," in which every cosmetic or soap applied to the face produces itching, burning, or stinging sensations.

The condition is somewhat analogous to "status asthmaticus," in which patients acquire allergic bronchitis in response to seemingly every possible airborne allergen. It must be emphasized, however, that "status cosmeticus" is an irritant and not an allergic reaction.[33]

Patients who have "status cosmeticus" typically have an unremarkable clinical picture initially. They may have a mild erythema of the "butterfly" area of the face with slight edema of the eyelids. Occasionally there is a follicular eruption. However, the signs are not as vivid as the patients' bitter complaints of burning, stinging sensations. These persons usually claim to have tried at least 20 different cosmetics, all of which "disagree" with them.

Results of patch tests using the various implicated cosmetics and soaps are negative, as are results of "use" tests performed on the antecubital fossa. Undoubtedly, the facial skin differs from that of other areas of the body in its irritant sensitivity to cosmetics.

A similar constellation of findings has been reported to occur in pityriasis folliculorum. Malar erythema and a prominent follicular accentuation may give a slightly sandpaper-like texture to the face accompanied by stinging, burning, or itching. A skin scraping examined with oil or potassium hydroxide demonstrates many Demodex organisms often packing into follicles in tight columns. Topical lindane, pyrethrum, malathione, or sulfur may eradicate live organisms, and a follicular purge of remaining material should be performed with topical tretinoin.[34]

Frosch and Kligman[35] have confirmed that stinging from topically applied substances occurs mainly on the face. They found that substances that cause sustained stinging can be recognized by application to the nasolabial folds and cheeks during profuse sweating. The tests were carried out on preselected persons in whom a susceptibility to stinging had been demonstrated by exposure to 5% aqueous lactic acid. A predisposition to complaints of stinging was greater in women than in men and greater in whites than in blacks, especially in light-complexioned persons who tan poorly. The application of 10% lactic acid to the face elicited stinging almost equivalent to that produced by the application of 5% acid on sweating skin. It should also be noted that substances with a high capacity to induce stinging can do so in the absence of sweating.

Calnan[36] described one type of nonallergenic cosmetic complaint as an immediate stinging sensation that occurred when the product was applied to the face. However, because the stinging is transient and the product can subsequently be tolerated, a customer who has this experience does not usually complain to the manufacturer. Nevertheless, it is a reaction commonly mentioned in consumer surveys and market research studies of individual products. In Calnan's patient, a severe, stinging sensation developed from a powder containing 2-ethoxyethyl-p-methoxycinnamate. This adverse sensation was enhanced by sweating when the skin surface was damaged (e.g., from sunburn or dermatitis).

Lahti[37] also showed that cinnamic acid compounds used in cosmetics can produce nonspecific redness and itching when applied to human skin. This is probably related to prostaglandin synthesis and is blocked by prostaglandin inhibitors, such as indomethacin and aspirin.[38,39]

A review of the literature and personal experience would indicate that "ideal" cosmetics would be free of the compounds shown in Table 6.2.[13,33,35–37] This is particularly true of patients who have "status cosmeticus."

Table 6-2 "Stinging" Cosmetic Agents that Can Produce "Status Cosmeticus"
Benzoic acid
Bronopol
Cinnamic acid compounds
Dowicel 200
Formaldehyde
Lactic acid
Nonionic emulsifiers
Propylene glycol
Quaternary ammonium compounds
Sodium lauryl sulfate
Sorbic acid
Urea

Table 6-3 "Anti-Irritant" Cosmetic Components
Carboxyl compounds
Hydroxy compounds
Polysorbate 20
Aloe vera gel
Imidazole compounds
Germall-115—imidazolidinyl urea allantoin
Imidazoline amphoteric surfactants (used in "no tears" shampoos)

THE ROLE OF ANTI-IRRITANTS IN COSMETICS

Goldenberg and Safrin[40] suggested that the "stinging" effects of cosmetic irritants may be neutralized by "anti-irritants." They proposed three possible mechanisms of action by which the anti-irritants may function: (a) complexing of the irritant, (b) blocking otherwise chemically reactive sites of skin keratin, and (c) preventing complete physical contact with the skin.

The anti-irritant chemicals are grouped in the following chemical categories: carboxyl, hydroxy, and imidazole compounds (Table 6.3). Miscellaneous anti-irritant compounds are listed in Table 6.4. Ongoing investigations will determine whether the inclusion of any of these anti-irritants in cosmetics will help eliminate stinging and burning sensations from cosmetic use and will be tolerated by those with "status cosmeticus."

PIGMENTED FACIAL CONTACT DERMATITIS

Brown or bluish pigmentation of the face has been described as a dermatosis of great cosmetic significance in Japanese women since the 1950s.[41] Many of the cases resemble the melanosis described by Riehl in Vienna in 1917, and the term "Riehl's melanosis" is commonly used by Japanese dermatologists for the condition.[42]

Table 6-4 Miscellaneous "Anti-Irritant" Compounds
Amine acid surfactant (acyl glutamate)
Amine oxides
Heavy mineral oils
High-molecular-weight polypropylene glycols
Lauroyl cycloimidinium amphoteric surfactants
N-lauroyl sarcosinates
Phthalate esters
Polyvinyl pyrrolidone
Protein-fatty acid condensates (amides)
Sorbitan esters
Tertiary amine oxide surfactants
Thiodiglycolic acids

At the International Conference on Dermatology and Cosmetic Science in Tokyo, the subject of facial melanosis was discussed extensively. The concept of Riehl's melanosis was considered, and the condition was defined in the perspective of recent progress in contact dermatitis.[43]

In Japan, where facial melanosis has been quite common, allergic contact dermatitis to scents, such as hydroxycitronella, benzyl-salicylate, ylang-ylang oil, and jasmine, as well as to bactericides such as carbanilides, has been demonstrated as the cause of the pigmentation. Most Japanese dermatologists use the term "Riehl's melanosis" for both inflammatory and noninflammatory forms.[41] Brilliant Lake Red R (widely used in cheek rouges and lipsticks until 1976) has been described as a common cause of sensitization.[44] A study showed that Brilliant Lake Red R, which has been described as the most important cause of Riehl's melanosis, contains Sudan 1 as a major impurity.[45] Investigations on the pattern of cross-sensitivity indicated that Sudan 1 is a potent sensitizer and that Brilliant Lake Red R itself is a weak sensitizer.

The dominant symptom of Riehl's melanosis is facial hyperpigmentation, most pronounced on the forehead and in the zygomatic or temporal regions. Riehl could find no explanation for the condition but suggested that certain foods used during the war could be responsible. Riehl's melanosis later was observed in dark-complexioned persons, in whom hyperpigmentation with pigment incontinence may be the main sign of contact dermatitis caused by certain allergens.

Today Riehl's melanosis is almost synonymous with pigmented contact dermatitis of the face. The most common cause has been sensitizing chemicals in cosmetics.

FACIAL DERMATITIS DUE TO RUBBER COMPOUNDS

The following rubber articles have produced facial dermatitis in rubber-sensitive persons:
- scuba diver face mask[46]
- bathing cap
- rubber cosmetic sponges[47]
- rubber-edged eyelash curlers[48]
- balloons[49]
- flubber (children's toys)[50]

FACIAL DERMATITIS DUE TO METALLIC COMPOUNDS

Nickel-plated objects used on the hair, such as bobby pins and curlers, may produce facial dermatitis in nickel-sensitive persons.

POSTOPERATIVE FACIAL DERMATITIS

The use of nickel-plated objects that make contact with the face during surgery or dentistry can produce facial dermatitis. Face masks sterilized with ethylene oxide may produce severe facial dermatitis.

PERIORAL DERMATITIS

Perioral dermatitis can occur from inhalers used to treat asthma. Such was the case of a woman who reacted to beclometasone dipropionate in her inhaler 20% aqueous and the commercial cream form of this corticosteroid. The exposure did not affect her asthma, and stomatitis did not occur, both of which suggest that the mucosal surfaces behave immunologically in a different manner.[51]

Scalp

The scalp is particularly resistant to contact dermatitis. Allergens applied to this area often produce dermatitis of the eyelids, ears, neck, and hands, whereas the scalp remains uninvolved. Persons who have exquisite sensitivity to paraphenylenediamine or glyceryl thioglycolate, however, may show a marked scalp reaction with edema and crusting. Permanent wave solutions of ammonium thioglycolate applied improperly may produce severe irritant reactions and burns of the scalp.

COSMETIC DAMAGE TO THE SCALP IN BLACK PATIENTS

McDonald[52] pointed out that most hair care products for black people are used to change the physical appearance of hair from naturally curly to some degree of straightness. When used improperly, they may cause severe damage to the hair and scalp.

The most potent hair straighteners (relaxers) are those containing the alkali sodium hydroxide. Sodium hydroxide straighteners, unlike thioglycolates, cause irreversible changes in the hair. When used improperly at home or by inexperienced beauticians, either on hair with small, weak fibers or on hair that has previously been abused by straighteners, these sodium hydroxide straighteners can cause devastating damage to the scalp and hair. A single, prolonged application of these products to normal hair may also result in damage to hair and scalp. Hair breakage, either immediate or removed, is the most common abnormality observed after the use of hair straighteners. Often, when remotely observed 4 to 6 months after application of the straightener, the patient may not associate hair breakage with the use of hair straighteners. As the relaxer is applied excessively, pooling on the scalp provides a greater degree of damage to the disulfide bonds that give the hair shaft its resistance to breakage. As this weak area grows away from the scalp surface, it loses the added support provided by the intrafollicular support structures and becomes increasingly "weathered" by combing, shampooing, and other treatments. The frictional injury of combing is also magnified by the added leverage exerted as the hair moves away from the scalp at a rate of about 12 to 14 mm per month. Thus, breakage occurs a month or more after a treatment.

The most severe damage caused by straightening with a hot comb occurs after severe burns to the scalp. This type of reaction may progress beyond the simple irritant type of skin reaction seen with many hair care products, including bleaching and coloring agents. In this case, the scalp sustains severe second- and third-degree burns that heal with permanent scarring. Hair follicles are thus destroyed, and hair loss becomes permanent. Alopecia not resulting from an overt burn was critically reviewed, and the original concept of its being caused by use of a hot comb was found wanting. The patchy vertex and coronal cicatricial alopecia most commonly seen in black patients has been reclassified from hot-comb alopecia to follicular degeneration syndrome, which is believed to be related to loss of the internal root sheath in sharply curved hair follicles.[53]

Nickel-sensitive patients may develop localized scalp dermatitis from prolonged contact with hairpins, curlers, and bobby pins. Ill-fitting wigs, as well as some adhesives used with wigs, may irritate the scalp.

The insertion of "artificial" hairs for the treatment of male alopecia has resulted in many cases of severe dermatitis, infections, and granulomas. Vioform preparation applied to the scalp may give white or silver hair a reddish hue,[54] and the use of Capitrol shampoo may produce a strawberry-blond tone.

Forehead

Pomade acne, so-called "Vaselinoderma," resulting from greasy applications to the scalp, affects the forehead. Pomades are the simplest of hair straighteners. They contain primarily paraffin and petrolatum mixtures with gums and perfumes added. They are the least damaging of all hair care products, but they often cause acneiform facial lesions (pomade acne). This is a unique form of acne characterized by the presence of uniform, localized, follicular comedones and occasionally papulopustules on the forehead and temples.

Forehead dermatitis may occur as a square dermatitis of the forehead in Orthodox Jews who place phylacteries on their foreheads during prayer ("Phylactery dermatitis"). Such a phylactery is a small, black leather cube containing a piece of parchment.

Bathing caps, rubber hair nets, and hat bands can also cause forehead dermatitis.

The Hindu practice of wearing a central forehead dot of color known as a *bindi* may lead to leukoderma associated with paratertiary butylphenol resin in the adhesive, with or without a related dermatitis or positive patch test.[55,56]

Ears

CONTACT OTITIS: DERMATITIS OF EXTERNAL EAR AND CANAL

The ear, particularly the helix, may be the site of the disease due to hair sprays, shampoos, and dyes. Earlobe dermatitis is a cardinal sign of nickel sensitivity in persons wearing costume jewelry earrings. Otitis externa may be caused by sensitizing medications applied to the ear canals, particularly neomycin (Figure 6-3). Habitual insertion of metallic objects (hairpins, pens, and pencils) into the canals may produce dermatitis in nickel-sensitive persons. The piercing of earlobes is often a precipitating factor in nickel and gold sensitivity.

The auricle and external ear canal, covered entirely by skin, are subjected to contact irritants and sensitizers just as is the skin elsewhere.[57,58] Furthermore, the inflamed, occluded ear canal is as readily sensitized by topical medicaments as are stasis eczemas and ulcers.

Allergic dermatitis of either the entire auricle or a portion of it may occur in sensitized individuals. Plastic helmets or bathing caps affect the entire auricle. Nail polish, on the other hand, may produce dermatitis of any portion of the ear that sensitized persons touch before the nail polish is dry. This is an example of "ectopic" cosmetic dermatitis.[59]

The site where the contact otitis originates often gives a clue to the causative contactant. Arnold[60] described "sugarcane" ears, resembling cauliflower ears, in workers who carry bundles of burned stalks of sugar. The lesions are unilateral, depending on whether the worker is right- or left-handed.

A study of 179 patients with a variety of ear conditions such as otitis externa, seborrheic dermatitis, atopic dermatitis, and psoriasis found that one-fourth of the patients had become allergic to one or more of their medications. Three-quarters of the medication-allergic patients were reactive to neomycin (76%), followed by framycetin (62%), gentamicin (31%), quinoline mix (18%), caine mix (11%), tixocortol pivalate (4%), and budesonide (2%).[61]

EARLOBE OTITIS

Like nickel sensitivity, gold sensitivity may similarly affect the earlobes. The piercing of earlobes is a common precipitating cause of nickel sensitivity. By having their ears pierced and then wearing nickel-containing jewelry, many persons develop a generalized nickel sensitivity that persists indefinitely. For this reason, it is advisable to insert stainless steel earrings, under sterile conditions, for 3 weeks following ear piercing.[62] Injury to the skin from ear piercing followed by intimate contact with metallic nickel favors the development of allergic eczematous dermatitis, which may be complicated by infection and hepatitis.[63] Other complications of earlobe dermatitis include split earlobes,[64] fissured granulomas,[65] cyst formation, and keloids (Figure 6-4).

Shore and Berger[66] described a case in which large hooped earrings produced dermatitis of the neck but not of the earlobes. Fur neck pieces and collars may also produce dermatitis of the earlobes.

POSTAURICULAR OTITIS

The metal or plastic frames of eyeglasses, plastic hearing aids, and telephone operator headsets can produce dermatitis in this area. Perfume-sensitive individuals who habitually place perfume behind their ears may also produce a postauricular otitis.

RETROAURICULAR DERMATITIS AND TRAUMA DUE TO SPECTACLES

Jirasek and colleagues[67] reported retroauricular dermatitis from nickel in eyeglass frames. Barnes and colleagues[68] stated that mechanical trauma from eyeglass frames can cause a fissured acanthoma behind the ear.

CONTACT OTITIS OF THE HELIX

Allergenic preparations applied to the scalp or hair, such as hair dyes, sprays, and shampoos, may primarily affect the helices. Many persons who have mild hypersensitivity to hair dyes may acquire allergic dermatitis of the helices and eyelids without affecting the scalp or other facial areas. Earmuffs and hairnets may also produce dermatitis, principally of the helices.

EXTERNAL CANAL OTITIS

The habitual insertion of metallic objects, such as hairpins, pens, and pencils, into the canals may produce dermatitis in nickel-sensitive persons. Hearing aid inserts may also produce allergic reactions of the canal.

Once the canal becomes inflamed, occluded, and excoriated by scratching, the stage is set for ready sensitization to topical therapeutic agents, such as neomycin, benzocaine, sulfonamides, mercurials, the parabens, and even corticosteroid preparations.

The combination of dermatitis and infection may produce an infectious eczematoid contact otitis similar to that which occurs following middle ear and mastoid surgery. A chronic discharge accompanied by severe pruritus and edema of the external canal are cardinal signs of this condition.

Otitis externa is one of the most frequent conditions with which neomycin sensitivity is associated; therefore, the use of this antibiotic should be avoided in ear canal therapy.[69] Unlike benzocaine dermatitis, which may be quite explosive, neomycin sensitivity is often subtle, consisting merely of an exacerbation of the otitis externa for which the neomycin was applied.

Antiseptics and antibiotics containing erythromycin (Ilotycin ointment), Terramycin, or Betadine are much less sensitizing than neomycin.

Local anesthetic topical agents containing xylocaine (Lidocaine) may be used instead of benzocaine.

"Sulfa" topical medication should also be avoided in benzocaine-sensitive persons because cross-reactions may occur.

McKelvie and McKelvie[70] stated that it is not unusual for patients to use match heads for cleaning or scratching their ears, and otitis externa caused by a contact dermatitis from a "strike-anywhere" match head may occur.

HEARING AID DERMATITIS

Guill and Odom[70] reported a patient who developed a dermatitis from a cold-cured, acrylate hearing aid but tolerated a heat-cured variety. Jordan and Dahl[71] described retroauricular dermatitis due to resorcinol monobenzoate in a component of a patient's hearing aid. Hearing aids may be made of the following plastics: acrylate, vinyl, polyethylene, and silicone (see Chapter 20).

Neck

The neck, like the eyelids and genitalia, is a highly reactive site. Cosmetics or topical acne medications applied to the face, scalp, or hair often initially affect the neck. Berloque and nail-polish dermatitis also commonly involve this area.

Nickel-sensitive patients may acquire dermatitis from necklaces, zippers, and the metallic neck pieces of stethoscopes. Necklaces made of various woods may also produce dermatitis. Tanita and Tagami[73] described a bizarre linear granuloma around the neck in a child who had placed a rubber band in the area. The neckline of tight leotards may produce a fine linear dermatitis of the neck, as can rubber hair nets. Rough-starched collars may also produce a dermatitis. Permanent wave solutions applied on the scalp and spilled accidentally on the neck have produced instances of allergic and irritant dermatitis of the neck.

"Fiddler's neck" is a common occupational mark among violin and viola players. It is an area of localized lichenification of the skin on the left side of the neck, just below the angle of the jaw, where the chin rest of the violin is in contact with the side of the neck. Additional signs are erythema, scaling, cyst formation, and papules or pustules within the area.

Lachapelle and colleagues[74] stated that a worsening of pseudofolliculitis of the beard has not been described as a clinical sign of "fiddler's neck."

Chest

Medallions, crosses, zippers, nickel-plated buttons, and wires in brassière cups have all produced dermatitis of the chest and breast. Perfume dermatitis of the upper chest and breast area is not uncommon. Sensitizing medications applied to eczematous nipples may produce an infiltrated dermatitis resembling a malignancy.

Lactating women may use herbal remedies for nipple eczema, and oil of chamomile contained in such remedies has caused contact dermatitis, which may be exacerbated by drinking chamomile tea.[75]

Beltline

Many men develop dermatitis at the tops of their underwear shorts. This dermatitis is an allergic reaction to either a rubber chemical or an oxidized chlorine-bleached chemical. In either case, the patient may purchase rubber-free men's boxer shorts that are fastened with a button and free of elastic (Whitehall Mfg. Co., 180 Madison Avenue, New York, NY 10016).

Umbilicus

Nickel-sensitive persons may acquire periumbilical dermatitis from metallic buttons of blue jeans. A study of 20 patients who were nickel sensitive and whose exposure was to nickel-containing belt buckles or buttons found that the periumbilical dermatitis initially seen evolved into a dermatitis that spread to the sides of the neck and flexures of the extremities. Avoidance of the belt buckle exposure resolved local and distant dermatitis.[76]

DERMATITIS OF THE RAW UMBILICAL STUMP

Antiseptics, such as thimerosal (merthiolate), and antibiotics, such as neomycin, applied soon after the cord is tied, may produce allergic contact dermatitis.

UMBILICAL GRANULOMAS

Treatment of the raw umbilical stump with talc or starch may produce granulomas.[77]

UMBILICAL STONE

Ehring[78] stated that, in rare instances, a hard, smooth, almost black bolus "omphalolith" is found in the umbilicus, resembling a malignant melanoma. After removal by tweezers, it reveals on its reverse side a colorless lamellar epithelium. Microscopic examination shows that it also consists of stratified corneocytes. Differential diagnosis of the omphalic stone includes the so-called umbilical cholesteatoma, an accumulation of crumbling, fetid masses in the umbilicus, often accompanied by seborrhea, that may lead to abscess formation.

Trunk, Periaxillary Region, and Antecubital Spaces

The trunk, periaxillary region, and antecubital spaces may be the sites of perfume dermatitis or a symmetrical type of dermatitis owing to the finishes and dyes in clothing.

Axillae

Deodorants, antiperspirants, and perfumes may cause contact dermatitis. "Consort" contact dermatitis may occur from resting of the head on the axilla when the consort has freshly-dyed hair or has put brilliantine on the scalp. Unilateral axillary dermatitis from zippers may occur in nickel-sensitive patients.

Forearms and Hands

The forearms also may be the site of dermatitis due to sensitizers that splash above protective gloves. It must not be forgotten that loose bracelets may have considerable excursion on the forearm and thereby can produce dermatitis from the wrist to the antecubital spaces.

While prolonged exposure to water causes the palms to wrinkle, tingling and pain on exposure to water accompanied by flesh-colored papules may be seen in aquagenic syringeal acrokeratoderma. This condition is treated with aluminium chloride hexahydrate 20%. It has also been reported under several other names: aquagenic palmoplantar keratoderma, transient reactive papulotranslucent acrokeratoderma, and aquagenic keratoderma. The condition usually resolves within 30 minutes untreated.[79]

Thighs

Gomez-Orbaneja and colleagues[80] reported that two men sensitized by the striking surfaces of match boxes developed thick, indurated plaques, first on the thighs, then on the face and other sites. These plaques fluctuated in severity and were initially identified clinically and histologically as mycosis fungoides. Another two men had patches confined to the thighs. Patch testing revealed that the four men tested positive to the striking surface of match boxes that they kept in their pockets.

Other objects in pockets that may cause thigh dermatitis include coins and keys. Police officers have acquired an irritant dermatitis of the thighs from leaking Mace canisters used in antiriot maneuvers.

Genital Region

VULVITIS DUE TO CONTACTANTS

Douches, feminine hygiene sprays, cleansers, deodorants, and medications used on the vulva and in the vagina may be possible causes of contact vulvitis. In addition, medications, cosmetics such as nail polish, and other sensitizers may be conveyed by the hands to the vulva. Frequently, sensitizing medications or douches well tolerated by the vaginal mucosa produce vulvitis and dermatitis of the thighs.[81] An evaluation of 92 women with vulvar complaints found that 35 (38%) had one or more positive patch tests and 15 of the cases were deemed relevant. Reactions to topical pharmaceutical products were common. Three of the women had contact urticaria syndrome from latex and two others had protein contact dermatitis from human seminal plasma.[82]

IRRITANTS AND SENSITIZERS IN DOUCHES

Most over-the-counter douches are prepared by the user. Douches containing acid or alkalis that are not properly diluted may produce an irritant vulvitis. The principal acid irritants are alum, citric acid, and lactic acid. Alkalis, such as sodium bicarbonate or sodium borate, in too high a concentration may also produce vulvitis.

Britz and Maibach[83] have shown that the vulvar skin is more readily irritated than the forearm. Often low-grade erythema of the vulva is not readily apparent because of pigmentation of the skin of the vulva. The patient may complain of burning and stinging of the vulva, but examination may not readily reveal dermatitis.

Table 6.5 lists the principal causes of allergic vulvitis from douches, as proved by positive patch test reactions.

Table 6-5 Sensitizers in Douches
Aromatics (perfumes)
Benzethonium chloride
Methyl salicylate
Oil of eucalyptus
Oxyquinoline
Phenylmercuric acetate
Thymol

Because practically all douches are irritants under a closed patch test, testing should be performed with the individual ingredients of the douche.

VULVITIS FROM FEMININE HYGIENE SPRAYS (DEODORANT SPRAYS)

Feminine hygiene sprays consist of perfume, an emollient, and a propellant. With the ban on hexachlorophene, most sprays no longer contain any antibacterial agents. Allergic reactions to spray ingredients are rare, usually occurring in patients who have miliaria, intertrigo, moniliasis, or seborrheic eczema in the inguinal or perineal area. Two cases of allergic reactions to the bacteriostat benzethonium chloride were encountered. Perfume in one instance and the emollient isopropyl myristate in another produced an allergic contact vulvitis.[84]

Preservatives and antibacterial agents in medications, as well as in feminine hygiene sprays, may produce allergic reactions.[85–88]

Irritant reactions from the chilling effect of fluorinated hydrocarbon propellants due to application too close to the vulvar area are much more common than reactions of the allergenic variety.[89–91] Such allergic reactions appear to occur particularly on skin that has been previously injured by some type of nonallergic dermatitis, such as miliaria, seborrheic dermatitis, or moniliasis.

CHEMICAL CONTRACEPTIVES

Vaginal spermicides rarely irritate the vulva but may occasionally produce allergic vulvitis. Table 6.6 is a list of the principal sensitizers in vaginal spermicides.

Patch tests with chemical contraceptives must be interpreted with care because some contain soapy substances

Table 6-6 Sensitizers in Vaginal Spermicides
Hexylresorcinol
Nonoxyl
Oxyquinoline sulfate
Phenylmercuric acetate and borate
Quinine hydrochloride

that may show nonspecific irritant reactions under a closed patch. A positive patch test reaction should be followed by testing with the individual ingredients of the product.

Many vaginal spermicides contain foaming agents and emulsifiers that may be irritating. Contact urticaria and anaphylaxis can occur as a response to exposure to seminal fluid (see Chapters 5 and 33). Severe irritant dermatitis of the vulvar and suprapubic area may occur with the use of depilatories.

RUBBER PRODUCTS PRODUCING VULVITIS

Rubber Support Pessaries and Contraceptive Diaphragms

Vaginitis and vulvitis may be produced by such rubber articles in rubber-sensitive individuals. For rubber-sensitive persons, plastic pessaries and contraceptive devices are now available as substitutes.

Rubber Condoms

These products may produce an acute dermatitis of the vulva and inner aspect of the thighs in a rubber-sensitive woman.

MISCELLANEOUS CAUSES OF VULVITIS

1. *Nickel-plated* objects (pins, fasteners, zippers, and clasps) on sanitary napkins may produce vulvitis in nickel-sensitive persons.
2. *Cosmetics* may be the cause of vulvitis. For example, nail polish dermatitis will, on occasion, manifest itself on the vulvar or anal area because of contact with fingernails on which the nail polish is not yet dry. The vulva may also be the site of perfume dermatitis from perfume or perfumed toilet tissue.
3. *Medicated soaps* containing sensitizing antiseptics can cause vulvitis.
4. *Wearing apparel.* Dyes and synthetic resins in underclothing may produce dermatitis in sensitized women. The wearing of close-fitting undergarments, such as panty hose, panty girdles, and tight sanitary napkins, may produce vulvar irritation.
5. *Bubble baths.* Prolonged immersion in bubble baths, particularly in children, may produce an irritant vulvitis.
6. *Medications.* Neurodermatitis of the vulva is often complicated by an allergic reaction to sensitizing medications, particularly benzocaine.
7. *Urine.* Incontinent patients, whether adults or infants, may acquire an ammoniacal vulvitis from the irritant effect of ammonia in the urine.

VULVAR DERMATITIS, PRURITUS, AND DYSESTHESIA

The value of patch testing patients with vulvar symptoms versus vulvar signs and symptoms has been investigated. Vulvar itching without rash was investigated with patch testing in a group of 69 such patients.[92] One or more allergic reactions were noted in 45 (65%), of which 40 (58%) were relevant. Most of the relevant substances were medications. Of the 69 patients, 31 (45%) had either complete resolution or significant improvement by avoiding the identified allergen. Lewis and colleagues[93] extended their series in a 1997 report. They tested 121 patients with vulvar pruritus without signs of skin disease and 32 patients with other vulvar dermatoses. The researchers found that 56 (46%) had relevant positive reactions. Medications and excipients were the most frequent source of difficulty. Seven of 16 patients with lichen sclerosis et atrophicus had positive patch tests, and 6 of these benefited from avoiding the identified allergen. Overall 67 (55%) improved.

In contrast to pruritus vulvae, vulvodynia is a burning rather than an itching sensation. Erythema or signs of dermatitis are absent. In a study of 18 vulvodynia patients, no relevant allergens were found by patch testing.[94] Vulvar vestibulitis is part of the vulvodynia complex; the condition is characterized by burning, stinging, and dyspareunia. Patch tests in 30 women with this diagnosis were also unrewarding, as no relevant reactions were found.[95] The presence of visible skin changes appears to be important in predicting whether patch testing will be valuable. Patch tests were conducted on 201 women with a variety of anogenital symptoms, of which eczema was the most common, followed by unknown diagnosis, then psoriasis, lichen planus, vestibulitis, and lichen sclerosis. One or more positive patch tests were noted in 79 (39%) of the women. Of the group, 56 (28%) had relevant patch test reactions. If the signs and symptoms were confined to the vulva only, 19% of patients had relevant reactions. If the reactions were confined to perianal skin, 33% had relevant reactions, but if both vulva and perianal skin were involved, 43% of the reactions were relevant.[96] Patients with vulvodynia were evaluated with an ultraviolet-light–killed *Candida albicans* patch test. The yeast was suspended in petrolatum at 0.4, 4.0, and 40%. The higher concentration was found to be immunosuppressive, and positive reactions occurred in 10 (37%) of 27 patients with vulvodynia but no reactions occurred in 13 atopic female control subjects. The 4% concentration was favored. The higher concentration was thought to signal toll-like receptor 2 resulting in fewer reactions; ie, immunosuppression.[97]

Patch tests were conducted on 44 women with vulval lichen simplex chronicus; 12 (27%) had relevant reactions.[98]

However, routine screening allergens were not particularly helpful. Medicaments and excipients were the most frequently encountered allergens. In a study of vulval dermatitis, nickel allergy was overrepresented.[99] However, avoidance of nickel or a move to a low-nickel diet was felt to be helpful, leading the authors to recommend that if dermatitis is present and a positive nickel patch test is found as well, relevance might be present. Other studies have suggested that nickel is not relevant in this setting. If no dermatitis was present (vulvodynia rather than dermatitis), patch tests were not helpful.[99]

CONTACT BALANITIS

The glans penis and prepuce may acquire contact dermatitis from douches, contraceptive jellies, feminine hygiene sprays, and other medicaments used by a sexual partner.

After intercourse, some men may cleanse the genital area with strong detergents that may produce severe irritant dermatitis and even superficial erosions. Traumatic balanitis may occur from certain sexual practices (see Chapter 5). Poison ivy may cause a severe balanitis and produce such marked swelling of the foreskin as to cause urinary retention. Numerous other exposures in work and play may also be factors in producing balanitis.

Sensitizing topical applications for dermatoses, such as psoriasis and lichen planus, may produce a superimposed contact balanitis.

RUBBER CONDOMS

These are popularly called "sheaths," "French letters," "prophylactics," "protectives," "rubbers," "skins," and "safes."

Edema of the prepuce may be the first sign of an allergic rubber condom reaction. The eruption may spread to the shaft of the penis, the scrotum, inguinal areas, and inner aspects of the thighs. Occasionally, the reaction is confined to the glans penis.

Rubber condom dermatitis is usually due to sensitivity to one or more rubber antioxidants or accelerators or natural rubber latex. Occasionally, a preservative powder dusted onto the condom is the actual cause of the dermatitis. In one instance, the powder contained 10% monobenzyl ether of hydroquinone (agerite alba), which produced balanitis, penile dermatitis, and eventually leukoderma.

Some men have found by trial and error that only certain brands of rubber condoms produce reactions, whereas others are well tolerated.

Patch Tests for Rubber Condom Sensitivity

Patch tests should be performed with the actual condom suspected of producing the reaction. If a powder or lubricant is present on the condom, tests should also be performed with these substances.

Patients allergic to tetramethyl thiuram in a rubber condom may develop a violent reaction and widespread dermatitis when given disulfuram for treatment of alcoholism.

If natural rubber latex sensitivity is suspected, prick tests or radioallerogsorbent test (RAST) rather than patch tests are indicated. In such cases, symptoms of itching and swelling are usually immediate (ie, within minutes of skin contact).

NONRUBBER CONDOMS

Fourex and Lambskin, which are made of processed lamb cecum, are available for persons who cannot tolerate any rubber contraceptives. Such preparations are popularly called "fishskins."

Polyurethane condoms have become available for men under the name Avanti by Durex.[100] Female condoms have also become available under names such as Femidom, Reality, Bikini, and Woman's Choice. The Reality condom is made of polyurethane.[101]

FEMALE CONTRACEPTIVES

Contact with rubber diaphragms, douching solutions, and feminine hygiene sprays may produce balanitis in sensitized males.

SCROTUM

A 69-year-old man developed redness and edema confined to the scrotum and sparing the thighs and inguinal folds. Patch testing indicated that he was allergic to disperse orange 3, paraphenylenediamine, and para-aminoazobenzene. When he followed the advice to wear only white cotton underwear, his formerly recalcitrant eruption dramatically improved.[102]

PENILE TOURNIQUET SYNDROME

Swelling of the penis may be caused by infection, allergy, trauma, or entrapment by a foreign body. In children, the latter may be due to human hair wrapped around the penis.

Garty and colleagues[103] reported a 2½-year-old boy who had been circumcised and presented with discoloration and severe swelling of the penis of 6 weeks' duration. The child had had difficulties in voiding and cried while urinating. The swelling of the penis had been attributed to allergy and later to infection, and he was treated with various antihistamine drugs, antibiotics, and warm baths but without any improvement.

Physical examination showed constriction at the proximal part of the penis, whereas its distal part was swollen and erythematous. Several hairs buried under the epithelium caused the constriction and were removed using fine forceps and scissors. Questioning of the parents failed to reveal the circumstances under which the hair had become wrapped around the penis. Healing was complete within 15 days.

Entrapment of the penis by hair is an example of the tourniquet syndrome, which may also affect the fingers, toes, or clitoris.[104–106] Foreign bodies, such as thread, metal rings, rubber bands, and hair, are usually involved in this condition. The penis becomes swollen, and difficulties in urination might arise, but surprisingly, the pain may not be severe. When the entrapment is caused by hair, as in the case reported, it may be buried under the skin and covered with epithelium. This phenomenon is attributed to the stretchable quality of moist hair. In cases of swelling of the penis in children, careful inspection for buried objects, sometimes under mild sedation, is indicated. The hair may remain undetected for a long time, and a delay of several weeks in the diagnosis is not unusual. In some cases, late diagnosis can be associated with serious sequelae, such as partial or complete transection of the urethra, deformity of the penis, or amputation of the glans.[107,108] In other patients, recovery is without serious complications despite the delay. This is most likely due to the multiple blood supply of the penis and the slow progression of constriction, which allows the development of deep collateral circulation. Entrapment of the penis is usually accidental; however, the possibility of child abuse should be investigated because such cases have been reported to be caused by parents in attempts to prevent nocturnal enuresis.[109]

Buttocks

Prolonged contact with wet bathing suits may produce a follicular-type dermatitis on the buttocks. There is also that unpleasant experience for swimmers commonly referred to as "bikini bottom" and scientifically known as occlusive folliculitis. This condition, marked by the development of annoying wet blisters all over the buttocks, can be caused by wearing a swimsuit all day.

ROLE OF CONTACTANTS IN PRURITUS ANI AND PROCTITIS

In patients with pruritus ani or proctitis, a list of all medicaments the patient has used in the past should be made, and particular inquiry should be focused on the use of sensitizers, such as benzocaine, neomycin, and balsam of Peru. Patch tests with these topical remedies may help rule out a contact dermatitis superimposed on the original pruritus.

The presence of hemorrhoids or fissures should lead one to inquire about special treatments used and to determine whether such treatments produced contact dermatitis. If the patient is using medicated dressings for anal hygiene, such as Tucks, medicated rectal wipes, or Balneol, one must be certain these preparations do not contain agents to which the patient is sensitized. In such instances, the patient who prefers a cooling, drying agent may use witch hazel, whereas the patient who prefers an oily cleanser may use cold mineral oil.

Perfumed and colored toilet paper should be avoided because of the remote possibility that the dyes or essences in it may be sensitizers.

The ingestion of spices, food with seeds, antibiotics, or laxatives that cause a slow leakage of oil or paraffin products may cause anal itching.

Foreign bodies inserted into the rectum and rectal intercourse may produce anal irritation that may be made worse by the use of anesthetic medications containing benzocaine.

Legs

The most common cause of allergic contact dermatitis of the legs is application of sensitizing medications to stasis eczemas and ulcers (see also Chapter 16). A study of venous leg ulcer patients found that 68% reacted to patch tests performed with the European standard series, antimicrobials and medicaments. Multiple allergies were found in 102 of 200 patients tested. The sensitizers were fragrances in 30%, antimicrobials in 20%, vehicle ingredients in 20%, rubber accelerators in 13%, and topical corticosteroids in 8%.[110] Salim and Shaw have pointed out that the evaluation of leg ulcer patients may be incomplete if rosin is tested without the additional use of ester gum resin, as rosin alone would have missed 40% of leg ulcer patients who had relevant patch tests. Ester gum resin is tested at 25% in petrolatum.[111] Soccer shin guard dermatitis was investigated with extensive patch testing in 8 children ranging in age from 9 to 16. In all cases, the patch tests, which included pieces of the shin guards, proved negative. An irritant dermatitis due to sweat and friction was considered the correct diagnosis.[112]

Nails

CONTACTANTS PRODUCING ONYCHIA AND NAIL DISCOLORATION

Ronchese[113] stated that nails are more important than teeth or hair. Thinness, fragility, splitting, separation into layers, detachment from the nail bed, and long-standing infections are serious handicaps to jewelers, weavers, metal platers, and printers. Occupational chemicals and trauma are common causes of onychia, koilonychia, nail dystrophy, and discoloration of the nail (see Table 6.7).

OCCUPATIONAL KOILONYCHIA

Spoon-shaped deformity of the nails may be produced by organic solvents (thinners) in cabinetmakers and by motor oils.[114,115] Trauma can produce koilonychia of the toenails in barefoot rickshaw pullers.[116]

Occupationally induced nail changes, such as koilonychia, traumatic onycholysis in poultry pluckers, and broadening and shortening of the nail plate in association with acro-osteolysis in workers exposed to vinyl-chloride monomer indicate that nail abnormalities as manifestations of occupational injury are not uncommon.[117]

Food handlers may develop contact urticaria to food, such as garlic, tomato, eggplant, chicory, kiwi fruit, egg yolk, bean, wheat flour, onion, and figs. Nine of 20 food handlers with contact urticaria of the proximal nail fold had a chronic paronychia.[118]

ACUTE ONYCHOLYSIS FROM CHEMICALS

Hydrofluoric burns have an apparent predilection for subungual tissues.[119,120] Acute onycholysis can also occur from detergent enzymes.[121] Hair cosmetics, such as dicyandiamide (especially useful to restore split and thin hair), depilatories, and thioglycolates used by hairdressers for permanent waving may produce occupational onychia.

Trauma to the nails on the job accompanied by quaternium-15 sensitivity (but not formaldehyde) leads to onycholysis without proximal nail fold changes. The quaternium-15 exposure was to an industrial liquid soap, and the nails returned to normal in 4 months.[122]

"ATHLETIC" NAILS

Scher[123] reviewed the subject of the "athletic nail." Nail changes occurring either in professional athletes or in those who participate occasionally in weekend sports activities have not been described extensively. Ronchese[124] spoke of the "worn down" fingernails of the frequent bowler, and Pardo-Costello and Pardo[125] referred to wearing down of the nails of the third and fourth

Table 6-7 Variety of Nail Discolorations Produced by Topical Agents

Orange-Brown Nails	*Yellow Nails*
Anthralin	Amphotericin
Arning's tincture	Amphotericin B
Burnt sugar	Dinitro-orthocresol
Chromium salts	Dinubuton
Chrysarobin	Fluorescein
Dinitrotoluene	Hatter's chemicals
Dithranol	Hydrofluoric acid
Formaldehyde	*Gray-Blue Nails*
Glutaraldehyde	Ammoniated mercury
Henna	Mercuric chloride (plus sunshine)
Hydroquinone	*Purple Nails*
Iodohydroxyquinolene	Gentian violet
Iron	*Red Nails*
Mepacrine	Carbol-fuchsin paint
Nicotine	*Dark Blue Nails*
Paraquat	Oxalic aci
Pecans	Silver and cyanide (galvanizers)
Picric acid	*Black Nails*
Potassium permanganate	Photographic developers (phenol sulfate hydroquinone)
Pyrogallol	Red wine
Resorcin combined with nail lacquer	Silver nitrite
Rivano	*Green Nails*
Roasted coffee	Chlorophyll (prophylline)
Thermal injury	Copper salts
Vioform	
Walnuts	

fingers and black discoloration of the nails in riflemen and hunters. Samman[126] mentioned periodic shedding of the great toenails of football players as a result of repeated minor injuries even in the absence of hematoma. Schwartz and colleagues[127] alluded to traumatic injuries sustained by amateur fishermen from fish scales and hooks, as well as to paronychia secondary to frequent water contact. Nail changes also have been reported to be associated with tennis and jogging,[128–131] and splinter hemorrhages were reported in cricket players in England.[132]

Scher[123] attributed a case of leukonychia to karate. The mechanism of formation of the white nail bed is not well understood. DeNicola and colleagues,[133] however, attribute it to a temporary anemia of this site. Because this may result from both systemic and local causes, it is conceivable that the vigorous trauma of karate, secondary to a period of hypoxia, could produce the transverse whiteness of the nail bed observed in this patient.

SUBUNGUAL HEMATOMA (JOGGER'S TOE, TENNIS TOE, AND SOCCER TOE)

Subungual hematoma has many causes, both local and systemic.[134–136] This discussion focuses only on local traumatic factors that produce hemorrhage beneath the nail plate in specific types of athletes. Examples include tennis and soccer players as well as joggers. In all three, the toes hit persistently against the shoe and the ground. In the runner or jogger, the hitting is constant and tends to involve the fourth and fifth toes predominantly. On the other hand, the tennis player's intermittent stopping and going, with sudden short stops and sprints, tends to produce subungual hematoma mainly in the big toe. Finally, in the soccer player, who kicks the ball close to and somewhat distal to the instep area, the second and third digits tend to be the ones that blacken.

It must be stated, however, that variations of all these patterns occur, so that the toe involved is not a pathognomonic indication of the sport involved. Likewise, these changes seem to be more likely to occur in persons whose second toe is longer than the first—approximately 25% of the population. This configuration apparently increases the incidence of subungual hematoma of the great toe, although, in other cases, it also renders the second toe more susceptible.

In all of these cases, acral lentiginous melanoma must always be considered in the differential diagnosis. Therefore, it is incumbent on the physician to prove that the blackness is due to blood, not to melanin. This is usually a simple matter, but occasionally the diagnosis may be more difficult, requiring partial or complete avulsion or histologic examination by nail biopsy.[137]

Microbiologic studies are also required to rule out both fungal and bacterial causes. Therapy for these patients is difficult, although keeping the nails cut short and wearing better fitting shoes may be of some benefit.

REACTIONS TO "SCULPTURED" ACRYLATE NAILS

"Sculptured" artificial nails are a popular method of improving the cosmetic appearance of natural nails. They are made by mixing a liquid monomer with a powder polymer, then molding this acrylic compound onto the natural nail.

The first reported case of a severe reaction to acrylic "sculptured" nails described a dermatologist with a severe, disfiguring onychomycosis of all his fingernails in the days before griseofulvin was available.[138] In an attempt to improve the appearance of his nails, he applied a mixture of methyl methacrylate monomer and acrylic polymer and fashioned artificial nails. An excruciatingly painful onychia and paronychia of all his fingers developed, requiring strong opiates. The pain and discomfort persisted for several weeks.

The United States Food and Drug Administration received so many complaints of severe reactions to methyl methacrylate monomer from consumers that, after litigation, in 1974, the District Court in Chicago issued an injunction prohibiting the further manufacture or interstate shipment of a product called Long Nails, which contained a methyl methacrylate monomer.[139] In order to comply with this injunction, the manufacturers of artificial nail products are now using ethyl or isobutyl methacrylate monomers. One preliminary study seemed to indicate that these "newer" monomers did not cross-react with the methyl methacrylate. However, Marksand colleagues[140] have shown that cross-reactions definitely do occur among the various methacrylate monomers.

The newer reformulated artificial nail products seem likely to cause as many problems as the old methyl methacrylate–containing formulations. It has been shown both in animals and in humans that various acrylate monomers used in nail products are sensitizers that may crossreact.

Fisher[141] reported permanent loss of fingernails from sensitization and reactions to acrylic monomer in a preparation designed to make artificial nails. There was marked erythema, edema, and pain of the eponychial and paronychial tissues with persistent paresthesia of the fingertips. Gradual destruction of the nail plates developed, and, because no regrowth of the nails resumed in 10 years, the loss of the fingernails was permanent.

REACTIONS TO "NAIL HARDENERS" CONTAINING FORMALDEHYDE

Although formaldehyde is still used in Canada as a "nail hardener," it is rarely used in the United States for this purpose at present. The United States Food and Drug Administration received so many complaints of reactions from this chemical that such nail hardeners were mostly withdrawn from the market.

Ronchese[113] reported a case of onycholysis due to a nail hardener imported from Canada and correctly predicted that, "with tighter limitations on nail hardener production in the United States, this foreign production might be the only source of this agent in the future."

Although Mitchell's patient[142] suffered only a simple onycholysis without inflammation, other reports detail much more severe reactions from the formaldehyde component of "nail hardeners." Such reactions include subungual hemorrhages, discoloration of the nail plate, subungual hyperkeratosis, and even lip hemorrhages in nail biters.[143–146]

Some so-called nail hardeners now available in the United States may contain various types of "protein," collagen, nylon acetates, toluene, and nitrocellulose.

PREFORMED PLASTIC NAILS

Preformed plastic nails are made with completely cured plastic and do not cause allergic reactions. The adhesives used to allow adhesion of the plastic nails to the nail plate, however, may produce changes similar to those produced by "nail hardeners."

STICK-ON NAIL DRESSINGS ("PRESS-ON NAILS")

These nail dressings consist of thin, colored synthetic film with an adhesive that makes them adhere to the nail. Nail dressings, such as "press-on nails," may produce onycholysis, paronychia, and loss of the cuticle.

NAIL WRAPPING

The free edge of the nail is splinted with cotton, wool, or plastic film and fixed with nitrocellulose glues. After drying, the edge is shaped and the nail coated with enamel. Nail damage can occur if the entire nail is occluded.

CONTACT CHROMONYCHIA

Color changes in the nails may occur with or without inflammatory changes from exposure to certain contactants.

Discoloration and Nail Damage from Insecticides and Weed Killers

Weed killers and insecticides, paroquat, diquats, and dinitrocresol may produce nail damage that may be preceded by several weeks of a noninflammatory distinctive nail discoloration in which the proximal part of the nail plate becomes yellow or whitish.[147,148]

Several grades of severity of nail damage were recognized:

Grade 1. Localized discoloration of transverse band of white discoloration affecting nail plate only.
Grade 2. Transverse bands of white discoloration affecting two or more nails (the most common lesions).
Grade 3. Nail deformity of the nail surface; irregularity of surface; transverse ridging and furrowing.
Grade 4. Grossly irregular deformity of nail plate, loosening, or both and beginning onycholysis.
Grade 5. Loss of nail.

Chromonychia from Thermal Injury

Brodkin and Bleiberg described nail changes from exposure to heat from a microwave oven.[149]

Table 6.7 lists the various colors that local agents can produce on the nails. As a rule, the range of color changes in the nail is wider than the primary colors. For example, ochreous discoloration induced by the chromium salts is intermediate between yellow and brown.

Discoloration of the Nails from Nail Enamels and Nail Hardeners

Nail enamels are responsible for a yellow-brown discoloration of the nail plate surface. This discoloration does not seem to be due to the coloring agents of the enamel but to a pigment deposit that penetrates the nail plate. It does not disappear when the varnish is washed off by a solvent and gradually disappears while the nail is growing.

Nail hardeners may be responsible for a discoloration varying in color from yellow to red-blue and brown affecting the extremity of the nail, associated with small punctate subungual hemorrhages, subungual hyperkeratosis, and distal onycholysis. A formaldehyde component of the hardener might be particularly responsible.

Rycroft[150] described nail dystrophy and dermatitis of the nail fold with discoloration of the nails in a patient who became allergic to paratertiary butylphenol resin in an artificial nail adhesive used to affix artificial nails to the fingers.

Nail Staining Due to Hydroquinone

Mann and Harman[151] reported nail staining due to hydroquinone skin-lightening creams. They reported two cases of women in whom brown discoloration developed after the use of cosmetic skin-lightening creams containing hydroquinone and for actinic lentigines of the hands.

This seemingly paradoxical nail darkening from bleaching creams was reported by Arndt and Fitzpatrick[152] in three patients who had discolored fingernails following the use of 2% and 5% hydroquinone-containing creams in the treatment of vitiligo, chloasma, freckles, and post-inflammatory hyperpigmentation. Garcia and collagues[153] noted diffuse orange-brown nail staining after the use of Esoterica cream by several patients. These investigators suggested that the color change was due to the oxidation products of hydroquinone and that a similar color change could be seen on the surface of the cream after exposure to air.

Hydroquinone is readily oxidized to quinone, a yellow compound, and quinone subsequently undergoes oxidation to hydroxyquinone. The oxidation of quinone is a photosensitive reaction. Hydroxyquinone, another yellow compound, is unstable and polymerizes to products that are dark brown. This reaction is also photosensitive. These oxidation and polymerization products are also probably the cause of the brown pigmentation that affects the cornea and conjunctiva of workers involved in the manufacture of hydroquinone, in which quinone is an intermediate.154

Orange-Brown Iron Nail Pigmentation from Well Water

Olsen and Jatlow[155] reported that an orange-brown chromonychia developed on the toenails of a woman from exposure to rural well water. Samples of the water and qualitative and quantitative examination of nail clippings confirmed that the source of the discoloration was contact exposure to elemental iron. Installation of water purification equipment resulted in resolution of the nail stain over a 6-week period.

A positive Prussian blue stain following the traumatic removal of the patient's nails and the results of quantitative iron analysis of the various nail clippings confirmed the diagnosis. Although the Prussian blue iron stain cannot provide precise quantitative data, its ease of application and usage should be emphasized in clinical situations in which the clinician is looking for the presence of tissue iron.

Exogenous versus Endogenous Chromonychia

Zais[156] stressed that gross inspection of the nail plate sometimes permits the clinician to separate an exogenous from an endogenous source. Chromonychias, following the shape of the lunula, tend to be endogenous in origin,

whereas discolorations following the proximal nail fold indicate a contact environmental source. Ionizing radiation, however, may produce longitudinal red streaks beginning in the lunula.

Daniel and Osment[157] suggest that several important points concerning examination of abnormal nails are worthy of mention. One should study the nails with the fingers completely relaxed and not pressed against any surface. Failure to do so may alter nail hemodynamics and change the appearance of the nail. The observer should then blanch the fingertip to see if the pigmented abnormality is grossly altered. This may help differentiate discoloration of the nail plate from that of the nail vascular bed. In addition, one may illuminate the nail by placing a penlight against the finger pulp and shining it up through the nail. If the discoloration is in the vascular bed, it usually disappears. If it is in the matrix or soft tissue, the exact position can be more easily identified. Furthermore, if scraping the nail plate surface, local cleansing, or using a solvent (such as acetone) removes the discoloration, a topical agent is likely to be the cause. If the substance is impregnated more deeply into the nail or subungually, the use of potassium hydroxide preparations, nail composition studies, special stains, or examination of a biopsy specimen with a light microscope or possibly an electron microscope may be indicated.

References

1. Amin KA, Belsito DV. The aetiology of eyelid dermatitis: a 10-year retrospective analysis. Contact Dermatitis 2006;55:280.

2. Ayala F, Fabbrocini G, Bacchilega R, et al. Eyelid dermatitis: an evaluation of 447 patients. Am J Contact Dermat 2003;14:69.

3. Herbst RA, Uter W, Pirker C, et al. Allergic and non-allergic periorbital dermatitis: patch test results of the Information Network of the Departments of Dermatology during a 5-year period. Contact Dermatitis 2004;51:13.

4. Guin JD. Eyelid dermatitis: a report of 215 patients. Contact Dermatitis 2004;50:87.

5. Pascher F. Adverse reactions to eye area cosmetics and their management. J Soc Cosmet Chem 1982;33:249.

6. Mathias TCG, Maibach HI. Cutaneous irritation: factors influencing the response to irritants. Clin Toxicol 1978;13:333.

7. Mohajerin AH. Common cutaneous disorders of the eyelids. Cutis 1972;10:279.

8. Le Coz C-J, Leclere J-M, Arnoult E, et al. Allergic contact dermatitis from shellac in mascara. Contact Dermatitis 2002;46:149.

9. Gallo R, Marro I, Pavesi A. Allergic contact dermatitis from shellac in mascara. Contact Dermatitis 2005;53:238.

10. Sacena M, Warshaw E, Ahmed DDF. Eyelid allergic contact dermatitis to black iron oxide. Am J Contact Dermat 2001;12:38.

11. Fisher AA. The paraben paradoxes. Cutis 1973;12:830.

12. Jordan WP Jr, Sherman WI, King SE. Threshold responses in formaldehyde-sensitive subjects. Am Acad Dermatol 1979;1:44.

13. Fisher AA. Allergic contact dermatitis from germall-115: a new cosmetic preservative. Contact Dermatitis 1975;2:126.

14. Fisher AA. Cutaneous reactions to sorbic acid and potassium sorbate. Cutis 1980;25:350.

15. Cronin E. Di-isopropanolamine in an eyeshadow. Contact Dermatitis Newsletter 1973;13:364.

16. Calnan CD. Ditertiarybutyl hydroquinone in eyeshadow. Contact Dermatitis Newsletter 1973;13:368.

17. Fisher AA. Allergen replacements in allergic dermatitis. Int J Dermatol 1977;16:319.

18. Guin JD. Eyelid dermatitis from benzophenone used in nail enhancement. Contact Dermatitis 2000;43:308.

19. Moffitt DL, Sansom JE. Allergic contact dermatitis from phthalic anhydride/trimellitic anhydride/glycols copolymer in nail varnish. Contact Dermatitis 2002;46:236.

20. Dejobert Y, Delaporte E, Piette F, et al. Eyelid dermatitis with positive patch test to coconut diethanolamide. Contact Dermatitis 2005;52:173.

21. Zuckerman BD. Conjunctival pigmentation due to cosmetics. Am J Ophthalmol 1966;62:672.

22. Jervey JH. Mascara pigmentation of the conjunctiva. Arch Ophthalmol 1969;81:124.

23. Forman WG, McDowell RV, Shivers JA, Steele JR. Cosmetic eye shadow mimicking orbital calcification [Letter]. JAMA 1977;235:2695.

24. van Ketel WG, Melzer-van Riemskijk FA. Conjunctivitis due to soft lens solutions. Contact Dermatitis 1980;6:321.

25. Steele MC, Ive FA. Recurrent facial eczema in females due to "strike anywhere" matches. Br J Dermatol 1982;106:477.

26. Burge SM, Powell SM. Contact urticaria to phosphorus sesquisulphide. Contact Dermatitis 1984;10:424.

27. Ive FA. Studies in Contact Dermatitis XXI: matches. Trans St Johns Hosp Dermatol Soc 1967;53:135.

28. Calnan CD. Quinazoline yellow SS in cosmetics. Contact Dermatitis 1975;2:160.

29. Mancuso G, Berdondini RM. Eyelid dermatitis and conjunctivitis as sole manifestations of allergy to nickel in an orthodontic appliance. Contact Dermatitis 2002;46: 245.

30. De Groot AC, Poelhuis JWK. Ectropion caused by periocular dermatitis. J Am Acad Dermatol 2001;44:385.

31. Bhat J, Smith AG. Xanthelasma palpebrarum following allergic contact dermatitis from para-phenylenediamine in a black eyelash-tinting product. Contact Dermatitis 2004;49:311.

32. Brasch J, Bruning H, Paulke E. Allergic contact dermatitis from chironomids. Contact Dermatitis 1992;26:317.

33. Fisher AA. Cosmetic actions and reactions: therapeutic, irritant and allergic. Cutis 1980;26:22.

34. Dominey A, Dominey A, Tschen J, Rosen T et al. Pityriasis folliculorum revisited. J Am Acad Dermatol 1989;21:81.

35. Frosch PJ, Kligman AM. A method for appraising the stinging capacity of topically applied substances. J Soc Cosmet Chem 1977;28:197.

36. Calnan CD. Stinging sensation from ethoxyethylmethoxy cinnamate. Contact Dermatitis 1978;4:294.

37. Lahti A. Skin reactions to some antimicrobial agents. Contact Dermatitis 1978;4:302.

38. Lahti A, Lahti A, Oikarinen A, et al. Prostaglandins in contact urticaria induced by benzoic acid. Acta Derm Venereol (Stockh) 1983;63:425.

39. Lahti A, Vaananen A, Kokkonen EL, Hannuksela M. Acetylsalicylic acid inhibits non-immunologic contact urticaria. Contact Dermatitis 1987;16:133.

40. Goldenberg RL, Safrin L. Reduction of topical irritation. J Soc Cosmet Chem 1977;28:667.

41. Sugai T, Takahashi Y, Takagi T. Pigmented cosmetic dermatitis and coal tar dyes. Contact Dermatitis 1977;3:249.

42. Nakavama H, Hanaoka H, Ohshiro A. Allergen controlled system (ACS). Tokyo: Kanehara Shuppan Co., 1974.

43. Rorsman H. Riehl's melanosis. Int J Dermatol 1982;21:75.

44. Kozuka T, et al. Brilliant Lake Red R as a cause of pigmented contact dermatitis. Contact Dermatitis 1979;5:297.

45. Kozuka T, Kozuka T, Tashiro M, Sano S. Pigmented contact dermatitis from azo dyes. Contact Dermatitis 1980;6:330.

46. Maibach HI. Scuba diver facial dermatitis: allergic contact dermatitis to N-isopropyl-N-phenylparaphenylenediamine. Contact Dermatitis 1975;1:330.

47. Furman D, Fisher AA, Leider M. Allergic eczematous contact-type dermatitis caused by rubber sponges used for the application of cosmetics. J Invest Dermatol 1950;15:223.

48. Curtis GH. Contact dermatitis of eyelids caused by an anti-oxidant in rubber fillers of eyelash curlers. Arch Dermatol 1945;52:262.

49. Gaul LE. Results of patch testing with rubber antioxidants and accelerators. J Invest Dermatol 1957;29:105.

50. Sauer GC. Flubber dermatitis. Arch Dermatol 1965;91:465.

51. Tani A, Miyoshi H , Kanzaki T. Allergic contact dermatitis due to beclometasone dipropionate in an inhalant for asthma. Contact Dermatitis. 2000;43:363.

52. McDonald CJ. Special requirements in cosmetics for people with black skin. In: Frost P, Horwitz SN, eds. Principles of cosmetics for the dermatologist. St. Louis: Mosby, 1982:302.

53. Sperling LC, Sau P. The follicular degeneration syndrome in black patients. "Hot comb alopecia" revisited and revised. Arch Dermatol 1992;128:68.

54. Bandmann HJ, Speer U. Red hair after application of chinoform. Contact Dermatitis 1984;10:113.

55. Mathur AK, Srivastava AK, Singh A, Gupta BN. Contact depigmentation by adhesive material of bindi. Contact Dermatitis 1991;24:310.

56. Bajaj AK, Gupta SC, Chatterjee AK. Contact depigmentation from free paratertiary-butylphenol in bindi adhesive. Contact Dermatitis 1990;22:99.

57. Fisher AA. Contact otitis: a dermatitis of the external ear and canal. Cutis 1975;15:311.

58. Jones EH. Allergy of the external ear canal. In: Allergy in otorhinolaryngology. Philadelphia: WB Saunders, 1974:735.

59. Fisher AA. Unique features of nail polish sensitization. Cutis 1974;14:327.

60. Arnold HK. In: Ronchese F, ed. Occupational marks and other physical signs. New York: Grune & Stratton, 1948:116.

61. Millard TP, Orton DI. Changing patterns of contact allergy in chronic inflammatory ear disease. Contact Dermatitis 2004;50:83.

62. Gaul LE. Development of allergic nickel dermatitis from earrings. JAMA 1967;200:176.

63. Johnson CJ, Anderson H, Spearman J, Madson J. Clinical notes; ear piercing and hepatitis: nonsterile instruments for ear piercing and the subsequent onset of viral hepatitis. JAMA 1974;227:1165.

64. Munro-Ashman D, MacDonald A, Feiwel M. Split ear lobe syndrome. Contact Dermatitis 1975;1:393.

65. Ayala F. Granuloma fissurato dell'orecchio associato a dermatite da contatto dan nichel. Giornale Italiano Dermatol Minerva Dermatol 1976;111:581.

66. Shore RN, Berger BJ. Earring dermatitis sparing the ears. Arch Dermatol 1974;109:95.

67. Jirasek L, Kobikova M, Jiraskova M. Retroauricular eczema caused by the nickel of celluloid-rimmed spectacles. Cesk Dermatol 1976;51:369.

68. Barnes HM, Calnan CD, Sarkany I. Spectacle frame acanthoma (granuloma fissuratum). Trans St John's Hosp Dermatol Soc 1974;60:99.

69. Jensen CO, Allen HJ, Mordecai LR. Neomycin contact dermatitis superimposed on otitis externa. JAMA 1966;195:175.

70. McKelvie M, McKelvie P. Some aetiological factors in otitis externa. Br J Dermatol 1966;78:227.

71. Guill MA, Odom RB. Hearing aid dermatitis. Arch Dermatol 1978;114:1050.

72. Jordan WP, Dahl MV. Contact dermatitis from cellulose ester plastics. Arch Dermatol 1972;105:880.

73. Tanita Y, Tagami H. Pericervical granuloma in a child due to constricting rubber bands [Letter]. Arch Dermatol 1984;120:709.

74. Lachapelle JM, Tennstedt D, Cromphaut P. Pseudofolliculitis of the beard and "Fiddler's Neck." Contact Dermatitis 1984;10:247.

75. McGeorge BCL, Steele MC. Allergic contact dermatitis of the nipple from Roman chamomile ointment. Contact Dermatitis 1991;24:139.

76. Dou X, Liu L-L, Zhu X-J. Nickel-elicited systemic contact dermatitis. Contact Dermatitis 20003;48:126.

77. McCallum DI, Hall GFM. Umbilical granulomata with particular reference to talc granuloma. Br J Dermatol 1970;83:151.

78. Ehring F. The umbilical stone. Hautarzt 1979;30:494.

79. Suchak R, Lawlor F. Water-induced palmar tingling and swelling. Clin Exp Dermatol 2006;32:119.

80. Gomez-Orbaneja J, Inglesias Diez L, Sanchez Lozano JL, Conde Salazar L. Lymphatoid contact dermatitis. Contact Dermatitis 1976;2:139.

81. Fisher AA. Vulvitis due to contactants. Cutis 1974;13:725.

82. Nardelli A, Degreef H, Goossens A. Contact allergic reactions of the vulva: a 14-year review. Dermatitis 2004;15:131.

83. Britz MB, Maibach HI. Human cutaneous vulvar reactivity to irritants. Contact Dermatitis 1979;5:375.

84. Fisher AA. Allergic reaction to feminine hygiene sprays. Arch Dermatol 1973;108:801.

85. Fisher AA, Fisher AA, Pascher F, Kanof NB. Allergic contact dermatitis due to ingredients of vehicles. Arch Dermatol 1971;104:286.

86. Fisher AA, Stillman MA. Allergic contact sensitivity to benzalkonium chloride. Arch Dermatol 1972;106:169.

87. Shmunes E, Levy EJ. Quaternary ammonium compound contact dermatitis from a deodorant. Arch Dermatol 1972;105:91.

88. Ljunggren B, Moller H. Eczematous contact allergy to chlorhexidine. Acta Derm Venereol (Stockh) 1972;52:308.

89. Kaye BM. Hazards of feminine hygiene sprays for women. JAMA 1970;212:2121.

90. Davis BA. Irritancy from feminine hygiene sprays. Obstet Gynecol 1970;36:812.

91. Gowdy JM. Feminine deodorant sprays. N Engl J Med 1972;287:203.

92. Lewis FM, Harrington CI, Gawkrodger DJ. Contact sensitivity in pruritus vulvae: a common and manageable problem. Contact Dermatitis 1994;31:264.

93. Lewis FM, Shah M, Gawkrodger DJ. Contact sensitivity in pruritus vulvae: patch test results and clinical outcome. Am J Contact Dermat 1997;8:137.

94. Petersen CS. Lack of contact allergy in consecutive women with vulvodynia. Contact Dermatitis 1997;37:46.

95. Nunns D, Ferguson J, Beck M, Mandal D. Is patch testing necessary in vulval vestibulitis? Contact Dermatitis 1997;37:87.

96. Goldsmith PC, Rycroft RJ, White IR, et al. Contact sensitivity in women with anogenital dermatoses. Contact Dermatitis 1997;36:174.97.

97. Nedorost ST. Cutaneous hypersensitivity to Candida albicans in idiopathic vulvodynia. Contact Dermatitis 2005;53:214.

98. Virgili A, Corazza M, Bacilieri S, Califano A. Contact sensitivity in vulval lichen simplex chronicus. Contact Dermatitis 1997;37:296.

99. Lucke TW, Fleming CJ, McHenry P, Lever R. Patch testing in vulval dermatoses: how relevant is nickel? Contact Dermatitis 1998;38:111.

100. Fisher AA. The new female and male polyurethane condoms. Cutis 1995;56:82.

101. Bounds W. Female condoms. Eur J Contracept Reprod Health Care 1997;2:113.

102. Lucke TW, Fleming CJ, McHenry P. Clothing dye dermatitis of the scrotum. Contact Dermatitis 1998;38:224.

103. Garty BZ, Mimouni M, Varsano I. Penile tourniquet syndrome. Cutis 1983;31:431.

104. Alpert J, Filler RJ, Glaser H. Strangulation of an appendage by hair wrapping. N Engl J Med 1965;273:866.

105. Quinn N. Toe tourniquet syndrome. Pediatrics 1971;48:145.

106. Press S, Schachner L, Paul P. Clitoris tourniquet syndrome. Pediatrics 1980;66:781.

107. Thomas A, Timmons J, Perlmutter A. Progressive penile amputation: tourniquet injury secondary to hair. Urology 1977;9:42.

108. Farah R, Cerny J. Penis tourniquet syndrome and penile amputation. Urology 1973;2:310.

109. Kerry R, Chapman DD. Strangulation of appendages by hair and thread. J Pediatr Surg 1973;8:23.

110. Tavadia S, Bianchi J, Dawe RS, et al. Allergic contact dermatitis in venous leg ulcer patients. Contact Dermatitis 2003;48:261.

111. Salim A, Shaw S. Recommendation to include ester gum resin when patch testing patients with leg ulcers. Contact Dermatitis 2001;44:34.

112. Weston WL, Morelli JG. Dermatitis under soccer shin guards: allergy or contact irritant reaction? Pediatr Dermatol 2006;23:19.

113. Ronchese F. Occupational nails. Cutis 1965;5:164.

114. Ancona-Alayon A. Occupational koilonychia from organic solvents. Contact Dermatitis 1975;1:367.

115. Dawber R. Occupational koilonychia. Br J Dermatol 1974;91:10.

116. Bentley-Phillips B, Bayles AH. Occupational koilonychia of the toe nails. Br J Dermatol 1971;85:140.

117. Moulin G, et al. Aspects sclerodermiques de l'acro-osteolyse professionnelle (polymerisation du chlorure de vinyle). Ann Dermatol Syphil 1974;101:33.

118. Tosti A, Guerra L., Morelli R, et al. Role of foods in the pathogenesis of chronic paronychia. J Am Acad Dermatol 1992;27:706.

119. Shewmaker W, Anderson BG. Hydrofluoric acid burns: a report of a case and review of the literature. Arch Dermatol 1979;115:593.

120. Baran R. Acute onycholysis from rust-removing agents. Arch Dermatol 1980;116:382.

121. Hodgson G, Mayon-White RT. Acute onychia and onycholysis due to an enzyme detergent. Br Med J 1971;3:352.

122. Marren P, de Berker D, Dawber RPR, Powell S. Occupational contact dermatitis to quaternium 15 presenting as nail dystrophy. Contact Dermatitis 1991;25:253.

123. Scher RK. The athletic nail. Dermatology 1981;21:49.

124. Ronchese F. Occupational marks and other physical signs. New York: Grune & Stratton, 1948.

125. Pardo-Costello V, Pardo OA. Diseases of the nails. Springfield, IL: Charles C Thomas Publisher, 1960.

126. Samman PD. The nails in disease. London: Heinemann Medical Books, 1978.

127. Schwartz L, Tulipan L, Birmingham DJ. Occupational diseases of the skin. Philadelphia: Lea & Febiger, 1957.

128. Gibbs RC. Tennis toe. Arch Dermatol 1973;107:918.

129. Gibbs RC. Skin diseases of the feet. St. Louis: Warren H. Green, 1974.

130. Scher RK. Jogger's toe. Int J Dermatol 1978;17:719.

131. Yaffee HS. Jogging some more. Int J Dermatol 1979;18:319.

132. Monk BE. The prevalence of splinter hemorrhages. Br J Dermatol 1980;103:183.

133. DiNicola P, Morisiani M, Zavagli G. Nail diseases in internal medicine. Springfield, IL: Charles C Thomas Publisher, 1974.

134. Levine N. Dermatologic aspects of sports medicine. J Am Acad Dermatol 1980;3:415.

135. Shuster RO. Foot types and the influence of environment on the foot of long distance runners. Ann NY Acad Sci 1977;301:881.

136. Resnick SS, Lewis LA, Cohen BH. The athlete's foot. Cutis 1977;10:351.

137. Scher RK. Punch biopsy of nails: simple, valuable procedure. J Dermatol Surg Oncol 1978;4:528.

138. Fisher AA, Frank A, Glicks H. Allergic sensitization of the skin and nails to acrylic plastic nails. J Allergy 1957; 28:84.

139. UC v CEB Products, Inc., 380 F. Suppl. 664 (N.D. Ill., 1974).

140. Marks JF Jr, Bishop ME, Willis WP. Allergic contact dermatitis to sculptured nails. Arch Dermatol 1979;215:100.

141. Fisher AA. Permanent loss of finger nails from sensitization and reaction to acrylic in a preparation designed to make artificial nails. J Dermatol Surg Oncol 1980;6:70.

142. Mitchell JC. Non-inflammatory onycholysis from formaldehyde-containing nail hardener. Contact Dermatitis 1981;7:173.

143. Danto JL. Allergic contact dermatitis due to a formaldehyde finger nail hardener. Can Med Assoc J 1968;98:652.

144. Lazar P. Reactions to nail hardeners. Arch Dermatol 1966;94:446.

145. Donsky HJ. Onycholysis due to nail hardener. Can Med Assoc J 1967;96:1375.

146. March CH. Allergic contact dermatitis to a new formula to strengthen nails. Arch Dermatol 1966;93:270.

147. Baran RL. Nail damage caused by weed killers and insecticides. Arch Dermatol 1974;110:467.

148. Hearn CED, Keir W. Nail damage in spray operators exposed to paraquat. Br J Ind Med 1971;28:399.

149. Brodkin RH, Bleiberg R. Microwave injury to the nails. Acta Dermatol Venereol 1973;53:50.

150. Rycroft RJG. Contact sensitization to p-tertiary butylphenol (PTBP) resin in artificial nail adhesive. Paper presented at the Fifth International Symposium on Contact Dermatitis, Barcelona, Spain, March 1980.

151. Mann RI, Harman RRM. Nail staining due to hydroquinone skin-lightening creams. Br J Dermatol 1983;108:363.

152. Arndt KK, Fitzpatrick TB. Topical use of hydroquinone as a depigmenting agent. JAMA 1965;194:965.

153. Garcia RK, White JW, Willis WF. Hydroquinone nail pigmentation. Arch Dermatol 1978;114:1402.

154. Sterner JH, Oglesby FL, Anderson B. Quinone vapours and their harmful effects. J Ind Hygiene Toxicol 1947;29:60.

155. Olsen TG, Jatlow P. Contact exposure to elemental iron causing chromonychia. Arch Dermatol 1984;120:102.

156. Zais N. The nail in health and diseases. 1st ed. New York: Spectrum Publications, 1980;19:188.

157. Daniel CR, Osment LS. Nail pigmentation abnormalities. Cutis 1980;25:595.

NONECZEMATOUS CONTACT DERMATITIS

EXECUTIVE SUMMARY

Erythema multiforme has resulted from contact with plants, laboratory chemicals, many medications, and miscellaneous compounds. Purpuric contact dermatitis can occur from clothing, rubber, wool, and topical fepradinol hydrochloride. Pigmented eruptions have followed contact with optical brighteners, azo dyes, fragrances, bactericides, and paratertiary butylphenol formaldehyde resin.

Lichenoid reactions associated with contactants include lichen planus most commonly from paraphenylenediamine-related chemicals, oral lichen planus from various dental metals, and chronic *Primula* exposure. Lichenoid tissue reactions from contactants include lichen simplex chronicus and subacute cutaneous lupus erythematosus.

Acneiform eruptions and chloracne may follow the use of pomade and halogenated hydrocarbons, respectively. Granulomatous reaction may occur from use of potent corticosteroids on the skin of infants. Granulomas are also associated with cutaneous exposure to zirconium, talc, beryllium, aluminum, and silica.

Unusual patterns of contact dermatitis have included prurigo nodularis, erythema dyschromicum perstans, granuloma annulare, erythema annulare centrifugum, and acute generalized exanthematous pustulosis.

Irritant or allergic contact dermatitis usually begins as an eczematous process characterized by itching, redness, edema, and a tendency toward oozing and crusting (Figure 7-1). Occasionally, however, it may be noneczematous with urticarial, granulomatous, acneiform, lichen planus–like, or dry, hyperkeratotic lesions (Figure 7-2). In addition, erythema multiforme and purpuric eruptions may result from exposure to contact allergens. Pigmented contact dermatitis resembling Riehl's melanosis and the actinic reticuloid syndrome may occur. Contact dermatitis may be complicated by lymphangitis and persistent edema. Various types of acneiform eruptions owing to contactants are discussed here and in Chapter 25 (Figure 7-3).

Erythema Multiforme–Like Eruptions from Contact Allergens

Various exotic tropical woods and certain chemicals can produce erythema multiforme–like eruptions (Table 7.1).

TROPICAL WOODS

Holst and colleagues[1] described three carpenters who, after working for a short time with tropical woods, Rio rose-wood (*Dalbergia nigra*), pao ferro (*Mackerium scleroxylon*), and eucalyptus saligna, developed erythema multiforme–like eruptions. The antigen of pao ferro (the ironwood tree of Brazil) is R-3,4-dimethoxy-dalbergione, and the antigen of Rio rosewood is R-4-methoxy-dalbergione. They are both quinones and are closely related.

Fisher and Bikowski[2] reported a male who had an erythema multiforme eruption from an allergic reaction on the neck and presternal area from a wooden cross. A patch test with the cross was strongly positive after 48 hours. A patch test with sawdust from the cross showed a marked reaction within 6 hours. Both reactions were eczematous.

The wood in the cross was identified as *Dalbergia nigra* by the Center of Wood Anatomy Research (U.S. Forest Products Laboratory, Madison, WI). A search of the available literature revealed that all previous reports of allergic contact dermatitis from *Dalbergia nigra* have been concerned with occupational exposures in carpenters, foresters, and cabinetmakers. This is apparently the first report of "nonoccupational" dermatitis from *Dalbergia*.

Martin and colleagues[3] reported a case of erythema multiforme–like eruption from Brazilian rosewood in a 35-year-old carpenter who initially developed rhinitis

Table 7-1 Contact Allergens Producing Erythema Multiforme

Tropical Woods Plants	Ketoprofen
Capsicum	Lamotrigene
Inula helenium	Lincomycin
Poison ivy	Mafenide acetate
Primula	Mephenesin
Pyrethrum	Mephenesin (Europe)
St. John's wort (*Hypericum erectum*)	Mofebutazone
Terpenes	Neomycin
Thuja essential oil	Phenylbutazone
Common chickweed	Povidone-iodine solution
Dandelion	Proflavin
Field milk thistle	Promethazine
White clover	Pyrrolnitrin
Costus resinoid	Scopolamine
Laboratory Chemicals	Sulfonamides
Brominated compounds	Tetrazepam
Dinitrochlorobenzene	Triamcinolone acetonide
Diphenylcyclopropenone	Tribenoside
N-hydroxyphthalamide	Vitamin E
Phenyl sulfone derivatives	*Miscellaneous Compounds*
1,2-ethanedithiol	Disperse blue 124
Medications	Epoxy resin
Budesonide	Formaldehyde
Bufexamac	Hair dyes
Chloramphenicol	Oxybenzone
Econazole	Paratertiary butylphenol formaldehyde resin
Ethylenediamine	Soap
Idoxuridine	Spray cologne
Iodochlorhydroxyquin (Vioform)	Trichloroethylene

and conjunctivitis. This eruption was succeeded by a generalized erythema multiforme–like eruption. A patch test with the wood dust produced a strong positive eczematous reaction, as did R- and S-methoxy-dalbergione. Table 7.2 lists some common names for *Dalbergia nigra*.

With regard to plants other than tropical woods, Hjorth[4] reported an erythema multiforme eruption from an allergic reaction to primula. Other plants and plant substances, such as *Artemesia*,[5,6] poison ivy,[7] and terpenes, can produce such eruptions.[8] The initial dermatitis may resemble a traditional eczematous morphologic pattern with a subsequent distant, noncontacted area demonstrating erythema multiforme morphologic patterns. This was the case with a patient who applied an

Table 7-2 Common Names for *Dalbergia nigra*

Bahia rosewood

Brazilian rosewood

Caviuana

Jacaranda (pardo)

Palissandre bresic

Rio rosewood

aqueous solution of Saint John's wort to treat a buttocks eczema only to subsequently develop distant erythema multiforme.[9] The allergen was Hypercin from the *Hypericum erectum* (Thunb).

Other plants or plant materials have caused contact dermatitis that evolved into erythema multiforme. A homemade dressing using tincture of capsicum caused an erythema multiforme–like eruption in a 65-year-old woman who applied this to her knee for arthritis.[10] Application of an "herbal bag" to the chest as a folk treatment for back pain led to eczema followed by an erythema multiforme–like eruption 2 weeks later.[11] The *Inula helenium* present in the bag was found responsible, and both sesquiterpene lactone mix and alantolactone were positive. Application of Thuja essential oil for hemorrhoids was followed by an erythema multiforme–like reaction.[12] Thuja oil is a distillate of *Thuja occidentalis* and contains fenchone, thujic acid, pinene, pinipicrine, borneol esters, and tannins. A patient with a 13-year history of episodes of erythema multiforme following home gardening and exposure to weeds was eventually patch tested. She had eczematous patch test reactions to common chickweed (*Stellaria media*), dandelion (*Taraxacum officinale*), field-milk thistle

(*Sonchus arvensis*) and white clover (*Trifolium repens*). By day 4 of the patch test procedure, erythema multiforme developed and was believed to be due to the patch test procedure. Other allergens that have been incriminated in producing erythema multiforme when patch tested include 9-bromofluorene, nickel sulfate, colophonium, and fragrance mix.[13]

HALOGENATED AND MISCELLANEOUS CHEMICAL COMPOUNDS

DeFeo[14] as well as Powell and colleagues[15] reported that chemists exposed to dimethyl allyl bromide and other brominated compounds, particularly 9-bromofluorene, acquired an erythema multiforme–type reaction. Roed-Petersen[16] stated that a 22-year-old male chemistry student's eruption started when he had to synthesize a new phenylsulfone derivative compound in the laboratory. Fregert and colleagues[17] reported that N-hydroxyphthalimide produced an erythema multiforme by contact. When 7.5% Povidone-iodine aqueous solution was applied to an operative wound, a dermatitis at the application site was followed by a distant erythema multiforme.[9] Similarly, a 2% dinitrochlorobenzene (DNCB) solution applied to the entire scalp for 4 days to treat alpaca areata produced an erythema multiforme reaction pattern on the back, arms, and hands. A patch test of 0.1% DNCB in acetone produced an eczematous response; 0.01% was negative.[18]

Magnusson and Gilje[19] stated that alkyl ether sulfates contaminated dishwashing detergents, and Bjornberg and Mobacken[20] found that benzene compounds can produce erythema multiforme–like contact dermatitis.

Nethercott and colleagues[21] reported that four men manufacturing printed circuit boards were exposed to palladium chloride, copper sulfate, formaldehyde, epoxy fiberglass, lead trichloroethylene, and ammonium persulfate. They developed erythema multiforme major after 6 to 12 weeks of exposure. Liver involvement was documented in three cases. On the basis of positive patch tests in two of the four workers, formaldehyde was presumed to cause the reactions.

Phoon and colleagues[22] reported five cases of Stevens-Johnson syndrome (erythema multiforme major) owing to exposure to trichloroethylene. All of these patients had liver involvement.

Vincenzi and colleagues[23] add to the list of erythema multiforme–causing agents disperse blue 124, hair dyes, and paratertiary butylphenol formaldehyde resin.

Oxybenzone produced an erythema multiforme–like eruption 1 week after the initial photoallergic contact dermatitis in a 44-year-old woman from Japan.[24] Photo-patch tests showed oxybenzone to be the sunscreen ingredient responsible.

A pyrethrum insecticide caused an airborne erythema multiforme–like eruption in a Spanish farmer detected by a 2% pyrethrum in petrolatum patch test.[25] No cross reactivity to lichens or sesquiterpene lactones was found.

The following contactants have been implicated as the cause of contact erythema multiforme: insecticides,[26] spray colognes,[27] metals,[28,29] and soaps.[30] Erythema multiforme–like dermatitis developed in a chemistry student exposed to costus resinoid. Upon re-exposure some months later to vapors of beta-cyclocostunolide, she experienced an erythematous and edematous dermatitis in areas previously involved in the erythema multiforme pattern. Patch tests were positive with sesquiterpene lactone mix 0.1% and 0.1% beta-cyclocostunolide. The flare-up on exposure to the vapors presented as an incomplete baboon syndrome.[31] Another chemistry student was exposed to 1,2-ethanedithiol and after limited skin contact, developed widespread erythema multiforme-like lesions. The histology was compatible with erythema multiforme and the patch test was positive.[32]

MEDICATIONS

Degreef and colleagues[33] described five patients (all using a mephenesin-containing ointment) who had acute contact dermatitis with an idlike spread and features resembling erythema multiforme. Patch tests were performed in four patients, and because mephenesin was the common allergen in each case, the investigators assumed this allergen was also the cause of the erythema multiforme–like lesions.

In Europe, mephenesin is taken orally as a muscle relaxant and is applied locally. It is used primarily by young people after injuries from sports. With local application, a vasodilating agent (methyl nicotinate and glycol salicylate) is usually added to promote skin penetration. This agent can cause hyperemia and sometimes even purpura. The increased permeability of the skin seems to contribute to sensitization to other materials (e.g., rubber in elastic bandages, dyes, and shoe materials) and promotes an idlike spread that can take on the aspect of exudative erythema multiforme.

Meneghini and Angelini[34,35] reported that the following topical medications produced erythema multiforme: ethylenediamine, neomycin, promethazine, iodochlorhydroxyquin (Vioform), and pyrrolnitrin. Other topical medications that have produced contact erythema multiforme include mafenide acetate,[36] scopolamine,[37] and sulfonamides.[38,39]

Saperstein and colleagues[40] stated that topical use of vitamin E on scar tissue resulted in a generalized erythema multiforme reaction in two patients. Patch tests with vitamin E oil showed positive local reactions in both patients.

Topical use of a phenylbutazone-containing cream caused an erythema multiforme–like eruption, which was patch test positive to 2% phenylbutazone in petrolatum.[41] No reaction was seen with oxyphenbutazone at 5% in petrolatum.

An erythema multiforme–like eruption may follow localized allergic contact dermatitis to bufexamac. This nonsteroidal anti-inflammatory drug (NSAID) has been used to treat a variety of disorders, including atopic dermatitis and localized leg lesions and ulcers. No epidermal necrosis was seen in four cases, as might be expected in true erythema multiforme.[42]

Mofebutazone is closely related to phenylbutazone. Its use topically and then orally resulted in a severe drug eruption.[43] This was documented by positive prick and patch tests to mofebutazone. This agent is used to treat thrombophlebitis in Germany and is known under the trade name Vasotonin.

More widespread erythema multiforme–like lesions in two cases reported from Italy followed use of topical budesonide to treat contact dermatitis.[44] In one case the administration of oral triamcinolone was thought to have caused extension of the eruption.

Intra-articular injection of triamcinolone acetonide was followed by an erythema multiforme–like eruption, which was treated with budesonide with acute worsening.[45] Resolution was achieved with 3% boric acid dressings. The only corticosteroids positive on patch testing were triamcinolone acetonide 1% in petrolatum and budesonide 1% in petrolatum. Tribenoside is an anti-hemorrhoidal sold in more than 20 countries and can be taken orally or in suppository forms. Erythema multiforme was reported after oral ingestion and patch tests with 1% and 10% in petrolatum were positive. Tribenoside is excreted as benzoic acid and this has been suggested as the antigenic determinant.[46] Cutaneous reactions to the anticonvulsant, lamotrigine, can be serious and include Stevens Johnson syndrome, a syndrome of generalized dermatitis, adenopathy, hepatitis, eosinophilia, and exfoliative dermatitis. Patch tests at 10% lamotrigine in petrolatum may detect the sensitivity as was reported by Monzon and colleagues.[47] Erythema multiforme and Steven-Johnson syndrome were caused by tetrazepam in two patients and two other patients experienced morbilliform eruptions. All four patients reacted to 10% tetrazepam in petrolatum on patch testing and 3 of the patients who agreed to oral challenge were confirmed to be sensitive. No crossreactions were found to diazepam by either patch testing or oral challenge.[48]

It appears that erythema multiforme–like reactions are not allergen specific but rather a biological response to delayed-type hypersensitivity to topical agents. Erythema multiforme is commonly seen as a sequela of herpes simplex infections.

In an effort to understand the difference between erythema multiforme from herpes simplex virus and contactants, a study was undertaken of cytokine expression in three cases of the former and two cases of the latter.[49] Epidermal expression of intercellular adhesive molecule (ICAM-1) was more prominent in the erythema multiforme–like contact dermatitis, and a greater percentage of cells in the inflammatory infiltrate was CD4+. There was a lower percentage of CD69+ cells in the cases caused by contactants.

Purpuric Contact Dermatitis

Purpura in patients with normal blood counts may be from various textile fabrics, rubber and antioxidants, other chemicals, or pressure (Figure 7-4). Some physicians recommend rubbing cocoa butter into scars to produce an improved cosmetic outcome; this concept is also endorsed in some folklore. The solid blocks of cocoa butter rubbed over lower-leg scars can produce a pressure-induced, nonallergic purpuric eruption (Figure 7-5).

CLOTHING PURPURA

Petechial and purpuric eruptions from woolen garments have been described.[50] So-called pigmented purpuric eruptions of the lower extremities, including Schamberg disease, often occur in areas exposed to woolen underwear, but the role of these garments is unclear (Figure 25*).

In addition, a water-soluble formaldehyde urea finish applied to woolen khaki shirts worn by British soldiers has been implicated as the cause of a purpuric eruption. The sedatives apronalide (Sedormid) and carbromal, both of which are capable of producing purpuric dermatitis medicamentosa, are also urea compounds.[51]

Contact with fiberglass may produce purpura, telangiectasia, folliculitis, urticaria, and linear erosions in the skin creases. Clothing washed with fiberglass curtains may become contaminated with the particles and produce a purpuric contact dermatitis in the wearer.[52]

Osmundsen[53] described a dermatitis of epidemic proportions that appeared in Europe from an optical whitener in washing powders. The eruption, a reticulate pattern of faint red-brown spots with a few petechiae and dilated small vessels, may suggest a reticulosis.

Flexural areas treated with clioquinol (Vioform) may develop a distinctive reticulated red-purple eruption with little scale. Patch tests in such cases are negative, and it is felt that this is an irritant contact dermatitis.[54]

PANTS PRESSURE PURPURA

Petrozzi and Lockshin[55] stated that mechanical trauma may produce purpuric eruptions in young patients.

Explanation of the problem occurred only after the patient disclosed he had slept overnight in a pair of tight-fitting dungarees. The instructive element in this case was the degree of trauma necessary to produce the purpura. It could not be reproduced under an inflated blood pressure cuff, nor did the number of petechiae distal to the cuff increase.

RUBBER PURPURA

Rubber or elasticized underwear may produce an allergic contact eczematous dermatitis associated with a secondary eruption resembling lichenoid pigmented dermatitis, eczematoid purpura, or a variant of pigmented purpuric dermatitis.[55]

Calnan and Peachey[56] reported that isopropylaminodiphenylamine, an antioxidant used in the manufacture of some types of rubber, can cause an allergic contact dermatitis. Some cases are associated with a widespread purpuric capillaritis similar to the eruption produced by sensitivity to carbromal and meprobamate.

Fisher[57] reported reactions in three patients involving a rubber diving suit, elasticized shorts, and a rubberized support bandage for the leg, respectively. All had itching petechial and purpuric eruptions at the sites of contact with a rubber article containing N-isopropyl-N-phenyl-paraphenylenediamine (IPPD), a rubber antioxidant. One patient had previous dermatitis underneath the elastic portions of her undergarments. It was determined that IPPD is added to elastic material used in some elastic strips on undergarments in the United States. All patients had positive patch tests to IPPD. Fisher reported that IPPD is manufactured by five American companies under the trade names Cyzone, Eastozone, Fleezwx, Flexazone 3C, and Santoflex 36. It is of interest that the substance also has been listed as a stabilizer in a Japanese insecticide formulation. Romaguera and Grimalt[58] similarly confirmed a pruritic purpuric eruption in a woman in the pattern of her brassiere. She was patch-test positive to IPPD (0.1% pet) with purpura.

Shmunes[59] described a 59-year-old saleswoman of black hats who had a severe purpuric eruption on the exposed areas of the face, neck, and arms. Patch testing to paraphenylenediamine produced a purpuric test reaction.

WOOL DUST AND WOOL RESIDUES PURPURA

Agarwal[60] reported that a patient acquired purpura from collecting raw wool from sheep breeders and selling it to textile mills. Although a patch test was negative, the application of wool dust on the patient's body reproduced the eruption. Agarwal emphasized that contact allergens can lead to purpura without systemic involvement and that a more vigilant search might reveal more contact allergens in the pathogenesis of intractable cases of allergic purpura. Romaguera and colleagues[61] implicated formaldehyde resins in wool residues as causing purpura in a man who was in charge of a special section for the recovery of the wool residues obtained from other sections of the same factory. In this case, the wool was not pure but was mixed with synthetic fibers.

PURPURIC ERUPTION FROM TOPICAL OXYQUINOLINE

A purpuric eruption on the extremities following application of medication containing oxyquinoline has also been reported.[62]

PURPURA FROM FEPRADINOL

Use of a 6% nonsteroidal anti-inflammatory drug, fepradinol hydrochloride, resulted in a purpuric papulonecrotic eruption on the lumbosacral region. The product, Dalgen spray, is sold in Spain and used to relieve musculoskeletal pain. Patch tests were positive to the spray and to fepradinol 0.1, 1, and 2% ethanol with 30 negative controls. Biopsy of both the patch test and the clinical eruption showed thrombotic vasculopathy accompanied by epidermal necrosis, but no leucocytoclastic vasculitis. A lymphoctic perivascular infiltrate with eosinophils was seen in adjacent dermis. While other cases of allergy to fepradinol have been reported, those cases were either eczematous or photoallergic in nature.[63]

PURPURIC PATCH TEST REACTIONS

Apronalide (Sedormid) and quinidine have produced purpuric patch test reactions in persons with purpuric drug eruptions from ingestion of these medicaments.[64] Apronalide (Sedormid) was tested as a saturated solution in propylene glycol. The patch test with quinidine consisted of a paste made of a crushed tablet of quinidine sulfate in a small volume of water. The material was left in contact with the patient's arm or back for 24 to 48 hours. The reaction is considered positive if the area of contact shows numerous small petechial hemorrhages.

COBALT

Schmidt and colleagues[65] stated that a total of 132 patch-tested patients reacted with petechial reactions to 1% cobalt chloride in petrolatum; 23 patients were retested with various concentrations of cobalt. In about 60% of those retested, the petechial reaction could be reproduced. A histopathologic examination showed slight perivascular-lymphocytic infiltration, swollen endothelium, and extravasation of erythrocytes but no signs of vasculitis. About 5% of patients tested with 1% cobalt chloride in petrolatum show this petechial hemorrhage, which has been localized to the acrosyringium.

Pigmented Contact Dermatitis

Pigmented contact dermatitis may occur from optical whiteners in washing powders and from azo dyes.[66]

OPTICAL WHITENERS

The term "pigmented contact dermatitis" was used by Osmundsen,[67] who, in a series of excellent observations and investigations, has contributed more than anyone else to our understanding of melanosis as a feature of contact dermatitis. In light of Osmundsen's studies and the observations of others, all types of Riehl's melanosis can be comprehended as a single disease entity. Osmundsen[53] described an epidemic in Copenhagen caused by optic whiteners in washing powder. The chemical responsible was a mixture of two pyrazoline derivatives that seem to have a marked tendency to induce pigmented contact dermatitis. Pigmentation developed at the site of several patch tests with the compounds responsible.

In another epidemic of contact dermatitis from optical whiteners of the same type, Pinol-Aguade and colleagues[68] reported strong hyperpigmentation in nearly half of their patients. Some had pigmentation compatible with Riehl's melanosis. The different genetic conditions for pigment formation in the Spanish and Danish populations probably explain the much higher incidence of hyperpigmentation in the Spanish material, in which the heaviest pigmentation occurred in patients who had dark complexions.

AZO DYES

A study of occupational pigmented contact dermatitis in a textile mill from an azo dye–coupling component[69] has further stressed the importance of the pigment-genetic predisposition for the development of pigmented contact dermatitis. Hyperpigmentation was most pronounced in persons with dark complexions, whereas more fair-skinned patients also showed "classic" eczematous symptoms, including pruritus.

Kgzuka and colleagues[70] reported that pigmented contact dermatitis in 23 patients was caused by cosmetics containing Brilliant Lake Red R. A strong allergen in all patients was 1-phenylazo-2-naphthol, but no patients showed a positive reaction to azobenzene.

PIGMENTATION FROM FRAGRANCES AND BACTERICIDES

In Japan, where facial melanosis has been quite common, allergic contact dermatitis from scents, such as hydrocitronellal, benzylsalicylate, ylang-ylang oil, and jasmine, and from bactericides, such as carbanilides, has been demonstrated to be the cause of pigmentation.[71]

Mathias[72] studied a patient who experienced repeated episodes of facial dermatitis with subsequent development of facial hyperpigmentation. A positive patch test to potassium dichromate strongly implicated chromium hydroxide, used as a pigment in a commercial toilet soap, as the contact allergen. Prurigo pigmentosa has been reported mainly from Japan and the eruption is truncal and flares in spring and summer resolving with reticulated pigmentation. Contact dermatitis has been reported to cause this eruption due to the presence of chrome in detergent. However, the authors did not show that the amount of chrome found in detergent (3.4ppm) could cause a reaction in their patient, so this is not a condition that can be definitively linked to such exposures.[73]

PARATERTIARY-BUTYLPHENOL-FORMALDEHYDE RESIN

A non-eczematous pigmented dermatitis occurred in a 51 year old white woman who wore a leather watch strap to which she reacted on patch testing. She also was positive to paratertiary-butylphenol-formaldehyde resin, the putative allergen in the strap. While her patch tests were strong to both the strap and allergen, her dermatitis was not eczematous and a biopsy showed a lichenoid dermatitis with an interface dermatitis that accounted for the prominent pigmentation.[74]

RIEHL'S MELANOSIS—A VARIANT OF PIGMENTED CONTACT DERMATITIS

Melanosis with incontinence of pigment may be the result of many inflammatory reactions in the skin. There are three subdivisions: (a) pigment abnormalities as an effect of irradiation, (b) pigment abnormalities after mechanical and chemical irritation, and (c) hyperpigmentation after exanthemas. Riehl's melanosis falls into Group 2 and is similar to melanodermatitis toxica caused by tar or oils. Riehl's melanosis, as originally described, was a pigmented contact dermatitis in which the inflammatory component was slight in many cases. These studies suggest that a pigmented variant of contact dermatitis is most common in persons with strong pigmentation.[67,68]

It also seems that hyperpigmentation may be the only macroscopic sign of a dermatitis. Persons with dark complexions who have a tendency to react with hyperpigmentation seem less likely than fair people to develop typical eczematous changes when exposed to certain chemicals.

Hyperpigmentation is not a common feature of contact dermatitis, and marked pigment-forming capacity is not the only explanation for the appearance of a pigmented contact dermatitis. Photo-contact dermatitis more often leads to hyperpigmentation, but abnormal pigmentation may also be absent.

Role of Chronic Contact Dermatitis in Actinic Reticuloid Syndrome (Persistent Light Reactors)

Addo and colleagues[75] stated that contact allergic sensitivity to allergens, such as plants of the Compositae family, is a feature of the chronic skin reaction seen in the photosensitivity dermatitis with actinic reticuloid syndrome. In 50 patients who have this syndrome, an increased incidence of contact allergic sensitivity to some common fragrance materials was demonstrated. Evidence is also presented, from in vitro and in vivo studies, that indicates a phototoxic mechanism is involved. The relevance of continued exposure to common allergens and their involvement in photosensitization mechanisms has been a theory for the state of "persistent light reaction."

These allergens include Compositae and allied compounds, rubber factors, and potassium dichromate. It therefore seems probable that the persistence of the skin reaction throughout the year is in part due to the perennial presence of such contact allergens. It also is possible that the pseudolymphomatous changes found in association with maximum skin reactivity may be explained by persistent antigen stimulation. Fragrance materials are also common environmental contactants.[76,77]

The persistence of chronic dermatitis year-round in many affected subjects is thus not simply from an ability to react to a broad-action spectrum of radiation present at any time of the year, but also (and this may be an important feature) from perennial exposure to relevant contact allergens. In addition, results indicate that some of these same allergens may involve photosensitivity mechanisms and that repeated phototoxic responses are therefore also likely to be an important feature in the chronicity of the reaction.

Chronic actinic dermatitis, which includes actinic reticuloid, was studied in 86 patients by du Peloux and colleagues,[78] who reported at the European Contact Dermatitis Society in Brussels, October 1992, that 74% of such patients had a positive patch or photopatch test: Twenty percent were fragrance sensitive, 20% colophony sensitive, 14% rubber sensitive, and 36% allergic to a mixture of sesquiterpene lactones (SLs). These investigators from St. John's Institute of Dermatology in London found only about 22% of SL-sensitive patients to be photosensitive. Most of the 114 relevant SL-allergic patients had hand (36%) or hand and face eczema (36%), whereas 20% had generalized dermatitis. This would indicate that multiple environmental allergens may account for persistent eczematous states. Because a reliable SL patch test allergen was not available previously, it is easy to understand how difficult it can be to exclude other environmental antigens when treating an ongoing eczema. The responsible allergen would simply go undetected.

Possible Role of Chronic Contact Dermatitis in Mycosis Fungoides

PREVALENCE OF NICKEL AND OTHER CONTACT ALLERGIES AMONG PATIENTS WITH MYCOSIS FUNGOIDES

Schlenzka and colleagues, at the International Contact Dermatitis Symposium in East Berlin in 1983, stated that 20 patients with the clinical and histologic diagnosis of mycosis fungoides were subjected to patch tests with chromate, nickel, and cobalt between 1971 and 1982. Positive results occurred in 12 patients (60%). The prevalence of such contact allergies is consequently much higher than among other people tested in recent years. These results could support the hypothesis that mycosis fungoides is an "immunoma."

Case-controlled studies have not verified an association between occupational exposures or chronic antigen stimulation and cutaneous T-cell lymphoma, despite these interesting observations.[79]

Contact dermatitis to paraphenylenediamine was identified as the source of a body fold dermatitis with features of lymphomatoid changes histologically. CD 8+ cells predominated and suggested a type of cutaneous T cell lymphoma. PCR studies of the T-cell gamma gene rearrangement found the pattern to be polyclonal. Avoidance of dark clothing and occupational exposures to oils resolved the dermatitis.[80] A prolonged reaction to dinitrochlorobenzene (DNCB) developed on the arm of a woman sensitized to treat alopecia areata. The area was excised and a dense lymphocytic infiltrate with germinal center was seen in the dermis, leading to a diagnosis of lymphoadenosis benigna cutis. The authors noted that this had also been reported from squaric acid dibutyl ester.[81] Lymphomatoid contact dermatitis was also observed from para-tertyl-butyl phenol resin. The source of contact was a black leather glasses case carried in pants pockets. Gold, nickel, formalin, glutaraldehyde and ethylenediamine have also been reported to produce this pattern of contact dermatitis.[82]

Lichenoid Contact Dermatitis

LICHENOID ERUPTIONS FROM CONTACT WITH FILM DEVELOPERS

Certain substituted paraphenylenediamine (PPDA) compounds used as color film developers can produce a lichenoid eruption on skin that comes in contact with these chemicals.[83] In affected persons, acute or subacute allergic eczematous or papular dermatitis appears, fades, and is replaced by an eruption identical to that of lichen planus.[84] It subsides after several weeks, leaving marked pigmentation. Sensitization in exposed workers is fairly high and may take 1 month to 3 years to develop.

Patch test reactions to color developers, such as CD2 (2-amino-5-diethylamino-toluene monohydrochloride), are positive in sensitized persons who acquire lichenoid eruptions.[85] Patch tests with CD2 should be performed with a 1% aqueous solution. The same chemicals used in color development are also used in high-speed, black-and-white film processing and may cause lichen planus eruptions.[86]

The lichen planus eruption caused by color developers does not usually affect the buccal mucosa or the tongue, although lesions occasionally appear in the mouth.[87]

Color film developer chemicals based on PPDA are associated with lichenoid tissue reactions. This has not been commonly associated with PPDA itself. However, four cases of lichenoid dermatitis were traced to PPDA in hair dyes.[88]

PATCH TESTING FOR LICHENOID CONTACT DERMATITIS

The closed patch technique is the most convenient method of testing for lichenoid contact dermatitis. The patch is removed after 24 hours, and the underlying skin is washed gently with an acid-type cleanser. This removes excess chemical, which, because of its ability to become fixed to epidermal cells, might lead to sensitization. Skin reactions are read after 1 hour and again 24 and 48 hours after removal of the patch. Evolution of the lesion over the next few days produces the typical lichenoid eruption. The brownish stain remaining on the skin after removal of the patch and subsequent washing should not be confused with a positive skin reaction.

Patch tests with color developers are not always positive in patients with lichenoid eruptions. A positive reaction that is eczematous may later become lichenoid.

PPDA does not produce this type of lichenoid eruption and does not seem to cross-react with the substituted PPDA used as a color developer.

LICHEN PLANUS ERUPTIONS FROM METALS

Frykholm and colleagues[89] reported that a patient allergic to metallic copper developed lichen planus of the buccal mucosa and tongue. Replacement of the copper-containing amalgam fillings in her teeth eliminated the lichen planus lesions. Lombardi and colleagues[90] stated that a lichenoid dermatitis was caused presumably by nickel salts in a nickel-sensitive person. Oral lichen planus has been attributed to zinc in dental restorations and a zinc concentration in the restorations in one such case was determined to be 5.3%. The patch test used was zinc chloride 2% petrolatum.[91]

Epoxy resin has also been reported to cause dermatitis that is histologically lichen planus.[92] It is common for the patch test to be eczematous, whereas the clinical eruption is lichen planus–like with epoxy, metallic mercury, metallic copper, nickel salts, and even color film developer.

ORAL LICHEN PLANUS–LIKE CHANGES AND MERCURY

Of 18 patients with oral lichenoid lesions near amalgam fillings, 15 were found to be mercury sensitive, and partial or complete removal of the amalgam improved 13 of the 15.[93] Five patients had partial amalgam removal, and all showed incomplete resolution; 7 of 10 who had complete amalgam removal had complete resolution of signs and symptoms. Lichenoid changes were frequently adjacent to amalgam fillings.

PRIMULA AND LICHEN PLANUS

Exposure to *Primula obconica* over a 7-month period resulted in hand, wrist and forearm dermatitis that histologically was lichen planus and showed lichenoid clinical morphology.[94]

LUPUS ERYTHEMATOSUS AND CONTACTANTS

Patch tests to carvone and spearmint mix in a patient with subacute cutaneous lupus erythematosus provoked a reaction 19 days after application. The reaction was histologically proven to be subacute cutaneous lupus erythematosus, but there was no preceding visible reaction to account for this. Avoidance of these two patch test substances for a period of months had no effect on her skin disease. The authors concluded that a subclinical irritant reaction must have provoked the occurrence of lupus at the sites of the patches.[95]

Allergic contact dermatitis due to oleyl alcohol in pimecrolimus cream presented as subacute cutaneous lupus erythematosus. A 10% oleyl alcohol patch test produced an eczematous response.[96]

LICHEN SIMPLEX CHRONICUS AND CONTACTANTS

Patients with lichen simplex chronicus who had weak positive patch tests to paraphenylenediamine had improvement in or complete clearing of the lichen simplex chronicus when they stopped dyeing their hair. Patients with strong reactions to the allergen did not improve. About half of the 25 patients reported by Chey and colleagues demonstrated this connection between lichen simplex chronicus, mild paraphenylenediamine, and a benefit to discontinuation of hair dye use.[97]

Acneiform Eruptions from Contactants

It is widely believed that cosmetics may aggravate or precipitate acne and that this can be easily evaluated by the rabbit ear assay for comedogenicity. This belief and conventional wisdom have led to the concept that oil-containing cosmetics are bad and oil-free cosmetics are good. These beliefs are incorrect and have largely been discredited by a recent consensus conference of knowledgeable dermatologists and industry representatives.[98]

Two separate adverse effects of topical agents fall under the category of acnegenesis. The first is a slow process over several months' time that results in a true comedo or formation of new comedones in acne-prone persons. The second occurs within weeks and is a form of follicular irritation morphologically manifested as papules and pustules. Both events are believed to be uncommon with most available cosmetics save for some hair pomades.

In the occupational setting, more severe acnegens may be encountered (Table 7.3). Halogenated hydrocarbons and coal tar are the standard categories of chemicals associated with acne, particularly chloracne. Cosmetic products have not been associated with chloracne. Lists of individual chemicals previously have been published as a way for clinicians to check products for their acnegenic potential.[98] Unfortunately, both the lists and the concept that checking for individual ingredients will provide accurate information for patient instruction are incorrect. The consensus panel noted that the acnegenic potential of individual ingredients is modified by their concentrations and vehicle components, which can

Table 7-3 Causes of Occupational Acne

1. Petrolatum and its derivatives
  Crude oil and fractions
  Cutting oils
2. Coal-tar products
  Coal-tar oils
  Creosote
  Pitch
3. Chloracne
  Chlorobenzenes
  Crude trichlorobenzene
  Crude benzene hexachloride
  3,4,39,49-tetrachloroazoxybenzene
  2,4,39,49-tetrachloroazobenzene
  Chloronaphthalenes
  Contaminants of chlorophenols
  2,3,7,8-tetrachlorodibenzo-*p*-dioxin (TCDD)
  Hexachlorodibenzo-*p*-dioxin
  Tetrachlorodibenzofuran
  Polychlorinated dibenzofurans (PCFs)—especially tri-, tetra-, penta-, and hexachlorodibenzofuran
  Polychlorobiphenyls (PCBs)*
4. Miscellaneous
  Asbestos
  DDT
  Frictional acne
  Halothane?
  Heavy water distillate
  Tropical acne in soldiers

*The polychlorodibenzofurans and hexachloronaphthalenes may occur as contaminants and may actually be the chloracnegens in some PCBs.

increase or decrease the actual acnegenic potential of a given product.[98] Meaningful patient information comes only from testing with the finished product. Furthermore, oiliness alone does not predict whether a product will aggravate acne. The features of acne-genesis are found in Table 7.4.

POMADE ACNE

Pomades used as hair straighteners contain primarily a paraffin and petrolatum mixture with gums and perfumes added. They often produce acneiform facial lesions characterized by uniform, localized papulopustules and follicular papulopustules on the forehead and temples. Such acneiform eruptions are common in people with black skin.[99]

OCCUPATIONAL ACNE

According to Taylor,[100] the chemicals listed in Table 7.3 are the principal causes of occupational acne.

Table 7-4 Acnegenic Responses to Topical Agents

Acnegenic response	Time course	Morphologic features	Potential sources
Mild	Months	True comedone increase	Cosmetics and medications
Mild	Weeks	Papules and pustules (follicular irritation)	Cosmetics and medications
Severe	Weeks/days	Comedones and straw-colored cysts	Coal-tar chlorinated hydrocarbons

Occupational acne is a type of acne venenata in which contact with a wide variety of substances can produce an acneiform and follicular eruption. Outbreaks of severe, generalized acne occurred in certain manufacturing plants in the 1920s and 1930s. In the intervening years, although advances have been made in industrial hygiene and acnegenic chemicals can be identified by the rabbit's ear test, sporadic epidemics of acne (especially chloracne) have occurred. Most recent reports[101] have come from Europe, because many US firms are unwilling to release or publish data on outbreaks among their employees.

Among the known causative agents of occupational acne are components of crude petrolatum, cutting oils, coal tar and some of its products, chlorinated aromatic chemicals, and various miscellaneous agents. Workers in oil fields and refineries who have prolonged skin contact with crude oil or the heavier oil fractions may develop the spectrum of acne lesions. By far, the most common sources of acneiform eruptions are cutting oils employed in machine tool operations. Low-level exposure to o-dichlorobenzene in a laboratory setting led to the development of chloracne in a graduate student with frequent exposure to this chemical. The air levels were 0.8 to 2.2 ppb. This level was well below the safety limit of 25 ppb. Cutaneous contact may have also been a factor.[102]

The insoluble (straight) oils and semisynthetic fluids are the most frequent culprits. Oil acne seems to start as an inflammatory folliculitis, especially in areas in contact with contaminated clothing. Comedones are also present.

Coal-tar oils, creosote, and pitches can produce extensive acneiform eruptions in coal-tar plant workers, roofers, and road building and construction workers. Comedones are typical of this form of acne. Phototoxic reactions may complicate the picture and produce coal-tar melanosis and exacerbations of the acne.

Chlorinated aromatic hydrocarbon compounds are among the most potent acnegenic materials known. These chemicals produce chloracne, an extremely refractory form of acne venenata that may be accompanied by serious systemic toxicity. The cutaneous eruption is characterized by straw-colored cysts and closed comedones, but inflammatory cysts and open comedones may abound. Chloracne

serves as a marker of the medical and environmental impact of contamination of technical-grade chemicals with highly toxic extraneous intermediates. Several new outbreaks of chloracne have occurred from exposure to two chlorobenzene compounds and from contaminants of chlorophenol compounds.

Pustular Allergic Contact Dermatitis

Burkhart[103] presented a case of acute allergic dermatitis in which the predominant lesions were pustules developing in a patient after the application of a topical antibiotic cream containing nitrofurazone.

The pustules noted in the patient were clinically similar to those from a reaction to heavy metals; however, the erythema and pruritus displayed by the patient were not features of such a reaction. The predominantly lymphocytic pustules characteristic of an ammonium-fluoride reaction are analogous histologically to the pathologic findings in this case; however, the acantholysis and ballooning degeneration associated with a pustular patch test reaction to ammonium fluoride were not features in this case.

In a study performed by Stone and Johnson,[104] 5% nickel sulfate was patch tested on patients who were not sensitive to nickel on areas previously injected with heat-killed *Corynebacterium acnes* organisms. As a result, multiple, small, asymptomatic pustules developed at the patch test sites. Histologically, the pustules contained equal parts of mononuclear cells and neutrophils. The investigators concluded that nickel sulfate produced this reaction by enhancing preexisting inflammation caused by the injection of heat-killed bacteria. Thus, they believed the reaction was an enhancement phenomenon of prior inflammation rather than an irritant or allergic reaction.

Pustules usually are associated with irritant reactions, but pustular allergic reactions have been reported to metals, nitrofurazone, and topical fluorouracil.[105] A woman who used 2% minoxidil solution (Lacovin) developed a mixture of vesicles and pustules on her forehead. Histologically, perifollicular lymphocytes, histocytes, and eosinophils were found. Her patch test reaction was 2+ and consisted of a mixture of vesicles and pustules.

Pustular contact dermatitis has also been reported from isoconazole nitrate.[106] The patch test was strongly eczematous.

PUSTULAR PATCH TEST REACTIONS

Hjorth[107] stated that such reactions are most likely to occur in atopic persons. Fisher and colleagues[108] found that metallic salts, particularly nickel, copper, arsenic trioxide, and mercuric chloride, produced such reactions, which usually dry promptly before disappearing completely. Pustular patch test reactions are usually irritant in nature but may sometimes accompany allergic reactions.[109]

Pustular reactions to standard patch tests with nickel sulfate (5%) were found to be the rule when patients with atopic dermatitis were tested on skin bearing follicular papules, erythema, or lichenification or when the skin integrity was disturbed by minor trauma, such as a pinprick.[110] This further supports the nonallergic (irritant) nature of the phenomena.

Dyshidrosiform Contact Dermatitis

In a personal communication, Martin, Piette, Boegoend, Huriez, and Desmons of France were concerned with the following questions: (a) Do dyshidrotic eczemas related to a contact allergy exist? and (b) Can dyshidrotic lesions be reproduced by patch tests?

Their study covered five patients affected by dyshidrotic eczema that had been developing for at least 4 years. Having obtained positive test results on the back, they reproduced the lesions by applying selected allergens to the palm in patch tests. These allergens were potassium dichromate (two cases), PPDA (two cases, of which one also was tested on the soles), and mercaptobenzothiazole (MBT, one case, with a sole test also positive).

Patients were tested as follows: (a) In a cement worker who since 1971 had dyshidrotic eczema of the palm with positive chromate and cobalt patch test results, patch testing of the palm and the back was positive for chromium but not for cobalt. (b) In a concrete worker with eczema on the backs of the hands who was allergic to dichromate and who had severe dyshidrotic dermatitis on the heels related to an allergy to rubber in his shoes, patch testing on the back was positive for MBT. Results of patch tests with MBT on the soles were also positive. (c) In a window cleaner with pompholyx of the palms and soles who was "intolerant" of rubber gloves and shoes, a patch test to PPDA on his back was positive. Patch testing on the palm with PPDA produced a positive reaction resembling a dyshidrotic eruption.

In this study, the allergen concentrations were identical for the patch tests on the back and on the palms or soles. These authors believed that perhaps penetration of the allergen is made easier by changes in the palms or soles in persons affected by dyshidrotic eczema, even after an apparent cure.

These authors commented that contact allergy is seldom proposed as a precursor of dyshidrotic eczema. They cited investigators[111] who claim that, in patients with allergy to nickel and pompholyx, intimate contact with nickel objects in no case induces an exacerbation of the hand eruption.

However, some authentic cases of dyshidrotic eczema of the palm and sole appear to improve when an "external" contact with nickel is removed. Fisher and Shapiro[112] cited positive results of patch tests on the palms with nickel.

Dyshidrotic eczema or pompholyx might better be thought of as a reaction pattern with many possible causes. Internal and external allergies have been capable of producing this pattern of eczema, as noted in the references cited. Irritant contact dermatitis induced by metal-working fluids has also produced dyshidrotic eczema in workers who had neither an atopic diathesis nor positive patch tests.[113] Therefore, it seems that the morphologic pattern associated with pompholyx is not specific for a route of exposure or a currently well-understood mechanism. Pompholyx is probably not a disease sui generis.

Contact "Halogenosis" from Topical, Fluorinated, or "Strong" Corticosteroids

In the past, the fluorinated corticosteroids have been implicated in the etiology of certain cases of perioral dermatitis, rosacea-like eruptions in both children and adults, and skin atrophy.[114,115] More recently, European and Japanese dermatologists[116–118] have reported apparently new entities under such terms as "granuloma gluteale infantum" and "Kaposi sarcoma–like granulomatous diaper dermatitis," in which fluorinated topical corticosteroids may be causative factors.

Malkinson and Pearson[119] posed the following question: Should these cases of infantile gluteal granuloma or Kaposi-like sarcomas occurring in the diaper area be considered as contact dermatitis vegetans or infant halogenosis? A brief description of these new entities complicating diaper dermatitis follows.

GRANULOMA GLUTEALE INFANTUM

Tappeiner and Pfleger[116] reported an apparently new entity, granuloma gluteale infantum, in six infants. All infants had painless firm nodules that resembled large angiomas or hematomas initially. The lesions were on the buttocks and the inner aspect of the thighs and consisted of symmetrical, round, or oval plum-sized, bluish-red or maroon nodules. The surrounding skin was normal. The infants were otherwise normal, as were their blood studies and X-ray examinations. The nodules resolved spontaneously in several months without sequelae.

The histologic examination did not correspond with any known dermatologic condition. No evidence of infection was present. Although the cause remained obscure, some "exogenous noxious factor" was considered the most likely.

"VEGETATING" HALOGENOSIS

Bazex and colleagues[117] reported a 3-month-old boy, seen because of a diaper rash, who had been treated with eosin, permanganate baths, and Mycolog Cream. The eruption disappeared in about 1 month, but 1 month later violet nodules resembling hematomas of traumatic origin appeared on the inside of the thighs and pubis. The hypothesis of "vegetating bromidism" was considered, but the infant had received no bromide treatment. The nodules disappeared spontaneously without treatment after approximately 1 month without sequelae.

KAPOSI SARCOMA–LIKE GRANULOMATOUS DIAPER DERMATITIS

Uyeda and colelagues[118] in Japan described five cases of Kaposi sarcoma–like granuloma occurring in areas of diaper dermatitis in infants age 2 to 8 months, who had worn paper diapers. These infants had had diaper dermatitis, and in each case, synthetic corticosteroid hormones were applied topically.

The granulomas appeared in the genitocrural region, the lower abdomen, and the inner thighs and bore a clinical and histologic resemblance to the early stage of Kaposi sarcoma. No evidence of infection was present. The lesions of diaper dermatitis disappeared, but the granulomas remained for several months, then cleared spontaneously and never recurred.

The authors, referring to the report of Tappeiner and Pfleger,[116] stated that the clinical features and histologic findings of granuloma gluteale infantum were similar to their Japanese cases, except that the gluteal region was not affected. The lesions were instead in the genitocrural region, the thigh, and the penile region. Thus, because the Japanese investigators believed the term "granuloma gluteale infantum" would be unsuitable, they described their cases as "Kaposi sarcoma–like granuloma on diaper dermatitis."

Malkinson and Pearson[119] stated that the suggestion by Bazex and colleagues[117] that this condition may be associated with halogen is supported to some extent by the histologic changes; however, beyond that, the evidence is very thin and highly speculative. These authors believed it was more reasonable that, rather than being directly related to the halogen contents in corticosteroids, the condition is secondary to the great potency of these corticosteroids, even though the pathogenic mechanism is obscure. A somewhat analogous situation is present in perioral dermatitis, in which some patients acquire the characteristic eruption after using potent fluorinated corticosteroids.

A recent report of Kaposi-like acroangiodermatitis from the friction and negative pressure of a suction prosthesis may shed light on a feature overlooked in the previously cited cases.[120] This patient with this condition was patch test negative to the prosthesis, had no arteriovenous fistula, and was negative for human immunodeficiency virus (HIV). A lighter, larger prosthesis was therapeutic. Most cases of granuloma gluteale infantum and Kaposi sarcoma–like granuloma have occurred in areas of friction, which may be a cofactor in their development.

OROFACIAL GRANULOMATOSIS

Contact allergy to gold and mercury in dental metals resulted in orofacial granulomatosis. The clinical disease was granulomatous but the patch tests were spongiotic dermatitis.[121]

ROSACEA-LIKE ERUPTION OF CHILDREN AND ADULTS

Although the etiology of perioral dermatitis remains controversial, many observations and reports in the literature continue to implicate strong topical corticosteroids, particularly the fluorinated variety. Savin and colleagues[122] reported 11 cases of children who had strong corticosteroids applied to the face; a bright malar flush was produced that was accompanied at times by small superficial papules, pustules, and scaling. The clinical picture was variable, sometimes closely resembling rosacea and sometimes perioral dermatitis, taking an average of 1 year to clear. Seven of the 11 children had a family history of atopy, and 2 had a family history of rosacea. These authors stated that potent topical corticosteroids may have played a role in the cause of these rashes and, on withdrawal, a pustular exacerbation was sometimes present. They speculated that a relationship exists between rosacea and perioral dermatitis.

"TOPICAL DRUG ADDICTION"— ADVERSE EFFECTS OF FLUORINATED CORTICOSTEROID CREAMS AND OINTMENTS

Under this eye-catching title, Burry[123] discussed the adverse effects that the anti-inflammatory powers of topical fluorinated corticosteroids have on acne rosacea, seborrheic complexions, and tinea infections of the skin as illustrated by eight cases. They stated that these steroids cause local atrophy, purpura, telangiectasia, and ulceration by interfering with skin-collagen metabolism, and that many patients are afraid to stop using locally applied corticosteroids because of the uncomfortable rebound inflammation that follows their withdrawal. Both the skin and the patient can therefore become readily "hooked" on these topical drugs.

Almeyda and Burt[124] concurred with Burry, stating it is now recognized that topically administered fluorinated compounds are just as likely to cause unwanted side effects as are systemically administered compounds.

Earlier, Sneddon[125] had drawn attention to the effects of fluorinated compounds on patients with rosacea, who seem to become addicted because corticosteroids initially suppress the soreness and inflammatory papular and pustular lesions. Each time application is stopped, however, the eruption exacerbates acutely, tempting the patient to apply more corticosteroid. With prolonged application, there is loss of dermal connective tissue, which exposes the subpapillary venous plexus and causes increasing erythema and telangiectasia. The process is slow, and the patients do not notice the deterioration in their appearance for some time. Weber[126] agreed that the rosacea-like condition and perioral dermatitis may well result from the use of fluorinated corticosteroids on the face.

Addiction to topical steroids can cause a chronic red face or eyelid dermatitis that can only be cured by withdrawal of the corticosteroid. However, a severe and prolonged rebound of facial erythema and edema is part of the pathway to a cure. This complication of topical steroid use has been detailed by Rapaport and Rapaport.[127]

Epstein and colleagues[128] pointed out that potent topical corticosteroids can produce striae and extensive bruising and ecchymoses with minor trauma owing to wasting of dermal connective tissue. Extreme soft tissue atrophy in the diaper area in an infant treated for diaper rash with fluorinated steroids for some months has also been reported by Johns and Bower.[129] Growth of vellus hair, delayed healing of ulcerated areas, and systemic absorption with depression of endogenous corticosteroid secretions have all been observed with use of potent fluorinated steroids.[130,131]

Contact Epilating Folliculitis

The popular depilatories include the thioglycolates, the sulfides, and the mechanical depilatories. These agents may produce a marked follicular reaction with a pustular reaction when they are not used properly.[132]

A similar type of folliculitis is produced by the penetration of sharp needles of sugarcane bark into the hair follicles of sugarcane workers.[133] An inflammatory, follicular, pustular eruption is produced, particularly on the extremities. The borders of the scalp, the pubic area, and the chest and back may also be involved. Pruritus is severe, and the involved follicle atrophies, causing permanent hair loss.

Contact Granulomas

Certain chemicals elicit a local sarcoid granuloma when introduced within the skin. Zirconium, talc, stearate, silica, magnesium, and beryllium may produce granulomas once they pierce the skin.[134] In addition, the pigments of tattoos, particularly chrominum oxide, may cause a granulomatous reaction in sensitized individuals.

ALLERGIC CONTACT GRANULOMAS

Zirconium Granuloma

This skin lesion, seen originally following use of zirconium compounds in deodorants, continues to occur following use of these compounds for the treatment of *Toxicodendron* dermatitis.[135]

The lesions usually appear 4 to 6 weeks after initial use of the zirconium preparation and are limited to the sites of contact. They appear as persistent, firm, shiny, erythematous papules the color of flesh or apple jelly, and they may be solitary, grouped, or coalescent. Eczematous changes are also usually present. Pruritus is minimal or absent. The histologic picture may be indistinguishable from sarcoid.

Any defect in the protective layer of the skin enhances the development of hypersensitivity.[136–138]

In the axillae, minute abrasions from shaving as well as from excess friction and sweating enhance penetration of the zirconium salts in deodorants. The preparations containing zirconium salts used to treat *Toxicodendron* dermatitis readily penetrate acutely inflamed skin, denuded areas, vesicles, and bullae.[139]

Zirconium granulomas, composed of epithelioid cells, represent an acquired, delayed-type allergic reaction to zirconium in sensitized individuals.[140]

The granulomas produced by soluble zirconium salts usually disappear within a few months, whereas those produced by insoluble salts may last indefinitely. Intralesional injections of corticosteroids may be effective in resolving these granulomas.

Tests for Zirconium Hypersensitivity

Either patch or intracutaneous testing may be employed to determine allergic hypersensitivity to zirconium salts.[141]

Patch Test The zirconium preparation suspected of causing a granulomatous reaction may be rubbed into a test site previously prepared by multiple scratches or denuding with a dermal curet. The test site is then covered with an occlusive dressing for 2 days. In sensitized persons, a positive reaction is the development of reddish-brown papules in about 4 weeks. Such papules show a sarcoid granulomatous infiltrate histologically.

Intracutaneous Test   A small wheal is produced by intracutaneous injection of a 1:10,000 dilution of sodium zirconium lactate. A positive reaction consists of a discrete papule that appears in 8 to 14 days. In about 1 month, the papule clinically and histologically resembles a sarcoid lesion. The papule may persist for 6 to 24 months.

Prognosis of Zirconium Granulomas   Axillary granulomas produced by the soluble zirconium lactate in deodorants usually disappear within a few months. Lesions produced by the insoluble zirconium oxide preparations used for poison ivy (*Toxicodendron*) dermatitis usually remain unchanged for several months to years and are refractory to therapy. Temporary improvement is obtained with corticosteroids administered systemically or intralesionally.

Aluminum Granulomas

Patients may occasionally become allergic to aluminum, which can be detected by reactions at all Finn chamber sites owing to their aluminum construction or by testing with 2% aqueous aluminum hydroxide. Vaccination with diphtheria-pertussis-tetanus vaccine is a potential problem for such allergic persons (usually children) because aluminum hydroxide is a component of the vaccine and has caused granulomas at the vaccination sites that can last for more than 1 year.[142] Of 21 cases followed, 5 cleared, 11 improved, and 5 remained unchanged. Aluminum was demonstrated in the granulomas by X-ray defraction analysis.

Nonallergic Contact Granulomas

SODIUM STEARATE

The granulomatous response to sodium stearate is not based on allergic reactivity. It can be contrasted with the allergic granulomatous responses in patients who have zirconium deodorant granulomas and who are prepared immunologically as a result of their allergic hypersensitivity to zirconium. Thus, relatively few people develop granulomas after skin tests with zirconium salts.

Large quantities of sodium stearate are required to elicit the granulomatous response, whereas unusually dilute preparations of zirconium produce it in susceptible individuals. Often even 0.0001-ML solutions of zirconium salts stimulate formation of a granuloma in an allergic person. Concentrations of sodium stearate or sodium palmitate more dilute than 0.1 ML do not induce such reactions.

Stearate granulomas resolve clinically within a few weeks, but allergic granulomas usually reach their peak at 3 to 6 weeks and persist for months to years. In general, allergic granulomas are still evolving when stearate granulomas have completely resolved.

Talc Granulomas

McCallum and Hall[143] stated that treatment of the raw umbilical stump can produce pyogenic granulomas and umbilical polyps. They recommend that treatment with talc or starch should be discontinued and replaced by a nonirritant, sterile substance.

Tye and colleagues[144] described hundreds of talc granulomas of the skin that developed in a 45-year-old woman. It is postulated that the talcum powder gained entrance through the skin at the sites of draining or incised furuncles.

Oil Granulomas

Bergeron and Stone[145] observed two cases of multiple perifollicular granulomas of the scalp produced by Egyptian Oil, a proprietary hair conditioner. Upon discontinuation of the hair conditioner, the lesions regressed in both patients.

Granuloma Fissuratum

Chronic irritation from eyeglasses or dentures can produce granulomas at sites of pressure from the hard object. Such granulomas usually have a crease down the middle of the lesion.

Dry, Lichenified, or Hyperkeratotic Contact Dermatitis

Airborne allergens and dust tend to form dry, lichenified eruptions.

AIRBORNE ALLERGENS AND IRRITANTS

Contact dermatitis from prolonged, repeated exposure to relatively small quantities of airborne allergens, such as pollens, dusts, and vapors, produces diffuse, dry, and lichenified eruptions with vesication. The exposed portions of the body as well as wrinkles and folds are most markedly involved.

RAGWEED DERMATITIS

This type of dermatitis rarely is frankly vesicular unless the patient actually comes in contact with the plant. Exposure to the oleoresin through airborne pollen may result in a dry, leathery dermatitis with skin so infiltrated that a cutaneous lymphoma is suspected.

DERMATITIS FROM DUST

Dusts and their contents may produce mechanical effects, primary irritant eruptions, and allergic reactions.[146]

Dust that contains glass fibers can produce cuts from sharp glass fragments. Exposed surfaces may sustain an intensely pruritic, papular eruption. The penetrating spicules of asbestos, a fibrous, silicate mineral, are mechanical irritants that can produce asbestos "corns," particularly on the palmar aspects of the fingers. Coal, rock, and stone dust have an abrasive effect on the skin and can produce a lichenified, papular eruption that may be complicated by folliculitis. Dust collecting about a collar, belt line, or sleeve end may be rubbed into the skin by friction, producing lichenified eruptions.

The dust from relining a blast furnace has been found to cause an irritant dermatitis with frequently follicular patterns. Hydroxides of calcium, sodium, and potassium were found to produce a pH of approximately 12, and skin moisture was sufficient to exacerbate the problem.[147]

Dermatitis from cement dust is also dry and lichenified, primarily because of its alkalinity, hygroscopic properties, and abrasive effects. In addition, even when cement dermatitis results from allergic hypersensitivity to the chromium or cobalt content, the eruption tends toward dryness rather than frank vesiculation.

Sawdust from teak, redwood, mahogany, and rosewood may contain sensitizers that produce a dry dermatitis, particularly on the face, penis, and scrotum among carpenters and woodworkers. A lichenified eruption may also appear on the penis and scrotum when sawdust falls inside the clothes or is conveyed to these areas by the hands.

Other chemical dusts, fumes, and vapors produce eruptions similar to sawdust dermatitis. In addition, dust and air pollutants containing pitch or tar produce follicular, keratotic, and acneiform eruptions, as well as melanosis and photosensitivity reactions.

A dermatitis resembling ichthyosis caused by a quaternary ammonium compound in an ointment has been reported in Japan.[148] The compound implicated is alkyl benzyl trimethyl ammonium chloride.

Contact Hyperkeratotic Eruptions of Fingers, Palms, and Soles

The thick, horny layer of the fingers, palms, and soles modifies the appearance of allergic contact dermatitis by minimizing the eczematous element. The dry, fissured eruptions may resemble those from primary irritants, psoriasis, hyperkeratotic fungal infections, or atopic dermatitis. In dentists, allergic contact dermatitis from procaine hydrochloride (Novocain) or acrylic monomer is scaly, thickened, and fissured. Affected nails may become thickened, dystrophic, and separated from the nail bed.

So-called tulip bulb fingers (seen both with tulip bulbs and with *Alstromeria* contact among florists), in which the affected skin is dry, fissured, and hyperkeratotic, may resemble procaine hydrochloride (Novocain) and acrylic dermatitis. Onions, garlic, and formaldehyde and its resins may produce similar eruptions on the palms and palmar surfaces of the fingers.

In nickel-sensitive persons, pressure and prolonged contact with nickel-plated handlebars or door handles may produce dry, fissured eruptions of the palm. Similarly, nickel-plated arch supports may produce such changes on the soles.

"Contact" Psoriasis: Koebner Phenomenon

Fisher[149] showed that pressure, trauma, and friction from occupational procedures may produce psoriasis of the hands, particularly the palms and volar surfaces of the fingers. This psoriasis, called Koebner phenomenon, occurred in a pharmacist (from the pressure of opening and closing containers with child-resistant caps), a surgeon, a dentist (from the pressure of various instruments), a bus driver (from the pressure of the steering wheel), and an office worker (from pounding a stapler), a bartender, a seamstress, an optician, a paperhanger, a pushcart peddler, and a cellist.

Stable psoriasis may become pustular when contact dermatitis is superimposed on the stable plaque-type disease. This occurred in a patient with scalp psoriasis who became sensitive to the shampoo ingredient zinc pyrithione.[150] Only areas of contact dermatitis developed the pustular form of the disease. A nearly identical case has been reported. Allergic contact dermatitis to zinc pyrithione in a shampoo lead to a "koebnerization" of psoriasis into the area of contact dermatitis. The morphologic presentation was that of pustular psoriasis. Patch tests with 1% zinc pyrithione in petrolatum were positive.[151]

Often the patient does not show obvious psoriasis elsewhere. One may have to examine the scalp carefully and the intergluteal area to discover if the patient has psoriasis.

Adams[152] believed that the fact that fresh lesions of psoriasis appear following trauma from scratching, abrasions, lacerations, folliculitis, and acne has led many workers to press for compensation in the belief that the disease was caused or brought to activity by their occupation. If a "koebnerized" lesion is followed quickly by a severe flare of the disease, the idea of occupational causation seems even more likely to the worker. Trauma undoubtedly may incite the development of new lesions of psoriasis, but this occurs only in persons who already have the disease, if only in latent form. For this reason, careful consideration should be given to the job placement of persons with active psoriasis and even to those with a history of the disease. Thus, the Koebner phenomenon is medicolegally important when it follows industrial injuries.

Irritant Dermatitis Without Erythema

At the 1983 International Contact Dermatitis Symposium in East Germany, Nakayama and colleagues discussed "nonerythematous irritant reactions detected by the microscopic relief method." They stated:

Erythema has been regarded as a necessary sign in irritant dermatitis. Chronic irritant dermatitis, however, provoked by repeated contact to diluted detergents often shows a scaly rough skin without accompanying marked erythema. Linear alkylbenzene sulfonate and sodium lauryl sulfate have been known to produce erythema and edema when closed patch tested at 2% in aqueous solution for 48 hours. The reactions were negative macroscopically when closed patch tested at less than 1% for 24 hours. Then, didn't these irritants actually produce a reaction under such conditions?

Even though erythema was not discernible, the reliefs of the patch-tested skin surfaces were found to have been markedly disturbed when the replicas of the reliefs were taken and microscopically examined. The replicas were taken using celluloid plates (1.5 cm in diameter) whose surfaces were dissolved by painting n-butyl acetate before pressed on the patch-tested sites for two minutes.

The most striking findings obtained by this method were the disappearance of normal triangle skin furrow patterns. They were replaced by rounded, flattened, or deepened skin furrows at the sites where these irritants had been applied.

Frictional Contact Dermatitis

In 1993, at the International Contact Dermatitis Symposium in East Germany, Torkil Menné of Copenhagen reported as follows:
Experimentally, friction in the palms may give rise to callosities, bullae or dermatitis-like changes. For the development of frictional dermatitis the following factors are important; individual, intensity of frictional trauma and architecture of the surfaces. The skin changes are confined to the thenar or hypothenar region and the fingertips. The lesions may heal by changing irregular surfaces to smooth ones.

CONTACT LYMPHANGITIS AND LYMPHEDEMA

Many solvents entering a fissure or abrasion may produce a "chemical" lymphangitis, distinguishable from bacterial lymphangitis by the lack of constitutional symptoms. In addition, lymphangitis and lymphedema may follow allergic contact dermatitis.[153]

Worm and colleagues[154] reported that two patients with allergic contact dermatitis developed gross edema of the upper and lower extremities following recurrent bacterial infections. It is unlikely that the specific allergens responsible for the dermatitis have had any influence on the development of edema, because patients described previously with edema of the hands had positive patch tests to other allergens. In cases of severe dermatitis, leakage of plasma proteins from the vessels of the involved skin is abnormally increased.[155] Increased drainage of lymphatic protein from the interstitium of involved skin can compensate for this leakage and thus counteract edema formation.

In the cases described, many years elapsed in which the lymphatics compensated for the increased leakage of microvascular protein without resulting edema. Recurrent bacterial skin infections, however, may have compromised the lymphatic function, causing an increased extravascular concentration of plasma proteins. We therefore suggest that a local increase in the volume of interstitial fluid in the skin elicited by colloid osmotic forces can explain the clinically manifest edema in our and in similar patients.

Benzopyrones diminish edema from experimentally induced protein-rich rat leg.[156] The mechanism by which this occurs is probably increased proteolysis, which facilitates the removal of proteins from the interstitial space. Theoretically, therefore, this treatment should have an effect in the patients described. However, a more exact characterization of the protein content of edema fluid before and during such treatment is mandatory to evaluate the clinical and the physiologic response.

Prurigo Nodularis

There have been reports of contact dermatitis to the oral antibiotic nifuroxazide, which is used to treat acute and chronic diarrhea.[157] A Polish pharmaceutical worker was exposed to nifuroxazide in a packaging operation, but her lesions resembled prurigo nodularis rather than contact dermatitis. She was sensitive to this antibiotic from 1% to 0.001% aqueous and cleared when not occupationally exposed. She did not cross-react to nitrofurazone.

ERYTHEMA DYSCHROMICUM PERSTANS

A study in Panama of banana plantation workers with an erythema dyschromicum perstans–like eruption found that almost all were sensitive to a 0.001% chlorothalonil patch test.[158] This finding was present in 34 of 39 such cases. Chlorothalonil is a fungicide, which is widely used on banana plantations. None of 41 controls showed a reaction. Although not proof of cause and effect, the strong possibility that sensitivity to chlorothalonil is responsible for some cases of erythema dyschromicum perstans remains.

Erythema Annulare Centrifugum

Erythema annulare centrifugum lesions occurred in areas of skin contact with metal hooks and studs of clothing. Avoidance of such metal-containing clothing resolved the eruption and when 3 months later, patch test to nickel and cobalt produced strong eczematous reactions, the erythema annulare centrifugum reappeared.[159]

Granuloma Annulare

Contact dermatitis developed in a radiology department maintenance worker exposed to TroubleShooter (3M, St. Paul, MN) and FAZ a Kodak DryView laser imaging film (Eastman Kodak Co., Rochester, NY). The histology of the eruption was that of granuloma annulare. FAZ is an exhaust product from the Dry View, and is a powdery wax deposited on the machine. This material was used for patch testing and photopatch testing. The patient reacted to both TroubleShooter and FAZ and had positive photopatch tests to FAZ. The TroubleShooter reaction was believed to be irritant and the FAZ to be the true source of this unusual eruption.[160]

Acute Generalized Exanthematous Pustulosis

While acute generalized exanthematous pustulosis (AGEP) is most commonly a drug eruption, AGEP was the clinical presentation of allergy to Class D corticosteroids. The histology was spongiform pustules within the superficial layers of the epidermis and beneath the stratum corneum.[161] In acute generalized exanthematous pustulosis patch tests are able to identify the cause in about half of the cases. Positive patch tests have been reported in AGEP induced by the following drugs: amoxicillin, augmentin, chloramphenicol, pristinamycin, propicillin, spiramycin, streptomycin, virginiamycin, buphenine, carbamazepine, diltiazem, dihydroquinidine, isoniazid, metronidazole, nustatin, nifuroxazide, paracetamol, phenobarbital, terbinafine, ticlopidine and dexamethasone.[162]

Poikiloderma of Civatte

A role for contact dermatitis in the initiation or perpetuation of poikiloderma of Civatte was proposed in a case where a moisturizer containing methylchloroisothiazolinone/methylisothiazolinone was shown to be an allergen. However, the interventions included extensive sun protection and not just allergen avoidance, so it is difficult to evaluate the role of allergy in this disorder.[163]

Pyoderma Gangrenosum

Contact dermatitis to rubber components of an ostomy bag produced peristomal dermatitis in a patient who had undergone proctocolectomy for ulcerative colitis.[164] He had been in remission with no active colitis, but the dermatitis around his stoma ulcerated and took on the characteristics typical of pyoderma gangrenosum. There was no flare of underlying bowel disease in this case, and he responded to oral minocycline combined with intralesional triamcinolone.

Desquamative Gingivitis

Inflammation of both the free and attached gingiva was seen in a 27-year-old woman evaluated at a dental school in Scotland.[165] A clinical diagnosis of desquamative gingivitis was made. However, the woman was extremely sensitive to the nail polish ingredient tosylamide/formaldehyde resin, and she was a nail-biter. She was cured by changing to a nail polish without the allergen.

Lymphocytoma Cutis

Persistent lower lip dermatitis that histologically proved to be lymphocytoma cutis was traced to a dental metal.[166] The patient had a strong positive reaction to zinc chloride 2% aqueous that was present in one rusted filling. Zinc was confirmed to be present in the filling. Lymphocytoma cutis and urticaria, lichen planus, stomatitis, and generalized dermatitis are forms of dental metal allergy.

Lymphocytoma cutis of the earlobes has also been reported due to contact dermatitis resulting from gold and nickel earlobe exposure.[167]

Persistent Urticarial Plaques

Persistent urticaria, rather than transient urticaria or chronic dermatitis as seen in the contact urticaria syndrome, is another morphologic presentation for contact dermatitis. A persistent urticarial axillary eruption was reported due to an emulsifier in a deodorant.[168] The emulsifier, commercially known as Eumulgin L, had not previously been reported to be an allergen. Patch tests were strongly positive at 30% in petrolatum and weakly positive at 1% aqueous. This compound is also known as cetyl stearyl alcohol 2 (OP) 9(OE). No cross-reactivity was found to cetyl stearyl alcohol+sodium cetyl stearyl sulfate (Lanette N) or cetyl alcohol (Lanette 16).

Chronic Urticaria

In a provocative study from Italy, patch tests were used to evaluate patients with chronic urticaria. Of 121 patients with chronic urticaria, 71 were patch test negative. However, 50 of the 121 (41%) had positive patch tests. None of the 50 had urticarial type patch tests, but 23 experienced an exacerbation of urticaria on patch testing. Metals were the most commonly identified allergens (20/50). In all 50 the avoidance of the identified patch test allergen led to remission within 10 to 30 days. Verification of this study is needed before this type of testing can be recommended as part of the evaluation of chronic urticaria.[169]

Anaphylaxis

Anaphylaxis usually does not result from topical allergen exposure to intact skin. Mucosal surfaces, abraded skin, or skin ulceration is more fertile ground for anaphylactoid reactions.

Skin contact has resulted in anaphylaxis from latex, black rubber mix, carba mix, bacitracin, neomycin, streptomycin, cephalosporin, rifamycin, chlorhexidine, mercurochrome,

Emulgade F (an emulsifying agent), chlorothalonil, formaldehyde, lidocaine, milk, rice mechlorethamine, and labetalol (Table 7.5).[170]

References

1. Holst R, Kirby J, Magnusson B. Sensitization to tropical woods giving erythema multiforme–like eruptions. Contact Dermatitis 1976; 2:295.

2. Fisher AA, Bikowski J. Allergic contact dermatitis due to a wooden cross made of *Dalbergia nigra*. Contact Dermatitis 1981;7:45.

3. Martin P, Bergoend H, Piette F. Erythema multiforme–like eruption from Brazilian rosewood. Paper presented at the Fifth International Symposium on Contact Dermatitis, Barcelona, March 28, 1980.

4. Hjorth N. Primula dermatitis. Trans St John's Hosp Dermatol Soc 1966;52:207.

5. Kurz G, Rapaport MJ. External/internal allergy to plants (Artemesia). Contact Dermatitis 1979;5:407.

6. Moschella SL. Erythema multiforme. In: Dermatology. Vol. 1. Philadelphia: WB Saunders, 1975:387.

7. Shelley W. The Duhring conferences: poison ivy with marked edema. Skin and Allergy News, November 2, 1979, p. 30.

8. Kirby JS, Darley CR. Erythema multiforme associated with a contact dermatitis to terpenes. Contact Dermatitis 1978;4:238.

9. Torinuki W. Generalized erythema multiforme–like eruption following allergic contact dermatitis. Contact Dermatitis 1990;23:202.

10. Raccagni AA, Bardazzi F, Baldari U, Righini MG. Erythema-multiforme-like contact dermatitis due to capsicum. Contact Dermatitis 1995;33:353.

11. Mateo MPG, Velasco M, Miquel FJ, de la Cuadra J. Erythema-multiforme-like eruption following allergic contact dermatitis from sesquiterpene lactones in herbal medicine. Contact Dermatitis 1995;33:449.

12. Puig L, Alomar A, Randazzo L, et al. Erythema multiform like reaction caused by topical application of Thuja essential oil. Am J Contact Dermat 1994;5:94.

13. Jovanovic M, Mimica-Dukic N, Poljacki M, et al. Erythema multiforme due to contact with weeds: a recurrence after patch testing. Contact Dermatitis 2003;48:17.

14. DeFeo CP Jr. Erythema multiforme bullosum caused by 9-bromofluorene. Arch Dermatol 1966;94:545.

15. Powell EW. Skin reactions to 9-bromofluorene. Br J Dermatol 1968;80:491.

16. Roed-Petersen J. Erythema multiforme as an expression of contact dermatitis. Contact Dermatitis 1975;1:270.

17. Fregert S, Gustafsson K, Trulsson L. Contact allergy to N-hydroxyphthalimide. Contact Dermatitis 1983;9:84.

Table 7-5 Causes of Anaphylaxis from Topical Exposure

Natural rubber latex
Rubber antioxidants: black rubber mix
Rubber accelerators: carba mix
Antibiotics: bacitracin, neomycin, streptomycin, cephalosporin, rifamycin
Antiseptics: chlorhexidene, mercurochrome
Foods: milk, rice
Anesthetics: lidocaine
Other medications: mechlorethamine, labetalol
Miscellaneous chemicals: chlorothalonil, formaldehyde, Emulgade F

18. Viraben R, Labrousse JL, Bazex J. Erythema multiforme due to DNCB. Contact Dermatitis 1990;22:179.

19. Magnusson B, Gilje O. Allergic contact dermatitis from a dishwashing liquid containing lauryl ether sulphate. Acta Derm Venereol (Stockh) 1973;53:136.

20. Bjornberg A, Mobacken H. Sensitization to benzene compounds. Berufsdermatosen 1972;21:245.

21. Nethercott JR, et al. Erythema multiforme exudativum linked to the manufacture of printed circuit boards. Contact Dermatitis 1982;8:314.

22. Phoon WH, et al. Stevens-Johnson syndrome associated with occupational exposure to trichloroethylene. Contact Dermatitis 1984;10:270.

23. Vincenzi C, Stinchi C, Guerra L, et al. Erythema multiforme–like contact dermatitis: report of 4 cases. Am J Contact Dermat 1994;5:90.

24. Zhang XM, Nakagawa M, Kawai K, Kawai K. Erythema-multiforme–like eruption following photoallergic contact dermatitis from oxybenzone. Contact Dermatitis 1998;38:43.

25. Garcia-Bravo B, Rodriguez-Pichardo A, de Pierola SF, Camacho F. Airborne erythema-multiforme-like eruption due to pyrethrum. Contact Dermatitis 1995;33:433.

26. Bhargave RK, Singh V, Soni V. Erythema multiforme resulting from insecticide spray. Arch Dermatol 1977;113:686.

27. Thompson JA, Wansker BA. A case of contact dermatitis, erythema multiforme and toxic epidermal necrolysis. J Am Acad Dermatol 1981;6:666.

28. Cook LJ. Associated nickel and cobalt contact dermatitis presenting as erythema multiforme. Contact Dermatitis 1982;8:280.

29. Calnan CD. Nickel dermatitis. Br J Dermatol 1956;68:229.

30. Agrup G, Cronin E. Contact dermatitis (X). Br J Dermatol 1970;82:428.

31. Le Coz C-J, Lepoittevin J-P. Occupational erythema-multiforme-like dermatitis from sensitization to costus resinoid, followed by flare-up and systemic contact dermatitis from B-cyclostunolide in a chemistry student. Contact Dermatitis;44;310.

32. Tjiu J-W, Chu C-Y, Sun C-C. 1,2-ethanedithiol-induced erythema multiforme-like contact dermatitis. Acta Dermatol-Venereol 2004;84:393.

33. Degreef H, Bonamie A, van Derheyden D, Dooms-Goossens A. Mephenesin contact dermatitis with erythema multiforme features. Contact Dermatitis 1984;10:220.

34. Meneghini CL, Angelini G. Secondary polymorphic eruptions in allergic contact dermatitis. Dermatologica 1981;163:63.

35. Meneghini CL, Angelini G. Contact dermatitis from pyrrolnitrin. Contact Dermatitis 1982;8:55.

36. Yaffee H, Dressler DP. Topical application of mafenide acetate: its association with erythema multiforme and cutaneous reactions. Arch Dermatol 1969;100:277.

37. Guill MA, et al. Erythema multiforme and urticaria: eruptions induced by chemically related ophthalmic anticholinergic agents. Arch Dermatol 1979;115:742.

38. Gottschalk HR, Stone OJ. Stevens-Johnson syndrome from ophthalmic sulfonamide. Arch Dermatol 1976;112:513.

39. Rubin Z. Ophthalmic sulfonamide-induced Stevens-Johnson syndrome. Arch Dermatol 1977;113:235.

40. Saperstein H, Rapaport M, Rietschel RL. Topical vitamin E as a cause of erythema multiforme–like eruption. Arch Dermatol 1984; 120:906.

41. Kerre S, Busschots A, Dooms-Goossens A. Erythema-multiforme– like contact dermatitis due to phenylbutazone. Contact Dermatitis 1995;33:213.

42. Koch P, Bahmer FA. Erythema-multiforme-like, urticarial papular and plaque eruptions from bufexamac: report of 4 cases. Contact Dermatitis 1994;31:97.

43. Walchner M, Rueff F, Przybilla B. Delayed-type hypersensitivity to mofebutazone underlying a severe drug reaction. Contact Dermatitis 1997;36:54.

44. Stingeni L, et al. Erythema-multiforme-like contact dermatitis from budesonide. Contact Dermatitis 1996; 34:154.

45. Valsecchi R, et al. Erythema-multiforme-like lesions from triamcinolone acetonide. Contact Dermatitis 1998; 38:362.

46. Endo H. Kawada A, Yudate T, et al. Drug eruption due to tribenoside. Contact Dermatitis 1999; 41:223.

47. Monzon S, Garces MM, Reichelt C, et al. Positive patch test in hypersensitivity to lamotrigine. Contact Dermatitis 2002;47:361.

48. Pirker C, Misic A, Brinkmeier T, et al. Tetrazepam drug sensitivity – usefulness of the patch test. Contact Dermatitis 2002;47:135.

49. Puig L, et al. Erythema-multiforme-like eruption due to topical contactants: expression of adhesion molecules and their ligands and characterization of the infiltrate. Contact Dermatitis 1995;33:329.

50. Greenwood K. Dermatitis with capillary fragility. Arch Dermatol 1960;81:947.

51. Hellier FF. Dermatitis purpura after contact with textiles. Hautarzt 1960;11:173.

52. Abel RR. Washing machine and fiberglass. Arch Dermatol 1966; 93:78.

53. Osmundsen PE. Contact dermatitis from an optical whitener in washing powders. Cutis 1972;10:59.

54. Beck MH, Wilkinson SM. A distinctive irritant contact reaction to Vioform (clioquinol). Contact Dermatitis 1994;31:54.

55. Petrozzi JW, Lockshin NA. Pants pressure purpura. Cutis 1974;13:799.

56. Calnan CD, Peachey RDG. Allergic contact purpura. Clin Allergy 1971;1:287.

57. Fisher AA. Allergic petechial and purpuric rubber dermatitis: the PPP syndrome. Cutis 1974;14:25.

58. Romaguera C, Grimalt F. PPPP syndrome. Contact Dermatitis 1977;3:102.

59. Shmunes E. Purpuric allergic contact dermatitis to paraphenylenediamine. Contact Dermatitis 1978;4:225.

60. Agarwal K. Contact allergic purpura to wool dust. Contact Dermatitis 1982;8:281.

61. Romaguera C, Grimalt F, Lecha M. Occupational purpuric textile dermatitis from formaldehyde resins. Contact Dermatitis 1981;7:152.

62. Ackroyd JF. The role of sedormid in the immunological reaction that results in platelet lysis in sedormid purpura. Clin Sci 1954;13:409.

63. Santos-Briz A, Antunez P, Munoz E, et al. Vascular-occlusive contact dermatitis from fepradinol. Contact Dermatitis 2004;50:44.

64. Friedman AL, Brody EA, Barr PS. Immunothrombocytopenic purpura due to quinidine: report of four new cases with special observations on patch testing. J Lab Clin Med 1956;48:205.

65. Schmidt H, Larsen FS, Larson PO, Sogaard H. Petechial reaction following patch testing with cobalt. Contact Dermatitis 1980;6:91.

66. Rorsman H. Riehl's melanosis. Int J Dermatol 1982;21:76.

67. Osmundsen PE. Pigmented contact dermatitis. Br J Dermatol 1970;83:296.

68. Pinol-Aguade J, et al. Dermatitis por blanquedores opticos. Med Cutan 1971;5:249.

69. Ancona-Alayon A, et al. Occupational pigmented contact dermatitis from Naphthol AS. Contact Dermatitis 1976;2:129.

70. Kgzuka T, Tashiro M, Sano S, et al. Pigmented contact dermatitis from azo dyes. I. Cross-sensitivity in humans. Contact Dermatitis 1980;6:330.

71. Nakayama H, Hanaoka H, Ohshiro A. Allergen controlled system (ACS). Tokyo: Kanehara Shuppan Co., 1974.

72. Mathias CGT. Pigmented cosmetic dermatitis from contact allergy to a toilet soap containing chromium. Contact Dermatitis 1982;8:29.

73. Kim M-H, Choi Y-W, Choi H-Y, et al. Prurigo pigmentosa from contact allergy to chrome in detergent. Contact Dermatitis 2001;44:289.

74. Ozkaya-Bayazit E, Buyukbabani N. Non-eczematous pigmented interface dermatitis from para-tertiary-butylphenol-formaldehyde resin in a watchstrap adhesive. Contact Dermatitis 2001;44:45.

75. Addo HA, Ferguson J, Johnson BE, Frain-Bell W. The relationship between exposure to fragrance materials and persistent light reaction in the photosensitivity dermatitis with actinic reticuloid syndrome. Br J Dermatol 1982;107:261.

76. Frain-Bell W, Johnson BE. Contact allergic sensitivity to plants and the photosensitivity dermatitis and actinic reticuloid syndrome. Br J Dermatol 1979;101:503.

77. Ive FA, Magnus IA, Warin RP, Jones EW. "Actinic reticuloid"; a chronic dermatosis associated with severe photosensitivity and the histological resemblance to lymphoma. Br J Dermatol 1969;81:469.

78. Ross JS, du Peloux Menage H, Hawk JL, White IR. Sesquiterpene lactone contact sensitivity: clinical patterns of Compositae dermatitis and relationship to chronic actinic dermatitis. Contact Dermatitis 1993;29:84–87.

79. Abel EA. Mycosis fungoides and occupational exposures: is there an association? Derm Clin 1990;8:169.

80. Calzavara-Pinton P, Capezzera R, Zane C, et al. Lymphomatoid allergic contact dermatitis from para-phenylenediamine. Contact Dermatitis 2002;47:173.

81. Yoshida Y, Duan H, Nakayama J, et al. Lymphadenosis benigna cutis induced by iatrogenic contact dermatitis from dinitrochlorobenzene. Contact Dermatitis 2004;49:165.

82. Evans AV, Banerjee P, McFadden JP, et al. Lymphomatoid contact dermatitis to para-tertyl-butyl phenol resin. Clin Exp Dermatol 2003;28:272.

83. Buckley WR. Lichenoid eruptions following contact dermatitis. Arch Dermatol 1958;78:454.

84. Canizares O. Lichen planus–like eruption caused by color developer. Arch Dermatol 1959;80:81.

85. Mandel EH. Lichen planus–like eruptions caused by a color-film developer. Arch Dermatol 1960;81:516.

86. Roed-Peterson J, Menne T. Allergic contact dermatitis and lichen planus from black and white photographic developing. Cutis 1976;18:699.

87. Knudsen EA. Lichen planus–like eruption caused by color developer. Arch Dermatol 1964;89:357.

88. Sharma VK, Mandal SK, Sethuraman G, Bakshi NA. Para-phenylenediamine-induced lichenoid eruptions. Contact Dermatitis 1999;41:40.

89. Frykholm KO, et al. Allergy to copper derived from dental alloys as a possible cause of oral lesions of lichen planus. Acta Derm Venereol (Stockh) 1969;49:268.

90. Lombardi F, Campolmi P, Sertoli A. Lichenoid dermatitis caused by nickel salts? Contact Dermatitis 1983;9:520.

91. Ido T, Kumakiri M, Kiyohara T, et al. Oral lichen planus due to zinc in dental restorations. Contact Dermatitis 2002;47:51.

92. Lichter M, Drury D, Remlinger K. Lichenoid dermatitis caused by epoxy resin. Contact Dermatitis 1992;26:275.

93. Laine J, Kalimo K, Forssell H, Happonen RP. Resolution of oral lichenoid lesions after replacement of amalgam

restorations in patients allergic to mercury compounds. Br J Dermatol 1992;126:10.

94. Lapiere K, Matthieu L, Meuleman L, et al. Primula dermatitis mimicking lichen planus. Contact Dermatitis 2001;44:199.

95. Deleuran M, Clemmensen O, Andersen KE. Contact lupus erythematosus. Contact Dermatitis 2000;43:169.

96. Andersen KE, Broesby-Olsen S. Contact Dermatitis 2006; 55: 354.

97. Chey WY, Kim KL, Yoo T-Y, et al. Allergic contact dermatitis from hair dye and development of lichen simplex chronicus. Contact Dermatitis 2004; 51: 5.

98. Strauss JS, Jackson EM. American Academy of Dermatology Invitational Symposium on Comedogenicity. J Am Acad Dermatol 1989;20:272.

99. Plewig G, Fulton JE, Kligman AM. Pomade acne. Arch Dermatol 1974;101:580.

100. Taylor JS. Chloracne—a continuing problem. Cutis 1974;13:585.

101. Taylor JS. Environmental acne: update and review. Ann NY Acad Sci 1979;320:295.

102. Violante FS, Milani S, Malenchini G, et al. Chloracne due to o-dichlorobenzene in a laboratory worker. Contact Dermatitis 2005;52:108.

103. Burkhart CG. Pustular allergic contact dermatitis: a distinct clinical and pathological entity. Cutis 1981;27:630.

104. Stone OJ, Johnson DA. Pustular patch test—experimentally induced. Arch Dermatol 1967;95:618.

105. Sanchez-Motilla JM, Pont V, Nagore E, et al. Pustular allergic contact dermatitis from minoxidil. Contact Dermatitis 1998;38:283.

106. Lazarov A, Ingber A. Pustular allergic contact dermatitis to isoconazole nitrate. Am J Contact Dermat 1997;8:229.

107. Hjorth N. Diagnostic patch testing. In: Marzulli F, Maibach HI, eds. Dermatoxicology and pharmacology. New York: John Wiley and Sons, 1977:344.

108. Fisher AA, Chargin L, Fleischmajer R, Hyman A. Pustular patch test reactions: with particular reference to those produced by ammonium fluoride. Arch Dermatol 1959;80:742.

109. Wahlberg JE, Maibach HI. Sterile cutaneous pustules—a manifestation of primary irritancy? J Invest Dermatol 1981;76:381.

110. Uehara M, Takahashi C, Ofuji S. Pustular patch test reactions in atopic dermatitis. Arch Dermatol 1975;111:1154.

111. Christensen OB, Moller H. External and internal exposure to antigen in hand eczema of nickel allergy. Contact Dermatitis 1975;1:136.

112. Fisher AA, Shapiro A. Allergic eczematous contact dermatitis due to metallic nickel. JAMA 1956;161:717.

113. de Boer EM, Bruynzeel DP, van Ketel WG. Dyshidrotic eczema as an occupational dermatitis in metal workers. Contact Dermatitis 1988;19:184.

114. Fisher AA. Contact halogenosis due to fluorinated corticosteroids. Cutis 1975;15:475.

115. Fisher AA. Facial papular dermatitis due to topical fluorinated steroids (so-called perioral or rosacea-like dermatitis). Cutis 1972;10:459.

116. Tappeiner J, Pfleger L. Granuloma gluteale infantum. Hautarzt 1971;22:383.

117. Bazex A, et al. Vegetating granulomas in childhood. Ann Derm Syph (Paris) 1972;99:121.

118. Uyeda K, Nakayasu K, Takaishi Y, Sotomatsu S. Kaposi sarcoma–like granuloma on diaper dermatitis. Arch Dermatol 1973;107:605.

119. Malkinson FD, Pearson RW. Infantile gluteal granuloma (Tappeiner and Pfleger: Should it be considered as "contact dermatitis vegetans or infant halogenosis?"). In: The Yearbook of Dermatology. Chicago: Year Book Medical Publishers, 1973:26.

120. Santucci B, et al. Kaposi-like acro-angiodermatitis of amputation stump caused by suction socket prosthesis. Contact Dermatitis 1992; 7:131.

121. Lazarov A, Kidron D, Tulchinsky Z, et al. Contact orofacial granulomatosis caused by delayed hypersensitivity to gold and mercury. J Am Acad Dermatol 2003;49:1117.

122. Savin JA, Alexander S, Marks R. A rosacea-like eruption of children. Br J Dermatol 1972;87:425.

123. Burry JN. Topical drug addiction: adverse effects of fluorinated corticosteroid creams and ointments. Med J Aust 1973;1:393.

124. Almeyda J, Burt BW. Double-blind controlled study of treatment of atopic eczema with a preparation of hydrocortisone in a new drug delivery system versus betamethasone 17—valerate. Br J Dermatol 1974;91:579.

125. Sneddon I. Adverse effect of topical corticosteroids in rosacea. Br Med J 1969;1:671.

126. Weber G. Rosacea-like dermatitis: contraindication or intolerance reaction to strong steroids. Br J Dermatol 1972;88:253.

127. Rapaport MJ, Rapaport V. Eyelid dermatitis to red face syndrome to cure: clinical experience in 100 cases. J Am Acad Dermatol 1999; 41(3 Pt 1):435.

128. Epstein NN, Epstein WL, Epstein JB. Atrophic striae in patients with inguinal intertrigo. Arch Dermatol 1963;87:450.

129. Johns AM, Bower BD. Wasting of napkin area after repeated use of fluorinated steroid ointment. Br Med J 1970;1:347.

130. Scoggins RB, Kligman AM. Relative potency of percutaneously absorbed corticosteroids in suppression of pituitary-adrenal function. J Invest Dermatol 1965;45:347.

131. Feiwel M, James VHT, Barnett ES. Effect of potent topical steroids in plasma-cortisol levels of infants and children with eczema. Lancet 1969;1:485.

132. Foussereau J, Beneczra C. Les eczemas allergiques professionels. Paris: Masson et Cie, 1970.

133. Pardo-Castello V. Epilating folliculitis. Derm Trop 1965;2:235.

134. Shelley WB, Hurley HJ, Mayock RL, et al. Intradermal tests with metals and other inorganic elements in sarcoidosis and anthraco-silicosis. J Invest Derm 1958;31:301.

135. Sheard G. Granulomatous reactions due to deodorant sticks. *JAMA* 1957;164:1085.

136. Rubin L. Granulomas of axillae caused by deodorants. *JAMA* 1956;162:953.

137. Williams RM, Skipworth GB. Zirconium granulomas of glabrous skin following treatment of rhus dermatitis. Arch Dermatol 1959;80:273.

138. Epstein WL, Allen JR. Granulomatous hypersensitivity after use of zirconium-containing poison oak lotions. JAMA 1964;190:162.

139. Baler GR. Granulomas from topical zirconium in poison ivy dermatitis. Arch Dermatol 1965;91:145.

140. Shelley WB, Hurley HJ. Allergic origin of zirconium deodorant granuloma. Br J Dermatol 1958;70:75.

141. LoPresti PJ, Hambrick GW. Zirconium granuloma following treatment of rhus dermatitis. Arch Dermatol 1965;92:188.

142. Kaaber K, Nielsen AO, Veien NK. Vaccination granulomas and aluminum allergy: course and prognostic factors. Contact Dermatitis 1992;26:304.

143. McCallum DI, Hall GFM. Umbilical granulomata—with particular reference to talc granuloma. Br J Dermatol 1970;83:151.

144. Tye MJ, Hashimoto K, Fox F. Talc granulomas of the skin. JAMA 1966;198:120.

145. Bergeron JR, Stone OJ. Multiple granulomas of the scalp of exogenous origin. Cutis 1969;5:57.

146. Sneddon I_B. Dust and the skin. Med Presse 1958;21:1102.

147. Rycroft RJG, Calnan CD. Irritant dermatitis during the relining of a blast furnace. Contact Dermatitis 1977;3:75.

148. Skevi M, Mizuno F. Unusual cornification in ichthyosis-like dermatitis. Arch Dermatol 1970;50:388.

149. Fisher AA. Occupational palmar psoriasis due to safety prescription container caps. Contact Dermatitis 1979;5:56.

150. Nielsen NH, Menne T. Allergic contact dermatitis caused by zinc pyrithione associated with pustular psoriasis. Am J Contact Dermat 1997;8:170.

151. Jo J-H, Jang H-S, Ko H-C, et al. Pustular psoriasis and the Koebner phenomenon caused by allergic contact dermatitis from zinc pyrithione-containing shampoo. Contact Dermatitis 2005; 52:142.

152. Adams RM. Occupational contact dermatitis. Philadelphia: JB Lippincott Co., 1969.

153. Lynde CW, Mitchell JC. Unusual complication of allergic contact dermatitis of the hands—recurrent lymphangitis and persistent lymphoedema. Contact Dermatitis 1982;8:279.

154. Worm A-M, Staberg B, Thomsen K. Persistent oedema in allergic contact dermatitis. Contact Dermatitis 1983;9:516.

155. Worm A-M. Exchange of macromolecules between plasma and skin interstitium in extensive skin disease. J Invest Dermatol 1981;76:489.

156. Piller NB, Casley-Smith JR. The effect of coumarin on protein and PVP clearance from rat legs with various high protein oedemas. Br J Exp Pathol 1975;56:439.

157. Kiec-Swierczynska M, Krecisz B. Occupational contact allergy to nifuroxazide simulating prurigo nodularis. Contact Dermatitis 1998;39:93.

158. Penagos H, et al. Chorothalonil, a possible cause of erythema dyschromicum perstans (ashy dermatitis). Contact Dermatitis 1996;35:214.

159. Sambucety PS, Agapito PG, Prieto MAR. Contact erythema annulare centrifugum. Contact Dermatitis 2006;55:309.

160. Marty CL, Cheng JF. Granuloma annulare presenting as contact dermatitis. Dermatitis 2005;16:34.

161. Chavarria Mur E, Ballesteros M G-C, Fernandez RS, et al Generalized exanthematous reaction with pustulosis induced by topical corticosteroids. Contact Dermatitis 2005;52:114.

162. De Thier F, Blondeel A, Song M. Acute generalized exanthematous pustulosis induced by amoxicillin with clavulanate. Contact Dermatitis 2001;44:114.

163. Sahoo B, Kumar B. Role of methylchloroisothiazolinone/methylisothiazolinone (Kathon CG) in poikiloderma of Civatte. Contact Dermatitis 2001;44:249.

164. Lenane P, McKenna D, Murphy GM. Pyoderma gangrenosum secondary to allergic contact dermatitis from rubber. Contact Dermatitis 1998;38:238.

165. Staines KS, Felix DH, Forsyth A. Desquamative gingivitis, sole manifestation of tosylamide/formaldehyde resin allergy. Contact Dermatitis 1998;39:90.

166. Komatsu H, Aiba S, Mori S, et al. Lymphocytoma cutis involving the lower lip. Contact Dermatitis 1997;36:167.

167. Zemtsov A, Cameron GS, Montalvo-Lugo V. Nickel-induced lymphocytoma cutis of the earlobe. Contact Dermatitis 1997;36:266.

168. Corazza M, Lombardi AR, Virgili A. Non-eczematous urticarioid allergic contact dermatitis due to Eumulgin L in a deodorant. Contact Dermatitis 1997;36:159.

169. Guerra L, Rogkakou A, Massacane P, et al. Role of contact sensitization in chronic urticaria. J Am Acad Dermatol 2007;56:88.

170. Skinner SL, Fowler JF Jr. Contact anaphylaxis: a review. Am J Contact Dermat 1995;6:133.

SYSTEMIC CONTACT-TYPE DERMATITIS

EXECUTIVE SUMMARY

The concept of systemic contact-type dermatitis includes flare-up of earlier patch test reactions, pompholyx, generalized maculopapular eruptions, erythema multiforme, vasculitis, the baboon syndrome, urticaria, and anaphylaxis.

Medications that cause systemic-type reactions include many antibiotics, nystatin, acyclovir, phenothiazines, benzodiazepines, salicylates, piroxicam, anticonvulsants, corticosteroids, halogenated hydroxyquinolines, resorcinol, and chloral hydrate. Cardiovascular agents such as nitroglycerin, mexiletine, captopril, pseudoephedrine, and salbutamol have produced this type of reaction. Also on the list are vitamins B1, B5, B12, hydrazine, parabens, sorbic acid, thimerosal, phenoxyethanol, cinnamon oil, balsam of Peru, garlic, *Toxicodendron*, disulfiram, quinine, quinidine, hydroxyzine, 5-fluorouracil, and fluoride. Dental metals and ingested metals have also been confirmed to produce this reaction.

Allergic eczematous contact dermatitis is produced ordinarily by external exposure of the skin to an allergen. Occasionally, however, in sensitized individuals a systematically administered allergen may reach the skin through the circulatory system and produce a hematogenous contact-type dermatitis. Although the eczematous condition is produced by systemic administration, the first sensitizing exposure to the allergen may have been by topical application. In such instances, an eczematous contact type of eruption may be produced not only by the sensitizing allergen but also by allergens that are related immunochemically.[1]

Ingestion of an allergen by a person sensitized previously by contact may result in a variety of reactions. Most frequent reactions are focal flares at sites of previous dermatitis or occasionally dyshidrotic eruptions, but generalized eruptions may occur. Sometimes such flares may occur also from *inhalation* of the allergen.

This type of endogenic contact eczema from ingestion or systemic administration of an allergen may be accompanied occasionally by systemic effects.

In relation to positive oral provocation with nickel and medicaments, general symptoms, such as headaches, fever, and malaise, may occur. In neomycin- and chromate-sensitive patients, oral provocation with hapten may produce nausea, vomiting, and diarrhea.[2,3]

Types of Systemic Contact Dermatitis

POMPHOLYX, DYSHIDROTIC HAND ECZEMA

This consists of recurring itching eruptions with deeply seated vesicles with some or no erythema, localized on the palms, volar aspects, and sides of the fingers. Exacerbations come at weekly to monthly intervals without obvious, external reasons. Patch testing may not be the best predictive test to identify all the patients who have dyshidrosiform hand dermatitis related to ingested materials. Veien[4] studied 202 patients with vesicular hand eczema and negative patch tests and found 58 to be reactive to oral provocation tests to substances, such as nickel (2.5 mg), cobalt (1 mg), and chromate (2.5 mg). However, oral provocation tests were more frequently positive when patch tests were also positive.

FLARE-UPS OF EARLIER PATCH TEST REACTIONS

This phenomenon has been observed experimentally in provocation studies with nickel and chromium in patients sensitized to these metals, medicaments, and poison ivy. The specificity with which skin reacts to topical and systemic exposure can be seen in the case of a patient with a fixed drug eruption to ibuprofen reported by Kuligowski and colleagues.[5] Systemic exposure to ibuprofen produced several lesions of a fixed drug eruption pattern. A 1% petrolatum patch test to one prior lesion flared all the other prior lesions, but a 10% patch test on normal skin produced no reaction.[4]

GENERALIZED MACULOPAPULAR-VESICULAR RASH

This rash consists of a symmetric eruption localized to the elbow flexures, axillae, eyelids, side of the neck, and genital area. This pattern seems characteristic of the systemic contact dermatitis reaction.

ERYTHEMA MULTIFORME AND VASCULITIS

Dissemination of allergic contact dermatitis in the form of erythema multiforme, such as purpura and vasculitis, has been observed in patients sensitive to topically applied drugs.[6] An example of the value of patch testing in suspected vasculitis can be found in the report of the benzodiazepine tetrazepam that caused a leukocytoclastic vasculitis of the legs and was patch test positive to a 1% petrolatum concentration.[7]

Unusual routes of exposure occasionally have been associated with induction of erythema multiforme patterns, andHayakawa and colleagues[8] reported a patient who had been sensitized to amlexanox (2-amino-7-isopropyl-5-oxo-5H-[1] benzopyrano [2,3-b]-3-carboxylic acid) in an ophthalmic solution. Oral ingestion of 50 mg of amlexanox subsequently for otitis media produced an erythema multiforme–like eruption. Occupational exposure to ethyl ethyoxymethylene cyanoacetate (EEMC), which is an intermediate in the synthesis of allopurinol, caused contact dermatitis.[9] Subsequent exposure to vapors of EEMC produced an erythema multiforme–like eruption in the sites of former dermatitis, and a 0.01% petrolatum patch test of EEMC was eczematous.[9] Contact allergens associated with erythema multiforme have been summarized by O'Donnell and Tan (Table 8.1).[10]

Circular excoriations on the back, buttocks, and thighs have been observed in nickel-sensitive women.[11] Similar excoriations have been noticed in two nickel-sensitive patients treated with a nickel-chelating drug. Histopathology shows superficial allergic vasculitis.

BABOON SYNDROME

The baboon syndrome involves an eruption that is most prominent on the buttocks and is bright red, resembling

Table 8-1 Contact Allergens Producing Erythema Multiforme

Tropical woods	Mofebutazone
Plants	Budesonide
Poison ivy	Triamcinolone acetonide
Primula	Bufexamac
Terpenes	Chloramphenicol
Saint John's wort *(Hypericum erectum)*	Econazole
Pyrethrum	Idoxuridine
Inula helenium	Ketoprofen
Thuja essential oil	Lincomycin
Capsicum	Mafenide acetate
Laboratory chemicals	Mephenesin
Brominated compounds	Neomycin
N-hydroxyphthalamide	Proflavin
Phenyl sulfone derivatives	Pyrrolnitrin
Deflazacort	Phenylbutazone
Dinitrochlorobenzene	*Miscellaneous compounds*
Diphenylcyclopropenone	Epoxy resin
Medications	Formaldehyde
Ethylenediamine	Soap
Iodochlorhydroxyquin (Vioform)	Spray cologne
Mephenesin (Europe)	Trichloroethylene
Promethazine	Oxybenzone
Scopolamine	Disperse blue 124
Sulfonamides	Hair dyes
Povidone-iodine solution	Paratertiary butylphenol formaldehyde resin
Vitamin E	

the buttocks of a baboon. Agents incriminated in the baboon syndrome include penicillin V, aminophylline, nickel, cimetidine, erythromycin, ampicillin, mercury, and amoxicillin. The term "baboon syndrome" has been challenged as culturally problematic and is a less-than-complete descriptive term for eruptions that favor the buttocks and other flexural areas. In their review, Haeusermann and colleagues point out that most of these cases arise from orally administered drugs and not from cutaneous sensitization followed by a subsequent systemic exposure. Because other flexural areas are commonly involved, they prefer the term SDRIFE, an acronym for "symmetrical drug-related intertriginous and flexural exanthema." Their review covered 42 cases in which orally ingested drugs were responsible for the eruption and 8 in which prior contact dermatitis set the stage for the clinical presentation. The topical exposures included ampicillin, neomycin, aminophylline (2 cases), 5-aminosalicylic acid, bufexamac, and cinchocaine (2 cases).[12]

URTICARIA AND ANAPHYLAXIS

Eczematous systemic contact dermatitis may be accompanied occasionally by urticaria. Rapid absorption through either intact skin or open wounds may rarely lead to anaphylaxis. Such was the case when rifamycin SV was applied on gauze to a leg ulcer. Contact urticaria outlined the shape of the gauze, and anaphylaxis and shock followed in 40 minutes.[13] The patient recovered, and a 0.05% aqueous open test was positive at 20 minutes, as was a Prausnitz-Küstner test, suggesting the reaction was IgE mediated. A patch test has rarely been reported to cause anaphylaxis. The nonselective beta-adrenergic blocking agent labetalol tested at 0.1% aqueous solution caused anaphylaxis within 90 to 150 seconds without contact urticaria.[14]

A patient who had high levels of IgE to formaldehyde and delayed hypersensitivity to formaldehyde underwent root canal treatment. The root-canal disinfectant contained paraformaldehyde, which slowly released formaldehyde over a period of several hours, resulting in a delayed onset of anaphylaxis. Patch tests showed reactions to formaldehyde, paraformaldehyde, and eugenol. Prick tests to 1% aqueous formaldehyde and paraformaldehyde were positive at 20 minutes. The authors found 15 similar cases in the literature, 7 of which showed a delay of allergic symptoms of up to 12 hours after root canal treatment.[15] Anaphylactoid reactions from patch tests are rare. A nurse developed signs and symptoms of immediate hypersensitivity manifested by a wheal-and-flare reaction after skin contact with cefotiam hydrochloride. After continued exposure she experienced cough, nausea, abdominal pain, and diarrhea. When patch tested with cefotiam hydrochloride 20% in physiologic saline, she developed a wheal at the patch test site and then total body whealing and abdominal pain. Intravenous antihistamine and corticosteroid resolved the symptoms, and a lymphocyte stimulation test was found to be positive with a stimulation index of 315%. This is considered a case of stage 3 contact urticaria syndrome. In separate prick testing, immediate hypersensitivity was confirmed without systemic complications.[16]

Patch Testing in Systemic Contact Dermatitis

Patch testing with the chemicals mentioned in this chapter may be valuable not only in determining the cause of an allergic contact dermatitis, but also in serving as a warning that the systemic administration of a related drug may produce an eczematous contact-type dermatitis medicamentosa. In addition, the epidermal contact type of sensitivity may be accompanied by the urticarial, anaphylactoid variety, particularly when penicillin is the cause. A positive patch test reaction to penicillin usually precludes its systemic use. Occasionally, the reactions to patch tests with penicillin and other drugs are positive when the scratch and intracutaneous test reactions are negative.

It is much safer to perform a patch test with a drug suspected of producing an eczematous dermatitis medicamentosa than to re-administer even a tiny fractional dose of the drug to prove that it is the culprit. Such proof may result in a widespread, disabling eruption.

In evaluating the significance of a positive patch test reaction to a medication, one must have knowledge of immunochemically related agents. Such considerations may explain an allergic (contact-type) eczematous eruption after an exposure to one or more compounds to which an individual has never previously been exposed. The cross-reaction phenomenon may also explain the persistence of allergic reactions in some patients long after the original agent has been avoided.

When several drugs have been administered concurrently or in combination and the patient has experienced an eczematous flare-up, patch tests may be of value in determining the culprit. For example, if the patient develops an eruption following the administration of a penicillin-streptomycin combination, the drug that causes a positive patch test reaction would be implicated. Such patch tests are safer than scratch or intracutaneous tests.

Mechanism of Systemic Contact Dermatitis

The clinical observation of rapid onset (within hours) of the effect of oral exposure to haptens in sensitized individuals suggests that mechanisms other than an allergic type 4 reaction are involved. It is not unusual for the nickel-sensitive patient who is provoked with nickel to develop a systemic eruption within hours, and after 12 to 48 hours to exhibit a flare in hand dermatitis. There is evidence that the systemic reaction to ingested haptens can be mediated by both a type 3 and a type 4 immunologic reaction. The immunologic reactivity, judged from a rise in the lymphocytic transformation test, can be maintained by oral ingestion of a hapten.[17]

Medicaments

Systemic contact dermatitis resulting from medicaments has been reviewed by Fisher[18] and Cronin.[19] Usually, sensitization has taken place by topical application of the drug; later, the patient has a systemic reaction when the drug or immunochemically related allergen is taken orally or parenterally. The opposite situation can occur, in which a patient first has an exanthema owing to an antibiotic and later develops a localized dermatitis when the drug is applied topically. Pirila[20] termed this phenomenon "primary endogenic contact eczema."

At the European Contact Dermatitis Society Meeting in Brussels in 1992, Bruynzeel and Camarasa[21] reported that their highest yield in patch testing drug eruptions actually came from testing morbilliform and even urticarial patterns rather than eczematous dermatitis cases. They recommend testing 6 to 12 weeks after the eruption clears, preferably with a pure drug in powder form with a concentration of 1% to 5% in a vehicle known to solubilize the drug. The latter information is available in pharmaceutical texts. Tablets or capsules can be used when pure drugs are not available. They also found the best concentration for penicillin, amoxicillin, aminoglycocides, and cephalosporins to be 20%. A safe way to proceed is to perform a 20-minute open test, then a 48-hour closed test.[21]

Antibiotics

Topical use of penicillin and streptomycin should be avoided because of the high sensitization potential.[22] Although neomycin has been reported to produce many instances of allergic contact dermatitis, it is still used widely. The other antibiotics, such as the tetracyclines, erythromycin, and chloramphenicol, rarely produce allergic contact dermatitis.

PENICILLIN

Topical use of penicillin is largely avoided at present because many individuals would develop contact sensitivity to the drug. Allergic contact dermatitis from penicillin occurs particularly in physicians, nurses, and pharmacists who handle this antibiotic. Systemic administration of penicillin to such "externally" sensitized individuals may produce an eczematous, contact-type dermatitis, which may be accompanied by urticarial, anaphylactic sensitivity. Penicillin in milk was the cause of attacks of eczema in two patients, both of whom were sensitive to penicillin on patch testing.[23]

STREPTOMYCIN

Although topical application of streptomycin is now avoided, members of the medical, nursing, and pharmaceutical professions who handle the drug readily become sensitized, and subsequent systemic administration may produce a severe eczematous contact-type dermatitis medicamentosa. Because streptomycin may crossreact with neomycin, systemic administration of streptomycin may produce the eczematous contact-type dermatitis in individuals who had become sensitized to neomycin but had never been exposed to streptomycin. Streptomycin may also crossreact with kanamycin sulfate (Kantrex).

Streptomycin may be administered alone or in combination with penicillin in preparations such as Strep-Combiotic (Pfizer), Bivillimycin (Wyeth), and Wycillin (Wyeth). Desensitization procedures by subcutaneous injection of streptomycin may be accompanied by urticaria or flares of dermatitis.

NEOMYCIN SULFATE

Not only is this antibiotic present in a host of ointments, creams, and other topical medications, but it also has been added to cosmetics, soaps, and deodorants.[24] It has a significant capacity to produce allergic contact sensitivity.[25] Once sensitization to neomycin from topical exposure has been established, systemic administration of either streptomycin or kanamycin, both of which may crossreact with neomycin, may cause an eczematous contact-type dermatitis medicamentosa.[26]

In addition, although neomycin and bacitracin are not related chemically, in many instances there is a combined sensitivity to these two drugs. Such occurrences represent coincidental simultaneous sensitization rather than true cross-sensitivity.[27]

Pirila and Rantanen[28] gave an account of repeated eruptions in a patient sensitive to neomycin and bacitracin because of their topical use on an amputation stump. Later, the patient developed a severe stomatitis from throat tablets containing bacitracin and from a paste containing both antibiotics used to fill an infected root canal. Oral administration of neomycin produced diarrhea and dermatitis. Ekelund and Moller[29] also produced dermatitis by the oral administration of neomycin in sensitized patients. Previous patch test sites flared.

Neomycin may be administered systemically in Baci-mycin, Cremomycin, Kaomycin, Mycifradin, Paremycin, Prednicidin, Sorboquel with Neomycin, and Sulfacidin.

Neomycin shows strong cross-sensitization with par-omomycin and ambutyrosin (CL-642) because of the presence of neosamine sugars in all three (W. Schorr, personal communication).

TETRACYCLINES

These antibiotics are safe to apply topically, because allergic contact dermatitis occurs rarely from such usage. Eczematous eruptions of the fixed type do result occasionally from systemic administration.[30] Furthermore, cross-fixed drug eruptions from systemic use of chlortetracycline (Aureomycin), tetracycline (Achromycin), and oxytetracycline (Terramycin) have been described.[31]

In rare instances in which allergic contact dermatitis does occur from use of Aureomycin or Achromycin ointment, the sensitizer may be the parabens added as preservatives or the certified azo dyes.

ERYTHROMYCIN (ILOTYCIN, ILOSONE, ERYTHROCIN, AND PEDIAMYCIN)

Topical sensitization to this antibiotic is rare. Ilotycin ointment does not contain parabens or coloring matter.

CHLORAMPHENICOL

The report by Schwank and Jirasek[32] that there was cross-sensitization between 2,4-dinitrochlorbenzene and chloramphenicol was not confirmed by Palacios and colleagues.[33] Dr. J. E. Rasmussen (personal communication) has also failed to find such cross-sensitization.

BACITRACIN

Roupe and Strannegard[34] stated that a case of anaphy-lactic shock followed topical administration of an ointment containing bacitracin and neomycin. Antiba-citracin reagins were demonstrated in sera from the patient who had atopic dermatitis. There is strong evidence that the anaphylactic shock was due to hypersensitivity to bacitracin.

CEPHALOSPORINS

A morbilliform eruption was traced to cefuroxime by patch testing with 0.1 mL of a 100 mg/mL solution in normal saline. The same concentrations of cephalothin and cephaloridine were also positive.[35] There was no sign of immediate hypersensitivity to cephalosporins or either major or minor penicillin determinants. Bruynzeel and Camarisa[21] report that in their experience crossreactions among cephalosporins are infrequent.

Sulfonamides

Crossreactions can occur between the antibacterial sulfo-namides and chemically related sulfonamides used as diuretics, oral hypoglycemics, and sweetening agents. Topical application of a sulfonamide may sensitize the patient, and subsequent systemic administration of a sulfonamide may produce eczematous contact-type der-matitis medicamentosa.[36]

SULFANILAMIDE

The systemic administration of this older sulfonamide preparation has largely been discarded. Exposure to sul-fanilamide, however, may still take place from topical application of the medications shown in Table 8.2.

Compounds containing sulfanilamide may be sensi-tizers and photoallergic agents and may crossreact with chemicals with a para-amino group and with diuretics such as hydrochlorothiazide (hydro-diuril) and thiazide antihypertensive drugs, which may be photosensitizers.[37]

THE ROLE OF SULFONAMIDE DRUGS IN DIABETICS

Many adult diabetics receive oral "para-amino" hypogly-cemic sulfonyl-urea drugs, such as tolbutamide (Orinase) and chlorpropamide (Diabinese). These diabetic patients may become sensitized to widely used topical para-amino compounds, such as hair dyes, particularly para-phenyle-nediamine, sunscreens containing para-aminobenzoic acid (PABA) or its esters, and local anesthetics, such as benzocaine. In addition, sensitization to the less widely used topical para-amino sulfanilamide compounds poses the threat of a systemic contact dermatitis to the ingestion of the closely related antidiabetic drugs and sulfonamide-sweetening agents (Tables 8.3 and 8.4).

Table 8-2 Sulfanilamide Topical Agents Still in Use
AVC Cream (Merrell-National)
AVC Suppositories (Merrell-National)
Cervex Vaginal Cream (Medics)

Table 8-3 Sulfonamide Oral Hypoglycemic Agents
Carbutamide (Nadisan)*
Diabinese (chlorpropamide)
Orinase (tolbutamide)

*Still used in Europe.

Table 8-4 Sulfonamide Sweetening Agents
Calcium cyclamate
Saccharin
Sodium cyclamate
Sucaryl
Sweeta

Thus, a patient sensitized to a topical sulfanilamide cream may acquire a systemic contact dermatitis from tolbutamide (Orinase) or other oral sulfonamide hypoglycemic drugs or by sulfonamide-sweetening agents. It should be noted that all of the oral hypoglycemic compounds and sweetening agents are para-amino sulfonamide compounds (Tables 8.3 and 8.4).

It has long been known that topical agents containing an amino group in the para position of the benzene ring are sensitizers. Such agents include paraphenylenediamine, PABA and its esters, certain local anesthetics (e.g., benzocaine), and sulfanilamide.

These para-amino compounds may crossreact with one another and with azo and aniline dyes. Allergic contact dermatitis may occur readily from exposure to paraphenylenediamine in hair and fur dyes. Of the topical anesthetics in this group, benzocaine is the most notorious sensitizer. The salts of para-aminobenzoic acid used in sunscreens occasionally sensitize, but the acid is not as potent a sensitizer as its esters. Although sulfanilamide is used sparingly as a topical medication at present, exposure to the topical agents shown in Table 8.2 may still take place.

Once a diabetic patient is sensitized to a topical sulfanilamide medication or other para-amino compound, the systemic administration of sulfanilamide-containing compounds, such as tolbutamide (Orinase) and chlorpropamide (Diabinese), may produce a systemic contact dermatitis. Tolbutamide [Orinase; 1-butyl-3-(p-tolylsulfonyl) urea] and chlorpropamide [Diabinese; 1-(p-chlorophenylsulfonyl)-3-propylurea], are widely used hypoglycemic drugs that are photosensitizers (38–40). The fact that they can produce a systemic contact dermatitis in patients sensitized to topical para-amino compounds is not so well known.[41]

Angelini and Meneghini[42] reported that a group of 34 patients who had contact allergy to para-amino compounds (sulfanilamide, paraphenylenediamine, and benzocaine) underwent a series of peroral tests using the structurally related substances sulfonyl ureas (carbutamide, tolbutamide, and chlorpropamide), diaminodiphenylsulfone, saccharin, and salicylazosulfapyridine. They found that these sulfonyl urea drugs given orally produced a widespread dermatitis in 11 subjects who had contact sensitivity to sulfanilamide, but not in those sensitized to paraphenylenediamine and benzocaine.

The positive results in 11 of 34 inpatients who reacted were as follows: (a) itching in all 11 patients, (b) the reappearance of erythema and vesicles at the site of the primary contact dermatitis in six patients, and (c) the relapse of the primary contact dermatitis with a moderate secondary vesicular eruption together with a reactivation of the patch test reaction in five patients. The provocative oral tests were considered positive when at least one of the following was produced: pruritus with recurrence of the primary dermatitis, spread of eczematous lesions, or reactivation of the patch test reactions.

In Italy, where topical sulfanilamide is apparently still used on leg ulcers and wounds, it was found that patients who were sensitized to such topical application had a positive response to the oral provocative tests with the hypoglycemic drugs, whereas those who were sensitized to other substances of the para-amino group, such as paraphenylenediamine and benzocaine, did not react.

Angelini and Meneghini[42] further state that none of the patients who were sensitized to sulfanilamide, paraphenylenediamine, or benzocaine reacted to the ingestion of saccharin. Although the sweetening agents shown in Table 8.4 are all sulfanilamide compounds, there are as yet no reports of "systemic" contact dermatitis in individuals using these agents who have been sensitized to topically applied para-amino compounds.

NYSTATIN

Oral nystatin is generally regarded as an oral agent that is not absorbed. However, fixed drug eruption and generalized systemic contact dermatitis have occurred with oral ingestion, and as little as 125,000 IU can cause generalized dermatitis.[43] A patch test with 30,000 IU in polyethylene glycol was positive in a patient after oral ingestion of nystatin, and no crossreaction was found to amphotericin B. The range of reactions to nystatin includes maculopapular eruption, maculopapular eruption accompanied by fever and arthralgia, acute generalized exanthematous pustulosis (AGEP), fixed drug eruption, and Stevens-Johnson syndrome. Positive patch tests to 20% nustatin in petrolatum confirm this sensitivity.[44]

ACYCLOVIR

Systemic contact dermatitis occurred on oral administration of acyclovir in a patient who previously had been sensitized to topical acyclovir. The reaction to oral acyclovir was urticarial, and on challenge with famciclovir an erythematous dermatitis of the trunk and extremities developed. Oddly, patch tests to famciclovir were negative but those to acyclovir were positive.

The patient also reacted to valacyclovir and propylene glycol.[45]

Phenothiazines

All phenothiazines are potential photosensitizers. Medical and nursing personnel who inject these drugs and those handling the compounds in the pharmaceutical industry readily acquire allergic eczematous contact dermatitis from such exposure. Often a photoallergic reaction occurs in combination with the contact dermatitis.[46] Systemic administration of the phenothiazine drugs may produce an eczematous contact-type dermatitis medicamentosa in individuals sensitized by topical application. Crossreactions take place readily between phenothiazines and related antihistamines such as promethazine (Phenergan), isothipendyl (Theruhistin), and pyrathiazine (Pyrrolazotte). Methylene blue, a phenothiazine dye, is also a powerful photosensitizer. Nurses sensitized to chlorpromazine have been desensitized by taking the drug orally. Positive patch test reactions have been reported to become negative after such procedures.[47]

Because chlorpromazine in particular is excreted almost unchanged in the urine, sensitized hospital personnel who handle urine-contaminated bed linen unprotected may acquire allergic contact dermatitis.

CROSSREACTIONS BETWEEN THE PHENOTHIAZINE ANTIHISTAMINES AND OTHER PHENOTHIAZINE COMPOUNDS

The phenothiazine drugs listed in Table 8.5 are all capable of crossreacting with the phenothiazine antihistamines, and all of these compounds are potential sensitizers. Often a photoallergic reaction occurs in combination with allergic eczematous contact dermatitis. The systemic administration of the phenothiazine drugs shown in Table 8.5 may produce an eczematous contact-type dermatitis medicamentosa in individuals sensitized by such topical exposure. Crossreactions take place readily between these phenothiazines and the related antihistamines.

Benzodiazepines

A generalized dermatitis occurred in two patients as a result of ingestion of tetrazepam given as a muscle relaxant. A 1% aqueous patch test to pure powder proved positive in both patients and negative in 30 controls.[48]

Table 8-5 Phenothiazine Antihistamines

Generic name	Trade name
Methdilazine hydrochloride	Tacaryl
Promethazine hydrochloride	Phenergan
Trimeprazine tartrate	Temaril

Drugs that Crossreact with Phenothiazine Antihistamines

Generic name	Trade name
Chlorpromazine	Thorazine
Prochlorperazine	Compazine
Trifluoperazine hydrochloride	Stelazine
Trifluopromazine	Vesprin
Trimeprazine tartrate	Temaril

Similarly, clobazepam was suspected of causing a generalized drug eruption. A crushed tablet in petrolatum caused a positive patch test and 36 hours later a generalized eruption.[49]

Anticonvulsants

Anticonvulsants are associated with dermatitis, fever, lymphadenopathy, eosinophilia and liver abnormalities. This is sometimes referred to as the DRESS syndrome (drug reaction with eosinophilia and systemic symptoms). Reactivation of human herpesvirus 6 and other herpes viruses occurs as a component of this syndrome. The anticonvulsants sodium valproate and ethosuximide were incriminated in a case involving a 6-year-old boy and confirmed oral rechallenge and positive patch tests to 20% aqueous mixes of the drugs. The positive patch test to sodium valproate was followed by a generalized eruption.[50]

Salicylates and Aspirin

Acetylsalicylic acid is a rare contact sensitizer. One patient sensitized to methyl salicylate developed a systemic contact dermatitis when treated with aspirin. A patch test with aspirin was negative but with sodium salicylate was positive. Hindson[51] suggests that the common intermediate metabolite was the cause of the systemic reaction.

PIROXICAM

The nonsteroidal anti-inflammatory drug piroxicam causes photosensitivity. Animals sensitized to thimerosal develop both contact and photocontact dermatitis on exposure to piroxicam alone or to piroxicam plus ultraviolet A (UVA) light.[52] Because piroxicam photosensitivity begins rapidly after ingestion, it was initially thought to be a phototoxic drug. Later it was learned that the rapid onset of photodermatitis could be explained by a crossreaction to thimerosal.[53] Studies found that no new photo product was produced when piroxicam was exposed to light, but when L-cysteine was added to piroxicam and UVA light, a product capable of causing a positive patch test in those patients clinically photosensitive to piroxicam was produced.[53] The thiosalicyclate portion of thimerosal, as well as thimerosal itself, produces positive reactions in patients with clinical piroxicam photodermatitis, and it is felt that these are photoallergic reactions.[54]

CORTICOSTEROIDS

It is helpful to remember that erythroderma (covered elsewhere in this book) has been produced by as little as 1 mg of several corticoids: hydrocortisone sodium phosphate, hydrocortisone butyrate, and budesonide.[55] In this case, adrenocorticotrophic hormone (ACTH) did not reproduce the systemic reaction.

Several cases of systemic dermatitis from oral ingestion of deflazacort, a corticosteroid sold in Spain, have been reported, including one of toxic epidermal necrolysis. An additional case presented with the baboon syndrome and a histology of erythema multiforme, and after patch testing, this individual experienced a widespread eruption. Crossreaction with other corticosteroids was not observed or predicted based on the unique chemical structure of deflazacort.[56]

Halogenated Hydroxyquinolines

These therapeutic agents include iodochlorhydroxyquin (Vioform), iodoquinol (Diodoquin), chlorquinaldol (Sterosan), and halquinol (Quinolor). Such preparations are commonly used topical agents. In addition, Vioform and Diodoquin may be administered systemically. Cross-sensitization between these compounds may exist. Vioform and Diodoquin administered orally may lead to an eczematous dermatitis medicamentosa in patients sensitized by topical application of any one of this group of compounds.[57]

QUINOLOR COMPOUND

This ointment consists of chlorhydroxyquinoline, benzoyl peroxide, menthol, methyl salicylate, and eugenol in a Plasti-base vehicle. When dermatitis occurs from its use, the chlorhydroxyquinoline is not necessarily the culprit; the benzoyl peroxide, eugenol, and Plastibase (a polyethylene compound related to Carbowax) can all cause allergic reactions.

Resorcinol (Resorcin)

Individuals sensitized to resorcin are usually also sensitized to resorcinol monoacetate (Euresol), which is present in Ar-Ex RMS Lotion and Scalp Lotion, Resulin-F, and Sulforcin Lotion.

Hexylresorcinol, which may crossreact with resorcinol[58] (resorcin), is present in ST37, Sucrets, Tetrazets, Caprokol, and Crystoids Anthelmintic. The ingestion of Crystoids or Caprokol could produce a contact-type dermatitis in patients sensitized to topical application of resorcin or hexylresorcinol. Some troches, including Iso-Thirium, Listerine, and Nymore, also contain hexylresorcinol.

Chloral Hydrate

Sensitization to chloral hydrate in topical medications may occur from exposure to hair tonics and other scalp medications. Rectules and Calmitol ointment contain chloral hydrate. Chlorbutanol (chlorbutol), a local anesthetic and preservative for parenteral solutions, is a chloral derivative. Chloral hydrate is also used in the manufacture of DDT, which is 1,1,1-trichloro-2–2-bis(p-chlorophenyl)ethane.

Chloral hydrate may be administered as a sedative in Aquachloral Supprettes, Beta-Chlor, EnChlor, Fello-Sed, Felsules, Loryl, Noctagetic, Noctec, and Somnos.

The ingestion of chloral hydrate by patients sensitized to it by topical exposure may result in an eczematous contact-type dermatitis medicamentosa.[59,60] Placidyl (ethchlorvynol), a condensation product of chloral hydrate, may produce a fixed drug eruption, with a flare-up upon patch testing with the drug.[61]

Cardiovascular Agents

NITROGLYCERIN

Nitroglycerin is another example of a medicament that when employed systemically (sublingually) did not produce any allergic reaction. Its recent use topically, however, has resulted in allergic contact dermatitis in several patients sensitized to topical nitroglycerin. Sublingual or oral use of nitroglycerin may produce an allergic systemic contact dermatitis.[62,63]

MEXILETINE HYDROCHLORIDE

The antiarrhythmia agent mexiletine hydrochloride produced a drug eruption that was confirmed by patch tests at 6.25%, 12.5%, and 25% in petrolatum. These tests were positive only on skin that initially developed dermatitis and were negative or equivocal on noninvolved normal or even noninvolved scarified skin at the same concentrations.[64]

CAPTOPRIL

The ACE inhibitor captopril produced a drug eruption confirmed by a 10% aqueous patch test, whereas patch tests to other ACE inhibitors were negative.[65]

PSEUDOEPHEDRINE

Two days after a patient took oral vasoconstrictor containing pseudoephedrine, an eczematous dermatitis of the neck, arms, and trunk occurred. Patch tests of skin previously involved in the rash were positive by day 4 to 1% and 3% concentrations of pseudoephedrine with concomitant crossreactions to ephedrine and phenylephrine.[66] Over-the-counter cold medicines commonly contain pseudo-ephedrine, which produced acute exanthematous pustulosis in one patient and a generalized papulovesicular eruption with palmoplantar involvement and mucosal erosions. Patch tests were positive to 10% pseudoephedrine. The most common reactions to pseudoephedrine are fixed drug eruption, scarlatiniform, or eczematous patterns of dermatitis.[67]

SALBUTAMOL

Salbutamol used in a nebulizer to treat chronic obstructive pulmonary disease caused central facial dermatitis with systemic spread of dermatitis to the arms and legs.[68] This compound is an adrenergic agent that selectively stimulates beta-receptors. A 5% concentration in petrolatum was positive in the patient but negative in 30 controls.

Thiamine Hydrochloride (Vitamin B_1, Betabion Hydrochloride, and Aneurin Hydrochloride)

Hypersensitivity to various vitamins has been reported, with thiamine accounting for the largest number of such cases.[69] Allergic contact dermatitis may occur in workers who fill vials during its manufacture.[70] The injection or ingestion of this vitamin in such sensitized individuals may produce an eczematous relapse in the form of a contact-type dermatitis.[71]

Thiamine may crossreact with coenzyme B (diphosphothiamin) and cocarboxylase.

Vitamin B_5

Dexpanthenol is a component of topical products such as hair care cosmetics, baby lotions, sunscreens, and topical medications. It is an alcoholic derivative of pantothenic acid, which is better known as vitamin B_5. Sensitization topically about the face and scalp margin was traced to use of a baby lotion in a 33-year-old woman.[72] She subsequently developed a flare of this dermatitis and a nummular eczema pattern of systemic dermatitis after ingesting a capsule containing Ca-D-pantothenate. A diet low in vitamin B_5 was found helpful, whereas a diet high in vitamin B_5 caused worsening of face and hand eczema within 1 week.

Vitamin B_{12} (Cobione and Berubigen)

Young and colleagues[73] reported a case of sensitivity to B_{12} concentrate in which there was a delayed tuberculin-type reaction to the intradermal injection of B_{12}. Subcutaneous and intramuscular injections did not produce a flare-up of the dermatitis.

Fisher[74] observed a patient with cobalt sensitivity who acquired a pruritic eruption at the site of injection of vitamin B_{12} (Berubigen, cyanocobalamin). This area flared when vitamin B_{12} was taken orally. The patient had a strongly positive patch test reaction to cobalt chloride and a delayed positive scratch and intradermal test reaction to vitamin B_{12} (Berubigen). Most surprising of all, the patient had a positive patch test reaction to vitamin B_{12} (Berubigen) alone.

Hydrazine Hydrobromide

A large percentage of individuals who are exposed to this compound in solder flux become sensitized.[75] It is the parent chemical of isoniazid (INH, Niconyl, Nydrazid, Rimifon, Tyvid), hydralazine (Apresoline), and phenelzine (Nardil), an antidepressant drug. The systemic administration of these drugs in individuals sensitized to hydrazine hydrochloride may produce eczematous contact-type dermatitis medicamentosa.

Preservatives

PARABENS

Fourteen patients who were sensitive to paraben mixture took oral capsules containing 100 mg of methyl-*p*-hydroxybenzoate and 100 mg of propyl-*p*-hydroxybenzoate in a study to determine whether oral parabens can cause systemically induced dermatitis.[76] Only two patients reacted, and both exhibited vesicular hand eruptions. One had a flare of a previous paraben patch test. A low paraben diet was of no value to these two individuals, and therefore oral challenge testing of paraben-sensitive patients was not recommended.

SORBIC ACID

Perianal and buttock dermatitis was traced to sorbic acid ingestion in a 50-year-old man in whom the positive patch test seemed irrelevant until his dietary intake of sorbic acid was restricted.[77] The presentation was "baboon syndrome" like, and this morphology has repeatedly been linked to systemic reactions.

Sorbic acid on moist towelettes caused dermatitis on the hands of a one year old child which cleared on avoidance of the towelettes, but later reappeared as a generalized eruption thought to be due to ingestion of foods that naturally contain sorbic acid, such as red fruits. A sorbic acid free diet improved the dermatitis without the need for additional treatment.[78] A low sorbic acid diet restricts:

Fruits:	Chestnuts, plums, prunes, strawberries, currants, cranberries
Candies:	Almond base, jellied candy, chocolates, ice cream and sherbet made with the above noted fruits
Dairy products:	Margarine and light butter, cheese spreads, fruit yogurt
Drinks:	Grape- and apple-flavored beverages
Other:	Refrigerated salads with meats or shellfish.

THIMEROSAL

Nummular eczema and dyshidrosiform eczema occurred in two children who were repeatedly exposed to oral and intranasal vaccines preserved with thimerosal.[79]

PHENOXYETHANOL

The diphtheria-pertussis-tetanus (DPT) vaccine was administered to an 18-month-old child on several occasions, and each time the child experienced generalized eczema.[80] A patch test to 2-phenoxyethanol 2% in petrolatum was the only reaction seen from testing of the vaccine ingredients (Infanrix). Use of a thimerosal preserved vaccine (Merioux) was successful. Phenoxyethanol is a component of Eurxyl K 400 that also contains methyldibromoglutaronitrile.

Flavoring Agents

CINNAMON OIL

This oil is used for flavoring foods, cakes, toothpaste, chewing gum, tobacco, vermouth, aperitifs, bitters, and beverages of the cola type. Cassia oil is a type of Chinese cinnamon. Occupational dermatitis from oil of cinnamon may occur in bakers, candy makers, cooks, and housewives.

Cinnamon may crossreact with balsam of Peru.

Ingestion of oil of cinnamon may produce an eczematous contact-type flare-up in individuals previously sensitized by contact with the oil.[81]

Fisher[74] observed a patient sensitized to cinnamon in a toothpaste whose dermatitis flared after drinking vermouth containing cinnamon.

OTHER FLAVORINGS

Hjorth[82] reported two children who were sensitive to balsam of Peru and orange peel and whose eczema flared after eating fruits and ices. Hjorth[83] also described a man with a severe hand eczema who was allergic to balsam of Peru and whose eczema flared when he ate some orange marmalade. After he avoided perfumes, cola drinks, vermouth, throat tablets, and cinnamon, his hand eczema cleared. Eating vanilla sugar has also caused a flare of eczema in a patient sensitive to balsam of Peru.[20] It is possible that garlic may also have this effect.[84] Veien[4] reported that 47% of patients placed on a low-balsam diet reported long-term improvements.

BALSAM OF PERU

Oral challenges of patients who were patch test positive to balsam of Peru were carried out in double-blind, placebo-controlled fashion by Niinimaki.[85] Spices such as cloves, cinnamon, Jamaica pepper, and vanilla, as well as balsam of Peru, were used for challenges. The only adverse reaction observed from the challenges was an increase in the number of palmar vesicles. This occurred with active as well as placebo challenges, but was more common with the active challenges. Neither the challenges nor the patch tests were predictive of who might benefit from an avoidance diet.

GARLIC

Contact dermatitis to garlic has been associated with fingertip dermatitis but caused a pompholyx pattern of dermatitis when ingested orally as a commercially available garlic extract to treat hyperlipidemia.[86] A 5% aqueous patch test to garlic extract was positive. Cooked garlic did not cause a reaction, as this denatures the allergens diallyldisulfide, allylpropyldisulfide, and allicin.

TOXICODENDRON

Rhus, or more properly *Toxicodendron*, is used as a folk medicine in Korea. A study of 42 patients who experienced an eruption from ingestion of this plant found that half of the cases developed a generalized maculopapular eruption,

29% experienced erythroderma, 14% had a vesiculobullous dermatitis, and 7% showed erythema multiforme-like changes. It was believed that only 14 of the patients had prior contact with the plant. Therefore most were not sensitized, but still experienced an eruption, which led the authors to speculate that this was a toxic rather than immunologic event. They did not identify a lymphocyte subset profile that distinguished between the sensitized and nonsensitized patients. However, leukocytosis did occur in 57% of cases during the eruption and 2 patients showed liver enzyme elevations.[87]

Disulfiram (Antabuse, Tetraethylthiuram Disulfide)

Antabuse is used as adjunctive treatment in alcoholism to help the patient remain in the state of self-imposed sobriety. When on Antabuse therapy, patients ingesting even small amounts of alcohol experience a highly unpleasant reaction, consisting of flushing, palpitations, dyspnea, hyperventilation, tachycardia, nausea, and vomiting. Antabuse implants are being used in the treatment of alcoholism (see Chapter 20).

Antabuse (disulfiram) and thiram (tetramethylthiuram) are used as rubber accelerators and may show crossreactions. Thiram is used widely as an insecticide and germicide and is present in Rezifilm (Squibb), a surgical wound dressing. Sensitization by contact with thiram may make the patient susceptible to an eczematous dermatitis medicamentosa if Antabuse is given.[84]

A patient sensitized to dipentamethylene thiuram disulfide from a rubber condom developed a violent reaction and a widespread eczema when given Antabuse (tetraethylthiuram disulfide) for the treatment of alcoholism.[88] A similar patient was described by Pirila.[89] The reaction occurred within 4 hours, and a thiuram patch test reaction that had faded was reactivated.

Quinine and Quinidine

It has long been known that quinine can sensitize the skin, particularly when inflammation is present. Topical sensitization may take place from hair preparations containing quinine. Quinamm (National) contains quinine sulfate, as do many over-the-counter cold and headache remedies. The ingestion of such remedies and even of quinine water may produce eczematous contact-type dermatitis in sensitized individuals. Quinidine contact dermatitis has been reported in a patient who worked in the pharmaceutical industry and whose exposure

resulted from grinding the drug.[90] Quinidine and quinine apparently do not crossreact.[91]

Hydroxyzine

Crossreactivity between hydroxyzine and ethylenediamine has been reported. Ash and Scheman[92] encountered a patient who was patch test positive to ethylenediamine and on oral challenge with hydroxyzine on three occasions developed pruritus and abdominal rash within 2 days. The ethylenediamine patch test did not flare, and the patient was completely clear after discontinuing hydroxyzine.

5-Fluorouracil

Extensive topical use of 5-fluorouracil led to allergic contact dermatitis due to this agent.[93] When the patient developed adenocarcinoma, intravenous 5-fluorouracil was administered. Within 1 day the patient developed severe head and neck erythema and edema that ultimately led to discontinuation of intravenous use of 5-fluorouracil.

Dibucaine

Application of dibucaine (also known as cinchocaine) to the perianal area resulted in a dermatitis of the face, axillae, antecubital fossae, and upper inner thighs in a baboon syndrome-like picture. A 5% dibucaine in petroleum patch test was positive and there were no crossreactions to either ester or amide anesthetics. The authors of the study point out that it is not always necessary to avoid all other anesthetics of the same class when sensitivity to one member of the ester or amide class of anesthetics is identified.[94]

Fluorides

Shea and colleagues[95] reported seven individuals who had urticaria, exfoliative dermatitis, atopic dermatitis, stomatitis, and gastrointestinal and respiratory allergy, apparently due to fluorides in a fluoride-containing toothpaste and vitamin preparations. One individual had a positive patch test reaction to fluoride.

Metals that Cause Systemic Contact Dermatitis

The role of dietary restriction of metal salts such as nickel, cobalt, and chromate, as well as oral balsams, has been investigated in Denmark.[4] Of 7,887 patients evaluated for eczema, oral challenge led to a final diagnosis in 122 (1.5%). Of 675 patients on diets restricting metal salts, balsams, and food allergens in general, 262 reported improvement. Seventy percent of those available for a follow-up questionnaire reported long-term benefit from diets of this type (144 of 206). Atopic patients with vesicular hand eczema were more likely to benefit.[4]

Exposure of the oral cavity to dental metals can result in recurrent vesicular hand eczema.[96]

Patch tests did not accurately predict all the patients who would benefit from removal of the dental metal. Rather, oral provocation with 2.5 mg of nickel and 1 mg of cobalt caused the dermatitis to flare. Of the five patients studied, one was chromate sensitive and one nickel sensitive by patch test, but four of the five had a positive oral challenge to chromate, nickel, or cobalt. Two of the cases had features of atopic dermatitis, as well as hand eczema. Oral symptoms were present in only one case.

Dermatitis of the face, neck, scalp, and arms developed 40 days after orthodontic brackets, bands, and wires were applied in a 15-year-old atopic female. She proved strongly allergic to nickel, but did not experience intraoral inflammation. Removal of the orthodontic appliances resulted in complete resolution of all symptoms.[97]

In a related study of chromate-sensitive patients, oral challenge proved provocative in 17 of 30 subjects who did not react to placebo. Most had hand and foot eruptions.[98] Veien and colleagues[98] used 2.5 mg of chromate for the oral challenge.

Systemic ingestion of nickel by nickel-sensitive individuals can result in flare-up of prior sites of nickel exposure and/or new areas of dermatitis. The amount of nickel required for this phenomenon to occur has been hotly debated, as many studies have used doses that far exceed what might be ingested in a normal diet. In order to establish information on the dose-response relationship of oral nickel ingestion, nickel sulfate hexahydrate was administered in the following doses: 0.3 mg (as would be found in a normal diet); 1.0 mg (as would be found in a high-nickel diet) and 4.0 mg (10 times what might be found in a normal diet). Four out of 10 individuals reacted to the 0.3 and 1.0 mg doses, and 7 of 10 reacted to the 4.0 mg dose. The study was placebo controlled and one individual reacted to the placebo. There were no reactions among 20 nonsensitized individuals to any of the nickel challenges or the placebo.[99] The mechanism by which a systemic response occurs when a cutaneous allergen is ingested was investigated by looking at the lymphocyte subtypes and their changes with increasing allergen concentration. Nickel-sensitive patients were orally challenged with increasing doses of nickel, and nonsensitive patients served as controls. Two major changes occurred, in the nickel-sensitive individuals only.

Memory cells bearing the markers CD3+CD45RO+CLA+ and CD8+CD45RO+CLA+ moved from the general circulation into peripheral tissues and IL-5 serum levels increased. The IL-5 increase is representative of a type 2 T lymphocyte response.[100]

Metals that cause systemic contact dermatitis are further discussed in Chapter 32.

References

1. Fisher AA. Allergic dermatitis medicamentosa: the "systemic contact-type variety." Cutis 1976;18:637.

2. Menne T, Hjorth N. Reactions from systemic exposure to contact allergens. Semin Dermatol 1982;1:15.

3. Menné T, Veien N, Sjolin K, Maibach HI. Systemic contact dermatitis. Am J Contact Dermat 1994;5:1.

4. Veien NK. Systemically induced eczema in adults. Acta Derm Venereol (Stockh) 1989[Suppl];147:1.

5. Kuligowski ME, Chang A, Rath A. Multiple fixed drug eruption due to ibuprofen. Contact Dermatitis 1991;25:259.

6. Meneghini CL, Angelini G. Secondary polymorphic eruptions in allergic contact dermatitis. Dermatologica 1981;163:63.

7. Collet E, Dalac S, Morvan C, et al. Tetrazepam allergy once more detected by patch test. Contact Dermatology 1992;26:281.

8. Hayakawa R, Ogin Y, Aris K, Matsunaga K. Systemic contact dermatitis to amlexanox. Contact Dermatitis 1992;27:122.

9. Hsu C-K, Sun CC, Su MS, et al. Systemic contact allergy from occupational contact with ethyl ethoxymethylene cyan oacetate. Contact Dermatitis 1992;27:58.

10. O'Donnell BF, Tan CY. Erythema multiforme reaction to patch testing. Contact Dermatitis 1992;27:230.

11. Hjorth N. Nickel vasculitis. Contact Dermatitis 1976;2:356.

12. Haeusermann P, Harr T, Bircher AJ. Baboon syndrome resulting from systemic drugs: is there strife between SDRIFE and allergic contact dermatitis syndrome? Contact Dermatitis 2004;51:297.

13. Mancuso G, Masara N. Contact urticaria and severe anaphylaxis from rifamycin SV. Contact Dermatitis 1992;27:124.

14. Bause GS, Kugelman LC. Contact anaphylactoid response to labetalol. Contact Dermatitis 1990;23:51.

15. Kunisada M, Adachi A, Asano H, et al. Anaphylaxis due to formaldehyde released from root-canal disinfectant. Contact Dermatitis 2002;47:215.

16. Yoshiyuki C, Takahashi S, Yamakawa Y, et al. Contact urticaria syndrome caused by patch testing with cefotiam hy drochloride. Contact Dermatitis 1999;41:234.

17. Veien NK, Svejgaard E, Menne T. In vitro lymphocyte transformation to nickel: a study of nickel-sensitive

patien ts before and after epicutaneous and oral challenge with nickel. Acta Derm Venereol (Stockh) 1979;59:447.

18. Fisher AA. Allergic reactions due to metals used in dentistry. Cutis 1974;14:797.

19. Cronin E. Contact dermatitis XVII: reactions to contact allergens given orally or systemically. Br J Dermatol 19 72;86:104.

20. Pirila V. Endogenic contact eczema. Allerg Asthma 1970;16:15.

21. Rietschel RL. Selected highlights of the European Contact Dermatitis Society Meeting, Brussels, Belgium, October 8–10, 1992. Am J Contact Dermat 1993;4:66.

22. Rees BR. Cutaneous reactions to antibiotics. JAMA 1964;189:685.

23. Vickers HR, Bagratuni L, Alexander S. Dermatitis caused by penicillin milk. Lancet 1978;61:351.

24. Shelley WB, Cahn MM. Effect of topically applied antibiotic agents on axillary odor. JAMA 1957;159:1736.

25. Epstein S. Dermal contact dermatitis from neomycin: observations on forty cases. Ann Allergy 1958;16:268.

26. Epstein S, Wenzel FJ. Cross-sensitivity to various "mycins. Arch Dermatol 1962;86:183.

27. Epstein S, Wenzel FJ. Sensitivity to neomycin and bacitracin, cross sensitization or coincidence? Acta Derm Vene reol (Stockh) 1963;43:1.

28. Pirilä V, Rantanen AV. Root canal treatment with bacitracin-neomycin as cause of flare-up of allergic eczem a. Oral Surg Oral Med Oral Pathol 1960;13:589.

29. Ekelund AG, Moller H. Oral provocation in eczematous contact allergy to neomycin and hydroxy-quinolines. Acta De rm Venereol (Stockh) 1969;49:422.

30. Welsh AL. The fixed eruption: a possible hazard of modern drug therapy. Arch Dermatol 1961;84:1004.

31. Welsh AL, Ede H. Cross-fixed drug eruption from three antibiotics. Arch Dermatol 1955;71:521.

32. Schwank R, Jirasek L. Contact allergy to chloramphenicol with special reference to group sensitization. Hautarzt 1963;14:24.

33. Palacios J, Nemuth MG, Blaylock WK. Lack of cross sensitization between 2,4-dinitrochlorbenzene and chlorampheni col. South Med J 1968;61:243.

34. Roupe G, Strannegard O. Anaphylactic shock elicited by topical administration of bacitracin. Arch Dermatol 1969; 100:450.

35. Romano A, Pietrantonio F, DiFonso M, Venuti A. Delayed hypersensitivity to cefuroxime. Contact Dermatitis 1992;2 7:270.

36. Sulzberger MB, et al. Sensitization by topical application of sulfonamides. J Allergy 1947;18:92.

37. Harber LC, Lashinsky AM, Baer RL. Photosensitivity due to chlorothiazide and hydrochlorothiazide. N Engl J Med 1 959;261:1378.

38. Seale E. Saccharin - A factor in sunlight sensitivity: current news in dermatology. The Schoch Letter, Dallas, T exas, July 1965.

39. Hitselberger JF, Fosnaugh RP. Photosensitivity due to chlorpropamide. J Am Acad Dermatol 1962;180:62.

40. Kennedy B, O'Quinn S, Perret WJ, et al. Phototoxic and photoallergic skin reactions resulting from modern drug therapy. J La State Med Soc 1961;113:367.

41. Fisher AA. Systemic contact dermatitis from Orinase and Diabinese in diabetics with para-amino hypersensitivity. Cutis 1982;29:551, 556, 565 passim.

42. Angelini G, Meneghini CL. Oral tests in contact allergy to para-amino compounds. Contact Dermatitis 1981;7:311.

43. Quirce S, Parra F, Lazaro M, et al. Generalized dermatitis due to oral nystatin. Contact Dermatitis 1991;25:197.

44. Cooper SM, Reed J, Shaw S. Systemic reaction to nystatin. Contact Dermatitis 1999;41:345.

45. Vernassiere C, Barbaud A, Trechot PH, et al. Systemic acyclovir reaction subsequent to acyclovir contact allergy: which systemic antiviral drug should then be used? Contact Dermatitis 2004;49:155.

46. Epstein S. Allergic photocontact dermatitis from promethazine (Phenergan). Arch Dermatol Syphilol 1960;81:175.

47. Morris-Owen RM. "Cover-dose" management of contact sensitivity to chlorpromazine. Br J Dermatol 1963;75:167.

48. Camarasa JG, Serra-Baldrich E. Tetrazepam allergy detected by patch test. Contact Dermatitis 1990;22:246.

49. Machet L, et al. Patch testing with clobazam: relapse of generalized drug eruption (published erratum appears in Contact Dermatitis 1992;27:351). Contact Dermatitis 1992;26:347.

50. Conilliau V, Dompmartin A, Verneuil L, et al. Hypersensitivity syndrome due to 2 anticonvulsant drugs. Contact Dermatitis 1999;41:141.

51. Hindson C. Contact eczema from methyl salicylate reproduced by oral aspirin (acetyl-salicylic acid). Contact Dermatitis 1977;3:348.

52. Kitamura K, Osawa J, Ikezawa Z, et al. Crossreactivity between sensitivity to thimerosal and photosensitivity to piroxicam in guinea pigs. Contact Dermatitis 1991;25:30.

53. Cirne de Castro JL, Freitas F, Menezes Brandao R, Themido R. Sensitivity to thimerosal and photosensitivity to piroxicam. Contact Dermatitis 1991;24:187.

54. Ikezawa Z, Kitamura K, Osawa J, et al. Photosensitivity to piroxicam is induced by sensitization to thimerosal and thiosalicylate. J Invest Dermatol 1992;98:918.

55. Wilkinson SM, Smith AG, English JS. Erythroderma following the intradermal injection of the corticosteroid budes-onide. Contact Dermatitis 1992;27:121.

56. Garcia-Bravo B, Repiso JB, Camacho F. Systemic contact dermatitis due to deflazacort. Contact Dermatitis 2000;43:359.

57. Leifer W, Steiner K. Studies in sensitization to halogenated hydroxyquinolines and related compounds. J Invest Dermatol 1951;17:233.

58. Caron GA, Calnan CD. Studies in contact dermatitis: XIV: resorcin. Trans St John's Hosp Dermatol Soc 1962;48:149.

59. Baer RL, Sulzberger MB. Eczematous dermatitis due to chloral hydrate (following both oral administration and topical application). J Allergy 1938;9:519.

60. Christianson HB, Perry HO. Reactions to chloral hydrate. Arch Dermatol 1956;74:232.

61. Auerbach R. Fixed drug eruption: ethchlorvynol: report of a case. Arch Dermatol 1965;92:184.

62. Chandraratna PAN, O'Dell RE. Allergic reactions to nitroglycerin ointment: report of five cases. Curr Ther Res 1979;25:481.

63. Sausker WF, Frederick FD. Allergic contact dermatitis secondary to topical nitroglycerin [Letter]. JAMA 1978;239:1743.

64. Kikuchi K, Tsunoda T, Tagami H. Generalized drug eruption due to mexiletine hydrochloride: topical provocation on previously involved skin. Contact Dermatitis 1991;25:70.

65. Cnudde F, Leynadier F, Dry J. Cutaneous reaction to captopril: value of patch tests. Contact Dermatitis 1990;23:375.

66. Tomb RR, Lepoittevin JP, Espinassouze F, et al. Systemic contact dermatitis from pseudoephedrine. Contact Dermatitis 1991;24:86.

67. Assier-Bonnet H, Viguier M, Dubetret L, et al. Severe adverse drug reactions due to pseudoephedrine from over-the-counter medications. Contact Dermatitis 2002;47:165.

68. Smeenk G, Burgers JA, Teunissen PC. Contact dermatitis from salbutamol. Contact Dermatitis 1994;31:123.

69. Combes FC, Groopman J. Contact dermatitis due to thiamine: report of 2 cases. Arch Dermatol Syphilol 1950;61:858.

70. Dalton JE, Pierce JD. Dermatological problems among pharmaceutical workers. AMA Arch Dermatol Syphilol 1951;64:667.

71. Hjorth N. Contact dermatitis from Vitamin B_1 (thiamine): relapse after ingestion of thiamine: cross-sensitization to cocarboxylase. J Invest Dermatol 1958;30:261.

72. Hemmer W, Bracun R, Wolf-Abdolvahab S, et al. Maintenance of hand eczema by oral pantothenic acid in a patients ensitized to dexpanthenol. Contact Dermatitis 1997;37:51.

73. Young WC, Ulrich CW, Fouts PJ. Sensitivity to vitamin B_{12} concentrate. JAMA 1950;143:893.

74. Fisher AA. Contact Dermatitis. 3rd ed. Philadelphia: Lea & Febiger, 1986.

75. Wheeler CE Jr, Penn SR, Cawley EP. Dermatitis from hydrazine hydrobromide solder flux. Arch Dermatol 1965;91:235.

76. Veien NK, Hattel T, Laurberg G. Oral challenge with parabens in paraben-sensitive patients. Contact Dermatitis 1996;34:433.

77. Giordano-Labadie F, Pech-Ormieres C, Bazex J. Systemic contact dermatitis from sorbic acid. Contact Dermatitis 1996;34:61.

78. Raison-Peyron N, Meynadier JM, Meynadier J. Sorbic acid: an unusual cause of systemic contact dermatitis in an infant. Contact Dermatitis 2000;43:247.

79. Zenarola P, Gimma A, Lomuto M. Systemic contact dermatitis from thimerosal. Contact Dermatitis 1995;32:107.

80. Vogt T, Landthaler M, Stolz W. Generalized eczema in an 18-month-old boy due to phenoxyethanol in DPT vaccine. Contact Dermatitis 1998;38:50.

81. Leifer W. Contact dermatitis due to cinnamon: recurrence of dermatitis following oral administration of cinnamon oil. AMA Arch Dermatol Syphilol 1951;64:52.

82. Hjorth N. Eczematous allergy to balsams, allied perfumes and flavoring agents. Copenhagen: Munkgaard, 1961:134.

83. Hjorth N. Allergy to balsams. Spectrum 1971;8:97.

84. Burks JW Jr. Classic aspects of onion and garlic dermatitis in housewives. Ann Allergy 1954;12:592.

85. Niinimaki A. Double-blind placebo-controlled peroral challenges in patients with delayed-type allergy to balsam of Peru. Contact Dermatitis 1995;33:78.

86. Burden AD, Wilkinson SM, Beck MH, Chalmers RJ. Garlic-induced systemic contact dermatitis. Contact Dermatitis 1994;30:299.

87. Oh S-H, Haw C-R, Lee M-H. Clinical and immunologic features of systemic contact dermatitis from ingestion of Rhus (*Toxicodendron*). Contact Dermatitis 2003;48:251.

88. Shelley WB. Golf-course dermatitis due to thiram fungicide. JAMA 1961;198:415.

89. Pirila V. Dermatitis due to rubber. Proc 11th Int Cong Derm 1957;2:252.

90. Klaschka F. Discussion of high grade quinine contact-allergy. Derm Wschr 1964;149:4.

91. Fernstrom AI. Occupational quinidine contact dermatitis: a concept apparently not yet described. Acta Derm Venereol (Stockh) 1965;45:129.

92. Ash S, Scheman AJ. Systemic contact dermatitis to hydroxyzine. Am J Contact Dermat 1997;8:2.

93. Nadal C, Pujol RM, Randazzo L, et al. Systemic contact dermatitis from 5-fluorouracil. Contact Dermatitis 1996;35:124.

94. Erdmann SM, Sachs B, Merk HF. Systemic contact dermatitis from cinchocaine. Contact Dermatitis 2001;44:260.

95. Shea JJ, Gillespie SM, Waldbott GL. Allergy to fluoride. Ann Allergy 1967;25:388.

96. Veien NK, Borchorst E, Hattel T, Laurberg G. Stomatitis or systemically-induced contact dermatitis from metal wire in orthodontic materials. Contact Dermatitis 1994;30:210.

97. Pigatto PD, Guzzi G. systemic contact dermatitis from nickel associated with orthodontic appliances. Contact Dermatitis 2004;50:100.

98. Veien NK, Hattel T, Laurberg G. Chromate-allergic patients challenged orally with potassium dichromate. Contact Dermatitis 1994;31:137.

99. Jensen CS, Menne T, Lisby S, et al. Experimental systemic contact dermatitis from nickel: a dose-response study. Contact Dermatitis 2004;49:124.

100. Jensen CS, Lisby S, Larsen JK, et al. Characterization of lymphocyte subpopulations and cytokine profiles in peripheral blood of nickel-sensitive individuals with systemic contact dermatitis after oral nickel exposure. Contact Dermatitis 2004;50:31.

CHAPTER 9

Medications and Medical Devices, and Implications for the Medical Community

EXECUTIVE SUMMARY

Topical agents in medications that can cause contact dermatitis include both active agents and inactive ingredients. Inactive agents discussed include aluminum and its salts, petrolatum, olive oil, sesame oil, castor oil, and lanolin. Active agents reported to cause contact dermatitis include common dermatologic drugs such as anthralin, crotamiton, ichthammol, sulfur, halogenated hydroxyquinolines, silver nitrate, phenol, salicylic acid, resorcinol, lindane, methyl salicylate, tretinoin, vitamin D_3, selenium sulfide, captan, coal tar, fluorouracil, glutaraldehyde, cantharidin, boric acid, minoxidil, many topical ophthalmic drugs, 8-methoxypsoralen, diclofenac, and clindamycin. Drugs may be applied to the skin for intended systemic activity or may come into contact with skin in the course of handling, causing contact dermatitis. Such drugs include phenylbutazone, diethylstilbestrol, epinephrine, ephedrine, phenylephrine, thiamine, vitamin B_6, vitamin B_{12}, vitamin K, nitroglycerin, heparin, transdermal estrogen, transdermal testosterone, transdermal nicotine, mitomycin C, interferon, spironolactone, phenoxybenzamine, diazepam, tetrazepam, piroxicam, statins, lansoprazole, ranitidine, insulin, ticlopidine, azathioprine, heroin, and others.

Agents that are involved in the care of patients and that cause contact dermatitis include mucolytics, anesthetics such as halothane, hydrocolloid dressings, radiographic contrast agents, technetium, transcutaneous electrical nerve stimulation (TENS) units and gels, identification bands, marking pens, adhesive remover, gowns, grounding plates, casts, stoma bags, and insulin pumps.

Contact hazards for surgeons include surgical scrub solutions, rubber gloves, and acrylic bone cement. Additional concerns for nurses include the medications handled such as streptomycin, penicillin, chlorpromazine, maclofenoxate, and famotidine. For dentists, special consideration is given to local anesthetics, acrylic monomers, formaldehyde, mercury, impression materials, and essential oils.

Veterinarians may encounter mercaptobenzothiazole in some veterinary medications, and additional antibiotics such as spiramycin and penethamate hydrochloride. They also may have contact with other causative agents such as animal feed additives, animal saliva, and dander. Pharmacists and laboratory workers may come into direct contact with final or intermediate forms of drugs.

Cutaneous adverse drug reactions may be evaluated by patch test, prick test, or intradermal test. Suggested guidelines for patch testing drugs to identify the source of the eruption have been published, and include:

1. Waiting 6 weeks to 6 months after the eruption has resolved
2. Testing of commercialized drugs at 30% petrolatum and/or aqueous.

125

3. Testing of a pure drug at 10% petrolatum or aqueous, but at a lower concentration if the reaction was severe
4. Taking of readings at days 1 and 7, in addition to traditional readings
5. Application of the test over the most affected area.[1]

A study of 826 patients who received patch tests to evaluate suspected drug hypersensitivity found 89 (10.8%) had a positive patch test. The most frequent of these drugs were beta-lactams, clindamycin and trimethoprim. A positive skin-prick test was found in only 10 of 935 patients (1.1%). Rechallenge with the drug identified by the positive skin test in 17 patients showed that 13 of 16 patch-test–positive patients developed an exanthema and one prick-test–positive patient developed urticaria.[2]

Aluminum and its Salts

Aluminum compounds are used extensively in cosmetic and medicinal preparations. In these preparations, advantage is taken of their astringent, antacid, antibacterial, and antiperspirant properties. The irritant effect of aluminum salts on the skin varies considerably; the chloride and nitrate have greater irritant properties than the chlorhydrate, allantoin, and citrate. Aluminum salts are also used as styptic agents for hemostasis and for aluminum-precipitated allergens.

ALLERGIC CONTACT SENSITIVITY

Sensitivity reactions to aluminum are rare. Desensitization of hay fever patients who have an aluminum-precipitated allergen, however, has been found to cause contact sensitivity to aluminum,[3] When such sensitivity occurs, the patients may show an allergic reaction to the aluminum-disc Finn chamber used for patch testing. Fischer and Rystedt[4] pointed out that if all patches in a Finn chamber test show red, infiltrated papular rings, contact sensitivity to aluminum ought to be suspected; irritant factors, however, may also be the cause of the reactions.

The patient of Fischer and Rystedt[4] had an axillary dermatitis that cleared up when she stopped using an antiperspirant stick. This was followed by attacks of more widespread eczema while she was receiving desensitizing hay-fever injections made up in an aluminum vehicle. There were no local eczematous reactions, but the eczema disappeared when the injections stopped. On patch testing, she reacted to the rims of the aluminum Finn chamber and later was strongly positive (+++) to aluminum sulfate (2% aq), aluminum chloride (2% aq), and aluminum subacetate (1% aq). An intradermal test

with 0.05 mL aluminum hydroxide in 0.5% sodium chloride was also positive. It was not certain whether she was sensitized by the deodorant or the injections.

ALLERGIC ALUMINUM HYDROXIDE GRANULOMAS FROM VACCINES

Slater and colleagues[5] described three children in whom painful subcutaneous nodules developed 1 to 2 years after the injection of absorbed diphtheria-pertussis-tetanus (DPT) vaccine. The diagnosis of aluminum hydroxide granuloma was established by ultrastructural examination with X-ray microanalysis.

Vaccination with aluminum hydroxide containing DPT in patients allergic to aluminum (as confirmed by reactions to Finn chamber or 2% aq aluminum chloride) can produce granulomas lasting more than 1 year.[6] Aluminum was confirmed in the granulomas by X-ray defraction analysis, and of 21 such cases followed, 5 cleared, 11 improved, and 5 remained unchanged.

FALSE-POSITIVE REACTIONS WHEN TESTING MERCURY SALTS ON ALUMINUM DISCS

Dr. K. J. Kalveram and G. Forck of Munster, Germany, at the Fifth International Symposium on Contact Dermatitis, Barcelona, March 1980, reported nonspecific skin irritant reaction when using the aluminum Finn chamber to patch test mercury salts. They explained the irritation as being due to a chemical reaction between the aluminum of the Finn chamber and the tested mercury salt solution.

Allantoin

Certain cosmetics and many over-the-counter topical medications, particularly those advocated for use in psoriasis, contain allantoin as one of their ingredients.[7]

NATURE OF ALLANTOIN

Allantoin (5-ureido-hydantoin), a uric acid derivative known chemically as the diureide of glyoxylic acid, is a product of purine metabolism. It is prepared synthetically by the oxidation of uric acid with alkaline potassium permanganate with dichloroacetic acid.

SAFETY OF ALLANTOIN

The Food and Drug Administration reported that a search of the literature has not produced any reports of adverse reactions to the topical use of allantoin.[8,9] Moreover, the Schwartz patch test on 200 persons has shown that allantoin is nontoxic, nonirritating, and nonallergenic. The

Draize technique in rabbits has shown that allantoin is nonirritating even when applied to the conjunctival sac of the eye. The repeated insult test on 12 human subjects has shown that allantoin is not a primary skin irritant or a primary sensitizer.

Anthralin (Dithranol)

This topical medication used for psoriasis may sensitize occasionally.[10,11]

Anthralin Cream is available at present as Dithocreme (American Dermal Company) and Anthra-Derm (Dermik). Staining of clothes, skin, nails, and hair is frequent. An unusual cutaneous anthralin-like staining of the perineum may follow the use of danthron as a laxative. Danthron (1,8-dihydroxyanthroquinone) is reduced in the bowel to 1,8-dihydroxyanthron, which is the purgative, and can produce an irritant contact dermatitis.[12] Anthralin ointment is a strong irritant when covered. Covered patch tests may be made with 1/30 strength in petrolatum.

Benzyl Benzoate

Wranicz and Czernielweski[13] reported a 79-year-old female patient who was treated for scabies with Novoscabin, which contains 30% benzyl benzoate. She developed an erythematous-bullous eruption on the sites to which the drug had been applied. The presence of circulating antibodies and of antibodies bound to the basement membrane could be demonstrated immunologically. The authors discussed the possibility of provoking "pemphigoid" by topical application of Novoscabin.

Phenylbutazone (Butazolidin)

This medication is not used topically to any extent in the United States. It may cause dermatitis from its use as a cream,[14] as an ointment,[15] and in suppositories.[16] Cross-reactions may occur with phenylbutazone.

Diethylstilbestrol

This hormone is present in such proprietary medications as Aquarant "E" (Webster), Furestrol suppositories (Eaton), and Diethylstilbestrol Suppositories (Lilly) and is used as pellets in veterinary medications. It may crossreact with dienestrol, hexestrol, bisphenol A, monobenzylether of hydroquinone, eugenol, stilbene benzophenone, and benzestrol.[17,18]

Epinephrine (Adrenalin)

Several investigators have reported allergic contact reactions to epinephrine with positive patch tests from its use in ophthalmic solutions and as a spray treatment for asthma.[19–22]

Inasmuch as Aaronson and Jamamoto[23] reported circulating antibodies to epinephrine following ocular hypersensitivity, an opinion as to the safety of injectable epinephrine was sought in those patients who had a delayed type of allergic contact hypersensitivity. The following communication from Dr. Philip S. Norman (Baltimore, MD) is helpful:

> The question calls attention to several reports of contact reactions to topically applied epinephrine preparations usually in the form of eyedrops. Although it is possible that some of the reactions reported were due to preservatives or chemicals in the vehicle, at least some of the reactions were reproduced with crystalline epinephrine dissolved in water. Such reactions are unlikely to have much relation to immediate systemic symptoms after injection of epinephrine, although the subject has not of course been thoroughly explored. While one might look for an alternative to epinephrine in the treatment of asthma in individuals with a history of contact dermatitis after exposure to epinephrine solutions, I would not withhold epinephrine in an emergency such as systemic anaphylaxis.

Dipivefrin chloride, which is used to treat glaucoma, is in fact a prodrug that is de-esterified to epinephrine, and contact dermatitis with crossreactivity to epinephrine has been reported. That crossreactivity was not confirmed in a report by Vilaplana and colleagues. Their patient reacted only to dipivefrine chlorhydrate 1% aqueous and not epinephrine 1% aqueous.[24]

Ephedrine

A systemic eruption of the trunk and arms due to ephedrine HCl in a cough medicine was reported.[25] A 5% aqueous solution of ephedrine HCl was used for diagnosis.

Phenylephrine

Phenylephrine has usually been reported to cause contact dermatitis from an ophthalmic product, but it has also been reported from an eardrop.[26] There was a positive reaction to a 5% petrolatum concentration of phenylephrine. When a 2-day closed patch test to phenylephrine hydrochloride was negative, although the clinical findings strongly suggested that the results should have been positive, Akita and colleagues[27] performed closed scratch-patch tests. The result was positive scratch-patch tests at concentrations of phenylephrine from 5% to 0.1% petrolatum noted at days 2, 3, and 7, lasting for 3 months. Since the phenylephrine was in an eyedrop, the different percutaneous penetration dynamics of the eye versus the skin were felt to require a different type of testing.[27]

Crotamiton (Eurax)

Crotamiton (Eurax) used topically as a scabicide and antipruritic is a rare sensitizer.[28,29] However, allergic contact dermatitis was reported from crotamiton (Eurax) after 6 days of an application three times per day. A 5% petrolatum concentration was used for diagnosis. Other cases have usually been from use on chronic eczemas, such as stasis dermatitis.[30]

Ichthammol (Ichthyol)

Ichthammol, a sulfonated bitumen, is derived from mineral deposits containing the remains of fish, consisting of sulfur (about 10%), ammonium sulfate (5 to 7%), hydrocarbons, nitrogenous bases, acids, and derivatives of thiophene. It has slight antiseptic and analgesic properties. Ichthammol is a weak antigen. A few scattered reports from Europe indicate allergic reactions to this medication.[31–34]

Sulfur

Sensitivity to sulfur, particularly when it is used as a topical agent, is rare. There are two reports in the literature of allergic hypersensitivity to sulfur.[35,36]

Whitfield's Ointment

This ointment, containing 6% salicylic acid and 12% benzoic acid petrolatum, is a rare sensitizer. The benzoic acid occasionally may produce a nonallergic contact urticaria that may cause a stinging sensation, particularly in the intertriginous areas. Such stinging sensations may decrease if the Whitfield's ointment is mixed with equal parts of zinc oxide ointment.

Halogenated Hydroxyquinolines

These therapeutic agents include iodochlorhydroxyquin (Vioform, Clioquinol), iodoquinol (Diiodohydroxyquinoline, Diodoquin), chlorquinaldol (Sterosan), and chlorhydroxyquinoline (Quinolor). Such preparations are commonly used topical agents. In addition, Vioform and Diodoquin may be administered systemically.[37] Cross-sensitization between these compounds may occur.[38] Vioform and Diodoquin administered orally may lead to an eczematous dermatitis medicamentosa in patients sensitized by topical application of any one of this group of compounds.

QUINOLOR COMPOUND

This ointment consists of chlorhydroxyquinoline, benzoyl peroxide, menthol, methyl salicylate, and eugenol in a Plastibase vehicle. When dermatitis occurs from the use of quinolor compound, chlorhydroxyquinoline is not necessarily the culprit, because the benzoyl peroxide, eugenol, and Plastibase, which is a polyethylene compound related to Carbowax, can all cause allergic reactions.

Kero and colleagues[39] reported irritant dermatitis from Vioform, particularly in men in the inguinal and scrotal areas. The topical use of Vioform and Diodoquin, iodine-containing compounds, may increase the protein-bound iodine of the blood. Such an increase may be mistaken for thyroid disease.[40,41]

Sodium Perborate

Vilanova and Camarasa[42] found that this oxidizing agent was a common sensitizer in Spain. In the United States, it is a rare sensitizer. Sodium perborate is present in Kleenite (Vick), a denture-cleansing preparation.

Sodium perborate, like other oxidizing agents, is a strong irritant.[43] Fisher[44] noted irritant stomatitis when Kleenite is not thoroughly washed off a denture before it is inserted into the mouth.

Silver Nitrate

Gaul and Underwood[45] described a man who developed a vesicular reaction to the 10% silver nitrate used for marking patch tests. On patch testing, he reacted to 5% and 10% aged silver nitrate but not to 10% fresh silver nitrate; a test with silver foil was positive, but one with silver chloride powder was negative.

Silver nitrate is kept in an amber bottle because on exposure to air and light it decomposes, forming small amounts of nitric acid, silver nitrite, and colloidal silver, which liberate silver ions. The ionized silver was considered the sensitizer in this patient, and its effect explained the discrepancy between the results of testing with old and fresh solutions.

Marcussen[46] stated long ago that silver nitrate, used therapeutically, occasionally sensitized.

The prolonged use of topical silver nitrate can lead to systemic argyria[47]

Phenol

IRRITANT AND TOXIC EFFECTS OF PHENOL

The inclusion of phenol in such medications as Castellani's (Carbol-fuchsin) paint, Carbolated Vaseline, P & S Liquid, and Panscol Lotion has proved to be an irritant in certain persons.[48]

Rogers and colleagues[49] proved that phenol was toxic in infants when it was applied in the form of magenta (Carbol-fuchsin) paint.

IRRITATION FROM PHENOL IN CASTELLANI'S (CARBOL-FUCHSIN PAINT) NATURAL FORMULA 13

This original Carbol-fuchsin paint has caused irritant dermatitis in so many individuals, particularly when used in the intertriginous areas, that several years ago it was decided at the New York Skin and Cancer Unit of New York University to remove the phenol and use the formula shown in Table 9.1. Removal of the phenol has not impaired the efficacy of the paint.

Table 9-1 Phenol-Free Modified Carbol-Fuchsin Solution*

	cc
Combine	
Alcohol	20.0
Fuchsin	2.6
Water	190.0
Filter and add	
Boric acid	2.0
Let stand 2 hours and add	
Acetone	10.0
Resorcinol (resorcin)	20.0
Filter solution	

*NY Skin and Cancer Formulary. This paint has proved useful in chronic intertriginous dermatitis, otitis externa, stasis ulcers, and eczema.

It has been observed that children who have fair complexions or those who have applied the paint immediately after bathing become mildly shocked and drowsy.

Estimations of phenol and methyl alcohol in the urine of 16 infants who had seborrheic eczema treated with magenta (Castellani's) paint BPC were made by Rogers and colleagues[49] to determine the degree of absorption. Phenol was detected in four patients and methyl alcohol in none.

LACK OF ALLERGIC SENSITIVITY TO PHENOL

There has been only a single report of allergic dermatitis to phenol in the past three decades.[50]

IRRITANT DERMATITIS FROM PHENOL IN CARBOLATED VASELINE

Carbolated Vaseline contains 0.2% phenol and 0.5% para-chloro-meta-xylenol (PCMX) in a petrolatum base.

Rubin and Pirozzi[51] reported that Carbolated Vaseline, a widely employed self-medication in the black community, is used to acquire a "shiny" complexion. In their study of 28 patients who had dermatitis from Carbolated Vaseline, acute reactions occurred in eight (28%) patients, all of whom had an underlying eczematous dermatitis. These reactions were due either to allergic contact sensitization to PCMX (four patients) or to a primary irritant response to phenol (four patients). Chronic reactions occurred in 20 (72%) patients and developed over a period of weeks. A low-grade primary irritant reaction to phenol was responsible for the chronic reactions.

PRECAUTIONS IN THE USE OF P & S LIQUID

P & S Liquid is a specially prepared mixture of liquid paraffin, oil, sodium chloride, and phenol, less than 1%. It is stated that "P & S Liquid provides safe and effective management of scaling conditions of the scalp resulting from psoriasis or seborrhea." There is a warning, however, stating that P & S Liquid should not be applied to large portions of the body.

Salicylic Acid

Salicylic acid is used widely in prescribed medications and in over-the-counter medications.

It is used for wart removal as a 2% to 20% solution in collodion or as a 10% to 40% plaster for plantar warts and plantar hyperkeratosis, in a salicylic acid soap for tinea versicolor, and as a 6% salicylic acid preparation in a 60% propylene gel for hyperkeratotic diseases. Low concentrations of salicylic acid are present in shampoo and other medications in which they would be used to cause desquamation.

Whitfield's ointment with 6% salicylic acid and 12% benzoic acid in wool fat and petrolatum is used occasionally for desquamation and as a nonspecific antifungal agent. Gels with 8.7% choline salicylate have been used for symptomatic relief of painful aphthous ulcers. Topical salicylates are bacteriostatic and photo-protective.

Salicylic acid–mercury combinations may form bichloride of mercury or other severe mercury irritants, particularly under a closed patch test.

USE OF SALICYLIC ACID IN PSORIASIS

Goldsmith[52] states that psoriatic patients receiving topical salicylates and methotrexates are at potential risk of methotrexate toxicity. Taylor and Halprin[53] state that Keralyt (6 salicylic acid, 20% alcohol in 60% propylene glycol) is safe to use under occlusion over widespread areas of the body for psoriasis. Soyka and Soyka,[54] however, report that salicylate intoxication can occur as a result of the Keralyt-occlusive regimen.

Birmingham and colleagues[55] studied the systemic absorption of salicylic acid in humans following topical application. Drug absorption was minimal following application to intact skin. Experimentally, however, measurable salicylate plasma levels were obtained if the stratum corneum was removed before the salicylic acid was applied. This finding indicates that the use of salicylic acid in psoriasis is safe.

ALLERGIC REACTIONS TO SALICYLIC ACID

Although allergic reactions to salicylic acid are rare, Rudzki and Koslowska[56] reported five patients who had allergic reactions to salicylic acid. In four cases, the source of salicylic acid was 2% salicylic acid in alcohol. Three patients themselves noticed that the use of this preparation was responsible for the reactions. In none of the patients did aspirin cause exacerbation or relapses of the dermatitis.

Resorcinol (Resorcin)

Allergic reactions to resorcinol are rare and have been reported mainly from its use in Castellani's Carbol-fuchsin paint.[57]

DISCOLORATION FROM RESORCINOL

Unless alcoholic solutions of resorcinol and resorcinol monoacetates are kept in dark bottles, they may produce a yellow-orange discoloration of the fingernails. In addition, the discolored resorcinol may act as an irritant.

Table 9-2 Acne Preparations Containing Resorcinol
Acne Dome Creme and Lotion (Dome)
Acnomel Cream and Cake (Menley and James)
Bensulfoid Lotion (Poythress)
Exzit Medicated Creme and Lotion (Dome)
Rezamid Acne Lotion (Dermik)

TOXIC EFFECT OF RESORCINOL

Acute resorcinol poisoning is rare. The application of an ointment containing 12.5% resorcinol to the diaper area of an infant produced dusky cyanosis, a maculopapular eruption, hemolytic anemia, and hemoglobinuria.

Resorcinol has an antithyroid activity similar to that of methyl thiouracil. The continued application of ointment containing resorcinol to large leg ulcers has given rise to myxedema, which may be associated with ochronosis. Hydroquinone, which is an isomer of resorcinol, can also produce ochronosis.[57]

RESORCINOL IN ACNE PREPARATIONS

In the United States, the most common exposure to resorcinol is probably in its use in acne preparations as a keratolytic agent and mild antiseptic. Table 9.2 lists acne preparations containing resorcinol. Because such preparations are usually applied to noneczematous skin, allergic reactions to resorcinol from such therapy are rare.

RESORCINOL IN COSMETICS

In eyedrops, skin "fresheners," freckle creams, hair "tonics," hair dyes, and certain lipsticks, as Caron and Calnan[59] point out, resorcinol allergic contact dermatitis is a very uncommon occurrence.

RESORCINOL IN SUPPOSITORIES

In 1933, Mitchell[60] reported the first case of anal dermatitis from resorcinol in Anusol suppositories.

OTHER THERAPEUTIC AGENTS THAT CONTAIN RESORCINOL

Table 9.3 lists resorcinol-containing products that also contain benzocaine, a common and potent sensitizer.

Table 9-3 "Anti-itch" Preparations Containing Resorcinol and Benzocaine
Bi Cozene Creme (Creighton Products)
Lanacane Medicated Creme (Combe)
Vagisil Feminine Itching Medication (Combe)

Table 9-4 Industrial Exposures to Resorcinol

Celluloid manufacturers
Duplicating fluid
Dyes and dye intermediates
Explosives
Mildew-proofing agents
Photocopy machines
Photographic developers
Plastic manufacture
Rubber additives
Tanning agents

INDUSTRIAL EXPOSURE TO RESORCINOL

Resorcinol (*m*-dihydroxybenzene, $C_6H_6O_2$) is an important compound in the preparation of numerous dyestuffs, especially those of the azo, fluorescein, and oxazine series. Styphnic acid (2,4,6-trinitroresorcinol) is used, like picric acid, as an explosive, as well as for the separation and characterization of organic bases, which frequently form well-crystallized styphnates. Table 9.4 lists the industrial uses of resorcinol.

RESORCINOL CROSSREACTIONS

Caron and Calnan[59] studied cross-sensitivity reactions to resorcinol and found that the most clinically significant crossreactions were to resorcinol monoacetate (Euresol) (Table 9.5) and to hexylresorcinol (Table 9.6). Keil[61] reported that "milder" crossreactions are occasionally encountered between resorcinol, pyrocatechol, hydroquinone, phenol, pyrogallol, and hydroxyhydroquinone, and orcinol.

RELATION OF RESORCINOL TO ORCINOL (5-METHYLRESORCINOL)

Orcinol, a homologue of resorcinol, is a constituent of many substances occurring in lichens of the *Rocella* and *Lecanora* series. It is obtained synthetically from P-toluidine. Orcinol becomes blue-violet in the presence of ferric chloride. With chloroform and alkali it becomes

Table 9-5 Resorcinol Monoacetate (Eurosol) Products that May Crossreact with Resorcinol

AR-EX-RMS Scalp Lotion (AR-EX)
Hil Cortac Lotion (Hill Dermaceuticals)
Resulin-F (Schiefflien)
Sulforcin Lotion (Texas Pharmacal)

Table 9-6 Hexylresorcinol-Containing Products that May Crossreact with Resorcinol

Oil-O-Sol Liquid (Health Care)
S.T. 37 (Beecham Products)
Sucret Lozenges (Beecham Products)

red, and, when then diluted with water, it becomes yellow with a green fluorescence.

Orcinol is the parent substance of the orseille and litmus dyes and is used in chemistry as a reagent for pentoses, lignin, beet sugar, saccharoses, and arabinose.

Petrolatum

Very few cases have been reported of allergic hypersensitivity to petrolatum, which is a rare sensitizer.[62–65]

NATURE OF PETROLATUM (SOFT PARAFFIN)

Petrolatum (C_nH_{2n+2}), a mixture of semisolid hydrocarbons chiefly of the methane series, is a colloidal system of non-straight-chain solid hydrocarbons and high-boiling liquid hydrocarbons. Petrolatum is also known as petroleum jelly, paraffin jelly, vasoliment, Vaseline, Saxoline, Cosmoline, and stonolene. Its various trade names are listed in Table 9.7.

There are three types of petrolatum. The first type, natural petrolatum, is a purified mixture of semisolid hydrocarbons obtained from petroleum. The purification is usually done with sulfuric acid and percolation through bone black or adsorptive clays. This removes odors and modifies the color. The second type, artificial petrolatum, is manufactured by

Table 9-7 Trade Names for Petrolatum

Amber (Penreco)
Amojell Petrolatum Cream (Amoco)
Amojell Petrolatum Snow White (Amoco)
Cream White (Penreco)
Extra Amber (Penreco)
Fonoline (Witco)
Fybrene (Witco)
Lilly White (Penreco)
Mineral Jelly (Penreco)
Pennsoline (Penreco)
Penreco White (Penreco)
Peffecta (Witco)
Petrolatum Snow White (Penreco)
Protopel (Witco)
Sonojell (Witco)
Ultima White (Penreco)

mixing natural hydrocarbon waxes with refined mineral oils. It is also purified by the aforementioned process. The third type, synthetic petrolatum, is made of synthetic hydrocarbons obtained by hydrogenation.

WHITE VERSUS YELLOW PETROLATUM

White petrolatum is prepared in the same manner as yellow petrolatum. The only difference is that the purification process is extended until practically all of the yellow color is removed. Fisher[62] had a patient allergic to both white and yellow petrolatum. Malten's[63] patient reacted only to yellow petrolatum, and the patient of Grimalt and Romaquera[64] was allergic to both the white and yellow varieties.

Dooms-Goossens and Degreef[65] reported on two patients who were allergic to yellow petrolatum but not to the white variety. These authors tested their patients with several brands of yellow petrolatum, and two of these tests gave positive results. Further patch testing with white soft paraffins and related products, such as liquid paraffin, ozokerite, ceresin, and hard paraffin, yielded negative results. The authors concluded that:

1. Natural petrolatum is a biologic product whose chemical composition may vary greatly. If yellow petrolatum is considered as an ideal vehicle for patch testing, then a thoroughgoing standardization must be implemented as regards both its purity and the use of additives. In any event, it seems always necessary to test the vehicle.
2. White petrolatum should be used as a vehicle instead of yellow petrolatum because it is purer.
3. Synthetic petrolatum might be better than natural petrolatum because a synthetic mixture of hydrocarbons is controlled more easily.
4. If contact allergic reactions to a topical preparation occur, patch tests should be performed with the same quality of ingredients that the patient has used.

PETROLATUM AS A THERAPEUTIC AGENT

Penneys and colleagues[66] reported that petrolatum preparations that contain no known pharmacologically active ingredients frequently produce partial or complete resolution of skin inflammation and burns. The beneficial effects, however, of a commonly applied "banal" substance, such as petrolatum, are difficult to explain. Clinical improvement has been ascribed generally to the physical effect of removing scale, crust, and debris and giving protection from irritants, thus allowing natural recuperative functions to operate. It also seems likely that complex biochemical mixtures, such as petrolatum, lanolin, and mineral oil from organic sources, would contain fractions that are active in various biochemical systems. Ghadially and colleagues[67] found that petrolatum enhanced recovery of human skin from acetone-induced irritation. This was accomplished by petrolatum occupying the intercellular spaces during recovery of barrier function.

IRRITATION, ACNE, AND PIGMENTATION IN BLACK SKIN FROM PETROLATUM

Maibach[68] reported on a black patient who acquired a chronic dermatitis and hyperpigmentation from white and yellow petrolatum, and Plewig and colleagues[69] studied 735 black men who had allergic reactions to scalp creams and oils. About 70% of these long-term users of pomades had a recognizable acneiform eruption of the forehead and temples. This eruption consisted mainly of uniformly closed comedones with occasional papulopustules. The more elaborate formulations (Noxzema, Dixie Peach, and Wildroot) induced pomade acne more frequently and more intensively than simpler preparations, such as mineral oil and petrolatum. Moreover, the application of five pomades to black skin under continuous occlusion for 8 weeks produced microscopic signs of early comedone formation. Pomade acne was indistinguishable histologically from acne vulgaris.

"VASELINOMAS" AND "PARAFFINOMAS" DUE TO INJECTION OF PETROLATUM

Aronete and Grupper[70] issued a warning against intralacrimal injections of medication with pure petrolatum. Such injections are likely to cause complications manageable only by complicated surgical procedures. In the past, certain so-called dermatologic institutes have injected the skin with paraffin or petrolatum to remove wrinkles, form dimples, and otherwise change the normal contour of the face to suit the fancy of the patient. Tumors following such injections may occur as late as 3 years after the original injection.

PETROLATUM AS A PATCH TEST VEHICLE

Generally, it is agreed that petrolatum (USP), also known as Vaseline or yellow soft paraffin, is the best vehicle for most test substances used in patch tests. Petrolatum is nonsensitizing, nonirritating, and so occlusive that it is possible to fix the patch test with nonocclusive, nonirritant adhesive tape. In many cases, this prevents adhesive reactions from interfering with test readings. In addition, test substances dissolved in petrolatum remain allergenic for at least 1 year.

When solvents are used instead of petrolatum as vehicles, there is the possibility they may evaporate, making the dissolved allergens irritant in nature. Because formaldehyde and propylene glycol do not dissolve well in petrolatum, they are tested in aqueous solution. In general, Fisher[62] found that metals such as nickel, cobalt, dichromates, and gold present better patch test results when dissolved in aqueous solutions than when dissolved in petrolatum. Alcohol, acetone, methyl ethyl ketone, and butyrlolactone have to be used as vehicles for patch testing organic chemicals, liquid resins, and resin components.

In 1983, Dooms-Goossens and DeGreef,[71] using several chromatographic and spectrometric procedures, established that the allergens present in pharmaceutical and cosmetic petrolatums are probably polycyclic aromatic hydrocarbons. These substances are impurities, and the quantity present is largely a function of the source of the petrolatum and the purification procedures. Because the aromatic portion in petrolatum is a complex and unstable mixture of chemically related agents, only two out of the several possible allergens present could be identified; they were most probably phenanthrene derivatives with molecular weights of 230 and 244.

Olive Oil

Van Joost and colleagues[72] state that sensitization to olive oil is seldom reported in the literature. By use of epicutaneous tests, a delayed type of hypersensitivity to pure, freshly prepared olive oil could be demonstrated in two patients. Patch tests with certain major constituents of olive oil, the methyl ester of linoleic acid, the glyceryl ester of palmitic acid, the glyceryl ester of stearic acid, glyceryl trioleate, and glycerides of arachidic acid, appeared to be negative. In one patient, a weak reaction to balsam of Peru was found. It is concluded that sensitization to olive oil must be taken into consideration, especially when it is used as a vehicle in patch testing.

Sesame Oil

"Immediate" urticarial reactions may occur from use of this oil.[73] Several patients who applied a zinc oxide "liniment" to stasis ulcers were sensitized to sesame oil.[74]

The principal allergens of sesame oil are sesamin and sesamolin.[75] Patch testing may be done with sesame oil 100% "as is."

Castor Oil

This oil may be used in cosmetics, particularly lipsticks, and may rarely produce allergic contact dermatitis.[76,77]

Lindane (Kwell)

This gamma benzene hexachloride product is used for scabies and pediculosis. The toxic effects from topical application have been reviewed by Matsum.[78] No reports of allergic contact sensitivity have appeared.

Methyl Salicylate

Methyl salicylate, the active ingredient in oil of wintergreen, is present in many over-the-counter liniments used for the treatment of muscle aches and bursitis but is usually not formulated into prescription drugs (Table 9.8). Hindson[79] reported that an ointment containing methyl salicylate sensitized a man whose eruption flared when he took aspirin.

Cerumenex (Xerumenex)

This solvent preparation to dissolve ear wax contains 10% triethanolamine polypeptide condensate, which may produce allergic contact dermatitis.[80,81]

Vitamin A Acid (Tretinoin, Retinoic Acid)

Tretinoin produces an irritant dermatitis and scaling in most individuals, particularly in high concentrations. Several instances of allergic reactions have been reported.[82–85]

Table 9-8 Uses of Methyl Salicylate
Ben-Gay External Analgesic Products (Leeming)
Bensulfoid Lotion (Poythress)
Black-draught Syrup (Chattem)
Deep-down Pain Relief Rub (JB Williams)
Heet Analgesic Liniment (Whitehall)
Heet Spray Analgesic (Whitehall)
Icy Hot Balm (Searle Consumer Products)
Icy Hot Rub (Searle Consumer Products)
Listerine Antiseptic (Warner-Lambert Co.)
Mentholatum Deep Heating Lotion (Mentholatum)
Mentholatum Deep Heating Rub (Mentholatum)
Panalgesic (Poythress)
Sinex Decongestant Nasal Spray (Vicks)
Soltice Quick-Rub (Chattem)
Vatronol Nose Drops (Vicks)
Vicks Inhaler (Vicks Health Care)
Vicks Sinex Decongestant Nasal Spray (Vicks)
Vicks Vatronol Nose Drops (Vicks)

Jordan and colleagues[85] found that two men on patch testing were sensitive to transretinoic acid. They were positive to 0.05% in petrolatum base and to 0.00625% in the commercial lotion diluted with alcohol. A cross-sensitivity was presumed, because neither man had had previous exposure, but the primary allergen was not identified.

Nordqvist and Mehr[82] reported a woman who had been sensitized by Retin-A liquid 0.05%, which she had used to treat a folliculitis of her legs.

Patch testing with tretinoin may be performed 0.05% petrolatum or 0.01% in alcohol.

Tosti and colleagues[86] reported the sudden development of facial erythema and swelling after 1 year of Retin A cream 0.05% use. Patch tests were positive to tretinoin at 0.1% petrolatum and 0.005% in alcohol.

Balato and colleagues[87] used tretinoin 0.05% petrolatum and eth. to identify sensitization to this retinoid best known for its irritant properties. Ten control subjects were negative, and they found nine other case reports in the literature.

Vitamin A Acetate

Exposure to vitamin A manufacturing led to contact dermatitis to retinyl acetate or vitamin A acetate.[88] Patch tests were positive from 10% down to 0.1% petrolatum Retinol palmitate has previously been reported to cause contact dermatitis in cosmetics.

Thiamine Hydrochloride (Vitamin B$_{19}$, Betabion Hydrochloride, and Aneurine Hydrochloride)

Hypersensitivity to various vitamins has been reported, with thiamine accounting for the largest number of such cases. Allergic contact dermatitis may occur in workers who fill vials in its manufacture. The injection or ingestion of this vitamin in such sensitized individuals may produce an eczematous relapse in the form of a contact-type dermatitis.[89,90]

Thiamine hydrochloride may crossreact with coenzyme B (diphosphothiamin) and cocarboxylase.

Vitamin B$_6$

Vitamin B$_6$ is actually three different substances: pyridoxine, pyridoxal, and pyridoxamine. When a disulfide bridge joins two molecules of pyridoxine, the compound pyritinol is formed. Pyritinol has been reported to cause pemphigus-like eruptions, lichen planus–like eruptions, and photosensitive and erythema multiforme–like eruptions. Contact dermatitis from pyritinol can occur during its manufacture. It is marketed in Europe as Encephabol tablets, which have also caused airborne contact dermatitis.[91] Pyridoxine hydrochloride caused widespread contact dermatitis and photosensitivity in a paramedical worker who injected vitamin B preparations. A 10% propylene glycol vitamin B$_6$ patch test was positive and an oral challenge with 100 mg caused reactivation of his dermatitis and his patch test site to B$_6$.[92]

Vitamin B$_{12}$ (Cobione and Berubigen)

When a patient has an allergic reaction to B$_{12}$, there are two possibilities: (a) The patient is allergic to vitamin B$_{12}$ itself, as reported by Young and colleagues,[93] who described a case of sensitivity to Cobione, a B$_{12}$ concentrate, in which there was a delayed tuberculin-type reaction to the intradermal injection of B$_{12}$; and (b) the reaction is due to cobalt sensitivity. In one patient that Fisher[94] studied, a positive patch test reaction to cobalt was correlated with an allergic reaction to vitamin B$_{12}$ in injectable Berubigen (1 mL of Berubigen contains 43.4 µg of cobalt). This cobalt-sensitive patient gave a positive patch reaction to 2% aqueous solution of cobalt chloride and to the vitamin B solutions in strengths of 100 and 1,000 µg/mL. In addition, there were positive delayed scratch and intradermal reactions to the vitamin B$_{12}$ solutions. The patient noted that after each injection of vitamin B$_{12}$, the injected area became red, tender, and pruritic but not eczematous. Oral ingestion of vitamin B$_{12}$ produced similar flares in the sites of previous injections. She also had an intractable hand eczema.

Rostenberg and Perkins[95] reported that a sensitive patient injected intradermally with crystalline vitamin B$_{12}$ gave a tuberculin-type action.

Vitamin D$_3$

The use of 1,25(OH)$_2$D$_3$ for psoriasis is increasing. A report of a positive patch test noted only at the day 4 (delayed) reading with a negative test to the vehicle confirmed allergic contact dermatitis to this medicament.[96]

The irritant properties of calcipotriol make it a challenging substance to evaluate for delayed hypersensitivity. De Groot[97] reported what he believes is the third clearly identified case of allergic contact dermatitis to this vitamin D$_3$ derivative. He used both 10 and 2 µg/mL in isopropanol for patch testing and had reactions at both concentrations. Studies of controls found that 3 of 26 had transient weak reactions to the 10 μg concentration. Frosch and Rustemeyer[98] endorsed the 2 μg/mL calcipotriol patch test in isopropanol as the most suitable for identifying true allergy to this vitamin D derivative.

Contact sensitivity to calcipotriol was noted after 18 months of uneventful use in a patient with palmoplantar psoriasis.[99] Positive patch tests were found down to 0.4 μg/mL. This patient was not sensitive to the closely related tacalcitol, which is another vitamin D derivative. Crossreaction between tacalcitol and calcipotriol has been reported, but apparently it is not obligate.

Vitamin E (Alpha-Tocopherol)

Vitamin E acts as an antioxidant. The natural vitamin E_1 obtained from plants such as germ oil and synthetic vitamin E (alpha-tocopherol) is incorporated into many cosmetics. There are several reports of allergic reactions to the vitamin in cosmetics and deodorants.[100–102]

A vitamin E aerosol deodorant produced so many instances of widespread allergic dermatitis that it had to be withdrawn from the market. Many women pierce vitamin E capsules to rub the vitamin oil into their faces to "improve" the skin. Many such patients have had an allergic contact dermatitis from this procedure.

Mitchell[103] reported that severe contact urticaria occurred in siblings who had been treated with a vitamin E preparation for burns.

A generalized dermatitis was caused by vitamin E in a soapy oats lotion. One percent tocopherol acetate in aqueous solution produced a positive reaction.[104]

Thus, vitamin E is another product that practically never produces allergic reactions when ingested; when applied to the skin, it frequently produces allergic contact dermatitis and urticaria.

Allergy to nicotinic acid ester of vitamin E has been reported from use of a hand cream. No cross reactivity to other forms of vitamin E such as D-alpha-tocopherol or DL-alpha-tocopherol were noted. Nicotinic acid ester of vitamin E is tested at 1% petrolatum.[105]

Vitamin K

Two types of adverse cutaneous reactions occur with vitamin K_1 (phytomenadione or phytonadione). The more common reaction consists of erythematous plaques at the injection sites that resolve in a few weeks after the injection. Scleroderma-like lesions known as Texier syndrome can develop without antecedent inflammation. In a report by Guidetti and colleagues,[106] the sclerodermatous plaque developed over the buttock

injection site, and patch tests with vitamin K_1 were negative while an intradermal test with 0.1 mL of vitamin K_1 was positive. Results of the intradermal test were negative in 10 control patients, suggesting that delayed hypersensitivity was involved in the scleroderma-like lesion. Intramuscular injection of vitamin K_1 led to a persistent and relapsing dermatitis at the injection site that lasted over 2 years. The patient had cystic fibrosis but no liver disease. Patch test reactions were positive to lipid-soluble vitamin K_1 2 mg/mL and also to water-soluble vitamin K_4 1% in aqueous solution. This crossreaction is rare and suggested that sensitization was to the active 1,4-naphthoquinone ring.[107]

In a review of the literature on vitamin K reactions, Bruynzeel and colleagues[108] found 52 cases and reported 2 more of their own. Reactions were not dose related and occurred with or without the presence of liver disease.

A 9-year-old child developed vesicular dermatitis of the buttock at the site of intramuscular vitamin K injections (10 mg/mL). Phytomenadione (vitamin K) at 10% and the injectable preparation both produced positive patch tests, whereas vitamins K_2 and K_3 were negative. Interestingly, sublingual administration of 10 drops per day of the 10 mg/mL intramuscular preparation was tolerated without side effects.[109]

Selenium Sulfide

Various "Selsun" preparations, which are used for seborrhea and tinea versicolor, contain this compound. No allergic reaction to this compound has been reported. Toxic effects, however, may occur if use is prolonged on acutely inflamed areas of the scalp.[110,111]

Captan -Trichloromethylthio-4-Cyclohexene-1,2-Dicarboximide)

Captan derived from the mercaptans is used in over 300 products, particularly as a fungicide for agricultural crops, house plants, and nursery businesses. Captan is also used extensively in veterinary shampoos to treat animals for ticks and fleas.

In aqueous solutions, the captans release sulfur-containing compounds. Captan is also used as a bacteriostat in cosmetic formulations, especially for the hair, including Selsun, Selsun Blue, Vancide 89, and Vancide 89 RE. Captan is present in Dangard, used almost exclusively by barbers and hairdressers. Table 9.9 shows the numerous uses of Captan.

Marzulli and Maibach,[112] using a concentration of 1%, both for induction and for challenge, sensitized 9 of 205

Table 9-9 Exposure to Captan
Agricultural antifungal agent
Barbers and hairdressers
Dangard
Q. E. D. Shampoo
Cosmetic bacteriostat in shampoos
Selsun
Selsun Blue
Vancide
Veterinary medicine
Ticks and fleas

subjects (4.4%). Fregert[113] described a farmer who had allergic contact dermatitis from Captan.

Epstein[114] reported an instance of photoallergic contact dermatitis due to Dangard, which is a trade name for the antimicrobial-antiseborrheic ingredient used in Q.E.D. Hair Groom and Q.E.D. Shampoo, which are sold exclusively by barbers. Dangard is a trade name for Vancide 89 RE, which is used in cosmetic and pharmaceutical preparations.

Coal Tar

Coal tar used as a topical therapeutic agent is a rare cause of allergic contact dermatitis and skin cancer.[115]

Tar and pitch (the residue after the distillation of tar) are phototoxic agents, which, in industry, can produce diffuse burning and erythema of the exposed skin. Edema and hyperpigmentation may develop later. "Tar itch" produces pruritus, folliculitis, and comedones on the trunk from oil-soaked clothes.

Emmett and colleagues[116] found that roofers working with coal-tar pitch develop a phototoxic keratoconjunctivitis that is enhanced markedly by ultraviolet exposure. Photosensitizing chemicals present in tar include anthracene, acridine, methylanthracene, pyrene, fluoranthene, and 3,4-benzpyrene.

As exposure to tar continues, poikilodermatous changes appear on the skin that are manifested by irregular areas of atrophy, loss of pigment with patch areas of hyperpigmentation, and diffuse telangiectasis on the neck, cheeks, and scrotum. Tar warts and multiple keratoacanthomas may develop.[117–119]

Fluorouracil

Leyden and Kligman[120] evaluated 1% and 5% formulations of 5-FU in the Kligman maximization procedure for inducing contact sensitization, and were unable to induce contact allergy to 5-FU. On the basis of these experiments, they concluded that contact allergy to 5-FU is unlikely to be as common as suggested by others, and they classified 5-FU as a weak sensitizer at best.

Mansell and colleagues[121] and Sams[122] have reported allergic responses to 5-FU. Goette and colleagues[123] describe several patients who have acquired allergic contact dermatitis owing to 5-FU. Because irritant reactions are common with 5-FU, Goette and colleagues[123] suggested the following criteria for one differentiation of an allergic from an irritant contact dermatitis to topical fluorouracil: (a) development of a severely pruritic eczematous eruption at the site of contact with a topical fluorouracil preparation, (b) development of a widespread pruritic dermatitis away from the treated area during fluorouracil treatment or the occurrence of a flare phenomenon at a site exposed previously to the drug, (c) development of a positive epicutaneous skin test reaction to preservative-free test materials of fluorouracil in concentrations of 5% or 10%, (d) development of a pruritic indurated erythema with papules or vesicles at the site of the intracutaneous injections (0.1-mL injections of 50 mg/mL, 25 mg/mL, 10 mg/mL of fluorouracil in sterile water), (e) excellent correlation of the intracutaneous and epicutaneous reactions, and (f) compatible histologic findings.[122]

The development of a severely pruritic eczematous dermatitis at the site of fluorouracil application in a fluorouracil-experienced patient should alert the clinician to the possibility of an acute allergic contact dermatitis to the drug. The simple testing methods outlined in this article can readily confirm or negate this diagnosis. Sometimes a patch test to 5% fluorouracil will produce equivocal results even on delayed readings to day 4. In such cases, an intradermal test with 0.1 mL of 10 mg/mL fluorouracil can produce reactions at days 2 and 4 of over 10 mm of erythema, edema, and vesiculation which confirm sensitization.[124]

ECDYSIS DUE TO FLUOROURACIL

Yaffee and Grots[125] found that the use of fluorouracil in three patients who had basal-cell carcinoma was followed by a peculiar necrosis, which, when curetted, shelled out completely like a snake skin. They have termed this "ecdysis." Histologic examination revealed tumor necrosis, leukocytes, and fibrin. There have been no recurrences to date.

Yaffee and Grots[125] commented that the appearance of a swollen, discolored lesion in the site of the original basal-cell tumor is alarming. It contrasts with the usual erythematous and necrotic reaction seen in the response of basal-cell carcinoma to topical fluorouracil. It may be reassuring to the clinician to recognize the "ecdysis" of the necrotic tumor, which casts out the entire noxious lesion.

NONALLERGIC ADVERSE REACTIONS TO FLUOROURACIL

The most frequently encountered local reactions are pain, pruritus, hyperpigmentation, and burning at the site of application. Other local reactions include scarring, soreness, tenderness, suppuration, scaling, and swelling. Also reported are alopecia, insomnia, stomatitis, irritability, medicinal taste, photosensitivity, lacrimation, telangiectasia, and urticaria.

Topical Nitroglycerin

Nitroglycerin administered sublingually or systemically almost never produces allergic reactions. Since nitroglycerin became available in ointment form, however, there have been several reports of allergic reactions to nitroglycerin administered in this form.[126–128] Most individuals tolerate sublingual nitroglycerin after having been sensitized by the ointment.

Contact dermatitis among those who are engaged in the manufacture of nitroglycerin has been reported.[129] Chandraratna and O'Dell[127] reported that one patient experienced an anaphylactoid reaction with oral mucosal and conjunctival edema within 6 hours of cutaneous application. Because of the possibility of a nitroglycerin withdrawal reaction, sublingual nitrate therapy should be instituted before discontinuing nitropaste treatment.

Hendricks and Dec[126] reported that topical nitroglycerin ointment is among the most effective long-acting vasodilators currently available. They reported two cases of contact dermatitis in which patch testing showed allergy to nitroglycerin-containing compounds. The severity of this dermatitis necessitated the discontinuation of topical nitroglycerin therapy in both patients. A potent corticosteroid cream applied once to previous nitroglycerin application sites prevented or minimized this dermatitis and enabled continuation of topical nitroglycerin therapy.

Topical nitroglycerin is now available in a transdermal system in which the nitroglycerin is incorporated into a disc. Three types are available: (a) Nitro-Dur (Key). This transdermal system contains nitroglycerin in a gel-like matrix composed of glycerin, water (purified), lactose, polyvinyl alcohol, providene, and sodium citrate to provide a continuous source of the active ingredient. Each unit is sealed in a polyester-foil-polyethylene laminate. The bandage portion consists of a medical-grade non-woven, heat-sealable, microporous tape, which contains an acrylate adhesive. (b) Nitrodisc (Searle). This contains nitroglycerin (on lactose) polyethylene glycol, water, silicone, rubber, plasticizers, aluminum foil laminate, polyethylene foam, and acrylic adhesive. (c) Transderm-Nitro (CIBA). This system comprises four layers. Proceeding from the visible surface toward the surface attached to the skin, these layers are (i) a tan-colored backing layer (aluminized plastic) that is impermeable to nitroglycerin; (ii) a drug reservoir containing nitroglycerin adsorbed on lactose, colloidal silicon dioxide, and silicone medical fluid; (iii) an ethylene-vinyl acetate copolymer membrane that is permeable to nitroglycerin; and (iv) a layer of hypoallergenic silicone adhesive. Before use, a protective peel strip is removed from the adhesive surface.

Two patients were observed who were allergic to acrylate adhesive in the disc. In such cases, the silicon adhesive may be used.[44]

Adverse cutaneous reactions to transdermal therapeutic systems (TTS) of nitroglycerin are said to occur in 10% to 70% of users. A prospective study[130] found that 15% of nitroglycerin TTS patients experienced an irritant reaction, which was transient. None of the 33 patients studied developed allergic contact dermatitis, and none had to stop treatment. A 0.5% aqueous or 2% petrolatum was recommended for nitroglycerin patch testing to identify the allergic cases.

Glutaraldehyde (Pentanedial)

NATURE OF GLUTARALDEHYDE

Glutaraldehyde (1,5-pentanedial), an aliphatic dialdehyde that forms colorless crystals, is soluble in water, alcohol, ether, and similar organic solvents. It is available most frequently as a 50% aqueous solution. It is used in a 2% water solution as a cold sterilizer, especially in hospital-medical work for sterilizing instruments, bronchoscopes, cystoscopes, and anesthetic equipment; in renal dialysis units for sterilizing forceps; and by patients at home for sterilizing their artificial kidney. Health care workers are more 8 times more likely to be allergic to glutaraldehyde than non-health care workers. Health care workers are also more likely to be allergic to thimerosal, benzalkonium chloride, methyl methacrylate, and formaldehyde.[131]

Relation of Cidex to Glutaraldehyde

Cidex is a 2% acidic glutaraldehyde, which is stable for long periods if stored in a cool place. When the buffering agent sodium bicarbonate is added, the resultant alkaline solution undergoes polymerization and loses its antimicrobial activity within 2 to 3 weeks. This alkaline Cidex is more active and is quicker to take effect than the acidic glutaraldehyde.

Unbuffered solutions of glutaraldehyde are stable for long periods of time, have a mildly acid pH, and a negligible odor, and are not potently antimicrobial; however, when Cidex becomes buffered to an alkaline pH of 7.5 to 8.0 upon the addition of sodium bicarbonate, glutaraldehyde is "activated" and its antimicrobial (sporocidal, bactericidal, viricidal, fungicidal) activity is greatly enhanced for periods of up to 14 days.[132]

Activated glutaraldehyde (Cidex) retains skin-sensitizing properties of pure glutaraldehyde. Furthermore, the relatively strong irritant effect of pure glutaraldehyde on the eyes, nasal passages, upper respiratory tract, and skin is enhanced slightly when this dialdehyde is activated.

GLUTARALDEHYDE AS A THERAPEUTIC AGENT

Use of Glutaraldehyde as an Antifungal Agent

Glutaraldehyde has been shown to have antifungal properties. Jordan and colleagues[133] reported a case of acute contact dermatitis in a man who used glutaraldehyde for onychomycosis.

Glutaraldehyde in Waterless Hand Cleaners

Waterless hand cleaners are commonly used by machinists. Storrs[134] reported hand dermatitis among machinists from glutaraldehyde found in several brands of waterless hand cleaners.

Glutaraldehyde as a Therapeutic Agent for Warts

The use of glutaraldehyde for warts has occasionally been marked by irritation, but apparently no allergic reactions have been encountered from such use.

Glutaraldehyde as a Therapeutic Agent for Bullous Disease

Comaish[135] reported that topical glutaraldehyde decreased skin friction and enhanced resistance to friction injury produced at a given load in short-term experiments. A single application produces a detectable effect for up to 31 days. These observations partly explain glutaraldehyde's known antiperspirant action; however, similar observations have been made with dead skin in vitro. It is suggested that glutaraldehyde and similar substances may be useful when a reduction in friction trauma is necessary, such as in the case of epidermolysis bullosa and porphyria cutanea tarda.

Des Grosseilliers and Brisson [136] stated that in two patients who had localized epidermolysis bullosa (recurrent bullous eruption of the hands and feet or Weber-Cockayne syndrome), experimentally induced blisters were studied histopathologically. The blisters showed cleft formation in the suprabasal layers of the epidermis. Therapy with topically applied 10% glutaraldehyde was beneficial, but the irritant and skin-sensitizing side effects of this chemical proved a limiting factor for its use.

These authors concluded that the therapeutic use of topical glutaraldehyde presents three general shortcomings: (a) the solution causes brown discoloration of the soles; (b) because of its chemical composition and instability, the preparation must be kept refrigerated in order to remain therapeutically effective for a 1-month period, and a new supply of the solution must be prepared every month; and (c) glutaraldehyde is an irritant and a potential skin sensitizer, and the development of an allergic contact dermatitis in a patient precludes further extensive use of therapy.

Gordon,[137] in commenting on Des Grosseliers and Brisson's article, stated that because allergic reactions to glutaraldehyde are quite rare, and because there is no specific treatment for localized bullous epidermolysis, the treatment with glutaraldehyde should not be discarded. Furthermore, the brown discoloration can be minimized by use of a 2% solution of glutaraldehyde, and three baths will remove the stain.

Gordon[138] has also advocated the use of glutaraldehyde for herpes zoster and simplex and pseudomonas infections. Gordon stated that he has received many requests for information on where to get glutaraldehyde and commented: "Any large hospital with an inhalation therapy department may be using buffered glutaraldehyde (Cidex) as a sterilant."[139] Union Carbide, Ethicon, and the Arbrook Companies provide it. It is supplied as a 25% solution, by Matheson, Coleman, Bell, in 1-kg volume bottles, to which sodium bicarbonate is added to a pH of 7.5, as reported by London.[140]

The fumes from glutaraldehyde may act as an irritant to the bronchial and laryngeal mucous membranes, and prolonged exposure could produce localized edema and symptoms suggestive of an allergic response.

USE OF GLUTARALDEHYDE IN HYPERHIDROSIS OF THE SOLES

Maibach and Prystowsky[141] found that glutaraldehyde is effective for hyperhidrosis of the soles. A usage test was performed on the soles and antecubital fossae of six previously documented glutaraldehyde-sensitive subjects. All subjects had negative-usage test reactions when 25% glutaraldehyde was applied to the soles. However, when tested on the antecubital fossae with 2.5% glutaraldehyde, these same patients developed severe dermatitis within 48 hours. These data demonstrate a striking variation by which glutaraldehyde-sensitive patients tolerate or react to its use in two diverse anatomic sites. Glutaraldehyde is not recommended for axillary hyperhidrosis.

Jordan and colleagues[133] reported on a man who developed an allergic contact hypersensitivity from the use of glutaraldehyde for hyperhidrosis of the soles.

ALLERGIC GLUTARALDEHYDE DERMATITIS IN MEDICAL AND ALLIED PROFESSIONS

Table 9.10 shows the exposure to glutaraldehyde in medical and allied professions. Certain X-ray film-developing solutions contain glutaraldehyde. Fisher[142] reported allergic contact dermatitis in radiologists and technicians handling such films.

There are several reports of nurses who acquired allergic glutaraldehyde dermatitis from handling instruments sterilized with this compound.[143–145] Also, a technician handling a renal dialysis unit and an inhalation therapy assistant acquired allergic contact dermatitis from contact with glutaraldehyde used as a cold sterilizing agent.

SAFETY OF GLUTARALDEHYDE-TANNED LEATHER SHOES

There are no reports of shoe dermatitis developing from glutaraldehyde-tanned leather shoes. Jordan and colleagues[133] studied three patients who had allergic hypersensitivity to glutaraldehyde. Although all of them had positive patch test reactions to glutaraldehyde-tanned leather, none of them had shoe dermatitis. Even the patient who had hyperhidrosis was not sensitized by the use of glutaraldehyde.

DOES GLUTARALDEHYDE CROSSREACT WITH FORMALDEHYDE?

In a report by Neering and van Ketel,[146] test results with formaldehyde were negative in all of the glutaraldehyde-sensitive patients but one, a renal dialysis assistant who was in contact with both formaldehyde and glutaraldehyde and had positive reactions on patch testing. Maibach[147] found that 20 patients with positive patch test reactions to 1% aqueous glutaraldehyde all had negative reactions to 2% aqueous formaldehyde.

Glutaraldehyde is prone to irritant reactions even when tested at 1% petrolatum; 9 of 13 reactions were found to be irritant when evaluated by Hansen and Menné.[148] They further studied 0.1% petrolatum and detected allergy in 2 of 884 but could not speculate on how many other cases might have been missed. They did not conclude what the ideal patch test concentration for glutaraldehyde should be.

Garcia[149] reported on a man who had positive reactions to both glutaraldehyde and formaldehyde. This was not unusual, because he was exposed extensively to formaldehyde in his work as a prosecutor's assistant; apparently, however, he had never been exposed to glutaraldehyde.

GLUTARALDEHYDE RARELY CROSS-REACTS WITH FORMALDEHYDE

Belani and Priedklans[150] described an "epidemic" of serious laryngeal injury associated with endotracheal intubation. Glutaraldehyde used for sterilization was suspected. Since the introduction of single-use disposable endotracheal tubes, there have been no further cases of "pseudomembranous laryngotracheitis."

EFFECT OF GLUTARALDEHYDE VAPORS

Zach[151] suspected that several radiologists and X-ray technicians have developed asthma and laryngeal edema from the inhalation of the glutaraldehyde present in certain X-ray film emulsions.

Hansen[152] emphasized that glutaraldehyde used as a hospital disinfectant is an occupational hazard. Table 9.11 lists industrial exposures to glutaraldehyde.

Cantharidin (Spanish fly)

Spanish fly, or cantharides, is a powder derived from certain crushed beetles that contain cantharidin, which

Table 9-10 Exposure to Glutaraldehyde in Medical and Allied Professions
Buffered (Cidex)
Renal dialysis
Pulmonary apparatus
Cold sterilizing solutions
Embalming
Tissue fixative
X-ray solution

Table 9-11 Industrial Exposure to Glutaraldehyde
Clothing
Hardening of photographic gelatin
Increase in water resistance in wallpaper
Intermediate in resin and dyes
Liquid fabric softener
Tanning of leather

is a vesicant and a potent irritant to the gastrointestinal and genitourinary mucosa.[153] The local application of cantharidin is used for treatment of resistant plantar and periungual warts (Cantharone, Cantharone Plus, Verr-Canth, and Verrusol). Two patients seen by Dilaimy developed a severe reaction with edema, redness, and tenderness accompanied by lymphangitis.[154] The reaction started about 30 hours after therapy. According to the author, this reaction is not uncommon.

Boric Acid

Although most cases of borism are due to accidental ingestion of boric acid, many have been traced to its topical application. Valdes-Dapena and Arey,.[155] in a review of the literature on boric acid poisoning, found that 53 of 172 patients had been treated externally for burns, wounds, or an eruption. A detailed account of boric acid intoxication via a transcutaneous route appeared in the Archives of Dermatology some years ago.[156] A dusting powder, with an undisclosed concentration of boric acid but nevertheless advertised as "safe for baby's sensitive skin," was applied several times daily to a 3-year-old boy who had diaper rash. Edema of the eyelids, exfoliation of the axillary areas, and bullae with exfoliation of the suprapubic area and along the inner aspect of the thighs appeared after 3 months of use. The child was febrile, restless, and irritable. Culture showed no bacterial growth. The diagnosis of borism was confirmed by the finding of high levels of boron in the blood (5.4 mg/dL as compared to a norm of 0.08 mg/dL). The findings suggest toxic epidermal necrolysis resulting from percutaneous absorption of the drug.

Topically applied drugs that have associated systemic effects are shown in Table 9.12.

Mechlorethamine (Nitrogen Mustard)

CONTACT ALLERGIC DERMATITIS

Approximately 50% of patients who apply topical mechlorethamine develop cutaneous sensitization of the delayed cell-mediated type. The sensitization is much less frequently of the immediate anaphylactoid (urticarial) type.[157–159] The probability of a delayed hypersensitivity reaction depends on many factors, including age of the patient, type and extent (stage) of disease, and previous or concurrent administration of immunosuppressant agents.[157] Attempts to prevent allergic sensitization by administering preliminary small doses of mechlorethamine (HN_2) intravenously for induction of specific immunologic tolerance or by administering ultraviolet radiation with or without psoralen for their inhibitory effects on Langerhans cell function have been incompletely successful.[160,161]

Contact allergic dermatitis usually develops between 2 and 4 weeks after initiation of topical therapy and may rarely manifest initially at lesion sites only or as an eczematous hand dermatitis. Distinction from a simple irritant dermatitis may be clinically difficult, and open patch testing may be required to clarify the nature of the reaction. For this purpose, fresh HN_2 solution, which is diluted to provide 10 mg in 0.1 mL, is applied uniformly over a $3 \times 2 \times 5$-cm area of normal skin, usually on the back. For patients who have positive skin tests, both topical and systemic procedures have been used for desensitization.

CONTACT IRRITANT DERMATITIS

Substantial irritation from the usual dose of HN_2 (10 mg/50 mL applied once daily) may be encountered in some patients, particularly in those who have generalized erythroderma or atrophic skin from advanced age or prior radiotherapy. In such sensitive patients, the concentration or frequency of topical HN_2 applications may be reduced temporarily until the skin becomes "hardened" to the irritant effects. Concurrent administration of a topical corticosteroid preparation also is useful in this circumstance. Optionally, the physician may prepare the HN_2 in a water-free vehicle.[162]

Table 9-12 Topical Drugs and Associated Systemic Effects

Drug	Systemic Effect
Boric acid	Bullae, exfoliation
Corticosteroids	Adrenocortical suppression
? Gamma benzene hexa-	Neurotoxicity chloride
Hexachlorophene	Neurotoxicity
	Vacuolar encephalopathy
Lomustine	Pancytopenia
Mercurials	Acrodynia
	Nephrotic syndrome
Phenol	Dizziness, collapse
Podophyllin	Coma, acute toxicity
Resorcinol	Chronic myxedema
	Exogenous ochronosis
	Hemoglobinuria
	Hemolytic anemia
	Methemoglobinemia
Salicylic acid	Deep, rapid breathing
	Dizziness, tinnitus
	Purpura
	Scarlatiniform rash
? Selenium sulfide	Tremor, GI distress
	Garlic breath

DRYING EFFECT

Daily applications of aqueous solutions of HN_2 to the skin may aggravate preexisting xerosis and cause pruritus. This effect can usually be counteracted by adding 1 to 3 tsp of an emulsified bath oil or propylene glycol to the HN_2 mixture. If necessary, additional emollient preparations may be applied to the skin after the HN_2 solution has dried.

HYPERPIGMENTATION

Lesion sites heal frequently with hyperpigmentation, but normal skin also may darken dramatically, indicative of a direct melanogenic influence. Such pigmentation is reversible and decreases gradually in most patients even if topical therapy is continued.

EPIDERMAL CARCINOGENESIS

This remains a potential risk as with other therapeutic modalities used to treat mechlorethamine. In patients treated for extended periods of time, an increased frequency (10%) of squamous cell carcinomas and keratoacanthomas has been noted on sun-exposed areas in whites, indicating at least a promoting activity of HN_2 on epidermal neoplastic development. Therefore, patients who have clinical evidence of solar damage and patients previously treated with ultraviolet or ionizing radiation should be monitored carefully. In addition, a few patients have developed epidermal neoplasms in areas not usually associated with solar-induced cancer, particularly the genital skin, indicating that HN_2 has initiating as well as promoting activity. These observations are quite consistent with animal studies that show topically applied HN_2 to be a potent carcinogen. No apparent increase has been made in the frequency of malignant melanomas, internal malignancies, or any demonstrable mutagenic effect on the reproductive system of patients treated with topical HN_2.

CONCLUSIONS

After a quarter century of use, topical HN_2 chemotherapy for mycosis fungoides has been shown to have an excellent therapeutic profile (benefit/risk ratio) that compares favorably with other treatment modalities. The major issues that must be addressed in the future concern the mechanism of action on malignant lymphoid infiltrates in the skin, the determination of the curative potential of topical HN_2 chemotherapy in mycosis fungoides, and the modification of existing therapeutic procedures to minimize potential adverse effects, particularly epidermal carcinogenesis.

Price and colleagues[162] state that the use of topical mechlorethamine hydrochloride in the treatment of skin disease has been restricted because of the frequent development of contact dermatitis. A series of 24 patients who had mycosis fungoides in stages 1A (8 patients), 1B (15 patients), and 2 (1 patient) were treated with ointment-based mechlorethamine prepared by an anhydrous method. This preparation was therapeutically effective. Complete clearing occurred in 15 of 18 patients who had the active disease over evaluation periods of up to 27 months, and 1 patient had partial clearing. Two patients showed a partial relapse during their evaluation periods. The incidence of contact dermatitis was very low: 8% in individuals who had a history of hypersensitivity to mechlorethamine and 0% in patients who were exposed to the medication for the first time. This new preparation is effective therapy for mycosis fungoides. Patient use is associated with minimal side effects.

Thomsen and Mikkelsen[163] stated that rubber gloves do not protect nurses who apply nitrogen mustard to patients. They found that one type of glove made of polyvinyl chloride (PVC) protected the nurse against penetration of nitrogen mustard. Rubber gloves did not give protection, and a polyethylene glove also permitted penetration of nitrogen mustard.

Fisher[44] observed several dermatologists who became allergic to nitrogen mustard, which they applied to patients while wearing rubber gloves.

Coumarin

The coumarins are used in over 300 products in the United States in acne preparations, fungal solutions, antiseptics, deodorants, "skin fresheners," hair dyes, and shampoos. They encompass a large class of synthetics, as well as naturally occurring substances. Exposure to these agents is common. Coumarin itself is present in several plants and essential oils (e.g., balsam of Peru) and has been in extensive use as a fragrance commonly incorporated into soaps, detergents, toiletries, cosmetics, sunscreens, and perfumes. Other coumarin derivatives, such as limettin (5,7-dimethoxycoumarin), occur naturally in bergamot oil. Several other coumarin derivatives have been synthesized for use as optical bleaches and as fragrances.

Allergic contact dermatitis was reported in a patient who applied a coumarin-containing ointment to a foot ulcer.[164]

Kaidbey and Kligman[165] report that coumarin and several of its derivatives were investigated for their photosensitizing properties. With a few exceptions, the coumarins are potentially strong photocontact sensitizers but do not evoke phototoxic reactions. Substitution at the six or seven positions of the benzopyrone ring confers photoallergic capability, whereas hydrogenation abolishes activity. Photo crossreactions among closely related derivatives can develop.

Kwong and colleagues[166] reported that the systemic administration of warfarin may produce generalized erythema. Schleicher and Fricker[167] reported that necrosis of the skin developed soon after the initiation of coumarin therapy in an elderly woman. Inadvertent rechallenge resulted in similar lesions. Coumarin necrosis has been found to relate to low levels of protein C rather than an allergic mechanism and is reversed by protein C concentrate administration.[168]

Heparin

There are several types of heparin and related anticoagulants. Unfractionated heparin refers to high-molecular-weight heparins such as Liquemin N 25000 and Thrombophob 25000. Fractionated heparins refer to low-molecular-weight heparins that have once a day dosing for easier patient use. Examples of low-molecular-weight heparins include dalteparin (Fragmin), enoxaparin (Lovenox), reviparin (Clavarine), andeparin (Normiflu), and nadroparin (Fraxiparine). Heparinoids include danaparoid (Orgaran) and pentosan polysulfate (Fibrezym). Hirudin is an anticoagulant derived from leeches and is available in a recombinate form: lepirudin (Refludan).

Although heparin allergy is rare, one patient with such an allergy who developed an eczematous reaction to subcutaneous heparin was able to tolerate 2,600 units of anti-factor Xa low-molecular-weight heparin when coadministered with 250 mg of methylprednisolone and 2 mg of clemastine hydrogen fumarate. The patient also tolerated subcutaneous glycosaminoglycan polysulfate. This treatment was not recommended for patients with skin necrosis.[169]

Eczematous plaques can occur around sites of subcutaneous injection of heparin due to delayed hypersensitivity. Topical application of low-molecular-weight heparin in gel form can also cause contact dermatitis. Crossreactions between fractionated and nonfractionated heparins have occurred.[170] Moreau and colleagues[171] reported a case of delayed hypersensitivity to three low-molecular-weight heparins and unfractionated subcutaneous calcium heparin but not to intravenous sodium heparin.

Koch and colleagues[172] reported a case of heparin sensitivity in a patient in whom pentosan polysulfate had to be used as an alternative due to broad crossreactivity among various types of heparin. Even this agent became problematic and required simultaneous administration of topical corticosteroids to the injection sites, as reactions occurred after about 2 weeks of use. Eczematous plaques rather than skin necrosis are the hallmark of allergy to heparin. In their case, unfractionated heparins from three suppliers and low-molecular-weight heparins from four companies all produced reaction. The latter group included dalteparin-sodium, enoxaparin-sodium, and reviparin-sodium. Even the heparinoid, danaparoid-sodium, was positive on patch and intradermal testing. Contrary to the experience in the case of Koch and colleagues, tolerance of intravenous heparin and heparinoid in the face of cutaneous reactions to subcutaneous injections of heparins was reported by Boehncke and colleagues.[173]

The need for heparin in patients who are developing adverse subcutaneous reactions led to a study of the safety of intravenous heparin in this setting. Eight patients who tested positive to either high- or low-molecular-weight heparin were given intravenous Liquemin N 25000 without any adverse reactions. The high-molecular-weight heparins Liquemin N 25000 and Thrombophob 25000 and the low-molecular-weight heparins Fragmin P, Fraxiparine, and the heparinoid Orgaran, as well as sodium pentosan polysulfate (Fibrezym), were the agents that had caused the subcutaneous reactions.[174]

Allergy to the heparin alternative pentosan polysulfate was found in a patient who was positive to multiple heparins but had never had exposure to pentosan polysulfate. This patient was sensitive to certoparin, dalteparin, enoxaparin, nadroparin, and reviparin, all proven by patch tests. She was also sensitive to danaparoid, heparin-calcium, and heparin-sodium by intracutaneous testing. In this case, hirudin was tolerated.[175]

At times cutaneous reactions occur from both high- and low-molecular-weight heparins and heparinoids. In one such case, intravenous challenge with high molecular-weight heparin which has been reported to be safe, proved problematic and produced a generalized delayed-type skin response. The recombinant hirudin, desirudin, was tolerated.[176] A series of 5 patients who reacted to various forms of low and high molecular weight heparin when evaluated by prick test, patch test, intradermal test or subcutaneous injection were subjected to an intravenous challenge with 5000 IE of heparin sodium in 500 mL of normal saline infused over 4 days. None of the 5 reacted to the intravenous challenge when followed for 2 days. Subcutaneous injection produced the most reactions. Tested substances that caused reactions included nadroparin calcium, enoxaprain sodium and danaparoid sodium. Pentosanpolysulfate heparinoid did not cause reactions on skin testing. While the authors acknowledge that there are reports of systemic reactions to intravenous heparin in this setting, their series argues that the more likely response is tolerance.[177] When lowmolecular-weight heparin and unfractionated heparin both cause reactions, lepirudin (recombinant hirudin) is frequently considered as an alternative. In one such instance, a subcutaneous challenge with lepirudin produced an Arthus reaction manifested by leucocytoclastic vasculitits. In this case, intravenous heparin was tried and found to be well tolerated.[178]

Fondaparinux

A patient who reacted to unfractionated heparin, low-molecular-weight heparins, and pentosan polysuphate was able to safely use fondaparinux, which is a pentasaccharide. Because fondaparinux is a short molecule, it was reasoned that protein binding might not occur, thus avoiding formation of a complete hapten.[179] Koch also found fondaparinux to be an acceptable anticoagulant in 3 patients who exhibited delayed-type hypersensitivity unfractionated heparins and low-molecular-weight heparins. Recombinant hirudins were also an alternative.[180] Jappe and colleagues reported that fondaparinux was a safe alternative agent in 6 of 7 patients with allergy to unfractionated and low-molecular-weight forms of heparin. The one patient who did not tolerate fondaparinux showed typical delayed-type hypersensitivity.[181] A case of fondaparinux reactivity in a patient sensitive to multiple low-molecular-weight heparins was reported by Hohenstein and colleagues.[182]

Hirudin

Perhaps the most reliable alternative is hirudin. Hallai and colleagues reported a patient who developed both immediate and delayed hypersensitivity to multiple low-molecular-weight heparins but was able to tolerate recombinant hirudin.[183]

A hirudin-containing ointment was used to treat hemorrhoids, but a 64-year-old man applied it to thrombophlebitis of his arm and developed contact dermatitis. A positive patch test produced by 20% raw hirudin in ethanol was confirmed with recombinant hirudin. Hirudin is the anticoagulant-antiinflammatory agent extracted from leeches. Twenty controls did not react to hirudin, and in vitro tests were also positive.[184]

Lanolin

Lanolin (wool fat, wool grease, wool wax, wool alcohol, and adeps lanae anhydrous) and its various esters, fatty acids, and aliphatic alcohols are used in many topical medicaments and cosmetics.

Lanolin is a natural product obtained from the fleece of sheep. Its constituents vary from time to time and place to place.

COMPOSITION

Lanolin contains sterols, fatty alcohols, and fatty acids. The lanolin sterols (lanolin alcohols or wool alcohols) include principally cholesterol, lanosterol, and agnesterol and are built from one or more benzene rings.

Commercially, these wool alcohols are called Cerolan, Type HO, Hartolan, Golden Dawn, and Nimco. Cholesterol is the major ingredient of lanolin alcohol, and commercial lanolin products list the cholesterol content. Further studies are required to establish whether these lanolin alcohols are the sole or main sensitizers in lanolin.[185]

The fatty alcohols are long-chained and include the closely related stearyl and cetyl alcohols. The fatty acids, the other ingredients of lanolin, have not been found to be sensitizers.

MODIFICATIONS

Acetylated lanolin (Modulan), according to Cronin,[185] is less of a sensitizer than plain lanolin. Dewaxed lanolin (Lantrol), formed by a solvent crystallization process, is also claimed to cause less sensitization than lanolin.

Another modification is hydrogenated lanolin. Vollum[186] reported that it is being used more frequently in the pharmaceutical and cosmetic industry because it is colorless, odorless, free from tackiness, and more hydrophilic than lanolin.

Hydrogenation is carried out by heating lanolin with a catalyst to 330°C at a pressure of 180 atmospheres. The absorption of hydrogen is complete within a half hour, and the hydrogenated lanolin contains dihydrocholesterol, other hydrogenated steroids, and some saturated alcohol. It was hoped originally that hydrogenated lanolin, or a modification, could be used in cases of lanolin sensitivity, but some patients show a marked sensitivity to hydrogenated lanolin and not to the plain lanolin. Dermatitis owing to hydrogenated lanolin may be missed if patients are patch tested with wool alcohols or plain lanolin and not the hydrogenated variety.

PATCH TESTS FOR LANOLIN SENSITIVITY

Many investigators routinely test with 30% wool alcohol petrolatum, but because it may not be the sensitizing substance in lanolin, patch testing should be performed with lanolin. Thune's[187] investigation indicates that the addition of salicylic acid to lanolin or Eucerin may cause false-positive reactions. Patch tests for wool fat sensitivity should be performed with lanolin without the addition of salicylic acid.

Newcomb[188] emphasizes that lanolin is a complex natural material, which is never completely identified because of the wide variations in purity. The development of new derivatives and further purification may contribute to lowering the incidence of skin reactions to this emollient.[189]

Oleffe and colleagues[190] emphasized that lanolin is a complex mixture of esters and polyesters of 33 alcohols with high molecular weights and 36 fatty acids. He made the following points: (a) The response of tested patients varies greatly within the same individual; thus, a patient may react to one brand of lanolin and not to another. (b) The lanolin alcohols are plainly responsible for allergy to lanolin. (c) The Trolab wool alcohol test is reliable for detecting lanolin allergy. (d) A positive reaction to wool alcohols should prompt the dermato-allergist to test the patient with the lanolin preparation that he or she actually will use. (e) The hydrogenated lanolin that was tested in the US had a very slight allergenic capacity, whereas in Japan, hydrogenated lanolin appears to be a strong sensitizer.

The exact allergenic fraction awaits clarification. It is still unknown whether or not lanolin-sensitive patients can tolerate modified or purified lanolin and its derivatives.

The results of Giorgini and colleagues[191] confirm the sensitizing action of lanolin alcohols and the fact that acetylation, ethylenation, and transesterification eliminate the allergenic activity of lanolin.

One must stress, however, that the various chemical treatments capable of reducing the sensitizing potential of lanolin may prejudice its use as an excipient and that Sulzberger and colleagues[192] pointed out that a considerable reduction in the emulsifying powers of acetylated derivatives compromises their usefulness in pharmacocosmetic preparations.

SENSITIZING POTENTIAL OF LANOLIN

The incidence of lanolin sensitivity is a controversial subject. Kligman[193] concludes that "[l]anolin is an extremely weak sensitizer. Its reputation as an allergen has been vastly inflated by reports emanating from European clinics where patients with chronic eczema have been treated with lanolin-based medicaments for many years. In the healthy population, the incidence is vanishingly small. Lanolin exposure takes place in many ways besides skin care products" (refer to Table 9.13). "I was not able to discover a single reported case among workers engaged in recovering wool wax, in refining it, in transporting it, or among wool sorters."

There is general agreement, however, that lanolin frequently produces allergic contact dermatitis when applied to stasis eczemas and ulcers.

Breit and Bandmann[194] found that 13.2% of 326 cases of leg eczema were sensitive to wool alcohols. Of the 43 Eucerin-positive patients of Bandmann and Reichenberger,[195] about 70% had stasis eczemas. Thus, stasis dermatitis patients are at unusually high risk.

Table 9-13 Lanolin: Noncosmetic and Industrial Exposure
Fur
Furniture polishes
Leather
Metallic corrosion preventatives
Paper
Printing inks
Shoe polishes
Textile finishes

Lanolin allergy is rare in patients who have chronic skin diseases that are not of the eczematous type (e.g., psoriasis, lichen planus, and bullous diseases).

Cronin and colleagues[196] showed that the proportion of atopic patients reacting to wool alcohols was comparable to that of other eczematous patients, except those patients who had stasis eczema.

Transdermal Estrogen

The Estraderm TTS delivers 0.05 mg of estrogen per 24 hours. About 17% of patients have cutaneous reactions, but only about 2% stop because of the reaction. The exact nature of the adverse reactions has been difficult to pinpoint.[197] Ethanol was incriminated in some cases[198] and estrogen (estradiol) in others.[199] Robert Adams (personal communication) observed patients who could tolerate the Estraderm TTS if they let about 1 minute elapse between opening the patch and placing it on the skin.

Most reactions to transdermal estradiol are irritant, but allergies to the adhesive, hydroxypropyl cellulose and ethanol, as well as one case of allergy to estradiol itself, have been reported (1990). A second case due to 17-beta-estradiol proven by a positive patch test to 4% in ethanol was reported by Boehncke and Gall.[200] Their patient was tolerant of the oral use of this agent before and after contact sensitization, as has been seen with clonidine and occasionally other agents (Figure 9-1).

Not all patients with a sensitivity to estradiol induced by Estraderm TTS are tolerant of oral estrogen. Two such cases were reported from Portugal.[201] Diffuse morbilliform erythema occurred 5 to 16 days after resumption of oral estrogen therapy. As the eruption is not life threatening, a trial of oral estrogen was not considered to be contraindicated when cutaneous sensitization is proven.

Transdermal hormonal patches used for postmenopausal symptoms can cause contact dermatitis from ethanol, hydroxypropylcellulose, colophony, and, at times, the involved hormones. True allergic contact dermatitis from 17-β-estradiol and norethisterone acetate was identified by patch tests with 0.1% in ethanol; both produced extreme reactions. When estradiol was tested at 0.5% petrolatum, no reaction was seen, indicating the importance of ethanol as the patch test vehicle.[202]

Transdermal Testosterone

Contact dermatitis to transdermal testosterone patch (Andropatch) was traced to a positive patch test reaction to testosterone propionate 1% in ethanol 90%.[203] The patient also reacted to progesterone and testosterone undecenoate, the latter of which was tested at 2.5% in oil. He tolerated intramuscular injections of a preparation containing testosterone propionate (Sustanon 250).

Jordan[204] compared the testosterone patch (Androderm, SmithKline Beecham) with a scrotal system (Testoderm Testosterone Transdermal System, Alza Corp.) and found less topical irritation with the scrotal system. His patients had reactions using the nonscrotal system, but no reaction was seen when they switched to the scrotal system. This suggested that testosterone was not the responsible substance.

Androgen patch use resulted in contact allergy to testosterone confirmed by positive reactions to 1% in 90% eth. testosterone enanthate and 1% in 90% eth. testosterone undecanoate. Interestingly, the patient also reacted to estradiol, which is formed by the action of aromatase on testosterone. Pretreatment of the skin with clobetasone butyrate 0.05% cream allowed continued use of the testosterone patch.[205]

Transdermal Nicotine

In addition to nicotine itself causing contact dermatitis in transdermal systems, a variety of acrylates may be present in these patches and can cause allergic contact dermatitis.[206]

About 7% of patients using a nicotine TTS experience skin reactions. A 10% aqueous nicotine base concentration can be used for patch test purposes. Fourteen patients intolerant of the device were evaluated; 5 proved allergic, and 9 acquired irritant dermatitis.[207]

Although allergy to nicotine can be a cause for adverse reactions to the transdermal nicotine patches, von Bahr and Wahlberg[208] point out that vasodilation is a normal pharmacologic effect of nicotine that can be confused with allergy. In their patient it occurred at from 10% to 30% nicotine levels but not at lower levels.

Nicotinic Acid Esters

Nicotinic acid esters have been used as topical rubefacients and generally produce erythema lasting from 2 to 4 hours. Benzyl nicotinate and bitoxyethyl nicotinate pro-

duced delayed (72-hour) reactions confirmed by 2.5% concentrations in petrolatum as patch tests.[209]

Mitomycin C

Instillation of mitomycin C, an antineoplastic antibiotic produced by *Streptomyces caespitosus,* into the bladder is followed by an acral eruption that may also affect the skin of the genitals or buttocks. A 0.1% petrolatum concentration is used for patch testing.[210,211] Up to 9% of patients receiving the treatment may experience this side effect, which usually follows five to eight bladder instillations.[212]

Minoxidil

Topical minoxidil at 2% concentration in a vehicle of propylene glycol, ethanol, and water has been used to partially reverse androgenetic alopecia in men and women. Allergic contact dermatitis (35 cases) and photoallergic contact dermatitis (1 case) have been reported from an occupational exposure.[213] Patient use for alopecia has also been associated with allergic contact dermatitis. In some cases, patch tests in petrolatum were negative and were found positive only with the addition of propylene glycol to facilitate percutaneous absorption.[214,215]

Ophthalmic Topical Products

Patch tests done with commercial ophthalmic medications may be negative due to the different barrier characteristics of skin compared to the eye. To overcome this, Corazza and Virgili pretreated the skin to be patch tested with an ophthalmic preparation with 40 μg of sodium lauryl sulfate 0.5% in aqueous solution on a filter paper disk in a 12 mm Finn chamber for 24 hours. When the sodium lauryl sulfate containing chamber was removed, a standard 8 mm Finn chamber with the eyedrops was left in place for 72 hours and read 1 hour after removal. By using this technique, 6 of 15 patients who had findings highly suggestive of contact dermatitis to their eyecare products had positive tests, whereas standard tests were negative.[216]

CYCLOPLEGICS

An ophthalmic preparation used before eye examinations to dilate the pupil was found to cause contact dermatitis.[217] The agent was cyclopentolate hydrochloride 0.5%. Patch tests with this concentration were positive in the patient and negative in 20 controls.

The mydriatic tropicamide is used diagnostically at a 1% concentration. It is sold under the name Mydriacyl and is used to obtain mydriasis and cycloplegia. Boukhman and Maibach[218] had no trouble eliciting a positive patch test to 1% tropicamide petrolatum, and this was negative in 20 controls. The patient had experienced dermatitis of the face, eyelids, and periorbital skin after this agent had been used for diagnostic purposes.

Eyelid and facial dermatitis occurred in a 43-year-old woman who applied eyedrops to patients in an ophthalmology clinic in her capacity as a nurse.[219] Homatropine 1% aqueous was strongly positive on patch testing. This cycloplegic is a semisynthetic tertiary amine antimuscarinic. The patient also reacted to phenylephrine 10% aqueous, which was also a component of eyedrops that she instilled in patients' eyes.

BETA-BLOCKERS

Contact dermatitis has been reported from the following beta-blockers: practolol, timolol, metoprolol, oxprenolol, metipranolol, befunolol, levobunolol, betaxolol, and propranolol.[220]

Beta-adrenergic receptor antagonists (beta-blockers) are used to treat glaucoma. These ophthalmic preparations cause dermatitis of the eyelids and periorbital areas. Koch[221] reported three such cases. In two of the cases the sensitizer was timolol maleate, and in one both levobunolol and pilocarpine. No crossreactivity to other beta-blockers was seen. Skin stripping before patch testing was helpful in identifying these cases.

Beta-blockers in eyedrops produced allergic contact dermatitis after years of safe use in a 68-year-old woman who had used both befunolol and timolol. Befunolol 1% in aqueous solution proved to be the culprit, and a crossreaction with carteolol was found.[222] Carteolol hydrochloride is a beta-blocker used to lower intraocular pressure. Contact allergy was confirmed by patch tests at both 1% and 2% concentrations and no crossreactivity to timolol was found.[223]

ALPHA 2-ADRENERGIC AGENTS

Eyedrops of apraclonidine, a selective alpha 2-adrenergic agent, are used to treat glaucoma in patients who are intolerant of beta-blockers. Adverse reactions to topical 0.5% and 0.1% apraclonidine range from 21% to 48%, and two cases with positive patch tests reported from Spain support the mechanism as being delayed hypersensitivity.[224] Positive patch test reactions may be seen with the commercial product, but it took a 10% aqueous concentration of apraclonidine to cause a positive patch test. Since benzalkonium chloride is in the commercial product

and may be a source of contact dermatitis, such testing is indicated. Other alpha-1-adrenergics including brimonidine and clonidine have not been noted to cross react.[225]

MYDRIATICS

In a study of mydriatic eyedrops (phenylephrine, tropicamide, and cyclopentolate hydrochloride), it was determined that patch tests were not as sensitive as direct instillation into the conjunctival sac in the detection of allergy.[226] In 31 subjects studied, 94% were sensitive to phenylephrine. Patch tests detected only 68% of those allergic using 1% and 10% concentrations in both aqueous and petrolatum vehicles. Twenty-four percent of phenylephrine-allergic subjects were detected only by conjunctival challenge.

The mydriatic agent atropine was found to be a source of contact allergy in a patient shortly after ophthalmologic surgery. A 1% aqueous patch test was positive and additional related belladonna alkaloids were positive. Scopolamine 0.2% in aqueous solution, homatropine HBr 1% in aqueous solution, and belladonna extract 5% petrolatum were all positive, as was the non-structurally related tropicamide 0.5% aq. Non-crossreacting agents proved to be phenylephrine HCl 1% aqueous and cyclopentolate HCl 0.5% aqueous.[227]

CARBONIC ANHYDRASE INHIBITORS

Carbonic anhydrase inhibitors are used for glaucoma therapy. A topical carbonic anhydrase inhibitor, dorzolamide, has caused eyelid dermatitis when used to treat glaucoma. Dorzolamide is a sulfonamide, and conjunctivitis and lip eczema are estimated to occur in about 4% of users.[228] Dorzolamide hydrochloride in Trusopt eyedrops caused eyelid dermatitis after 6 weeks of use in a patient with glaucoma. This is a carbonic anhydrase inhibitor and is a rare cause of contact dermatitis. Patch tests were positive at 5% aqueous or petrolatum[229] A second case of dorzolamide sensitivity which presented as blepharoconjunctivitis has been reported with patch tests positive down to 0.01% in aqueous solution.[230]

MISCELLANEOUS OPHTHALMIC AGENTS

Ketotifen fumarate used as an eyedrop to treat allergic conditions has caused contact dermatitis of the periorbital skin.[231]

Pilocarpine produced both allergic and photoallergic conduct allergy, and on patch testing the reaction was first noticed at day 7, which is quite late. A use test took 3 weeks to become positive. Pilagan 2% (pilocarpine nitrate) and Pilocar 4% (pilocarpine HCl) may be used for patch testing.[232]

Rubidium iodide is thought to interact with lens opacification and is used to prevent cataracts. Contact dermatitis was reported and confirmed with a 1% concentration in petrolatum.[233]

To prevent fibrosis of the cornea after chemical trauma, topical *d*-penicillamine was used. This can crossreact with penicillin and cause contact dermatitis, even in the absence of penicillin allergy. This was confirmed with 1% and 3% aqueous patch tests in a patient who used *d*-penicillamine eyedrops.[234]

β-Interferon eyedrops produced contact conjunctivitis and dermatitis at a 1:32 dilution. There was a prior report of allergy to interferon-a 2 C, but the *β*-interferon patient did not crossreact with *α*- or *γ*-interferon.[235]

Hard contact lenses that were cleaned with Aersolv produced eyelid dermatitis due to cocamidopropyl betaine present at 1.8%. A 1% petrolatum concentration was positive, as was the product tested "as is."[236]

Herbst and Maibach[237] reviewed the many reports of ophthalmic sensitivity and suggested the patch test concentrations. To their list of ophthalmic allergens Herbst and Maibach added prednisolone, diclofenac, tetracaine, ketotifen fumarate, resorcinol, tobramycin sulfate, dipivalyl epinephrine hydrochloride, cyclopentolate hydrochloride, and betaxolol.[238]

Latanoprost, a prostaglandin analog used in ophthalmology to treat open-angle glaucoma and ocular hypertension, is a prodrug of prostaglandin F2alpha. It is marketed as Xalatan. Contact dermatitis was reported from this source and confirmed by patch tests with the commercial product and negative tests to the product minus the active agent. The concentration in the commercial product is 0.005%.[239]

Bimatoprost is used to treat glaucoma and a report of contact dermatitis from this component of Lumigan, an Allergan product, was accompanied by some unusual additional symptoms. These included conjunctival hyperemia, foreign body sensation, blepharitis, and increased pigmentation of the periocular skin. The commercial product was diluted to achieve a 0.003% bimatoprost concentration and the patch test also showed hyperpigmentation. Other components of the commercial product were negative, and brimonidine 0.2% was found to be a safe alternative drug.[240]

Epsilon-aminocaproic acid is present at 1% concentration in eyedrops used to treat cataracts in Japan. Miyamoto and Okajima cite 11 other cases, all from Japan. They point out that this compound is also used to make nylon 6, but that only one case from that source has been reported.[241]

N-acetylcysteine is a mucolytic agent that may be added to eyedrops. Contact allergy detected by a 10% aqueous patch test can be used to identify this rare source of reactivity to eye drops.[242]

Trometamol, which is 2-amino-2-(hydroxymethyl)1, 3-propanediol, is a tris-buffer that has caused contact dermatitis in ophthalmologic gels. It is also used in cardioplegic solutions, liver transplantation, and lysis of renal calculi. It is patch tested at 0.5% in aqueous solution.[243]

An eye ointment sold as Noviform was used to treat atopic eyelid dermatitis, but the condition worsened and a patch test to the product was positive. This agent contains 5% bibrocathol, which is a bismuth oxide-tetrabromocatechol complex. A patch test to the tetrabromocatechol component 5% petrolatum was negative and bismuth oxide was positive down to 0.5% petrolatum.[244]

Interferon

Reactions to injections of interferon (*α* and *β*) are common and may occur in up to 65% of patients. Erythema and infiltration are most common, but necrosis can also occur. Injections of less than 200,000 IU/mL are used to try to check for allergy with *β*-interferon. Depth of injection appears to be the prime determinant of whether a reaction will occur, with deeper reactions being less problematic.[245]

Spironolactone

Topical spironolactone has been used to treat androgenetic alopecia, hirsutism, and acne. In this form, contact dermatitis has occurred with concentrations ranging from 2% to 5% solutions or creams. The onset of dermatitis usually occurs within 1 month of starting the application.[246]

Alpha-Adrenergic Blocking Agents

The alpha-adrenergic blocking agent phenoxybenzamine hydrochloride is used to treat hypertension. Nurses who mix the injectable medication may become sensitized. Contamination of work surfaces is another route of exposure. The correct patch test concentration is 0.1% aqueous.[247]

Benzodiazepams

A mother rendering care to her daughter with cerebral paralysis was required to handle powdered forms of several medications, including diazepam, and developed fingertip dermatitis.[248] A positive patch test to diazepam was observed with a 1% aqueous patch test. A positive test was also found to tetrazepam but not to lorazepam.

Tetrazepam

Photosensitivity to tetrazepam occurred from systemic administration and was proven by photopatch testing.[249] In this case, no crossreaction to diazepam was seen.

Piroxicam and Thimerosal

A link has been established between allergy to thimerosal and photosensitivity to piroxicam. The link is strongest for those thimerosal-sensitive patients who are allergic to the thiosalicylate portion of the molecule. In one study,[250] the overall crossreactivity between thimerosal allergy and piroxicam photosensitivity was found to be only 8%. A form of piroxicam with enhanced bioavailability is used in Portugal: piroxicam-β-cyclodextrin.[251] Photosensitivity was commonly found with this form of piroxicam and attributed in part to a high sensitization rate to thimerosal in Portugal. A non-photosensitizing oxicam, tenoxicam, is recommended as an alternative drug. Another study of thimerosal-sensitive patients found that 45% were sensitive to thiosalicylic acid and thus at risk for photosensitivity to piroxicam.[252]

Ampiroxicam, the prodrug of piroxicam, is available in Japan. It is metabolized to piroxicam and causes photosensitivity in individuals who are also thimerosal sensitive. The same restrictions that apply to the thimerosal-piroxicam story are appropriate for ampiroxicam.[253] Additional cases of ampiroxicam photosensitivity were confirmed by Toyohara and colleagues.[254]

8-Methoxypsoralen

The drug 8-methoxypsoralen has been used to treat alopecia areata, psoriasis, vitiligo, and chronic dermatitis, and reports of contact dermatitis or photocontact dermatitis have occurred in each setting. The commercially available 1% solution can be diluted 1:100 to 1:1,000 for patch test purposes. Protection from inadvertent light exposure is necessary to assess contact dermatitis as opposed to phototoxic reactions. These reactions are thought to be rare.[255]

Cholesterol-Lowering Agents

Nummular eczematous plaques developed on a 59-year-old man who was taking multiple medications.[256] The medications were pulverized and applied as patch tests. A positive reaction to pravastatin occurred; this same pro-cedure in 20 controls was negative. A prick test was also positive with pulverized pravastatin in a drop of saline. This same method for prick testing pravastatin was negative in 10 controls. Simvastatin has previously been associated with generalized dermatitis.

Photosensitivity in the ultraviolet A (UVA) range was detected in a 50-year-old woman treated with simvastatin to treat hypercholesterolemia.[257] A 10% solution of simvastatin in petrolatum exposed to 4.5 J/cm^2 gave a positive photopatch test. Persist photosensitivity with a lowered minimal erythema dose to ultraviolet B (UVB) over 7 months after stopping simvastatin was found as a form of chronic actinic dermatitis in a Spanish man.[258] His minimal erythema dose (MED) was decreased within 5 days of taking simvastatin, but his photopatch test with UVA was negative. When the photopatch test with simvastatin (Zocor) was repeated with UVB light at suberythemagenic doses, a photopatch test was positive at 24 hours.

Proton Pump Inhibitors

Exposure to lansoprazole at a manufacturing facility led to contact dermatitis to this proton pump inhibitor. The patient also reacted to omeprazole. Patch tests to both were positive at 10% in petrolatum. As the patient had no prior exposure to omeprazole, a true crossreaction between the two proton pump inhibitors was expected.[259]

Ranitidine

Contact dermatitis to ranitidine hydrochloride occurs primarily in manufacturing facilities and not in patients using this drug for gastric hypersecretory syndromes. A 1% petrolatum patch test identified 7 of 8 such cases.[260]

Insulin

Insulin allergy can be specific to insulin itself and can present as urticaria or angioedema, Arthus or serum sickness type reactions, or local delayed type reactions. False insulin allergy is a reaction to a vehicle ingredient. Metacresol is present in almost all commercially available insulins. Allergy to metacresol can be detected with 3 mg/mL metacresol in a medium of glycerol 16 mg/mL. This can be used for patch testing. Systemic symptoms may accompany local injection site reactions to metacresol, including nausea, headache, sweating, and diarrhea.[261] A local eczematous reaction to injected insulin (Protaphane insulin HM NovoLet) was traced to the protamine content of the product rather than to insulin itself. Protamine is complexed to insulin to delay absorption and is derived from the sperm of salmon or related fish. Intradermal testing was required to confirm the reaction.[262]

Diclofenac

Strong reactions to treatment of actinic keratoses can be a sign of allergic contact dermatitis rather than just a desirable treatment effect. Solaraze gel contains diclofenac, and allergy to this ingredient can be tested with 2.5% or 5% petrolatum. Contact dermatitis from this source was reported by Kerr and colleagues.[263]

Ticlopidine

The platelet aggregation inhibitor ticlopidine produced a fixed drug eruption which was confirmed by patch tests at 1% and 5% tested over previously lesional skin. No cross reactivity was detected by oral challenge with clopidogrel.[264]

Azathioprine

It is always a surprise when a drug that is supposed to suppress immune responsiveness produces the opposite reaction. Azathioprine tablets were prescribed for a child with leukemia after bone marrow transplantation, but as he had trouble swallowing the tablets his mother crushed the tablets and developed eczema of the hands, face, neck, and soles. A tablet crushed and diluted to 1:333 in water produced a positive patch test.[265]

Antifungals

Lanoconazole and neticonazole ointment have caused at least 10 cases of contact dermatitis each in Japan. These are vinyl imidazoles, used to treat dermatophyte infections. Patch tests at 1% of both are adequate to detect sensitization. Crossreactions are not common. However, Umebayashi and Ito reported a patient who was initially positive to lanoconazole and negative to neticonazole, but after a few months of use he became sensitive to neticonazole as well.[266]

Thiocolchicoside

The topical muscle relaxant, thiocolchicoside, has been reported to cause allergic contact dermatitis rarely. This may occur occupationally in physiotherapists, or in non-

occupational use. A 1% concentration in petrolatum is used for patch testing. This agent can also be administered orally or parenterally.[267]

Clindamycin

Acute generalized exanthematous pustulosis (AGEP) developed from orally administered clindamycin. Patch tests with 1% clindamycin in petrolatum were positive and pustular at day 2 and day 4.[268]

Mucolytics

The mucolytic, mesna, is found in Mistabron. Contact dermatitis may result from cutaneous exposure and this can be confirmed with a patch test of Mistabron 1% aqueous. Inhalation of mesna may not trigger an allergic respiratory reaction, but one day later an eruption of the face and neck may occur.[269]

Heroin

A medical facility that dispensed inhalable heroin was found to have work-related problems in half the nurses, and exposure to heroin was believed to be the source of difficulty. About one-third of the symptomatic nurses had a positive patch test to heroin and eyelid or facial dermatitis. Patch tests were done with diacetylmorphine (heroin) at 0.3%, 1%, 3%, and 5% petrolatum. The 3% concentration seemed to identify most cases.[270]

Hemorrhoidal Preparations

A Spanish hemorrhoidal preparation sold under the name Proctolog contains trimebutine [2-dimethylamino-2-phenylbuty 3,4,5-trimethoxybenzoic acid]. Trimebutine was tested in water at multiple concentrations and reacted down to 0.15 mg/mL. This ingredient has been used an an antispasmodic orally and for anal fissures and hemorrhoids, applied rectally.[271]

Contact Dermatitis from Agents Used to Care for Patients

RESPIRATORY AGENTS AND GASES

Tiopronin [N(2-mercaptopropionyl)glycine] is a sulfhydryl compound used in aerosol therapy as a mucolytic. It has caused contact dermatitis, erythema multiforme, and lichen planus–like eruptions, and the similar sulfhydryl, stepronin, has also caused contact dermatitis. The eruption is usually in the perioral region due to the mask worn during administration.[272]

Airborne dermatitis resulted from exposure to meta-proterenol (Alupent) used by a respiratory therapist to treat patients.[273] A 2.5% aqueous concentration was used for patch testing, and 50 controls were negative.

Sleep apnea is treated with nasal continuous positive air pressure (CPAP). The device is secured with elastic bands around the scalp and lateral aspects of the face. Bands containing thiourea compounds produced eczematous changes in a patient allergic to diethylthiourea.[274] These lesions were eczematous on the face and in the scalp. However, in the scalp, circular patches of alopecia followed the eczema, and this was accompanied by the regrowth of depigmented hair. It was not clear if the contact dermatitis had triggered alopecia areata, but because contact dermatitis is used to correct alopecia areata, this seems less likely. Alternatively, depigmentation may have been a sequela of the thiourea allergy and unique for scalp melanocytes, as no pigment alteration occurred on the face.

An anesthetist who had worked in that capacity for 25 years developed dermatitis on exposed surfaces when using isoflurane (Halothane) anesthesia.[275] Open applications repeated five times produced a nummular erythematous patch. This test was negative in 10 controls. Facial eczema in anesthetists can be a manifestation of contact allergy to volatile anesthetics such as isoflurane. Due to the volatile nature of the isoflurane (1-chloro-2,2,2-trifluoroethyl difluoromethyl ether), closed patch tests and single open application tests are negative. Repeated open application tests (ROATs) are needed; 1 mL of the suspect anesthetic is applied twice daily to the volar forearm to conduct the ROAT, which may be positive in as little as 3 days.[276]

Contact dermatitis can occur from volatile gases such as ethyl chloride, which is used as a local anesthetic. Cross-reactivity with dichlorodifluoromethane (CFC 12) has been seen in such cases.[277] Patch tests with volatile gases requires a ventilated chamber, and Bircher and colleagues[277] constructed a device of a 16-mm pad covered by a plastic membrane on silk tape (Leukotest) that was punctured several times with a thick injection needle.

HYDROCOLLOID DRESSING

Hydrocolloid dressings are a popular form of wound management. One such device is known as DuoDERM CGF, or in the United Kingdom, Granuflex E. One component of this dressing has been identified as a cause of dermatitis: pentaerythritol ester of rosin. This allergen is tested at either 10% or 20% in petrolatum.[278]

Hydrocolloid dressings sold under the name DuoDERM E, as well as DuoDERM CGF, contain pentaerythritol ester of hydrogenated rosin, to which colophony-sensitive patients will react.[279] The same dressing is available under the names Granuflex E and Verihesive E.

Polyisobutylene has been found to be a potential source of allergic contact dermatitis in hydrocolloid dressings. This material is also found in chewing gum, insulating tapes, and wound plasters. However, in a series of eight cases, most of the dermatitis cases were patch test negative, raising the possibility that the reactions were either irritant or unpolymerized contaminants.[280]

Carboxymethylcellulose (CMC) has caused contact urticaria in hydrocolloid dressings. It has also been an allergen contained within injectable corticosteroid preparations. In this exposure, anaphylactic shock can result. The presence of CMC in barium radiocontrast material has also caused anaphylaxis.[281]

CONTRAST

Nonionic contrast medium used for coronary angiography can produce delayed reactions 1 to 2 days after a procedure. The delay makes some physicians suspect causes other than the contrast. Systemic symptoms of nausea, flulike illness, asthma, or abdominal pain have been part of these delayed reactions, and patch tests can produce positive reactions in these individuals. Iopromid is an example of one such substance proven to give positive patch test reactions.[282] Reactions to X-ray contrast media usually develop 3 hours to 2 days after administration and resolve in a week. A Norwegian study identified four risk factors for such reactions: previous contrast reactions; a history of allergy; IL-2 treatment and being of Japanese descent.[283] A study of 142 atopic patients given either ionic contrast (ioxaglate) or nonionic contrast (iopamidol) found that 8 of 68 given nonionic and 19 of 74 given ionic contrast had an allergic-type event, however there was more flushing (38/68) with iopamidol than ioxaglate (24/74).[284]

A Japanese study of reactions to ionic and nonionic contrast found equal numbers of reaction to both. The nonionic agents were iopamidol and iohexol and the ionic were iothalamate and diatrizoate. There were adverse reactions to 5.0% of the ionic group and 4.9% of the nonionic group.[285]

Reactions to X-ray contrast medium that occur hours after injection are termed late reactions as compared to immediate reactions. Patch tests can at times identify allergy of the late type. Visipaque and its component iodixanol produced positive patch test reactions in one such patient and 5% iodixanol in aqueous solution was negative in 35 controls, indicating that it is an acceptable patch test concentration.[286] Iodixanol (Visipaque) is a water-soluble, low-osmolar, nonionic dimeric, hexaiodinated contrast agent. A study of 12 patients who experienced a maculopapular exanthema between 2 hours and 3 days after receiving this X-ray contrast medium found that patch tests were positive in only three cases and were deemed to be of little use in confirming the cause. Readministration of the medium was more diagnostic.[287]

TECHNETIUM

Bone scans with technetium Tc 99m may be followed by an eruption beginning from 4 to 24 hours after the injection. Previously it was thought that methylene diphosphonate, which is part of the preparation, was responsible, but Mooser and colleagues[288] demonstrated that it is the technetium Tc 99m that is at fault. Intravenous methylene diphosphonate was negative in their patient, and a patch test to technetium 99m was positive after 2 and 3 days.

TENS GEL

Patch test reactions that occur to TENS units have been traced to the gels that are placed in the electrical field between the skin and electrode. Patch testing with the individual ingredients in these gels has frequently been negative, whereas a reaction occurs to either the finished product or the gel only after subjected to electrical stimulation by the TENS device. The cause for these reactions remains elusive, and some authors have invoked compound allergy to try to explain the phenomena.[289] Transcutaneous electrical nerve stimulators can cause dermatitis, which appears to be specifically due to the electromagnetic radiation. This diagnosis requires exclusion of possible contactants such as nickel, rubber chemicals, and propylene glycol in the conductive gel.[290]

PHOTODYNAMIC THERAPY

Use of topical delta aminolevulinic acid (d-ALA) produced dermatitis that was a spreading reaction beyond the area of application.[291] The application was to the vulva as part of photodynamic therapy for Bowen's disease. A photoprotected patch test to a 20% aqueous preparation was positive in the patient to d-ALA and negative in 10 controls.

DEVICES

ID Bands

Identification bands placed on all patients admitted to the hospital are usually constructed of polyvinyl chloride. Tung and Taylor[292] had a patient who reacted to three of four types of these bands and also to resorcinol mono-

benzoate and benzoyl peroxide. They were unable to confirm the presence of these additives in the bands.

Pens

Fluorescent marking pens are commonly used to highlight the location of patch tests, as the ink can be seen under black light examination. Such use can sometimes lead to contact dermatitis if the patient is allergic to any of the ingredients in the marking pen. Triethanolamine has been identified as a cause of marking pen reactions.[293]

Adhesive Remover

Adhesive remover contact dermatitis occurred around the stoma of two patients who used ConvaCare stoma bag adhesive remover.[294] In one of the cases sensitivity to d-limonene was demonstrated, and this sensitizer was found to be present in the adhesive remover.

Gowns

Fiber gowns used to provide a barrier against water or blood are treated with epoxy-based materials to bind the waterproof plastic film to the fibers. Use of such gowns can result in unexpected exposure to epoxy allergens in a medical setting. Contact dermatitis to this processing was discovered in the production of such gowns. In the case reported by Tarvainen and colleagues,[295] an epoxy hardener rather than resin was the allergen. Isophoronediamine (IPDA) was the epoxy hardener found responsible, and a 1% patch test concentration was positive. IPDA is also known as 3-amino-methyl-3,5,5-trimethylcyclohexylamine and is considered a cycloaliphatic epoxy resin hardener. IPDA has also caused occupational asthma and contact dermatitis in epoxy floor-laying, painting, tennis racket manufacture, and floor coatings.

Grounding Plate

Acrylates are being used to adhere grounding plates for electrosurgical devices to skin. Both 2-hydroxyethyl acrylate and 2-hydroxyethyl methacrylate are confirmed to be present in the pressure-sensitive adhesive of these devices.[296,297]

Electrodes

Patients who react to cardiac monitoring electrodes may be allergic to components of the electrode gel or the electrode adhesive. In a study of three patients allergic to Red Dot2239 3M TM electrodes, it was learned that p-tert-butylphenol-formaldehyde was present in both the electrode gel and the electrode adhesive.[298]

Cedar Oil

Oil is used with dermatoscopic examination of skin lesions. Three days after her dermatoscopic examination, a woman with atypical nevi developed discs of eczema, which were traced to cedarwood oil.[299] This oil has the same refractive index as glass and is derived from *Juniperus mexicana* and *virginiana*.

Casts

Reactions to plaster of Paris are rare and almost always due to benzalkonium chloride present in the plaster of Paris. The lining material of plaster casts has been another potential source of contact dermatitis due to dioctyl sodium sulfosuccinate in the lining material.[300] Scotch Soft Casts (3m, Glostrup, Denmark) used in orthopedic clinics expose health care personnel to diisocyanates. A study of 10 members of an outpatient orthopedic department found no cases of allergy to diaminophenylmethane or isophorene diisocyanate, but irritant reactions were observed.[301]

Stoma Bags

Stoma-related contact dermatitis reactions have been reported from epoxy resin and stoma adhesive, as well as rubber. The hydrocolloid used to make the bags adhere is polyisobutylene, which proved to be the source of dermatitis in a 48-year-old woman.[302]

Insulin Pump

Acrylates used to attach infusion needles for insulin pumps, commonly known as butterfly catheters, have caused contact dermatitis at the site of skin introduction.[303] Epoxy resins have also caused problems in this setting. The Pureline Basic, also known as the Disetronic Plus, has been recommended as an alternative because the needle is attached by heat rather than by glue.

Allergic contact dermatitis can arise from the acrylates used to assemble insulin pumps. Commercially available acrylate series generally do not contain the appropriate test substances to detect this sensitivity. Phenoxyethoxy ethylacrylate and 2-phenoxy ethylacrylate were found to cause the reaction, with a patch test concentration of 0.01% in petrolatum.[304] In contrast, Saccabusi and colleagues found multiple positive patch tests to acrylates in commercially available series in an insulin pump infusion set case. In their case, the tubing (rather than the adhesive used to attach the needle to the tubing) was the causative agent. They demonstrated by chemical extraction that methyl methacrylate was present in the tubing.[305]

Cannula

Epoxy resin can cause reactions around hemodialysis cannulas, and this presents as dermatitis over the shunt used for vascular access.[306]

Suture

Prolene suture is a polypropylene monofilament, and in its colorless form it produced a positive patch test in a patient who underwent a corneal transplant. Ethilon, a polyamide 6 monofilament, was negative and proved a suitable alternative. This is considered a very rare occurrence.[307]

SURGICAL PREPARATION AGENTS

Povidone-iodine surgical "preps" may contain colophony, and four cases of contact dermatitis from this source were reported form France. A history of reaction to adhesive tapes should alert the surgeon to avoid this type of surgical prep.[308]

Contact Dermatitis in Health Personnel

Physicians, nurses, dentists, veterinarians, pharmacists, and laboratory workers in histology and biologic chemistry are included in this group. The most common type of contact dermatitis in this group is an irritant dermatitis from frequent hand washing with various harsh, alkaline soaps, detergents, and disinfectant solutions. Such frequent washing produces a dry, fissured, pruritic dermatitis that readily becomes secondarily infected and eczematized. Persons with an atopic background in this group often develop intractable hand dermatitis (see Chapter 17). Health care personnel with hand dermatitis should use a mild, unscented soap free of all antiseptics and deodorants.

Reports of occupational dermatitis in hospital workers vary from 12% to 21% of workers affected. In one such study in Italy, the primary problem was found to be irritant contact dermatitis 95% of the time.[309] Younger women were most likely to have hand eczema, and the most common irritants were chlorhexidine gluconate, glutaraldehyde, and glove powder. As is common in occupational contact dermatitis, atopy was a significant risk factor for the development of hand eczema.

Benzalkonium chloride (alkylbenzyldimethylammonium chloride), a quaternary ammonium cationic detergent, is widely used as a preoperative skin disinfectant and sometimes for the disinfection of surgical instruments. It is used in the treatment of burns, ulcers, wounds, and infected dermatoses. Benzalkonium chloride is also present in many cosmetics, deodorants, mouthwashes, dentifrices, lozenges, and ophthalmic preparations. It has produced allergic contact dermatitis in surgical personnel who handle instruments soaked in the antiseptic and who apply it as a preoperative skin disinfectant.[310] Table 9.14 lists commercially available solutions containing

Table 9-14 Benzalkonium Chloride in Over-the-Counter Preparations
Bactine Antiseptic/Anesthetic First-Aid Spray (Miles Laboratories)
Clens (Alcon/BP)
Mediconet (Medicone)
Medi-Quik (Lehn amp; Fink)
Mercurochrome II (Becton-Dickinson)
NTZ (Consumer Products Division, Winthrop)
Prefrin Liquifilm (allergen)
Prescription preparations
Amino-Cerv (Milex)
Cetylcide Solution (Cetylite)
Florida Foam Improved (Hill Dermaceuticals)
Ivy-Chex (nonaerosol) (Bowman)
Zephiran Chloride 1:750 (Winthrop)
Zephiran Chloride Spray (Winthrop)
Zephiran Chloride Tinted Tincture (Winthrop)

benzalkonium chloride that must be avoided by surgeons and others sensitized to this chemical.

Two physicians were reported to have become sensitized to benzalkonium chloride from handling instruments soaked in the disinfectant for cold sterilization. They developed allergic conjunctivitis subsequently from the presence of benzalkonium chloride in ophthalmic solutions. The detergent is the most commonly used preservative in ophthalmic medications, solutions for contact lenses, and "artificial tears."[311]

Huriez and colleagues[312] reported that allergic contact sensitivity to topically applied quaternary ammonium compounds is not uncommon in France. These investigators suggested that such allergic sensitivity may produce generalized reactions from the systemic administration of drugs chemically related to topically applied quaternary ammonium compounds. Such medications include the cholinergic agents, hypotensive drugs (e.g., tetraethylammonium chloride), neuromuscular blocking agents (e.g., decamethonium bromide), or heparin antagonists (hexadimethrine bromide).

Patch testing with benzalkonium chloride should be performed with a 1:1,000 aqueous solution because higher concentrations may produce nonspecific irritant reactions.[313]

Surgeons

Surgical "scrubs" of the hands often precipitate atopic dermatitis with superimposed contact dermatitis of the hands in surgical personnel who have been free of atopic dermatitis since childhood.

Hexachlorophene is still a popular preoperating scrubbing agent. Many surgeons complain of dryness of the skin from this agent, which is a primary irritant reaction.

Allergic reactions to hexachlorophene are rare. Cross-contact sensitivity and photocontact sensitivity to hexachlorophene have been observed in guinea pigs with primary photosensitivity to tetrachlorosalicylanilide and tribromosalicylanilide. It is not yet generally accepted that hexachlorophene is a primary photosensitizer, although such photosensitivity has been reported.[314]

VITAMIN E

Several physicians and surgeons have developed allergic contact dermatitis from the use of so-called "vitamin E" soaps and hand lotions. There is a mistaken notion that topical vitamin E can somehow "improve" the skin. Although the systemic administration of vitamin E almost never produces any allergic reaction, various topical preparations can cause allergic dermatitis.

BETADINE

Betadine Skin Cleanser and Surgical Scrub (Purdue Frederick) are rarely the cause of allergic contact dermatitis in health care personnel and may be substituted for hexachlorophene or deodorant soaps by physicians.[315]

Patients have experienced chemical burns from povidone-iodine, usually after prolonged skin contact.[316] Immediate hypersensitivity manifests as generalized urticaria, and angioedema can occur after application to wounds.[317] Contact dermatitis has also been reported from povidone-iodine, although it is very uncommon.[318]

RUBBER GLOVES

Any hand dermatitis that stops abruptly above the wrists should be considered as stemming from sensitization to ingredients in rubber gloves until proved otherwise.[319]

Allergic hypersensitivity to such rubber chemicals as mercaptobenzothiazole, tetramethylthiuram, and isopropyl paraphenylenediamine present in the standard series are among the most common causes of allergic contact dermatitis in surgeons.[320] Latex itself has become a problem as well and is discussed in Chapter 29 (rubber allergy) and briefly reviewed here.

Natural Rubber Latex

The prevalence of natural rubber latex (NRL) occupational allergy ranges from 8% to 17% and latex-induced asthma from 2.5% to 6%.[321] Contact urticaria from natural rubber latex has been reported in 2.8% to 10.7% of European health care workers. In Finland, incidence rates are available rather than prevalence rates. Among laboratory assistants, the incidence of NRL allergy is 1.0 per 10,000 employed workers. Among cleaners who commonly wear rubber gloves, the incidence is only 0.5 per 10,000 workers. NRL allergy is found in 0.12% of unselected Finns prior to surgery. The incidence of NRL allergy in Finland among medical and nursing personnel was found to be 1.8 per 10,000. This figure was broken down to 3.9 per 10,000 physicians, 2.2 per 10,000 for nurses, and 6.0 and 11.8 per 10,000 dentists and dental assistants, respectively.[322]

The recent epidemic of latex sensitivity has led to surveys of health workers as to glove-related problems (glove-related problems are discussed in detail in Chapter 29). In one such study, 37% of health workers reported skin symptoms with glove use.[323] Of this group, 2% described contact urticaria–like symptoms, 10% eczematous dermatitis, and 24% an unclassifiable skin intolerance from gloves. These same investigators carefully evaluated patients with glove complaints by prick tests with multiple latex extracts as well as radioallergosorbent testing (RAST).[324] Less than 10% of medical workers reporting intolerance of latex gloves proved to be latex sensitive. Some patients identified as RAST positive were accepted as being latex sensitive even though they exhibited no symptoms on direct exposure to latex.

Part of the difficulty of understanding NRL allergy is the complexity of latex sap. More than 240 separate proteins have been identified by electrophoresis.[325] Fewer than 25% of latex proteins are immunogenic, and the proteins that cause reactions are different in different populations.[326] Among medical professionals, prohevein (20 kd) and hevein (4.7 kd) are the prevalent antigenic proteins, whereas children with multiple operations more frequently react to a 27 kd protein and rubber elongation factor (14 kd).

The reactions to NRL include urticaria, conjunctivitis, rhinitis, asthma, abdominal cramping, diarrhea, hypotension, and anaphylaxis.[325] The most severe reactions have occurred with mucosal exposure. Glove powder can act as a carrier for NRL, giving rise to airborne elicitation of symptoms.[327]

Presently, 19 new cases of contact urticaria/100,000 health care workers per year is occurring.[328]

In her comprehensive review, Warshaw[329] has proposed a diagnostic algorithm.

A lack of standardized skin prick test materials and RAST tools that do not detect all cases make establishing a rapid and certain diagnosis challenging. To establish the presence of immediate hypersensitivity, the physician can cut a finger off a latex glove and have the patient moisten the finger and wear the dampened latex for 15 to 30 minutes to check for reactions. If no reaction occurs, the exercise can be repeated with a whole glove. Some authors have expressed concern about the safety of such testing, but patient history as to the nature of symptoms normally experienced when wearing gloves can guide the level of risk that wear testing actually poses.

A strong history of latex glove intolerance manifested by rapid onset of pruritus within minutes of donning gloves suggests immediate hypersensitivity. This is not always the case. Armstrong and colleagues[330] reported such a patient, a nurse, who did not develop respiratory symptoms when exposed to latex gloves. Her prick test to high-protein latex and to her gloves specifically was negative. A wet latex glove was tolerated with only pruritus and no whealing, except that when the patient was allowed to rub her hands in response to the pruritus, then and only then did whealing occur. A diagnosis of dermographism was made. Vinyl gloves did not provoke dermographism. Physical urticaria can closely mimic latex allergy. Thomson and Wilkinson[331] reported three additional cases of dermographism mimicking latex glove allergy. These cases highlight the need for an accurate diagnosis when a health care worker's career is at stake.

The cost of health facilities changing to nonlatex glove use is considerable. However, the costs to the institution of 1% of health care workers becoming fully disabled or 2% partially disabled has been estimated to exceed the cost of changing to a nonlatex environment.[321]

HAND DERMATITIS IN ORTHOPEDIC SURGEONS FROM ACRYLIC BONE CEMENT

Acrylic bone cement, a mixture of polymethyl methacrylate and methyl methacrylate (acrylic monomer), is used for fixation of prostheses to bone in surgical procedures on the hip joint. The brochure describing the bone cement contains the following statement: "The liquid component (methyl methacrylate monomer) is a powerful lipid solvent. It should not be allowed to come into direct contact with sensitive tissues or be absorbed by the body. Also, it should not be permitted to come in contact with rubber, including rubber gloves."

Ironically, a surgeon cannot prevent the cement from coming into contact with rubber gloves, because rubber gloves are the only type of gloves used regularly in the operating room.[332] The manufacturer of the bone cement recommends, "The surgeon [should] wear two pairs of rubber gloves when handling the cement directly and discard these for a fresh pair immediately after he [or she] has finished putting the cement in place." It is thought that this is sufficient protection for an operator unless he or she is sensitive to the methyl methacrylate monomer. If, however, sensitization to acrylic monomer has occurred, sufficient cement penetrates the gloves to produce allergic contact dermatitis.[333]

Some surgeons who have become sensitized to the bone cement have an assistant perform the part of an operation requiring handling of bone cement; the sensitized surgeon then completes the operation.

Allergic contact dermatitis of the hands from acrylic bone cement is accompanied usually by marked dryness and fissuring of the skin.[334]

Another unique feature of allergic contact dermatitis caused by acrylic monomer is a distressing paresthesia of the fingertips in the form of a burning sensation, tingling, and slight numbness. The paresthesia may persist for several weeks after the dermatitis has subsided. Fisher[335] also saw this type of paresthesia in two orthodontists who became sensitized to acrylic monomer in bonding cement. The prolonged paresthesia caused by the monomer may be due to the fact that acrylic monomer is a powerful solvent that readily penetrates damaged skin and thus produces inflammation of the nerve endings in the fingers.[336] One report described paresthesia persisting for at least 3 months in a patient who was allergic to a hydroxyethyl methacrylate compound.[337]

Because the gloves currently available do not protect the hands from acrylic monomer, only the development of a "no-touch" technique will enable the orthopedic surgeon to utilize bone cement with instruments. Sufficient protection will be provided by avoiding direct contact of the gloved hands with the cement. A new potential problem in orthopedic personnel and patients was reported from plaster casts reinforced with melamine-formaldehyde resin. These casts are waterproof, but technicians applying them may become sensitized, as may patients. A 10% melamine-formaldehyde resin in petrolatum patch test is used diagnostically.[338]

Nurses

Aside from exposures while in pursuit of their medical duties, nurses may be exposed to detergents, other cleansers, and alcohol that can lead to dryness and eczematization of their hands. Such irritated skin may be more readily sensitized than nonirritated skin to the medications and chemicals that nurses handle in their work.

When a nurse has intractable hand dermatitis, patch tests should be performed with the chemicals and medications listed under housewife's eczema and under eczema in the professional group. In addition, it may be useful to perform patch tests with streptomycin, penicillin, and chlorpromazine.

STREPTOMYCIN

This drug is an especially important occupational hazard to nurses and a frequent cause of allergic contact sensitization.[339] The allergic dermatitis may first be noted at the tips of the thumb and the index and middle fingers where there is contact with streptomycin from a leaking syringe or needle. Prolonged contact in the sensitized individual may produce deep fissures and hyperkeratoses with superimposed eczematization. Once dermatitis has developed, several weeks of treatment may be required before the hands return to normal, even if contact with streptomycin is avoided.

For patch test purposes, a 2.5% aqueous solution of streptomycin is used. In most instances, sensitized individuals show a strongly positive patch test reaction. Occasionally the reaction is negative, but a scratch test may produce an urticarial wheal within 15 minutes, which may remain for 1 hour or so and be replaced by a papule or vesicle after 24 to 48 hours. Although scratch testing with streptomycin is a relatively safe procedure, the intracutaneous test is hazardous and may cause a generalized urticaria and anaphylactoid shock. Desensitization to streptomycin is dangerous and usually fails.

PENICILLIN

Allergic sensitization to penicillin may be initiated by external contact with various forms of penicillin, and dermatitis may be produced in sensitized individuals by contact with penicillin used for injections or by handling syringes contaminated with it. Allergic contact sensitivity to penicillin is combined usually with the immediate anaphylactic variety. Inhalation of penicillin from powder or aerosols or molds may produce asthma and anaphylactoid shock in individuals with contact sensitivity.

Patch tests may be performed with penicillin powder, ointment (500 U/g) or topical medications. The usual positive reaction occurs in 24 to 48 hours. In sensitive individuals, however, within a half hour an immediate reaction may occur consisting of an erythematous wheal, sometimes with pseudopods.[340] A positive patch test reaction of the delayed type may be significant, because the allergic eczematous contact sensitivity is accompanied frequently by the immediate anaphylactic reaction. If there is a compelling need for penicillin in a patient who has a positive patch test reaction to it, scratch and intracutaneous tests must be performed to determine the presence or absence of the immediate type of sensitivity before systemic administration is attempted. Furthermore, systemic administration to an individual with a positive patch test reaction can produce a severe eczematous contact-type dermatitis medicamentosa, which may be widespread and disabling.

Nurses and others with known sensitivity to penicillin must avoid handling all preparations containing this drug. Desensitization is hazardous and should be attempted with caution.

CHLORPROMAZINE (THORAZINE)

This drug is a common cause of contact dermatitis in nurses who inject it.[341] Pharmacists and others who handle chlorpromazine powder or tablets may also become sensitized.[342,343] Three types of sensitivity are seen with the phenothiazine drugs[344]:

1. The usual allergic contact eczematous variety in which the covered patch test reaction is positive.
2. A photoallergic reaction in which the covered patch reaction is negative when the drug is used alone but becomes positive when the patch test site is irradiated.
3. A photoallergic reaction in combination with an allergic eczematous contact-type sensitization in which the patch test reaction is positive with the phenothiazine derivative alone, but a stronger response is elicited if the site is irradiated with a suberythematous dose of ultraviolet rays or exposed to strong sunlight for 20 minutes.

The increased sensitivity of the skin to light sometimes persists for months. The patient sensitized to chlorpromazine, therefore, should avoid exposure to sunlight for at least several weeks after recovering from the dermatitis. If exposure is unavoidable, a sunscreen should be used to protect the involved skin.

Sensitivity to chlorpromazine may cause crossreactions with other phenothiazine drugs, such as prochloroperazine, chlorpromethazine, pramazine, and promethazine hydrochloride (Phenergan).

MACLOFENOXATE

This injectable analeptic central nervous system stimulant can produce allergic contact dermatitis in nurses who inject their patients with the medication known as Lucidril in France.[345]

FAMOTIDINE

Contact dermatitis of the hands occurred in a nurse handling famotidine, an H_2-receptor antagonist. An aqueous 10 mg/mL patch test was positive, and there were no cross reactions to ranitidine or cimetidine.[346]

REQUIRED VACCINATIONS AMONG MEDICAL PERSONNEL

US Occupational Safety and Health Administration regulations require personnel who handle body fluids to be offered hepatitis B immunization. Pruritic nodules lasting 1 to 2 years have occurred after subcutaneous injections of hepatitis B vaccine (Hevac B). An allergic reaction to aluminum hydroxide present in Hevac B leads

to these granulomatous reactions, which contain aluminum crystals. A 1% aluminum chloride acetate or acitotartrath patch test is superior to aluminum hydroxide.[347]

Prolonged reactions to Heptavac containing thimerosal have also been reported in health personnel receiving subcutaneous injections.[348] It has been noted that thimerosal-sensitive patients tolerated intramuscular immunization without incident in contradistinction to subcutaneous injections.[349] It has been estimated that 16% of Japanese who receive vaccinations containing 0.01% thimerosal will become sensitized.[350] These individuals will be at risk for piroxicam photosensitivity via thiosalicylate allergy induction.[350]

Dentists

Dentists frequently have combined irritant and allergic hand dermatitis.[351] The tips and volar aspects of the fingers and the palms may become dry, fissured, and hyperkeratotic from exposure to both irritants and sensitizers. The fingers may become leathery, with loss of fine tactile perception. When the dorsal aspect of the fingers and hands become involved, erythema, edema, and vesiculation may occur. Patch tests are valuable not only in distinguishing between an allergic and an irritant hand dermatitis, but also in quickly pinpointing responsible allergens.[352]

A strongly positive patch test reaction alerts the dentist to the risk of contacting even minute amounts of a material. Dentists protest frequently that they hardly touch or rarely use a chemical that produces a positive reaction, but it must be emphasized that a single exposure in a sensitized individual may produce a dermatitis that persists for a week or more. Even exposure once weekly may produce a chronic dermatitis. The dentist must not only avoid contact with the sensitizer but also become aware of the guises under which it may appear and the chemicals that crossreact with it.

TOPICAL (SURFACE) AND INJECTABLE LOCAL ANESTHETICS

Dentists, in particular, are frequently sensitized to local anesthetics because they are exposed in two ways: (a) by rubbing on the gum surface with the finger before the era of glove wearing, a solution, spray, or ointment containing a "caine," before the injection of the local anesthetic or for treating various conditions in the mouth, such as relief of ulcers or traumatic injury; and in the form of gauze packs or ointment for postextraction sockets (more than half of the agents listed for surface application in currently accepted dental remedies contain benzocaine and many contain tetracaine; benzocaine and tetracaine are both p-aminobenzoic acid derivatives, which are sensitizers) and (b) by injecting a "caine" compound into the buccal areas. Skin contact occurs due to the leakage of the solution spilling over on the fingers used in retraction or holding the syringe.

IRRITANT DERMATITIS IN DENTISTS

Probably the most common causes of dermatitis among dentists are soaps, detergents, and other cleaners. In addition, the acids used in direct bonding agents and preventive fluoride treatments expose the dentists to strong irritants.

The grinding, polishing, and buffing of metal alloys may release chromium that can produce a characteristic lesion, which is the chrome node appearing over the joints of fingers, eyelids, and face. Usually small painless ulcers, 2 to 4 mm in diameter, deep and firm, with slow healing, are apparent.

DENTAL ALLERGENS

Dental personnel are exposed to many contact allergens, as shown in Table 9.15.

Table 9-15 Contact Allergen Exposure in Dental Personnel
Acrylates
Amalgrams (mercury)
Anesthetics, local
Antibiotics
Bonding agents
Acrylic
Epoxy
Disinfectants
Cresol
Formaldehyde
Halogenated salicyanilides
Hexachlorophene
Mercury
Thymol
Essential oils
Eugenol
Peppermint
Wintergreen
Impression compounds
Rosin
Soldering fluxes
Hydrazine
Rosin
Wax (carnauba)

Dental Technicians

Skin problems related to work were reported by 36% of dental technicians, and most suspected plastic based materials in a survey of 1,132 such workers.[353] Patch tests were performed on 55 examined workers, and allergic contact dermatitis was diagnosed in 64%, with irritant contact dermatitis seen in 24%. The most common allergen was 2-hydroxyethyl methacrylate, followed by ethylene glycol dimethacrylate and methyl methacrylate. Fingertip dermatitis was present in almost all of the allergy cases, and dorsal hand eczema was the most common presentation in irritant reactions.

ACRYLIC MONOMER

In the United States, 95% of dentures are made of acrylic resin by mixing the acrylic liquid monomer methyl methacrylate with polymethyl methacrylate powder.[354] Polymerization and hardening of the resin may take place by heating or by self-curing at room temperatures. For selfcuring acrylic resins, polymerization of the mixture of liquid monomer and polymethyl powder is induced with an organic peroxide and an accelerator or promoter. The self-cured resin normally contains much more residual monomer than does the heat-cured resin.

As a rule, dentures are cured by heat, but when the dentist has to repair or build up a portion of the denture, the self-curing acrylic resin is used. In addition, self-curing acrylic material is used extensively in creating small temporary bridges, crowns, and fillings.

Acrylic monomer alone is a powerful sensitizer, but the polymer and the heat-cured resin are not. Enough residual acrylic monomer is present in the self-cured portion of a denture, however, to cause reactions on the skin and the oral mucosa in sensitized individuals.

Excessive exposure of the dentist to acrylic monomer may cause not only an allergic contact eczematous reaction but also dryness and fissuring of the fingertips by a defatting action on the skin. It is, therefore, advisable for dentists with hand dermatitis to avoid direct contact with liquid acrylic monomer and self-cured dentures and acrylic teeth. Dentists with marked allergic sensitivity to the acrylic monomer, proved by strong patch-test reactions may, nevertheless, wear heat-cured acrylic dentures.

It must be remembered, however, that the acrylic monomer is a strong solvent that readily penetrates rubber gloves.

Acrylic resin sealers and adhesives may produce hand dermatitis in sensitized individuals.

Patch Tests with Acrylic Monomer

Patch tests may be performed with 10% acrylic monomer in olive oil. Because some monomers contain benzoyl peroxide (test 10% pet) and hydroquinone (test 2% pet), patch tests with these chemicals should also be done to determine whether a positive reaction is due to the monomer or these additives.

Methyl methacrylate monomer usually produces a delayed eczematous patch test reaction in sensitized dental personnel. Occasionally, however, an allergic contact urticaria is produced, in which case an urticarial wheal will be produced at the patch test site within an hour.

FORMALDEHYDE

Exposure to this disinfectant occurs during sterilization of dental instruments and is used for the reduction of ammoniacal silver nitrate.

Members of the medical and allied professions may be exposed to formaldehyde when it is used for sterilizing purposes, as a disinfectant, or as a fixing solution for tissues. Formaldehyde is not only a powerful sensitizer but also a potent primary irritant. A strong solution of formaldehyde can coagulate the protein of the skin and produce necrosis and scarring. Prolonged contact, even with weak solutions, may cause extreme dryness of the skin with fissuring. Formaldehyde solution (formalin) may cause the nails to become discolored, soft, or brittle. Paronychia and even suppuration of the matrix may follow exposure to this chemical.

When an allergic sensitization to formaldehyde solution occurs, the dermatitis may become widespread. In sensitive individuals, the mere presence of formaldehyde gas in a room in which a bottle of it was previously opened is sufficient to cause dermatitis. A minute amount of formaldehyde on thermometers, instruments, slides, and biopsy containers is also sufficient to produce dermatitis in sensitized individuals. Few patients are this exquisitely sensitive to formaldehyde. Flyvholm and colleagues[355] found most lose their reactivity between 5,000 and 10,000 ppm formaldehyde. They did not find any formaldehyde-sensitive patients who reacted to less than 250 ppm.

MERCURY

Aside from producing eczematous dermatitis, metallic mercury from a mercury amalgam can produce a granulomatous response.

DENTAL BONDING AGENTS

Dental "bonding" is now popular. The bonding employs the use of an epoxy resin and a methacrylate. At present, BIS-GMA (2,2 bis (4(2-hydroxy-3 methacryloyoxy-propyloxy) phenyl-)-propane is the chemical generally used for almost all bonding. The term "BIS-GMA" refers to the reactants bisphenol A and glycidyl methacrylate.

Unless the dentist practices a "no touch" technique, he or she will readily become sensitized to the epoxy resin or the methacrylate.

The bonding plastic is generally combined with quartz, lithium aluminum silicate, glass, or silicon dioxide to modify the physical properties of the resin. The size of these particles is generally 0.04 to 40 mm.

Contacto (bonding material) is free of methyl methacrylate and epoxy resin. Contacto contains hydroxyl groups and acrylic resins; it may be obtained from General Orthodontic Labs. Inc., P.O. Box 298, W.O.B., West Orange, NJ 07052.

DENTAL IMPRESSION MATERIALS

Allergic reactions to dental impression materials have been reported by van Ketel,[356] Cronin,[357] Nally and Storrs,[358] and van Groeningen and Nater.[359] Dentists handling these materials may develop allergic contact dermatitis, and patients may develop stomatitis after impressions taken with Impregum material. The sensitizers appear to be the Impregum catalyst, methyl dichlorobenzene sulfonate.

Van Ketel[356] reported that a dentist with a contact dermatitis of his hands was allergic to these catalysts as shown by the fact that tests with 1% Impregum catalyst in acetone was strongly positive, whereas five other catalysts showed no positive reactions. The dentist did not react to Permlastic (Kerr-Sybron Corp., Romulus, MI 48174), an impression compound.

SCUTAN—USED IN CROWNS AND FOR TOOTH SEALING

Scutan is an irreversible, stiff epimin plastic that polymerizes in the cold and hardens quickly; it is used for sealing teeth. The catalyst is methyl p-toluenesulfonate, and the solvent is dibenzyltoluene.

The catalyst may produce contact dermatitis in dentists' fingers.[360] Testing may be done with 1% in acetone.

As an alternative for Scutan, Texton (SS White Ltd., 51 St. Arms Road, Harrow, Middlesex HA1 lLR, England) may be used. Texton, however, contains methyl methacrylate, which may be sensitizing.

ESSENTIAL OILS

In dentistry, essential oils are used chiefly as pharmaceutical aids and as mild antiseptics and anodynes. Those oils to which the dentist is exposed and which are sensitizers include:

1. *Eugenol.* This pale-yellow liquid with a strong smell of carnation is employed in the widely used zinc oxide–eugenol dental cement. It may also be

combined with rosin and zinc oxide. It is the essential chemical constituent of clove oil and is also present in cinnamon oil, perfumes, soaps, and bay rum. Individuals sensitized to eugenol should avoid exposure to such products. Eugenol is both a primary irritant and a sensitizer. For patch testing, a 5% solution in olive oil or petrolatum is used.

2. *Clove oil.* This oil is used mainly in dentistry as an anodyne. For patch tests, a 25% concentration in castor oil is used.

3. *Cinnamon oil* (cassia oil). This oil is an antiseptic and a flavoring agent. For testing, a 5% solution in olive oil is used. Vermouths that are flavored with it are also possible sources.

4. *Flavoring agents.* Oils of spearmint, peppermint, wintergreen (methyl salicylate), and menthol. These flavoring agents may be tested 2% in olive oil.

5. *Balsam of Peru.* This substance is used in dentistry as a component of cement liquids. It is tested as a 10% petrolatum solution.

6. *Eucalyptus oil.* This oil is used mainly as a solvent for gutta percha in root canal fillings. It is tested as a 1% solution in alcohol.

Essential oils, particularly eugenol, cinnamon oil, and clove oil, may crossreact with balsam of Peru, benzoin, rosin, and vanilla and may be present in or crossreact with perfumes in soap and toilet water.

Veterinarians and Animal Feed Handlers

Veterinarians are exposed to many contact allergens that not infrequently produce contact dermatitis. Contact dermatitis, which is uncommon for veterinarians, may be due to exposure to bovine tuberculin and Tylosin, which is restricted to veterinary use.[361,362] In addition, veterinarians are exposed to the numerous contactants listed in Table 9.16.[363]

SPIRAMYCIN

This antibiotic is given intramuscularly to cows for mastitis, to pigs for enteritis, and to cats for respiratory infections. Dogs may be treated with capsules. Both spiramycin and Tylosin are added to the drinking water given to pigs with enteritis.

PENETHAMATE HYDROIODIDE (BENZYL PENICILLIN-DIETHYLAMINOETHYLESTER)

This antibiotic is used for local treatment of mastitis in cows as a 25% suspension in oil injected into the teat of

Table 9-16 Patch Test "Series" for Veterinarians[a]
Antibiotics
Benzyl penicillin
Bezathine penicillin
Dihydrostreptomycin 0.1% pet
Erthromycin 1% pet
Oxytetracycline 10% pet
Penethamate hydroiodide 1% pet
Penicillin G 10,000 IU G pet
Procaine penicillin
Spiramycin (Rovamycin) 10% pet
Streptomycin 1% pet
Tylosin tartrate (Tylan) 10% pet
Benzocaine 5% pet
Bovine tuberculin 10% aq
Formaldehyde 1% aq
Mercaptobenzothiazole 1% pet
(rubber gloves and antiseptic)
Merthiolate 0.1% pet
Piperazine 1% aq
Procaine 2% aq
Rubber gloves
Tuberculin 10% aq

[a]Aq, aqueous; pet, in petrolatum.

the cow's udder. Penethamate crossreacts with penicillin in about 50% of the cases.[364]

MERCAPTOBENZOTHIAZOLE

Adams[365] reported that mercaptobenzothiazole is found in the following veterinary medications:

    Analan Ointment (Diamond Labs.) 2%
    Caladerm Ointment (Diamond Labs.) 1.25%
    Delcreo Penetram Skin Balm (Delson) 1%
    Dr. Merrick's Sulfodene Preparation (Westchester) 1.25%
    Happy Jack Skin Balm 1%
    Legear Flea and Tick Powder (Le Gear) 1%
    Mercaptocaine (Pitman-Moore) 2%

"IMMEDIATE" CONTACT URTICARIA IN VETERINARIANS

Hjorth[364] suggested that veterinarians should have scratch tests done with a cow's hairs, horse dander, and a pig's bristles. These allergens can produce dermatitis, hay fever, and asthma in sensitized veterinarians.

In addition, obstetric work with cattle is not unusual among veterinarians. Specific IgE and positive scratch tests to cow placenta extract have been demonstrated in veterinarians with hand eczema after delivering a calf.[366]

Table 9-17 Animal "Pet" Medications
Anesthetics
Antibiotics
Antihistamines
Antimycotic agents
Antiparasiticides
Alugan
Benzyl benzoate
Carbaryl
Dichlorphos
Fenchlorphos
Fenithrothion
Lindane
Mesulphen
Piperonyl butoxide
Propoxur
Pyrethrin I
Rotenone
Tetrachloruinphos
Antiseptics
Eye medications

Rudzki and colleagues[367])summarized occupational dermatitis in veterinarians, stating that the most common causes of such dermatoses are antibiotics, procaine, bovine tuberculin, and irritation from obstetric work.

Malten[368] listed the numerous "pet" medications that can produce contact dermatitis in veterinarians and others who apply them to animals (Table 9.17).

ANIMAL FEED ADDITIVES

Commercially prepared animal feed may contain several growth stimulants, hormones, vitamins, anti-infection agents, minerals, antioxidants, and metals that may lead to allergic contact dermatitis from the handling of these additives.[369] The following feed additives have been reported to produce allergic contact dermatitis.

Tylosin

Neldner[370] described a 13-year-old girl with an allergic contact dermatitis from Tylosin acquired by feeding this antibiotic to a pig. Tylosin is used as a growth promoter in feed for cattle and swine.

Additives to animal feed can cause allergic contact dermatitis. In this setting, vitamin B_{12} has been identified as a cause with a negative reaction to cobalt.[371]

Dinitolmide (Zoalene)

Bleumink and Nater[372] reported a worker in a poultry food factory with an allergic dermatitis of the hands due to dinitolmide, which is added to chicken food to control outbreaks of coccidiosis. Dinitolmide is a dinitrobenzene derivative.

Nitrofurazone (Furacin)

Neldner[370] found that the cause of an allergic contact dermatitis in a hog rancher was due to nitrofurazone, which he used to treat a pig infected with salmonella. Nitrofurazone is also used as a growth promoter in feed, especially for cattle and swine. Nitrofurazone was once a popular remedy for the treatment of burns and stasis ulcers. So many instances of allergic sensitivity to this remedy occurred that its use has largely been abandoned.

Furazolidone and Furaltadone

Furazolidone is used both as an antibiotic in veterinary medicine and as an animal feed additive. When patch tested at 2% petrolatum, false-negative reactions occur. The correct vehicle for testing is either PEG-400 or alcohol.[373] No crossreactions have been reported between furazolidone and nitrofurazone, nitrofurantoin, and furfural.[373] A 1% petrolatum patch test to furaltadone tartrate was successful in detecting allergy to this feed additive.[374]

Ethoxyquin (Santoquin)

Melhom and Beetz[375] recorded an allergic contact dermatitis due to sensitization to ethoxyquin used as an antioxidant in animal feeds. The patient was employed in the manufacture of compounded animal feed.

Burrows[376] pointed out that vitamins A and D_3, as supplied by the manufacturer, contain 5% ethoxyquin (6-ethyl-1,2-dihydro-2,2,4-trimethylquinoline) as an antioxidant preservative. These vitamins are usually diluted with cereal in a premix that dilutes the ethoxyquin to between 0.2% and 0.15%. Further dilution in the final meal would end with a finished product containing 0.0001% ethoxyquin from the vitamin sources. It should be remembered that ethoxyquin also appears in the meal from two other sources. Fish, bonemeal, and tallow have an antioxidant that is likely to be ethoxyquin.

Quindoxin

Burrows[376] reported that quindoxin (Grufas) is used in Great Britain and Ireland as an antioxidant preservative in vitamin additives and animal feed. Burrows showed that quindoxin is capable of inducing a photodermatitis at a low concentration.

Scott and Dawson[377] reported 17 farmers who acquired a photocontact dermatitis from exposure to quindoxin in animal feed as a growth-promoting factor. The patients all showed a dry, lichenified, fissured dermatitis of the exposed parts of the body "resembling a cement dermatitis." Photopatch tests were positive with quindoxin 0.1% petrolatum Quindoxin is also capable of producing allergic contact dermatitis in the absence of light.

Halquinol

This chemical is added to feeds for prevention and treatment of scours in pigs caused or complicated by *Escherichia coli* and Salmonella. The people who add the chemical are exposed to a high concentration. Halquinol is a chlorinated derivative of 8-hydroxyquinoline (oxine) consisting of the following three constituents, added in a 0.1% concentration to meal: 5,7-dichloro-8-hydroxyquinoline, 5-chloro-8-hydroxyquinoline, and 7-chloro-8-hydroxyquinoline.

Caplan[378] noted that animal feed additives can provoke not only irritant, allergic eczematous dermatitis and photodermatitis, but also dermatitis that is urticarial in nature. Direct contact with the animal feed is not necessary because a diffuse dermatitis through the airborne route can occur in farmers and mill workers.

Fisher[369] reported a patient who was allergic to ethylenediamine hydroiodide who also showed a crossreaction to ethylenediamine hydrochloride, to which he had become sensitized by using original formula Mycolog cream.

Burrows[376] listed the numerous chemicals that may be added to animal feed (Table 9.18).

Dawson and Scott[379] reviewed the contact dermatitis in agricultural workers due to animal feed additives.

Pharmacists

Pharmacists have acquired an unusual type of "contact" psoriasis owing to the trauma of the friction of closing and opening "childproof" prescription container caps. In several instances that Fisher observed,[335] such friction has localized psoriasis in the area of friction in pharmacists who have psoriasis elsewhere on their body: this is termed Koebner phenomenon.[380]

Laboratory Workers

Table 9.19 lists the allergens in workers in chemistry and histology laboratories.[381,382]

An unusual source of epoxy resin is immersion oil. Leicat immersion oil uses modified cyclohexyl epoxy resin, which can cause airborne contact dermatitis affecting the face and neck.[383] An epidemic of immersion oil dermatitis with the new Leica formula was confirmed to be due to epoxy resin, and the presence of diglycidyl ether of bisphenol A was confirmed by HPLC.[384]

An electron microscopy technician was found to be allergic to three epoxy components: diglycidyl ester of hexahydrophthalic acid, epichlorohydrin, and an allergen not previously reported—epoxy propane. Epoxy propane is a transition solvent and chemically similar to epichlorhydrin.[385] A 1% concentration in acetone was positive in a patient but negative in 20 controls.

A water laboratory worker developed hand, arm, and face dermatitis from exposure to hydroxylammonium chloride.[386] This chemical is used in the manufacture of pharmaceuticals, in the production of surface coatings, in photography, and in rubber, textile, and plastics

Table 9-18 Commonly Used Animal Feed Additives[a]

Drug	Uses
Amprolium 10% aq sol	Growth promoter in feed (poultry); coccidostat
Arsanilic acid, 3-nitro-4-hydroxyphenyl-arsonic acid 10%	Organic arsenicals; growth promoters in feed (cattle,mineral oil swine, and poultry)
Bacitracin zinc test as is	Growth promoter in feed (swine)
Chlortetracycline hydrochloride, oxytetracycline 3% pet	Growth promoter in feed (swine and sheep); prevention of bacterial enteritis
Diethylstilbestrol 0.1% ethyl alc	Feed additive used in fattening cattle or treatment of anestrus
Ethoxyquin 1% pet	Antioxidant preservative in vitamins A and D_3 and many foods
Ethylenediamine, ethylenediamine dihydroiodide 1% pet	Feed additive; especially for cattle with "foot rot" or "lumpy jaw"
Medroxyprogesterone acetate 1% pet	Feed additive (cattle, dogs, and sheep); threatened abortion and synchronizing estrus and ovulation
Neomycin sulfate 20% pet	Feed additive (swine), especially in sow farrowing to prevent dysentery
Nitrofurazone, furazolidone (Furacin) 1% pet	Growth promoter in feed (cattle and swine); also for *Salmonella*
Penicillin (powder or ointment) test as is	Seldom used in feed; mainly for variety of diseases, especially mastitis in lactating cows[b]
Phenothiazine,[c] piperazine citrate, and thiabendazole 1% aq sol	Feed additive (cattle and swine) for worm control
Sulfacetamide, sulfamethazine test as is	Growth promoter in feed, especially pig starter; to prevent bacterial enteritis
Tylosin (Tylan) 1% aq sol	Growth promoter in feed (cattle and swine): for gram-negative infection, *Leptospira*, and coccidiosis

[a]Aq, aqueous; pet, in petrolatum; sol, solution; alc, alcohol.
[b]Used intramuscularly.
[c]Photosensitizer.

Table 9-19 Allergens in Laboratory Workers in Biologic Chemistry and Histology[a]

Allergens	Test	Use
Acrylamide	5% pet	Polyacrylamide gel electrophoresis
Aniline (amino benzol)[b]	1% pet	Ziehl staining
Benzidine (para-diamino-diphenyl)[b]	1% pet	Demonstration of blood in feces
Congo red	2% pet	Amyloid
N,N'-dimethylpara phenylenediamine	1% pet	Neisseria gonorrhea staining
Epoxy resin	1% pet	Electronic microscope
Epoxy resin hardener	1% pet	Electronic microscope
Formaldehyde	2% aq	Fixator (bouin liquid)
Glutaraldehyde	0.5% aq	Fixator (bouin liquid)
Mercury ammoniated	2% pet	Chloremia titration
Methyl orange	2% pet	Determination of pH
Paraphenylenediamine	2% pet	Glucidograms coloring
Phenylhydrazine	2% pet	Research of osazones in urine
Picric acid (trinitrophenol)	2% pet	Creatine titration
Potassium dichromate	0.5% pet	Cleaning of glassware
Sudan III	2% pet	Lipid staining
Sudan IV	2% pet	Lipid staining

[a]Aq, aqueous; pet, in petrolatum.
[b]May crossreact with paraphenylenediamine.

industries. It has been reported to be a sensitizer in diazo copy paper, and from chemical and photographic facilities.

ACRYLAMIDE

Individuals working with polyacrylamide gel electrophoresis may become sensitized even if latex or polyvinyl chloride gloves are worn, as the acrylamine goes through these glove types.[387]

ALCOHOL

Although it is widely recognized that alcohol can dry and irritate the skin, the possibility of alcohol being a cutaneous sensitizer is usually overlooked. Externally applied alcohol is usually ethyl alcohol, which for this purpose is denatured or is unfit for drinking because of the addition of chemicals. For industrial use, 5% methyl alcohol or acetone is often added to denatured ethyl alcohol; for ordinary or medicinal use, about 40 chemicals are available for denaturing it. Most of these substances have a bitter taste or cause emesis. Rubbing alcohol is 70% ethyl

alcohol with a denaturing agent. In alcohol used in cosmetics, the added chemicals are odorless and non-toxic. Denatured alcohols used for perfumes and other cosmetics often contain diethyl phthalate.

The most popular denaturing agents in rubbing alcohol include tartar emetic, salicylic acid, quinine sulfate, colchicum extract, brucine (an alkaloid resembling strychnine), quassia (the bitter principle of a Jamaica wood), and sucrose octa-acetate (an anhydrous adhesive used in lacquers). Isopropyl alcohol, which has a slight odor resembling that of acetone, may also be used as a denaturing agent. Pure ethyl alcohol is used in some hospitals, but coloring matter, such as methylene blue or amaranth pink (an azo dye used to color elixir phenobarbital), is added to discourage drinking it. Some individuals who have allergic contact sensitivity to alcohol may react to the ingestion of alcohol with a generalized erythema. Reports indicate that allergic reactions to the alcohols are not as rare as formerly believed.[388–392]

Richardson and colleagues[392] reported an allergic eczematous contact dermatitis to a commercially available prepackaged alcohol sponge (Preptic Swab). The dermatitis appeared on the hands of nurses and at the sites of electrocardiogram electrode placement (where the sponges were used as conductors) on cardiac patients. Patch tests indicated that the allergen is probably a volatile substance added to sterilize the swab. The actual sensitizer was not discovered.

Contact Dermatitis Caused by Alcohol

Allergic contact dermatitis is caused occasionally by pure ethyl alcohol, and the allergic sensitivity extends usually to amyl, butyl, methyl, and isopropyl alcohols. The dermatitis may take the form of an eczematous eruption or, rarely, an erythematous flush or contact urticaria at the exposed sites.[393,394] Alcohols, however, are usually irritant.

Systemic Contact Dermatitis

The ingestion of alcohol or even beer or wine by individuals sensitized by external contact to alcohol may be accompanied by extensive stomatitis, aphthous stomatitis, urticaria, angioedema, morbilliform eruptions, or a flare of eczematous dermatitis at sites affected previously by the external exposure to alcohol.

Van Ketel and Tan-Lim[395] reported an allergic eczematous contact dermatitis from alcohol. This patient also had positive reactions to beer, red wine, sherry, and acetone. Van Ketel and Tan-Lim also stated that an external reaction to alcohol does not necessarily mean that systemic contact dermatitis will develop after drinking alcoholic beverages.

Testing for Allergic Alcohol Hypersensitivity

Alcohol may be tested undiluted. Two types of reactions may occur: (a) an immediate urticarial contact reaction, which occurs usually within 15 minutes after the topical application of alcohol in the form of a bright red erythema with or without urticarial elements, which may persist for 2 hours or more (it is advisable to test for contact sensitivity to alcohol first by the open patch test method and to keep the patient under observation for an hour or so); and (b) a delayed reaction, which may take place after 24 or 48 hours with the formation of an erythematous, eczematous patch at the patch test site. Occasionally, there is a combination of the immediate and delayed reaction.[395]

Additional discussions on reactions to alcohol are detailed in Chapter 28.

Allergic Glutaraldehyde Dermatitis in Medical and Allied Professions

There are several reports of nurses who acquired allergic glutaraldehyde dermatitis from handling instruments sterilized with this compound.[396–399] Also reported were a technician handling a renal dialysis unit and an inhalation therapy assistant who acquired allergic contact dermatitis from contact with glutaraldehyde used as a cold sterilizing agent.[400,401] Table 9.20 lists the exposure to glutaraldehyde in medical, nursing, dental, and allied personnel.

Cases have been reported of X-ray technicians and radiologists with allergic glutaraldehyde dermatitis due to the presence of glutaraldehyde in X-ray film solution.[402,403]

Belani and Priedklans[404] described an "epidemic" of serious laryngeal injury associated with endotracheal intubation. Glutaraldehyde used for sterilization was suspected. Since the introduction of single-use disposable endotracheal tubes, there have been no further cases of "pseudomembranous laryngotracheitis." Cidex may be obtained from any large hospital that uses it for sterilization, particularly for inhalation therapy. The following companies produce Cidex: Union Carbide, Ethicon,

Table 9-20 Exposure to Glutaraldehyde in Medical and Allied Professions

Cold sterilizing solution
Buffered (Cidex)
Renal dialysis
Pulmonary apparatus
Embalming
Tissue fixative
X-ray film solution

Arbrook, Matheson, Coleman, and Bell. Patch testing may be performed with 1% Cidex or 1% unbuffered glutaraldehyde in aqueous solution.

References

1. Barbaud A, Goncalo M, Bruynzeel D, et al. Guidelines for performing skin tests with drugs in the investigation of cutaneous adverse drug reactions. Contact Dermatitis 2001;45:321.

2. Lammintausta K, Kortekangas-Savolainen O. The usefulness of skin tests to prove drug hypersensitivity. Brit J Dermatol 2005;152:968.

3. Clemmensen O, Knudsen HE. Contact sensitivity to aluminum in a patient hyposensitized with aluminum precipitated grass pollen. Contact Dermatitis 1980;6:305.

4. Fischer T, Rystedt R. Case of contact sensitivity to aluminum. Contact Dermatitis 1982;8:343.

5. Slater DN, Underwood JC, Durrant TE et al. Aluminium hydroxide granulomas: light and electron microscopic studies and X-ray microanalysis. Br J Dermatol 1982;107:103.

6. Kaaber K, Neilsen AO, Veien NK. Vaccination granulomas and aluminum allergy: course and prognostic factors. Contact Dermatitis 1992;26:304.

7. Fisher AA. Allantoin: a non-sensitizing topical medication: therapeutic effect of the addition of 5% allantoin to Vaseline. Cutis 1981;27:5.

8. Mecca SB. The function and applicability of the allantoins. Proc Scientific Section Toilet Goods Association 1963;39:7.

9. Mecca SB. Allantoin and the newer allantoinates. Proc Scientific Section Toilet Goods Association 1959;31:31.

10. Lawlor P, Hindson C. Allergy to dithranol. Contact Dermatitis 1982;8:137.

11. DeGroot AC, Nater JP. Contact allergy to dithranol. Contact Dermatitis 1981;7:5.

12. Harland CC, Mortimer PS. Laxative-induced contact dermatitis. Contact Dermatitis 1992;27:268.

13. Wranicz A, Czernielweski A. Pemfigoid sprowokowany nowoskabina. Preg Dermatitis 1974;61:693.

14. Krook G. Contact sensitivity to oxyphenbutazone (Tanderil) and cross sensitivity to phenylbutazone (butazolidin). Contact Dermatitis 1975;1:385.

15. Thormann J, Kaaber K. Contact sensitivity to phenylbutazone ointment (Butazolidin). Contact Dermatitis 1978;4:235.

16. Valsecchi R, Tornaghi G, Falgheri G, et al. Drug reaction from oxyphenbutazone. Contact Dermatitis 1983;9:419.

17. Fregert S, Rorsman H. Hypersensitivity to diethylstilboestrol. Acta Derm Venereol (Stockh) 1960;40:206.

18. Fregert S, Rorsrnan H. Hypersensitivity to diethylstilbestrol with cross-sensitization to Benzestrol. Acta Derm Venereol (Stockh) 1962;42:290.

19. Romaguera C, Grimalt F. Contact dermatitis from epinephrine. Contact Dermatitis 1980;6:364.

20. Gibbs RC. Allergic contact dermatitis to epinephrine. Arch Dermatol 1970;101:92.

21. Alani SD, Alani MD. Allergic contact dermatitis and conjunctivitis from epinephrine. Contact Dermatitis 1976;2:147.

22. Colldahl H, Fagerberg E. Conjunctivitis and eyelid eczema due to hypersensitiveness to adrenalin solution employed by spray treatment for asthma. Acta Allergy 1956;10:77.

23. Aaronson SB, Jamamoto EA. Ocular hypersensitivity to epinephrine. Invest Ophthalmol Vis Sci 1960;5:75.

24. Vilaplana J, Zaballos P, Romaguera C. Contact dermatitis by dipivefrine. Contact Dermatitis 2005;52:169.

25. Audicana M, Urrutia I, Echechipia S, et al. Sensitization to ephedrine in oral anticatarrhal drugs. Contact Dermatitis 1991;24:223.

26. Bardazzi F, Tardio M, Mariani R, et al. Phenylephrine in eardrops causing contact dermatitis. Contact Dermatitis 1991;24:56.

27. Akita H, Akamatsu H, Matsunaga K. Allergic contact dermatitis due to phenylephrine hydrochloride, with an unusual patch test reaction. Contact Dermatitis 2004;49:232.

28. Bereston ES. Contact dermatitis due to N-ethyl-o-crotonotoluide ointment (Eurax). Arch Dermatol 1952;65:100.

29. van Dijk E, Manen K. Allergic contact dermatitis from Eurax. Contact Dermatitis Newsletter 1972;12:334.

30. Baptista A, Barros MA. Contact dermatitis to crotamiton. Contact Dermatitis 1992;27:59.

31. Bandmann H-J. Ichthyol dermatitis. Contact Dermatitis Newsletter 1971;10:224.

32. Calnan CD. Ichthyol. Contact Dermatitis Newsletter 1971;9:218.

33. Cooke MA, Hocken Robertson DE. Ichthammol dermatitis. Contact Dermatitis 1981;7:335.

34. Lawrence CM, Smith AG. Ichthammol sensitivity. Contact Dermatitis 1981;7:335.

35. Schneider HG. Allergy to sulphurs. Hautarzt 1978;29:340.

36. Wilkinson DS. Sulphur sensitivity. Contact Dermatitis 1975;1:58.

37. Ekelund A, Moeller H. Oral provocation in eczematous contact allergy to neomycin and hydroxyquinolines. Acta Derm Venereol (Stockh) 1969;49:422.

38. Van Ketel WG. Cross-sensitization to 5.7-di-bromo-8-hydroxy quinoline (D.B.O.) (a compound of Synalar + D.B-O- Cream). Contact Dermatitis 1975;1:385.

39. Kero M, Hannuksela M, Sothman A. Primary irritant dermatitis from topical clioquinol. Contact Dermatitis 1979;5:115.

40. Boe A, Knut W. Increased protein-bound iodine in the serum from the topical use of iodochloro-hydroxy-quinoline (Vioform). Acta Dermatol 1970;50:397.

41. Hodgson-Jones IS. Clioquinol (Vioform) and iodine metabolism. Trans St Johns Hosp 1970;56:53.

42. Vilanova S, Camarasa G. Present importance of the so-called cutaneous tests in the diagnosis of contact eczema. Acta Derm Venereol (Stockh) 1959;50:243.

43. Phillips B. Occupational dermatitis. Practitioner 1954;172:531.

44. Fisher AA. Contact dermatitis. 3rd ed. Philadelphia: Lea & Febiger, 1986.

45. Gaul LE, Underwood GB. The effect of aging a solution of silver nitrate on its cutaneous reaction. J Invest Dermatol 1948;11:7.

46. Marcussen PV. Variations in the incidence of contact hypersensitivities. Trans St John's Hosp Dermatol Soc 1962;48:40.

47. Marshall JP, Schneider BP. Systemic argyria secondary to topical silver nitrate. Arch Dermatol 1977;113:1077.

48. Fisher AA. Irritant and toxic reactions to phenol in topical medications. Cutis 1980;26:363.

49. Rogers SCF, Burrows D, Neill D. Percutaneous absorption of phenol and methyl alcohol in magenta patient BPC. Br J Dermatol 1978;98:559.

50. Baer RL, Serri F, Weissenbach-Vial C. Studies on allergic sensitization to certain topical therapeutic agents. Arch Dermatol 1955;72:19.

51. Rubin MB, Pirozzi DJ. Contact dermatitis from carbolated Vaseline. Cutis 1973;12:52.

52. Goldsmith LA. Salicylic acid. Int J Dermatol 1979;18:38.

53. Taylor RP, Halprin RM. Percutaneous absorption of salicylic acid. Arch Dermatol 1975;111:740.

54. Soyka P, Soyka L. Absorption of salicylic acid. [Letter]. JAMA 1980;224:7.

55. Birmingham BK, Greene DS, Rhodes CT. Systemic absorption of topical salicylic acid. Int J Dermatol 1979;18:228.

56. Rudzki E, Koslowska A. Sensitivity to cylic add. Contact Dermatitis 1976;2:178.

57. Fisher AA. Resorcinol-A rare sensitizer. Cutis 1982;29:331.

58. Findlay GH, DeBeer HA. Chronic-hydroquinone poisoning of the skin from skin lightening cosmetics: a South

African epidemic of ochronosis of the face in dark-skinned individuals. S Afr Med J 1980;57:187.

59. Caron GA, Calnan CD. Studies in contact dermatitis: 14. Resorcin. Trans St Johns Hosp Dermatol Soc 1962;48:149.

60. Mitchell JH. Resorcin anal dermatitis due to resorcin in anusol suppositories. JAMA 1933;101:1067.

61. Keil H. Group reactions in contact dermatitis due to resorcinol. Arch Dermatol 1962;86:212.

62. Fisher AA. Cutaneous reactions to petrolatum. Cutis 1981;28:23.

63. Malten KE. A case of contact eczema to yellow soft paraffin. Contact Dermatitis 1978;4:62.

64. Grimalt F, Romaquera C. Sensitivity to petrolatum. Contact Dermatitis 1978;4:377.

65. Dooms-Goossens A, Degreef H. Sensitization to yellow petrolatum used as a vehicle for patch testing. Contact Dermatitis 1980;6:146.

66. Penneys NS, Eaglestein W, Ziboh V. Petrolatum: interference with the oxidation of arachidonic acid. Br J Dermatol 1980;103:257.

67. Ghadially R, Halkier-Sorensen L, Elias PM. Effects of petrolatum on stratum corneum structure and function. J Am Acad Dermatol 1992;26:387.

68. Maibach H. Chronic dermatitis and hyperpigmentation from petrolatum. Contact Dermatitis 1978;4:62.

69. Plewig G, Fulton JE, Klisman AIM. Pomade acne. Arch Dermatol 1970;101:580.

70. Aronete J, Grupper C. Vaselinoma of the eyelid (second reported case). Bull Soc Fr Dermatol Syphiligr 1970;77:808.

71. Dooms-Goossens A, Degreef H. Contact allergy to petrolatums: attempts to identify the nature of the allergens. Contact Dermatitis 1983;9:247.

72. Van Joost R, Sillevis Smitt JH, Van Ketel WG. Sensitization to olive oil (olea europea). Contact Dermatitis 1981;7:309.

73. Tomsey PJ. Hypersensitivity to sesame seed. J Allergy 1964;35:514.

74. Van Dijk E, Neering H, Vitanyi BEJ. Contact hypersensitivity to sesame oil in patients with leg ulcers and eczema. Acta Derm Venereol (Stockh) 1973;53:133.

75. Neering H, Vitanyi BE, Malten KE, et al. Allergens in sesame oil contact dermatitis. Acta Derm Venereol (Stockh) 1975;55:31.

76. Brandle I, Boujnah-khouadja A, Foussereau J. Allergy to castor oil. Contact Dermatitis 1983;9:121.

77. Sais I. Contact dermatitis to castor oil in a lipstick. Contact Dermatitis 1983;9:75.

78. Matsum LY. Convulsions following application of gamma benzene hexachloride. J Am Acad Dermatol 1981;5:98.

79. Hindson C. Contact eczema from methyl salicylate reproduced by oral aspirin (acetyl salicylic acid). Contact Dermatitis 1977;3:348.

80. Grice K, Johnson CL. Contact dermatitis from Xerumenex. Br Med J 1972;1:508.

81. Boxlev JD, Dawber RPR. Contact dermatitis from one ingredient in Xerumenex Ear Drops. Contact Dermatitis 1976;2:233.

82. Nordqvist B, Mehr K. Allergic contact dermatitis to retinoic acid. Contact Dermatitis 1977;3:55.

83. Romaguera C, Grimalt F. Sensitization to benzoyl peroxide, retinoic acid and carbon tetrachloride. Contact Dermatitis 1980;6:442.

84. Rudzki E, Grzywa A. Dermatitis from retinoic acid. Contact Dermatitis 1978;4:305.

85. Jordan WP, Higgins M, Dvorak J. Allergic contact dermatitis to all-trans-retinoic acid: epicutaneous and leukocyte migration inhibition testing. Contact Dermatitis 1975;1:306.

86. Tosti A, Guerra L, Morelli R, Piraccini BM. Contact dermatitis due to topical retinoic acid. Contact Dermatitis 1992;26:276.

87. Balato N, Patruno C, Lembo G, et al. Allergic contact dermatitis from retinoic acid. Contact Dermatitis 1995;32:51.

88. Heidenheim M, Jemec GBE. Occupational allergic contact dermatitis from vitamin A acetate. Contact Dermatitis 1995;33:439.

89. Dalton IE, Pierce ID. Dermatological problems among pharmaceutical workers. Arch Dermatol Syphilol 1951;64:667.

90. Hjorth N. Contact dermatitis from vitamin B (thiamine): relapse after ingestion of thiamine cross-sensitization to co-carboxylase. J Invest Dermatol 1958;30:261.

91. Wigger-Alberti W, Elsner P. Occupational contact dermatitis due to pyritinol. Contact Dermatitis 1997;37:91.

92. Bajaj AK, Rastogi S, Misra A, et al. Occupational and systemic contact dermatitis with photosensitivity due to vitamin B6. Contact Dermatitis 2001;44:184.

93. Young WC, Ulrich CW, Fouts PI. Sensitivity to B_{12} concentrate. JAMA 1950;143:893.

94. Fisher AA. Contact dermatitis at home and abroad. Cutis 1972;10:719.

95. Rostenberg A, Perkins AJ. Nickel and cobalt dermatitis. J Allergy 1952;22:466.

96. Yip J, Goodfield M. Contact dermatitis from MC 903, a topical vitamin D_3 analog. Contact Dermatitis 1991;25:139.

97. de Groot AC. Contact allergy to calcipotriol. Contact Dermatitis 1994;30:242.

98. Frosch PJ, Rustemeyer T. Contact allergy to calcipotriol does exist: report of unequivocal case and review of the literature. Contact Dermatitis 1999;40:66.

99. Zollner TM, Ochsendorf FR, Hensel O, et al. Delayed-type reactivity to calcipotriol without cross-sensitization to tacalcitol. Contact Dermatitis 1997;37:251.

100. Aeling JL, Panagotacos PJ, Andreozzi RJ. Allergic contact dermatitis to vitamin E aerosol deodorant. Arch Dermatol 1973;108:579.

101. Brodkin RH, Bleiberg J. Sensitivity to topically applied vitamin E. Arch Dermatol 1965;92:76.

102. Minkin W, Cohen HJ, Frank SB. Contact dermatitis from deodorants. Arch Dermatol 1973;107:774.

103. Mitchell J. Contact urticaria from a vitamin E preparation (vitamin E–vegetable oil) in two siblings. Int J Dermatol 1975;14:246.

104. Garcia-Bravo B, Mozo P. Generalized contact dermatitis from vitamin E. Contact Dermatitis 1992;26:280.

105. Oshima H, Tsuji K, Oh-I T, et al. Allergic contact dermatitis to DL-alpha-tocopheryl nicotinate. Contact Dermatitis 2003;48:167.

106. Guidetti MS, Vincenzi C, Papi M, Tosti A. Sclerodermatous skin reaction after vitamin K_1 injections. Contact Dermatitis 1994;31:45.

107. Sommer S, Wilkinson SM, Peckham D, et al. Type IV hypersensitivity to vitamin K. Contact Dermatitis 2002;46:94.

108. Bruynzeel I, Hebeda CL, Folkers E, Bruynzeel DP. Cutaneous hypersensitivity reactions to vitamin K: 2 case reports and a review of the literature. Contact Dermatitis 1995;32:78.

109. Pigatto PD, Bigardi A, Fumagalli M, et al. Allergic dermatitis from parenteral vitamin K. Contact Dermatitis 1990;22:307.

110. Pascher F. Systemic reactions to topically applied drugs. Int J Dermatol 1978;17:269.

111. Ransome JW, Scott NM, Knoblock EC. Selenium sulfide intoxication. N Engl J Med 1961;264:384.

112. Marzulli FN, Maibach HI. Antimicrobials: experimental contact sensitization in man. J Soc Cosmet Chem 1973;24:399.

113. Fregert S. Allergic contact dermatitis from the pesticides captan and phaltan. Contact Dermatitis Newsletter 1967;2:28.

114. Epstein S. Photoallergic contact dermatitis—report of case due to Dangard. Cutis 1968;4:856.

115. Jacobs PH, Farber EM, Nall ML. Psoriasis and skin cancer. In: Farber EM, Cox A, eds. Second International Symposium on Psoriasis. New York: Yorke Medical Books, 1977:350.

116. Emmett EA, Stetzer L, Taphorn B. Phototoxic keratoconjunctivitis from coal tar pitch volatiles. Science 1977;198:841.

117. Goetz H. Tar keratosis. In: Andrade R et al, eds. Cancer of the skin. Philadelphia: WB Saunders, 1976:495.

118. DeMoragas JM. Multiple keratoacanthomas: relation to jamarsan therapy of pemphigus foliacens. Arch Dermatol 1966;93:679.

119. Colomb DJ, Descos L, Gauthier D. Multiple keratoacanthomas and coal tar disease. Rev Lyon Med 1966;15:449.

120. Leyden JJ, Kligman AM. Studies on the allergenicity of 5-fluorouracil. J Dermatol Surg Oncol 1977;3:518.

121. Mansell PWA, Litwin MS, Ichinose H, Krementz ET. Delayed hypersensitivity to 5-fluorouracil following topical chemotherapy of cutaneous cancers. Cancer Res 1975;35:1288.

122. Sams WM. Untoward response with topical fluorouracil. Arch Dermatol 1968;97:14.

123. Goette DK, Odom RB, Owens R. Allergic contact dermatitis from topical fluorouracil. Arch Dermatol 1977;113:196.

124. Sanchez-Perez J, Bartolome B, Jesus del Rio M, et al. Allergic contact dermatitis from 5-fluorouracil with positive intradermal test and doubtful patch test reactions. Contact Dermatitis 1999;41:106.

125. Yaffee HS, Grots I. "Ecdysis" secondary to 5-fluorouracil. Cutis 1980;25:649.

126. Hendricks AA, Dec GW Jr. Contact dermatitis due to nitroglycerin ointment. Arch Dermatol 1979;115:853.

127. Chandraratna PAN, O'Dell RE. Allergic reactions to nitroglycerin ointment: report of five cases. Curr Ther Res Clin Exp 1979;25:481.

128. Zugerrnan C, Zheutlin T, Giacobetti R. Allergic contact dermatitis secondary to nitroglycerin in Nitro-Bid ointment. Contact Dermatitis 1979;5:270.

129. Bressler RR. Nitroglycerin reactions among pharmaceutical workers. Ind Med Surg 1949;18:519.

130. Vaillant L, Biette S, Machet L, et al. Skin acceptance of transcutaneous nitroglycerine patches: a prospective study of 33 patients. Contact Dermatitis 1990;23:142.

131. Shaffer MP, Belsito DV. Allergic contact dermatitis from glutaraldehyde in health-care workers. Contact Dermatitis 2000;43:150.

132. Stonehill AA, Krop S, Borick MP. Buffered glutaraldehyde a new chemical sterilizing solution. Am J Hosp Pharm 1963;20:458.

133. Jordan WP, Dahl MV, Albert HL. Contact dermatitis from glutaraldehyde. Arch Dermatol 1972;105:94.

134. Storrs FJ. Technical and ethical problems associated with patch testing. Clin Rev Allergy Immunol 1996;14:185.

135. Comaish S. Glutaraldehyde lowers skin friction and enhances skin resistance to acute friction injury. Acta Derm Venereol (Stockh) 1973;53:455.

136. Des Grosseilliers JP, Brisson P. Localized epidermolysis bullosa: report of two cases and evaluation of therapy with glutaraldehyde. Arch Dermatol 1974;109:70.

137. Gordon HH. Glutaraldehyde therapy for epidermolysis bullosa. [Letter]. Arch Dermatol 1974;110:297.

138. Gordon HH. Herpes zoster and simplex: local therapy with glutaraldehyde. Cutis 1973;12:918.

139. Gordon HH. Pseudomonas infections. Arch Dermatol 1974;109:261.

140. London ID. Buffered glutaraldehyde solution for warts. Arch Dermatol 1971;104:96.

141. Maibach HL, Prystowsky SD. Glutaraldehyde (pentanedial) allergic contact dermatit is. Arch Dermatol 1977;113:170.

142. Fisher AA. Reactions to glutaraldehyde with particular reference to radiologists and X-ray technicians. Cutis 1981;28:113.

143. Sanderson KV, Cronin E. Glutaraldehyde and contact dermatitis. Br Med J 1968;3:820.

144. Skog E. Sensitivity to glutaraldehyde. Contact Dermatitis Newsletter 1968;4:79.

145. Lyon TC. Allergic contact dermatitis due to Cidex. Oral Surg 1971;32:895.

146. Neering H, van Ketel WG. Glutaraldehyde and formaldehyde allergy. Contact Dermatitis Newsletter 1874;16:518.

147. Maibach H. Glutaraldehyde: cross reaction to formaldehyde. Contact Dermatitis 1975;1:326.

148. Hansen EM, Menné T. Glutaraldehyde: patch test, vehicle and concentration. Contact Dermatitis 1990;23:369.

149. Garcia RL. Delayed hypersensitivity reaction to glutaraldehyde and formaldehyde. Bull Assoc Military 1972;21:11.

150. Belani KG, Priedklans J. An epidemic of pseudomembranous laryngotracheitis. Anaesthesia 1977;47:530.

151. Zach RG. How prevalent is glutaraldehyde sensitivity? Consultant 1980(May):116.

152. Hansen KS. Glutaraldehyde occupational dermatitis. Contact Dermatitis 1983;9:81.

153. Presto AJ III, Muecke EC. A dose of Spanish fly. JAMA 1970;214:592.

154. Dilaimy M. Lymphangitis caused by cantharidin. Arch Dermatol 1975;111:398.

155. Valdes-Dapena MA, Arey JB. Boric add poisoning: three fatal cases with pancreatic inclusions and a review of the literature. J Pediatr 1962;61:531.

156. Skipworth GB, Goldstein N, McBrite WP. Boric acid intoxication from "medicated talcum powder." Arch Dermatol 1967;95:83.

157. Vonterheid EC, Van Scott EJ, Grekin DA. Topical chemotherapy and immunotherapy of mycosis fungoides: intermediate-term results. Arch Dermatol 1977;133:454.

158. Daughters D, Zackheim H, Maibach H. Urticaria and anaphylactoid reactions after topical applications of mechlorethamine. Arch Dermatol 1973;107:429.

159. Grunnet E. Contact urticaria and anaphylactoid reaction induced by topical application of nitrogen mustard. Br J Dermatol 1976;94:101.

160. Leshaw S, Simon RS, Baer BL. Failure to induce tolerance to mechlorethamine hydrochloride. Arch Dermatol 1977;113:1406.

161. Monk BE, Vollum DI, Du Vivier AWP. Combination nitrogen mustard and photochemotherapy for mycosis fungoides: effects on sensitization and treatment. Br J Dermatol 1982;107(Suppl 22):25.

162. Price NM, Deneau DG, Hoppe RT. The treatment of mycosis fungoides with ointment based mechlorethamine. Arch Dermatol 1982;228:234.

163. Thomsen K, Mikkelsen HI. Protective capacity of gloves used for handling of nitrogen mustard. Contact Dermatitis 1975;1:268.

164. van Ketel WG. Allergy to coumarin and coumarin derivatives. Contact Dermatitis Newsletter 1972;13:355.

165. Kaidbey C, Kligman, A. Photocontact allergy to coumarins. Arch Dermatol 1981;217:259.

166. Kwong P, Roberts P, Prescott SM, Tikoff G. Dermatitis induced by warfarin. JAMA 1978;239:1884.

167. Schleicher SM, Fricker MP. Coumarin necrosis. Arch Dermatol 1980;116:444.

168. Schramm W, Spannagl M, Bauer KA, et al. Treatment of coumarin-induced skin necrosis with a monoclonal antibody purified protein C concentrate. Arch Dermatol 1993;129:753.

169. Koch P, Bahmer FA, Schäfer H. Tolerance of intravenous low-molecular-weight heparin after eczematous reaction to subcutaneous heparin. Contact Dermatitis 1991;25:205.

170. Krasovec M, Kammerer R, Spertini F, Frenk E. Contact dermatitis from heparin gel following sensitization by subcutaneous heparin administration. Contact Dermatitis 1995;33:135.

171. Moreau A, Dompmartin A, Esnault P, et al. Delayed hypersensitivity at the injection sites of a low-molecular-weight heparin. Contact Dermatitis 1996;34:31.

172. Koch P, Hindi S, Landwehr D. Delayed allergic skin reactions due to subcutaneous heparin-calcium, enoxaparin-sodium, pentosan polysulfate and acute skin lesions from systemic sodium-heparin. Contact Dermatitis 1996;34:156.

173. Boehncke WH, Weber L, Gall H. Tolerance of intravenous administration of heparin and heparinoid in a patient with delayed-type hypersensitivity to heparins and heparinoids. Contact Dermatitis 1996;35:73.

174. Trautmann A, Brocker EB, Klein CE. Intravenous challenge with heparins in patients with delayed-type skin reactions after subcutaneous administration of the drug. Contact Dermatitis 1998;39:43.

175. Hunzelmann N, Gold H, Scharffetter-Kochanek K. Concomitant sensitization to high and low molecular-weight

heparins, heparinoid and pentosanpolysulfate. Contact Dermatitis 1998;39:88.

176. Schiffner R, Glaessl A, Landthaler M, et al. Tolerance of desirudin in a patient with generalized eczema after intravenous challenge with heparin and a delayed-type skin reaction to high and low molecular weight heparins and heparinoids. Contact Dermatitis 2000;42:49.

177. Irion R, Gall H, Peter R-U. Delayed-type hypersensitivity to heparin with tolerance of its intravenous administration. Contact Dermatitis 2000;43:249

178. Jappe U, Reinhold D, Bonnekoh B. Arthus reaction to lepirudin, a new recombinant hirudin, and delayed-type hypersensitivity to several heparins and heparinoid, with tolerance to its intravenous administration. Contact Dermatitis 2002;46:29.

179. Ludwig RJ, Beier C, Lindhoff-Last E, et al. Tolerance of fondaparinux in a patient allergic to heparins and other glycosaminoglycans. Contact Dermatitis 2004;49:158.

180. Koch P. Delayed-type hypersensitivity skin reactions due to heparins and heparinoids. Tolerance of recombinant hirudins and of the new synthetic anticoagulant fondaparinux. Contact Dermatitis 2004;49:276.

181. Jappe U, Juschka U, Kuner N, et al. Fondaparinux: a suitable alternative in cases of delayed-type allergy to heparins and semisynthetic heparinoids? A study of 7 cases. Contact Dermatitis 2004;51:67.

182. Hohenstein E, Tsakiris D, Bricher AJ. Delayed-type hypersensitivity to the ultra-low-molecular weight heparin fondaparinux. Contact Dermatitis 2004;51:149.

183. Hallai N, Hughes TM, Stone N. Type I and Type IV allergy to unfractionated heparin and low-molecular-weight heparin with no reaction to recombinant hirudin. Contact Dermatitis 2004:51:153.

184. Zollner TM, Gall H, Volpel H, Kaufmann R. Type IV allergy to natural hirudin confirmed by in vitro stimulation with recombinant hirudin. Contact Dermatitis 1996;35:59.

185. Cronin E. Lanolin dermatitis. Br J Dermatol 1966;78:617.

186. Vollum DI. Sensitivity to hydrogenated lanolin [Letter]. Arch Dermatol 1969;100:774.

187. Thune P. Allergy to wool fat: the addition of salicylic acid for patch test purposes. Acta Derm Venereol (Stockh) 1969;49:282.

188. Newcomb EA. Lanolin allergy. J Soc Cosmet Chem 1966;17:_149.

189. Peter C, Schropl F, Franzwa H. Experimental investigation regarding allergenic effects of wool wax alcohols. Hautarzt 1969;20:450.

190. Oleffe JD, Blondeel A, Boschmans L. Patch testing with lanolin. Contact Dermatitis 1978;4:233.

191. Giorgini S, Melli MC, Sertoli A. Comments on the allergenic activity of lanolin. Contact Dermatitis 1983;9:425.

192. Sulzberger MB, Warshaw T, Herrmann F. Studies of skin hypersensitivity to lanolin. J Invest Dermatol 1953;20:33.

193. Kligman AM. Lanolin allergy: crisis or comedy. Contact Dermatitis 1983;9:99.

194. Breit R, Bandmann H-J. Dermatitis from lanolin. Br J Dermatol 1973;88:414.

195. Bandmann H-J, Reichenberger M. Beobachtungen und Untersuchungen zur Frage der durch Eucerin Bedingten seltenen Allergies. Hautarzt 1957;8:11.

196. Cronin E, Bandmann HJ, Calnan CD, et al. Contact dermatitis in the atopic. Acta Derm Venereol (Stockh) 1970;50:183.

197. McBurney EI, Noel SB, Collins JH. Contact dermatitis to transdermal estradiol system. J Am Acad Dermatol 1989;20:508.

198. Pecquet C, Pradalier A, Dry J. Allergic contact dermatitis from ethanol in a transdermal estradiol patch. Contact Dermatitis 1992;27:275.

199. Carmichael AJ, Foulds IS. Allergic contact dermatitis from oestradiol in oestrogen patches. Contact Dermatitis 1992;26:194.

200. Boehncke WH, Gall H. Type-IV hypersensitivity to topical estradiol in a patient tolerant to it orally. Contact Dermatitis 1996;35:187.

201. Goncalo M, Oliveira HS, Monteiro C, et al. Allergic and systemic contact dermatitis from estradiol. Contact Dermatitis 1999;40:58.

202. Koch P. Allergic contact dermatitis from estradiol and norethisterone acetate in transdermal hormonal patch. Contact Dermatitis 2001;44:112.

203. Buckley DA, Wilkinson SM, Higgins EM. Contact allergy to a testosterone patch. Contact Dermatitis 1998;39:91.

204. Jordan WP Jr. Allergy and topical irritation associated with transdermal testosterone administration: a comparison of scrotal and nonscrotal transdermal systems. Am J Contact Dermat 1997;8:108.

205. Should J, Shum KW, Gadour M, et al. Contact allergy to testosterone in an androgen patch: control of symptoms by pre-application of topical corticosteroid. Contact Dermatitis 2001;45:124.

206. Dwyer CM, Forsyth A. Allergic contact dermatitis from methacrylates in a nicotine transdermal patch. Contact Dermatitis 1994;30:309.

207. Bircher AJ, Howald H, Rufli T. Adverse skin reactions to nicotine in a transdermal therapeutic system. Contact Dermatitis 1991;25:230.

208. von Bahr B, Wahlberg JE. Reactivity to nicotine patches wrongly blamed on contact allergy. Contact Dermatitis 1997;37:44.

209. Audicana M, Schmidt R, Fernandez de Corres L. Allergic contact dermatitis from nicotinic acid esters. Contact Dermatitis 1990;22:60.

210. Giorgini S, Martinelli C, Sertoli A. Delayed type sensitivity reaction to mitomycin. Contact Dermatitis 1991;24:378.

211. Arregui MA, Aquirre A, Gil N, et al. Dermatitis due to mitomycin C bladder instillations: study of 2 cases. Contact Dermatitis 1991;24:368.

212. de Groot AC, Conemans JM. Systemic allergic contact dermatitis from intravesical instillation of the antetumor antibiotic mitomycin C. Contact Dermatitis 1991;24:201.

213. Veraldi S, Benelli C, Pigatto PD. Occupational allergic contact dermatitis from minoxidil. Contact Dermatitis 1992;26:211.

214. Whitmore SE. The importance of proper vehicle selection in the detection of minoxidil sensitivity. Arch Dermatol 1992;128:653.

215. Rietschel RL. The patch test as an exercise in cutaneous pharmacokinetics. Does compound allergy exist? [Editorial; comment]. Arch Dermatol 1992;128:678.

216. Corazza M, Virgili A. Allergic contact dermatitis from ophthalmic products: can pre-treatment with sodium lauryl sulfate increase patch test sensitivity? Contact Dermatitis 2005;52:239.

217. Camarasa JG, Pla C. Allergic contact dermatitis from cyclopentolate. Contact Dermatitis 1996;35:368.

218. Boukhman MP, Maibach HI. Allergic contact dermatitis from tropicamide ophthalmic solution. Contact Dermatitis 1999;41:47.

219. Marcos ML, Garces MM, Alonso L, et al. Occupational allergic contact dermatitis from homatropine and phenylephrine eyedrops. Contact Dermatitis 1997;37:189.

220. Valsecchi R, Leighissa P, Piazolla S, et al. Occupational contact dermatitis from propranolol. Contact Dermatitis 1994;30:177.

221. Koch P. Allergic contact dermatitis due to timolol and levobunolol in eyedrops, with no cross-sensitivity to other ophthalmic beta-blockers. Contact Dermatitis 1995;33:140.

222. Nino M, Suppa F, Ayala F, et al. Allergic contact dermatitis due to the B-blocker befunolol in eyedrops, with cross-sensitivity to carteolol. Contact Dermatitis 2001;44:369.

223. Sanchez-Perex J, Cordoba S, Bartolome B, et al. Allergic contact dermatitis due to the B-blocker carteolol in eyedrops. Contact Dermatitis 1999;41:298

224. Armisen M, Vidal C, Quintans R, et al. Allergic contact dermatitis from apraclonidine. Contact Dermatitis 1998;39:193.

225. Silvestre JF, Carnero L, Ramon R, et al. Allergic contact dermatitis from apraclonidine in eyedrops. Contact Dermatitis 2001;45:251.

226. Villareal O. Reliability of diagnostic tests for contact allergy to mydriatic eyedrops. Contact Dermatitis 1998;38:150.

227. Decraene T, Goosens A. Contact allergy to atropine and other mydriatic agents in eye drops. Contact Dermatitis 2001;45:309.

228. Aalto-Korte K. Contact allergy to dorzolamide eyedrops. Contact Dermatitis 1998;39:206.

229. Shimada M, Higaki Y, Kawashima M. Allergic contact dermatitis due to dorzolamide eyedrops. Contact Dermatitis 2001;45:52.

230. Mancuso G, Berdondini RM. Allergic contact blepharo-conjunctivitis from dorzolamide. Contact Dermatitis 2001;45:243.

231. Niizeki H, Inamoto N, Nakamura K, et al. Contact dermatitis from ketotifen fumarate eyedrops. Contact Dermatitis 1994;31:266.

232. Helton J, Storrs FJ. Pilocarpine allergic contact and photocontact dermatitis. Contact Dermatitis 1991;25:133.

233. Cameli N, Bardazzi F, Morelli P, Tosti A. Contact dermatitis from rubidium iodide in eyedrops. Contact Dermatitis 1990;23:377.

234. Conraads PJ, Woest TE, Blanks LJ, Houtman WA. Contact allergy to d-penicillamine. Contact Dermatitis 1990;23:371.

235. Pigatto PD, Bigardi A, Legori A, et al. Allergic contact dermatitis from beta-interferon in eyedrops. Contact Dermatitis 1991;25:199.

236. Cameli N, Tosti G, Venturo N, Tosti A. Eyelid dermatitis due to cocamidopropyl betaine in a hard contact lens solution. Contact Dermatitis 1991;25:261.

237. Herbst RA, Maibach HJ. Contact dermatitis caused by allergy to ophthalmic drugs and contact lens solution. Contact Dermatitis 1991;25:305.

238. Herbst RA, Maibach HI. Allergic contact dermatitis from ophthalmics: update 1997. Contact Dermatitis 1997;37:252.

239. Jerstad KM, Warshaw E. Allergic contact dermatitis to latanoprost. Am J Contact Dermatitis 2002;13:39.

240. Sodhi PK, Verma L, Ratan SK. Contact dermatitis from topical bimatoprost. Contact Dermatitis 2004;50:50.

241. Miyamoto H, Okajima M. Allergic contact dermatitis from epsilon-aminocaproic acid. Contact Dermatitis 2000;42:50.

242. Davison SC, Wakelin SH. Allergic contact dermatitis from N-acetylcysteine eyedrops. Contact Dermatitis 2002;47:238.

243. Bohn S, Hurni M. Bircher AJ. Contact allergy to trometamol. Contact Dermatitis 2001;44:319.

244. Wictorin A, Hansson C. Allergic contact dermatitis from a bismuth compound in an eye ointment. Contact Dermatitis 2001;45:318.

245. van Rengen A, Goossens A. Local reactions after subcutaneous injections of b-interferon. Contact Dermatitis 1998;39:209.

246. Fernandez-Vozmediano JM, Gil-Tocados G, Manrique-Plaza A, et al. Contact dermatitis due to topical spironolactone. Contact Dermatitis 1994;30:118.

247. Sommer S, Wilkinson SM. Contact dermatitis caused by phenoxybenzamine hydrochloride. Contact Dermatitis 1998;38:352.

248. Garcia-Bravo B, Rodriguez-Pichardo A, Camacho F. Contact dermatitis from diazepoxides. Contact Dermatitis 1994;30:40.

249. Quinones D, Sanchez I, Alonso S, et al. Photodermatitis from tetrazepam. Contact Dermatitis 1998;39:84.

250. Stingeni L, Lapomarda V, Lisi P. What risk of piroxicam photodermatitis in thimerosal-positive patients? Contact Dermatitis 1996;34:60.

251. Varela P, Amorim I, Massa A, et al. Piroxicam-beta-cyclodextrin and photosensitivity reactions. Contact Dermatitis 1998;38:229.

252. Goncalo M, Figueiredo A, Concalo S. Hypersensitivity to thimerosal: the sensitizing moiety. Contact Dermatitis 1996;34:201.

253. Kurumaji Y. Ampiroxicam-induced photosensitivity. Contact Dermatitis 1996;34:289.

254. Toyohara A, Chen KR, Miyakawa S, et al. Ampiroxicam-induced photosensitivity. Contact Dermatitis 1996;35:101.

255. Korffmacher H, Hartwig R, Matthes U, et al. Contact allergy to 8-methoxypsoralen. Contact Dermatitis 1994;30:283.

256. de Boer EM, Bruynzeel DP. Allergy to pravastatin. Contact Dermatitis 1994;30:238.

257. Morimoto K, Kawada A, Hiruma M, et al. Photosensitivity to simvastatin with an unusual response to photopatch and photo tests. Contact Dermatitis 1995;33:274.

258. Granados M, de la Torre C, Cruces MJ, Pineiro G. Chronic actinic dermatitis due to simvastatin. Contact Dermatitis 1998:38:294.

259. Vilaplana J, Romaguera C. Allergic contact dermatitis due to lansoprazole, a proton pump inhibitor. Contact Dermatitis 2001;44:47.

260. Ryan PJJ, Rycroft RJG, Aston IR. Allergic contact dermatitis from occupational exposure to ranitidine hydrochloride. Contact Dermatitis 2003;48:67.

261. Clerx V, Van Den Keybus C, Kochuyt A, et al. Drug intolerance reaction to insulin therapy caused by metacresol. Contact Dermatitis 2003;48:162.

262. Raap U, Liekenbroecker T, Kapp A, et al. Delayed-type hypersensitivity to protamine as a complication of insulin therapy. Contact Dermatitis 2005;53:57.

263. Kerr OA, Kavanagh G, Horn H. Allergic contact dermatitis from topical diclofenac in Solaraze ® gel. Contact Dermatitis 2002;47:175.

264. Garcia CM, Carmena R, Garcia R, et al. Fixed drug eruption from ticlopidine, with positive lesional patch test. Contact Dermatitis 2001;44:40.

265. Lauerma AI, Koivuluhta M, Alenium H. Recalcitrant allergic contact dermatitis from azathioprine tablets. Contact Dermatitis 2001;44:129.

266. Umebayashi Y, Ito S. Allergic contact dermatitis due to both lanoconazole and neticonazole ointments. Contact Dermatitis 2001;44:48.

267. Mancuso G, Berdondini RM. Occupational allergic contact dermatitis from thiocolchicoside. Contact Dermatitis 2000;43:180.

268. Valois M, Phillips EJ, Shear NH, et al. Clindamycin-associated acute generalized exanthematous pustulosis. Contact Dermatitis 2003;48:1169.

269. Kiec-Swierczynska M, Krecisz B. Occupational airborne allergic contact dermatitis from mesna. Contact Dermatitis 2003;48:171.

270. Esch AJH, van der Heide S, van den Brink W, et al. Contact allergy and respiratory/mucosal complaints from heroin (diacetylmorphine). Contact Dermatitis 2006;54:42.

271. Reyes JJ, Farina MC. Allergic contact dermatitis due to trimebutine. Contact Dermatitis 2001;45:164.

272. Romano A, Pietrantonio F, diFonso M, et al. Contact allergy to tiopronin: a case report. Contact Der matitis 1995;33:269.

273. Fung MA, Geisse JK, Maibach HL. Airborne contact dermatitis from metaproterenol in a respiratory therapist. Contact Dermatitis 1996;35:317.

274. Reynaerts A, Bruze M, Erikstam U, Goossens A. Allergic contact dermatitis from a medical device, followed by depigmentation. Contact Dermatitis 1998;39:204.

275. Caraffini S, Ricci F, Assalve D, Lisi P. Isoflurane: an uncommon cause of occupational airborne contact dermatitis. Contact Dermatitis 1998;38:286.

276. Finch TM, Muncaster A, Prais L, et al. Occupational airborne allergic contact dermatitis from isoflurane vapour. Contact Dermatitis 2000;42:46.

277. Bircher AJ, Hampl K, Hirsbrunner P, et al. Allergic contact dermatitis from ethyl chloride and sensitization to dichlorodifluoromethane (CFC 12). Contact Dermatitis 1994;31:41.

278. Mallon E, Powell SM. Allergic contact dermatitis from Granuflex hydrocolloid dressing. Contact Dermatitis 1994;30:110.

279. Sasseville D, Tennstedt D, Lachapelle JM. Allergic contact dermatitis from hydrocolloid dressings. Am J Contact Dermat 1997;8:236.

280. Schliz M, Rauterberg A, Weiss J. Allergic contact dermatitis from hydrocolloid dressings. Contact Dermatitis 1996;34:146.

281. Johnsson M, Fiskerstrand EJ. Contact urticaria syndrome due to carboxymethylcellulose in a hydrocolloid dressing. Contact Dermatitis 1999;41:344.

282. 282..Schick E, Weber L, Gall H. Delayed hypersensitivity reaction to the non-ionic contrast medium iopromid. Contact Dermatitis 1996;35:312.

283. Christiansen C, Pichler WJ, Skotland T. Delayed allergy-like reactions to X-ray contrast media: mechanistic considerations. Eur Radiol 2000;10:1965.

284. Simon MR. Allergic-type adverse reactions to low osmolality contrast media in patients with a history of allergy or asthma. Invest Radiol 1995;30:285.

285. Yamaguchi K, Takanashi I, Kanauchi T, et al. A retrospective survey of delayed adverse reactions to ionic and nonionic contrast media. Nippon Igaku Hoshasen Gakkai Zasshi. 1992:52:1565.

286. Sanchez-Perez J, F-Villalta MG, Ruiz SA, et al. Delayed hypersensitivity reaction to the non-ionic X-ray contrast medium Visipaque ® (iodixanol). Contact Dermatitis 2003;48:167.

287. Delgado-Jimenez Y, Perez-Gala S, Aragues M, et al. Late skin reaction to iodixanol (Visipaque (R)): clinical manifestations, patch test study, and histopathological evaluation. Contact Dermatitis 2006;55:348.

288. Mooser G, Gall H, Peter RU. Delayed-type allergy to technetium Tc 99m. Contact Dermatitis 1998;39:269.

289. Dwyer CM, Chapman RS, Forsyth A. Allergic contact dermatitis from TENS gel. Contact Dermatitis 1994;30:305.

290. Strobos MA, Coenraads PJ, De Jongste JL, et al. Dermatitis caused by radio-frequency electromagnetic radiation. Contact Dermatitis 2001;44:309.

291. Gniazdowska B, Rueff F, Hillemanns P, Przybilla B. Allergic contact dermatitis from delta-aminolevulinic acid used for photodynamic therapy. Contact Dermatitis 1998;38:348.

292. Tung RC, Taylor JS. Contact dermatitis from polyvinyl chloride identification bands. Am J Contact Dermat 1998;9:234.

293. Hamilton TK, Zug KA. Triethanolamine allergy inadvertently discovered from a fluorescent marking pen. Am J Contact Dermat 1996;7:164.

294. Lazarov A, Trattner A. Allergic contact dermatitis from the adhesive remover wipe of stoma bags. Contact Dermatitis 1998;39:48.

295. Tarvainen K, Jolanki R, Henriks Eckerman ML, Estlander T. Occupational allergic contact dermatitis from isophoronediamine (IPDA) in operative-clothing manufacture. Contact Dermatitis 1998;39:46.

296. Miranda-Romero A, Martinez M, Sanchez-Sambucety P, et al. Allergic contact dermatitis from the acrylic adhesive of a surgical earthing plate. Contact Dermatitis 1998;38:279.

297. Jagtman BA. Contact dermatitis from acrylates in an electrosurgical earthing plate. Contact Dermatitis 1998;38:280.

298. Avenel-Audran M, Goossens A, Zimerson E, et al. Contact dermatitis from electrocardiograph-monitoring electrodes : role of p-tert-butylphenol-formaldehyde resin. Contact Dermatitis 2003;48:108

299. Franz H, Frank R, Rytter M, Haustein UF. Allergic contact dermatitis due to cedarwood oil after dermatoscopy. Contact Dermatitis 1998;38:182.

300. Stanford D, Georgouras K. Allergic contact dermatitis from benzalkonium chloride in plaster of Paris. Contact Dermatitis 1996;35:371.

301. Larsen TH, Gregersen P, Jemec GBE. Skin irritation and exposure to diisocyanates in orthopedic nurses working with Soft Casts. Am J Contact Dermatitis 2001;12:211.

302. Parslew R, Evans S, King CM. Allergic contact dermatitis from polyisobutylene in stoma bags. Contact Dermatitis 1996;35:178.

303. van den Hove J, Jacobs MC, Tennstedt D, Lachapelle JM. Allergic contact dermatitis from acrylates in insulin pump infusion sets. Contact Dermatitis 1996;35:108.

304. Jolanki R, Kanerva L, Estlander T, et al. Allergic contact dermatitis from phenoxyethoxy ethylacrylates in optical fiber coating, and glue in an insulin pump set. Contact Dermatitis 2001;45:36.

305. Saccabusi S, Boatto G, Asproni B, et al. Sensitization to methyl methacrylate in the plastic catheter of an insulin pump infusion set. Contact Dermatitis 2001;45:47.

306. Ng PPL, Leow YH, Ng SK, Goh CL. Allergic contact dermatitis to epoxy resin in a hemodialysis cannula. Am J Contact Dermat 1998;9:55.

307. Sanchez-Morillas L, Reano Martos M, Rodriguez Mosquera M, et al. Delayed sensitivity to Prolene ®. Contact Dermatitis 2003 ;4 8 :338.

308. Reichert-Penetrat S, Barbaud A, Penetrat E, et al. Allergic contact dermatitis from surgical paints. Contact Dermatitis 2001;45:116.

309. Stingeni L, Lapomarda V, Lisi P. Occupational hand dermatitis in hospital environments. Contact Dermatitis 1995;33:172.

310. Afzelius H, Thulin H. Allergic reactions to benzalkonium chloride. Contact Dermatitis 1979;5:60.

311. Fisher AA, Stillman MA. Allergic contact sensitivity to benzalkonium chloride. Arch Dermatol 1972;106:169.

312. Huriez C, et al. Frequence des sensibilisations aux ammoniums quaternaires. Semin Hop Paris 1965;72:106.

313. Wahlberg JE. Two cases of hypersensitivity to quaternary ammonium compounds. Acta Derm Venereol (Stockh) 1962;42:230.

314. Morikawa F, Kobayashi T, Nakayama Y, et al. Some problems on the appraisal of the skin safety of hexachlorophene. J Soc Cosmet Chem 1974;25:113.

315. Marks Jr JG. Allergic contact dermatitis to povidone-iodine. J Am Acad Dermatol 1982;6:473.

316. Corazza M, Bulciolu G, Spisani L, Virgili A. Chemical burns following irritant contact with povidone-iodine. Contact Dermatitis 1997;36:115.

317. Lopez Saez MP, de Barrio M, Zubeldia JM, et al. Acute IgE-mediated generalized urticaria-angioedema after topical application of povidone-iodine. Allergol Immunopathol (Madr) 1998;26:23.

318. Erdmann S, Hertl M, Merk HF. Allergic contact dermatitis from povidone-iodine. Contact Dermatitis 1999;40:331.

319. Fisher AA. Contact dermatitis in surgeons. J Derm Surg 1975;1:3.

320. Rudzki E. Occupational dermatitis among health service workers. Dermatosen 1979;27:112.

321. Phillips VL, Goodrich MA, Sullivan TJ. Health care worker disability due to latex allergy and asthma: a cost analysis. Am J Public Health 1999;89:1024.

322. Jolanki R, Estlander T, Alanko K, et al. Incidence rates of occupational contact urticaria caused by natural rubber latex. Contact Dermatitis 1999;40:329.

323. Wrangsjo K, Osterman K, Van Hage-Hamsten M. Glove-related skin symptoms among operating theatre and dental care unit personnel (I). Interview investigation. Contact Dermatitis 1994;30:102.

324. Wrangsjo K, Osterman K, van Hage-Hamsten M. Glove-related skin symptoms among operating theatre and dental care unit personnel (II). Clinical examination, tests and laboratory findings indicating latex allergy. Contact Dermatitis 1994;30:139.

325. Ownby DR. Manifestations of latex allergy. Immunol Allergy Clin North Am 1995;15:31.

326. Kurup VP, Murali PS, Kelly KJ. Latex antigens. Immunol Allergy Clin North Am 1995;15:45.

327. Truscott N. The industry perspective on latex. Immunol Allergy Clin North Am 1995;15:89.

328. Kujala V. A review of current literature on epidemiology of immediate glove irritation and latex allergy. Occup Med (Lond) 1999;49:3.

329. Warshaw EM. Latex allergy. J Am Acad Dermatol 1998;1.

330. Armstrong DKB, Smith HR, Rycroft RJG. Glove-related hand urticaria in the absence of Type I latex allergy. Contact Dermatitis 1999;41:42.

331. Thomson KF, Wilkinson SM. Localized dermographism: a differential diagnosis of latex glove allergy. Contact Dermatitis 1999;41:103.

332. Fisher AA. Hypoallergenic surgical gloves and gloves for special situations. Cutis 1975;15:797.

333. Pegum J, Medhurst FA. Contact dermatitis from penetration of rubber gloves by acrylic monomer. Br Med J 1971;2:141.

334. Fries JB, Fisher AA, Salvati EA. Contact dermatitis in surgeons from methylmethacrylate bone cement. J Bone Joint Surg 1975;57a:547.

335. Fisher AA. Contact dermatitis, 3rd ed. Philadelphia: Lea & Febiger, 1986.

336. Bohling HG, Borchard U, Drouin H. Monomeric methyl-methacrylate acts on desheathed myelinated nerve and on node of Ranvier. Arch Toxicol 1977;38:307.

337. Fisher AA. Paresthesia of the fingers accompanying dermatitis due to methylmethacrylate bone cement. Contact Dermatitis 1979;5:56.

338. Ross JS, Rycroft RJG, Cronin E. Melamine-formaldehyde contact dermatitis in orthopaedic practice. Contact Dermatitis 1992;26:203.

339. Sidi E, Longueville R, Hincky M. Occupational eczema in therapists. Springfield, IL: Charles C Thomas Publisher, 1958.

340. Blanton WB, Blanton FM. Unusual penicillin hypersensitivities. J Allergy 1953;24:405.

341. Calnan CD, Frain-Bell W, Cuthbert JW. Occupational dermatitis from chlorpromazine. Trans St John Hosp Derm Soc 1962;48:49.

342. Lewis GM, Sawicky HH. Contact dermatitis from chlorpromazine. JAMA 1955;157:909.

343. Goodman D, Cahn MM. Contact dermatitis to phenothiazine drugs. J Invest Dermatol 1959;33:27.

344. Epstein S. Allergic photo contact dermatitis from promethazine (Phenergan). Arch Dermatol Syph 1960;81:175.

345. Fousseraeu J, Lantz JP. Allergy to maclofenoxate in nurses. Contact Dermatitis Newsletter 1972;6:231.

346. Monteserín J, Conde J. Contact eczema from famotidine. Contact Dermatitis 1990;22:290.

347. Cosnes A, Flechet M-L, Revuz J. Inflammatory nodular reactions after hepatitis B vaccination due to aluminum sensitization. Contact Dermatitis 1990;23:65.

348. Rietschel RL, Adams RM. Reactions to thimerosal in hepatitis B vaccines. Dermatol Clinics 1990;8:161.

349. Aberer W. Vaccination despite thimerosal sensitivity. Contact Dermatitis 1991;24:6.

350. Osawa J, Kitamura K, Ikezawa Z, Nakajima H. A probable role for vaccines containing thimerosal in thimerosal hypersensitivity. Contact Dermatitis 1991;24:178.

351. Samitz MH, Schmunes E. Occupational dermatoses in dentists and allied personnel. Cutis 1969;5:180.

352. Calnan CD, Stevenson CJ. Studies in contact dermatitis (XV). Dental materials. Trans St John Hosp Derm Soc 1963;18:24.

353. Rustemeyer T, Frosch PJ. Occupational skin diseases in dental laboratory technicians (I). Clinical picture and causative factors. Contact Dermatitis 1996;34:125.

354. Fisher AA. Allergic sensitization of the skin and oral mucosa to acrylic denture materials. JAMA 1954;156:238.

355. Flyvholm MA, Hall BM, Agner T, et al. Threshold for occluded formaldehyde patch test in formaldehyde-sensitive patients: relationship to repeated open application test with a product containing formaldehyde releaser. Contact Dermatitis 1997;36:26.

356. van Ketel WG. Reactions to dental impression materials. Contact Dermatitis 1977;3:55.

357. Cronin E. Impregum (dental impression material). Contact Dermatitis Newsletter 1973;13:362.

358. Nally FS, Storrs J. Hypersensitivity to dental impression material. Br Dental J 1973;134:244.

359. van Groeningen G, Nater J. Reaction to dental impression materials. Contact Dermatitis 1975;1:373.

360. Malten KE. Recently reported causes of contact dermatitis due to synthetic resins and hardeners. Contact Dermatitis 1979;5:11.

361. Hjorth N, Schonning L. Occupational dermatitis from tuberculin among veterinary surgeons. Contact Dermatitis Newsletter 1968;4:64.

362. Hjorth N, Weismann K. Occupational dermatitis among veterinary surgeons caused by spiramycin and Tylosin. Contact Dermatitis Newsletter 1972;12:320.

363. Hjorth N. Battery for testing veterinary surgeons. Contact Dermatitis 1975;1:122.

364. Hjorth N. Occupational dermatitis among veterinary surgeons caused by penethamate. Berufsdermatosen 1967;15:163.

365. Adams RM. Mercaptobenzothiazole in veterinary medications. Contact Dermatitis Newsletter 1974;16:514.

366. Prahl P, Roed-Petersen J. Type I allergy from cows in veterinary surgeons. Contact Dermatitis 1979;5:33.

367. Rudzki E, Rebandel P, Grzywa Z, et al. Occupational dermatitis in veterinarians. Contact Dermatitis 1982;8:72.

368. Malten KE. Therapeutics for pets as neglected causes of contact dermatitis in housewives. Contact Dermatitis 1978;4:296.

369. Fisher AA. Allergic contact dermatitis in animal feed handlers. Cutis 1975;16:201.

370. Neldner KH. Contact dermatitis from animal feed additives. Arch Dermatol 1972;106:722.

371. Rodriguez A, Echechipia S, Alvarez M, Muro MD. Occupational contact dermatitis from vitamin B_{12}. Contact Dermatitis 1994;31:271.

372. Bleumink E, Nater JP. Allergic contact dermatitis to dinitolmide. Arch Dermatol 1973;108:423.

373. deGroot AC, Conemans JMH. Contact allergy to furazolidone. Contact Dermatitis 1990;22:202.

374. Vilaplana J, Grimalt F, Romaguera C. Contact dermatitis from furaltadone in animal feed. Contact Dermatitis 1991;22:232.

375. Melhom HC, Beetz D. Das Antioxydans Aethoxyquin als berufliches Ebenzatogen bil einer futtermitteldosierer. Berufsdermatosen 1971;19:84.

376. Burrows D. Contact dermatitis in animal feed mill workers. Br J Dermatol 1975;92:167.

377. Scott KW, Dawson TAJ. Photo contact dermatitis arising from the presence of quindoxin in animal feeding stuff. Br J Dermatol 1974;90:543.

378. Caplan RM. Contact dermatitis from animal feed additives. Arch Dermatol 1973;107:18.

379. Dawson TAJ, Scott KW. Contact eczema in agricultural workers. Br Med J 1972;1:469.

380. Lorenzetti OJ. Occupational dermatitis-prescription container caps. Contact Dermatitis 1975;1:53.

381. Cronin E. Picric acid dermatitis. Contact Dermatitis 1975;1:64.

382. Grimalt F, Romaguera C. Cutaneous sensitivity to benzidine. Dermatosen 1981;29:95.

383. Downs AMR, Sansom JE. Airborne occupational contact dermatitis from epoxy resin in an immersion oil used for microscopy. Contact Dermatitis 1998;39:267.

384. Le Coz C-J, Coninx D, Van Rengen A, et al. An epidemic of occupational contact dermatitis from an immersion oil for microscopy in laboratory personnel. Contact Dermatitis 1999;40:77.

385. Morris AD, Ratcliff J, Dalziel KL, English JS. Allergic contact dermatitis from epoxy propane. Contact Dermatitis 1998;38:57.

386. Estlander T, Jolanki R, Kanerva L. Hydroxylammonium chloride as sensitizer in a water laboratory. Contact Dermatitis 1997;36:161.

387. Dooms-Goossens A, Garmyn M, Degreef H. Contact allergy to acrylamide. Contact Dermatitis 1991;24:71.

388. Wasilewski C. Allergic contact dermatitis from isopropyl alcohols. Arch Derm Venereol (Stockh) 1968;98:502.

389. Fregert S, Groth O, Hjorth N, et al. Alcohol dermatitis. Arch Dermatol 1969;49:493.

390. Fregert S, Groth O, Gruvberger B, et al. Hypersensitivity to secondary alcohols. Acta Derm Venereol (Stockh) 1971;51:271.

391. Hicks R. Ethanol, a possible allergen. Ann Allergy 1968;26:64.

392. Richardson D, et al. Allergic contact dermatitis to "alcohol" swabs. Cutis 1969;5:1115.

393. Fregert SK, Rorsman H, Tryding N, Ovrum P. Dermatitis from alcohols. J Allergy 1963;34:404.

394. Martin-Scott I. Contact dermatitis from alcohol. Br J Dermatol 1960;72:372.

395. van Ketel WG, Tan-Lim KN. Contact dermatitis from ethanol. Contact Dermatitis 1975;1:7.

396. Sanderson KV, Cronin E. Glutaraldehyde and contact dermatitis. Br Med J 1968;3:820.

397. Skog E. Sensitivity to glutaraldehyde. Contact Dermatitis Newsletter 1968;4:79.

398. Harman RRM, O'Grady KJ. Contact dermatitis due to sensitivity to Cidex (activated glutaraldehyde). Contact Dermatitis Newsletter 1972;11:279.

399. Lyon TC. Allergic contact dermatitis due to Cidex. Oral Surg 1971;32:895.

400. Neering H, van Ketel WG. Glutaraldehyde and formaldehyde allergy. Contact Dermatitis Newsletter 1974;16:518.

401. Gordon HH. Glutaraldehyde contact dermatitis. Contact Dermatitis Newsletter 1974;15:442.

402. Zach RG. How prevalent is glutaraldehyde sensitivity? Consultant 1980;6:116.

403. Fisher AA. Reactions to glutaraldehyde with particular reference to radiologists and x-ray technicians. Cutis 1981;28:113.

404. Belani KC, Priedklans J. An epidemic of pseudo membranous laryngotracheitis. Anesthesia 1978;47:530.

MEDICATIONS FROM PLANTS

EXECUTIVE SUMMARY

Some commonly tested allergens are derived from plants and have use as medications. Included in this category are balsam of Peru, rosin, and benzoin. Not tested as often as in decades past are turpentine and tars (wood, juniper, pine, birch, and coal). Common dermatologic treatments from plants include podophyllum resin and psoralens. Folk treatments and alternative therapies from plants with implications for contact dermatitis are aloe vera, propolis, chamomile, tannins, jojoba oil, tea tree oil, and black cumin oil.

Less commonly reported contact dermatitis-associated plants include ergot, rue, verbena, Krameria, Elecampane, Centella, rosemary, sandalwood, Ginkgo biloba, burdock, goldenrod, curcuminoids, spearmint, guava, Boswellia, kudzu, Astronium, gordolobo, butcher's broom, white flower embrocation, members of the ginger family, prickly pear cactus, and some grasses.

Balsam of Peru

Balsam of Peru is used widely in topical medicines for wounds, burns, hemorrhoids, and scabies and in sunscreening agents (Tables 10.1 and 10.2). It is an effective capillary-bed stimulant used to increase circulation in a wound-site area. Also, balsam of Peru has a mild, bacteriocidal action; toothpastes, medicated cough lozenges, dental cements, and liquids may also contain this balsam.[1]

EXPOSURE TO BALSAM OF PERU IN INFANCY AND CHILDHOOD

The following "baby care" medicaments containing balsam of Peru have produced dermatitis in infants: Balmex Baby Powder, Emollient Lotion and Ointment; Diaprex Ointment; and A&D Pediatric Ointment. This reaction to balsam of Peru in infants is described in a report by Fregert and Möller,[2] who tested 101 children under age 15 and found that 24% reacted to balsam of Peru 25% petrolatum, which was much higher than the 6% found in more than 2,000 adults tested. This sensitization was thought to occur by exposure to compounds related to balsam of Peru in medicaments.

In addition, Ebner[3] tested 51 patients under age 20 who had contact allergy. Balsam of Peru was the most frequent cause of contact allergy in children and young persons attending the clinic.

About 30% of persons who apply balsam of Peru medicaments obtain an immediate red flare, which lasts about 1 hour. Such a flare is a nonspecific, urticarial-type reaction.[4,5]

Olholm-Larsen and Heydenreich[6] stated that the increased use of perfumes produces an increasing allergy to balsam of Peru and wood tars. Veien and colleagues[7] reported that certain patients with chronic eczema were challenged by administration of two capsules containing 450 mg of balsam of Peru. Several patients had flares of eczema after ingesting the substance. Later, 45 of 210 patients with various eczemas were found to have flares after challenge with oral balsam of Peru.[8] In further studies of 64 patients placed on a diet restricting oral sources of balsams, 37 derived long-term benefit. Generally, benefit was evident by 1 to 2 months. While a 1-g oral challenge was used to evaluate some cases, this was not found to be a reliable predictor of the benefits of a dietary restriction of balsam of Peru.[9] The restricted foods are listed in Table 10.3.

In further studies, Veien and colleagues[10] extended their work with 1-g oral challenges of balsam of Peru. They did not find the oral challenge sufficiently predictive of who might benefit from a low-balsam diet to recommend such testing. However, the diet did provide long-term benefit to 28 of 46 patients. The foods most often identified as causing dermatitis were wine, candy, chocolate, cinnamon, citrus fruit, and flavorings. Personal observations (Robert L. Rietschel) on this type of diet suggest that usually only one or two items are critical, and the rest of the restrictions are unnecessary. Identifying the critical item requires some trial and error.

Table 10-1 Trade Names of Products That May Contain Balsam of Peru

Product	Product
A and D Hemorrhoidal Suppositories with Hydrocortisone	Kurlene (eyelash pomade)
Anusol Suppositories	Manhatten Drug Rectal Ointment
Benzoin (Tincture of)	Marlock Hemorrhoidal
Bonaseptic Foot Lotion	M-D-C Rectal Ointment
Bonate Suppositories	Medicone Rectal Suppositories
B.Q.R. (for colds)	Medicone Rectal Unguent
Calmol 4 Suppositories	Moava Rectal Suppositories
Carson Scarlet Wound Spray	Nap-ol Ointment (for nipples during nursing)
Castroid Inj. Unguentum	N.J.F. Hemorrhoidal Suppositories
Chap Balm	Obtundia Calamine Lotion
Codallate Suppositories	Obtundia Cream
Consin Rectal Suppositories	Obtundia Liniment
Derma Zemo Ointment	Obtundo bulbs (analgesic)
Dermo-o-creme	Obtundorrhoid (for hemorrhoids)
Desitin Hemorrhoidal	Pad Kote—astringent (external veterinary)
Diaprex Ointment	Palmer's Antiseptic Lotion
Doctient Suppositories	Pearsons Suppositories
Ergozide (for boils and burns)	Pilodyne Ointment
Ferol Rectal Ointment	Recreo Powder Plain (dusting)
Fort Dodge Scarlet Oil (wound dressing)	Rectodyne Ointment
Granulex	Rectone Improved Suppositories
Hance Improved Rectone Suppositories	Resicaine Suppositories
Hemasthesia Ointment (for hemorrhoids)	Soothe Salve
Hemasthesia Suppositories	Thoroughbred Heel Ointment (veterinary)
Hemoid Ointment	TO-NE-KA Brand Ointment
Husk Dressing (antiseptic)	Tuf-foot (for tender feet of dogs)
Itchybalm (antiseptic veterinary)	Wyanoid Suppositories (for hemorrhoids)

Turpentine

Turpentine is the ingredient in many "liniments," cold remedies, and veterinary medications. Some of these "liniments" and "rubs" for human use are listed in Table 10.4.

Turpentine oil is regarded as a local irritant. Medically, it is used externally as a counterirritant. Cronin[11] reported that turpentine oil has become an infrequent allergen because of its replacement by the petroleum product white spirit and its deliberate exclusion from

Table 10-2 Balsam of Peru in Sunscreening Agents

Beach Party Tanning Cream
Bronze Lustre Moisturizing Tan Cream
Bronze Lustre Moisturizing Tan Gelee
Glamomour Tan Sun Cream
Golden Gaby Suntan Lotion
Hypoallergic Suntan Lotion
Moon Drops Bronze Lustre Moisturizing Tanning Lotion and Gelee
RVPaque
Sundare Lotion
Sun Foam
Sun Lo
Sunbath Moisturizing Tanning Lotion
Sunbath Spray with Insect Repellent
Suntan Glee

Table 10-3 Low-Balsam Diet

Foods to Be Restricted

Products containing the peel of citrus fruits (oranges, lemons, grapefruit, bitter oranges, tangerines, mandarin oranges, etc.), for example, marmalade, juice, baked goods, cocktails

Products flavored with essences, for example, baked goods, candy, chewing gum

Perfumed products, for example, perfumed teas, tobacco

Various types of cough medicine and lozenges

Ice cream

Cola and other spiced soft drinks

Spices such as cinnamon, cloves, vanilla, curry (and products made with these spices), for example, tomato ketchup, chili sauce, chutney, pickled herring, pickled vegetables such as beets and cucumbers, baked goods, liver paste, paté, vermouth, bitters, and other similarly spiced beverages

Table 10-4 Turpentine in Over-the-Counter Preparations
Cloverine Salve
Johnson's Anodyne
Mentholatum
Minard Liniment
Penetro Analgesic Rub
Sloan's Liniment
Vicks Vaporub

Table 10-5 Rosin in Topical Medications
Ace Adherent
Amlab Drawing Salve
Boilex Drawing Salve
Drawex Salve
Dr. Daniels Hoof Ointment and Softener
Dr. Naylor's Red-Kote
Falk's Nu Salve
Gilkey's Blister
Griswold's Family Salve
Larson's Podiatry Pre-tape, Formula JC-6
Larson's Trainer's Pre-tape, Formula JC-4
Legulo
Mollimentus
Severa's First Aid Ointment
Udderkream
Wonderful Dream Brand Salve

industrial products, and because the balsam oils used now do not contain the sensitizer α-carene.

Dooms-Goossens and colleagues[12] reported a case of turpentine-induced hypersensitivity to peppermint oil owing to the sensitizing properties of three ingredients, d-pinene, limonene, and phellandrene. These compounds are also found in turpentine oil.

Peppermint oil is used widely for its aromatic properties in confections (chewing gum, candies), cosmetics, toothpaste, and pharmaceutical products such as mouthwashes. Fisher[13] and Andersen[14] have reported contact allergy to peppermint oil from certain toothpastes.

Rosin (Colophony)

This natural resin is used widely in topical medications, particularly the veterinary variety. A list of these medications is shown in Table 10.5.

In dentistry, rosin in chloroform solution has been used as a varnish for pulp protection in deep cavities. It has been added to zinc oxide or to eugenol as an ingredient of pulp-capping preparations, surgical packs, impression pastes, dental and periodontal dressings, dental cement, and liquid and cavity varnishes, and as an antiseptic for sealing pulp canals. Denture adhesive powder may also contain rosin. Such dental exposure to rosin can produce stomatitis.[15,16]

Rasmussen and Fisher[17] reported two patients in whom allergic eczematous contact dermatitis developed to salicylic acid plaster used to treat plantar warts. Both patients were shown subsequently to be allergic to dehydroabietic acid present in the rosin contained in the plaster.

Hambly and Wilkinson[18] described a dermatitis from physiotherapy wax "contaminated" with rosin. Ducombs[19] reported a patient who was allergic to many adhesive tapes because of his allergic hypersensitivity to rosin. He had a crossreaction to a lubricant prepared from pine resin used on the leather belts of an electric saw.

Newer adhesives such as Dermicel, Scanpor, and Blenderm are free of rosin.

Yellow soft laundry soap owes its consistency to the presence of rosin.

Tiger Balm

Tiger balm is a popular Chinese proprietary ointment now used in the United States. Three patients that Fisher[20] observed acquired contact dermatitis from this ointment. They all had crossreactions to balsam of Peru.

Agathos[21] stated, "Tiger balm seems to be an allergen of increasing importance. In Bavaria, a similar ointment is used; we have occasionally seen severe allergic contact dermatitis to this substance, which is sold by a 'healer' on written demand." Agathos's patient had a positive reaction to rosin.

An additional Chinese herbal medicine is known as musk and tiger bone plaster. It is used as a medical plaster for treatment of rheumatic disease, arthralgias, neuralgias, aches, and sprains. The contents include musk, tiger bone, evodia fruit, bornelone, rhizome, monkshood, kusnezoff monkshood, camphor, menthol, and zinc resinate. Zinc resinate is a mixture of zinc oxide and colophony and thus is more akin to "Bavarian" tiger balm in this respect.[22]

Benzoin Tincture (Gum Benzoin)

Benzoin tincture contains 10% benzoin in alcohol, whereas the compound formulation also contains 2% aloes, 8% storax (styrax), and 4% tolu balsam in alcohol. Benzoin may be present in adhesives, water-repellent barrier creams, lozenges, benzoinated lard, and cosmetics.

Spott and Shelley[23] reported that a student developed acute eczematous contact dermatitis in response to the application of benzoin tincture to the skin under a cast. This finding was followed within 48 hours by the appearance of a generalized, noneczematous exanthem. Analysis led to the conclusion that absorption of benzoin through the skin was responsible for both the contact dermatitis and the exanthem. Patch tests demonstrated an eczematous reaction to benzoin with cross-sensitivity extending to the gums of myrrh, locust, galbanum, gamboge, and oblibanum.

Cullen and colleagues[24] reported a patient who had allergic contact dermatitis to compound benzoin-tincture spray under a cast.

Coskey[25] had one patient who developed allergic contact dermatitis after applying benzoin tincture for pruritus ani. Another patient developed dermatitis from applying the tincture to his leg.

Crossreactions may occur to balsam of Peru, storax (styrax), eugenol, vanilla, pinene, benzyl alcohol, and benzyl cinnamate. Many athletes apply benzoin tincture to toughen various parts of their skin, particularly the feet, in order to prevent the formation of blisters.

In a personal communication, Dr. W. D. James (Walter Reed Army Medical Center, Washington, DC) reported that five military cadets acquired allergic dermatitis from benzoin tincture. All five were allergic to storax (styrax). Mastic also proved to be a much less potent sensitizer than benzoin tincture.

MEDICATIONS RELATED TO BENZOIN

Arning's Tincture

This compound contains benzoin, ammonium tumenol, anthrarobin, and ether.

Mastic (Mastisol, Balsam Tree, Pistachia Galls, Mastiche, Mastix, and Lentisk)

Mastic is a resin derived from certain varieties of *Pistacia lentiscus* trees growing in Mediterranean countries. It is used in dentistry to secure surgical dressings and in chewing gums, incense, and varnish.

Contact dermatitis from Mastisol, which contains gum mastic, styrax liquid, methyl salicylate, and alcohol, was reported by Mitchell and Dupuis.[26] The patient reacted to styrax 2% in petrolatum, benzoin 10% in ethanol, and balsam of Peru 10% in petrolatum.

Smith's Cremolia Cream

This British preparation, which contains benzoin, produced allergic contact dermatitis, as reported by Mann.[27]

Greasepaint Makeup

One patient acquired allergic contact dermatitis from benzoin in a makeup.[28]

Storax (Styrax)

Storax is the purified balsam from the Turkish tree *Liquidambar orientalis*; it is a component both of benzoin inhalation and compound benzoin tincture and has been used as a parasiticide. Storax may crossreact with benzoin, balsam of Peru, and styrene, which is used in polyester resins. Storax is present in Plexoderm in a 6% concentration with 1% allantoin and 1% salicylic acid.

Fregert and Rorsman[29] reported that a woman sensitive to diethylstilbestrol also reacted to storax and balsam of Peru.

Wood Tars

The wood tars include pine tar, beech tar, juniper tar (oil of Cade), and birch tar (oleum rusci). They are present in shampoos, deodorants, cough syrups, counterirritant veterinary liniments, pyorrhea and tooth pulp treatments, tooth powders, disinfectants, and insecticides.

Hjorth[1] stated that of 230 patients sensitive to balsam of Peru, 79 (34%) had positive reactions to wood tar and 37 (16%) had positive reactions to coal tar. Some of these patients were sensitive to both wood tar and coal tar. Positive reactions to coal tar and wood tar are much more frequent among patients sensitive to balsam of Peru than among other patients with eczema. Patients sensitive to balsam of Peru have positive reactions to wood tars twice as frequently as they have positive reactions to coal tar.

Van Andel and colleagues[30] found that 9% of 650 persons tested positive to wood tar, whereas 7% reacted to coal tar. Many had crossreactions to balsam of Peru, rosin (colophony), and turpentine. Juniper tar was the most active sensitizer.

Olholm-Larsen and Heydenreich[6] believed that this increase in positive reactions to balsam of Peru and wood tars may indicate an increased frequency of allergy to perfumes in toilet soaps and cosmetics in Denmark.

In Spain, Alomar and colleagues[31] found that in 10.3% of patients the wood tars produced an irritant response with mild erythema and edema at 48 hours, which disappeared at 96 hours. The reactions were considered allergenic in only 1.8% of patients.

JUNIPER TAR (OIL OF CADE)

Mathias and colleagues[32] suspected that juniper extract is an irritant in many instances and probably should be tested at half its commercial strength or possibly at a lower concentration.

Rothe and colleagues[33] reported a case of contact dermatitis and asthma from occupational exposure to oil of juniper, which is used for spicing sausage and as a smoking additive. The allergy to oil of juniper was proved by patch tests, intracutaneous tests, and a respiratory allergen test.

PINE OIL

Pine oil is a mixture of terpene alcohols, hydrocarbons, and ethers. Products containing pine oil include Breath-O-Pine Disinfectant, Black Flag Disinfectant, Go-Fecto Disinfectant, Pinuseptol, West Pine Deodorant, Whitepine Disinfectant, and Wilbert's Fresh Pine Deodorant. This oil is capable of producing serious toxic effects if ingested or aspirated.

BIRCH TAR OIL, EMPYREUMATIC (OLEUM RUSCI)

Lahti and Hannuksela[34] reported that fresh sap and crushed leaf of birch (*Betula verrucosa*) were tested with the scratch-chamber method in 117 atopic persons, 74 of whom were allergic and 43 of whom were nonallergic to birch pollen.

Immediate positive reactions to birch sap were seen in 39% of the patients, and positive reactions to birch leaf were seen in 28% of the patients allergic to birch pollen. These investigators stated that birch leaves may cause contact urticaria in Finnish saunas, where bath whisks made of birch sprigs are traditionally used.

Rothenborg and Hjorth[35] found that positive patch test reactions to a mixture of wood tars consisting of pine, juniper, beech, and birch often produce false-positive reactions. When a mixture of wood tars is positive, each tar should be tested individually.

RELATIONSHIP OF WOOD TARS TO COAL TARS

Whereas wood tars and coal tars may crossreact occasionally, it must be emphasized that, although coal tars are phototoxic, wood tars are not.

Rothenborg and Hjorth[35] stated that most patch test reactions to coal tars are irritant reactions and that allergic reactions are rare. Rudzki and Grzywa[36] reported that a pharmacist who prepared coal-tar ointments became allergic to coal tar.

The solution of coal tar (Liquor Carbonis Detergens), which consists of coal tar, quilla bark, and alcohol, is probably the least phototoxic coal-tar preparation.[37]

PRECAUTIONS REGARDING USE OF MEDICINAL COAL TAR

All patients using coal-tar products (with the possible exception of shampoos) should be cautioned that their exposure to the sun should be limited. No more than 15 minutes of direct exposure to midday summer sun should be tried the first time. Exposure can be increased gradually as patients define their own responses. All patients using tar products should be warned of the carcinogenic potential of tar used alone and in combination with the sun.[38]

Podophyllum Resin

Podophyllum resin remains a common treatment for condylomata acuminata (venereal warts). As a rule, an intense inflammatory reaction occurs that may become quite painful for a few days. The treatment is usually successful, and no local or systemic sequelae occur. Occasionally, however, severe systemic and local reactions do occur.[39]

SYSTEMIC EFFECTS FROM TOPICAL USE OF PODOPHYLLUM RESIN

Although many dermatologists have used topical podophyllum resin for many years without encountering systemic reactions in their patients, a review of the literature reveals several reports of severe systemic reactions. Among the various systemic effects that have been reported from the use of topically applied podophyllum resin are paresthesia, polyneuritis, paralytic ileus, pyrexia leukopenia, thrombocytopenia, coma, and death.

Grabbe[40] described a 19-year-old female patient who developed weakness and polyneuritis of the legs 2 days after a single application of a 25% podophyllum solution. On the sixth day she developed a paralytic ileus. The patient recovered after approximately 10 weeks. An 18-year-old female patient studied by Ward and colleagues[41] became comatose approximately 24 hours after the application of 25% podophyllum ointment on vulvar warts. She died 8 days later.

Schirren[42] observed a 25-year-old man whose extensive condylomata acuminata on the prepuce and perianal area were treated with a 16% solution of podophyllum in alcohol. Two hours after treatment, the patient vomited and became unconscious and cyanotic. It should be mentioned that this patient had consumed a large amount of alcohol immediately after the local treatment. According to Schirren, this may have increased the absorption of podophyllum.

Cormaine[43] reported a 20-year-old woman who was treated for extensive condylomata acuminata of the labia majora, labia minora, and vaginal mucosa. A 10% podophyllum solution in collodion was applied with a tampon and left in place for 6 hours. The patient became febrile and experienced paresthesia and weakness of the toes and fingers. The paresis from polyneuritis disappeared after 14 days.

Hasler and Standish[44] stated that vomiting and an acute confused state occurred from the use of podophyllum in the treatment of hairy tongue. Chamberlain and colleagues[45] described a case of severe intoxication in a woman in the 32nd week of pregnancy who had subsequent delivery of a stillborn infant. According to the authors, podophyllum resin should never be used during pregnancy or in circumstances in which the genital warts are either florid with a large surface area or so hemorrhagic that absorption of the toxin resin is probable.

Larsson[46] reported two patients who developed urticaria and transient fever after the use of podophyllum resin. Stoehr and colleagues[47] observed a case of leukopenia and thrombocytopenia resulting from podophyllum-resin treatment of condylomata acuminata. Montaldi and colleagues[48] and Balucani and Zellers[49] stated that systemic toxicity may produce nausea, vomiting, respiratory stimulation, peripheral neuropathy, fever, acute confused states, tachycardia, oliguria, anuria, adynamic ileus, coma, and death.

PREVENTION OF SYSTEMIC REACTIONS TO PODOPHYLLUM RESIN

Stoehr and colleagues[47] stated that systemic toxicity from local podophyllum treatment occurred when the drug was applied to extensive areas or was allowed to remain in contact with the skin for an extended period. To avoid toxicity, they recommend that applications be limited to small areas of intact skin. Although most dermatologists allow the podophyllum to remain on the skin for 4 to 6 hours, Stoehr and colleagues recommend that the drug should be allowed to remain in contact with the skin for no longer than 1 hour.

Schirren[42] suggested that because ingestion of alcohol shortly after local therapy may increase the absorption of podophyllum, alcoholic beverages should be avoided by patients for several hours following this treatment. Also, the use of podophyllum resin on the buccal mucosa or tongue and during pregnancy should be avoided.[44,45,50]

UNUSUALLY SEVERE LOCAL REACTIONS TO TOPICAL PODOPHYLLUM RESIN

Usually the application of podophyllum resin causes an acute inflammatory reaction and the subsequent development of yellowish necrosis over the treated area. The drug induces arrest of mitosis in metaphase and epithelial cell death. Vacuolation, nuclear degenerations, and swelling of the cell give rise to the podophyllum cell. The cytotoxic principles in podophyllum resin are podophyllotoxin and its derivatives.

Sullivan and King[51] were among the first to warn that podophyllum can produce "bizarre forms of epithelial cells" that can be mistaken for carcinoma cells. Maxwell and Lamb[52] described a hyperplastic infiltrated reaction to the application of podophyllum, simulating epithelioma in two patients.

Wade and Ackerman[53] stated that it has been suggested that podophyllum can induce changes in condylomata acuminata that are indistinguishable from those of squamous cell carcinoma in situ. These investigators have shown that these two conditions can be differentiated histologically. They found that podophyllum induces necrosis and mitosis in keratinocytes, but not cytologic atypia or multinucleated cells. Cytologic atypia is the sine qua non for squamous cell carcinoma in situ.

Fisher[20] became aware of severe necrosis and scarring of the anogenital area in two patients from the use of podophyllum resin. In one instance, a fistula-in-ano developed. Additional local reactions to podophyllum resin include paraphimosis, requiring circumcision, and pseudoepitheliomatous hyperplasia.

PREVENTION OF LOCAL COMPLICATIONS FROM PODOPHYLLUM RESIN

The United States Pharmacopeia (USP) podophyllum-resin topical solution is 25% podophyllum resin and benzoin in alcohol. Although the USP calls for the use of "native" American podophyllum resin, in actual practice it has been found that the practitioner may be using a mixture of the American and Indian resins. The Indian resin is stronger and more irritating than the American variety (see Table 10.6). In addition, some resins on the market are contaminated with guaiacium wood, which may be a sensitizer.[54]

Arnica Tincture

This volatile oil obtained from the composite plant *Arnica montana* is applied as a rubefacient for sprains, bruises, and painful swellings. Self-medication with arnica tincture has produced many cases of allergic contact dermatitis.[55] The sequiterpene lactones (helanalin) and methacrylate esters have proved to be the primary sensitizers.[56]

Table 10-6 Differences between American and Indian Podophyllum

	American	Indian
Scientific name	*Podophyllum pelatatum*	*Podophyllum emodi*
Common name	May apple, Mandrake	
Habitat	Eastern US	Tibet, Afghanistan
Resin content	2% to 8%	6% to 12%
Podophyllotoxin	20%	36% to 39%
Reaction to copper acetate	Bright green color	Brown color
Addition of alcohol and potassium hydroxide	Does not gelatinize	Gelatinizes

Hausen[57] stated that arnica tincture is a strong sensitizer that has caused dermatitis in hundreds of persons.

Arnica (*Arnica montana* L.) and marigold (*Calendula officinalis* L.) are used as alternative medicines. Contact allergy to arnica was found in 5 of 443 patients and marigold in 9 of 443. Only of about half of these cases would have been detected by the commercially available Compositae mix.[58]

Good data on the frequency of allergic reactions from topical or systemic exposure to Compositae plants used as herbal medications are difficult to come by. Paulsen[59] reviewed this subject and made an estimate based on the literature. Arnica (*Arnica montana*) and Elecampane (*Inula helenium*) were considered to be frequent allergens, due to multiple reports in the literature. Marigold (*Calendula officinalis)* and Costus (*Saussurea lappa*) were frequent allergens in some literature, in the case of Costus from prior use in perfume. Other Compositae were considered rare problems, and include dandelion (*Taraxacum officinale*); feverfew (*Tanacetum parthenium*); French marigold (*Tagetes patula*); sticky elecampane (*Inula viscosa*); purple coneflower (*Echinacea purpurea*); dog fennel (*Anthmis cotula*); Roman chamomile (*Chamaemelum nobile*); German chamomile (*Chamomilla recutita*); mugwort (*Artemisia vulgaris*); great burdock (*Arctium lappa*), and yarrow (*Achillea millefolium*).

Psoralen

Topical 8-methoxypsoralen is phototoxic and may also occasionally be photoallergic.[60] In addition, ordinary allergic contact dermatitis may occur from its topical use. Thus, Weissmann and colleagues[61] reported that a 20-year-old male patient was treated topically with 8-methoxypsoralen and long-wave ultraviolet light (UVA) for alopecia areata. After the sixth treatment (day 17), he developed contact allergy to 8-methoxypsoralen verified by patch testing and histopathology.

Aloe Vera

The gelatinous material inside the leaf of aloe vera has been recommended from ancient times for the alleviation of inflammatory changes in the skin. More recently, it has been advocated in the treatment of radiodermatitis and leg ulcers.[62–64]

Aloes consist of a variable mixture of aloin, aloe-emodin, and other substances. Aloin is an anthraquinone that may be regarded as a potential sensitizer. Crossreactions may occur with benzoin and balsam of Peru.

At present, Dermaide Aloe Ointment is listed as an over-the-counter product (Dermaide Research Corporation). Dermaide Aloe Ointment has as an active ingredient 70% gel of the aloe vera plant in a special white, homogenous base of mineral oil, stearic acid, petrolatum, triethanolamine, beeswax, synthetic spermaceti, propylparaben, methyl paraben, and fragrance.

Morrow and colleagues[65] described a case of hypersensitivity to aloe manifested by generalized nummular eczematous and papular dermatitis, and presumably by contact urticaria, that developed in a 47-year-old man after 4 years' use of oral and topical aloe. Patch tests for aloe were positive in this patient.

Aloe vera is a popular folk treatment for a variety of skin conditions. The safety of the plant extracts was evaluated in 702 patients. Patch tests with the oily extract of the leaves, pulverized whole plant, and a concentrated gel were negative in all 702 cases, attesting to the safety of the plant extracts.[66]

Propolis (Bee Glue) and Beeswax

Propolis (bee glue) is a dark yellow-brown adhesive resin that bees mix with wax to form a cementing substance in their hives. The purified wax from the honeycomb, beeswax, is used widely in cosmetics. Beeswax may be used as cera alba (bleached) or as cera flava (unbleached).

PROPOLIS (BEE GLUE)

Propolis (bee glue), derived mainly from poplar and other tree resins, contains, among other things, well-known sensitizers such as cinnamic acid and vanillin. It may crossreact with balsam of Peru. Allergic contact dermatitis from propolis is an occupational hazard for beekeepers.[67,68] In rare instances, a beekeeper may be allergic to beeswax. Beekeepers who have dermatitis may be tested with the contactants shown in Table 10.7.

Table 10-7 Beekeepers Patch Test Series	
Allergens	Test
Balsam of Peru	25% pet
Pine balsam	10% pet
Pine bud	As is
Poplar resin	10% pet
Propolis (bee glue)	As is
Wax (beeswax)	As is

Propolis is sold in many health food stores in various forms for ingestion as a "cure-all" for numerous diseases and as a topical agent in ointments, powders, and cosmetic creams. Solid propolis, which can be chewed, may produce a perioral dermatitis and stomatitis. Thus, Wanscher[69] described two patients who had contact dermatitis and stomatitis from chewing so-called natural propolis products, which are sold without prescription as tablets or as solid propolis in large or small chunks.

Petersen[70] predicted that, with the increasing employment of propolis for self-medication, a growing number of cases of allergic contact eczema from exposure to this preparation should be anticipated.

BEESWAX

Beeswax is secreted by bees. Camasara[71] reported a woman who was employed in molding art objects from beeswax who developed chronic palmar dermatitis. A strongly positive patch test to natural beeswax was obtained. A beekeeper described by Rothenborg[68] reacted to raw, unpurified beeswax but not to purified beeswax. The raw wax was considered contaminated by poplar tree resins, to which he was sensitive.

Honey is a saccharin substance deposited in the honeycomb by the honeybee. It is used as an excipient, as a flavor in gargles and cough medicine, and as a food.

Chamomile (Camomile)

Chamomile is a yellow dye extracted from the dried flower heads of *Chamaemelum nobile* (Roman source) and *Matricaria recutita* (German source), both of which are of the Asteraceae family. The Roman product is thought to be more allergenic.[72]

Chamomile is used in shampoos, hair rinses, and as a vegetable hair dye. Allergic contact dermatitis has occurred in persons who have handled the plant or who have used compresses of chamomile or chamo-mile ointment.[73,74] Chamomile may crossreact with the *Compositae* group of plants. Oil of chamomile has been added to nipple eczema cream used by nursing mothers, and contact dermatitis has been confirmed with 0.1% petrolatum of the oil of chamomile. Drinking chamomile tea was found to flare the original contact dermatitis.[72]

GERMAN CHAMOMILE

Allergy to chamomile is most commonly reported from Roman chamomile (*Anthemis nobilis*), but Pereira and colleagues[75] had a patient who used chamomile tea compresses to treat an eczema of the forearms and became sensitive to both Roman and German chamomile (*Matricaria chamomilla*). The allergen in the German chamomile is sesquiterpene lactone desacetyl matricarin.

German chamomile tea used to treat a facial dermatitis resulted in contact dermatitis to the tea.[76] In this case, sesquiterpene lactone mix was positive and Roman chamomile negative. Subsequent ingestion of German chamomile tea caused flare-up of the facial dermatitis, as well as eczema of the arms and trunk and anal pruritus.

HERBAL TEAS

The fact that herbal teas share ingredients with topical herbal remedies caused Lundh and colleagues[77] to question how commonly patients allergic to sesquiterpene lactones might react to herbal tea. To investigate this question, they tested 20 sesquiterpene lactone-sensitive patients to herbal teas prepared for patch testing by boiling 1.5 g of dried tea in 50 mL of water, filtering it, removing the water in a rotary evaporator, and suspending the residue in 1 mL of water. This stock solution was tested at 100%, 10%, and 1%. Eighteen of 20 patients reacted to teas of the Asteraceae family, ie, mainly those containing German chamomile, dandelion, and wormwood. Ingestion of the teas was not studied.

Tannin

Some hemorrhoid ointments contain up to 10% tannin, a rare sensitizer. Two cases from hemorrhoid ointments were reported by van Ketel and Bruynzeel,[78] which brings to four the number of reported cases of tannin sensitivity. A 1% to 10% petrolatum or aqueous tannin patch test is positive.

Natural Oils

JOJOBA OIL

Jojoba oil is a liquid-wax ester extracted from the jojoba bush, which grows wild in the southwestern United States and in northern Mexico. It is now grown commercially in the United States and Israel.

The oil is used in cosmetics as a skin lubricant, hair conditioner, and wrinkle "remover." Jojoba oil was first reported as a sensitizer by Markin[79] and later by Scott.[80]

TEA TREE OIL

Topical use of tea tree oil has been a source of allergic contact dermatitis. De Groot[81] reported a patient who developed facial dermatitis from vapors of tea tree oil used to treat bronchitis. He noted that while the allergen most frequently sited in tea tree or melaleuca oil is *d*-limonene, the sensitizing components include aromadendrene, alpha terpinene, 1,8-cineole (eucalyptol), terpinen-4-ol, *p*-cymene, and alpha-phellandrene. In a study of botanical extracts, tea tree oil was found to have caused the most relevant positive reactions.[82]

Tea-tree oil from the *Melaleuca alternifolia* tree has enjoyed increased use as an antimicrobial agent. As its use has expanded, so have reports of adverse reactions to it. These have included allergic contact dermatitis, systemic contact dermatitis, linear immunoglobulin A disease, erythema multiforme-like reactions, and systemic hypersensitivity reactions. Antimicrobial properties have been attributed to terpinen-4-ol from the plant. The anti-inflammatory effects of tea tree oil have been related to alpha-pinene, alpha-terpinene, terpinen-4-ol, alpha-terpineol, and linalool.[83]

BLACK CUMIN OIL

Therapeutic use of black cumin (*Nigella sativa*) oil, which is promoted in Germany for skin diseases of many divergent types, has led to contact dermatitis.[84] The oil is sold as an herbal remedy under the name Schwedenkreuther, or Swedish herbs. A 1:200 dilution in olive oil can be used for patch testing. Black cumin has been used for digestive disorders, gynecologic disease, and respiratory conditions due to its bronchodilatory and anticholinergic effects. It has been added to some skin care products, exposure to which can cause contact dermatitis.[85]

LAUREL OIL

Laurel oil is used as an analgesic. Application to the knees to relieve joint pain, on the advice of a herbalist, resulted in allergic contact dermatitis. Laurel comes from the *Laurus nobilis* and it is used in aromatherapy as well as in perfumes and soaps.[86]

Vegetable Gums

These gums are resinous plant exudates. Karaya, acacia, and tragacanth are probably the most common sensitizers among them.[87] They may be used "as is" for patch tests.

Karaya is an ingredient in many cosmetics, particularly hair-waving lotions. It is used in toothpastes, powders, adhesives, and cement substances to make ileostomy and colostomy bags adhere to the skin. Fasteeth, a denture adhesive, contains karaya gum, sodium borate, and peppermint flavoring.

Acacia (gum arabic)is used in cosmetics and in offset sprays in the printing industry.

Gum tragacanth (tragacanth), an insoluble vegetable gum that absorbs water to form a jelly, may crossreact with acacia. Tragacanth is used in cosmetics, particularly gum-based hair dressings, and in troches, toothpastes, depilatories, and other topical medications. Exposure may take place from contact with textile finishes and sizing papers or in printing operations or enameling.

Gum resins are naturally occurring mixtures of gum, oil, and resin. There is probably wider exposure to benzoic gum resin than to other gum resins. Acacia (gum arabic), which is used in adhesives, may be a sensitizer.[88] Other gums (plant exudates consisting of high-polymer polysaccharides, some with a low nitrogen content) such as karaya, acacia (gum arabic), and gum tragacanth, may act occasionally as sensitizers.

Ergot

The principal medical use of ergot is via systemic administration; however, nicergoline (1,6-dimethyl-8-b-5-bromonicotinyl-oxymethyl-10-a-methoxyergoline) is used in the manufacture of a calcium channel blocker derived from ergot. Nicergoline caused an airborne contact dermatitis in a factory worker exposed to the product. A 7% concentration in ethyl alcohol produced a positive patch test.[89]

Rue

In some parts of the world, members of the Rutaceae family are used as folk remedies and to protect against mosquito bites. Unfortunately, this leads to photocontact dermatitis and intense hyperpigmentation, as members of this family contain 5- and 8-methoxypsoralen. Reports of this type of reaction include *Ruta montana, R. graveolens,* and *R. chalenpensis.*[90]

Verbena

An "omelette" made from *Verbena officinalis* (wild verbena) and egg whites is used as a folk medicine for sinusitis, bronchitis, ocular diseases, and dermatitis.[91] This mixture may facilitate contact dermatitis, as the allergenic fraction of the plant is thought to be oil soluble, and mere handling of the plant was not sufficient to cause dermatitis.

Krameria

Krameria triandra is also known as Peruvian rhatany, red rhatany, rhatanhia, and rhatania. It is a member of the Krameriaceae family and is a low shrub native to South America. It has been used as a botanical medication due to its astringent, antidiarrheic, and anti-inflammatory properties. When compounded into an antihemorrhoidal gel, it caused allergic contact dermatitis, proven by a positive patch test to rhatany tincture 1% petrolatum.[92]

Elecampane

Elecampane is the common name of a herb used systemically and topically as a supplement in phytotherapy. The scientific name is *Inula helenium,* a member of the *Compositae* family, which contains both isoalantolactone and alantolactone. This herb was added to a massage liniment and caused contact dermatitis in a woman who had taken this herb orally 1 year previously.[93] Although taking the oral form of this botanical, she experienced facial dermatitis.

Centella

Slow-healing wounds and chronic ulcers are treated with a cream containing the triterpenic fraction of *Centella asiatica,* a member of the Umbelliferae family. This is commercially available as Centelase cream. The plant is thought to be of low sensitization potential based on guinea pig tests of the sensitizing constituents: asiaticoside, asiatic acid, and madecassic acid.[94]

Rosemary

Use of rosemary leaves as a topical anti-inflammatory plaster caused contact dermatitis, confirmed by patch testing with the leaves[95] Rosemary (*Rosmarinus officinalis L.*) is a member of the Labiatae family. Other members of Labiatae include thyme, origanum, and mint. Patch tests to these three plants were negative. Contact dermatitis and photoaggravated contact dermatitis to rosemary were reported by Serra and colleagues.[96]

Rosemary in an alcohol solution was applied to the chest to try to improve breathing. Contact dermatitis resulted. The patient reacted to other Lamiacea family members. Thyme, sage, and lavender leaves (both fresh and dried) produced positive patch tests. Fresh plants produced the stronger reaction.[97]

Sandalwood

Traditional sandalwood is *Santalum album,* whereas red sandalwood is *Pterocarpus santalinus.* Red sandalwood bark is used as a folk remedy in India to treat postacne scarring and when used this way has caused allergic contact dermatitis. The allergens are santalin A (9,10,12-tri-o-methylsantalin) and santalin B (9,10,12,49-tetra-o-methylsantalin), and the allergens in *S. album* are alpha and beta santalol.[98]

Ginkgo Biloba

Dietary supplements containing *Ginkgo biloba* are popular for cerebral function enhancement. Because these are similar to *Toxicodendron,* the possibility of systemic contact dermatitis exists. Hausen[99] attempted to quantify the risk that these supplements hold. He found that pure ginkgolic acids could sensitize guinea pigs but that extracts of the *Ginkgo biloba* leaves could not. He found that leaf extracts up to 1,000 ppm of ginkgolic acids would be safe.

Burdock

Burdock (*Arctium lappa*) is used as an herbal supplement in the United States, and it is applied topically in Spain as burdock root plasters for an anti-inflammatory effect. Burdock is a member of the Compositae family, and three cases of contact dermatitis to the plasters were reported from Spain.[100]

Goldenrod

Oral ingestion of a medication (Urodyn) that contains goldenrod resulted in a systemic contact dermatitis.[101] Patch tests confirmed reactions to goldenrod (*Herba solidaginis*) and related Compositae tansy and yarrow.

Curcuminoids

Curcuminoids are used to treat peptic ulcers and wounds and have antioxidant properties which have led to their inclusion in sunscreens and cosmetics. Tetrahydracurcumin from the rhizome of *Curcuma longa* (turmeric root) has been identified as a contact allergen in its use in a sunscreen product. 1% petrolatum was used to patch test.[102] Curcuminoids are also used in some skin care products for their antioxidant properties and anti-inflammatory properties. Tetrahydracurcumin (1% pet) in Avon Age Block cream caused contact dermatitis.[103]

Guava Tea

Guava tea made from *Psidium guajava* has been introduced into Japan as a treatment for atopic dermatitis. A 45 kD protein and tannin have been identified as the allergenic components in a 17-year-old atopic patient who developed allergic contact dermatitis from this source.[104]

Spearmint

An infusion of fresh leaves of spearmint (*Mentha spicata*) was used to treat knee pain. This resulted in acute allergic contact dermatitis confirmed by commercial patch tests to spearmint oil. Peppermint oil was also positive. Spearmint is more commonly associated with contact cheilitis, and carvone and limonene have been found in the plant.[105]

Boswellia Serrata

A woman treated a second-degree burn with a naturopathic cream composed of resin extract of *Boswellia serrata*, rosemary oil, olive oil, and virgin beeswax. The resulting contact dermatitis was traced to the *Boswellia serrata* extract. which reacted at 0.1% in both petrolatum and alcohol. This is a common folk medicine in India. It is thought that the mechanism of its anti-inflammatory properties come from inhibition of 5-lipoxygenase.[106]

Kudzu

Kakonto is a Japanese herbal medicine used to treat influenza, allergic rhinitis and early polio or encephalitis. It is known as kudzu or arrowroot decoction and it can cause a generalized dermatitis which was confirmed with a 30% petrolatum patch test.[107]

Astronium Urundeuva

In northeastern Brazil, *Astronium urundeuva*, of the Anacardiaceae family is used for treatment of dermatologic and gynecologic conditions. Contact dermatitis has been detected with 10% eth. extracts of the bark.[108]

Gordolobo

Gordolobo is the Spanish common name for *Verbascum densiflorum*, a folk medicine used as an infusion of leaves and stems to treat cough, bronchitis, asthma, anemia, and gastroenteritis. A worker involved in mixing medical herbs became sensitized to gordolobo, by patch tests to the dried herb.[109]

Butcher's Broom

Butcher's broom (*Ruscus aculeatus*) is used medicinally as a laxative and a diuretic. Ruscogenin and neuroruscogenin are components thought to improve capillary flow and blood vessel tone. Ruscogenins that were present in the commercial product Proctolog caused allergic contact dermatitis, and the patch test was 3+ (concentration not stated). Ruscogenin is also found in some anticellulite creams.[110]

White Flower Embrocation

The Chinese herbal remedy known as white flower embrocation, sometimes used to treat insect bites, can cause contact dermatitis. The ingredients include wintergreen oil 40%, menthol crystal 30%, eucalyptus oil 18%, camphor 6%, and lavender oil 6%.[111]

Ginger Family

Alpinia galanga is a member of the ginger family. Application of slices of the fresh plant to relieve pain produced a local dermatitis and, 10 days later, a generalized erythema multiforme-like eruption. Patch tests with powdered and fried forms of the plant at 2%, 10%, and 100% petrolatum were positive. The major ingredients are 1.8-cineole, a-fenchyl acetate, camphor, methyl cinnamate, guaiol, and sesquiterpenes.[112]

Prickly Pear Cactus

Prickly pear cactus (*Opuntia ficus-indica*) has been used in Mexico as a folk medicine for systemic conditions such as diabetes, gastritis, and arteriosclerosis. In Korea,

Opuntia ficus-indica var. saboten is used both as a food and as a topical folk remedy. The latter use produced contact dermatitis (tested as the fruit, "as is").[113]

Grasses

Grasses that are members of the Gramineae family have been associated with a variety of reactions, ranging from contact dermatitis and anaphylaxis to gastroenteritis, rhinoconjunctivitis, and asthma. A pet-shop assistant was occupationally exposed to the seed of canary-grass (*Phalaris aquatica,* a member of the Gramineae family), which caused an allergic contact dermatitis. Patch tests with extracts of canary-grass seed proved positive, with negative results in 12 control subjects.[114]

References

1. Hjorth N. Eczematous allergy to balsams. Acta Dermatol Venereol Suppl (Stockh) 1961;41:34.

2. Fregert S, Möller H. Contact allergy to balsam of Peru in children. Br J Dermatol 1963;75:218.

3. Ebner H. Contact allergy to Peru balsam in children and adolescents. Tagl Prax 1976;17:155.

4. Rudzki E, Grzywa Z. Immediate reactions to balsam of Peru, cassia oil and ethyl vanillin. Contact Dermatitis 1976;2:360.

5. Forsbeck M, Skog E. Immediate reactions to patch tests with balsam of Peru. Contact Dermatitis 1977;3:201.

6. Olholm-Larsen P, Heydenreich G. Allergy to balsam of Peru and wood tars: an increasing problem? Contact Dermatitis 1976;2:293.

7. Veien NK, Hattel T, Justesen O, Norholm A. Oral challenge with balsam of Peru in patients with eczema: a preliminary study. Contact Dermatitis 1983;9:75.

8. Veien NK, Hattel T, Justesen O, Norholm N. Oral challenge with balsam of Peru. Contact Dermatitis 1985;12:104.

9. Veien NK, Hattel T, Justesen O, Norholm N. Reduction of intake of balsams in patients sensitive to balsam of Peru. Contact Dermatitis 1985;12:270.

10. Veien NK, Hattel T, Laurberg G. Can oral challenge with balsam of Peru predict possible benefit from a low-balsam diet? Am J Contact Dermat 1996;7:84.

11. Cronin E. Oil of turpentine—a disappearing allergen. Contact Dermatitis 1979;5:30.

12. Dooms-Goossens A, Degreef H, Holvoet C, Maertens M. Turpentine induced hypersensitivity to peppermint oil. Contact Dermatitis 1977;3:304.

13. Fisher AA. Contact stomatitis, glossitis, and cheilitis. Otolaryngol Clin North Am 1971;7:82.

14. Andersen KE. Contact allergy to toothpaste flavors. Contact Dermatitis 1978;4:195.

15. Lysell L. Contact allergy to rosin in a periodontal dressing: a case report. J Oral Med 1976;31:24.

16. Dawson TJ. Colophony sensitivity in dentistry. Contact Dermatitis 1977;3:342.

17. Rasmussen IE, Fisher AA. Allergic contact dermatitis to a salicylic acid plaster. Contact Dermatitis 1976;2:237.

18. Hambly EM, Wilkinson DS. Dermatitis from contaminated physiotherapy wax. Contact Dermatitis 1975;1:53.

19. Ducombs G. Allergy to colophony. Contact Dermatitis 1978;4:118.

20. Fisher AA. Contact dermatitis. 3rd ed. Philadelphia: Lea & Febiger, 1986.

21. Agathos M. Bavarian tiger balm. Contact Dermatitis 1982;8:215.

22. Barbaud A, Mougeoll JM, Tang JQ, Protois JC. Contact allergy to colophony in Chinese musk and tiger bone plaster. Contact Dermatitis 1991;25:324.

23. Spott DA, Shelley WB. Exanthem due to contact allergen (Benzoin) absorbed through skin. JAMA 1970;214:1881.

24. Cullen SI, Tonkin A, May FE. Allergic contact dermatitis to compound tincture of benzoin spray. J Trauma 1974;14:348.

25. Coskey RJ. Contact dermatitis owing to tincture of benzoin. Arch Dermatol 1978;114:128.

26. Mitchell IC, Dupuis G. Allergic contact dermatitis from storax (styrax). Contact Dermatitis Newsletter 1972;11:274.

27. Mann RJ. Benzoin sensitivity. Contact Dermatitis 1982;8:263.

28. Hoffman TE, Adams RM. Contact dermatitis to benzoin in greasepaint makeup. Contact Dermatitis 1982;4:379.

29. Fregert S, Rorsman H. Hypersensitivity to diethylstilbestrol with cross-sensitization to benzestrol. Acta Derm Venereol (Stockh) 1962;42:290.

30. Van Andel P, Bleumink E, Nater IP. The significance of positive patch tests to wood tars. Trans St Johns Hosp Dermatol Soc 1974;60:94.

31. Alomar A, Camarasa JG, Garcia Perez A, Pascual M. Wood tar patch test. Contact Dermatitis 1977;3:220.

32. Mathias CGT, Maibach HI, Mitchell IC. Plant dermatitis—patch test results (1975–1978). Contact Dermatitis 1979;5:336.

33. Rothe A, Heine A, Rebohle E. Oil of juniper as an allergenic substance for skin and respiratory tract. Berufsdermatosen 1973;21:11.

34. Lahti A, Hannuksela M. Immediate contact allergy to birch leaves and sap. Contact Dermatitis 1980;6:464.

35. Rothenborg HW, Hjorth N. Allergy to perfumes from toilet soaps and detergents in patients with dermatitis. Arch Dermatol 1968;97:417.

36. Rudzki E, Grzywa A. Occupational dermatitis partly elicited by coal tar. Contact Dermatitis 1877;3:54.

37. Kaidbey KH, Kligman AM. Clinical and histological study of coal tar phototoxicity in humans. Arch Dermatol 1977;123:592.

38. Rasmussen JE. The crudeness of coal tar. Prog Dermatol 1978;12:23.

39. Fisher AA. Severe systemic and local reactions to topical podophyllum resin. Cutis 1981;28:233.

40. Grabbe W. Gefahren bei der Behandlung spitzer Kondylome mit Podophyllin beigleichzeitiger Neosalvarsan-Therapie. Hautarzt 1951;2:325.

41. Ward JW, Clifford WS, Monaco AR, Bickerstaff HJ. Fatal systemic poisoning following podophyllin treatment of condyloma acuminatum. South Med J 1954;47:1204.

42. Schirren CG. Schwere Allgemeinvergiftung nach ortlicher Anwendung von Podophyllin-Spiritus bein spitzen Kondylomen. Hautarzt 1966;17:321.

43. Cormaine RH. Condylomata acuminata en podofyllin. Ned Tijdschr Geneeskd 1968;112:2305.

44. Hasler JF, Standish SM. Podophyllin treatment of hairy tongue: a warning. J Am Dent Assoc 1969;78:563.

45. Chamberlain MJ, Reynolds AL, Yeoman WB. Toxic effect of podophyllum application in pregnancy. Br Med J 1972;3:391.

46. Larsson LG. Podophyllin treatment of skin carcinomas. Acta Derm Venereol (Stockh) 1952;32:56.

47. Stoehr GP, Peterson A, Taylor WJ. Systemic complications of local podophyllin therapy. Ann Intern Med 1978;89:362.

48. Montaldi DH, Giambrone JP, Courey NG, Taefi P. Podophyllin poisoning associated with the treatment of condyloma acuminatum: a case report. Am J Obstet Gynecol 1974;119:1130.

49. Balucani M, Zellers DD. Podophyllum resin poisoning with complete recovery. JAMA 1964;189:639.

50. Nelson LM. Use of podophyllin (podophyllum resin) in dermatology. Arch Dermatol Syphilol 1953;67:488.

51. Sullivan M, King LS. Effects of resin of podophyllum on normal skin: condylomata acuminata and verrucae vulgaris. Arch Dermatol Syphilol 1947;56:30.

52. Maxwell TB, Lamb JH. Unusual reaction to application of podophyllum resin. Arch Dermatol Syphilol 1954;70:510.

53. Wade T, Ackerman AB. The effects of resin of podophyllin on condyloma acuminatum. Am J Dermatopathol 1984;6:109.

54. Mitchell J, Rook A. Botanical dermatology—plants and plant products injurious to the skin. Vancouver: Greengrass, 1979:720.

55. Rudzki E, Grzywa Z. Dermatitis from *Arnica montana*. Contact Dermatitis 1977;3:281.

56. Hausen BM, Herman HD, Willuhn G. The sensitizing capacity of Composite plants (Arnica). Contact Dermatitis 1978;4:3.

57. Hausen BM. Identification of the allergens of *Arnica montana*. Contact Dermatitis 1978;4:308.

58. Reider N, Komericki P, Hausen BM, et al. The seamy side of natural medicines: contact sensitization to arnica (*Arnica montana* L.) and marigold (*Calendula officinalis* L.). Contact Dermatitis 2001;45:272.

59. Paulsen E. Contact sensitization from Compositae-containing herbal remedies and cosmetics. Contact Dermatitis 2002;47:189.

60. Plewig G, Hofmann C, Braun-Falco O. Photoallergic dermatitis from 8-methoxy psoralen. Arch Dermatol Res 1978;261:201.

61. Weissmann I, Wagner G, Plewig G. Contact allergy to 8-methoxypsoralen. Br J Dermatol 1980;102:113.

62. Gjerstad G, Riner TD. Current status of aloe as a "cure-all." Am J Pharm 1968;140:58.

63. El Zawahry M, Hegazy MR, Helal M. Use of Aloe in treating leg ulcers and dermatoses. Dermatol Int 1973;12:68.

64. Wright CS. Aloe vera in treatment of roentgen ulcers and telangiectasis. JAMA 1936;106:1363.

65. Morrow DM, Rapaport MJ, Strick A. Hypersensitivity to aloe. Arch Dermatol 1980;116:1064.

66. Reider N, Issa A, Hawranek T, et al. Absence of contact sensitization to *Aloe vera* (L.) Burm. f. Contact Dermatitis 2005;53:332.

67. Bunney MH. Contact dermatitis in beekeepers due to propolis (bee glue). Br J Dermatol 1968;80:17.

68. Rothenborg HW. Occupational dermatitis in a beekeeper due to poplar resins in beeswax. Arch Dermatol 1967;95:381.

69. Wanscher B. Contact dermatitis from propolis. Br J Dermatol 1976;94:451.

70. Petersen HO. Allergy to propolis (bee glue) in patients with eczema. Ugeskr Laeger 1977;139:2331.

71. Camasara G. Occupational dermatitis from beeswax. Contact Dermatitis 1975;1:124.

72. McGeorge BC, Steele MC. Allergic contact dermatitis of the nipple from Roman chamomile ointment. Contact Dermatitis 1991;24:139.

73. Mitchell JC, Rook A. Botanical dermatology. London: Henry Kimpton, 1979:187.

74. Beetz D, Cramer HJ, Mehlhorn C_H. Zur Haufigkeit der Epidermalen Allergie gegenuber Kamille in Kamillenhaltigen Arzneimitteln und Kosmetica. Dermatol Monatsschr 1971;157:505.

75. Pereira F, Santos R, Pereira A. Contact dermatitis from chamomile tea. Contact Dermatitis 1997;36:307.

76. Rodriguez-Serna M, Sanchez-Motilla J_M, Ramon R, Aliaga A. Allergic and systemic contact dermatitis from *Matricaria chamomilla* tea. Contact Dermatitis 1998;39:192.

77. Lundh K, Hindsen M, Gruvberger B, et al. Contact allergy to herbal teas derived from Asteraceae plants. Contact Dermatitis 2006;54:196.

78. van Ketel WG, Bruynzeel DP. Contact sensitivity to tannin. Contact Dermatitis 1991;25:75.

79. Markin LE. Boxwood sensitiveness. J Allergy 1930;1:346.

80. Scott MJ. Jojoba oil. J Am Acad Dermatol 1982;6:545.

81. De Groot AC. Airborne allergic contact dermatitis from tea tree oil. Contact Dermatitis 1996;35:304.

82. Simpson EL, Law SV, Storrs FJ. Prevalence of botanical extract allergy in patients with contact dermatitis. Dermatitis 2004;15:67.

83. Crawford GH, Sciacca JR, James WD. Tea tree oil: cutaneous effects of the extracted oil of *Melaleuca alternifolia*. Dermatitis 2004;15:59.

84. Steinmann A, Schatzle M, Agathos M, Breit R. Allergic contact dermatitis from black cumin (*Nigella sativa*) oil after topical use. Contact Dermatitis 1997;36:268.

85. Zedlitz S, Kaufmann R, Boehncke W-H. Allergic contact dermatitis from black cumin (*Nigella sativa*) oil-containing ointment. Contact Dermatitis 2002;46:188.

86. Ozden MG, Oztas P, Oztas MO, et al. Allergic contact dermatitis from Laurus nobilis (laurel) oil. Contact Dermatitis 2001;45:178.

87. Nilsson DS. Sources of allergenic gums. Ann Allergy 1960;18:518.

88. Cooke MA, Wilkinson J_F. Formalin sensitivity in gum arabic. Contact Dermatitis Newsletter 1973;13:379.

89. Fumagalli M, Bigardi AS, Legori A, Pigatto PD. Occupational contact dermatitis from airborne nicergoline. Contact Dermatitis 1992;27:256.

90. Ortiz-Frutos FJ, Sanchez B, Garcia L, et al. Photocontact dermatitis from rue (*Ruta montana* L.). Contact Dermatitis 1995;33:284.

91. Del Pozo MD, Gastaminza G, Navarro JA, et al. Allergic contact dermatitis *from Verbena officinalis* L. Contact Dermatitis 1994;31:200.

92. Goday Bujan JJ, Oleaga Morante JM, Yanquas Bayona I, et al. Allergic contact dermatitis from *Krameria triandra* extract. Contact Dermatitis 1998;38:120.

93. Pazzaglia M, Venturo N, Borda G, Tosti A. Contact dermatitis due to a message liniment containing *Inula helenium* extract. Contact Dermatitis 1995;33:267.

94. Danese P, Carnevali C, Bertazzoni MG. Allergic contact dermatitis due to *Centella asiatica* extract. Contact Dermatitis 1994;31:201.

95. Fernandez L, Duque S, Sanchez I, et al. Allergic contact dermatitis from rosemary (Rosmarinus officinalis L.). Contact Dermatitis 1997;37:248.

96. Serra E, Vila A, Peramiquel L, et al. Allergic contact dermatitis due to rosemary. Contact Dermatitis 2005;53:179.

97. Gonzalez-Mahave I, Lobesa T, Del Pozo MD, et al. Rosemary contact dermatitis and cross-reactivity with other labiate plants. Contact Dermatitis 2006;54:210.

98. Sandra A, Shenoi SD, Srinivas C_R. Allergic contact dermatitis from red sandalwood (*Pterocarpus santalinus*). Contact Dermatitis 1996;34:69.

99. Hausen BM. The sensitizing capacity of ginkgolic acids in guinea pigs. Am J Contact Dermat 1998;9:146.

100. Rodriguez P, Blanco J, Juste S, et al. Allergic contact dermatitis due to burdock (*Arctium lappa*). Contact Dermatitis 1995;33:134.

101. Schatzle M, Agathos M, Breit R. Allergic contact dermatitis from goldenrod (*Herba solidaginis*) after systemic administration. Contact Dermatitis 1998;39:271.

102. Lamb SR, Wilkinson SM. Contact allergy to tetrahydracurcumin. Contact Dermatitis 2003;48:227.

103. Thompson DA, Tan BB. Tetrahydracurcumin-related allergic contact dermatitis Contact Dermatitis 2006;55:254.

104. Obi M, Miyazaki Y, Yokozeki H, et al. Allergic contact dermatitis due to guava tea. Contact Dermatitis 2001;44:116.

105. Bonzmonte D, Mundo L, Daddabbo M, et al. Allergic contact dermatitis from *Mentha spicata* (spearmint). Contact Dermatitis 2001;45:298.

106. Acebo E, Baton JA, Sautua S, et al. Allergic contact dermatitis from *Boswellia serrata* extract in a naturopathic cream. Contact Dermatitis 2004;51:91.

107. Akita H, Sowa J, Makiura M, et al. Maculopapular drug eruption due to the Japanese herbal medicine Kakkonto (kudzu or arrowroot decoction). Contact Dermatitis 2003;48:348.

108. Vilar MDLL, Diogenes MJN, Vilar JL, et al. Contact dermatitis associated with *Astronium urundeuva* (allemao) Engl., a traditional medicinal plant from Brazil. Contact Dermatitis 2004;51:311.

109. Castro AI, Carmona JB, Gonzales FG, et al. Occupational airborne dermatitis from gordolobo (*Verbascum densilorum*). Contact Dermatitis 2006;55:301.

110. Ramirez-Hernandez M, Garcia-Selles J, Merida-Fernandez C, et al. Allergic contact dermatitis to ruscogenins. Contact Dermatitis 2006;54:60

111. Saary MJ, Holness DL. Contact dermatitis from white flower embrocation. Contact Dermatitis 2001;44:100.

112. Hong SJ, Chang CH. Erythema multiforme-like generalized allergic contact dermatitis caused by *Alpinia galanga*. Contact Dermatitis 2006;54:118.

113. Yoon HJ, Won CH, Moon SE. Allergic contact dermatitis due to *Opuntia ficus*-indica var. saboten. Contact Dermatitis 2004;51:311.

114. Monteseirin J, Perez-Formoso JL, Sanchez-Hernandez MC, et al. Occupational contact dermatitis from canary-grass seed. Contact Dermatitis 2002;47:247.

CHAPTER 11

ANTISEPTICS AND DISINFECTANTS

EXECUTIVE SUMMARY

Antiseptics are for use on living tissue and disinfectants on inanimate objects. Antiseptics covered here include thimerosal, mercurochrome, phenylmercuric salts, iodine, sodium hypochlorite, bromine, chloramine T, chlorhexidine, cetrimide, chloroxine, chloroxylenol, hexachlorophene, dichlorophene, the irgasans, Tego, and benzoyl peroxide.

Disinfectants causing contact dermatitis include quaternary ammonium compounds, triphenylmethane dyes, acriflavine dyes, eosin, glyoxal, alcohol, Gigasept AF, diethyl glycol monobutyl ether, and alkylpropylenediamineguanidium diacetate.

Antiseptics are chemicals applied to living tissue that kill or prevent the growth of micro-organisms. They must retain their activity in the presence of body fluids without being harmful locally or systemically.

Disinfectants, on the other hand, are used on inanimate objects. They must be effective in the presence of organic materials, such as blood, feces, and sputum, but nondestructive to the materials they contact, such as surgical instruments or counter tops.

Thimerosal (Merthiolate)

This compound, sodium ethylmercurithiosalicylate, is used as an antiseptic and a preservative in topical medicaments, cosmetics, and vaccines (Table 11.1).

Solution no. 45 Merthiolate is formulated to contain sodium borate in the current formulation but is colored with two dyes, fluorescein (D & C Yellow no. 70) and eosin yellowish-(YS) (D & C Red no. 22).[1]

NATURE OF SENSITIZATION TO THIMEROSAL (MERTHIOLATE)

It should be noted that thimerosal contains two distinct radicals: an organic mercury compound and a thiosalicylate. The allergic reactions may be from either compound. Ellis[2] and Gaul[3] were among the first to show that the thiosalicylate compound is a strong sensitizer. More recently, Takino[4] reported that almost all of 23 Japanese thimerosal-sensitive persons were allergic to the thiosalicylate radical.

Reports of cross-sensitivity of thimerosal with other mercury compounds are confusing because the investigators did not state whether they had tested the thimerosal-sensitive persons to both the mercury and the thiosalicylic acid radicals. Epstein[5] stated that one of his five thimerosal-sensitive patients had crossreactions to ammoniated mercury. Sertoli and colleagues[6] reported that a thimerosal-sensitive person had crossreactions to phenylmercuric nitrate, whereas Fisher and colleagues[7] found that none of their thimerosal-sensitive patients had crossreactions with organic mercury compounds. In addition, Möller[8] states that cross-sensitization occurs to a few organic mercurials, but not to inorganic and metallic mercury in thimerosal-sensitive persons.

Patients sensitive to thimerosal (Merthiolate) can be divided into three groups: (a) positive to thimerosal but negative to other mercurials and to thiosalicylic acid, (b) positive to thimerosal and to some other mercurials but negative to thiosalicylic acid, and (c) positive to thimerosal and to thiosalicylic acid but negative to other mercurials.

THIMEROSAL (MERTHIOLATE) AS A SENSITIZER IN EYE PREPARATIONS

There are numerous reports of allergic contact sensitization to thimerosal (Merthiolate) in various eye preparations and contact lens solutions. The allergic reaction may produce conjunctivitis alone or a combination of conjunctivitis and eyelid dermatitis. In one instance, a sensitized person had dermatitis of the hands without conjunctivitis.

Fregert and Hjorth[9] stated that allergic reactions to eyedrops often produce both conjunctivitis and eyelid

Table 11-1 Partial List of Agents Containing Thimerosal (Merthiolate)

Adapettes	Isotogen Ear Drops
Adapt	Jenkins Nasal Spray
Adsorbonac (2% and 5%)	Lauro Eye Wash
Aeroaid	LC-65 Daily Contact Lens Cleaner
Aerocauticals Aerosol Merthiolate	Loridine Cephaloridine
Allerest Eye Drops	McKesson's IBath and IDrops
Allergex (Concentrate)	Merthiolate (also contains ethylenediamine, fluorescin, and eosin dyes)
Amertan	Metycaine with Merthiolate Ophth.
Amlab Brite Eye Lotion and Eye-Care Drops	Munichem Mycobac
Biomydrin Nasal Spray/Drops	Murine
BoilnSoak	Mycostatin Cream
Bonmiotin	Neosporin Ophthalmic Solution, Sterile
Collyrium and Collyrium with Ephedrine	Ocusol Eye Drops
Coly-Mycin S Otic	Paredrine 1% with Boric Acid Ophthalmic Solution
Contact Nasal Mist	Phenspray Nasal Spray
Cortisporin Ophthalmic Suspension	Polyspectrin Ophthalmic Solution
Cortisporin Otic Suspension	Preflex
Del Staph 600	Prefrin-Z Liquifilm
Drilitol Spraypak Solution	Pyocidin-Otic Solution
Dristan Nasal Mist and Children's Dristan Mist	Quotane
Econochlor	Rexall Eye Drops
Elase Ointment	S.A.C. Nasal Spray
Elase-Chloromycetin Ointment	Soaclens
Elcide	Soltice Nasal Spray
Eppy 1/2%	Soothe Eye Drops
Esromiotin 1/4%	Stoxil Ophthalmic Ointment and Ophthalmic Solution
Estivin	Sulfa-Statin
Eye Drop Liquid	Sulf-10 Dropperette Ophthalmic Solution
Eye-Gene	Sulf-10 Ophthalmic Solution
Eyelo Eyedrops	Surfacaine
Florotit	Triscocort Spraypak
4-Way Long Acting Nasal Spray	20/20 Eye Drops
4-Way Mentholated Long Acting Nasal Spray	Vapocyn II Nasal Spray
4-Way Mentholated Nasal Spray	Vasocort Spraypak
4-Way Nasal Spray	Vicks Sinex Nasal Spray
Fungicin	Va-tro-nal Nose Drops
Impact Nasal Spray	V12

dermatitis, whereas van Ketel and Melzer-van Riemsduk[10] pointed out that thimerosal, present as a preservative in many soft-lens solutions, produced allergic conjunctivitis but no eyelid dermatitis in three of their patients. Pedersen[11] also described conjunctivitis without eyelid dermatitis.

Sertoli and colleagues[6] reported that a patient who had allergic thimerosal sensitization developed allergic contact dermatitis on the fingers and palms; however, when this same solution was applied to the eyes, it did not produce conjunctivitis or eyelid dermatitis. The patient in this case, a 20-year-old woman, had two small patches of dyshidrosiform vesicles which merged into blisters and contained clear fluid; one patch of vesicles was located in the center of the right palm, and the other was on the tip of the left index finger. She had worn soft contact lenses for 1 month before the eruption began. When not worn, the lenses were kept in a lens container with a preserving liquid; they were taken out for use individually (using the tip of the left index finger), put on the right palm, and there washed with a liquid (again using the tip of the left index finger) before being put into the eyes.

Rietschel and Wilson[12] reported that soft contact lenses cleaned and stored in thimerosal-containing solutions may produce an ocular inflammatory process and, if untreated, corneal neovascularization. They examined 38 patients who were using soft contact lenses and found that 31 had positive ocular provocation test results to a thimerosal-preserved, artificial-tears solution. Delayed hypersensitivity to thimerosal was demonstrated by positive patch tests in 27 patients. Avoidance of thimerosal and the use of unit-dose sterile saline solutions resulted in complete resolution of ocular symptoms.

LIFE-THREATENING REACTIONS TO THIMEROSAL (MERTHIOLATE)

Maibach[13] reported a case of marked reaction to thimerosal after treating a patient's slightly sore throat with a thimerosal first-aid spray. The next day, because of continued discomfort, he repeated the treatment. Laryngeal obstruction followed within hours. Emergency tracheotomy produced prompt improvement. Patch testing revealed an extreme spreading reaction to thimerosal. It was believed that the acute laryngeal obstruction developed as a delayed hypersensitivity reaction to this first-aid spray.

PATCH TEST WITH THIMEROSAL (MERTHIOLATE)

At present, most testing is done with 0.1% thimerosal in petrolatum. Although there has been controversy as to whether positive patch test reactions to thimerosal are irritant or allergic in nature, allergy is the most likely explanation because provocative product use tests are positive in most subjects who have patch test reactions to thimerosal. Occasionally, however, mercury salts may produce a false-positive reaction when the patch test is performed in a Finn chamber, because a chemical reaction between the aluminum of the chamber with the tested mercury salt may occur (Kalveram KJ and Forck G, Munster, Germany, personal communication).

THIMEROSAL (MERTHIOLATE) AS A SENSITIZER IN INJECTABLE BIOLOGIC SOLUTIONS

Thimerosal (Merthiolate) is used as a preservative in vaccines, antitoxins, parenteral medications, and diluting fluids used for preparations of antigens for scratch or intradermal testing.

Epstein[5] observed five patients within 1 year who showed consistently delayed-type reactions to intradermal tests with multiple antigens. The diluting fluid of these extracts contained thimerosal; all five patients were allergic to this preservative.

Reisman,[14] in the course of routine allergy investigation, found ten patients who had delayed hypersensitivity reactions to the thimerosal preservative in the testing solutions. Three patients had previous contact dermatitis from thimerosal. Five patients may have been sensitized through either direct contact or parenteral injections, and the mode of sensitization in at least two patients was unknown. Reisman stated that the availability of phenol, which rarely if ever sensitizes, indicates there is no reason to continue to use thimerosal as a preservative in allergy extracts.

Rietschel and Adams[15] reported that thimerosal was a limiting factor in Heptavax immunization against hepatitis B. Two patients, both working in the medical field, had intense local reactions to as little as 0.1 mg of intradermal Heptavax from the thimerosal preservative.[15] All current hepatitis B vaccines in the United States contain thimerosal.

Hansson and Möller[16] stated that thimerosal gives a high frequency of positive reactions when tested epicutaneously and intracutaneously in young adults. Thimerosal is added as a preservative to Swedish old tuberculin (OT). The reactions to intracutaneously injected OT thimerosal and purified protein derivative (PPD) have been compared in 412 healthy young adults, and a positive reaction to thimerosal was recorded in 15%. Thimerosal influenced the reactions in 63 of the 163 positive OT tests. Consequently, it was concluded that thimerosal should not be added to intracutaneous test solutions because this additive may interfere with the evaluation of positive reactions.

Although thimerosal is commonly found in vaccines such as hepatitis, tetanus, and meningoencephalitis, reports of significant adverse reactions to this type of exposure are rare. Only 10% of thimerosal sensitive patients reported slight to moderate adverse reactions to thimerosal-containing vaccines consisting mainly of painful swelling at the injection site.[17]

WORLDWIDE INCIDENCE OF THIMEROSAL (MERTHIOLATE) SENSITIVITY

The North American Contact Dermatitis Research Group (NACDG) reintroduced thimerosal in the "standard" or "screening" patch test tray because preliminary results indicate that thimerosal is a fairly common cause of allergic contact sensitization in the United States.

Möller[18] stated that, from laboratories in which patch testing is performed with a standard series including thimerosal, quite different figures emerge from the incidence of contact allergy to this compound. Apparently, there is a geographic variation. High figures of 8% to 15% have been reported from the United States and Brazil, but moderate figures of 3% to 4% from Denmark and Sweden.

When thimerosal was used as a disinfectant and sold over the counter for self-medication, a high degree of sensitization was recorded in several countries, including the United States and Brazil. A particular problem arose when remarkably high figures of thimerosal allergy (15% to 25%) were reported among healthy young Swedes from subpopulations of military recruits, nursing students, and medical students. The occurrence could not be explained on the basis of self-medication, because thimerosal had never been sold over the counter in Sweden, and the agent was no more readily available than in low-allergy countries. A national campaign against tuberculosis in Sweden, however, had suggested repeated tuberculin testing in children and young people. It was shown that the thimerosal contained in the tuberculin could sensitize when injected intracutaneously. This iatrogenic sensitization, however, did not induce any skin disease or other clinical manifestation.[19]

Also in Sweden, Hansson and Möller[20] reported that patch test results were positive in 16% of healthy young military service recruits tested with 0.1% thimerosal in petrolatum and in 15% tested intracutaneously with 0.01% thimerosal in saline. These reactions to thimerosal caused false-positive responses to tuberculin because thimerosal was present as a preservative in the tuberculin solution.

On the basis of their results, the authors stressed that thimerosal (Merthiolate) should not be used as a preservative in solutions for the detection of delayed-type hypersensitivity; however, if it is present, a control test with thimerosal should be included in the investigation.

In Japan, Takino[4] found 23 cases of thimerosal sensitivity in a 2-year period. In Czechoslovakia, Novak and Kvicalova[21] reported 38 positive thimerosal patch test results in 316 patients examined. These investigators found it difficult to correlate the patch test reactions with the clinical picture. The authors did not exclude the possibility that the reactions were caused by subcutaneous or intramuscular injections of biological preparations containing thimerosal (Merthiolate). This shows the importance of a search for thimerosal (Merthiolate) in the environment.

The significance of thimerosal allergy has expanded because it has been learned that piroxicam photosensitization occurs regularly in thimerosal-sensitive individuals.[22] Furthermore, animals sensitized to thimerosal develop contact and photocontact dermatitis on exposure to piroxicam (Feldene) alone or piroxicam plus ultraviolet A (UVA), respectively.[23] See Chapter 9 for additional information.

Merbromin (Mercurochrome, Flavurol)

This organic mercurial antiseptic may crossreact with inorganic mercurials. There are several reports of allergic contact dermatitis to merbromin.[24]

Camarasa[25] reported a man with injuries treated with merbromin who developed a violent, local reaction, a generalized eruption, and facial and laryngeal edema of such severity that he required treatment in an intensive care unit. Patch tests revealed that he was strongly positive to thimerosal (Merthiolate) (0.1% aqueous) and to mercuric chloride (0.05% aqueous). The response to Mercromina, containing 2% aqueous solutions of the sodium salt of dibromohydroxy mercuric resorcinolphthalein, precipitated an erythroderma and laryngeal edema that necessitated his return to the intensive care unit.

A similar case was reported by Pelaez Hernandez and colleagues.[26] Minutes after applying Mercurochrome, a 51-year-old man developed anaphylaxis consisting of generalized urticaria, dyspnea, dysphonia, and dizziness. His evaluation revealed both immediate and delayed hypersensitivity to Mercurochrome. He was prick test positive, PK test positive (but negative with serum heated to 56°C to destroy IgE antibodies), and patch test positive to multiple mercury compounds, but patch test negative to thimerosal.

Merbromin may be tested "as is," undiluted.

Mercurochrome and Merthiolate are not the same compound and will not crossreact unless the patient is sensitive to the mercurial component of Merthiolate (thimerosal).[27]

Phenylmercuric Salts (Acetate, Nitrate, Bromide, and Benzoate)

Phenylmercuric salts may be present in the products shown in Table 11.2. The US Food and Drug Administration (FDA) allows these salts in eye solutions and cosmetics used about the eyes because they are effective against pseudomonad infections.

PHENYLMERCURIC ACETATE

Morris[28] reported that a woman's vulva itched and burned when she used a contraceptive jelly containing 0.02% phenylmercuric acetate. A patch test with 0.06% phenylmercuric chloride was positive. Although Hjorth and Trolle-Lassen[29] indicated that patch tests with a 0.1% concentration of phenylmercuric acetate may give

Table 11-2 Phenylmercuric Salts	
Contraceptives	Ophthalmic solutions
Cosmetics	Shampoos
Emulsion paints	Shoe linings

false-positive irritant reactions, such reactions did not occur in our experience. In sensitized persons, however, patch test reactions may be obtained in concentrations from 0.01% to 0.16% in petrolatum.

Not infrequently, crossreactions occur between organic mercury compounds, such as phenylmercuric acetates, and the inorganic salts, such as ammoniated mercury and bichloride of mercury. Moreover, an allergic eczematous dermatitis from external sensitization by a mercurial compound may be exacerbated or reproduced by *systemic* administration of medication containing mercury, such as metalluride (Mercuhydrin), in sensitized persons.

An allergic contact dermatitis from phenylmercuric acetate and phenylmercuric oleate was reported by Hartung[30] in a worker who sewed tarpaulin treated with these chemicals. Three such patients were patch tested with each of these chemicals in concentrations of 0.025% and 0.026%, and all three reacted to both.

PHENYLMERCURY BORATE (PHENYLMERCURIC BORATE)

In Germany, phenylmercury borate is used for tinea pedis and preoperatively on the skin. Breit and Bandmann[31] reported that it was the cause of dermatitis in 116 of 1,094 patients sensitized by a topical medicament, and many of these patients had cross-sensitivity to other mercury compounds used as preservatives in creams and ointments. The use of phenylmercury borate as thermometer disinfectant also caused allergic contact dermatitis.

PHENYLMERCURIC NITRATE

This preservative contains 65% mercury. Morris[28] reported two patients sensitized by phenylmercuric nitrate. The first patient developed a contact dermatitis on his legs after putting a weed-killer powder containing this chemical on his lawn. A woman developed dermatitis of the face from the acetate in an ointment. Both patients reacted to patch tests with a 0.06% solution of phenylmercuric nitrate.

Relationship of Organic and Inorganic Mercury Compounds

The organic mercurials used as antiseptics include thimerosal (Merthiolate), merbromin (Mercurochrome), nitromersol (Metaphen), and mercocresol (Mercresin). The inorganic mercurials include metallic mercury, ammoniated mercury, yellow oxide of mercury, and the phenylmercuric salts (acetate, nitrate, bromide, and borate). Crossreactions between metallic mercury and the organic and inorganic mercurial compounds may occur. Sidi and Casalis[32] reported a case of chronic eczema of the face and arms of a patient who had positive patch test reactions to

dental amalgam, inorganic mercury, and merbromin (Mercurochrome). Hjorth and Trolle-Lassen[29] stated categorically, however, that "the mercury ion does not cross-sensitize to the organic compounds." In Fisher's experience,[33] three patients who had mercury sensitivity reacted to metallic mercury, as well as the organic and inorganic compounds. Furthermore, in patients who had allergic contact sensitivity to mercury, the skin lesions may be exacerbated or reproduced by systemic administration of mercurial compounds.[34]

Van Ketel and Roeleveld[35] reported a case of crossreactions among the following mercurial compounds: mercuric oxycyanide, thimerosal (Merthiolate), phenylmercuric nitrate, ammoniated mercury, and metallic mercury.

MERCURIC CHLORIDE

Other names for mercuric chloride are mercury bichloride, mercury perchloride, and corrosive sublimate. This mercury compound may be found in some antiseptic hair "tonics," such as Elm's Hair and Scalp Treatment, Scalpo Ointment, and Bar Soap, and is also used in embalming fluids.

Mercuric chloride is a strong sensitizer that may produce a nonspecific, pustular reaction or an irritant patch test reaction even when diluted to 0.05% solution.[36,37]

MERCUROUS CHLORIDE (CALOMEL)

Calomel, used in the past as an antiseptic, is still occasionally used at present as a laxative. In mercury-sensitive persons, the ingestion of Calomel may produce "systemic" contact dermatitis.[33]

PARA-CHLOROMERCURIPHENOL

This organic mercurial is used occasionally in soaps or topical medications as a disinfectant. Mathias and colleagues[38] reported a case of dermatitis of the hands and forearms from a woman's allergic hypersensitivity to this mercury compound used to treat her baby's diaper rash. There was a crossreaction to phenylmercuric acetate but not to thimerosal (Merthiolate).

Miscellaneous Antiseptic and Disinfectant Mercury Compounds

Table 11.3 lists several other mercury compounds used as antiseptics, disinfectants, fungicides, and wood preservatives. Table 11.4 lists the numerous antiseptic topical skin preparations that at one time have contained mercury compounds other than thimerosal

Table 11-3 Mercury Compounds
Mercuric chloride
Mercuric cyanide
Mercuric dimethyldithiocarbamate
Mercuric lactate
Mercuric oleate
Mercuric stearate
Mercurous chloride
Phenylmercuric acetate
Phenylmercuric benzoate
Phenylmercuric chloride
Phenylmercuric ethanolammonium acetate and lactate
Phenylmercuric hydroxide
Phenylmercuric lactate
Phenylmercuric naphthenate
Phenylmercuric nitrate
Phenylmercuric oleate
Red mercuric oxide
Yellow mercuric oxide

(Merthiolate), merbromin (Mercurochrome), or nitromersol (Metaphen).

The tables list other categories of topical preparations that have contained mercury compounds: Table 11.5,

Table 11-4 Topical Skin Preparations Containing Mercury Compounds
Antiseptic and first-aid
AAA Paste
Bag Balm
Dermacol Liquid
Dermato Ointment
Hermesol
Kay-Sen
Lanacane
Lubafax
Marsa
Massengill's Tanic Acid. Jelly, and Benzocaine
Mazon
Mercoseptic
Mertok
Metaphen
Mystacin Cream
Palmer's Antiseptic Lotion
Phillips Corona Ointment
Purepas Blue Ointment
Raleigh's Ointment
Rexall Skin Antiseptic
Sperti Ointment
Unguentine
Veterinary preparations
Bag Balm
McClellan's Eyelid Ointment
Mulrilicare
Stevens Ointment

Table 11-5 Acne Preparations Containing Mercury Compounds
Derma-Teen Skin Soap
Derma-Tone
Teen-Ac

acne preparations; Table 11.6, fungicides; Table 11.7, eye, ear, nose, and throat preparations; Table 11.8, vaginal medications and "prophylactic kits," Table 11.9, plant fungicides and antiseptics.

Iodine

Iodine USP is 2% iodine and 2.4% sodium iodide in alcohol, whereas strong iodine tincture NF is 7% iodine and 5% potassium iodide in alcohol.

Tincture of iodine is a primary irritant that should be tested by the "open" method. Old solutions of iodine are particularly irritating. Povidone-iodine (Betadine), iodine in a base of polyvinyl pyrrolidine, is not as irritating as tincture of iodine and may be tested "as is" by the usual patch test method. The irritancy of several antiseptics was evaluated in an open application of 30 minutes' exposure time twice a day for 4 days.[39] Normal use concentrations were studied. Sodium hypochlorite 0.25% and 1% iodine in 70% ethanol were both too irritating to complete the study. In this method 4% chlorhexidine, 0.5% chlorhexidine in 70% ethanol, and ethanol 70% were deemed nonirritating. Lee et al tested iodine in pet, iodine in isopropyl alcohol, and povidone-iodine in 24 subjects, and concluded that 1% iodine in pet, 0.5% iodine in isopropyl alcohol, and 10% povidone iodine were nonirritant.[40]

Povidone-iodine (Betadine) may produce allergic contact dermatitis.[41,42] Two recent cases of povidone-iodine contact dermatitis were positive at 10% concentration in petrolatum.[43] Povidone-iodine solution has both irritant and allergic properties. In a study of 500 patients patch tested to 10% povidone-iodine solution diluted with water tenfold, 14 patients reacted. When the 14 were

Table 11-6 Fungicides Containing Mercury Compounds
Amber Liquid
Athlete Ointment
Epidex
Gebauer's PMC Spray
Maseda Foot Powder
Melsan
Phe-Mer-Nite
Phytox-ointment

Table 11-7 Mercury Compounds in Ear, Nose, Eye, and Throat Preparations

Ear preparations
Clopane
Nasal preparations (drops and spray)
    Neotrol
    Otall Drops
    Privine
    Vasefrin
    Vasohist
Eye preparations
    Blinx Eye Wash
    Clean-N' Soak
    Coloptin
    Noxmol
    Wetting Solution
    Yellow Mercuric Oxide Ointments
Throat lozenges
    B & R Homeopathic Tablets no. 195A
    Phe-Mer-Caine
    Phe-Mer-Nite
    Thantis

Table 11-8 Mercury Compounds in Vaginal Medications and Prophylactic Kits

Prophylactic kits
Dough-Boy
Vaginal jellies, tablets, and douches
    Baculin
    Dorana
    Koromex
    Lorophyn
    Merpertogel
    Norforms
    Nylmerate
    Phe-Mer-Nite
    Servex
    Southern Pharmacal
    Tricho-San
    Triserts
    Vagagill

tested with a repeated open application of povidone-iodine solution, only 2 had a positive test indicating true allergic contact dermatitis.[44]

Table 11-9 Mercury Compounds in Plant Fungicides and Antiseptics

Seed fungicides, protectants, and disinfectants
Amacene
Gallotox
Gy-Treet SQS
Isotox Seed Treater
Merc-O-Dent
Mergamma "C"
Merlane Dust
Merlane Liquid
Panodrin
Panogen
Pantirra
Parson's Seed Saver Dust
Semesan
Turf fungicides and disinfectants
    Calocine
    Caloclor
    Calogreen
    Coromerc
    Corrosive sublimate
    Mersolite-8
    Mersolite-10
    Phenylmercuric acetate Phix
    PM Grain Protectant
    PMN Germicide
    Semesan
Plant fungicides
    Orchard Brand Mercury Spray
    Puratized Agricultural Spray

Puratized Apple Spray
Semesan Fungicide
Herbicides (crabgrass and weed killer)
    Blitz
    Dynaside Homelawn Crabgrass Killer
    PMAS
    Puraturf
Insecticides
    Green Cross
    Hubbard Cabbage Maggot Dust
    Magic Brand Bug Killer
    Mergamma
    P & P Cabbage Maggot Destroyer
    Real-Kill Bug Killer
    Real-Kill Moth Bomb
    Setrete Mist
Root, bulb, and grain treatments
    Mercan
    Merfendel 41
    Merfenel 51
    Merfenelope
    Merlane Dust
    Mer-Sol 48
    Mer-Sol 51
Soil conditioners
Fertilizers

Prolonged skin contact with povidone-iodine saturated drapes can occur during surgery, and the surgical team may be unaware of the pooling of povidone-iodine prep solution in this manner.[45] After 3 to 4 hours of exposure in this fashion, a chemical burn–like skin change can result. These reactions are commonly mistaken for electrical burns. A direct toxic effect is thought to be responsible.

Povidone-iodine is a rare cause of allergic contact dermatitis and has also caused irritant and systemic reactions.[46] A 10% aqueous solution of povidone-iodine is used for patch test purposes. After 1 month of applications of 10% povidone-iodine solution to a leg ulcer, dermatitis developed around the ulcer and generalized over the body. This was accompanied by systemic eosinophilia. Discontinuation of the povidone-iodine solution and systemic corticoids resolved the rash. Patch tests with povidone iodine 2% aqueous were positive and polyoxyethelene nonylphenyl ether at 0.2% was negative.[47]

Hjorth[48] reported that 1,3-di-iodo-2-hydroxypropane, a "white tincture of iodine" used in Denmark for first aid, caused contact dermatitis in one patient. He had a strong positive patch test, whereas 20 control subjects were negative.

Iodine may crossreact with iodoform, which is insoluble in water but readily soluble in alcohol and with thymol iodide. Both of these iodide preparations may be tested 25% in petrolatum. They may crossreact with radiopaque iodine and iodides in medications. Thus, crossreactions with the organic and inorganic iodides may occur.

Patch tests with iodine and potassium iodide may result in a nonspecific, papulopustular reaction that must be differentiated from a contact allergic response. Patch tests with potassium iodide have been used in the diagnosis of dermatitis herpetiformis (DH) but are nonspecific.

A positive patch test reaction to iodine may mean that the patient may react adversely if an iodine-containing contrast material is administered. Lieberman and colleagues,[49] however, stated that a review of the literature involving anaphylactoid reactions to iodinated contrast material suggests that the reactions are nonantibody-mediated but that a complex activation of inflammatory mediators occurs. Histamine release or complement activation has been demonstrated in experimental systems both in vitro and in vivo. It appears that pretreatment of selected cases (patients with a previous anaphylactoid reaction) with antihistamine and corticosteroids is effective in reducing the frequency and severity of subsequent reactions when readministration is necessary.

Rothe and colleagues,[50] reporting a case of contact dermatitis from a radiopaque iodine used in angiography and renography, stated that a difficulty with iodine-containing contrast material is the lack of a consistently reliable in-vitro test or a safe in-vivo test to predict whether a given patient is likely to have an adverse reaction. The generally adopted practice today is to regard all patients who have highly allergic backgrounds or histories of adverse reactions to contrast media as being at greater than average risk.

Chlorine and Chlorinated Products

CHLORINATED WATER

Neering[51] described a patient who acquired contact urticaria whenever he swam in chlorinated, swimming pool water disinfected with sodium hypochlorite. This patient also developed contact urticaria from contact with a cleansing powder containing Chlorox. Closed patch tests were negative, but a scratch test produced a strongly positive reaction.

SODIUM HYPOCHLORITE

This chlorinated product is present in the following products in the United States: eau de Javelle, Chlorox, Dazzle, and Dakin's Solution. Osmundsen[52] reported a case of severe allergic contact dermatitis from sodium hypochlorite in a patient who had avoided swimming pools for years because the heavy smell of chlorine made her feel ill. After an abortion in which chloramine-T (chloramine) was used, she developed severe dermatitis in the genital area. Osmundsen performed patch testing with a popular bleaching agent, 10% in water, corresponding to about 0.5% sodium hypochlorite. The patch test elicited a more than palm-sized, red, vesicular, strongly edematous, and infiltrated reaction.

Suspected contact dermatitis to bleach (sodium hypochlorite) can be tested with a 1% aqueous solution using 17 to 20 mL volume in the Finn chamber, provided that the concentration of sodium hydroxide in the bleach is not more than 1%.[53] The concentration of sodium hydroxide in bleach varies with different manufacturers and may cause irritant reactions.

Chlorine is commonly used to disinfect swimming pools. Sasseville and colleagues[54] report contact allergy to DiHalo, which is a 1-bromo-3-chloro-5,5-dimethylhydantoin and releases both bromine and chlorine. Their patient reacted to DiHalo, sodium hypochlorite, and lithium hypochlorite all of which are tested at 1% aqueous. They pointed out that DiHalo had caused a near-epidemic of dermatoses in the United Kingdom in the early 1980s which was blamed on irritant rather than allergy mechanisms due to negative patch tests. They found that polyhexamethylene biguanide, sold as Bacquacil or Softswim, was a suitable alternative.

BROMINE

Bromine-based disinfectants are used in pools and hot tubs to maintain water purity. Three cases of dermatitis were traced to bromine in the form of Halobrome, which is 1-bromo-3-chloro-5,5-dimethylhydantoin.[55] Patch tests with 0.1% aqueous were positive. Brominated tablets used to disinfect a spa tub sold under the name ProGuard were identified as the cause of eczema on the immersed body parts of a patient report by Sasseville and Moreau.[56] The pellets contain 1-bromo-3-chloro-5,5-dimethylhydantoin which was patch test positive at 1% and 2% aqueous. The patient did not react to sodium hypochlorite or DMDM hydantoin. Lithium hypochlorite pellets were used successfully as an allergen substitute. Another potential allergen substitute would be polyhexamethylene biguanide, sold as Bacquacil or Softswim. Another hot-tub disinfectant that has caused contact dermatitis is potassium peroxymonosulfate (5% pet). This disinfectant can also be found in oral hygiene products, paper recycling, printed circuit board etching, wool shrink proofing, and laundry bleaches. It is used as "shock" in hot tubs to kill algae and reduce chloramines. Cross reactions to ammonium persulfate may occur.[57]

CHLORAMINE-T (CHLORAMINE)

Chloramine is used commonly as a sterilizer, disinfectant, and chemical reagent. It has been described as an occupational hazard for pharmaceutical workers, nurses, butchers, cleaners, and brewers.[58]

Dooms-Goossens and colleagues[59] reported a case of contact urticaria from chloramine. Over several months, the patient had recurrent attacks of edema of the eyelids, accompanied by dyspnea, rhinitis, and a tingling sensation in her mouth and occasionally in her fingers whenever she came into contact with chloramine powder, which she frequently (two to three times a week) had to dissolve in water to make 0.5% solutions to disinfect bedpans. The symptoms appeared 15 to 20 minutes after contact with the chloramine powder and sometimes lasted for several days despite local treatment with a corticosteroid cream. She also had minor reactions after coming into contact with 0.5% chloramine solutions. An open test with chloramine "as is" on the patient's forearm yielded erythema and wheal formation after 20 minutes. A closed patch test with a 0.2% solution produced erythema and wheal formation at the 48-hour

patch test reading, which disappeared by the 96-hour reading.

There are several reports of asthma produced by chloramine in industrial use.[60–63] Kramps and colleagues[63] demonstrated the presence of specific IgE antibodies in the serum of asthmatic chloramine-allergic patients. Bourne and colleagues[60] stated that it is advisable to open chloramine powder under water or in a glove box, or with the operator fully protected by an air-fed hood or suit or a properly fitting, appropriate filter-type mask, preferably pressurized.

CHLORHEXIDINE

Chlorhexidine (1.1-hexamethylenebis [5(P chlorophenyl) biguanide]) is an antibacterial compound active against gram-positive and gram-negative bacteria even in the presence of body fluids. The chlorhexidine salts used most frequently in medicine are digluconate, acetate, and diacetate. The use of chlorhexidine as an antiseptic has increased in recent years at the expense of quaternary ammonium compounds. Chlorhexidine is used clinically for disinfection of hands and operation sites in the treatment of burns and scalds, in urology and gynecology, and by dentists in the treatment of caries and periodontitis.

Mobacken and Wengstrom[64] have suggested that, pending further knowledge, chlorhexidine be used with caution on wounds caused by disturbed circulation where additional tissue injury may be dangerous, and on tissue structures with function that may be restricted by excessive scar tissue, for example, exposed tendons and tendon sheaths. Occlusive dressings may increase penetration into the tissues and contribute consequently to the development of untoward effects. The use of chlorhexidine on mucous membranes has been discouraged as it poses a risk of anaphylaxis. Use of this disinfectant on wounds was thought to be safe. A woman cut her foot on broken glass and applied a chlorhexidine disinfectant to the broken skin site and within minutes developed generalized urticaria, angioedema, wheezing, dizziness, vomiting, and diarrhea. Application of 1% chlorhexidine to intact skin produced an immediate hypersensitivity reaction, but greater dilutions were negative. A sulfidoleukotriene stimulation test showed high stimulation with chlorhexidine.[65]

Although chlorhexidine is used widely, allergic reactions are rare.[66–68] Ljunggren and Möller[67] described a case of contact dermatitis resulting from the antiseptic chlorhexidine. The allergic nature of the reaction was proved by epicutaneous and intracutaneous testing with various salts and solvents. False-negative patch tests were obtained when chlorhexidine was applied in petrolatum, because chlorhexidine for physicochemical reasons is biologically and allergologically active in aqueous solutions only. Surfactants incorporated in emulsions may also interfere with the patch test response. Use of a chlorhexidine preparation for insertion of an intrauterine device (IUD) resulted in urticaria and dyspnea.[69] Prick tests to both diacetate (0.5% aq) and digurconate (0.5% aq) were positive.

The ideal test for chlorhexidine is uncertain. Acetate at 1% produces more reactions than gluconate at 1%, but many reactions are irritant.[70] Thirteen percent of patients with leg ulcers are sensitive to chlorhexidine; therefore, it is not recommended for use with such patients. A 0.05% aqueous concentration of acetate is probably acceptable for screening purposes.[70]

Application of chlorhexidine antiseptic to the buttocks led to anaphylactic shock in a 33-year-old man who had irritation after a riding lesson.[71] Prick tests were positive to 0.2% chlorhexidine in the patient and negative in three controls. Prior reports of anaphylaxis from chlorhexidine involved mucosal exposure or catheter insertion.

A woman used an antiseptic containing chlorhexidine digluconate after having an umbilical piercing, which resulted in a dermatitis that covered the whole abdomen. The reaction was traced to decyl glucoside, also known as decyl D-glucoside or decyl-beta-D-glucopyranoside. This is a nonionic surfactant with good foaming qualities. It is more commonly found in rinse-off products such as shampoo, hair dye, or soap, but is also found in some leave-on products such as sunscreens. It can be patch tested at 0.5% aqueous.[72] Curcumin is made from *Curcuma longa* root and is commonly used to color foods, but it is also used to provide a yellow color to some chlorhexidine solution used for skin disinfection prior to surgery. Reactions may be seen to curcumin 1% petrolatum or 0.05% in ethanol.[73]

CETRIMIDE

Patients occasionally use antiseptics improperly by applying them undiluted to skin disease. A series of 18 such patients used a product containing 3% cetrimide and 0.3% chlorhexidine.[74] Within 1 to 4 weeks dermatitis was seen, principally in the genital region and antecubital fossa. Patch tests revealed irritant reactions to cetrimide at 0.5%, 1%, or 2% aqueous. The morphology of the reactions was xerotic or chemical burn–like, and the histology showed ortho and parakeratosis without spongiosis.

CHLOROXINE

Chloroxine is a dichloro-hydroxyquinoline antiseptic compound that readily forms colored complexes with polyvalent metal ions but is not a sensitizer. This antiseptic, present in Capitrol shampoo, may produce a yellow tint on white or light-colored hair. Individuals working with Capitrol may acquire yellow skin on the hands and fingers. This discoloration disappears usually within 24 hours (Levy J, Westwood Pharmaceuticals Inc, personal communication).

It is known that greenish discoloration of light-colored hair has been traced to the use of copper-containing algaecides used in swimming pools and the presence of copper eluted from copper plumbing.[75,76] Because chloroxine complexes with copper, the use of Capitrol shampoo could increase the chance of greenish discoloration of the hair.[77]

Although Bhat and colleagues[78] have said that shampooing does not remove the green color, an acidic cream rinse or a "vinegar" rinse does readily remove the greenish color. A 3% solution of peroxide also removes the color.

CHLOROXYLENOL

This chlorinated phenol antiseptic is also known as parachlorometaxylenol (PCMX), *p*-chloro-*m*-xylenol, 4-chloro-3,5,-xylenol, ottasept, and benzytol.

Table 11.10 shows the products that may contain chloroxylenol. The related chlorinated phenols, 4-chloro-*m*-cresol* (chlorocresol) and parachlorometaxylenol, are used as preservatives in betamethasone

Table 11-10 Products Containing Parachloro-Metaxylenol*
Absorbine Junior (W.F. Young)
Acne Aid (Steifel)
Aveeno Baby Powder (Cooper)
Carbolated Vaseline
Cebum Shampoo (Dermik)
Cenathesin (Central)
Chloroxylenol (British Pharmacopea)
Desitin Baby Powder (Leeming)
Enden Shampoo Cream & Lotion (Curtis)
Natural Wonder Alive & Well Transparent Face Color (Revlon)
Natural Wonder Oil Free Makeup (Revlon)
Nu-Flow Shampoo
Nullo Foot Cream (De Pree)
Redux ECG Paste
Rezamid, Rezamid Cream, and Rezamid Lotion (Dermik)
Stopette Deodorant Roll-on Clear (Helene Curtis)
Top Brass (Revlon)
Unburn Spray (Leeming)
Unguentine Plus (Norwich)
Unguentine Spray (Norwich)
Vaseline Medicated First Aid Petroleum Jelly
Zeasorb Powder
Zetar Shampoo (Dermik)

*Also in some contraceptive douches.

cream, electrocardiogram paste, and in more than 30 over-the-counter products. Contact allergic eczema does occur sporadically. The two compounds may crossreact.[79,80]

According to Calnan,[66] chloroxylenol ranked second in his list of antibacterial agents (excluding antibiotics) in the incidence of allergic sensitivity produced. Of 220 cases of contact allergy to antibacterial agents, 53 were caused by chloroxylenol. Only mercury (60 cases) caused more disease than chloroxylenol. Hjorth and Trolle-Lassen[81] demonstrated cross-sensitization between chlorocresol and chloroxylenol in three patients. This finding means that the chemical structure of these two compounds is so close that the human body cannot tell them apart. As a result, a patient allergic to one compound may react to both.

4-Chloro-*m*-cresol (4-Chloro-3-Methylphenol, Ottafect, Parachlorometacresol, PCMC, Phenol, Chloro-3-Methyl)

Incidence of Sensitivity

Clinically, chlorocresol is an infrequent sensitizer. Of 1,000 patients who had contact dermatitis analyzed by Burry and colleagues[82] in southern Australia, only 11 reacted to chlorocresol.

Causes of Sensitivity

Dermatitis from chlorocresol in betamethasone creams was reported in 13 patients in Australia by Burry and colleagues.[82] Many were thought to have been primarily sensitized by chloroxylenol because, on patch testing, although all were positive to chloroxylenol, only eight were additionally positive to chlorocresol. It was suggested that, in the negative reactors, absorption of chlorocresol was dependent upon its incorporation into the corticosteroid cream. A woman who had been sensitized, possibly by betamethasone cream, was described by Park[83] in New Zealand. Oleffe and colleagues[84] also reported an allergic reaction to chlorocresol in a steroid cream.

Chlorocresol is used as a preservative in Valisone Cream and some cosmetics. It is also present in Royal Bond Pre-injection fluid. In veterinary medicine, it is used in pesticides and fungicides. Certain embalming fluids contain this antiseptic.

Hexachlorophene (G-11, AT-7, K-34)

This halogenated phenolic antiseptic, closely related to dichlorophene, was once widely used in cosmetics, soaps, and pharmaceutical vehicles as an antiseptic. At present, hexachlorophene is present in pHisoHex and Burdeo

(Hill). The results of testing with a vehicle series show that hexachlorophene is a rare sensitizer. Irritant reactions of the scrotum and the face from pHisoHex, which contains a soluble from hexachlorophene, have been reported, but in none was hexachlorophene implicated as a sensitizer.[85]

The FDA restriction of the use of hexachlorophene is related to toxic brain damage and not to marked skin toxicity or sensitivity.

Epstein[86] found cross-sensitivity between dichlorophene and hexachlorophene. Fisher and colleagues[7] found no such crossreactions. Fregert and Hjorth[87] reported a sensitization index of 0.3% in 660 patients, although acute primary irritant contact dermatitis occurred more frequently, especially in areas with susceptible skin, such as the scrotum.[88] Positive patch tests believed to be crossreactions to hexachlorophene were found in patients who had allergy to tetrachlorosalicylanilide, bithionol, and dichlorophene.

Hexachlorophene may crossreact to such halogenated photosensitizers as tetrachlorosalicylanilide and bithionol.[89] (Bithionol is not used in the United States.)

Dichlorophene (G-4, Cuniphen)

Dichlorophene is a fungicide and bactericide used in dentifrices, shampoos, antiperspirant and deodorant creams, powder, toilet waters, and preparations for dermatophytosis of the foot. Compound G-4 is used extensively as a mildewcide to treat and preserve cotton fibers, various fabrics, paper, synthetic leather lattices, and some adhesive tape backings.

Allergic stomatitis and cheilitis owing to G-4 in dentifrices have been reported, and it is now used rarely in such products.[90,91] Gaul and Underwood[92] reported allergic dermatitis from G-4 used as a fungicide. This compound is still present in numerous over-the-counter preparations for "athlete's foot."

Schorr[93] reported instances of allergic contact dermatitis from the presence of G-4 in Duke Gelocast Bandage for treatment of stasis ulcers. [*Note:* The Primer Medicated Bandage (Glenwood) contains glycerin, acacia, zinc oxide, white petrolatum, and amylum in a vegetable oil base and is free of preservatives.] Schorr also found instances of allergic dermatitis from the presence of G-4 in Jergens Lotion.

Irgasans

Two popular "irgasans" are chemically unrelated to each other:

Table 11-11 Products that Have Contained Irgasan DP 300
Bacterio Polyvinyl Gloves (Europe)
Calgon
Calm
Colgate P300
Commercial laundry products
Deodorant antiperspirant spray
Deodorant Foot Powder (Durope) (Cosmea)
Dial Soap
Disposable paper products
Irish Spring Soap
"Odor Eaters" Latex Insole (Combe)
"Odor Eaters" Men's Hose (Burlington Mills)
Palmolive
Paper linings for rodent cages
Right Guard

1. Triclosan (irgasan DP 300), a diphenyl ether (2,4,49-trichloro9-20-hydroxydiphenyl ether). Table 11.11 lists some products that have contained irgasan DP 300. There are reports of allergic contact dermatitis from a deodorant foot powder, a deodorant, and an antiperspirant spray.[94,95] Wahlberg[96] also reported an allergic reaction to irgasan DP 30 during routine screening. Irgasan DP 300, when incorporated into such footwear as men's hosiery and insoles of shoes, is called an "odor-eater" because it is claimed that this chemical can suppress the odor produced by foot organisms. Such hosiery and insoles may produce "odor-eater" dermatitis.[97]
2. Cluflucarban [irgasan CF 3(4,49-dichloro-3-(trifluoromethyl) carbanilide)] is a carbanilide unrelated chemically to irgasan DP 300. Safeguard soap, marketed in the United States, contains irgasan CF 3.

Triclocarban (TCC)

This antiseptic is used in several antiseptic soaps. Maibach and colleagues[98] found that the potential for allergic contact dermatitis was minimal following use of bar soap containing triclocarban. Freeman and Knox[99] studied photocontact dermatitis caused by the halogenated salicylanilides and related compounds, and found only one patient positive on photopatch testing to TCC alone. Triclocarban, however, has been described as a contact allergen from certain antiperspirants marketed in Europe.[100,101]

Tego

TEGO (dodecylic aminomethyl glycine hydrochloride, Nisson Anon, and Ampholyt G) is an antiseptic detergent used abroad in hospitals, food industries, and public baths and for cleaning machinery. Several cases of allergic dermatitis have occurred from its use in hospital operating room personnel.[102–104] Positive patch tests were obtained to 1:1000 and 1:100 aqueous solutions.

The workers cleaning milk tanks with TEGO 51 developed hand eczema and were patch test positive to 0.05% and 1% aqueous solutions, although ten control subjects were negative.[105] TEGO 51 is derived from glycine. Cleaning pipes in the milk industry with TEGO Diocto St[106] similarly caused contact dermatitis. This product is a blend of dioctyl-trioctyl-diethylenetriamine alcohol, acetic acid, and polyethylene glycol trioleate, and it may crossreact with triethanolamine. A 1% petrolatum concentration of TEGO Diocto St had been used. Alkyldiaminoethylglycine hydrochloride is also known as Tego, and is an antiseptic that enjoys wide use. Usually the individual who experiences contact dermatitis from this agent will be someone working directly with the product, but Ito and colleagues[107] reported that a hospitalized patient who required oxygen developed contact dermatitis from tubing that had been sterilized with it. She was patch test positive down to 0.01% aqueous. A nasal cannula that had not been exposed to the allergen was patch test negative.

Benzoyl Peroxide

Exposure to benzoyl peroxide may occur from its use in the products shown in Table 11.12.

TOPICAL ACNE PREPARATIONS

Whereas mild irritant reactions to benzoyl peroxide are common, allergic reactions are rare.108–112 Caro[113] reported that a physician acquired a "connubial" contact dermatitis to benzoyl peroxide, which his wife used for acne. Bushkell[114] stated that benzoyl peroxide used on the bearded area can bleach black hair to a "patchy orange."

BENZOYL PEROXIDE USED FOR LEG ULCERS

The use of benzoyl peroxide for the treatment of leg ulcers may be accompanied by sensitization dermatitis.[115,116]

Table 11-12 Benzoyl Peroxide
Acne preparations
Additive to self-curing acrylic
Bleach for flour and oils
Quinilor ointment
Stasis ulcer treatments
Unguentum benzoyl peroxide

BENZOYL PEROXIDE AS AN ACTIVATOR OF ACRYLIC BONE CEMENT

Jager and Balda[117] reported loosening of a total hip prosthesis due to an allergic reaction to benzoyl peroxide in the acrylic bone cement.

BENZOYL PEROXIDE AS A CAUSE OF BAKER'S DERMATITIS

On rare occasions, benzoyl peroxide has been used to bleach flour. Fisher[118] reported allergic hand dermatitis in a baker owing to such flour.

BENZOYL PEROXIDE AS AN AIRBORNE CONTACTANT

Benzoyl peroxide is used to bleach candles white. Intense exposure to burning candles in a church has caused facial dermatitis. The patch test was positive to benzoyl peroxide at 0.5% in petrolatum.[119]

Quaternary Ammonium Compounds

These compounds are the active ingredient in disinfectants and sanitizers for homes, farms, offices, and public transportation vehicles. They are also used as algaecides and slimicides for swimming pools, industrial water reservoirs, and farm ponds. They are included in the last rinse in laundering by some hospitals, diaper services, and various institutions.

Quaternary ammonium compounds are also used as surface active agents. These compounds are strongly absorbed by many substances. The positive charge imparts antistatic properties to wool, cotton, and other cellulosic fibers, as well as certain synthetic fibers. The compounds are used in hair conditioners, as softeners for textiles and paper products, and as pigment dispersers. It was for this latter reason that the manufacturer included a quaternary ammonium compound in a roll-on deodorant, which produced dermatitis in a patient reported by Shmunes and Levy.[120]

Even in solutions as dilute as 0.1%, the quaternary ammonium compounds are irritants under the closed patch technique. Several controls must always be used when a "positive" patch test reaction is obtained with a patch test procedure. In addition, the "use" test should be used to confirm patch test findings.[121]

BENZALKONIUM CHLORIDE

Benzalkonium chloride (BZK), a mixture of alkyl dimethyl benzyl ammonium chlorides, is a quaternary ammonium cationic detergent. It is used widely as a preoperative skin disinfectant, for disinfecting surgical instruments, and in the treatment of burns, ulcers, wounds, and infected dermatoses. It is also present in many cosmetics, deodorants, mouthwashes, dentifrices, lozenges, and ophthalmic preparations. It is used industrially in the fabrication of textiles and dyes and in metallurgy and agriculture.

BZK is present in such products as Zephiran Chloride, Zephirol, BTC, Rocca, Benirol, Enuclen, Germitol, Drapolene, Drapolex, Cequartyl, Paralkan, Germinol, Rodalon, and Osvan. It has produced allergic contact dermatitis in medical personnel from exposure to instruments soaked in it[122,123] and from its use in the treatment of ulcers, burns, and cutaneous infections.[124,125]

A bizarre ichthyosis-type dermatitis was reported in Japan to be caused by an ointment containing alkyl benzyl trimethylammonium chloride,[126] which differs from BZK only by an additional methyl group. Pandos and colleagues[127] reported an instance of combined cutaneous and mucous-membrane allergic contact reaction from BZK that complicated a tracheotomy procedure.

Theodore and Schlossman[128] stated that BZK in ophthalmic preparations may produce allergic reactions, but they did not cite specific cases with confirming patch test proof. Fisher and Stillman[129] reported that one of the authors (M.A. Stillman) developed conjunctivitis from acquired hypersensitivity to BZK in an ophthalmic medicament, which was then made worse when an unsuspecting ophthalmologist prescribed another preparation containing BZK.

Dabiez and colleagues[130] pointed out that the primary preservative of most contact lens soaking solutions is BZK, and in a personal communication Dabiez suggested the ophthalmic preparations shown in Table 11.13 for BZK-sensitive persons.

Huriez and colleagues[131] reported that allergic contact sensitivity to topically applied quaternary ammonium compounds is common in France, and that generalized reactions may result from systemic administration of chemically related drugs. Such medications include the cholinergic medicaments, hypotensive drugs (2 g-tetraethylammonium chloride), neuromuscular blocking agents (e.g., decamethonium bromide), and heparin antagonists (hexadimethrine bromide).

Ocular inflammation was suspected to be caused by airborne exposure to a quaternary ammonium

Table 11-13 Ophthalmic Preparations Free of Benzalkonium Chloride
Soaclens (Alcon)
Vasocon (Cooper)

compound (Lofarma) and a lauryl alkyl sulfonate (Firma) in an Italian nurse. The patch tests to 0.1% aqueous solutions of both compounds produced a vesicular reaction increasing at day 3 and 4 of the patch test readings.

Lovell and Staniforth[132] reported an unusual case of allergic contact dermatitis owing to the presence of benzalkonium chloride in plaster of Paris. Moreover, this patient showed crossreactions to cetrimonium bromide (cetrimide), another quaternary ammonium compound.

BENZOXONIUM CHLORIDE

Benzoxonium chloride is used in Spain in Cohortan cream and antibiotic. It is also known as D-301, dodecylbenzyldihydroxyethylammonium chloride, dodecyldi-(betaoxethyl) benzylammonium chloride, and benzyldodecylbis (2-hydroxyethyl) ammonium chloride. Topical use for seborrheic dermatitis led to scalp, forehead, and retroauricular dermatitis.[133] A patch test of 0.1% aqueous was positive, and no crossreactivity to benzalkonium chloride was seen. The quaternary ammonium compound, benzoxonium chloride, has caused contact dermatitis in veterinary products. In Spain, it is contained in topical formulations used to treat seborrheic dermatitis. It can be tested at 0.1% aqueous. While a crossreaction to benzalkonium chloride and domiphen bromide has been observed, other reports have not demonstrated crossreactivity with other quaternary ammonium compounds.[134]

DEQUALINIUM CHLORIDE

Dequalinium chloride is an ingredient of Micrin and Gargilon. Although it is a rare sensitizer, this quaternary ammonium compound has been reported as a cause of necrotic ulcers on the penis, in the vulva, the perineum, and the body folds.[135] Allergic hypersensitivity to this compound has been reported.[136]

Dental wipes used to disinfect equipment have caused contact dermatitis due to N-benzyl-N,N-dihydrosyethyl-N-cocsalkyl-ammonium chloride.[137] This quaternary ammonium compound is also found in dental mouthwashes used to reduce plaque and treat gingivitis. No crossreactivity to benzalkonium chloride was found.

A hospital worker became sensitive to a disinfectant used on the job and was relocated to another area. She was exposed to a room cleaned with the disinfectant and had a flare of her dermatitis even though 7 months had passed since the initial eruption. The allergens in the disinfectant were quaternary ammonium compounds:

didecyldimethylammonium chloride, which was positive at 0.01% aqueous, and bis-(aminopropyl)-laurylamine, which was positive at 0.1% aqueous. Didecyldimethylammonium chloride is used as a wood preservative against termites, as an algicide in swimming pools, and as a fungicide for wood.[138]

Cetyl pyridinium chloride (CPC) is a quaternary ammonium compound that is present in Biogelt latex gloves. It was found to be a cause of contact dermatitis in eight nurses in Norway who had positive patch test reactions to their gloves but negative latex prick tests and use tests.[128] CPC is used in cosmetics, antiseptics, and disinfectants. Biogelt gloves without CPC were tested and found negative in seven of the eight cases; in the remaining case only a doubtful reaction was encountered.[139]

Antiseptic Triphenylmethane Dyes

Triphenylmethane dyes such as gentian violet, crystal violet, methyl violet, rosaniline, malachite green, brilliant green, chrysoidine, and eosin are weak sensitizers. Sensitization to these dyes occurs especially when they are applied to statis ulcers or eczematous skin.

Bielicky and Novak[140] observed 11 patients who had eczema mainly on the legs due to allergic sensitization to brilliant green. A simultaneous sensitivity to gentian violet and crystal violet was found in 8 patients and to malachite green in 6 patients. Patch tests with various triphenylmethane dyes have shown the possibility of cross-sensitization between crystal violet (contained in gentian violet), brilliant green, and malachite green. The probable determinant groups of sensitization are $N(CH_3)_2$ or $2N(C_2H_5)_2$ in the para position of the benzene-ring structure. Crossreactions are limited only to substances with amino groups substituted with at least two alkyl groups. The test reactions to pararosaniline were all negative.

Bjornberg and Mobacken[141] described 3 patients in whom a necrotic, painful, and slowly healing skin reaction developed after topical treatment with 1% gentian violet in aqueous solution. The reaction could be reproduced in stripped but not in nonstripped skin in normal humans and in guinea pigs with both gentian violet and brilliant green. These adverse reactions to triphenylmethane dyes may be diagnosed erroneously as exacerbations of the underlying skin disease, with ensuing treatment. Treatment with 1% aqueous solutions of these dyes is not as harmless as supposed.

Epstein[142] studied a patient who was treated for a resistant stasis dermatitis of the lower part of her right leg. After a period of time, gentian violet seemed to irritate the skin. Patch tests with this drug were negative, but an intradermal test with 0.5 mL of a 1:5,000 dilution produced a positive delayed tuberculin-type reaction.

Gentian violet is also known as pyoctanin, and previous reports of contact dermatitis to this dye often blurred the irritant and allergic qualities of the weak and very rare sensitizer. Although some have patch tested with 1% to 2% concentration of gentian violet, 0.0025% to 0.05% is considered preferable to eliminate any toxicity issues and distinguish allergy from irritation. Two such cases were reported from Germany.[143]

Triphenylmethane dyes have produced anaphylactic reactions when used topically and during lymphography.[144] Thus, patent blue (PB), a triphenylmethane dye, is in common use for the visualization of the lymphatic vessels before lymphography. Severe complications in association with PB injections have been reported in 0.1% to 2.8% of procedures; these complications include hypersensitivity reactions from urticaria to cardiovascular collapse.[145] Inhalation of these dyes may produce asthma.[146]

The most widely used of these dyes, gentian violet, may produce not only allergic contact dermatitis but also necrosis in the intertriginous areas.[147,148] The concentration of dyes for patch testing is given in Table 11.14.

In instances in which the erythematous patch test reaction is obscured by the color of the tested dye and papules or vesicles are not evident, an intradermal test with 0.05 mL of a 1:500 dilution of the dyes may be performed. A delayed tuberculin-type reaction indicates sensitivity.

ACRIFLAVINE (ACRIDINE) DYES

Acriflavine and proflavine dihydrochloride, rarely used at present, have been reported in the past as the causes of allergic contact dermatitis.[149,150] Patch testing may be done with a 0.1% concentration in petrolatum.

Table 11-14 Patch Test Concentrations for Dyes
Brilliant green (2% in water)
Crystal violet (2% in water)
Gentian violet (2% in water)
Malachite green (2% in water)
Pararosaniline (saturated solution)
Rosaniline or basic fuchsin (2% in water)
Triphenylmethane (1% in petrolatum)

Acriflavine is an acridine derivative of proflavine and is bacteriostatic against gram-positive and some gram-negative organisms. It is sold over the counter in the tropics and developing countries and has been reported to be a potent sensitizer. Purpuric and erythema multiforme–like eruptions have also been seen.[151] A 0.1% aqueous concentration has been used for patch testing. Proflavine at 0.5% aqueous concentration has also been incriminated.[151]

EOSIN

Formerly a lipstick allergen in the 1950s, and tested at 50% in petrolatum, eosin is occasionally used as an antiseptic. It should be patch tested at the use concentration of 1% to 2% aqueous or alcoholic solution. A contaminant is suspected to be the true sensitizer.[152]

GLYOXAL

Glyoxal, which is also known as ethanedial, is a dialdehyde used in medical and dental offices as a disinfectant for surfaces and instruments. Crossreactions to formaldehyde and glutaraldehyde have been reported. An analysis of 20 cases of glyoxal allergy found that 5 individuals were in dental work, but 9 were machinists without any obvious exposure to glyoxal. Air samples revealed that glyoxal was present at 9.4-21 $\mu g/m^3$ in a machinist's environment. Since glyoxal was not identified in any of the metal working fluids, its formation by heating of fatty acids, microbial modifications of fluids, incomplete combustion of organic compounds, or due to reduction of oxalic acid in fluids was suspected. The recommended patch test concentration of glyoxal is 1 to 2% aqueous.[153]

OTHER AGENTS

The detergent-disinfectant Gigasept AF produced symptoms ranging from hand and arm eczema to burning eyes and coughing fits in 2 hospital workers who used this agent to clean instruments. Use of gloves and masks did not improve the symptoms. Positive patch tests to 0.1% aqueous dimethyldidecylammonium chloride and 1% aqueous N,N-bis(3-aminopropyl)dodecylamine were found as well as reactions to the whole product tested at 10% aqueous.[154]

Cocospropylenediamine-guanidinium diacetate and alkylpropylenediamine-guanidium diacetate are two names for the same compound, which is being used in multiple medical instrument disinfectants. Contact dermatitis has been detected with a 0.01% aqueous concentration. N-cocosprophylenediamin-ammonium borate is thought to cross react with this agent.[155]

Diethylene glycol monobutyl ether is an organic solvent which is one of a family of agents called Carbitols. It is patch tested at 1% aqueous and has been reported to cause dyshidrotic hand dermatitis in a podiatrist who used in the workplace. It can also be found in paints, cleaners, polishes as well as disinfectants.[156]

DISINFECTANTS AND GLOVES

Gloves made of latex, vinyl, and polyethylene are not impermeable to such disinfectants as PCMX and glutaraldehyde. Gloves of these types generally provide about 60 minutes of protection against permeation. The structural integrity of these glove types is lost in less than 10 minutes on exposure to ethanol and isopropanol.[157]

ALCOHOL

Alcohol can produce a variety of adverse topical reactions ranging from subjective irritation to irritant contact dermatitis and contact urticaria. In ten cases of contact urticaria from alcohol identified by patch test concentrations ranging from 0.5% to 100%, oral provocation was also positive in some of the cases. Allergic contact dermatitis to alcohol has also been reported and identified with patch test concentrations down to 1%. The allergen in alcohol has been found to be ethanol itself, impurities, or aldehyde metabolites. It is not common for primary alcohols to crossreact with secondary or tertiary alcohols.[158] Pigosept is a common skin preparative agent for blood draw in Korea and it contains 0.1% dodecyldiaminoethylglycine and 67% isopropyl alcohol. A patient who developed dermatitis from having her arm swabbed with Pigosept reacted to patch test concentrations ranging from 1% to 0.001% of both ingredients.

Dodecyldiaminoethylglycine is the principal ingredient in Tego, which is widely used in hospitals and other public places for purposes of disinfection.[159]

References

1. Fisher AA. Allergic reactions to Merthiolate (thimerosal). Cutis 1981;27:580.

2. Ellis FA. The sensitizing factor in Merthiolate. J Allergy 1947;18:212.

3. Gaul LE. Sensitizing component in thiosalicylic acid. J Invest Dermatol 1958;31:91.

4. Takino C. Thiomersal contact dermatitis (Japanese). Jap J Clin Dermatol 1971;25:1175.

5. Epstein S. Sensitivity to merthiolate: a cause of false delayed intradermal reactions. J Allergy 1963;35:225.

6. Sertoli A, Di Fonzo E, Spallanzani P, et al. Allergic contact dermatitis from thimerosal in a soft contact lens wearer. Contact Dermatitis 1980;6:292.

7. Fisher AA, Pascher F, Kanof NB. Allergic contact dermatitis due to ingredients of vehicles. Arch Dermatol 1971;204:286.

8. Möller H. Merthiolate allergy: a nationwide iatrogenic sensitization. Acta Derm Venereol (Stockh) 1977;57:509.

9. Fregert S, Hjorth H. Contact Dermatitis. In: Rook AJ, Wilkinson DS, Ebling JFG, eds. Textbook of dermatology. Oxford: Blackwell, 1972.

10. van Ketel WG, Melzer-van Riemsduk FA. Conjunctivitis due to soft lens solutions. Contact Dermatitis 1980;6:321.

11. Pedersen NB. Allergic conjunctivitis from Merthiolate in soft contact lenses. Contact Dermatitis 1978;4:165.

12. Rietschel RL, Wilson LA. Ocular inflammation in patients using soft contact lenses. Arch Dermatol 1982;118:147.

13. Maibach HI. Acute laryngeal obstruction presumed secondary to thiomersal (Merthiolate) delayed hypersensitivity. Contact Dermatitis 1975;1:221.

14. Reisman RE. Delayed hypersensitivity to Merthiolate preservative. J Allergy 1969;43:245.

15. Rietschel RL, Adams RM. Reactions to thimerosal in hepatitis B vaccines. Dermatol Clin 1990;8:161.

16. Hansson H, Möller H. Intracutaneous test reactions to tuberculin containing Merthiolate as a preservative. Scand J Infect Dis 1971;3:169.

17. Wantke F, Demmer CM, Gotz M, Jarisch R. Contact dermatitis from thimerosal: 2 years' experience with ethylmercuric chloride in patch testing thimerosal-sensitive patients. Contact Dermatitis 1994;30:115.

18. Möller H. Why thimerosal allergy? Int J Dermatol 1980;19:29.

19. Mannuksela M, Forstrom L, Hannuksela M, Kousa M, Lehmuskallio E. Merthiolate hypersensitivity and vaccination. Contact Dermatitis 1980;6:241.

20. Hansson H, Möller H. Patch test reactions to Merthiolate in healthy young subjects. Br J Dermatol 1970;83:349.

21. Novak M, Kvicalova E. The problem of contact reactions to Merthiolate. Cesk Dermatol 1978;53:313.

22. Cirne de Castro JL, Cirne de Castro JP, Freitas F, et al. Sensitivity to thimerosal and photosensitivity to peroxicam. Contact Dermatitis 1991;24:187.

23. Kitamura K, et al. Cross-reactivity between sensitivity to thimerosal and photosensitivity to piroxicam in guinea pigs. Contact Dermatitis 1991;25:30.

24. van Ketel WG. Sensitization to mercury from Mercurochrome. Contact Dermatitis 1980;6:499.

25. Camarasa G. Contact dermatitis from Mercurochrome. Contact Dermatitis 1976;2:120.

26. Pelaez Hernandez A, Braso Aznar JV, Jorro Martinez G, et al. Mercurochrome allergy: concurrence of 2 hypersensitivity mechanisms in the same patient. Contact Dermatitis 1994;30:48.

27. Bardazzi F, Vassilopoulou A, Valenti R, et al. Mercurochrome-induced allergic contact dermatitis. Contact Dermatitis 1990;23:381.

28. Morris GE. Dermatoses from phenylmercuric salts. Arch Environ Health 1960;1:53.

29. Hjorth N, Trolle-Lassen C. Skin reactions to preservatives in cream with special regard to paraben esters and sorbic acid. Am Perf 1962;77:43.

30. Hartung J. Phenyl-Quecksilberacetate und Phenyl-Quecksilberoleat in textilien. Berufs-dermatosen 1965;13:116.

31. Breit R, Bandmann H-J. The wide world of antimycotics. Br J Dermatol 1973;89:657.

32. Sidi E, Casalis F. Les intolérances de la muqueuse buccale. Presse Med 1951;59:730.

33. Fisher AA. Recent developments in the diagnosis and management of drug eruptions. Med Clin North Am 1959;43:787.

34. Foussereau J, Laugier P. Allergic eczema from metallic foreign bodies (tooth fillings and denture alloys). Clin Dermatol 1966;52:221.

35. van Ketel WG, Roeleveld CG. A curious case of allergy to mercuric compounds. Contact Dermatitis 1977;3:106.

36. Baer RL, Ramsey DL, Biondi E. The most common contact allergens. Arch Dermatol 1973;108:74.

37. Epstein E. Mercury allergy and patch testing. Arch Dermatol 1974;109:98.

38. Mathias CGT, Maibach HI, Chappler RR. Contact dermatitis to para-chloromercuriphenol. Contact Dermatitis 1981;7:117.

39. Tupker RA, Schuur J, Coenraads PJ. Irritancy of antiseptics tested by repeated open exposures on the human skin, evaluated by non-invasive methods. Contact Dermatitis 1997;37:213.

40. Lee SK, Zhai H, Maibach HI. Allergic contact dermatitis from iodine preparations: a conundrum. Contact Dermatitis 2005;52:184.

41. Feldtman RW, Andrassy RI, Page CP. Povidone iodine skin sensitivity observed with possibly altered immune status. JAMA 1979;242:239.

42. Marks JG, Jr. Allergic contact dermatitis to povidone-iodine. J Am Acad Dermatol 1982;6:473.

43. Tosti A, Vincenzi C, Bardazzi F, et al. Allergic contact dermatitis due to povidone-iodine. Contact Dermatitis 1990;23:197.

44. Lachapelle J-M. Allergic contact dermatitis from povidone-iodine : a re-evaluation study. Contact Dermatitis 2005;52:9.

45. Corazza M, Bulciolu G, Spisani L, Virgili A. Chemical burns following irritant contact with povidone-iodine. Contact Dermatitis 1997. 36:115.

46. Mochida K, Hisa T, Yasunaga C, et al. Skin ulceration due to povidone-iodine. Contact Dermatitis 1995;33:61.

47. Sowa J, Tsuruta D, Nakanishi T, et al Generalized dermatitis with eosinophilia resulting from allergic contact dermatitis due to povidone iodine. Contact Dermatitis 2006;54:174.

48. Hjorth N. Contact dermatitis from 1,3-di-iodo-2-hydroxypropane. Contact Dermatitis Newsletter 1972;12:322.

49. Lieberman P, Siegle RL, Raylor WW, Jr. Anaphylactoid reactions to iodinated contrast material. J Allergy Clin Immunol 1978;62:174.

50. Rothe A, Yousif S_H, Zschunke E. Allergic contact eczema from sodium amidotrizoate—a radiopaque substance in angiography and renography. Contact Dermatitis 1977;3:284.

51. Neering H. Contact urticaria from chlorinated swimming pool water. Contact Dermatitis 1977;3:279.

52. Osmundsen P. Contact dermatitis due to sodium hypochlorite. Contact Dermatitis 1978;4:177.

53. Hostynek JJ, Wilhelm KP, Cua AB, Maibach HI, et al. Irritation factors of sodium hypochlorite solutions in human skin. Contact Dermatitis 1990;23:316.

54. Sasseville D, Geoffrion G, Lowry RN. Allergic contact dermatitis from chlorinated swimming pool water. Contact Dermatitis 1999;41:347.

55. Fitzgerald DA, Wilkinson SM, Bhaggoe R, et al. Spa pool dermatitis. Contact Dermatitis 1995;33:53.

56. Sasseville D, Moreau L. Contact allergy to 1-bromo-3-chloro-5,5-dimethylhydantoin in spa water. Contact Dermatitis 2004;50:323.

57. Kagen MH, Wolf J, Scheman A, et al. Potassium peroxymonosulfate-induced contact dermatitis. Contact Dermatitis 2004;51:88.

58. Key M. Some unusual allergic reactions in industry. Arch Dermatol 1961;83:57.

59. Dooms-Goossens A, Gevers D, Mertens A, Vanderheyden D. Allergic contact urticaria to chloramine. Contact Dermatitis 9:319,1983.

60. Bourne M, Flindt M, Walker J. Asthma due to industrial use of chloramine. Br Med J 1979;7:10.

61. Charles T. Asthma due to industrial use of chloramine. Br Med J 1979;4:334.

62. Dijkman J, Vooren P, Kramps J. Occupational asthma due to inhalation of chloramine-T:1. Clinical observations and inhalation-provocation studies. Int Arch Allergy Appl Immunol 1981;64:422.

63. Kramps J, van Toorenenbergen AW, Vooren H, Dijkman JH. Occupational asthma due to inhalation of chloramine-T: 2. Demonstration of specific IgE antibodies. Arch Allergy Appl Immunol 1981;64:428.

64. Mobacken H, Wengstrom C. Interference with healing of rat skin incisions treated with chlorhexidine. Acta Derm Venereol (Stockh) 1974;54:29.

65. Krautheim AB, Jermann THM, Bircher AJ. Chlorhexidine anaphylaxis: case report and review of the literature. Contact Dermatitis 2004;50:113.

66. Calnan CD. Contact dermatitis from drugs. Proc R Soc Med 1962;55:39.

67. Ljunggren B, Möller H. Eczematous contact allergy to chlorhexidine. Acta Derm Venereol (Stockh) 1972;52:308.

68. Muston H_L, Boss JM, Summerly R. Dermatitis from Ammonyx 1.0, a constituent of Hibiscrub. Contact Dermatitis 1977;3:347.

69. Wong WK, Goh CL, Chan KW. Contact urticaria from chlorhexidine. Contact Dermatitis 1990;22:52.

70. Knudsen BB, Avnstorp C. Chlorhexidine gluconate and acetate in patch testing. Contact Dermatitis 1991;24:45.

71. Autegarden JE, Pecquet C, Huet S, et al. Anaphylactic shock after application of chlorhexidine to unbroken skin. Contact Dermatitis 1999;40:215.

72. Le Coz C-J, Meyer M-T. Contact allergy to decyl glucoside in antiseptic after body piercing. Contact Dermatitis 2003;48:279.

73. Fischer LA, Agner T. Curcumin allergy in relation to yellow chlorhexidine solution used for skin disinfection prior to surgery. Contact Dermatitis 2004;51:39.

74. Lee JY, Wang BJ. Contact dermatitis caused by cetrimide in antiseptics. Contact Dermatitis 1995;33:168.

75. Nordlund JJ, Hartley C, Fister J. On the cause of green hair. Arch Dermatol 1977;113:1700.

76. Lampe RM, Hendersen AL, Hansen GH. Green hair. JAMA 19:2092, 1977.

77. Goette DK. Swimmers' green hair [Letter]. Arch Dermatol 1978;114:128.

78. Bhat GR, Lukenbach, Kennedy, Parreira. The green hair problem: a preliminary investigation. J Soc Cosmet Chem 1979;30:1.

79. Burry JN, Kirk J, Reid JG, Turner T, Chlorocresol sensitivity. Contact Dermatitis 1975;1:41.

80. Storrs F. Para-chloro-meta-xylenol allergic contact dermatitis in seven individuals. Contact Dermatitis 1975;1:211.

81. Hjorth N, Trolle-Lassen C. Skin reactions to ointment bases. Trans St John Hosp Derm Soc 1963;49:127.

82. Burry JN, Kirk J, Reid JG, Turner T. Environmental dermatitis: patch tests in 1000 cases of allergic contact dermatitis. Med J Aust 1973;2:681.

83. Park RG. Chlorocresol sensitivity. Contact Dermatitis Newsletter 1970;7:152.

84. Oleffe JA, Blondeel A, de Coninck A. Allergy to chlorocresol and propylene glycol in a steroid cream. Contact Dermatitis 1979;5:53.

85. Baker H, Ive FA, Lloyd MJ. Primary irritant dermatitis of the scrotum due to hexachlorophene. Arch Dermatol 1969;99:663.

86. Epstein E. Dichlorophene allergy. Ann Allergy 1966;24:437.

87. Fregert S, Hjorth N. Results of standard patch tests with substances abandoned. Contact Dermatitis Newsletter 1969;5:85.

88. Morikawa F, Kobayashi T, Nakayama Y, et al. Some problems on the appraisal of the skin safety of hexachlorophene. J Soc Cosmet Chem 1974;25:113.

89. Epstein JH, Wuepper KD, Maibach HI. Photocontact dermatitis to halogenated salicylanilides and related compounds. Arch Dermatol 1968;97:236.

90. Fisher AA, Lipton M. Allergic stomatitis due to "baxin" in a dentifrice. Arch Dermatol 1951;64:640.

91. Fisher AA, Tobin L. Sensitivity to compound G-4 ("Dichlorophene") in dentifrices. JAMA 1953;151:998.

92. Gaul LE, Underwood GB. The cutaneous toxicity of dihydroxydichlordiphenylmethane: a new fungicide for athlete's foot. J Indian Med Assoc 1949;42:22.

93. Schorr WF. Dichlorophene (G-4) allergy. Arch Dermatol 1979;102:515.

94. Roed-Petersen J, Auken G, Hjorth N. Contact sensitivity to irgasan DP 300. Contact Dermatitis 1975;1:293.

95. Hindson TC. Irgasan DP 300 in a deodorant. Contact Dermatitis 1975;1:328.

96. Wahlberg JE. Routine patch testing with Irgasan DP 30D. Contact Dermatitis 1976;2:292.

97. Fisher AA. Irgasan DP 300 and Irgasan CF3. Contact Dermatitis Newsletter 1974;14:416.

98. Maibach HI, Calnan CD, Fregert S, et al. Triclocarban: evaluation of contact dermatitis potential in man. Contact Dermatitis 1978;4:283.

99. Freeman RG, Knox JM. The action spectrum of photocontact dermatitis. Arch Dermatol 1968;97:130.

100. Agren-Jonsson S, Magnusson B. Sensitization to propaniteline bromide, trichlorocarbanilide and propylene glycol in an antiperspirant. Contact Dermatitis 1976;2:79.

101. Osmundsen PE. Concomitant contact allergy to propantheline bromide and TCC. Contact Dermatitis 1975;1:251.

102. Foussereau J, Samsoen M, Hecht MT. Occupational dermatitis to Ampholyt G in hospital personnel. Contact Dermatitis 1983;9:233.

103. Lachapelle JM, Reginster JP. Occupational contact dermatitis from an ampholytic soap (TEGO). Contact Dermatitis 1977;3:211.

104. Suhonen R. Contact allergy to do-ecyldi-(aminoethyl) glycine-Desimex I. Contact Dermatitis 1980;6:290.

105. Valsecchi R, Leghissa P, Pazzolla S. TEGO allergy in the food industry. Contact Dermatitis 1990;23:188.

106. Piraccini BM, Peluso A, De Maria P, Tosti A, et al. Occupational contact dermatitis due to the disinfectant TEGO Diocto S[reg]. Contact Dermatitis 1991;24:228.

107. Ito H, Inui S, Sakurane J, et al. Contact dermatitis due to alkyl diaminoethylglycine hydrochloride. Contact Dermatitis 2003;48:233.

108. Vena GA, Angelini G, Meneghini CL. Contact dermatitis to benzoyl peroxide. Contact Dermatitis 1981;7:137.

109. Lindemayr H, Drobil M. Contact sensitization to benzoyl peroxide. Contact Dermatitis 1981;7:137.

110. Rietschel RL, Duncan SH. Benzoyl peroxide reactions in an acne study group. Contact Dermatitis 1982;8:323.

111. Romaguera C, Grimalt F. Sensitization to benzoyl peroxide, retinoic acid and carbon tetrachloride. Contact Dermatitis 1980;6:442.

112. Cunliffe WJ, Burke B. Benzoyl peroxide: lack of sensitization. Acta Dermatol 1982;62:458.

113. Caro I. Connubial contact dermatitis to benzoyl peroxide. Contact Dermatitis 1976;2:362.

114. Bushkell LL. Bleaching-benzoyl peroxide [Letter]. Arch Dermatol 1974;110:465.

115. Angelini G, Rantuccio F, Meneghini CL. Contact dermatitis in patients with leg ulcers. Contact Dermatitis 1975;1:81.

116. Jensen O, Petersen SH, Vesteroger L. Contact sensitization to benzoyl peroxide following topical treatment of chronic leg ulcers. Contact Dermatitis 1980;6:179.

117. Jager M, Balda BR. Loosening of a total hip prosthesis at contact allergy due to benzoyl peroxide. Arch Orthop Traumat Surg 1979;94:175.

118. Fisher AA. Hand dermatitis - A "baker's dozen." Cutis 1982;29:214.

119. Bonnekoh B, Merk HF. Airborne allergic contact dermatitis from benzoyl peroxide as a bleaching agent of candle wax. Contact Dermatitis 1991;24:367.

120. Shmunes E, Levy EJ. Quaternary ammonium compound contact dermatitis from a deodorant. Arch Dermatol 1972;105:91.

121. Norrlind R (cited by Wahlberg JE). Two cases of hypersensitivity to quaternary ammonium compounds. Acta Derm Venereol (Stockh) 1962;42:230.

122. Huriez C, Agache P, Martin P, et al. L'allergie aux sels d'ammonium quaternaire. Semin Hop (Paris) 1965;41:230.

123. Garcie-Perez A, Moran M. Dermatitis from quaternary ammonium compounds. Contact Dermatitis 1975;1:316.

124. Afzelius H, Thulin H. Allergic reactions to benzalkonium chloride. Contact Dermatitis 1974;5:60.

125. Wahlberg JE. Two cases of hypersensitivity to quaternary ammonium compounds. Acta Derm Venereol (Stockh) 1962;42:239.

126. Seiji M, Mizuno F. Unusual cornification in ichthyosis-like dermatitis. Acta Dermatol 1970;50:338.

127. Pandos E, Horowitz ID, Wunder G. Contact dermatitis complicating tracheostomy. Am J Dis Child 1965;109:90.

128. Theodore F, Schlossman A. Ocular allergy. Baltimore: Williams amp; Wilkins, 1958.

129. Fisher AA, Stillman MA. Allergic contact sensitivity to benzalkonium chloride (BAK): cutaneous, ophthalmic and general medical implications. Arch Dermatol 1972;106:169.

130. Dabiez OH, Naugle BS, Reich L. Evaluation of a stronger concentration of preservative (benzalkonium chloride) in contact lens soaking solution. Eye, Ear, Nose, Throat Monthly 1966;45:78.

131. Huriez C, et al. Frequences des sensibilisations aux ammoniums quaternaires. Bull Soc Franc Derm Syph 1965;72:106.

132. Lovell CR, Staniforth P. Contact allergy to benzalkonium chloride in plaster of Paris. Contact Dermatitis 1983;7:343.

133. Diaz-Ramon L, Aguirre A, Raton-Nieto JA, de Miguel M. Contact dermatitis from benzoxonium chloride. Contact Dermatitis 1999;41:53.

134. Diaz-Ramon L, Aguirre A, Raton-Neito JA, et al. Contact dermatitis from benzoxonium chloride. Contact Dermatitis 1999;41:53.

135. Coles RB, Wilkinson D_S. Necrosis and dequalinium: 1. Balanitis. Trans St. John Hosp Derm Soc 1965;51:46.

136. Wilkinson DS. Durch Dequalinium hervogerufene hautnergrosen. Hautarzt 1970;21:114.

137. Placucci F, Benini A, Guerra L, Tosti A. Occupational allergic contact dermatitis from disinfectant wipes used in dentistry. Contact Dermatitis 1996;35:306.

138. Dejobert Y, Martin P, Piette F, et al. Contact dermatitis from didecyldimethylammonium chloride and bis-(aminopropyl)-lauryl amine in a detergent-disinfectant used in hospital. Contact Dermatitis 1997;37:95.

139. Steinkjer B. Contact dermatitis from cetyl pyridinium chloride in latex surgical gloves. Contact Dermatitis 1998;39:29.

140. Bielicky T, Novak M. Contact-group sensitization to triphenylmethane dyes-gentian violet, brilliant green and malachite green. Arch Dermatol 1969;100:540.

141. Bjornberg A, Mobacken H. Necrotic skin reactions caused by 1 per cent gentian violet and brilliant green. Acta Derm Venereol (Stockh) 1972;52:55.

142. Epstein S. Dermal contact dermatitis. Dermatologica 1958;117:291.

143. Schoppelrey HP, Mily H, Agathos M, Breit R. Allergic contact dermatitis from pyoctanin. Contact Dermatitis 1997;36:221.

144. Koehler PR. Complications of lymphography. Lymphology 1968;1:116.

145. Kalimo K, Saarni H. Immediate reactions to patent blue dye. Contact Dermatitis 1983;7:171.

146. Keskinen H, Wagar G. Occupational asthma due to ECG ink. Presented at the annual meeting of the European Academy of Allergology and Clinical Immunology, Helsinki, 1979 (abstract).

147. Meurer M, Konz B. Necrotic skin reactions after treatment with crystal violet. GFR Hautarzt 1977;28:94.

148. Lawrence CM, Smith G. Ampliative medicament allergy: concomitant sensitivity to multiple medicaments including yellow soft paraffin, white soft paraffin, gentian violet and Span 20. Contact Dermatitis 1982;8:240.

149. Beare JM. Generalized skin sensitivity following local application of acriflavine: report of case. Lancet 1947;1:410.

150. Mitchell JC. Contact dermatitis from proflavine dihydrochloride. Arch Dermatol 1972;106:294.

151. Lim J, Goh CL, Lee CT. Perioral and mucosal oedema due to contact allergy to proflavine. *Contact Dermatitis* 1991;25:195.

152. Tomb RR. Allergic contact dermatitis from eosin. Contact Dermatitis 1991;24:27.

153. Aalto-Korte K, Makela EA, Huttunen M, et al. Occupational contact allergy to glyoxal. Contact Dermatitis 2005;52:276.

154. Dibo M, Brasch J. Occupational allergic contact dermatitis from N,N-bis(3-aminopropyl)dodecylamine and dimethyldidecylammonium chloride in 2 hospital staff. Contact Dermatitis 2001;45:40.

155. Komericki P, Kraenke B, Derhaschnig J, et al. Cocospropylenediamine-guanidium diacetate: synonym and cross-reactants. Contact Dermatitis 2002;46:176.

156. Schliemann-Willers S, Bauer A, Elsner P. Occupational contact dermatitis from diethylene glycol monobutyl ether in a podiatrist. Contact Dermatitis 2000;43:225.

157. Mellström GA, Lindberg M, Boman A. Permeation and destructive effects of disinfectants on protective gloves. Contact Dermatitis 1992;26:163.

158. Ophaswongse S, Maibach HI. Alcohol dermatitis: allergic contact dermatitis and contact urticaria syndrome: a review. Contact Dermatitis 1994;30:1.

159. Kwon JA, Lee MS, Kim MY, et al. Allergic contact dermatitis from dodecyldiaminoethylglycine and isopropyl alcohol in a commercial disinfectant swab. Contact Dermatitis 2003;48:339.

TOPICAL ANTIMICROBIALS

EXECUTIVE SUMMARY

Contact dermatitis to and crossreaction among antimicrobials are covered in this chapter.

Prominent agents include neomycin, penicillin, streptomycin, cephalosporins, bacitracin, polymyxin, gentamicin, pristinamycin, clindamycin, lincomycin, erythromycin, chloramphenicol, virginiamycin, kitasamycin, and tetracyclines. Other broad-spectrum antimicrobials discussed include nitrofurazone, the sulfonamides, acetarsone, metronidazole, quinolone, cloxyquin, rifamycin, and mupirocin.

Antifungal agents covered include nystatin, tolnaftate, haloprogin, undecylenic acid, clotrimazole, sertaconazole, croconazole, lanoconazole, neticonazole, and a host of imidazole derivatives, naftifine, amorolfine, and nifuratel.

Antiviral agents causing contact dermatitis discussed are idoxuridine, tromantadine, acyclovir, and valacyclovir.

Neomycin

Neomycin, the most widely used topical antibiotic in the United States, has become the most sensitizing of all topical antibacterial preparations since the use of topical penicillin was banned.[1] It has been found that 30% of persons who have stasis ulcers, 15% of patients who have chronic otitis externa, and 5% of those who have various chronic eczematous conditions become sensitized by treatment with neomycin (Figures 12-1 and 12-2)[2–4].

Wereide[3] did not find that atopic dermatitis predisposes patients to neomycin sensitivity when compared with other eczematous conditions. Patrick and colleagues,[4] however, stated that, in their study, the occurrence of neomycin sulfate sensitivity in the normal population was less than in a population of patients who have atopic dermatitis or those who have nonatopic dermatoses.

Leyden and Kligman[5] concluded that the intermittent use of neomycin on minor cuts and wounds is not associated with an excessive rate of sensitization. Prystowsky and colleagues[6] found that the prevalence of neomycin patch test sensitivity in the general population is approximately 1%. Such positive patch tests correlate closely with "use tests." These authors suggest wisely that the package instructions for topical neomycin-containing products should carry warnings to the effect that (a) people who have previously used products containing neomycin on inflammatory dermatoses, such as leg ulcers or otitis externa, for extended periods of time have

an increased chance of experiencing an allergic reaction; and (b) failure of acute minor lesions to heal or chronic lesions to improve within 7 days after treatment with such products indicates that the medication should be discontinued until the advice of a physician is sought.

In general, ointment vehicles are less sensitizing than creams or lotions because they do not usually contain preservatives, emulsifying agents, or solvents.[7,8] Hjorth and Thomsen,[9] however, stated that neomycin ointments are the major cause of sensitization to this antibiotic, and they recommended that neomycin should not be prescribed in ointments. The risk of inducing sensitization with neomycin in creams, lotions, or powders appears to be significantly less, according to these investigators.

CROSSREACTIONS WITH NEOMYCIN

There is general agreement that the drugs shown in Table 12.1 crossreact with neomycin.[10–12] Tobramycin (Nebcin) is an aminoglycoside antibiotic for prescription ophthalmologic use in the United States. Schorr and Ridgway[13] stated that tobramycin (ophthalmic) should not be used to treat known neomycin-allergic patients without first testing the patient with 20% tobramycin in white petrolatum. Crossreactions to neomycin among aminoglycosides have been evaluated, and Table 12.2[14] lists the frequency of crossreactions.

Table 12-1 Neomycin Crossreactors

Butirosin (ambutylosin)

Gentamicin (Garamycin)*

Kanamycin

Neomycin (framycetin)

Paromomycin

Spectinomycin

Streptomycin

Tobramycin (Nebcin)†

*Topical preparation.
†Ophthalmic preparation.

NEOMYCIN SYSTEMIC CONTACT DERMATITIS

The administration of a crossreacting drug, such as streptomycin, to a neomycin-sensitive person can produce a severe "systemic eczematous contact-type dermatitis." Also, Ekelund and Möller[15] have shown that the oral administration of neomycin sulfate to neomycin-sensitive persons may cause a flare-up of the original neomycin dermatitis in addition to a "toxicodermic" type of drug eruption. A flare-up of the positive patch test reaction to neomycin may occur infrequently. These authors stress that neomycin may be used occasionally in the treatment of hepatic cirrhosis and in preparative therapy for bowel surgery. Neomycin is given in daily doses of 6 to 8 g (and with good renal function 1% to 3% oral neomycin is excreted in the urine).

Panzer and Epstein[16] found that no percutaneous absorption was detected using a bioassay method sensitive to 0.033 mg/mL for serum following topical application of neomycin sulfate ointment in groups of normal male volunteers who had neomycin sulfate ointment applied to their bodies and that very little absorption has been found with neomycin sulfate administered orally. In fact, it is used frequently as a bowel preparation before gastrointestinal surgery because of its poor absorption from the bowel. According to Ekelund and Möller,[15] however, sufficient neomycin is absorbed to produce a systemic contact-type reaction in neomycin-sensitive persons.

CO-REACTIONS WITH BACITRACIN

Although bacitracin and neomycin are not related chemically, it is not unusual for patients to become sensitized to both antibiotics simultaneously from the use of Neosporin ointment. Thus, Polysporin ointment, which is free of neomycin but contains bacitracin, is not a safe alternative for neomycin-sensitive persons.

Pirila and Rouhunkosky[17] reported that all 99 patients who had positive patch tests to bacitracin also had positive neomycin patch tests. Bjorkner and Möller,[18] who patch tested 1,000 patients who had suspected contact dermatitis, found three patients allergic to bacitracin, all of whom also had positive tests to neomycin. Binnick and Clendenning[19] further point out that because bacitracin and neomycin are not chemically related, positive reactions are left to represent coincidental sensitization rather than cross-sensitization. This lack of cross-sensitization is also borne out by Epstein and Wenzel's[20] guinea pig studies showing that animals sensitized to neomycin did not react to bacitracin, and vice versa. However, within a 1-year period, Fisher and Adams[1] observed nine cases of bacitracin sensitivity without coexistent neomycin sensitivity and recommended that the North American Contact Dermatitis Group begin routinely screening for bacitracin allergy. Within the first year of routine patch testing with bacitracin ointment, this author (RLR) observed three cases of bacitracin allergy with negative reactions to neomycin, all relevant to the current dermatitis. It would appear that bacitracin is capable of inducing sensitization without co-reactivity, contrary to the report of Binnick and Clendenning.[19]

Pirila and Rantanen[21] gave an account of repeated eruptions in a patient sensitive to neomycin and bacitracin because of their topical use on an amputation stump. Later, the patient developed a severe stomatitis from throat tablets containing bacitracin and from a paste containing both antibiotics used to fill an infected root canal. Oral administration of neomycin produced diarrhea and dermatitis.

Table 12.3 lists topical medicaments containing neomycin that should be avoided in neomycin-sensitive persons. As alternatives to the medicaments in Table 12.3, Table 12.4 lists those free of neomycin, bacitracin, and polymyxin. Van Ketel[22] reported a patient who was allergic to both bacitracin and polymyxin and concluded that the sensitization to polymyxin and bacitracin may be cross-sensitization because both antibiotics are obtained from *Bacillus subtilis*. It would, therefore, be wise to use

Table 12-2 Neomycin Crossreactions

Substance	% Crossreacting
Gentamiycin	40–66
Paromomycin	66–97
Tobramycin	25–65
Kanamycin	43–60
Sisomycin	50
Amikacin	33
Amino sydin	91
Streptomycin	0

Table 12-3 Topical Medicaments Containing Neomycin

Alba-3 Ointment (Alba)
Bacimycin (Merrell-National)
Biotres Ointment (Central Pharmacal)
BPN Triple Antibiotic Ointment (Norwich-Eaton)
Cortisporin Cream and Ointment (Burroughs Wellcome)
Mycifradin Powder (Upjohn)
Myciguent Antibiotic Ointment (Upjohn)
Mycitracin Antibiotic Ointment (Upjohn)
Mycolog Cream and Ointment (Squibb)
Mycotriacet Cream and Ointment (Premo)
Mytrex Cream and Ointment (Savage)
Neo-Cortef Cream and Ointment (Upjohn)
Neo-Medrol Ointment (Upjohn)
Neo-Oxylone Ointment (Upjohn)
Neo-Polycin (Dow Pharmaceuticals)
Neosporin Aerosol (Burroughs Wellcome)
Neosporin G.U. Irrigant (Burroughs Wellcome)
Neosporin Powder and Ointment (Burroughs Wellcome)
Neosporin-G Cream (Syntex)
Neo-Synalar Cream and Ointment (Syntex)
Nyst-olone Cream (Schein)
Septa Ointment—Triple Antibiotic Ointment (Circle)

the numerous bacitracin-polymyxin topical medications with caution in neomycin-sensitive persons because of the possibility of "co-reactors" between these antibiotics.

Table 12.5 lists otic preparations that should be avoided by neomycin-sensitive persons. Table 12.6 lists alternative otic preparations that can be used by neomycin-sensitive persons. It should be noted that several of these alternative otic preparations contain acetic acid, which has proved quite effective for the treatment of otitis externa in neomycin-sensitive persons.[23–25] When all other different treatments of otitis externa fail, Fisher[26] has found that half-strength Carbol-fuchsin paint often succeeds in controlling the condition.

Table 12.7 shows ophthalmic preparations that should be avoided by neomycin-sensitive persons. It should be noted that ophthalmic preparations containing tobramycin may crossreact with neomycin. Table 12.8 lists ophthalmic preparations free of neomycin that can be used as alternatives in neomycin-sensitive persons. It has

Table 12-4 Alternative Antibiotics for Neomycin-Sensitive Persons

Betadine Solution and Ointment (Purdue Frederick)
Bactroban Ointment
Ilotycin Ointment (Dista)

These ointments may be combined with Nystatin Cream or ointment for Candida infections.

Table 12-5 Neomycin Otic Preparations to Be Avoided by Neomycin-Sensitive Persons

Coly-Mycin S Otic with Neomycin and Hydrocortisone (Parke-Davis)
Cortisporin Otic Solution (Burroughs Wellcome)
Cortisporin Otic Suspension (Burroughs Wellcome)
Otobione Otic Suspension (Schering)
Otocidin Otic Drops (Marin)
Otocort Ear Drops (Lemmon)

been found that the proper application of antibiotic ophthalmic ointments gives results superior to that of an aqueous vehicle, and that by placing the ophthalmic ointment on the fingertip and applying it medially and laterally to the lids and lashes, the medication can reach the conjunctival sac. This medication has an antibacterial effect lasting for several hours.[27]

Table 12.9 lists some miscellaneous methods by which individuals are exposed to neomycin. Neomycin-sensitive persons may acquire an allergic contact dermatitis from handling such products.

Penicillin

The topical use of penicillin is largely avoided at present because many individuals would develop contact sensitivity to the drug. Allergic contact dermatitis from penicillin occurs particularly in physicians, nurses, pharmacists, and veterinarians who handle this antibiotic. Allergic sensitization to penicillin may be initiated by

Table 12-6 Alternative Otic Preparations for Neomycin-Sensitive Persons

Castellani's Paint (Pedinol Pharmacal, Inc.)
Chloromycetin Otic (Parke-Davis)
Chloramphenicol in Propylene Glycol*
Lidosporin Otic Solution (Burroughs Wellcome)
Polymyxin B Sulfate,† Lidocaine Hydrochloride,
Propylene Glycol*
Orlex Otic Solution (Baylor)
Acetic Acid Propylene Glycol*
Orlex HC Otic Solution (Baylor)
Acetic Acid, Hydrocortisone, Propylene Glycol*
Otic Domeboro Solution (Dome)††
Acetic Acid in Aluminum Acetate (Modified Burow's) Solution
VoSOL and VoSOL-HC Otic Solution (Wallace)
Acetic Acid in Propylene Glycol,* Propylene
Glycol Diacetate Hydrocortisone

*Propylene glycol may be a sensitizer.
†The polymyxin may rarely "co-react" with neomycin.
††A nonsensitizing preparation.

Table 12-7 Ophthalmic Preparations to Be Avoided by Neomycin-Sensitive Persons

Cortisporin Ointment Ophthalmic (Burroughs Wellcome)

NeoDECADRON Sterile Ophthalmic Ointment (Merck Sharp & Dohme)

NeoDECADRON Sterile Ophthalmic Solution (Merck Sharp & Dohme)

Neo-Hydeltrasol Sterile Ophthalmic Ointment (Merck Sharp & Dohme)

Neo-Hydeltrasol Sterile Ophthalmic Solution (Merck Sharp & Dohme)

Neosporin Ophthalmic Ointment (Burroughs Wellcome)

Neosporin Ophthalmic Solution (Burroughs Wellcome)

Tobramycin* Solution (benzalkonium chloride) (Alcon)*

*Tobramycin (Nebcin) may crossreact with neomycin.

Table 12-9 Miscellaneous Exposure to Neomycin

In dentistry
   Tooth root canal work
In deodorants
   Hi and Dry
   Top Brass
In pet foods
In veterinary use
   Growth promoter in feeds (particularly for poultry)
   Systemic (Calf Drench)
   Topical medicaments

external contact with various forms of penicillin, and dermatitis may be produced in sensitized individuals by contact with penicillin used for injections or by cleaning syringes contaminated with it. Allergic contact sensitivity to penicillin is usually combined with the immediate anaphylactic variety. Inhalation of penicillin from powder, aerosols, or molds may produce asthma and anaphylactoid shock in individuals who have contact sensitivity. In Malaysia, where penicillin medicaments are available over the counter, penicillin is the most frequent cause of contact dermatitis from antibiotics.[28] The systemic administration of penicillin to such "externally" sensitized individuals may produce an eczematous contact-type dermatitis, which may be accompanied by urticarial anaphylactic sensitivity.

Girard[29] reported a patient who applied penicillin topically on a varicose ulcer. Two days later, a severe contact dermatitis developed around the ulcer. The immunologic investigations, which were done a few days later, failed to reveal specific IgG or IgE antibodies. The RAST test was negative, but the lymphocyte transformation test was highly positive.

Table 12-8 Alternative Ophthalmic Preparations Free of Neomycin

Achromycin Ophthalmic Ointment (Lederle)

Achromycin Ophthalmic Suspension 1% (Lederle)

Chloromycetin Ophthalmic Ointment 1% (Parke-Davis)

Gantrisin Ophthalmic Ointment (Roche)

Gantrisin Ophthalmic Solution (Roche)

Garamycin Ophthalmic OintmentSterile (Schering)

Garamycin Ophthalmic SolutionSterile (Schering)

Ilotycin Ophthalmic Ointment (Dista)

Metimyd Ophthalmic OintmentSterile (Schering)

Metimyd Ophthalmic Suspension (Schering)

Sodium Sulamyd Ophthalmic Ointment (Schering)

Sodium Sulamyd Ophthalmic Solution (Schering)

Terra-Cortril Ophthalmic Suspension (Pfizer)

Desensitization of penicillin sensitivity is hazardous and should be attempted with great caution.

Hjorth[30] stated that occupational dermatitis in veterinary surgeons is common and that in six veterinarians the dermatitis had been provoked or aggravated by penethamate hydriodide (benzyl-penicillin b-diethylaminoethyl ester hydriodide), used for local treatment of mastitis in cows. Penethamate is used as a 25% suspension in oil injected into the teat of the udder. In Denmark, it is the drug usually used for mastitis, not only because it achieves a high concentration but also because it is rapidly eliminated from the milk. Penethamate is a base, whereas benzyl penicillin is an acid.

Although the six patients were all sensitive to penethamate, only three had positive patch test reactions to benzyl penicillin, indicating that patch tests should also be performed with penethamate. This finding may explain why some patients who have a definite history of reaction after treatment with one penicillin have tolerated later treatment with another type of penicillin. Thus, the different types of penicillin do not necessarily crossreact when it comes to allergic contact sensitivity. Some individuals may be allergic to ampicillin, some to penicillin G, some to oxicillin, and some to dicloxacillin. One must not take for granted that cross-sensitivity occurs.

REPORTS WITH POSITIVE PENICILLIN PATCH-TEST REACTIONS

Blanton and Blanton[31] reported that patch tests may be performed with penicillin powder, ointment (500 units/g), or topical medications. The usual positive reaction occurs in 24 to 48 hours. In sensitive individuals, however, an immediate reaction consisting of an erythematous wheal, sometimes with pseudopods, may occur within a half hour.

A positive patch test reaction of the delayed type may be significant, because the allergic eczematous contact sensitivity is accompanied frequently by the immediate anaphylactic reaction. If there is a compelling need for penicillin in a patient who had a positive test reaction to it, scratch and intracutaneous tests must be performed to determine the presence or absence of the immediate type of sensitivity before systemic administration is attempted.

Valsecchi and colleagues[32] stated that a 14-year-old boy who had acute tonsillitis was treated for 1 week with ampicillin. The treatment was then stopped because of a widespread urticarial eruption with mucous membrane edema and itching. When treated again with ampicillin, the patient showed the same generalized cutaneous eruption and was hospitalized. Patch tests to ampicillin and cephalexin gave positive reactions. The patient had not had any previous known contact with topical compounds containing ampicillin or cephalexin. This finding indicates the value of patch testing in the diagnosis of adverse drug reactions and supports a possible crossreaction between penicillin, its derivatives, and cephalosporins; the latter compounds have the same antigenic determinant, namely the β-lactam ring.

The utility of patch tests to evaluate β lactams was undertaken in 101 patients who had either intentional or accidental re-exposure to the drug to which they were sensitive.[33] Therefore, confirmation of allergy was established by systemic means. In this group of patients, patch, prick, and intradermal tests were conducted. Patch tests were conducted with amoxicillin in 25%, sodium penicillin G 5%, ampicillin 25%, bacampicillin 25%, aztreonam 20%, and ceftriazone 20%, all in petrolatum. The type of systemic reactions experienced when challenged had been urticaria, angioedema, morbilliform eruptions, and anaphylactic shock. Intradermal tests were the most sensitive, and about half of the patients had one or more positive test. Patch tests were positive in 31% of morbilliform eruptions, 20% of urticarial/angioedematous eruptions, and none of the anaphylactic shock cases.

Vickers and colleagues[34] reported that penicillin in milk from cows treated for mastitis caused dermatitis in two patients. Both patients had positive patch tests. One reacted to penicillin at 200,000 units/mL and the other to procaine penicillin at 100,000 units/mL.

Ampicillin sensitivity is an occupational hazard among nurses. A 5% aqueous solution may be used for patch tests. Hand dermatitis developed in a nurse and continued for a 20-year period as vesiculation and erythema of the sides of the fingers of the right hand.[35] This was associated with handling ampicillin or amoxicillin vials for parenteral use. Patch tests with 50 mg/mL aqueous ampicillin and amoxicillin were strongly positive, whereas sodium benzylpenicillin at 100 U/mL aqueous was negative. Oral challenge with 250 mg of phenoxymethylpenicillin was negative. The difference in structure between these antibiotics is an aminogroup on the benzene ring. This minor difference in β-lactam side chains led to a very different immunologic response.

Schulz and colleagues[36] described 62 cases of occupational eczema occurring among members of the medical and allied professions. Sixty-one had an allergic contact dermatitis, principally from drugs. Ampicillin was the most frequent allergen, being the sensitizer in 24 of the patients, most of whom were nurses exposed occupationally. Patch tests revealed positive reactions to ampicillin 5% aqueous solution.

Inappropriate application of cloxicillin to the skin from vials intended for intravenous use led to contact dermatitis in two women.[37] No crossreactivity to other β-lactam antibiotic was found in these two cases, which is consistent with animal studies showing no crossreactivity.

Streptomycin

Streptomycin produced by actinomycetin *Streptomyces griseus* has its greatest application in the treatment of tuberculosis and may be administered alone or in combination with penicillin in preparations such as Wycillin (Wyeth).

Desensitization procedures by subcutaneous injection of streptomycin are dangerous and may be accompanied by urticaria or flares of dermatitis. Furthermore, such desensitization is rarely successful.

Although topical application of streptomycin is now avoided, members of the medical, nursing, and pharmaceutical professions who handle the drug become readily sensitized, and subsequent administration may produce a severe eczematous contact-type dermatitis medicamentosa. Because streptomycin may crossreact with neomycin, systemic administration of streptomycin may produce the eczematous contact-type dermatitis in individuals who had become sensitized to neomycin and had never been exposed to streptomycin. However, this was not observed by Menendez-Ramos and colleagues.[14] Streptomycin may also crossreact with kanamycin sulfate (Kantrex).

This drug is an important occupational hazard to nurses and a frequent cause of allergic contact sensitization. The allergic dermatitis may first be noted at the tips of the thumb and the index and middle fingers, where there is contact with streptomycin from a leaking syringe or needle. Prolonged contact in the sensitized individual may produce deep fissures and hyperkeratoses with superimposed eczematization.

For patch test purposes, a 2.5% aqueous solution of streptomycin is used. In most instances, sensitized individuals show a strongly positive patch test reaction. The reaction is negative occasionally, but a scratch test may produce an urticarial wheal within 15 minutes, which may remain for an hour or so and may be replaced by a papule or vesicle after 24 to 48 hours. Although scratch testing with streptomycin is a relatively safe procedure, the intracutaneous test is hazardous and may cause a generalized urticaria and anaphylactoid shock. Desensitization to streptomycin is dangerous and usually fails.

Contact dermatitis among nurses giving streptomycin to patients who have tuberculosis was first reported by Strauss and Warring.[38] Four of 12 nurses working in a sanatorium developed dermatitis of their hands and eyelids, and each had a positive patch test to 2% streptomycin. In a study of 18 sensitized nurses, Wilson[39] reported that the hands, arms, and eyelids were affected most frequently; 17 nurses had positive patch tests to streptomycin 5% in aqueous solution, and 1 reacted only to an intradermal injection. It was found that, on wards where gloves and masks were worn for giving injections, nurses escaped sensitization, whereas on other wards where nurses were not so protected, dermatitis occurred.

Adams[40] states that streptomycin is used to control bacterial disease in plants, such as fire blight of pears, apples, begonias, roses, and other flowers. The streptomycin is often combined with tetracycline, and allergic contact dermatitis from such exposure to streptomycin may take place.

Cephalosporins

Nursing can also lead to cephalosporin exposure and occupational contact dermatitis. A 24-year-old nurse was found reactive to cefazolin, cefoxitin, ceftriaxon, and cedfazidime on patch testing, and this explained her hand, forearm, and facial dermatitis.[41]

CEFTIOFUR

Ceftiofur sodium is a third-generation veterinary cephalosporin used in chicks to control *E. coli*. Chicken vaccinators are at risk for contact dermatitis to this agent, and two cases have been reported.[42] Other contact allergens seen in chicken vaccinators include tylosin, spectinomycin, and lincomycin. Other cephalosporins reported to cause contact dermatitis are listed in Table 12.10.

Table 12-10 Cephalosporins Reported to Cause Contact Dermatitis

Cephalexin	Cefoxitin
Cefuroxime	Ceftriaxone
Cephaloridine	Cefodizime
Cephamandol	Ceftazidime
Cephazolin	Cedfazidime
Cephazoline	Cephotaxime
Cefotiam	Ceftizoxime

Bacitracin

Bacitracin is a sensitizer. Topical application may produce anaphylactic shock. Comaish and Cunliffe[43] reported that soon after a woman applied bacitracin to a statis ulcer, she complained that she had a pricking sensation and swelling of her face, generalized itching, sweating, dyspnea, and hypotension. She then collapsed. Later, she remembered that twice in the past she had had urticaria after her ulcer had been treated with other preparations containing bacitracin. Three months later, because a prick test with bacitracin 1/1,000 was negative, 0.03 mL of the bacitracin 1/1000 (2.3 units) was injected intradermally, and within 4 minutes she suffered severe anaphylactic shock and lost consciousness.

It was stressed that the concentration for intradermal testing should be **1,000-fold less** than that for prick tests.

Roupe and Strannegard[44] described a 14-year-old atopic girl who collapsed with anaphylactic shock after an ointment containing bacitracin was applied to her atopic dermatitis. Two months previously, a similar application had caused irritation and swelling of her lip. Prausnitz-Kustner tests done on monkeys and one human were positive.

At the 1992 meeting of the American Contact Dermatitis Society, Dr. William James reported another case of anaphylactic shock in response to bacitracin. The patient was a healthy adolescent (his son) who applied bacitracin to an abrasion. James's case was subsequently reported by Farley and colleagues.[45] They collected nine cases from the literature and added two of their own. They recommended prick testing with 0.1 U/mL and if no reaction occurred, then increasing the concentration tenfold.

Van Ketel[22] stated that a woman who had contact dermatitis of her feet had positive patch test reactions to polymyxin B sulfate and bacitracin. It was thought these might be crossreactions rather than independent sensitizations.

Although bacitracin and neomycin are not chemically related, they often "co-react" because the patients may have become sensitized simultaneously to both antibiotics when they are used in combination in such preparations as Neo-Polycin and Neosporin (Table 12.11). At a meeting of the North American Contact Dermatitis Group (NACDG) in the mid-1980s, Alexander Fisher presented his experience with bacitracin sensitivity and suggested that it might be more prevalent than neomycin sensitivity, but, because routine testing for bacitracin was not done at that time, the issue was unanswerable. The NACDG began testing bacitracin after that presentation. A study of leg ulcer patients found Fisher's concern to be legitimate, as bacitracin was the most common antibiotic allergen among leg ulcer patients, slightly exceeding

Table 12-11 Bacitracin-Containing Antibiotics
Baciguent Antibiotic Ointment (Upjohn)
Bacitracin Ointment (American Pharm.)
Bacitracin Topical Ointment (Pfipharmecs)
BNP Ointment (Norwich-Eaton)
Cortisporin Ointment (Burroughs Wellcome)
Mycitracin Antibiotic Ointment (Upjohn)
Neo-Polycin (Merrell Dow)
Neosporin Aerosol, Ointment, Powder (Burroughs Wellcome)
Norwich Bacitracin Ointment (Norwich Eaton)
Polysporin Ointment (Burroughs Wellcome)

Table 12-12 Polymyxin-Containing Antibiotics
Aerosporin Powder (Burroughs Wellcome)
Chloromyxin (Parke Davis)
Cortisporin Cream (Burroughs Wellcome)
Cortisporin Ophthalmic Ointment and Suspension (Burroughs Wellcome)
Cortisporin Otic Suspension (Burroughs Wellcome)
Neo-Polycin (Merrell Dow)
Neosporin Aerosol and Ointment (Burroughs Wellcome)
Neosporin GU Irrigant (Burroughs Wellcome)
Neosporin Ophthalmic Ointment and Solution (Burroughs Wellcome)
Neosporin Powder and Cream (Burroughs Wellcome)
Ophthocort (Parke-Davis)
Otobiotic Sterile Otic Solution (Schering)
Otocidin Otic Drops (Marin)
Polymyxin B Sulfate (Burroughs Wellcome)
Polysporin Ophthalmic Ointment (Burroughs Wellcome)
Pyocidin-Otic Solution (Berlex)
Terramycin Ointment (Pfipharmecs)
Terramycin with Polymyxin B Sulfate Ophthalmic Ointment (Pfipharmecs)

neomycin.[46] This was attributed to the widespread use of a polymyxin/bacitracin mixture for the management of leg ulcers at the institution.

Thus, Bjorkner and Möller[18] patch tested 1,000 patients who had suspected contact dermatitis and found only 3 allergic to bacitracin, all of whom also had positive tests to neomycin. After intracutaneous injection of bacitracin, the three patients showed a delayed eczematous reaction. A strong, immediate wheal and flare reaction was induced by intracutaneously injected bacitracin. This was inhibited by a simultaneous local injection of the antihistamine mepyramine, which also abolished the vascular response to histamine and to the histamine liberator polymyxin B. Depletion of cutaneous histamine by pretreatment with polymyxin B diminished the wheal and flare induced by bacitracin. The vascular effects of bacitracin in human skin are due apparently to a release of histamine.

Binnick and Clendenning[19] reported a patient who had allergic contact dermatitis owing to bacitracin. As noted in the discussion of neomycin cosensitivity, isolated bacitracin sensitivity has been found increasingly when looked for by members of the NACDG.

Polymyxin

Polymyxin is used widely in topical medications, often in combination with neomycin and bacitracin (Table 12.12).

Van Ketel[22] pointed out that polymyxin B sulfate is used in patients who have ulcers of the legs contaminated with *Pseudomonas aeruginosa*. In contrast to bacitracin, which is also present in topically used preparations, polymyxin B sulfate and the related polymyxin E (Colistin) are used parenterally in cases of infection of the intestines and other organs, mainly in cases of *P. aeruginosa* infection. Thus, patients topically sensitized to polymyxin B sulfate could acquire a systemic contact dermatitis.

According to van Ketel,[22] topical polymyxin B sulfate crossreacts not only with Colistin (polymyxin E) but also with bacitracin, because both antibiotics are obtained from *B. subtilis*.

Möller[47] reported that patients who had stasis ulcers and eczema treated with Terramycin-polymyxin B ointment became sensitized to polymyxin B sulfate.

Gentamicin (Garamycin, Cidomycin, Gentalyn, Genticin, and Refobacin)

The topical antibiotics listed in Table 12.13 contain this antibiotic. Crossreactions between gentamicin (Garamycin) and neomycin have been reported several times. Thus, Pirila and colleagues[48] demonstrated that of 100 neomycin-sensitive individuals, 40 showed positive patch test reactions to gentamicin (Garamycin) despite lack of previous exposure to gentamicin. Bandmann and Mutzek,[49] Braun and Schutz,[50] and Schorr and colleagues[51] showed similar crossreactions between neomycin and gentamicin. Lynfield[52] described a patient who was so sensitive to gentamicin that he gave a positive patch test reaction to a cream containing 0.1% concentration of gentamicin. This patient also crossreacted with neomycin. Drake[53] reported that a woman developed tinnitus each time she applied Garamycin Cream 0.1% to a paronychia.

Table 12-13 Topical Garamycin (Gentamicin)
Garamycin Cream and Ointment (Schering)
Garamycin Ophthalmic Ointment and Sterile Solution (Schering)
Gentamicin Cream 0.1% and Ointment 0.1% (Schein)

Pristinamycin

Crossreactivity to pristinamycin administered orally occurred in patients who had previously been sensitized topically to virginiamycin ointment.[54] Features of both immediate and delayed hypersensitivity were present in these cases reported in France.

ALLERGIC SENSITIZATION TO TOPICAL CLINDAMYCIN

Allergic contact dermatitis owing to topical clindamycin is rare but should be suspected when patients using topical clindamycin complain of itching. Patch testing with the preparation and its separate ingredients should then be performed.

Mild, local, adverse reactions to topical clindamycin preparations, such as burning, stinging, excessive dryness, itching, and erythema, are not uncommon but are usually caused by the vehicle. Contact allergy to clindamycin seems to be rare, especially in relation to the widespread use of this antibiotic in topical formulations.

Coskey[55] and De Groot[56] have reported positive patch test reactions and dermatitis from topical clindamycin. Conde-Salazar and colleagues[57] described a patient who was exposed to both systemic and topical clindamycin for an atopic dermatitis. The patient developed a superimposed contact dermatitis and showed positive reactions to both clindamycin and lincomycin. Lincomycin is an antibiotic of the *Streptomyces* genus, and clindamycin is a semisynthetic derivative used as a phosphate, chlorhydrate, or palmitate. Yokoyama and colleagues[58])reported clindamycin sensitivity with positive patch tests to the hydrochloride form at 0.5% aqueous and the phosphate form at 0.1% aqueous. Their patient did not react to lincomycin.

Topical clindamycin (either as the hydrochloride salt or the phosphate ester) is used widely in the treatment of acne vulgaris.[59,60] Topical clindamycin has been used to treat acne for more than 20 years. Case reports of contact dermatitis to this antibiotic are rare. Vejlstrup and Menne[61] found three cases in the literature and reported one additional case of their own. They considered clindamycin to be a weak allergen.

NONALLERGIC ADVERSE REACTIONS TO TOPICAL CLINDAMYCIN

Several adverse reactions to topical clindamycin have been described that are similar to those described from systemic administration: diarrhea, abdominal pains, pseudomembranous colitis, migraine, and fatigue.

Feingold and colleagues,[62] after experimental topical application of clindamycin to the backs of hamsters, state: "The possibility of colitis from topical applications of antibiotics cannot be dismissed out of hand. In these hamsters, care was taken that no clindamycin could be ingested. In patients using clindamycin on the face, it is likely that some of the drugs would enter through the mouth."

Milstone and colleagues[63] reported that abdominal cramping and diarrhea developed in a 24-year-old woman 5 days after she started topical therapy with 1% clindamycin hydrochloride for treatment of facial acne vulgaris. A stool specimen contained a significant titer of a toxin produced by *Clostridium difficile*. Findings from sigmoidoscopy and a colonic biopsy specimen were consistent with pseudomembranous colitis. The patient became asymptomatic after 10 days of supportive care and oral vancomycin hydrochloride therapy. This case is presented as an example of pseudomembranous colitis associated with topical application of clindamycin. Milstone and colleagues[63] concluded that topical clindamycin is a safe and apparently effective therapy for some forms of acne vulgaris in many patients. Pseudomembranous colitis can be fatal, however, if not recognized and treated appropriately. All patients receiving topical clindamycin should be warned that they should discontinue therapy and consult their physicians if intestinal symptoms occur.

Percutaneous absorption does occur, however, and several other cases of associated diarrhea have been reported.[64,65] Another possible unwanted effect of topical antibiotic usage is the selection of a resistant gram-positive skin flora,[60] which may pose a drawback to this therapeutic approach, as the drugs used for acne are also utilized for other infections caused by gram-positive organisms. Some authors, however, consider this to be a theoretical rather than a practical problem.[66]

Lincomycin

Lincomycin, along with spectinomycin, has been implicated in causing hand and forearm rashes in chicken vaccinators. Lincomycin was tested at 5% in petrolatum and spectinomycin at 1% petrolatum.[67]

Erythromycin

Fisher's[66] experience with erythromycin base in a petrolatum ointment in more than 300 infected dermatoses and in a study of 60 patients who had infected stasis ulcers failed to produce even a single instance of sensitization. He was unable to find any reports in the literature of allergic reactions to the topical application of erythromycin base at that time.

Lombardi and colleagues[68] describe "delayed hypersensitivity to erythromycin." It should be emphasized that they patch tested with an erythromycin salt, erythromycin sulfate 25% in petrolatum. In addition, van Ketel[69] reported an allergic reaction to erythromycin stearate.

Although erythromycin is an extremely rare sensitizer, topical use followed by oral use caused both a local and generalized dermatitis.[70] In this case, erythromycin base at 2.5% in petrolatum was positive, as was the ethylsuccinate base.

Chloramphenicol

Table 12.14 lists some topical chloramphenicol preparations. Allergic contact sensitivity to this antibiotic is rare.

Schwank and Jirasek[71] reported much sensitivity to chloramphenicol applied to stasis ulcers and eczemas. Patch tests with chloramphenicol 1% in petrolatum or in alcohol elicited reactions in all the patients, but in only 9 of 149 controls. Six further patients, who worked in a plant making chloramphenicol, developed a contact dermatitis of the face and hands. The report of Schwank and Jirasek[71] concerning cross-sensitization between 2,4-dinitrochlorbenzene and chloramphenicol was not confirmed.[72,73]

Rudzki and colleagues[74] attributed a positive patch test reaction to 50% chloramphenicol to a previous drug eruption from intramuscular chloramphenicol. Kozakova[75] reported that a woman who had used chloramphenicol topically in the past was given the drug by mouth. She developed anaphylactic shock with edema of the face and generalized urticaria. A week later, a patch test with 1% chloramphenicol produced the same reaction, but to a lesser degree.

Bandmann[76] attributed the small number of case reports of chloramphenicol sensitivity to the fact that this antibiotic is used rarely for eczema.

Milkowski[77] presented a patient who had two episodes of contact conjunctivitis and dermatitis of the lids after application of chloramphenicol as drops into the conjunctival sac. Chloramphenicol is available in France only in topical form as an eyedrop preparation. In this form, it caused contact dermatitis of the face and conjunctivitis.[78] Crossreactivity with thiamphenicol was observed. Wereide[79] reported that azidamphenicol used as an antibiotic showed crossreactions with chloramphenicol.

Tetracyclines

Although fixed-drug eruptions from the systemic use of tetracycline are fairly commonly observed in the United States, allergic reactions to the topical application of tetracycline are rarely seen. European investigators, however, report that allergic reactions to tetracycline are not uncommon. Thus, Fontanot[80] reported in Italy that four patients were sensitized to ointments containing tetracycline compound. Bojs and Möller[81] reported in Belgium that, whereas neomycin is still the leading contact antibiotic allergen, the tetracyclines are not "harmless." They reported three cases of eczematous contact allergy in patients using oxytetracycline. Results of patch tests with six other tetracyclines showed that cross-sensitivity to tetracycline and methacycline could be demonstrated in two of the patients.

Calnan[82] stated that a woman who had used Aureomycin ointment on a dermabraded tattoo developed dermatitis. Another patient used Aureomycin ointment to treat her varicose ulcers. Patch tests revealed that the first patient reacted to the Aureomycin ointment, chlortetracycline, and demeclocycline, but not to tetracycline. The second patient reacted to Aureomycin 0.5% (in petrolatum).

It should be emphasized that these European reports do not deal with the topical application of tetracycline in lotion form for acne.

COSMETIC DRAWBACKS TO TOPICAL TETRACYCLINE

Standlee[83] emphasized that topical tetracycline preparations yellow the skin. The discoloration is noticeable, especially on patients who have fair complexions. Furthermore, patients complain about the fluorescence of the drug. Standlee states, "A patient on Topicycline was slightly shocked and embarrassed when visiting a display of fluorescent minerals in a museum. To her dismay, her face fluoresced as brightly as the minerals!"

Nystatin

Wasilewski[84] studied a patient who was allergic to nystatin following exposure to two topical medications

Table 12-14 Chloramphenicol
Chloromycetin Cream (Parke Davis)
Chloromycetin Ophthalmic and Otic Ointment (Parke Davis)
Chloromyxin Ointment (Parke Davis)
Ophthochlor Solution (Parke Davis)
Ophthocort Ointment (Parke Davis)

containing this antibiotic in combination with different ingredients. On patch testing, the patient reacted to Mycolog cream, Nystaform-HC ointment, and ethylenediamine. Although original Mycolog cream contained ethylenediamine, Nystaform-HC ointment does not. Nystatin is the only ingredient common to both preparations, and a subsequent patch test with nystatin (Mycostatin sterile powder for laboratory use) was strongly positive. The patch test material was prepared in a concentration of 100,000 units/mL (1 mg = approximately 3,000 units), and 70% ethanol was used as the vehicle. None of ten volunteers patch tested with this material showed any reaction.

Coskey[85,86] and Foussereau and colleagues[87] have also reported allergic contact sensitivity to nystatins.

Nitrofurazone (Furacin)

Topical nitrofurazone is available in the following forms:

Furacin Soluble Dressing (Norwich-Eaton), which contains 0.2% nitrofurazone (Furacin) in Solubase (a water-soluble base of polyethylene glycols 4,000, 1,000, and 300).

Furacin Soluble Powder (Norwich-Eaton), which contains 0.2% nitrofurazone (Furacin) in a water-soluble powder of polyethylene glycol 6,000.

Furacin Topical Cream (Norwich-Eaton), which contains nitrofurazone (Furacin) in a water-miscible base consisting of glycerin, cetyl alcohol, mineral oil, an ethoxylated fatty alcohol, methylparaben, propyl-paraben, and water.

Nitrofurazone is a well-known sensitizer, and many instances of severe allergic contact dermatitis occur where it is used extensively.

Hull and de Beer[88] state that patients who had stasis eczema and ulcers or injury to the skin of the leg are particularly prone to sensitization, whereas Braun and Schutz[50] reported that 58 patients (many of whom had stasis eczema or ulcers) were sensitized by medicaments containing 0.2% nitrofurazone (Furacin), and that re-exposure to it had caused a generalized eczema in some patients. Sensitization has also been reported by Bleumink and colleagues[89] in 14 patients who had leg ulcers. A positive patch test to Furacin ointment containing 0.2% nitrofurazone was obtained in each patient.

Nitrofurazone (Furacin) is also used in veterinary medicine and in animal feeds. Caplan[90] reported a man who worked in a feed shop and scooped chicken feed containing Furacin from storage bins into sacks. He developed acute attacks of dermatitis. On patch testing he reacted to 1% nitrofurazone. Neldner[91] also reported contact dermatitis from Furacin added to animal feed.

CONTACT DERMATITIS FROM POLYETHYLENE GLYCOL IN "SOLUBLE" FURACIN PREPARATIONS

Fisher[92] reported that Furacin Soluble Dressing (Eaton) applied to a second-degree burn of the leg produced a severe allergic contact dermatitis. Patch tests with Furacil Soluble Dressing, polyethylene glycol (PEG) 300 and 400, were strongly positive in the patient and negative in six controls. Patch tests to PEG 1,000 and 4,000 were negative.

A second patient was a 64-year-old man who had received cobalt radiation for carcinoma of the lung and had developed a severe second-degree burn of the irradiated skin of the chest for which he had been treated with a spray of Furacin Solution (Eaton). A severe, edematous vesicular and crusted contact dermatitis became superimposed upon the radiation burn. Patch tests with Furacin solution, PEG 400 and 300, were strongly positive. Patch tests with PEG 1,000 and 4,000 were negative.

Braun[93] studied 40 patients who showed a delayed allergic contact sensitivity to a medication containing nitrofurazone (nitrofural), which is a Furacin-like product. In 3 of 40 cases, the active ingredient nitrofurazone was not the cause of the dermatitis, but the solvent PEG 300 proved to be the culprit.

It should be emphasized that Furacin Soluble Dressing and Powder contain polyethylene glycols. Allergic reactions may occur either from Furacin or the polyethylene glycols.

NIFUROXAZIDE

The oral antibiotic nifuroxazide is used to treat acute and chronic diarrhea. There have been reports of contact dermatitis to this. A Polish pharmaceutical worker was exposed to nifuroxazide in a packaging operation, but her lesions resembled prurigo nodularis rather than contact dermatitis.[94] She was sensitive to this antibiotic from 1% to 0.001% aqueous and cleared when not occupationally exposed. She did not crossreact to nitrofurazone.

FURALTADONE

Furaltadone is an antibiotic most commonly associated with veterinary practice or use in animal feeds. It is a component of a Spanish eardrop and along with neomycin caused contact dermatitis. The product (Panotile) contains 4.5 mg/mL of furaltadone chlorhydrate, and a 1% concentration in petrolatum was positive in the patient but negative in 20 controls.[95]

Sulfonamides

Crossreactions can occur between the various antibacterial sulfonamides and chemically related sulfonamides used as diuretics, oral hypoglycemics, and sweetening agents. In addition, crossreactions may occur occasionally with para-amino compounds, such as paraphenylenediamine and para-aminobenzoic acid (PABA).

SULFANILAMIDE

The topical administration of this older sulfonamide preparation has largely been discarded. Exposure to sulfanilamide may still take place, however, from topical application of the compounds shown in Table 12.15.

Table 12-15 Topical Sulfanilamides
AVC Cream and Suppositories (Merrell Dow)
Vagimide Cream (Legere)
Vaginal Sulfa Suppositories (Schein)

In certain European countries, mafenide acetate (Sulfamylon Acetate Cream) (4-homosulfanilamide) is used particularly for burns. Bandmann and Breit[96] reported that 6.4% of the men and 5.4% of the women had positive patch tests to 10% mafenide, a popular antibiotic in Germany. Yaffee and Dressler[97] studied 400 patients treated with mafenide; although the incidence of skin complications was 9.5%, none of the 11 patients had positive patch test reactions to mafenide.

Velasco and Africk[98] reported three patients who developed an eruption at the site of application. All three reacted to mafenide acetate 8.5% and to mafenide hydrochloride 5%, but crossreactions to sulfanilamide 8.5% or to a mixture containing sulfadiazine, sulfamerazine, and sulfamethazine did not occur.

It is of interest to note that they believe that the critical antigenic site of the mafenide molecule is the methyl group in the para position.

The various topical sulfonamides shown in Tables 12.16 to 12.20 may all crossreact with one another. Because patch testing to one sulfonamide, however, does not necessarily detect sensitivity to the whole group, the specific sulfonamide that the patient has used should be used for patch test purposes.

Table 12-16 Topical Sulfabenzamides
Sultrin Triple Sulfa Cream (Ortho Pharmaceutical)
Triple Sulfa Vaginal Cream (Schein)
Trysul Cream (Savage)

Table 12-17 Topical Sulfacetamides
Sultrin Triple Sulfa Cream (Ortho)
Triple Sulfa Vaginal Cream (Schein)
Trysul Cream (Savage)

Sulzberger and colleagues[99] showed that prolonged use of topical sulfonamides can readily cause allergic sensitization. Gottschalk and Stone[100] reported a case of Stevens-Johnson syndrome from an ophthalmic sulfonamide preparation.

Table 12-18 N'-Acetylsulfanilamide_ (Sulfacetamide Sodium)
Sodium Sulamyd Ophthalmic Solution and Ointment (Schering)

SODIUM FUSIDATE

Sensitization to this antibiotic used abroad may occur from its use on stasis ulcers.[101,102] De Groot[103] reported a patient who had used an ointment employing sodium fusidate on a stasis ulcer with resulting superimposed allergic contact

Table 12-19 Sulfisoxazole
Cantri Vaginal Cream (Hauck)
Koro-Sulf Vaginal Cream (Youngs)
Vagilia Cream and Suppositories (Lemmon)

dermatitis. Positive patch tests to the ointment and sodium fusidate 1% in petrolatum were obtained. Sodium fusidate at 0.5% in petrolatum was used to diagnose a case caused by 2% Fucidin cream.[104] This drug is used widely in Europe, but not as yet in the United States.

Table 12-20 Sulfisoxazole Diolamine
Gantrisin Ophthalmic Ointment/Solution (Roche)

SYSTEMIC CONTACT DERMATITIS FROM SULFONAMIDE DRUGS

Topical sensitization to a sulfonamide compound may engender a systemic contact dermatitis when the following sulfonamide compounds are administered:

1. sulfonamide diuretics (Table 12.21)
2. sulfonamide oral hypoglycemic agents (Table 12.22)

Table 12-21 Sulfonamide Diuretics
Bendroflumethiazide (Naturetin)
Benzthiazide (Exna)
Chlorothiazide (Diuril)
Cyclothiazide (Anhydron)
Hydrochlorothiazide (Esidrix, Hydrodiuril, Oretic)
Hydroflumethiazide (Saluron)
Polythiazide (Renese)
Trichlormethiazide (Naqua)

3. sulfonamide sweetening agents (Table 12.23)

Fisher[105] has reported that many adult diabetics receive oral "para-amino" hypoglycemic sulfonyl urea drugs, such as Orinase and Diabinese. These diabetic patients may become sensitized to widely used topical para-amino compounds, such as hair dyes, particularly paraphenylenediamine, sunscreens containing PABA or its esters, and local anesthetics, such as benzocaine. In addition, sensitization to the sulfanilamide compounds poses the threat of a systemic contact dermatitis to the ingestion of the closely related antidiabetic drugs. Thus, a diabetic person sensitized to the topical vaginal sulfanilamide cream acquired a systemic contact dermatitis from the administration of Orinase, an oral antidiabetic compound.

Angelini and Meneghini[106] reported that a group of 34 patients who have contact allergy to para-amino compounds (sulfanilamide, paraphenylenediamine, and benzocaine) underwent a series of peroral tests using structurally related substances, sulfonyl ureas (carbuta-

Table 12-22 Sulfonamide Oral Hypoglycemic Agents
Carbutamide (Nadisan)*
Diabinese (Chlorpropamide)
Orinase (Tolbutamide)

*Still used in Europe.

mide, tolbutamide, and chlorpropamide), diaminodiphenyl sulfone, saccharin, and salicylazo-sulfapyridine. They found that these sulfonyl urea drugs given orally

Table 12-23 Sulfonamide Sweetening Agents
Calcium Cyclamate
Saccharin
Sodium Cyclamate
Sucaryl
Sweeta

produced a widespread dermatitis in 11 subjects who have contact sensitivity to sulfanilamide, but not in those sensitized to paraphenylenediamine and benzocaine.

The positive results in 11 of 34 inpatients who reacted were manifest as follows: (a) itching in all 11 patients; (b) the reappearance of erythema and vesicles at the site of the primary erythema and vesicles at the site of the primary contact dermatitis in 6 patients; and (c) the relapse of the primary contact dermatitis with a moderate secondary vesicular eruption, together with a reactivation of the patch test reaction in 5 patients.

The provocative oral tests were considered positive when at least one of the following was produced: pruritus with recurrence of the primary dermatitis, spread of eczematous lesions, and reactivation of the patch test reactions.

Angelini and Meneghini[106] state that none of the patients who were sensitized to sulfanilamide, paraphenylenediamine, or benzocaine reacted to the ingestion of saccharin. Although the sweetening agents shown in Table 12.23 are all sulfanilamide compounds, there are as yet no reports of "systemic" contact dermatitis in individuals using these agents who have been sensitized to topically applied para-amino compounds.

Acetarsone

Vaginal treatment for trichomonal vaginitis with acetarsone caused vulval and inner thigh urticaria and dermatitis.[107] Acetarsone is also known as acetarsol, acetphenarsine, and [3-(acetylamino)-4-hydroxyphenyl]-arsonic acid. It also can be found in toothpaste, mouthwashes, and treatments for proctitis.

Metronidazole

Facial contact dermatitis has been reported from 1% metronidazole gel.[108] This is chemically an imidazole. Although crossreaction with imidazoles commonly used as antifungals has not been reported, it is a potential issue for this widely used rosacea therapy.

Quinolone

A drug eruption due to norfloxacin presented with a genitocrural toxicoderma that resembled the baboon syndrome.[109] The quinoline mix patch test commonly included in European screening series of patch test materials was positive and resulted in a recall dermatitis in the genitocrural area 1 month after the initial rash had cleared. Because norfloxacin is a quinolone antibiotic, it may be possible to screen for this allergy with the quinoline mix.

Cloxyquin

Cloxyquin, which is closely related to clioquinol, caused dermatitis confirmed with a 5% patch test concentration.[110] The patient also reacted to clioquinol, and it was not certain whether induction of allergy came from the former or the later.

Virginiamycin (Staphlomycin), Stapolidex, and Pristinamycin (Stapyocine)

Baes[111] reported that a man sensitized to virginiamycin in a topical preparation took one tablet of pristinamycin and 4 hours later had an anaphylactic reaction with stupor, urticaria, and vomiting. Patch tests with virginiamycin, pristinamycin, and factors M and IIa, each 1% in petrolatum, were all positive. He developed transient edema of his eyes and lips and wheals adjacent to a positive patch test.

Pristinamycin, like virginiamycin, contains two fractions (Ia and IIa). Chemically, both antibiotics are very closely related, and all patients sensitized by virginiamycin have reacted to pristinamycin.

Bleumink and Nater[112,113] and Lachapelle and Lamy[114] also reported allergic contact dermatitis from these antibiotics when used for burns and other inflammatory dermatoses. Tennstedt and colleagues[115] state that these antibiotics are used as a food additive for pigs and poultry and pose an occupational hazard for individuals dispensing such feed.

Rifamycin

Three cases of contact dermatitis due to rifamycin occurred in patients using it to treat leg ulcers. A 2.5% concentration in petrolatum was used for patch testing.[116]

Kitasamycin and Midecamycin

Kitasamycin is a macrolide antibiotic from *Streptomyces ketasatoensis* and very similar to midecamycin from *S. mycarofaciens*. Occupational exposure to large quantities of dust caused an airborne allergic contact dermatitis. No co-reactions were observed to either erythromycin or triolendomycin.[117]

Mupirocin

Mupirocin, a very rare sensitizer, has caused contact dermatitis when applied to leg ulcers.[118] The reaction was confirmed to be due to the active ingredient in Bactroban by patch testing with calcium mupirocin—free base 10% in ointment base with a negative reaction to the ointment alone.

Topical Antifungal Agents

TOLNAFTATE (TINACTIN)

Gellin and colleagues,[119] reporting the first case of delayed hypersensitivity to Tinactin, stated that no other instances of tolaftate sensitivity have been reported in the past literature despite its use by several million persons in the past decade. Soon after, Emmett and Marrs[120] reported a similar case.

HALOPROGIN (HALOTEX)

Rudolph[121] described a case of allergic contact dermatitis from Halotex. Moss[122] and Berlin and Miller[123] state that ethyl sebacate, a solubilizer in both the cream and the lotion formulations of haloprogin, has caused contact dermatitis.

DESENEX OINTMENT

This "older" antifungal agent containing undecylenic acid rarely irritates or sensitizes. However, undecylenic acid used to treat onychomycosis produced allergic contact dermatitis confirmed by patch testing with 4% in petrolatum.[124]

CLOTRIMAZOLE

Sensitization by a connubial exposure was assumed to have occurred due to intravaginal clotrimazole used by the wife of a 35-year-old man.[125] When he was instructed to use topical clotrimazole at the same time that his wife was retreated intravaginally, a genital dermatitis appeared. No crossreaction was seen to miconazole, econazole, ketoconazole, bifonazole, or isoconazole.

A man who was known to have used only one imidazole antifungal, clotrimazole, was found to be allergic to it.[126] He also reacted to croconazole and itraconazole. Although both clotrimazole and croconazole are phenylmethyl imidazoles, itraconazole is a triazole.

SERTACONAZOLE

Sertaconazole is an imidazole used topically in Spain. Patch tests 1% and 5% in petrolatum were positive in a 26-year-old man who developed contact dermatitis from use of this product on his hand.[127] Crossreactivity with micronazole and econazole were seen but not to seven other closely related imidazoles.

CROCONAZOLE

Croconazole is promoted for both antifungal and anti-inflammatory properties. It is a phenoxyethyl imidazole derivative, but it has sensitized in as little as 4 weeks of use.[128] It has a distinct structure and does not crossreact with clotrimazole or bifonazole.

LANOCONAZOLE

A new member of the imidazole family introduced into Japan caused contact dermatitis within 1 month of use on the feet of a 79-year-old man.[129] The agent in this case was lanoconazole, and a 20% concentration in petrolatum was used to confirm the sensitivity. In a second report of lanoconazole, no crossreactivity to vinyl imidazoles such as croconazole and neticonazole was observed.[130] Lanoconazole and neticonazole ointment have caused at least 10 cases of contact dermatitis each in Japan. These are vinyl imidazoles and used to treat dermatophyte infections. Patch tests at 1% of both are adequate to detect sensitization. Crossreactions are not common, but Umebayashi and Ito reported a patient who was initially positive to lanoconazole and negative to neticonazole, but after a few months of use he became sensitive to neticonazole as well.[131]

NETICONAZOLE

The vinyl imidazole, neticonazole, caused contact dermatitis of the feet after 6 months of use.[132] This patient also reacted to econazole and sulconazole.

IMIDAZOLE DERIVATIVES

These antifungal agents include clotrimazole (Lotrimin) (Table 12.24), which Roller[133] reported caused an allergic reaction with a positive reaction to 1% in methyl ethyl ketone. Clotrimazole is present in Gyne-Lotrimin Vaginal Cream and Mycelex Cream and Solution, as well as Lotrimin AF.

Degreef and Verhoeve[134] reported one allergic reaction and many irritant reactions to Micatin. Such irritant reactions are most likely to occur when Micatin is applied to moist, intertriginous areas.[135]

The newer topical imidazole antifungals may crossreact. Two cases of contact dermatitis due to topical ketoconazole were both found to crossreact to miconazole and sulconazole (all tested at 1% in ethanol).[136] Baes[137] reported a pattern of crossreactivity among antifungals that were β-substituted 1-phenethyl imidazoles with an ortho-chlorine substitution and dubbed this "ortho-chloro crossreactivity." The group of antifungal agents includes isoconazole, tioconazole, oxiconazole, and miconazole. The non-β-substituted 1-phenethyl imidazoles include econazole, sulconazole, enilconazole, and ketoconazole.[138] Machet and colleagues[138] observed that crossreactions within groups were common (see Table 12.25), but crossreactions between groups occurred less frequently. Marren and Powell[139] reviewed 43 published cases of allergic contact dermatitis due to imidazoles from 1974 to 1992 and found 34 reports of crossreactions to other imidazoles. Their own case of tioconazole allergy crossreacted to ketoconazole but not miconazole, sulconazole, or clotrimazole. Tioconazole used on a paronychia led to contact dermatitis but without crossreactions to other imidazoles,[140] but Stubb and colleagues[141] found that 9 of 14 patients who were allergic to tioconazole crossreacted with

Table 12-24 Imidazole Classes

2,4-Dichlorophenylethyl imidazole derivatives	Chemically less similar imidazoles
Miconazole	Ketoconazole
Isoconazole	Clotrimazole
Tioconazole	
Oxiconazole	
Sulconazole	
Econazole	
Enilconazole	

Table 12-25 Antibiotic Patch Test Series

Ampicillin, 5% aq sol
Bacitracin, 20% in pet
Chloramphenicol, 5% in pet
Clindamycin, 1% aq
Erythromycin, 5% in pet
Furacin, 0.2% in pet
Garamycin (Gentamicin), 20% in pet
Lincomycin, 1% aq
Mafenide, 5% in pet
Neomycin, 20% in pet
Nystatin, 100,000 units/mL in alcohol
Penicillin, 100,000 units/mL
Polymyxin B, 3% in pet
Sodium fusidate, 2% in pet
Streptomycin, 2.5% aq sol
Sulfanilamide, 5% in pet
Tetracycline, 5% in pet
Tobramycin, 20% in pet

clotrimazole, econazole, miconazole, and ketoconazole. The introduction of a 28% tioconazole lotion for nail fungus was suggested as the cause for most of the recent case reports.[141] Patch testing with commercial products has been said to be more satisfactory than breakdown of the formulas.[138]

As an example of the somewhat unpredictable nature of crossreactions, Jones and Kennedy[142] reported a tioconazole-sensitive onychomycosis patient who crossreacted to ketoconazole but not miconazole, clotrimazole, or sulconazole. The pattern that has emerged does not allow for good generalizations about crossreactions, even though the work of Baes[137] and Marren and Powell[139] attempted to place this on a chemical conceptual framework. Instead, the emerging pattern seems idiosyncratic.

Dooms-Goossens and colleagues[143] have reviewed the literature and their experience with 15 cases of imidazole contact dermatitis with an eye toward making sense of the crossreaction patterns. They were able to identify three common patterns of crossreactivity. Isoconazole, miconazole, and econazole commonly are linked, as are sulconazole, miconazole, and econazole; the third linkage was isoconazole and tioconazole. This can be remembered as I-ME, S-ME, IT. Patients with these sensitivities can be treated with nonimidazoles or alternatively with ketoconazole, clotrimazole, bifonazole, or flutrimazole.

Imidazole Intermediate

The production of azathioprine has caused occupational contact dermatitis to the finished compound, but Jolanki and colleagues[144] reported a patient who manufactured azathioprine but was sensitive to an intermediate rather than the final product. The intermediate was 5-chloro-1-methyl-4-nitroimidazole. This patient showed sensitivity to other imidazoles commonly used to treat fungal infections including tioconazole, econazole, and miconazole.

Naftifine

The allylamine antifungal, naftifine, has caused contact dermatitis.[145] Because the risk of sensitization is estimated to be 1 in 100,000, the frequency of case reports makes this estimate suspect. Some have suggested that it has greater sensitizing potential than the imidazoles.

Amorolfine

Amorolfine 0.5 cream is marketed in Japan as an antimycotic and has caused contact dermatitis when applied to the leg of a 29-year-old woman.[146] A patch test concentration of 0.25% and 0.5% yielded positive results in the patient and negative results in 30 controls.

NIFURATEL

Corazza and colleagues[147] reported a case of vulvar contact dermatitis caused by a vaginal cream containing nifuratel. This substance, N-(5-nitro-2-furfurilidene)3-amino-5-methyl-mercaptom ethyl-2-oxazolidone, is considered both antimycotic and antitrichomonal. It was tested at 1% in acetone. A man whose wife used the product Macmiror complex ointment developed a genital rash through connubial contact.[148] Corazza and colleagues[147] cite other cases.

Antiviral Topical Agents

IDOXURIDINE (5-IODO-2-DEOXYURIDINE)

Idoxuridine, used widely for herpes simplex, is sold under the names Herplex, Stoxil, Dendrid, Emanil, Iducher, and Iduviran. Europeans or those traveling abroad may have used idoxuridine as Herpid (Britain), Iduridin (Denmark), or Zostrum and Viruquent (Germany).

Many instances of sensitivity occur from its use, particularly in genital herpes, but also in its use as eyedrops.[149–156]

Crossreactions may occur with pyrimidine analogues, such as trifluridine (trifluorothymidine) eyedrops.[157] Crossreactions, however, do not occur with 5-FU, which also has a pyrimidine structure but is a 5-fluorinated compound.[151] Trifluoridine eyedrops for herpetic eye infection sensitized two patients, and patch tests at 5% and 10% petrolatum were diagnostic.[158]

Amon and colleagues[151] reported that idoxuridine has been used for many years in the treatment of herpes simplex infections of the eye. Ophthalmologists have noted occasional conjunctival and corneal-irritant reactions, but no true delayed cutaneous hypersensitivity has been verified. Amon and colleagues[151] studied four cases of allergic contact dermatitis from idoxuridine, sensitized by both eye and skin applications. Crossreactivity to brominated and chlorinated, but not fluorinated, pyrimidine analogues was noted.

TROMANTADINE HYDROCHLORIDE

This synthetic antiviral compound, unrelated to idoxuridine, is used abroad in the form of Viru-Merz ointment for topical treatment of herpes simplex. Several instances of allergic sensitization have been reported.[159–161]

In the search for a "cure" for herpes, several Americans used this agent, one of whom acquired an allergic contact dermatitis from its use.

Tromantadine is derived from amantadine, with which it may crossreact. A 10% petrolatum concentration was used to diagnose a patient sensitized by Viruserol.[162]

ACYCLOVIR

Topical 5% acyclovir ointment (Zovirax) has been reported to cause contact dermatitis. Concentrations of this 9-[(2-hydroxyethoxy) methyl] guanine used for patch testing include 1%, 3%, and 5% in petrolatum[163] and 5% aqueous.[164]

Use of Zovirax cream produced cheilitis on sun exposure initially confused with recurrent herpes labialis.[165] Photopatch tests with 9 J of UVA light and the Zivirax cream were positive, but testing with the individual ingredients proved negative (compound allergy). Topical use of acyclovir on a herpetic lesion was followed by oral treatment with valacyclovir which caused a symmetrical eruption of the face, trunk, and extremities. Subsequent topical acyclovir use caused an eczematous reaction locally and an exanthema on the upper body. Patch test to 1% petrolatum and aqueous acyclovir and valacyclovir were positive as was a 20% concentration of ganciclovir aqueous. Famcyclovir was negative on patch testing at 20% and "as is" in both vehicles, but on oral administration of famcyclovir an eruption of the upper lip and upper body occurred.[166]

ANTIMICROBIAL COATINGS

An antimicrobial coating on a desk mat caused dermatitis of the forearms in a worker, and the substance was found to be 2,3,5,6-tertrchloro-4(methylsulfonyl)pyridine or TCMSP, which is tested at 10% in olive oil. TCMSP is also used in paints and adhesives, providing other environmental sources of exposure.[167]

References

1. Fisher AA, Adams RM. Alternative for sensitizing neomycin topical medicaments. Cutis 1981;28:491.

2. Fisher AA. Prevention of contact dermatitis. NY State J Med 1978;78:1739.

3. Wereide K. Neomycin sensitivity in atopic dermatitis and other eczematous conditions. Acta Derm Venereol (Stockh) 1970;50:114.

4. Patrick J, Panzer JD, Derbes VJ. Neomycin sensitivity in the normal (nonatopic) individual. Arch Dermatol 1970;102:32.

5. Leyden JJ, Kligman AM. Contact dermatitis to neomycin sulfate. JAMA 1979;242:1276.

6. Prystowsky SD, Nonomura JH, Smith MS, Allen AM. Allergic hypersensitivity to neomycin: relationship between patch test reactions and "use" tests. Arch Dermatol 1979;115:713.

7. Hannuksela M, Kousa M, Pinla V. Allergy to ingredients of vehicles. Contact Dermatitis 1976;2:105.

8. Fisher AA, Pascher F, Kanof NB. Allergic contact dermatitis due to ingredients of vehicles: a "vehicle tray" for patch testing. Arch Dermatol 1971;104:286.

9. Hjorth N, Thomsen K. Differences in the sensitizing capacity of neomycin in creams and in ointments. Br J Dermatol 1968;80:163.

10. Pirila V, Pirila L. Sensitization to the neomycin group of antibiotics: patterns of cross sensitivity as a function of polyvalent sensitization to different portions of the neomycin molecule. Acta Derm Venereol (Stockh) 1966;46:489.

11. Chung CW, Carson TR. Sensitization potentials and immunologic specificities of neomycins. J Invest Dermatol 1975;64:158.

12. Forstrom L, Pirila V, Pirila L. Cross-sensitivity within the neomycin group of antibiotics. Acta Derm Venereol (Stockh) 1979;59(Suppl):67.

13. Schorr WF, Ridgway HB. Tobramycin-neomycin cross-sensitivity. Contact Dermatitis 1977;3:133.

14. Menendez-Ramos F, Llamas Martin C, Zarco Olivo J, et al. Allergic contact dermatitis from tobramycin. Contact Dermatitis 1990;22:305.

15. Ekelund AG, Möller H. Oral provocation in eczematous contact allergy to neomycin and hydroxyquinolines. Acta Derm Venereol (Stockh) 1969;49:422.

16. Panzer JD, Epstein WL. Percutaneous absorption following topical application of neomycin. Arch Dermatol 1970;102:536.

17. Pirila V, Rouhunkosky S. On sensitivity to neomycin and bacitracin. Acta Derm Venereol (Stockh) 1959;39:470.

18. Bjorkner B, Möller H. Bacitracin: a cutaneous allergen and histamine liberator. Acta Derm Venereol (Stockh) 1973;53:487.

19. Binnick AN, Clendenning WE. Bacitracin contact dermatitis. Contact Dermatitis 1978;4:180.

20. Epstein S, Wenzel F. Cross-sensitivity to various "mycins." Arch Dermatol 1962;86:183.

21. Pirila V, Rantanen AV. Root canal treatment with bacitracin-neomycin as cause of flare-up of allergic eczema. Oral Surg 1960;13:589.

22. van Ketel WG. Polymixine 8-sulfate and bacitracin. Contact Dermatitis Newsletter 1974;15:445.

23. Dadagian AJ, Hicks JJ, Ordonez GE, Glassman JM. Treatment of otitis externa: a controlled bacteriological-clinical evaluation. Curr Ther Res 1974;16:431.

24. Jenkins BH. Simplified approach to otitis externa. Arch Otolaryngol 1963;77:442.

25. Kremer WF. Management of external otitis. West J Med 1961;2:15.

26. Fisher AA. Contact dermatitis. 3rd ed. Philadelphia: Lea & Febiger, 1986.

27. Nom MS. Eyelid ointment penetration into the conjunctival sac. Acta Ophthalmol 1972;50:206.

28. Nagreh DS. Contact dermatitis from proprietary preparations in Malaysia. Int J Dermatol 1976;15:34.

29. Girard JP. Recurrent angioneurotic oedema and contact dermatitis due to penicillin. Contact Dermatitis 1978;4:309.

30. Hjorth N. Occupational dermatitis among veterinary surgeons caused by penethamate (benzyl penicillin-beta-diethylaminoethyl ester). Berufs-Dermatosen 1967;15:163.

31. Blanton WB, Blanton FM. Unusual penicillin hypersensitiveness. J Allergy 1953;24:405.

32. Valsecchi R, Serra M, Pansera B, et al. Patch testing in adverse drug reactions to penicillin and cephalosporin. Contact Dermatitis 1981;7:158.

33. Lisi P, Stingeni L, Assalve D, et al. Skin tests in the diagnosis of eruptions caused by betalactams. Contact Dermatitis 1997;37:151.

34. Vickers HR, Bagratuni L, Alexander S. Dermatitis caused by penicillin milk. Lancet 1958;61:351.

35. Gamboa P, Jauregui I, Urrutia I. Occupational sensitization to aminopenicillins with oral tolerance to penicillin V. Contact Dermatitis 1995;32:48.

36. Schulz KH, Schopf E, Wex O. Allergische Berufsekzeme durch Ampicillin. Berufs-Dermatosen 1970;18:132.

37. Gamboa P, Jauregui I, Urrutia I, et al. Contact sensitization to cloxacillin with oral tolerance to other beta-lactam antibiotics. Contact Dermatitis 1996;34:75.

38. Strauss MJ, Warring FC. Contact dermatitis from streptomycin. J Invest Dermatol 1947;9:3.

39. Wilson HTH. Streptomycin dermatitis in nurses. Br Med J 1958;1:1378.

40. Adams RM. Occupational skin disease. New York: Grune & Stratton, 1983:367.

41. Filipe P, Almeida RS, Rodrigo FG. Occupational allergic contact dermatitis from cephalosporins. Contact Dermatitis 1996;34:226.

42. Garcia-Bravo B, Gines E, Russo F. Occupational contact dermatitis from ceftiofur sodium. Contact Dermatitis 1995;33:62.

43. Comaish JS, Cunliffe WJ. Absorption of drugs from varicose ulcers: a cause of anaphylaxis. Br J Clin Pract 1967;21:97.

44. Roupe G, Strannegard O. Anaphylactic shock elicited by topical administration of bacitracin. Arch Dermatol 1969;100:450.

45. Farley M, Pak H, Carregal V, et al. Anaphylaxis to topically applied bacitracin. Am J Contact Dermat 1995;6:28.

46. Zaki I, Shall L, Dalziel KL. Bacitracin: a significant sensitizer in leg ulcer patients? Contact Dermatitis 1994;31:92.

47. Möller H. Eczematous contact allergy to oxytetracycline and polymyxin B. Contact Dermatitis 1970;2:289.

48. Pirila V, Hirvonen ML, Rouhunkosh S. The pattern of cross-sensitivity to neomycin: secondary sensitization to gentamicin. Dermatologica 1968;236:321.

49. Bandmann H-J, Mutzek E. Contact allergy to gentamycin sulfate. Contact Dermatitis Newsletter 1973;13:371.

50. Braun W, Schutz R. Beitrag zur Gentamycin Allergie. Hautarzt 1969;20:108.

51. Schorr WF, Wenzel FJ, Hededus SI. Cross-sensitivity and aminoglycoside antibiotics. Arch Dermatol 1973;107:533.

52. Lynfield YL. Allergic contact sensitization to gentamicin. NY State J Med 1970;70:2235.

53. Drake TE. Reaction to gentamicin sulfate cream [Letter]. Arch Dermatol 1974;110:638.

54. Michel M, Dompmartin A, Szczurko C, et al. Eczematous-like drug eruption induced by synergistins. Contact Dermatitis 1996;34:86.

55. Coskey RJ. Contact dermatitis due to clindamycin [Letter]. Arch Dermatol 1978;114:446.

56. De Groot AC. Contact allergy to clindamycin. Contact Dermatitis 1982;8:428.

57. Conde-Salazar L, Guimaraens D, Romero LV, et al. Contact dermatitis from clindamycin. Contact Dermatitis 1983;9:225.

58. Yokoyama R, E Mizuno, M Takeuchi, et al. Contact dermatitis due to clindamycin. Contact Dermatitis 1991;25:125.

59. Becker LE, Bergstresser PR, Whiting DA, et al. Topical clindamycin therapy for acne vulgaris: a cooperative clinical study. Arch Dermatol 1981;217:482.

60. Eady EA, Holland KT, Cunliffe WJ. Topical antibiotics in acne therapy. J Am Acad Dermatol 1981;5:455.

61. Vejlstrup E, Menne T. Contact dermatitis from clindamycin. Contact Dermatitis 1995;32:110.

62. Feingold DS, Chen WC, Chou DL, Chang TW. Induction of colitis in hamsters by topical application of antibiotics. Arch Dermatol 1979;115:580.

63. Milstone EB, McDonald AJ, Scholhamer CE Jr. Pseudomembranous colitis after topical application of clindamycin. Arch Dermatol 1991;117:154.

64. Voron DA. Systemic absorption of topical clindamycin [Letter]. Arch Dermatol 1978;114:798.

65. Tedesco FJ, Barton RW, Alpers DH. Clindamycin-associated colitis: a prospective study. Ann Intern Med 1974;81:429.

66. Fisher AA. The safety of topical erythromycin. Contact Dermatitis 1976;2:43.

67. Vilaplana J, Romaguera C, Grimalt F. Contact dermatitis from lincomycin and spectinomycin in chicken vaccinators. Contact Dermatitis 1991;24:225.

68. Lombardi P, Campolmo P, Spallanzani P, Settoli A. Delayed hypersensitivity to erythromycin. Contact Dermatitis 1982;8:416.

69. van Ketel WG. Immediate and delayed-type allergy to erythromycin. Contact Dermatitis 1976;2:363.

70. Fernandez Redondo V, Casas L, Taboada M, Toribio J. Systemic contact dermatitis from erythromycin. Contact Dermatitis 1994;30:43.

71. Schwank R, Jirasek L. Contact allergy to chloramphenicol with special reference to group sensitization. Hautarzt 1963;14:24.

72. Palacios J, Nemuth MG, Blaylock WK. Lack of cross sensitization between 2,4- dinitrochlorobenzene and chloramphenicol. South Med J 1968;61:243.

73. Enksen K. Cross allergy between paranitro compounds with special reference to DNCB and chloramphenicol. Contact Dermatitis 1978;4:29.

74. Rudzki E, Grzywa Z, Maciejowska E. Drug reaction with positive patch test reaction to chloramphenicol. Contact Dermatitis 1976;2:181.

75. Kozakova M. Sub-shock state brought on by epidermic test for chloramphenicol (in Slovak; author's translation). Cesk Dermatol 1976;52:82.

76. Bandmann N-J. Sind Chloramphenikol-haltige extelna kontraindiziert. Hautarzt 1972;23:145.

77. Milkowski S. Contact conjunctivitis following local application of chloramphenicol. Wiad Lek 1971;24:695.

78. Le Coz C-J, Santinelli F. Facial contact dermatitis from chloramphenicol with cross-sensitivity to thiamphenicol. Contact Dermatitis 1998;38:108.

79. Wereide K. Sensitivity to azidamphenicol. Contact Dermatitis 1975;1:271.

80. Fontanot S. Tetracycline compounds and responsibility for allergic dermatitis after local use. G Ital Dermatol Venereol 1978;113:397.

81. Bojs G, Möller H. Eczematous contact allergy to oxytetracycline with cross-sensitivity to other tetracyclines. Berufs-Dermatosen 1974;22:202.

82. Calnan CD. Chlortetracycline sensitivity. Contact Dermatitis Newsletter 1967;1:16.

83. Standlee TL. Facial fluorescence. Schoch Lett 1979;29:7.

84. Wasilewski C Jr. Allergic contact dermatitis from nystatin. Arch Dermatol 1970;102:216.

85. Coskey RJ. Contact dermatitis due to nystatin. Arch Dermatol 1971;103:228.

86. Coskey RJ. Contact dermatitis due to multiple corticosteroid creams. Arch Dermatol 1978;114:115.

87. Foussereau J, Liman-Mestiri S, Khochnevis A, Basset A. L'Allergie a l'association therapeutique locale nystatine, neomycine et acetonide de triamcinolone. Bull Soc Fr Dermatol Syphilol 1971;78:457.

88. Hull PR, de Beer HA. Topical nitrofurazone, a potent sensitizer of the skin and mucosae. South Afr Med J 1977;52:189.

89. Bleumink E, te Lintum JC, Nater JP. Kontaktallergie durch Nitrohrazon (Furacin) und Nihrprazin (carohr). Hautarzt 1974;25:_403.

90. Caplan RM. Cutaneous hazards posed by agricultural chemicals. J Iowa Med Soc 1969;59:295.

91. Neldner KH. Contact dermatitis from animal feed additives. Arch Dermatol 1972;106:722.

92. Fisher AA. Immediate and delayed allergic contact reactions to polyethylene glycol. Contact Dermatitis 1978;4:135.

93. Braun W. Contact allergies to polyethylene glycols. Z Haut Geschlectskr 1969;44:385.

94. Kiec-Swierczynska M, Krecisz B. Occupational contact allergy to nifuroxazide simulating prurigo nodularis. Contact Dermatitis 1998;39:93.

95. Sanchez-Perez J, Cordoba S, del Rio MJ, Garcia-Dies A. Allergic contact dermatitis from furaltadone in eardrops. Contact Dermatitis 1999;40:222.

96. Bandmann HJ, Breit R. Die medikamentose allergische kontaktdermatitis. Internist 1974;15:47.

97. Yaffee HS, Dressler DP. Topical application of mafenide acetate: its association with erythema multiforme and cutaneous reactions. Arch Dermatol 1969;100:277.

98. Velasco JE, Africk JA. Contact dermatitis to mafenide acetate. Arch Dermatol 1971;103:61.

99. Sulzberger MD, Kanoff A, Baer RL, et al. Sensitization by topical application of sulfonamide. J Allergy 1947;18:92.

100. Gottschalk HR, Stone OJ. Stevens-Johnson syndrome from ophthalmic sulfonamide. Arch Dermatol 1976;112:513.

101. Verbov JL. Sensitivity to sodium fusidate. Contact Dermatitis Newsletter 1970;7:150.

102. Dave VK, Main RA. Contact sensitivity to sodium fusidate. Contact Dermatitis Newsletter 1973;14:398.

103. de Groot AC. Contact allergy to sodium fusidate. Contact Dermatitis 1982;8:429.

104. Baptista A, Barros MA. Contact dermatitis from sodium fusidate. Contact Dermatitis 1990;23:186.

105. Fisher AA. Systemic contact dermatitis from OrinaseTM and DiabineseTM in diabetics with para-amino hypersensitivity. Cutis 1982;29:551.

106. Angelini G, Meneghini CL. Oral tests in contact allergy to para-amino compounds. Contact Dermatitis 1981;7:311.

107. Sasseville D, Carey WD, Singer MI. Generalized contact dermatitis from acetarsone. Contact Dermatitis 1995;33:431.

108. Vincenzi C, Lucente P, Ricci C, Tosti A. Facial contact dermatitis due to metronidazole. Contact Dermatitis 1997;36:116.

109. Silvestre JF, Alfonso R, Moragon M, et al. Systemic contact dermatitis due to norfloxacin with a positive patch test to quinoline mix. Contact Dermatitis 1998;39:83.

110. Wantke F, Gotz M, Jarisch R. Contact dermatitis from cloxyquin. Contact Dermatitis 1995;32:112.

111. Baes H. Allergic contact dermatitis to virginiamycin. Dermatologica 1974;149:231.

112. Bleumink E, Nater JP. Allergic contact dermatitis to virginiamycin. Dermatologica 1972;144:253.

113. Bleumink L, Nater JP. Allergic contact dermatitis to virginiamycin (Staphlomycin) and pristinamycin (Stapyocin). Contact Dermatitis Newsletter 1972;12:337.

114. Lachapelle JM, Lamy F. On allergic contact dermatitis to virginiamycin. Dermatologica 1973;146:320.

115. Tennstedt D, Dumont-Fruytier M, La Chapelle JM. Occupational allergic contact dermatitis to virginiamycin, an antibiotic used as a food additive for pigs and poultry. Contact Dermatitis 1978;4:_133.

116. Guerra L, Adamo F, Venturo M, et al. Contact dermatitis due to rifamycin. Contact Dermatitis 1991;25:328.

117. Dooms-Goossens A, Bedert R, Degreef H, Vandaele M. Airborne allergic contact dermatitis from kitasamycin and midecamycin. Contact Dermatitis 1990;23:118.

118. Eedy DJ. Mupirocin allergy in the setting of venous ulceration. Contact Dermatitis 1995;32:240.

119. Gellin GA, Maibach HI, Wachs GN. Contact allergy to tolnaftate. Arch Dermatol 1972;106:715.

120. Emmett EA, Marrs JM. Allergic contact dermatitis from tolnaftate. Arch Dermatol 1973;108:98.

121. Rudolph RI. Allergic contact dermatitis caused by haloprogin. Arch Dermatol 1975;111:1487.

122. Moss HV. Allergic contact dermatitis due to Halotex solution [Letter]. Arch Dermatol 1974;109:572.

123. Berlin AR, Miller OF. Allergic contact dermatitis from ethyl sebacate in haloprogin cream. Arch Dermatol 1976;112:1563.

124. Anguita JL, Escutia B, Mari JI, et al. Allergic contact dermatitis from undecylenic acid in a commercial antifungal nail solution. Contact Dermatitis 2002;46:109.

125. Valsecchi R, Pansera B, di Landro A, Cainelli T. Connubial contact sensitization to clotrimazole. Contact Dermatitis 1994;30:248.

126. Erdmann S, Hertl M, Merk HF. Contact dermatitis from clotrimazole with positive patch-test reactions also to croconazole and itraconazole. Contact Dermatitis 1999;40:47.

127. Goday JJ, Yanguas I, Aguirre A, et al. Allergic contact dermatitis from sertaconazole with cross-sensitivity to miconazole and econazole. Contact Dermatitis 1995;32:370.

128. Steinmann A, Mayer G, Breit R, Agathos M. Allergic contact dermatitis from croconazole without cross-sensitivity to clotrimazole and bifonazole. Contact Dermatitis 1996;35:255.

129. Nakano R, Miyoshi H, Kanazaki T. Allergic contact dermatitis from lanoconazole. Contact Dermatitis 1996;35:63.

130. Tanaka N, Kawada A, Hiruma M, et al. Contact dermatitis from lanoconazole. Contact Dermatitis 1996;35:256.

131. Umebayashi Y, Ito S. Allergic contact dermatitis due to both lanoconazole and neticonazole ointments. Contact Dermatitis 2001;44:48.

132. Kawada A, Hiruma M, Fujioka A, et al. Contact dermatitis from neticonazole. Contact Dermatitis 1997;36:106.

133. Roller JA. Contact allergy to clotrimazole. Br Med J 1978;2:737.

134. Degreef H, Verhoeve L. Contact dermatitis to micronazole nitrate. Contact Dermatitis 1975;1:269.

135. Wade TR, Jones HE, Artis WA. Irritant and allergic reactions to topically applied Micatin cream. Contact Dermatitis 1979;5:168.

136. Santucci B, Cannistraci C, Cristaudo A, Picardo M. Contact dermatitis from ketoconazole cream. Contact Dermatitis 1992;27:274.

137. Baes H. Contact sensitity to miconazole with othrochloro cross-sensitivity to other imidazoles. (Published erratum appears in Contact Dermatitis 1991;25:79.) Contact Dermatitis 1991;24:89.

138. Machet L, Vaillant L, Muller C, et al. Contact dermatitis and cross-sensitivity from sulconazole nitrate. Contact Dermatitis 1992;26:352.

139. Marren P, Powell S. Contact sensitivity to tioconazole and other imidazoles. Contact Dermatitis 1992;27:129.

140. Brunelli D, Vincenzi C, Morelli R, Tosti A. Contact dermatitis from tioconazole. Contact Dermatitis 1992;27:120.

141. Stubb S, Heikkala H, Reitamo S, et al. Contact allergy to tioconazole. Contact Dermatitis 1992;26:155.

142. Jones SK, Kennedy CT. Contact dermatitis from tioconazole. Contact Dermatitis 1990;22:122.

143. Dooms-Goossens A, Matura M, Drieghe J, Degreef H. Contact allergy to imidazoles used as antimycotic agents. Contact Dermatitis 1995;33:73.

144. Jolanki R, Alanko K, Pfaffli P, et al. Occupational allergic contact dermatitis from 5-chloro-1-methyl-4-nitroimidazole. Contact Dermatitis 1997;36:53.

145. Willa-Craps C, Wyss M, Elsner P. Allergic contact dermatitis from naftifine. Contact Dermatitis 1995;32:369.

146. Kaneko K, Aoki N, Hata M, et al. Allergic contact dermatitis from amorolfine cream. Contact Dermatitis 1997;37:307.

147. Corazza M, Virgili A, Mantovani L. Vulvar contact dermatitis from nifuratel. Contact Dermatitis 1992;27:273.

148. Di Prima TM, De Pasquale R, Nigro MA. Connubial contact dermatitis from nifuratel. Contact Dermatitis 1990;22:117.

149. Lombardi P, Spallanzani P, Giorgini S, Seroli A. Allergic contact dermatitis from idoxuridine. Contact Dermatitis 1982;8:50.

150. Thormann J, Wildenhoff KE. Contact allergy to idoxuridine: sensitization following treatment of herpes zoster. Contact Dermatitis 1980;6:170.

151. Amon RB, Lis AW, Hanifin JM. Allergic contact dermatitis caused by idoxuridine. Arch Dermatol 1975;111:1581.

152. Osmundsen PE. Allergic contact dermatitis from idoxuridine. Contact Dermatitis 1975;1:251.

153. Calnan CD. Contact dermatitis to idoxuridine. Contact Dermatitis 1976;2:58.

154. Calnan CD. Allergy to idoxuridine ointment. Contact Dermatitis 1979;5:194.

155. Reiffers J. Allergy to 5-iodo-29-desoxyuridine. Contact Dermatitis 1981;7:125.

156. Van Ketel WG. Allergy to idoxuridine eyedrops. Contact Dermatitis 1977;3:106.

157. Cirkel PKS, van Ketel WG. Allergic contact dermatitis to trifluorthymidine eyedrops. Contact Dermatitis 1981;7:49.

158. Millan-Parrilla F, de la Cuadra J. Allergic contact dermatitis from trifluoridine in eyedrops. Contact Dermatitis 1990;22:289.

159. Brandao FM, Pecegueiro M. Contact dermatitis to tromantadine hydrochloride. Contact Dermatitis 1982;8:140.

160. Fanta D, Mischer P. Contact dermatitis from tromantadine hydrochloride. Contact Dermatitis 1976;2:282.

161. Mischer P, Fanta D. Das Tomantadin-Kontaktekzem. Hautarzt 1978;29:337.

162. Patruno C, Auricchio L, Mozzillo R, Brunetti B. Allergic contact dermatitis due to tromantadine hydrochloride. Contact Dermatitis 1990;22:187.

163. Valsecchi R, Imberti G, Cainelli T. Contact allergy to acyclovir. Contact Dermatitis 1990;23:372.

164. Goday J, Aguirre A, Ibarra NG, Eizaguirre X. Allergic contact dermatitis from acyclovir. Contact Dermatitis 1991;24:380.

165. Rodriguez-Serna M, Velasco M, Moquel J, et al. Photoallergic contact dermatitis from Zovirax cream. Contact Dermatitis 1999;41:54.

166. Lammintausta K, Makela L, Kalimo K. Rapid systemic valaciclovir reaction subsequent to acyclovir contact allergy. Contact Dermatitis 2001;45:181.

167. Gushi A, Kanekura T, Katahira Y, et al. Contact dermatitis from the antimicrobial coating of a desk mat. Contact Dermatitis 2003;48:347.

CHAPTER 13

ANTIHISTAMINES

EXECUTIVE SUMMARY

Antihistamines are classified by chemical groups as carbon-linked alkylamines, piperazines, nitrogen-linked ethylenediamines, oxygen-linked ethanolamines, phenothiazines, piperidines, and miscellaneous.

Nitrogen-linked ethylenediamines include hydroxyzine, which can crossreact with cetirizine.

Oxygen-linked ethanolamines include diphenhydramine, dimenhydrinate (Dramamine), and clemastine (Tavist), among others. Prominent phenothiazine antihistamines include promethazine (Phenergan) and trimeprazine (Temaril).

Carbon-linked alkylamine antihistamines are chlorpheniramine and brompheniramine, among others.

Examples of piperidine and miscellaneous antihistamines are cyproheptadine and doxepin.

It must be emphasized that, although the *systemic* administration of the antihistamines rarely engenders sensitization, *topical* applications, such as antihistamines, on occasion produce allergic contact sensitivity. Once the patient is sensitized by topical application of the antihistamine, an eczematous contact dermatitis may occur from the antihistamine or from immunochemically related compounds. As a rule, the systemic administration of an antihistamine to which there has been topical sensitization will not only reproduce the original allergic eczematous contact dermatitis but at times will also produce a generalized dermatitis with a resulting exfoliative dermatitis.[1,2] In some instances, "systemic" eczematous contact dermatitis is accompanied by urticarial elements. On rare occasions, systemic administration of an antihistamine can induce allergic hypersensitivity with production of urticaria, morbilliform and scarlatiniform eruptions, erythema multiforme, photosensitivity, and anaphylactic shock. In asthmatic patients, the antihistamine may lead to bronchial obstruction with anaphylactic reactions.

Eruptions from antihistaminic agents appear usually 6 to 12 hours after their ingestion. There may be an incubation period, or dermatitis may appear after ingestion of the first dose. The eruption is usually generalized and explosive. The lesions may resemble any of the acute drug eruptions. Skin tests are of little value in these reactions. The history of dermatitis occurring within 12 hours after the introduction of one of these agents suggests that the antihistamine is the cause of the eruption. Testing by readministering the drug is justifiable only in mild dermatoses and is contraindicated in severe reactions.

Nature and Classification of Antihistamines

For appropriate management of antihistamine dermatitis, knowledge of the nature and the classification of the various antihistamines is necessary. Most antihistamines are basically related at their structural core by a substituted ethylamine group that is also present in the histamine and has the following structure: X-CH$_2$-CH$_2$-N. This portion of the molecule presumably competes with histamine for cell receptors and thus blocks the action of histamine. To this substituted core, different arrangements of atoms can be added to make different antihistamines. X represents the element that links the ethylamine group to the rest of the compound. Depending on the nature of X, oxygen (O), nitrogen (N), or carbon (C), the antihistamine belongs to a specific class.

The two main reasons for becoming familiar with the various groups of antihistamines are the following: (a) It is generally agreed that if any antihistamine is not effective in a particular patient, the rest of the antihistamines in that group are not likely to be as effective as an antihistamine in a different group. This concept of choosing an antihistamine from a new group is one of the reasons certain pharmaceutical companies manufacture two different antihistamine compounds. (b) A patient who is allergic

Table 13-1 Classes of Antihistamines

Carbon-linked alkylamines
Cyclizines (piperazines)
Nitrogen-linked ethylenediamines
Oxygen-linked ethanolamines
Phenothiazine antihistamines
Piperidines
Miscellaneous

Table 13-3 Instructions for Ethylenediamine-Sensitive Patients

Avoid the following injections, tablets, creams, capsules, or suppositories:
1. Aminophylline
2. Antihistamine tablets, capsules, or creams:
   tripelennamine (Pyribenzamine), Histadyl, Fiogesic, Pyma, Hydroxyzine (Atarax, Vistaril), Durrax, and piperazine antihistamines: Fedrazil, Mantadil, Migral, Marezine, Bucladin-S, Bonine Antivert
   Avoid the following creams: Mycotriocet, Pyribenzamine, Surfadil, and Allergan

Avoid the following nose or eye solutions: Prefrin, Privine, and Vasocon-A

to an antihistamine in one group is very likely to also be allergic to every other antihistamine in that particular group. It is, therefore, important that the sensitized patient be informed of which antihistamines must be avoided and which can be used safely.

Table 13.1 lists the various classes of antihistamines. The antihistamines are useful primarily in the control of certain allergic disorders. Their effect in allergic conditions is purely palliative and largely due to the suppression of symptoms attributable to the action of histamine, which is but one of the chemicals released by the antigen-antibody reaction. In addition, they may diminish capillary permeability to substances other than histamine.

Topical antihistamine preparations are used because they are slightly antipruritic and may have a mild local anesthetic effect. Such topical antihistamines, however, are common and potent sensitizers. The use of topical antihistamines should be discouraged. Instead, topical corticosteroids or nonsensitizing local anesthetic preparations free of benzocaine, such as lidocaine (Xylocaine) and pramoxine (Pramosone), may be used to control pruritus.

Nitrogen-Linked Ethylenediamines

Table 13.2 lists the nitrogen-linked ethylenediamine antihistamines. It should be noted that ethylenediamine hydro-

chloride, the parent substance of this group of histamines, a component of aminophylline, and a stabilizer in the popular nystatin-neomycin sulfate-gramicidin-triamcinolone acetonide cream, has become such a common sensitizer that it is included in the "Screening" Patch Test Series of the North American Contact Dermatitis Group. (Nystatin-neomycin sulfate-gramicidin-triamcinolone acetonide *ointment* is free of ethylenediamine hydrochloride.)

Unless the sensitized patient is informed of how to avoid ethylenediamine hydrochloride and related chemicals, the ethylenediamine-sensitive individual is doomed not only to repeated attacks of dermatitis, but also to drug eruptions from the systemic administration of aminophylline and ethylenediamine-related antihistamines and from topical exposure to antihistamines derived from ethylenediamine.[3,4]

The ethylenediamine-sensitive individual should be given the written instructions listed in Table 13.3. The systemic administration of these antihistamines in an ethylenediamine-sensitive individual may cause a previous dermatitis to flare and may, in addition, produce a generalized drug eruption.

It should be emphasized that, fortunately, ethylenediamine hydrochloride does not crossreact with the ubiquitous ethylenediamine tetra-acetate (EDTA).

THE ASTHMATIC PATIENT AND ETHYLENEDIAMINE SENSITIVITY

The following facts must be taken into consideration by the practitioner should an asthmatic patient become sensitized to ethylenediamine hydrochloride:

1. Aminophylline is composed of theophylline and ethylenediamine.
2. Ethylenediamine renders theophylline soluble so that it can be injected.
3. The administration of aminophylline to an ethylenediamine-sensitive individual can produce a severe disabling "systemic" contact dermatitis with generalized exfoliative dermatitis.[5]

Table 13-2 Nitrogen-Linked Ethylenediamine Antihistamines

Trade name	Generic name
Atarax	Hydroxyzine hydrochloride
Fiogesic	Pyrilamine maleate
Histadyl	Methapyrilene hydrochloride
Pyma	Pyrilamine maleate
Pyribenzamine	Tripelennamine hydrochloride
Vistaril (intramuscular)	Hydroxyzine hydrochloride
Vistaril (oral)	Hydroxyzine pamoate

4. Although there are many theophylline medications without ethylenediamine that can be given orally, in an emergency, aminophylline cannot be given intramuscularly or intravenously. Travenol Labs, Inc., Deerfield, IL, has made available intravenous preparations of theophylline that are free of ethylenediamine.

5. Ethylenediamine-free theophylline for intramuscular injection is available as dyphylline (Lufyllin) (Wallace).

INDUSTRIAL DERMATITIS FROM ETHYLENEDIAMINE SENSITIVITY

In industry, ethylenediamine is used in the preparation of dyes, inhibitors, rubber accelerators, fungicides, synthetic waxes, resins, insecticides, and asphalt wetting agents. Industrial exposure, however, rarely leads to sensitization, probably because exposure is usually not prolonged or intimate, and normal rather than abnormal skin is exposed.

EPOXY RESIN DERMATITIS

Certain polyamines, such as triethylenetetramine, triethylenediamine, and ethanolamine, used as amine "curing" agents of "hardeners" in epoxy resin systems, may crossreact with ethylenediamine. Such crossreactions can produce epoxy resin dermatitis in ethylenediamine-sensitive individuals.[6,7]

MACHINE WORKER'S DERMATITIS

Synthetic coolants used in factories producing pistons can produce eruptions on the hands of machine tool operators.[8] In these cases, ethylenediamine sensitivity may be a major cause.[9]

RELATIONSHIP OF HYDROXYZINES TO ETHYLENEDIAMINE

Although the hydroxyzine ethylenediamines Atarax and Vistaril are not usually classified with the ethylenediamine antihistamines, it should be noted that the formula of Atarax (hydroxyzine hydrochloride) is 1-*p*-chlorobenzhydryl-4,2 (2 [2-hydroxyethoxy]ethyl) *diethylenediamine dihydrochloride*. It would be prudent to avoid the use of hydroxyzine antihistamines in individuals with ethylenediamine sensitivity. Dermatitis that worsened after oral hydoxyzine administration proved to be due to the antihistamine. A patch test with 2.5% petrolatum was positive. Because hydroxyzine is an ethylenediamine related material, patch tests to ethylenediamine dihydrochloride are commonly positive. The authors point out that crossreactions to cetirizine have also been reported.[10]

HYDROXYZINE AND CETIRIZINE

Three cases of systemic reactions to hydroxyzine allergy confirmed by patch testing were reported from France[11] In these individuals, there was no crossreactivity to piperazine, ethylenediamine, triethanolamine, dexchlorpheniramine, loratadine, chlorpromazine, mequitazine, terfenadine, and the hydroxyzine derivative cetirizine. A 2% aqueous solution of hydroxyzine was positive. In contrast, the following case shows broad crossreactivity.

A 70-year-old woman developed a morbilliform and urticarial eruption traced to the use of cetirizine.[12] This was confirmed by a positive patch test to cetirizine at 2.5% and 5% in petrolatum. She was also sensitive to ethylenediamine dihydrochloride and diethylenediamine, which is a piperazine. It has been suggested that crossreactions between ethylenediamine and piperazine-based antihistamines are dependent on sensitivity to diethylenediamine, which can be visualized as two molecules of ethylenediamine glued together to make a cyclic structure that is in fact piperazine. Because she was sensitive to not only ethylenediamine but also piperazine and diethylenediamine, it is not surprising that cetirizine, which contains a piperazine ring, was also capable of causing an allergic reaction.

A patient who developed a drug eruption to both cetirizine and hydroxyzine was found to have positive patch tests to 1% ethylenediamine in petrolatum and 1% piperazine in petrolatum as well as reactions to 2.5%, 5%, and 10% cetirizine and 1%, 2.5%, 5%, and 10% hydroxyzine. Cetirizine reactions in this case and 7 others cited by the authors were urticaria. It can be very challenging to differentiate the urticaria that is being treated with cetirizine from the urticaria that is being induced by cetirizine. The lack of a therapeutic benefit to cetirizine administration was considered a clinical clue. The authors also cite 10 additional cases of hydroxyzine allergy that presented as either a fixed drug eruption or a maculopapular eruption.[13]

RELATIONSHIP OF PIPERAZINE (CYCLIZINE) ANTIHISTAMINES TO ETHYLENEDIAMINE

The piperazine (cyclizine) antihistamines are listed in Table 13.4. The piperazine antihistamines, like the

Table 13-4 Piperazine Antihistamines

Trade name	Generic name
Bonine Antivert	Meclizine hydrochloride
Bucladin-S	Buclizine hydrochloride
Fedrazil, Mantadil	Chlorcyclinine hydrochloride
Marezine	Cyclizine hydrochloride
Migral	Cyclizine hydrochloride

hydroxyzines, are related closely to the ethylenediamine antihistamines. It is believed that, because ethylenediamine is on the metabolic pathway of both piperazine and hydroxyzine, it is advisable to avoid the use of piperazine antihistamines in ethylenediamine-sensitive individuals.

Thus, piperazine citrate used for the treatment of pinworms (threadworms) can produce an allergic drug eruption in ethylenediamine-sensitive individuals.[14] Crossreactions can occur in chemists and laboratory technicians who handle both of these chemicals.[15] Price and Hall-Smith[16] reported a patient who was sensitive to ethylenediamine hydrochloride and developed a generalized erythroderma after he took piperazine phosphate for treatment of threadworm infection. The patient had been exposed previously to Triadcortyl Cream, which is an English preparation identical to the original formula Mycolog cream. The original formula of Mycolog cream is only available from generic suppliers, as Mycolog II has been reformulated without ethylenediamine. The original formula is no longer made by Squibb-Westwood.

Oxygen-Linked Ethanolamine Antihistamines

Table 13.5 lists these antihistamines. Of this group of antihistamines, diphenylenediamine hydrochloride has been widely used both systemically and topically for 4 decades. The other ethanolamines are used only systemically.

The incidence of cutaneous reactions to topically applied diphenhydramine is difficult to assess.[17] In one series, 12 of 117 cases of dermatitis medicamentosa seen in England in 1 year were due to a lotion composed of diphenhydramine hydrochloride and calamine.[18] All 12 were confirmed by positive patch tests, although in 10 instances, closed patch tests were positive only when performed on areas that had undergone repeated cellophane-tape strippings.

Table 13-5 Ethanolamine Antihistamines

Trade name	Generic name
Ambenyl	Diphenhydramine hydrochloride
Benadryl	Diphenhydramine hydrochloride
Benylin	Diphenhydramine hydrochloride
Clistin	Carbinoxame maleate
Decapryn	Doxylamine succinate
Diphenadril	Diphenhydramine hydrochloride
Dramamine	Dimenhydrinate
Tavist	Clemastine fumarate

SYSTEMIC "ENDOGENIC" CONTACT DERMATITIS FROM ETHANOLAMINES

Individuals who have become sensitized by topically applied diphenhydramine can acquire a "systemic" eczematous contact dermatitis when diphenhydramine or any of the other ethanolamines listed in Table 13.5 are ingested or injected.

It is not generally realized that dimenhydrinate (Dramamine) is an ethanolamine (the chlorotheophylline salt of the antihistaminic agent diphenhydramine). Dimenhydrinate contains between 53% and 56% diphenhydramine and therefore should not be administered to any individual who has allergic hypersensitivity to the ethanolamine groups of antihistamines.

PHOTOALLERGIC DERMATITIS FROM DIPHENHYDRAMINE

Antihistamine photodermatitis to the *systemic* administration of such ethanolamines as diphenhydramine and carbinoxamine and to topical ethanolamines is rare.[19] Although topical promethazine therapy appears to be a relatively frequent cause of photoallergic contact dermatitis, for years only a single instance of photoallergy induced by topical diphenhydramine therapy was reported.[17] The diagnosis was confirmed by photopatch testing. This diphenhydramine photoallergy appeared to differ from most other forms of photoallergy in that it was elicited by ultraviolet light in the 290- to 320-nm wavelength range (UVB), rather than the more usual 320- to 400-nm range (UVA). This finding may be related to the photochemical properties of diphenhydramine, which absorbs in the UVB, but not in the UVA, the UVB absorption being associated with a distinctive fluorescence.

A case of diphenhydramine photosensitivity with the more customary UVA activation wavelength was reported from Japan.[20] A 1% diphenhydramine in petrolatum patch test irradiated with 4.85 J/cm2 was used to confirm the photoallergy.

Phenothiazines

Although topical phenothiazine antihistamine preparations, such as promethazine hydrochloride (Phenergan) cream, are no longer used in the United States, such topical antihistamine preparations are still widely used in Europe. Individuals who have become sensitized by such topical phenothiazine antihistamines often suffer a flare of the dermatitis when a phenothiazine antihistamine is taken, that is, a "systemic" eczematous contact dermatitis. In addition, many individuals acquire allergic sensitization to various phenothiazine drugs that show crossreactions with the phenothiazine antihistamines. Table 13.6 lists the phenothiazine antihistamine compounds.

PROMETHAZINE HYDROCHLORIDE

This antihistamine is used not only in tablet form but also as suppositories. Proctitis and perianal dermatitis have occurred from the use of such suppositories in sensitized individuals. This antihistamine can also produce phototoxic and photoallergic reactions.[21] In France, where Phenergan cream is used extensively as a topical antipruritic agent, many instances of photocontact dermatitis occur. Photosensitivity seems to be induced primarily by contact exposure to promethazine hydrochloride cream.[22] Systemic administration without topical sensitization does not appear to induce photosensitivity.[23]

CROSSREACTIONS BETWEEN PHENOTHIAZINE ANTIHISTAMINES AND OTHER PHENOTHIAZINE COMPOUNDS

The phenothiazine drugs listed in Table 13.6 are all capable of crossreacting with the phenothiazine antihistamine, and all of these compounds are potential photosensitizers.[24] Often a photoallergic reaction occurs in combination with the allergic eczematous contact dermatitis. The systemic administration of the phenothiazine drugs shown in Table 13.6 may produce an eczematous contact dermatitis medicamentosa in individuals sensitized by such topical exposure. Crossreactions take place readily between phenothiazines and the related antihistamines.[25]

EXPOSURE OF MEDICAL AND NURSING PERSONNEL TO PHENOTHIAZINES

Medical and nursing personnel who inject phenothiazine drugs or who handle phenothiazine tablets that are given to patients, as well as those who come into contact with the compounds in the pharmaceutical industry, readily acquire allergic eczematous contact dermatitis of the hands from such exposure; the dermatitis may flare when a phenothiazine antihistamine is given.[26] Because chlorpromazine, in particular, is excreted almost unchanged in the urine, sensitized nurses and orderlies who handle unwashed linen may experience flares.

EXPOSURE OF VETERINARIANS AND FARMERS TO PHENOTHIAZINES

The same phenothiazines or closely related compounds that are used as psychotropic drugs or as sedatives in humans are used by veterinarians and farmers as insecticides and anthelmintics for animals and birds. Table 13.7 lists some commercial phenothiazine insecticides and "wormers" used by veterinarians. Many individuals in these professions have acquired allergic contact dermatitis, photoallergic reactions, or both by spraying such phenothiazines for insect control or feeding these compounds as wormers. Such individuals must avoid using phenothiazine antihistamines because of the likelihood of producing flares of the phenothiazine dermatitis.

EXPOSURE TO METHYLENE BLUE

Methylene blue is 3,7-bis-(dimethyl-amino) phenozathionium chloride tetramethyl thionin chloride, a phe-

Table 13-7 Phenothiazines Used in Veterinary Medicine	
Anthelmintics	Worm Free Eddie
	Early Bird Wormer
Insecticides	Fly Free Eddie
	Bar-Fly Feed

nothiazine derivative used in various ways, as shown in Table 13.8. The administration of methylene blue urinary antiseptic produced a flare of photodermatitis in one observed individual who had acquired a photosensitivity from a phenothiazine compound.[27]

Table 13-6 Phenothiazine Antihistamines	
Trade name	Generic name
Phenergan	Promethazine
Tacaryl	Methdilazine
Temaril	Trimeprazine
Note: May crossreact with the following phenothiazine drugs:	
Compazine	Prochlorperazine
Stelazine	Trifluoperazine
Temaril	Trimeprazine
Thorazine	Chlorpromazine
Vesprin	Triflupromazine
Veterinary medications such as insecticides and anthelmintics	

Table 13-8 Sources of Exposure to Methylene Blue (a Phenothiazine Dye)
Antidotes for methemoglobinemia and cyanide poisoning
Biologic stains
Blue hair dyes
Photodynamic treatment of herpes
Urinary antiseptics
M-B tablets, Urolene Blue, TRA tablets, Urised

Dilute mixtures of methylene blue, acid violet, and nigrosine are used as a color rinse for gray hair. Such rinses should be used with great care in those who have become sensitized to the phenothiazines.

VARIETIES OF ALLERGIC REACTIONS TO PHENOTHIAZINE COMPOUNDS

Three types of allergic hypersensitivity are seen with the phenothiazine drugs. These reactions are:

1. The classical allergic contact eczematous variety, in which the covered patch test reaction is positive.
2. A photoallergic reaction, in which the covered patch reaction is negative but becomes positive when the patch test site is exposed to sunlight or ultraviolet radiation.[27]
3. A photoallergic reaction in combination with an allergic eczematous contact sensitization, in which the patch test reaction is positive with the phenothiazine derivative alone, but a stronger response is elicited if the site is irradiated with a suberythematous dose of ultraviolet rays or exposed to strong sunlight for 20 minutes. The increase in intensity of an ordinary patch test reaction on exposure to light must be carefully interpreted, because it may be a nonspecific irritating effect.

If possible, controls should be used as on other positive patch test reactions. Whenever an allergen can produce both photoallergic and allergic eczematous contact hypersensitivity, the photoallergic reaction appears to be more intense. At times, phenothiazine, capable of producing photoallergic and ordinary allergic eczematous contact dermatitis, will produce a photoallergic reaction in areas exposed to light, whereas the same concentration of the drug that reaches the skin from systemic administration will not produce a contact dermatitis on covered areas of the body. In many instances, however, both types of reactions occur simultaneously.

A unique feature of photoallergic reactions to the phenothiazines is that the wavelengths that produce the photoallergic reactions are not always identical to those absorbed by the phenothiazine drug. These drugs have a maximal absorption in the ultraviolet wavelengths below 310 nm. Having become photoallergic to them, however, the patient may also react to longer ultraviolet wavelengths and even visible light. This is called "widening of the action spectrum."

The increased sensitivity of the skin to light sometimes persists for months. The patient sensitized to a phenothiazine, therefore, should avoid exposure to sunlight for at least several weeks after recovering from the dermatitis. If sunlight exposure is unavoidable, a sunscreen preparation and protective clothing should be used to protect the involved skin; otherwise, the patient may become a "persistent light reactor." In one instance, a case of photosensitivity to Phenergan and chlorpromazine was described in which contact sensitivity originally could be demonstrated only to Phenergan; cross-photo-sensitivity existed at the same time, also to chlorpromazine (Thorazine.[28]

The following conclusions can be drawn:

1. In photoallergy to phenothiazine derivatives, such as Phenergan and chlorpromazine (Thorazine), both contact and photocontact sensitivity to these drugs may be found.
2. The allergen in this photoallergic reaction is different from the original drug, probably an oxidation or decomposition product.
3. Cross-photosensitivity between Phenergan and chlorpromazine may exist, even though plain contact sensitivity (without light) can be demonstrated only to Phenergan, and vice versa.
4. Photoallergy plays a role in only some cases of photosensitivity to phenothiazine derivatives.

Carbon-linked Alkylamine (Propylamine) Antihistamines

Fortunately, these carbon-linked alkylamine antihistamines (see Table 13.9) are not commonly used as topical agents. Urticaria and other allergic drug manifestations, however, may occur.

A topical eyedrop containing both cromolyn and chlorpheniramine was found to cause a facial dermatitis.[29] The cause was traced to a chlorpheniramine test at 5% in petrolatum. Oral ingestion of chlorphenamine resulted in a widespread rash within 5 hours and a patch test with chlorphenamine 20% in petrolatum produced a bullous eruption in the patient and no reaction in 20 controls. This alkylamine antihistamine allergy had no

Table 13-9 Carbon-Linked Alkylamine (Propylamine) Antihistamines

Trade name	Generic name
Actidil	Triprolidine
Chlor-Trimeton	Chlorpheniramine
Dimetane	Brompheniramine
Disomer	Dexbrompheniramine
Forhistal	Dimethindene
Histaspan	Chlorpheniramine
Polaramine	Dexchlorpheniramine
Teldrin	Chlorpheniramine

history of a cutaneous exposure to an agent such as chlorphenamine cream or eyedrops that had previously been sources of contact allergy to this agent.[30] In Japan, a product known as Makiron, sold over the counter for skin-wound management, contains both dibucaine and chlorpheniramine maleate. Contact dermatitis to both ingredients occurred in a man with use of this product on an injured leg. dl-chlorpheniramine maleate 1% in petrolatum was positive as well as dibucaine hydrochloride 1% in petrolatum.[31]

Antihistamines are used topically in eyedrops and are reported from Italy as frequent causes of allergic contact dermatitis. Parente and colleagues[32] reported a case that was caused by eyedrops in a patient who was patch tested and found allergic to pheniramine maleate (1% aq), dexchlorpheniramine maleate (1% aq), chlorphenira-mine maleate (1% aq), and diphenhydramine hydro-chloride (2% pet).

Miscellaneous and Piperidine Antihistamines

Topical use of antihistamines has been associated with sensitization and is generally not recommended. In China, cyproheptadine hydrochloride is available topically and has been reported to cause allergic contact dermatitis.[33] A patch test concentration of 1% petrolatum has been recommended.

These antihistamines generally are not used topically and are not associated with contact dermatitis, although LaChapelle[34] reported four cases of vasculitis at the Euro-pean Contact Dermatitis Society meeting, Brussels, October 1992, to oral ingestion of terfenadine that were not reproducible by topical exposure and thought to be from a metabolic product. Table 13.10 lists some repre-sentatives of these classes.

Doxepin

Greenberg[35] reported the active ingredient in Zonalon cream to be the source of contact dermatitis in a 68-year-old man who applied the product to his scalp. The patch test was positive to 5% doxepin in petrolatum. Doxepin

Table 13-10 Miscellaneous and Piperidine Antihistamines

Cyproheptadine	Astemizole
Phenindamine	Terfenadine
Diphenylpyraline	Loratadine
Azatadine	Azelastine
Ketotifen	Cetirizine

used topically was confirmed to be a sensitizer in a larger series from the Cleveland Clinic.[36]

Antihistamines that May Aggravate Urticaria

Aldridge and colleagues[37] reported a list of common anti-histamines used in England for the treatment of urticaria that contain dyes and preservatives not indicated in the usual formularies and that can exacerbate the condition.

The most commonly implicated substances that can aggravate urticaria when ingested are the azo dyes, benzoates, and salicylates. Tartrazine (FD&C Yellow No. 5), as a yellow coloring agent, is an azo dye used extensively in antihistaminic preparations, such as Dime-tane tablets (Robins), Atarax 25-mg tablets (Roerig), and Actifed syrup (Burroughs Wellcome). Other azo dyes implicated in the exacerbation of urticaria are New Coc-cine and Sunset Yellow; the latter is present in Actidil elixir (Burroughs Wellcome). Several antihistaminic pre-parations also contain benzoates as preservatives, for example, Dimetane elixir, Actidil elixir, Dimetapp elixir (Robins), and Actifed syrup.

The authors mention that exacerbations of urticaria with azo dyes and benzoates have been demonstrated in up to 50% of patients who have chronic urticaria; if aspirin is added, crossreactivity can occur with the azo dyes or preservatives.

Role of Tartrazine in Allergic Antihistamine Reactions

Like many other drugs, the antihistamines may be colored by various dyes that are allergenic.[38]. Tartrazine, the azo dye FD&C Yellow No. 5, has been implicated as a cause of urticaria and asthma.[39,40]

Tartrazine is most likely to produce urticaria in patients who have allergic hypersensitivity to aspirin and the salicylate drugs[34] It is, therefore, prudent to administer "white" antihistamines, free of dyes, to such aspirin-sensitive individuals. (The presence of color in a tablet or capsule does not imply that the FD&C Yellow No. 5 is used in its manufacture, however, a "white" antihistamine is free of all dyes.)

Juhlin and colleagues[40] showed that seven of eight aspirin-sensitive patients developed asthma, urticaria, or both after ingesting a test dose of tartrazine in water. The patients also reacted to some benzoic acid derivatives. Because tartrazine (FD&C Yellow No. 5), an azo dye, is used commonly as a food and drug color, and benzoic acid derivatives are used commonly as preservatives in food and drugs, the authors stressed the importance of properly identifying these additives to avoid untoward allergic reactions in sensitive patients. Further provocation tests done by Michaëlsson and Juhlin[39] showed that these additives could exacerbate urticaria even in patients who were not aspirin sensitive. They concluded that negative aspirin-provocation tests did not exclude sensitivity to the additives. Instituting a diet free of these additives for 6 months cleared the chronic urticaria in 13 of 16 patients.

Corroboration of some of these findings was reported[41] in a carefully controlled double-blind cross-over study in which aspirin-intolerant patients and normal controls were matched by age and sex. The authors showed that 15% of aspirin-intolerant individuals had significant adverse reactions to tartrazine challenge and not to the placebo, whereas none of the control subjects had any adverse reactions.

Because antihistamines are the standard therapeutic agents in the treatment of urticaria, it is important to realize that color additives and preservatives present in some of them could aggravate rather than relieve the original complaint.

Use of "White" Antihistamines

Because it is sometimes difficult to ascertain which colored antihistamines may contain tartrazine, the "white" antihistamines may be used.

References

1. Fisher AA. The antihistamines. J Am Acad Dermatol 1980;3:303.

2. Fisher AA. Antihistamine dermatitis. Cutis 1976;18:329.

3. Provost TT, Jullson OF. Ethylenediamine contact dermatitis. Arch Dermatol 1867;96:231.

4. Baer RL, Cohen HJ, Neidorff AH. Allergic eczematous sensitivity to aminophylline. Arch Dermatol 1959;79:647.

5. Petrozzi JW, Shore RN. Generalized exfoliative dermatitis from ethylenediamine. Arch Dermatol 1976;112:525.

6. Van Hecke E. Ethylenediamine sensitivity from exposure to epoxy resin hardeners and Mycolog cream. Contact Dermatitis 1975;1:344.

7. Fisher AA. Epoxy resin dermatitis. Cutis 1976;17:1027.

8. Angelini G, Meneghini CL. Dermatitis in engineers due to synthetic coolants. Contact Dermatitis 1977;3:219.

9. Crow KD, Peachey RDG, Adams JE. Coolant oil dermatitis due to ethylenediamine. Contact Dermatitis 1978;4:359.

10. Dalmau J, Serra-Baldrich E, Roe E, et al. Skin reaction to hydroxyzine (Atarax ®): patch test utility. Contact Dermatitis 2006;54:216.

11. Michel M, Dompmartin A, Louvet S, et al. Skin reactions to hydroxyzine. Contact Dermatitis 1997;36:147.

12. Stingeni L, Caraffini S, Agostinelli D, et al. Maculopapular and urticarial eruption from cetirizine. Contact Dermatitis 1997;37:249.

13. Lew B-L, Haw C-R, Lee M-H. Cutaneous drug eruption from cetirizine and hydroxyzine. J Am Acad Dermatol 2004;50:953.

14. Burry JN. Ethylenediamine sensitivity with a systemic reaction to piperazine citrate. Contact Dermatitis 1978;4:380.

15. Calnan CD. Occupational piperazine dermatitis. Contact Dermatitis 1975;1:126.

16. Price ML, Hall-Smith SP. Allergy to piperazine in a patient sensitive to ethylenediamine. Contact Dermatitis 1984;10:120.

17. Emmett EA. Diphenhydramine photoallergy. Arch Dermatol 1974;110:249.

18. Vickers CFH. Dermatitis meticamentosa. Br Med J 1961;1:1366.

19. Schreiber MM, Naylor LZ. Antihistamine photosensitivity. Arch Dermatol 1962;86:58.

20. Yamada S, Tanaka M, Kawahara Y, et al. Photoallergic contact dermatitis due to diphenhydramine hydrochloride. Contact Dermatitis 1998;38:282.

21. Camarasa G. Contact dermatitis to phenothiazines nemactil and decentan. Contact Dermatitis 1976;2:123.

22. Epstein JH, Brunsting LA, Petersen MC, et al. A study of photosensitivity occurring with chlorpromazine therapy. J Invest Dermatol 1957;28:329.

23. Cahn MM, Levy EJ. Ultraviolet light factor in chlorpromazine dermatitis. Arch Dermatol 1957;75:38.

24. Lewis GM, Sawicky HH. Contact dermatitis from chlorpromazine. JAMA 1955;157:909.

25. Mitchell JC, Ongley R. Photodermatitis presenting as universal exfoliative dermatitis ("phenothiazine contact allergy"). Contact Dermatitis Newsletter 1972;11:278.

26. Calnan CD, Frain-Bell W, Cuthbert JW. Occupational dermatitis from chlorpromazine. Trans St John Hosp Dermatol Soc 1962;48:49.

27. Epstein S. Allergic photocontact dermatitis from promethazine (Phenergan). Arch Dermatol 1960;81:175.

28. Epstein S, Rowe JR. Photoallergy and photocross sensitivity to Phenergan. J Invest Dermatol 1957;29:319.

29. Tosti A, Bardazzi F, Piancastelli E. Contact dermatitis due to chlorpheniramine maleate in eyedrops. Contact Dermatitis 1990;22:55.

30. Brown VL, Orton DI. Cutaneous adverse drug reaction to oral chlorphenamine detected with patch testing. Contact Dermatitis 2005;52:49.

31. Hayashi K, Kawachi S, Saida T. Allergic contact dermatitis due to both chlorpheniramine maleate and dibucaine

hydrochloride in an over-the-counter medication. Contact Dermatitis 2001;44:38.

32. Parente G, Pazzaglia M, Vincenzi C, Tosti A. Contact dermatitis from pheniramine maleate in eyedrops. Contact Dermatitis 1999;40:338.

33. Li LF, Sun XY, Li SY. Allergic contact dermatitis from cyproheptadine hydrochloride. Contact Dermatitis 1995;33:50.

34. Rietschel RL. Selected highlights of the European Contact Dermatitis Society Meeting: Brussels, Belgium, October 8–10, 1992. Am J Contact Dermatitis 1993;4:66.

35. Greenberg JH. Allergic contact dermatitis from topical doxepin. Contact Dermatitis 1995;33:281.

36. Taylor JS, Praditsuwan P, Handel D, Kuffner G. Allergic contact dermatitis from doxepin cream: one-year patch test clinic experience. Arch Dermatol 1996;132:515.

37. Aldridge RD, Main RA, Smith ME. Dyes and preservatives in oral antihistamines. Br J Dermatol 1980;102:545.

38. Lockey S. Reactions to hidden agents in foods and drugs can be serious. Ann Allergy 1975;35:239.

39. Michaëlsson G, Juhlin L. Urticaria induced by preservatives and dye additives in food and drugs. Br J Dermatol 1973;88:525.

40. Juhlin L, Michaëlsson G, Zetterstrum O. Urticaria and asthma induced by food and drug additives in patients with aspirin hypersensitivity. J Allerg Clin Immunol 1972;50:92.

41. Ros A, Juhlin L, Michaëlsson G. A follow-up study of patients with recurrent urticaria and hypersensitivity to aspirin benzoates and azo dye. Br J Dermatol 1976;95:19.

CHAPTER 14

LOCAL ANESTHETICS AND TOPICAL ANALGESICS

EXECUTIVE SUMMARY

Topical anesthetics are classified as amides (lidocaine, dibucaine), esters (benzocaine, tetracaine), benzoic acid esters (cocaine), and miscellaneous (dyclonine, pramoxine). Contact dermatitis can develop from all of the classes, and while crossreactions within each class can logically be expected, at times crossreactions occur across class lines.

Topical analgesics include salicylates, acetaminophen, and the nonsteroidal anti-inflammatory drugs (NSAIDs) indomethacin, ketoprofen, ibuproxam, suprofen, bufexamac, benzydamine, etofenamate, diclofenac, cinnoxicam, piketoprofen, aceclofenac, nimesulide, bendazac, and celecoxib. Topical NSAID use is widespread in Spain and many of the reports originate there. Additional analgesics that have been reported to cause contact dermatitis include enoxolone, mafenide, fepradinol, chlorproethazine, pyrazinobutazone, opium alkaloids, and belladonna.

The local anesthetics may be applied topically or by injection, and certain local anesthetics may be used in either fashion. Topical anesthetics may produce allergic contact dermatitis, whereas the injectable variety may also produce adverse reactions, some of which are allergic in nature. Such reactions may be mild or, if more serious, may produce anaphylactic shock, angioedema, urticaria, serum-sickness syndrome, or vasculitis.

Anesthetic allergy is commonly suspected when an unexplained perioperative collapse occurs. The epidemic of latex sensitivity added this concern in the setting of perioperative collapse. An investigation of 26 patients who experienced perioperative anaphylactoid reactions found that 84% were allergic to at least one anesthetic agent.[1] Only 7.7% were latex sensitive, and atopy was confirmed to be a risk factor for latex sensitivity. Both radioallergoabsorbent test (RAST) and skin-prick tests with raw latex were performed in this investigation. Oral reactions that begin within hours of dental procedures can suggest a problem with local anesthetics, but another possibility needs to be considered. Allergy to thiuram in gloves can occur within this time course and three such cases were reported from Switzerland. In each case the referring dentist was concerned about an anesthetic reaction, but sensitization to thiurams proved the cause.[2]

Topical Anesthetics

The topical anesthetic drugs comprise several chemically dissimilar structures, including alkaloids related to cocaine, and aminoalcohol esters of benzoic acid related to procaine, amides, anilides, phenylalkyl alcohols, and phenols.[3] Table 14.1 classifies topical anesthetics.

Because topical application may induce an allergy to a local anesthetic and a crossreaction to related drugs, dermatologists, allergists, and dental personnel should, insofar as possible, limit topical application of local anesthetics to drugs that are not used parenterally.

Although benzocaine, which is a sensitizer, is not used systemically, it may crossreact with anesthetics of the "ester" type that are administered parenterally. It must be emphasized that the parabens are *parahydroxy* compounds, which Fisher[4] did not find to crossreact with the para-amino compounds.

BENZOCAINE

Benzocaine is commonly used in many topical anesthetic compounds. The synonyms for benzocaine include ethyl aminobenzoate, Anesthesin, Anesthone, and Parathesin. Benzocaine is a para-aminobenzoic acid (PABA) derivative and is related chemically and immunologically to topical anesthetics based on benzoic acid, such as cocaine.

Table 14-1 Classification of Topical Anesthetics
Amides
Dibucaine hydrochloride (Nupercaine)
Lidocaine (Xylocaine)
Lidocaine hydrochloride (Xylocaine)
Esters
Aminobenzoate esters
Benzocaine (Americaine)
Benoxinate hydrochloride (Dorsacaine)
Butamben picrate (Butesin picrate)
Tetracaine hydrochloride (Pontocaine)
Benzoic acid esters
Cocaine hydrochloride
Hexylcaine hydrochloride (Cyclaine)
Piperocaine hydrochloride (Metycaine)
Proparacaine hydrochloride (Alcaine, Ophthaine)
Miscellaneous
Cyclomethycaine (Surfacaine)
Dimethisoquin (Quotane)
Diperodon monohydrate (Diothane)
Dyclonine (Dyclone)
Pramoxine (Tronolane, Tronothane)

Table 14-2 Benzocaine Crossreactors
Butacaine
Butethamine HCL (Monocaine)
Chloroprocaine HCL (Nesacaine)
Cocaine—topical
Isobucaine (Kinacaine)
Meapaine
Meprylcaine (Oracaine)
Metabutethamine (Unacaine)
Neo-Orthoform
Orthoform
Para-amino salicylic acid
Para-aminobenzoic acid and glyceryl PABA (sunscreens)
Paraphenylenediamine
Procainamide (Pronestyl) used for treating heart arrhythmias
Procaine hydrochloride (Novocain)
Propoxycaine hydrochloride (Ravocaine) with 2% procaine
Sulfonamides
Tetracaine hydrochloride (Pontocaine)

Because benzocaine is an effective topical anesthetic, it is used in at least 600 different products. Not only is it used in the treatment of pruritus and burns, but is also has been used as a smoke inhibitor, an appetite suppressant, and for the control of coughing. Benzocaine is used in every orifice of the body, including the ear, mouth (even in "teething lotions"), vagina, and rectum.

As a result of such wide exposure, benzocaine has become a common cause of allergic contact dermatitis. The International and North American Contact Research Groups have placed benzocaine on the "Screening" Patch Test Series. Benzocaine and procaine have been thought to crossreact. This finding has been disputed by Wilkinson and colleagues.[5] In an attempt to refine the crossreactions among benzocaine, tetracaine, and dibucaine, Sidhu and colleagues[6] found that a crossreaction between benzocaine and tetracaine was uncommon (3/22 cases, or 13.6%). Crossreactions between benzocaine and dibucaine were no more frequent. A stronger tendency was found for crossreactions between tetracaine and dibucaine (about one in three).

Benzocaine-sensitized patients occasionally may suffer urticarial reactions and anaphylaxis from procaine injections. Furthermore, benzocaine may show crossreactions with sulfonamides and certain dyes. The administration of "sulfa" drugs to a benzocaine-sensitive person may result in a widespread dermatitis, and exposure to paraphenylenediamine in hair and fur dyes may also cause a severe allergic contact dermatitis. Table 14.2 lists local anesthetics and various medications and chemicals that may crossreact with benzocaine.

About 14% of benzocaine-sensitive individuals are also sensitive to paraphenylenediamine, the most popular of hair dyes.[6] Some sunscreens that were labeled as containing glyceryl PABA actually contained benzocaine.[7]

Hjorth and colleagues[8] reported that benzocaine-reactive patients were patch tested to two commercial sources of glyceryl *p*-aminobenzoate containing varying concentrations of benzocaine as a contaminant. Eleven of 20 patients reacted to the source with 0.3% benzocaine; none reacted to the source with 0.001% benzocaine.

Benzocaine-sensitive patients may show crossreactions with the following injectable local anesthetics, which are based on PABA: procaine hydrochloride (Novocain), butethamine hydrochloride (Monocaine), tetracaine hydrochloride (Pontocaine) with 2% procaine, and propoxycaine hydrochloride (Ravocaine).

Metabutethamine (Unacaine), which is based on meta-aminobenzoic acid, and meprylcaine (Oracaine), which is based on benzoic acid, may also crossreact with benzocaine.

The injection of these local anesthetics into benzocaine-sensitive persons may lead to localized swelling of the oral mucosa at the site of injection. On rare occasions, generalized urticaria or anaphylaxis will result from the injection of procaine into benzocaine-sensitive patients. Unfortunately, although many crossreactions *may* occur, they also may not. Crossreactions have not been predictable, and a positive test for benzocaine with a negative test for paraphenylenediamine would suggest that broad allergy is not likely to be present. Because both compounds are routinely used in patch test screening series worldwide, it is possible to let these tests assist (but not dictate) the magnitude of crossreactions likely to occur. If both the benzocaine and the paraphenylenediamine tests are positive, the theoretical crossreactions become more likely.

BENZOCAINE AS SCREENING ALLERGEN

Wilkinson and colleagues[5] found that 5% benzocaine in petrolatum as a screen for local anesthetic allergy would have identified only 5 of 13 patients so sensitive. Among the anesthetic allergens missed were cinchocaine (2.5%) (Dibucaine) and amethocaine (2.5%).[5] Similarly, benzocaine was found not to detect allergy to butyl aminobenzoate (*n*-butyl-*p*-amino-benzoate), which in the United States is found in hemorrhoid suppositories under the names butamben picrate and butesin picrate.[9]

Wilkinson's group[6] further reviewed their data over a 10-year period and found that benzocaine was an inappropriate screening allergen for local anesthetic sensitivity. Rather, tetracaine and dibucaine made up 78.1% of reactions seen. This finding is consistent with the observations of Beck and Holden,[10] who found that only 0.63% of patients tested reactive to benzocaine. The recommended screening allergen of Sidhu and colleagues'[6] data is a mix of 5% benzocaine, 5% tetracaine hydrochloride (amethocaine), and 5% dibucaine hydrochloride (cinchocaine).

ALTERNATIVES FOR BENZOCAINE-SENSITIVE INDIVIDUALS

Safe *topical* anesthetics for benzocaine-sensitive individuals include lidocaine (Xylocaine), mepivacaine (Carbocaine), prilocaine hydrochloride (Citanest), pyrrocaine (Dynacaine), and pramoxine (Pramasone).

The following *injectable* local anesthetics do not crossreact with benzocaine because they are based on an "amide" structure: lidocaine (Xylocaine), mepivacaine (Carbocaine), prilocaine hydrochloride (Citanest), pyrrocaine (Dynacaine), and nupercaine (Dibucaine).

Table 14.3 lists products containing tetracaine that may need to be avoided by some benzocaine-sensitive persons. Kalveram and colleagues[11,12] showed that guinea pigs are readily sensitized to tetracaine and that tetracaine crossreacts with procaine and PABA. Crossreaction between proparacaine and tetracaine has been reported in ophthalmic use and was considered an occupational hazard for ophthalmologists and their technicians. Both proparacaine and tetracaine are benzoic acid esters and thus the crossreaction would be anticipated.[13]

Table 14-3 Products That Have Contained Tetracaine (Pontocaine)
Clean 'N Treat
Icy Kool Lotion (Daniels)
Isotraine Ointment (Phillips)
PNS Suppositories (Winthrop)
Pontocaine Cream and Ointment, Ophthalmic Liquid (Winthrop)
Rectodyne Ointment (SeMed)
Tycal Lotion (Daniels)
Vanocide Lotion, Cream Foam (Daniels)
Vertussin Loz-Tablets (Warren-Teed)
Products containing both benzocaine and tetracaine
Cetacaine Topical Anesthetic Ointment (Cetylite)
Novol-Benzocaine-Tetracaine Solution (Novocol)
in the topical, liquid, ointment and spray forms

Topical 4% tetracaine produced contact dermatitis in a woman who was applying Ametop prior to collagen injections. While she was sensitized by direct skin contact, the use of vinyl gloves subsequently did not provide adequate protection. The authors also point out that the beauty industry presents a further industry other than traditional medicine where such products are finding use.[14]

"Amide" Local Anesthetics

LIDOCAINE (XYLOCAINE)

Lidocaine (Xylocaine) is an "amide" compound that does not crossreact with benzocaine. It is used widely not only as a surface anesthetic and as an injectable local anesthetic, but also intravenously for cardiac arrhythmias. Allergic reactions to lidocaine (Xylocaine) are rare, but do occur.

Lignocaine is a synonym for lidocaine. The amide group of anesthetics includes lidocaine, bupivacaine, prilocaine, and cinchocaine. Crossreactions occur within the group but are most common between lidocaine and bupivacaine.[15]

Thus, Fregert and colleagues[16] reported two patients who had contact allergy to lidocaine (Xylocaine) who also reacted to chemically related anesthetics of the "amide" type. One reacted to bupivacaine, mepivacaine (Carbocaine) only. The patients also reacted to the chemically nonrelated dibucaine hydrochloride (Cincaine), an anesthetic of the ester type. Reactions to lidocaine (Xylocaine) metabolites *o*-toluidine, and *m*-xylidine were negative. These authors state that the patient who reacted to all four anesthetics of the amide type should avoid being treated with the usual anesthetics (e.g., those administered by a dentist). Tetracaine, which gave a negative reaction, could be used.

Roed-Petersen[17] reported that two patients were sensitized to an ointment containing betamethasone valerate 0.05%, metaoxedrine hydrochloride 0.1%, and lidocaine (Xylocaine) hydrochloride 2.5%. Results of a patch test in one patient showed a +2 reaction to lidocaine hydrochloride (Xylocaine).

Goransson's[18] patient suffered an anaphylactic reaction from a dental injection of the "amide" prilocaine. Black and colleagues[19] reported similarly that a patient sensitive to Xyloproct ointment (1% lignocaine) crossreacted with prilocaine but not to other members of the class, including bupivacine and mepivacaine.

Hofmann and colleagues[20] reported on a patient who had a generalized papular, pruritic eruption from a dental anesthetic injection of lidocaine (Xylocaine). The skin tests were performed as follows: (a) The results of patch tests with 20% lidocaine hydrochloride in petrolatum were negative at 72 and 96 hours after the test. (b) Intradermal test with 2% lidocaine hydrochloride was negative to 45 minutes. Eight hours after intradermal and patch testing, however, a papular, pruritic rash appeared on his upper extremities and shoulders.

Chin and Fellner[21] conclude that allergic hypersensitivity to lidocaine hydrochloride is rare. Only four such cases had been found in the literature in the past 18 years, and in these, symptoms ranged from urticaria to bronchospasms and hypotension with syncope. These symptoms were reversible usually with epinephrine and antihistamines. Skin testing with "as-is" lidocaine has been useful in some patients. Mackley et al safely tested 4 patients who were positive to lidocaine on patch testing with 0.1mL of preservative-free lidocaine and found this to be useful in sorting out the history and skin reactivity in a manner that replicates normal usage.[22]

Allergy to lidocaine or lignocaine, as it is known in Australia, is not rare. Many of the cases of contact dermatitis have been reported from Australia. This has been attributed to the wide availability of lignocaine-containing preparations in Australia. A total of 49 of the 62 cases reported worldwide were from Australia, according to Weightman and Turner.[23] They tested with lignocaine 15% in petrolatum and reported 29 cases seen from 1990 to 1998. For so many cases to have been found by one group would seem to suggest that the cases are not being picked up because testing for "amide" anesthetics is not routinely done.

Allergy to lidocaine was documented by intradermal patch and lymphocyte transformation tests.[24] Crossreactivity to other aminoacylamide local anesthetics was found. These crossreacting substances include bupivacaine, mepivacaine, and prilocaine. Articaine, which has a thiophen ring instead of a methylated phenyl ring, was safe for use in this patient, as was the case in one prior patient who was found to be allergic to mepivacaine. Because of the structural difference, articaine would seem the logical alternative when any of the other aminoacylamide anesthetics becomes an issue. Alternatively, the ester anesthetics (benzocaine, procaine, tetracaine) or the aminoalkylamide cinchocaine could be considered. A patient exhibiting sensitization to both raised the possibility that lidocaine and crotamiton crossreact[25] The structural formulas are similar, as both have a butanoyl toluidine moiety in common.

Some patients who are allergic to lidocaine have been found to tolerate procaine, prilocaine, or mepivacaine. Klein and Gall[26] had a patient who was allergic to both lidocaine and mepivacaine, but who was, however, able to use articaine. All the reactions were type 4 with erythema and itching 1 day after subcutaneous injection.[26] Breit and colleagues[27] reported a patient sensitive to lidocaine administered for epicondylitis and found patch test positive to a 15% lidocaine hydrochloride patch test, but not positive to intradermal testing at 10 mg/mL and also prick-test negative. Crossreactivity was seen to mepivacaine, but not to etidocaine or bupivacaine. The authors point out how difficult it is to predict crossreaction. The presence of both immediate hypersensitivity to lidocaine and delayed hypersensitivity that manifested as allergic contact dermatitis was reported in a woman who was also allergic to benzocaine and propolis. The authors felt that the benzocaine sensitivity was likely to have been separately acquired and not a crossreaction.[28]

A patient experienced postoperative cellulitis that was thought to represent a reaction to lignocaine (lidocaine). She also reacted to other amide anesthetics (prilocaine, mepivacaine, and bupivicaine) with delayed (not immediate) hypersensitivity. Coincidentally, she was also found photocontact allergic to oxybenzone.[29] Lidocaine used during the induction of general anesthesia produced an eruption from the neckline to below the knees in a patient undergoing cataract surgery. The patient had received 30 mg intravenously. Patch testing showed a positive reaction at day 4; an intradermal test with preservative-free 1% lidocaine was negative at 15 minutes, became positive at day 2, and expanded at day 4. No reactions were found to cinchocaine, tetracaine, procaine, prilocaine, benzocaine, or amylocaine.[30]

Fisher[31] reported a patient who acquired an allergic contact dermatitis from Xylocaine ointment. This patient showed a strongly positive patch test reaction to propylene glycol, which is present in the ointment. Results of patch tests with 20% lidocaine hydrochloride in petrolatum were negative. Dynexan is a local anesthetic gel, and when it was applied to the gums of a dental patient a life-threatening immediate reaction occurred. The anesthetic was not the source of the reaction, but rather the gelling agent Meyprogat 60, a derivative of guar gum. Guar or guar gum is obtained from *Cyamopsis tetragonoloba* beans to which the patient also reacted on prick testing. No reaction was seen to lidocaine.[32]

In this connection, it should be noted that both lidocaine (Xylocaine) 5% ointment and lidocaine (Xylocaine) 2.5% ointment contain propylene glycol, but that lidocaine (Xylocaine) hydrochloride 4% solution, lidocaine (Xylocaine) hydrochloride jelly, and lidocaine (Xylocaine) hydrochloride viscous solution do not.

Soesman-van Waadenoden Kernekamp and van Ketel[33] treated a patient whose contact allergy was apparently due to lidocaine itself and not to any of the ingredients in the base.

A mixture of 2.5% lidocaine and 2.5% prilocaine in a vehicle that keeps both anesthetics in solution at room temperature (rather than crystals) has been introduced for topical anesthesia under the brand name EMLA (Astra). A patient who was allergic to lignocaine (lidocaine), prilocaine, and pseudoephedrine led Downs and colleagues[34] to propose that structural similarity of the three compounds could account for the allergy. In their patient, EMLA cream was thought to be the source of the sensitization to the anesthetics. Prilocaine and lidocaine are known crossreactants as members of the amide group of anesthetics.

The prilocaine component of EMLA caused contact dermatitis in a 78-year-old man who applied the medication to a leg ulcer. No reaction was seen to the other active ingredient, which is lidocaine.[35] Use of EMLA cream resulted in contact urticaria, traced to the lidocaine component of EMLA. An open skin test with EMLA was urticarial in minutes. Five percent lidocaine produced a reaction within 20 minutes under a closed patch test. No crossreactions to other anesthetics were found.[36]

Topical application of EMLA cream with Tegaderm occlusion caused purpura in five patients within 30 to 60 minutes.[37] Immediate and delayed patch tests did not confirm sensitization, and a toxic effect on capillary endothelium is thought to be the explanation.

Table 14.4 lists some injectable "amide" local anesthetics, and Table 14.5 lists some topical anesthetics with the "amide" structure.

DIBUCAINE HYDROCHLORIDE (NUPERCAINE)

Dibucaine hydrochloride (Nupercaine), a local anesthetic, is also known as percaine, cincaine, sovcaine, and cinchocaine. Because it is a quinoline derivative, there is a possibility that it may crossreact with iodochlorhydroxyquin (Vioform), but not with the ester

Table 14-4 Injectable "Amide" Anesthetics
Bupivacaine HCl [Marcaine HCl (Breon) and Sensorcaine (Astra)]
Dibucaine (Nupercainal)
Etidocaine [Duranest Solution (Astra)]
Lidocaine HCl [Lidocaine Ups (Abbott) and Xylocaine (Astra)]
Lidopen auto-injector (Survival)
Mepivacaine [Carbocaine HCl (Breon)]
Prilocaine [Citanest Solution (Astra)]

types of local anesthetics, because it is an "amide" anesthetic.

Wilson[38] reported several patients who had allergic contact sensitivity to this medication. Application of dibucaine (also known as cinchocaine) to the perianal area resulted in a dermatitis of the face, axillae, antecubital fossae, and upper inner thighs in a baboon syndrome-like picture. A patch test of 5% dibucaine in petrolatum was positive and there were no crossreactions to either ester or amide anesthetics. The authors point out that it is not always necessary to avoid all other anesthetics of the same class when sensitivity to one member of the ester or amide class of anesthetics is identified.[39]

Table 14.6 lists some products containing this anesthetic.

As noted earlier in this chapter, Sidhu and colleagues[6] found crossreactions between dibucaine and tetracaine in about one-third of cases and between dibucaine and benzocaine about 14% of the time.

MEPIVACINE

A woman who was undergoing sclerotherapy with polidocanol and mepivacaine developed an eruption on her legs that was traced to mepivacaine. She had a positive intradermal test to a 1:1 dilution of mepivacaine and positive patch tests to 1%, 2%, and 3% mepivacaine and also positive patch tests to 2%, 5%, and 20% lidocaine.

Table 14-5 Topical "Amide" Anesthetics
Dibucaine [Corticaine Cream (Glaxo)]
Lidocaine [Anestacon (Webcon)]
Lidocaine HCl [Bactine First Aid Spray (Miles)]
Lidocaine HCl [Lidosporin Otic Solution (Burroughs Wellcome)]
Lidocaine 2.5% and Prilocaine 2.5% [EMLAt (Astra)]
Lidocaine HCl [Unguentine Plus First Aid and Burn Cream (Procter & Gamble)]
Lidocaine HCl [Xylocaine Jelly and Ointment (Astra)]

Table 14-6 Dibucaine Hydrochloride (Nupercaine)

Nupercainal Cream and Ointment (Ciba)

Nupercainal Suppositories (Ciba)

Nupercaine Heavy Solution (Ciba)

Nupercaine Hydrochloride 1:200 and 1:1,500 (Ciba) (for spinal anesthesia)

Since she had not used lidocaine, this was presumed to be a crossreaction. She did not react to other amide anesthetics, specifically bupivacaine and articaine.[40]

CYCLOMETHYCAINE (SURFACAINE)

Cyclomethycaine (Surfacaine) is a substituted piperidine alkyl benzoate and thus is not related to para-aminobenzoic acid. It closely resembles piperocaine (Metycaine). Although cyclomethycaine (Surfacaine) is a rare sensitizer, cyclomethycaine sulfate (Jelly Surfacaine) contains propylene glycol and thimerosal.

Over the years, Fisher[4] observed three patients who were allergic to Jelly Surfacaine. One patient was allergic to propylene glycol and two patients to thimerosal.

Aside from Jelly Surfacaine, Surfadil Cream and Surfadil Lotion (Lilly), both containing cyclomethycaine, are available as surface local anesthetic agents. Cyclomethycaine is also present in Surfadil (Lilly), Surfathesin, and Topocaine.

PRAMOXINE HYDROCHLORIDE (TRONOTHANE)

Pramoxine hydrochloride (Tronothane), 4-[3 (p-butoxyphenoxy) propyl], morpholine hydrochloride, is a surface anesthetic agent different from local anesthetics of the benzoate ester type, such as benzocaine and procaine. It is *not used* by injection.

Although Schmidt and colleagues[41] reported the virtues of pramoxine hydrochloride (Tronothane) more than 25 years ago, this surface anesthetic is not widely used as yet by dermatologists. These investigators stated that "Tronothane exhibits outstanding qualities as a topical local anesthetic agent. It combines high potency with low systemic toxicity. Also it possesses a low sensitizing potential and is well tolerated by tissues. Extensive laboratory and clinical testing have demonstrated the following properties of Tronothane: (1) it is equivalent to ethyl aminobenzoate in anesthetic activity; (2) its effective minimal concentration is greater than cyclomethycaine; (3) its duration of action is double that of cocaine; (4) it produces no apparent irritation to skin and mucous membranes; and (5) it possesses a low sensitizing potential."

Peal and Karp[42] confirmed its low sensitization and irritation potential in a study involving 71 adult volunteers. Several patients sensitive to other topical anesthetics showed no sensitization to Tronothane. The patch test sensitization reactions that did occur were of a mild and moderate character. The incidence of such reactions was approximately one-fifth that observed in similar tests on the same objects using cyclomethycaine.

COMBINED USE OF PRAMOXINE (TRONOTHANE) WITH HYDROCORTISONE ACETATE

Sladek[43] reported that a new foam preparation, containing 1% hydrocortisone acetate and 1% pramoxine hydrochloride, was clinically investigated in 118 postoperative and 5 nonsurgical proctologic patients with beneficial results. Excellent to good responses in terms of smooth and faster healing of surgical wounds and relief of discomfort were seen in 95% of patients. Eight patients showed fair to poor response to therapy. No untoward reactions were observed. This new mode of administration appears to offer significant advantages over hemorrhoidal suppositories, ointments, and other forms of therapy. Sladek[43] believed that the use of these two active ingredients was superior to either one alone. Presently, preparations containing pramoxine hydrochloride and hydrocortisone acetate together with their vehicles are available. Fisher[44] has reviewed the literature related to pramoxine and listed some available products in Tables 14.7 and 14.8.

Van Ketel[45] reported two patients who had allergic contact sensitivity to pramoxine (Tronothane) apparently from the application of a Dutch preparation called Nestosyl ointment, which reportedly contains pramoxine. This is the only report of allergic reaction that Fisher44 could find in the literature.

Table 14.9 lists miscellaneous topical anesthetics. Adverse reactions have been described in Chapter 9.

Table 14-7 Products Containing Pramoxine Hydrochloride

Anugesic Ointment (Warner/Chilcott)

Anugesic Suppositories (Warner/Chilcott)

F-E-P Creme (Boots)

Otall Ear Drops (Saron)

Perifoam (Rowell)

Pramosone Lotion and Ointment (Ferndale)[a]

Prax Lotion and Cream (Ferndale)[b]

ProctoFoam/nonsteroid (Reed & Carnrick)

Tronothane Hydrochloride Cream, Jelly (Abbott)

[a] Contains pramoxine hydrochloride and hydrocortisone. Note: Pramoxine used only for surface anesthesia and not for injections, so sensitization to this anesthetic does not entail any risk of future systemic reactions.

[b] Contains pramoxine hydrochloride alone.

Pramosone Cream and Ointment (Ferndale)
Pramosone Lotion (Ferndale)
Proctofoam (Reed & Carnrick)

Testing for Allergic Reactions to Local Anesthetics

Patch testing for allergic contact dermatitis caused by topical anesthetics is quite reliable. The reliability of skin tests for adverse reactions to injectable anesthetics, however, leaves much to be desired.

The unreliability of skin tests to decide what local anesthetic is safe for a patient who has a history of prior adverse reactions is illustrated by the findings of Incaudo and colleagues.[46] These investigators reported the following.

The clinical histories of 71 patients evaluated for suspected local anesthetic (LA) allergy were reviewed retrospectively. The clinical histories were classified as immediate generalized reactions (15%), localized swelling at the injection site (25%), nonspecific systemic symptoms (42%), and other histories (17%). Serial dilutional intradermal skin tests were performed in 59 patients using mepivacaine, lidocaine, and procaine. There were five skin-test positive patients, each with a positive reaction to an LA to which, according to their medical history, they had never reacted before. In 50 patients when an LA was subsequently required, a subcutaneous challenge was per-

formed, with an LA chosen for chemical nonsimilarity. No significant reactions were observed in this group. Three patients tolerated a challenge with an LA to which they were skin-test positive.

These data indicate the low incidence of reactions compatible with a systemic IgE-mediated mechanism by history in patients referred for evaluation of LA allergy, the lack of specific and clinically relevant information provided by dilutional skin tests, and the apparent safety and usefulness of careful challenge with an alternative LA.

Other in vivo tests, such as nasal and conjunctival tests, are not only unreliable but also risky. Thus, Adriani[47] reported a fatal reaction to the instillation of one drop of a local anesthetic into the conjunctival sac.

In vitro testing, such as the leucocyte histamine release test and the lymphocyte transformation test, may possibly be of some value.

Lehner[48] reported positive results for four patients who had suspected allergy to local anesthetics and for whom the intradermal test was negative.

Miscellaneous

PROPARACAINE (PROXYMETACAINE; OPHTHAINE, OPHTHETIC)

This ophthalmic topical anesthetic, with the formula 3-amino-4-propoxybenzoic acid 2(diethylamino) ethyl ester, may produce dermatitis of the hands in sensitized ophthalmologists and allergic conjunctivitis from its presence in eye preparations.[49,50]

DIPEROTON HYDROCHLORIDE (PROCTODON)

This topical anesthetic in the form of Diperodon cream is based on dicarbanalide, and thus does not crossreact with the PABA anesthetics. Diperodon cream is used as a lubricant and anesthetic for rectal examination and to alleviate pain of postoperative bowel movements. Calnan[51] reported an allergic reaction to this anesthetic.

PHENOLIC ANESTHETICS

The phenolic anesthetic preparations are listed in Table 14.9. The accompanying literature to these preparations stresses that they are free of "caines" and are anesthetic and antiseptic. These phenolic compounds are rare sensitizers.

PROPANIDID

Propanidid, which is not listed in the Physicians' Desk Reference, is a derivative of eugenol used in Europe as an intravenous anesthetic instead of barbiturates. Gastelain and Piriou[52] have reported a contact dermatitis due to

Table 14-9 Miscellaneous Topical Anesthetics

Topical anesthetics	Ingredients
Aspercreme (Thompson Medical)	Triethanolamine salicylate
Ben-Gay (Leeming)	Methyl salicylate, menthol
Chloraseptic Gel (Norwich Eaton)	Phenol, sodium phenolate
Deep Down Pain Relief Rub (Beecham)	Methyl salicylate, menthol, methyl nicotinate, camphor
Icy Hot Balm (Searle)	Methyl salicylate, menthol
Mentholatum Ointment, Rub (Mentholatum)	Methyl salicylate, menthol
Myoflex Creme (Adria)	Triethanolamine salicylate
Oraderm Lip Balm (Schattner)	Sodium phenolate, sodium tetraborate, phenol
Panalgesic (Poythress)	Methyl salicylate, aspirin, menthol, camphor
Proctodon (Rowell)	Diperodon hydrochloride
Soltice Quick-Rub (Chattem)	Menthol, methyl salicylate, camphor, eucalyptus oil
Thera-Gesic (Mission)	Methyl salicylate, menthol
Vicks Vaporub (Vicks Health Care)	Menthol, spirits of turpentine, eucalyptus oil, camphor, cedar leaf oil, thymol

propanidid in an anesthetic. Sneddon and Caldwell[53] reported a similar case previously.

Topical Analgesics

A wide variety of topical analgesic preparations are available in Europe but not the United States. Contact dermatitis and photocontact dermatitis have been reported from a variety of topical analgesic products.

SALICYLATES

Hydroxyethyl salicylate in topical analgesic gel has caused contact dermatitis and was detected by use of 0.1% in petrolatum.[54] No crossreactivity to salicylic acid, sodium salicylate, or acetylsalicylic acid was noted.

Methyl butetisalicylate is used topically for musculoskeletal pain. It is also known as methyl diethylacetylsalicylate, and the usual use concentration is 30% in a cream base. A 40-year-old woman developed contact dermatitis to methyl butetisalicylate used to treat a painful knee.[55] Oral acetylsalicylic acid (aspirin) up to 1,000 mg did not cause any reaction in this case.

Topical salicylates are rare contact allergens. Picolinamine salicylate used as a topical antiinflammatory cream in Spain was found to be a potential source of contact dermatitis.[56] A patch test with 2% concentration in oil was positive. Anti-rheumatic and anti-inflammatory gels containing 2-hydroxyethyl salicylate are used in Europe under various trade names and are rare sensitizers. Products containing this agent include Venosin gel (Klinge Pharma, Munich, Germany), Bayolin cream (Bayer Austria, Vienna, Austria), and Ambenat ointment (Merckle, Blaubeuren, Germany). Sensitivity can be detected with 2-hydroxyethyl salicylate 5% aqueous.[57]

ACETAMINOPHEN (PROPACETAMOL)

Nurses who do not wear gloves while mixing or handling the analgesic propacetamol may develop contact dermatitis on the hands and forearms. Four such cases were reported from France, where the drug is used commonly for postoperative pain.[58] The agent is a prodrug composed of diethylglycine linked to paracetamol. The patients tolerated oral paracetamol. Paracetamol is better known as acetaminophen.

Propacetamol is broken down by esterases or nonenzymatic mechanisms into acetaminophen and N,N-diethylglycine. Patch tests in propacetamol sensitive patients have found the allergenic determinant to reside in the N,N-diethylglycine, which is a phenyl ester, and these are known skin sensitizers.[59]

INDOMETHACIN

Topical indomethacin caused contact dermatitis in a 14-year-old boy within 10 days after he applied it to his right ankle.[60] A patch test of 1% pure indomethacin in petrolatum was positive, and there was no crossreaction to multiple other topical nonsteroidal anti-inflammatory drugs (NSAIDs) or to the excipients of Inacid gel.

KETOPROFEN

Topical ketoprofen is sold in Italy in both cream and gel bases. It is a propionic acid derivative categorized as an NSAID. Seven cases of both contact and photocontact allergy were reported by Tosti and colleagues[61] and confirmed by patch testing with the 2.5% gel formula, which was positive in all seven cases. A 10% petrolatum patch test was positive in only two of seven cases, demonstrating the importance of proper vehicle selection for patch testing with ketoprofen. However, a 2.5% petrolatum patch test plus 10J of UVA light confirmed contact and photocontact dermatitis in another study.[62] In this later case, crossreactivity with ibuproxam was observed. A study of 18 patients who were photoallergic to ketoprofen found that hyperphotosusceptibility to react to chemically unrelated compounds occurred. These reactions were not relevant. Positive photopatch tests occurred to fentichlor in 67% of cases, tetrachlorosalicylanilide in 28%, triclosan in 17%, tribromsalan in 11%, and bithionol in 11%. The authors speculate that compounds containing a benzene ring with an associated oxygen group produce these co-reactions.[63] A study of 20 patients with dermatitis from topical ketoprofen products found ketoprofen, and not the other vehicle ingredients, to be the cause in all cases. When tested with 2% ketoprofen in petrolatum, 17 of the 20 were photoallergic, 1 was contact allergic, and 2 were contact allergic with photoaggravation. Fewer than 30% of these patients were photoallergic to benzophenone-3 and none was allergic to benzophenone-4. However, 69% reacted to fragrance mix. This was explained by an aldehyde function on ketoprofen and the presence of cinnamic aldehyde in fragrance mix.[64]

Topical NSAIDs are popular in Spain, and two Spanish hospitals reviewed the use of such products and their records of adverse reactions. They reported 139 reactions to topical NSAIDs, of which 56 (40%) were allergic contact dermatitis and 83 (60%) were photoallergic contact dermatitis. While diclofenac was the most commonly used topical NSAID, ketoprofen (the third most commonly used product) caused the greatest number of reactions. Ketoprofen accounted for 28% of the contact allergy and 82% of the photoallergy.[65]

Six cases of photocontact allergy to dexketoprofen were reported from Spain. All were found to be photocontact allergy to ketoprofen. The authors point out that it is the benzophenone moiety of these agents, rather than their arylpropionic function, that leads to photoallergy. They believe that all dexketoprofen photoallergic patients should avoid fenofibrate, benzophenones, and ketoprofen. Dexketoprofen 2% in petrolatum can be used for testing.[66]

Ketoprofen is also available in Italy in a transdermal patch. A patient who developed a bullous eruption in reaction to this device proved allergic to glyceryl-hydrogenated rosinate (ester gum), rather than the active agent, in the patch. A 20% petrolatum patch test confirmed the allergy.[67]

Contact urticaria to ketoprofen in a poultice was confirmed by patch tests to 1%, 5%, and 10% etoprofen in petrolatum. The patient was found to also to react to loxoprofen sodium 10% in petrolatum and diclofenac sodium 10% in petrolatum, and since these all have a 2-phenyl acetate in common, cross-sensitivity was suggested.[68]

NSAID CROSSREACTIONS

An Italian study of topical NSAID crossreactions found most of the 123 patients tested to be monosensitive, and ketoprofen was the most common problem.[69] The investigators felt that a possible crossreaction between cinnamic aldehyde and ketoprofen might exist based on a common ketonic group and the frequency of co-reactivity between fragrance mix, cinnamic aldehyde, and ketoprofen. The most common linkage between topical NSAIDs was between ketoprofen and ibuproxam (10 contact dermatitis cases and 3 photocontact dermatitis cases). There were five ketoprofen-thiaprophenic acid cases.

Le Coz and colleagues[70] investigated the pattern of crossreactivity among photosensitizing NSAIDs. Ketoprofen photoallergic patients and tiaprofenic acid patients crossreacted in 12 of 12 cases. These are arylpropionic acid derivatives. These same patients reacted to fenofibrate in 8 of 12, oxybenzone in 3 of 12, and unsubstituted benzophenone in 11 of 12 cases. Ketoprofen has an unsubstituted benzophenone moiety that appears to be the basis for the crossreactions. In the case of tiaprofenic acid, the thiophene-phenylketone moiety is very similar to the benzophenone moiety and is the likely basis for crossreactions. The arylpropionic moiety does not appear to be part of the crossreaction problem.

Topical ketoprofen caused photosensitivity that recurred in the absence of reapplication but recurred from sun exposure up to 6 months after the last application of the drug.[71] Crossreactivity to benzophenone-3 was found in this patient.

Connubial contact led to photodermatitis from ketoprofen.[72] A husband was using topical ketoprofen, and his wife also frequented tanning salons. After UVA exposure, a handprint on her thigh appeared due to the connubial contact.

An erythema multiforme pattern of dermatitis occurred in an 82-year-old man following application of a ketoprofen-containing gel for diffuse rheumatic pain.[73] The patch test was positive to ketoprofen 1% in petrolatum at days 2 and 3.

IBUPROXAM

Both ibuproxam and ketoprofen are aryl-propionic acid derivatives that are possible but not obligate crossreacting molecules.[74] Contact dermatitis to topical ibuproxam cream has been confirmed with a 5% concentration in petrolatum.[75]

SUPROFEN

Topical 1% suprofen ointment is sold as an NSAID in Japan and has been reported to cause photocontact dermatitis.[76] In five patients, UVA elicited photoallergy in conjunction with patch tests of 0.1% to 0.01% in petrolatum. In three patients, UVB elicited photoallergy with 0.1% to 1.0% in petrolatum. All cases crossreacted with tiaprofenic acid but not with ketoprofen, piroxicam, bufexumac, bendazac, ibuprofen piconol, or ufenamate.[76]

BUFEXAMAC

Topical NSAIDs are in widespread use in Germany, where more than 130 such products are available. Routine testing with a group of NSAIDs in 371 consecutive patients found 17 sensitized individuals (4.6%). The most frequently encountered allergen was bufexamac, which was positive in 12 (3.2%) of patients.[77]

Bufexamac was found to be a common sensitizer when applied to treat eczema. Females seem more likely to be sensitized, as, in one series, 88% of the bufexamac cases were female.[78]

No crossreactivity between bufexamac and diclofenac was seen in 11 cases of bufexamac sensitivity.[79] Although both have benzene rings, the different side chains (acetamide for bufexamac and acetic acid for diclofenac) probably account for the lack of crossreactivity.

An erythema multiforme–like eruption may follow localized allergic contact dermatitis to bufexamac. This NSAID has been used to treat a variety of disorders, including atopic dermatitis and localized leg lesions and ulcers. No epidermal necrosis was seen in four cases, as might be expected in true erythema multiforme.[80]

BENZYDAMINE HYDROCHLORIDE

Topical application of the NSAID benzydamine hydrochloride caused both contact and photocontact dermatitis. The commercial ointment (Tantam) is a 5% concentration, and patch tests with 5% aqueous were positive.[81]

ETOFENAMATE

Etofenamate is 2-(2-hydroxyethoxy)-ethyl N-(aaa-trifluro-m-tolyl) anthranilate, and contact dermatitis has been reported and confirmed with 2% petrolatum[82] and 5% lanolin[83] patch tests. Application to the lumbosacral region has progressed to exfoliative erythroderma.[84]

Nine cases of contact allergy to etofenamate were reported by Hergueta and colleagues,[85] with onset of rash generally within 7 days of using the product (range 1–30 days). A 2% concentration in petrolatum identified all of the cases, with no reaction in 30 controls. Flogoprofen gel, a topical NSAID available in Spain, has etofenamate as its active agent. Etofenamate produced both contact and photocontact allergic dermatitis in a woman who applied the gel to her ankle. Etofenamate was tested at 0.05% in petrolatum.[86]

DICLOFENAC

This arylacetic NSAID was reported as the cause of three cases of contact allergy. A 2.5% petrolatum patch test concentration was used.[87]

Diclofenac sodium and diclofenac diethylamine tested at 10% in petrolatum produced delayed positive patch test reactions.[88] Diclofenac is in the arylacanoic acid group, which also includes bufexamac, mefenamic, meclofenamic, flufenamic, tolfenamic, and etofenamic acids.

Diclofenac has also caused contact dermatitis when used as an ophthalmic preparation.[89] Eyelid dermatitis and conjunctivitis were produced, but crossreactivity with bufexamac was not observed. Diclofenac, applied as Voltaren Emulgel in a Spanish patient, resulted in dermatitis in the areas of application. Those areas were sun exposed, and subsequent patch testing found that there were no reactions to 1% diclofenac or the commercial product, but photopatch tests of the same two items with 5J of UVA light produced strong reactions indicating photoallergic contact dermatitis.[90]

Jonker and Bruynzeel[91] reported a patient whom they considered to have developed anaphylactic symptoms after a patch test was applied to the arm with diclofenac 1% petrolatum. The patient had previously had anaphylactic shock from a sodium diclofenac 100 mg suppository. The symptoms from the suppository included swelling of the face and extremities, hypotension, and respiratory distress. However, the symptoms that began 15 minutes after patch test application were hoarseness, headache, sputum production, and hypertension. There was no reaction at the patch test site, but within 30 minutes of removal of the patch test, administration of salbutamol by inhalation, and 2 mg of clemastine intramuscularly, the symptoms resolved. Whether this can be classified as an anaphylactic reaction is arguable.

Kowalzick and Ziegler[92] report a patient who developed photoallergic contact dermatitis to diclofenac used to treat actinic keratoses. Patch tests with 1% diclofenac aqueous and various concentrations of the commercial product were negative, while photopatch tests with 10 J/cm UVA produced positive reactions to 1% diclofenac and various Solaraze gels. The authors cite another series in which 5 of 75 cases of photodermatoses were traced to diclofenac. In another patient treated for actinic keratoses with Solaraze gel, the offending agent proved to be the one of the ingredients in the vehicle, polyethylene glycol monomethyl ether 350, which was positive at 5% and 10% in petrolatum.[93]

CINNOXICAM

Cinnoxicam, an ester of piroxicam and cinnamic acid, is used topically in Italy and has caused contact dermatitis. It was not found to crossreact with other common NSAIDs.[94]

PIKETOPROFEN

Piketoprofen is used topically in Spain and caused contact dermatitis in a 27-year-old woman who applied it to treat back pain.[95] Patch tests with 1% and 5% in petrolatum were positive, and 5 controls were negative. No crossreactions were found to oxicams, phenylacetic, indole, fenamates, or propionic acid–derived NSAIDs. This arylpropionic acid group NSAID is sold in Spain in aerosol, cream, and gel forms. It has been reported as a rare cause of allergic and photoallergic contact dermatitis. A 1% patch test concentration in petrolatum is recommended.[96] Piketoprofen contact dermatitis was also seen in a Spanish patient who used Calmatel cream on stasis dermatitis at the direction of her physician. The patient was positive to both 1% and 2% piketoprofen in petrolatum.[97]

ACECLOFENAC

Aceclofenac, an NSAID of the phenylacetic acid group, is used orally, topically, and parenterally in Spain. It is metabolized to diclofenac. Aceclofenac caused photoallergic contact dermatitis confirmed by photo patch tests at 10% petrolatum. No crossreactivity was seen in an extensive series of other NSAIDs including diclofenac.[98] An additional case of contact dermatitis to aceclofenac developed after 8 days of topical use and without sun exposure in a patient with no prior history of topical NSAID use.[99]

NIMESULIDE

Nimesulide is an NSAID popular in some European countries. It can cause fixed drug eruption. Three such cases were reproduced with patch tests applied to the healed eruption site some 6 to 8 weeks after the eruption. Application to non-involved skin was negative. The patch test concentration was either 5% or 10% in petrolatum.[100]

BENDAZAC

In Japan, bendazac is sold as a topical nonsteroidal anti-inflammatory agent. Contact dermatitis to bendazac was confirmed with patch test concentrations down to 0.3% in a patient who also reacted to alclometasone dipropionate.[101]

FELBINAC

Vehicle ingredients in nonsteroidal topical anti-inflammatory agents can also cause contact dermatitis. A rare such case involved isopropanolamine in Traxam gel (felbinace). A test concentration of 1% aqueous was recommended for isopropanolamine, but occasional irritant reactions can be seen at day 2 with this.[102]

CELECOXIB

Celecoxib, a cyclo-oxygenase-2 inhibitor, was evaluated as a patch test substance. In undiluted form, celecoxib produced reaction both in patients allergic to other NSAIDS and in controls. Oral challenge was negative with up to 350 mg of drug and the reactions were considered irritant in nature. Dilutions of 5% and 10% in petrolatum proved non-irritating.[103]

ENOXOLONE AND MAFENIDE

Topical Pentalmicina produced contact dermatitis around a tracheostomy site.[104] This compound is 1.5% enoxolone and 7% mafenide. Enoxolone is a topical anti-inflammatory drug from glycyrrhizinic acid and was tested at 10% in petrolatum.

Mafenide, a sulfonamide (para-amino methylbenzyl-sulfonamide), also tested at 10% in petrolatum. No crossreactions between mafenide and other para-amino group compounds, such as paraphenylenediamine and sulfonanilamide, have been found.[104]

FEPRADINOL

A topical spray of fepradinol caused two cases of contact dermatitis confirmed by 0.1% to 5% aqueous patch tests.[105] Although 20 controls were negative at 5% aqueous, Izu and colleagues[105] do not recommend testing above 1% aqueous. No crossreactions to other NSAIDs were found, and this agent is not chemically an NSAID. Fepradinol is used topically as an anti-inflammatory agent, although it is an adrenergic compound more closely related to ephedrine, phenylephrine, and terbutaline.[106]

Two cases of contact dermatitis to fepradinol were studied to look for crossreactivity to phenylethanolamine compounds, such as adrenergics phenylephrine, ephedrine, and terbutaline. No crossreactivity was found.[107]

Fepradinol caused allergic contact dermatitis when applied to a 12-year-old boy for treatment of myalgia.[108] The application was in the form of a spray known as Flexidol. Patch tests were positive at 0.1 and 1.0% in both aqueous and petrolatum bases.

Photocontact dermatitis to fepradinol was reported from the use of a spray (Dalgen) that contained this anti-inflammatory.[109]

CHLORPROETHAZINE

An ointment containing chlorproethazine was used for chronic neck pain and subsequently incriminated in producing lip and eyelid edema after sun exposure,[110] Photocontact urticaria was reproduced by 0.1% patch tests for 24 hours of chlorproethazine and chlorpromazine followed by 10J of UVA light that produced immediate erythema.[110]

PYRAZINOBUTAZONE

Topical use of this compound, which is an equimolar salt of piperazine and phenylbutazone, produced a dermatitis in an individual sensitized through prior pharmaceutical industry exposure. Patch tests with 5% piperazine hexahydrate and 1% phenylbutazone were positive. Oral provocation produced a hand eczema.[111]

OPIUM ALKALOIDS

Occupational exposure to codeine and morphine was the cause of 11 cases of dermatitis, of which 7 reacted to para group chemicals, such as paraphenylenediamine.[112] Interestingly, the neutral alkaloid piocarpine was found to cause dermatitis from an eyedrop in a patient also paraphenylene-diamine sensitive.[113] A medical facility that dispensed inhalable heroin was found to have work-related problems in half the nurses, and exposure to heroin was believed to be the source of difficulty. About one-third of the symptomatic nurses had a positive patch test to heroin and eyelid or facial dermatitis. Patch tests were done with diacetylmorphine (heroin) at 0.3%, 1%, 3%, and 5% petrolatum. The 3% concentration seemed to identify most cases.[114]

BELLADONNA

A belladonna plaster used as a topical analgesic for back pain caused contact dermatitis traced to atropine. The product was 0.25% belladonna, and the patient was negative to a 2% hyoscine patch test and positive to a 1% atropine in petrolatum patch test.[115]

References

1. Tan BB, et al. Perioperative collapse: prevalence of latex allergy in patients sensitive to anesthetic agents. Contact Dermatitis 1997;36:47.

2. Yilmaz B, Courvoisier S, Bircher AJ. Thiuram-elicited contact dermatitis mistaken for local anesthetic intolerance. Contact Dermatitis 1999;41:301.

3. Mathewson HS. Structural forms of anesthetic compounds. Kansas City, MO: Charles C Thomas Publisher, 1961.

4. Fisher AA. Contact dermatitis. 3rd ed. Philadelphia: Lea & Febiger, 1986.

5. Wilkinson JD, et al. Preliminary patch testing with 25% and 15% "caine"-mixes. Contact Dermatitis 1990;22:244.

6. Sidhu SK, Shaw S, Wilkinson JD. A 10-year retrospective study on benzocaine allergy in the United Kingdom. Am J Contact Dermat 1999;10:57.

7. Fisher AA. The presence of benzocaine in sunscreens containing glyceryl PABA (Escalol 106). Arch Dermatol 1977;113:1299.

8. Hjorth N, et al. Glyceryl p-aminobenzoate patch testing in benzocaine-sensitive subjects. Contact Dermatitis 1978;4:46.

9. van Ketel WG, Bruynzeel DP. A "forgotten" topical anesthetic sensitizer: butyl aminobenzoate. Contact Dermatitis 1991;25:131.

10. Beck MH, Holden A. Benzocaine—an unsatisfactory indicator of topical local anesthetic sensitization of the UK. Br J Dermatol 1988;118:91.

11. Kalveram K, Semmelmann J, Forck G. Experimental animal study of the allergenicity of Tetracaine. Contact Dermatitis 1978;4:374.

12. Kalveram K, et al. Tetracaine allergy: cross-reactions with paracompounds? Contact Dermatitis 1978;4:376.

13. Dannaker CJ, Maibach HI, Austin E. Allergic contact dermatitis to proparacaine with subsequent cross-sensitization to tetracaine from ophthalmic preparations. Am J Contact Dermat 2001;12:177.

14. Connolly M, Mehat A, Sansom JE, et al Allergic contact dermatitis from tetracaine in the beauty industry. Contact Dermatitis 2004;51:95

15. Hardwick N, King CM. Contact allergy to lignocaine with cross-reaction to bupivacaine. Contact Dermatitis 1994;30:245.

16. Fregert S, Tegner E, Thelin I. Contact allergy to lidocaine. Contact Dermatitis 1979;5:185.

17. Roed-Petersen J. Contact sensitivity to metaoxedrine. Contact Dermatitis 1976;2:235.

18. Goransson K. Hypersensitivity to prilocaine. Dermatologica 1976;152:158.

19. Black RJ, Dawson TA, Strang WC. Cross-sensitivity to lignocaine and prilocaine. Contact Dermatitis 1990;23:117.

20. Hofmann H, et al. Presumed generalized exfoliative dermatitis to lidocaine [Letter]. Arch Dermatol 1976;111:266.

21. Chin TM, Fellner MJ. Allergic hypersensitivity to lidocaine hydrochloride. Int Soc Trop Derm 1980;19:147.

22. Mackley CL, Marks JG, Anderson BE. Delayed-type hypersensitivity to lidocaine. Arch Dermatol 2003;139:343.

23. Weightman W, Turner T. Allergic contact dermatitis from lignocaine: report of 29 cases and review of the literature. Contact Dermatitis 1998;39:265.

24. Bircher AJ, Messmer SL, Surber C, Rufli T. Delayed-type hypersensitivity to subcutaneous lidocaine with tolerance to articaine: confirmation by in vivo and in vitro tests. Contact Dermatitis 1996;34:387.

25. Kawada A, et al. Simultaneous contact sensitivity due to lidocaine and crotamiton. Contact Dermatitis 1997;37:45.

26. Klein CE, Gall H. Type IV allergy to amide-type local anesthetics. Contact Dermatitis 1991;25:45.

27. Breit S, Rueff F, Przybilla B. 'Deep impact' contact allergy after subcutaneous injection of local anesthetics. Contact Dermatitis 2001;45:296.

28. Jovanovic M, Karadaglic D, Brkic S. Contact urticaria and allergic contact dermatitis to lidocaine in a patient sensitive to benzocaine and propolis. Contact Dermatitis 2006;54:124.

29. Langas SM, Collins P. Photocontact allergy to oxybenzone and contact allergy to lignocaine and prilocaine. Contact Dermatitis 2006;54:173.

30. Hickey JR, Cook SD, Gutteridge G, et al. Delayed hypersensitivity following intravenous lidocaine. Contact Dermatitis 2006;54:215.

31. Fisher AA. Propylene glycol dermatitis. Cutis 1978;21:166.

32. Roesch A, Haegele T, Vogt T, et al. Severe contact urticaria to guar gum included as gelling agent in a local anaesthetic. Contact Dermatitis 2005;52:307.

33. Soesman-van Waadenoden Kernekamp A, van Ketel WG. Contact allergy to lidocaine (Xylocaine, Lignocaine). Contact Dermatitis 1979;5:403.

34. Downs AMR, Lear JT, Wallington TB, Sansom JE. Contact sensitivity and systemic reaction to pseudoephedrine and lignocaine. Contact Dermatitis 1998;39:33.

35. van den Hove J, Decroix J, Tennstedt D, Lachapelle JM. Allergic contact dermatitis from prilocaine, one of the local anesthetics in EMLA cream. Contact Dermatitis 1994;30:239.

36. Waton J, Boulanger A, Trechot PH, et al. Contact urticaria from EMLA ® cream. Contact Dermatitis 2004:51:284.

37. de Waard-van der Spek FB, Oranje AP. Purpura caused by Emla is of toxic origin. Contact Dermatitis 1997;36:11.

38. Wilson HTH. Dermatitis from anesthetic ointments. Practitioner 1966;197:673.

39. Erdmann SM, Sachs B, Merk HF. Systemic contact dermatitis from cinchocaine. Contact Dermatitis 2001;44:260.

40. Sanchez-Morillas L, Martinez JJL, Martos MR, et al. Delayed-type hypersensitivity to mepivacaine with cross-reaction to lidocaine. Contact Dermatitis 2005;53:352.

41. Schmidt JL, Blockus LE, Richards RK. The pharmacology of pramoxine hydrochloride: a new topical anesthetic. Anesth Anal 1953;32:418.

42. Peal L, Karp M. A new surface anesthetic agent: Tronothane. Anesthesiology 1954;15:637.

43. Sladek WR. Clinical evaluation of a new product for proctologic inflammatory conditions and postoperative use. Am J Clin Res 1970;1:33.

44. Fisher AA. Allergic reactions to topical (surface) anesthetics with reference to the safety of Tronothane (pramoxine hydrochloride). Cutis 1980;25:584.

45. van Ketel WG. Allergy to pramoxine (pramocaine). Contact Dermatitis 1981;7:49.

46. Incaudo G, Schatz M, Patterson R. Administration of local anesthetics to patients with a history of prior adverse reaction. J Allergy Clin Immunol 1978;61:339.

47. Adriani J. Etiology and management of adverse reactions to local anesthetics. Int Anesthesiol Clin 1972;10:127.

48. Lehner T. Lignocaine hypersensitivity. Lancet 1971;1:1245.

49. March C, Greenwood MA. Allergic contact dermatitis to proparacaine. Arch Ophthalmol 1968;79:159.

50. Bandman H-J, Breit R, Mutzeck E. Allergic contact dermatitis from proxymetacaine. Contact Dermatitis Newsletter 1974;14:451.

51. Calnan CD. Allergy to the local anesthetic Diperodon. Contact Dermatitis 1980;6:367.

52. Gastelain PY, Piriou A. Contact dermatitis due to propanidid in an anesthetist. Contact Dermatitis 1980;6:360.

53. Sneddon IB, Caldwell RG. Contact dermatitis due to propanidid in an anaesthetist. Practitioner 1973;211:321.

54. Reichert C, Gall H. Contact dermatitis from hydroxyethyl salicylate. Contact Dermatitis 1995;33:275.

55. Valsecchi R, et al. Contact dermatitis from methyl butetisalicylate. Contact Dermatitis 1998;38:360.

56. Gamboa P, et al. Contact sensitization to topical salicylate. Contact Dermatitis 1995;33:52.

57. Horak J, Hemmer W, Focke M, et al. Contact dermatitis from anit-inflammatory gel containing hydroxyethyl salicylate. Contact Dermatitis 2002;47:120.

58. Szczurko C, et al. Occupational contact dermatitis from propacetamol. Contact Dermatitis 1996;35:299.

59. Berl V, Barbaud A, Lepoittevin J-P. Mechanism of allergic contact dermatitis from propacetamol: Sensitization to activated N,N-diethylglycine. Contact Dermatitis 1998;38:185.

60. Pulido Z, et al. Allergic contact dermatitis from indomethacin. Contact Dermatitis 1999;41:112.

61. Tosti A, Gaddoni G, Valeri F, Bardazzi F. Contact allergy to ketoprofen: report of 7 cases. Contact Dermatitis 1990;23:112.

62. Mozzanica N, Pigatto PD. Contact and photocontact allergy to ketoprofen: clinical and experimental study. Contact Dermatitis 1990;23:336.

63. Durbize E, Vigan M, Puzenat E, et al. Spectrum of cross-photosensitization in 18 consecutive patients with contact photoallergy to ketoprofen : associated photoallergies to non-benzophenone-containing molecules. Contact Dermatitis 2003;48:144.

64. Matthieu L, Meuleman L, Van Hecke E, et al. Contact and photocontact allergy to ketoprofen. The Belgian experience. Contact Dermatitis 2004;50:238.

65. Diaz RL, Gardeazabal J, Manrique P, et al. Greater allergenicity of topical ketoprofen in contact dermatitis confirmed by use. Contact Dermatitis 2006;54:239.

66. Goday-Bujan JJ, Rodriguez-Lozano J, Martinez-Gonzalez MC, et al. Photoallergic contact dermatitis from dexketoprofen: study of 6 cases. Contact Dermatitis 2006;55:59.

67. Foti C, Bonamonte D, Consrva A, et al. Allergic contact dermatitis to glyceryl-hydrogenated rosinate in a topical plaster. Contact Dermatitis 2006;55:120.

68. Suzuki T, Kawada A, Hashimoto Y, et al. Contact urticaria due to ketoprofen. Contact Dermatitis 2003;48:284.

69. Pigatto P, et al. Cross-reactions in patch testing and photopatch testing of ketoprofen, thiaprophenic acid, and cinnamic aldehyde. Am J Contact Dermat 1996;7:220.

70. Le Coz CJ, et al. Photocontact dermatitis from ketoprofen and tiaprofenic acid: cross-reactivity study in 12 consecutive patients. Contact Dermatitis 1998;38:245.

71. Horn HM, Humphreys F, Aldridge RD. Contact dermatitis and prolonged photosensitivity induced by ketoprofen and associated with sensitivity to benzophenone-3. Contact Dermatitis 1998;38:353.

72. Mirande-Romero A, et al. Ketoprofen-induced connubial photodermatitis. Contact Dermatitis 1997;37:242.

73. Mastrolonardo M, Loconosole F, Rantuccio F. Conjugal allergic contact dermatitis from ketoprofen. Contact Dermatitis 1994;30:110.

74. Valsecchi R, Cainelli T. Contact dermatitis from ibuproxam: a case with cross-reactivity with ketoprofen. Contact Dermatitis 1990;22:51.

75. Molinini R. Contact allergy to ibuproxam. Contact Dermatitis 1991;24:302.

76. Kurumaji Y, et al. Allergic photocontact dermatitis due to suprofen: photopatch testing and cross-reaction study. Contact Dermatitis 1991;25:218.

77. Gniazdowska B, Rueff F, Przybilla B. Delayed contact hypersensitivity to non-steroidal antiinflammatory drugs. Contact Dermatitis 1999;40:63.

78. Kranke B, Derhaschnig J, Komericki P, Aberer W. Bufexamac is a frequent contact sensitizer. Contact Dermatitis 1996;34:63.

79. Barbaud A, et al. Bufexamac and diclofenac: frequency of contact sensitization and absence of cross-reactions. Contact Dermatitis 1998;39:272.

80. Koch P, Bahmer FA. Erythema-multiforme-like, urticarial papular and plaque eruptions from bufexamac: report of 4 cases. Contact Dermatitis 1994;31:97.

81. Vincenzi C, Cameli N, Tardio M, Piraccini BM. Contact and photocontact dermatitis due to benzydamine hydrochloride. Contact Dermatitis 1990;23:125.

82. Guerra L, et al. Contact dermatitis due to etofenamate. Contact Dermatitis 1992;26:199.

83. Götze A, Teikemeier G, Goerz G. Contact dermatitis from etofenamate. Contact Dermatitis 1992;26:209.

84. Correia O, Barros MA. Exfoliative dermatitis with etofenamate. Contact Dermatitis 1990;23:264.

85. Hergueta JP, Ortiz FJ, Iglesias L. Allergic contact dermatitis from etofenamate: report of 9 cases. Contact Dermatitis 1994;31:60.

86. Sanchez-Perez J, Sanchez TS, Garcia-Diez A. Combined contact and photocontact allergic dermatitis to etofenamate in Flogoprofen gel. Am J Contact Dermat 2001;12:215.

87. Schiavino D, et al. Delayed allergy to diclofenac. Contact Dermatitis 1992;26:357.

88. Gebhardt M, Reuter A, Knopf B. Allergic contact dermatitis from topical diclofenac. Contact Dermatitis 1994;30:183.

89. Valsecchi R, Pansera B, Leghissa P, Reseghetti A. Allergic contact dermatitis of the eyelids and conjunctivitis from diclofenac. Contact Dermatitis 1996;34:150.

90. Montoro J, Rodriguez M, Diaz M, et al. Photoallergic contact dermatitis due to diclofenac. Contact Dermatitis 2003;48:115.

91. Jonker MJ, Bruynzeel DP. Anaphylactic reaction elicited by patch testing with diclofenac. Contact Dermatitis 2004;49:114.

92. Kowalzick L, Ziegler H. Photoallergic contact dermatitis from topical diclofenac n Solaraze ® gel. Contact Dermatitis 2006;54:348.

93. Taibjee SM, Prais L, Foulds IS. Allergic contact dermatitis from polyethylene glycol monomethyl ether 350 in Solaraze ® gel. Contact Dermatitis 2004;49:170.

94. Valsecchi R, Pansera B, Di Landro A, Cainelli T. Contact allergy to cinnoxicam. Contact Dermatitis 1995;32:63.

95. Navarro LA, Jorro G, Morales C, Pelaez A. Allergic contact dermatitis due to piketoprofen. Contact Dermatitis 1995;32:181.

96. Bujan JJG, Morante JMO, Guemes MG, et al. Photoallergic contact dermatitis from piketoprofen. Contact Dermatitis 2000;43:315.

97. Rodriguez-Lozano J, Goday Bujan JJ, Del Pozo J, et al. Allergic contact dermatitis from topical piketoprofen. Contact Dermatitis 2005;52:110.

98. Bujan JJG, Alvarez-Erie GMG, Martinez W, et al. Photoallergic contact dermatitis from aceclofenac. Contact Dermatitis 2001;45:170.

99. Bort GP, de la Cuadra Oyanguren J, Aguilar AT, et al. Allergic contact dermatitis due to aceclofenac. Contact Dermatitis 2006;55:365.

100. Cordeiro MR, Goncalo M, Fernandes B, et al. Positive lesional patch tests in fixed drug eruptions from nimesulide. Contact Dermatitis 2000;43:307.

101. Iwakiri K, Hata M, Miura Y, et al. Allergic contact dermatitis due to bendazac and alclometasone dipropionate. Contact Dermatitis 1999;41:218.

102. Cooper SM, Shaw S. Contact allergy to isopropanolamine in Traxam gel. Contact Dermatitis 1999;41:233.

103. Kleinhans M, Linzbach L, Zedlitz S, et al. Positive patch test reactions to celecoxib may be due to irritation and do not correlate with the results of oral provocation. Contact Dermatitis 2002;47:100.

104. Fernandez JC, Gamboa P, Jauregui I. Concomitant sensitization to enoxolone and mafenide in a topical medicament. Contact Dermatitis 1992;27:262.

105. Izu R, et al. Allergic contact dermatitis from fepradinol. Contact Dermatitis 1992;27:266.

106. Schnuch A. Fepradinol allergy: possibly a case of unnoticed cross-reaction due to misclassification. Contact Dermatitis 1994;30:243.

107. Goday JJ, et al. No evidence of cross-reaction between fepradinol and other phenylethanolamines. Contact Dermatitis 1997;36:170.

108. Gomez A, Martorell A, dela Cuadra J. Allergic contact dermatitis from fepradinol in a child. Contact Dermatitis 1994;30:44.

109. Rodriguez Granados T, Pineiro G, de la Torre C, Cruces Prado MJ. Photoallergic contact dermatitis from fepradinol. Contact Dermatitis 1998;39:194.

110. Loesche C, Dejobert Y, Thomas P. Immediate wheal after topical administration of chlorproethazine. Contact Dermatitis 1992;26:278.

111. Bris JMD, Montanes MA, Candela MS, Diez AG. Contact sensitivity to pyrazinobutazone (Carudolt) with positive oral provocation test. Contact Dermatitis 1992;26:355.

112. Conde-Salazar L, et al. Occupational allergic contact dermatitis from opium alkaloids. Contact Dermatitis 1991;25:202.

113. Ortiz FJ, et al. Allergic contact dermatitis from pilocarpine and thimerosal. Contact Dermatitis 1991;25:203.

114. Esch AJH, van der Heide S, van den Brink W, et al. Contact allergy and respiratory/mucosal complaints from heroin (diacetylmorphine). Contact Dermatitis 2006;54:42.

115. Williams HC, duVivier A. Belladonna plaster—not as bella as it seems. Contact Dermatitis 1990;23:119.

TOPICAL CORTICOSTEROIDS

EXECUTIVE SUMMARY

Reactions to corticosteroids may be suspected when use of these agents leads to worsening of the treated condition. Efforts to simplify and standardize testing for corticosteroid allergy have led to development of various tests to screen for categories of corticosteroid allergens. Tixocortol pivalate 1% in petrolatum is widely used to test for hydrocortisone allergy which commonly links to prednisone and prednisolone allergy. Budesonide in concentrations of 1% to 0.1% in petrolatum is used to screen for allergy to two classes of commonly used corticosteroids referred to as Class B and D. This combination of tests is often supplemented with hydrocortisone-17-butyrate which is from Class D2. Narrow corticosteroid allergy may be missed by such limited testing, so testing with the actual corticoid used is required in such a case. Broad-based allergy to corticosteroids is more likely to follow a pattern predicted by the Class A, B, C, D1, and D2 characterization of corticosteroids.

Patch testing with estrogens and progesterones has not been as useful as testing with corticosteroids, with some exceptions. Inhaled corticosteroids used to treat asthma more commonly cause cutaneous reactions than mucosal reactions.

Vehicle ingredients have produced reactions, but they have not been reported as frequently as reactions to the active corticosteroid.

Reactions to topical corticosteroids or their vehicles should be suspected when the use of the topical corticosteroids either does not improve the existing dermatitis or makes it worse. One should be alerted particularly when a patient has used a topical corticosteroid with a good response but then no longer responds, or the existing dermatitis becomes worse. If a patient with a corticosteroid-responsive dermatosis does not respond appropriately, one could consider the possibility that corticosteroid allergy might be the reason for a lack of response. In a study of 41 such cases, 9 or 22% were found to be allergic to corticosteroids.[1]

Children with atopic dermatitis are exposed to topical corticosteroids over prolonged periods of time. A study of 71 children with atopic dermatitis and use of topical corticosteroids for greater than 6 months in the prior 2 years found that 18 (25.3%) reported aggravation or lack of improvement in the dermatitis with such treatment. While this might suggest corticosteroid allergy, only one child proved to be sensitive on patch testing with tixocortol pivalate, hydrocortisone-17-butyrate, and Locoidon cream.[2]

Superimposed contact dermatitis from the topical steroid may be due to allergic hypersensitivity to the corticosteroid itself or to one of the ingredients in the vehicle or base of the topical corticosteroid. Some patients are allergic to a single corticosteroid, whereas others may be sensitized to several corticosteroids. A rare consequence of patch testing with corticosteroids is the development of persistent telangiectasia, which can be ablated with laser treatment if unduly objectionable.[3]

Hydrocortisones

Soon after hydrocortisones were introduced, several cases of allergic contact sensitivity to these low-potency topical corticosteroids were reported (Figure 15-1).[4–7]

OVER-THE-COUNTER TOPICAL HYDROCORTISONE PREPARATIONS

The U.S. Food and Drug Administration has approved the use of over-the-counter preparations containing 0.5% and 1% hydrocortisone or hydrocortisone acetate.

It is a paradox, however, that, prescription-type corticosteroid preparations require the manufacturer to give details of the vehicles, but no such requirement is made for over-the-counter preparations. This creates difficulty in testing persons suspected of having superimposed allergic contact dermatitis from an

Table 15-1 Over-the-Counter Topical Corticosteroids Containing Parabens

Nonprescription hydrocortisone ½%

    Bactine Hydrocortisone Skin Care Cream (Miles Laboratories)

    Caldecort Hydrocortisone Cream (Pennwalt)

    Corticaine (Glaxo)

    Delacort (Medicon)

    Prepcort Hydrocortisone Cream (Whitehall)

    Resicort Cream (Mentholatum)

Nonprescription hydrocortisone acetate ½%

    Cortaid Cream, Lotion, Ointment (Upjohn)

    Cortef Feminine Itch Cream (Upjohn)

    Cortef Rectal Itch Ointment (Upjohn)

    Gynecort Antipruritic Cream (Combe)

    Lanacort Antipruritic Cream (Combe)

    Wellcortin Cream, Lotion (Burroughs Wellcome)[a]

[a]No longer manufactured.

ingredient in the vehicle of the OTC hydrocortisone preparations.

Table 15.1 lists those OTC topical corticosteroids that contain parabens often used as preservatives. It should be noted that most prescription-type topical corticosteroids do not contain parabens; however, most OTC nonprescription-type corticosteroids do.[8] Table 15.2 lists over-the-counter topical corticosteroid creams and lotions free of parabens.

Table 15.3 lists preparations that contain propylene glycol. Certain manufacturers of topical corticosteroid preparations state that a 25% concentration of propylene glycol in the vehicle may have sufficient bactericidal reactions to guarantee formulation stability without any of the usual preservatives, such as parabens.[9]

The only preparation sold in the United States that contains sorbic acid is Hytone Cream (Dermik), a nonprescription preparation with ½% hydrocortisone. Sorbic acid is a rare sensitizer, but, not uncommonly, it produces a slight stinging sensation and erythema in some persons.[10]

Several reports show that hydrocortisone sensitivity may be accompanied by hypersensitivity to more potent topical corticosteroids.[5,11–13]

Table 15-2 Paraben-Free Over-the-Counter Corticosteroid Lotions and Creams

Dermolate Anti-Itch Cream (Schering)

Dermolate Scalp Itch Lotion (Schering)

Hytone Cream (Dermik)

Rhulicort Cream and Lotion (Lederle)

Table 15-3 Over-the-Counter Corticosteroid Preparations Containing Propylene Glycol

Nonprescription hydrocortisone ½%

    Bactine Hydrocortisone Skin Care Cream (Miles Laboratories)

    Caldecort Hydrocortisone Cream, Spray, Ointment (Pennwalt)

    Cortef Feminine Itch Cream (Upjohn)

    Delacort (Medicon)

    Dermolate Anti-Itch Cream and Spray (Schering)

Hydrocortisone-17-butyrate has been reported to have produced allergic contact sensitivity in several patients in Europe.[14–16] Brandao and Camarasa[14] obtained a positive patch test with 0.1% in petrolatum, whereas Soesman-van Waadenoden Kernekamp and van Ketel[15] obtained a positive patch test with 1% in petrolatum. Corticosteroid allergy has been so commonly reported that 2.9% to 4.8% of patients screened in European clinics have been found to be allergic to one or more corticosteroids.[17]

The availability of corticosteroids not sold in the United States has aided in screening for hydrocortisone and other corticosteroid allergy. Tixocortol pivalate and budesonide in petrolatum (1%) detect most cases, but, just as petrolatum is not the ideal base for delivering corticosteroids through the stratum corneum, it has not always proven to be the correct base for patch testing.[17] A study of 127 patients allergic to one or more corticosteroids found that the combination of tixocortol pivalate and budesonide detected 91.3% of the cases.[18] In the study, a larger group of corticoids was used for patch testing, and the frequency of reactions was as follows: tixocortol, 96; hydrocortisone butyrate, 51; budesonide, 47; betamethasone valerate, 11; clobetasone butyrate, 11; clobetasol propionate, 8. Although some investigators recommend ethanol or mixtures of ethanol, propylene glycol, and isopropanol or higher concentrations of corticosteroid,[17] others have found the commercial preparations adequate for screening purposes.[19,20]

Freeman[21] found that the best way to screen for corticosteroid allergy was to use the patient's corticosteroid in cream base for patch testing. This had the highest yield, followed by commercially prepared corticosteroid ointment, and was more sensitive than pure corticosteroid in either petrolatum or alcohol. Delayed positive reactions were common and required late readings for proper detection. The repeat open application test proved a simple and useful diagnostic tool.

Tixocortol pivalate (Pivalone) has been shown to be both a sensitive and specific marker for hydrocortisone allergy confirmed by intradermal skin tests with hydrocortisone (Figures 15-2 and 15-3).[22] Pivalone was more accurate than hydrocortisone in tests with ethanol or a hydrocortisone/ethanol/-dimethylsulfoxide (DMSO) mixture.[22] An intradermal skin test with 1 mg of hydrocortisone sodium phosphate confirms the accuracy of tixocortol pivalate, and tests with precursors and metabolites of hydrocortisone do not appear to be the allergen.[23] Intradermal skin tests for corticosteroid allergy are thought to be more sensitive but less convenient than patch tests. However, this is only true for some corticosteroids. Tixocortol pivalate 1% in petrolatum detected all the cases of corticosteroid allergy to hydrocortisone that were detected by intradermal hydrocortisone succinate.[24] Likewise, budesonide 1% in petrolatum was as sensitive as intradermal budesonide. However. patch tests with hydrocortisone-17-butyrate missed 30% of cases due to this corticosteroid.

CORTICOSTEROIDS AS HAPTENS

The C17 position on the corticosteroid has been suggested as the site for protein binding to form a complete antigen.[23]

The mechanism by which corticosteroids become complete allergens rather than haptens has focused around binding to arginine. An alternative hypothesis involving the metabolism of the corticosteroid at the 21 position to form a 21-dehydroderivative, which is then converted to an alpha-ketoaldehyde, has been proposed and partially supported by patch test observations as a potential mechanism.[25]

EFFECT OF CONCENTRATION AND TIME

The standard recommended concentration for patch testing with budesonide is 0.1% in petrolatum. However, a lower dose was found to yield higher results in some patients.[26] Patch test concentrations down to 0.0002% were at times more sensitive in detecting allergy than higher concentrations. It was recommended that 0.02% to 0.002% be used based on cases from Sweden and Belgium in whom this dosage range proved most effective.[26] An investigation into whether 1% or 0.1% tixocortol pivalate is the better for detecting corticosteroid allergy found that 1.74% of tested patients reacted to 1% in petrolatum, while 0.95% reacted to 0.1% in petrolatum. The 1% concentration was considered preferable. This study also looked at budesonide at 0.1% and 0.01%, and found that 0.62% of tested patients reacted to the higher concentration and 0.43% to the lower concentration, both of which were in petrolatum. The authors did not feel that a clear choice was evident between the budesonide concentrations.[27]

A careful evaluation of the relationship between the pharmacologic and immunologic effects of the corticosteroid budesonide was undertaken to examine the time course, dose, and occlusion times on reactions.[28] A range of 2% to 0.002% was studied with occlusion times of 5, 24, and 48 hours and readings at days 2, 4, and 7. High concentrations tended to produce late reactions, and lower concentrations were seen at day 2. A 48-hour occlusion time was best. A phenomenon seen with corticosteroids known as the edge effect or a rim reaction, in which erythema occurs only around the circumference of the chamber, represents true sensitization (Figure 15-4). This can be demonstrated by lowering the concentration and repeating the test. A more traditional reaction is then seen. When testing with corticosteroids in ethanol, the optimum concentration for testing depends on when the reading will be taken. Day 4 readings are common end points and on that reading schedule the optimum concentration for budesonide was 0.002, triamcinolone acetonide 0.001, amcinonide 0.0001, hydrocortisone-17-butyrate 1.0 and prednicarbate 0.1, all v/v. These are lower concentrations than are commonly used.[29] A comparison of budesonide 1% in ethanol to 0.01% in petrolatum was conducted in 4033 patients to see if one proved more useful. The results were similar in terms of detecting allergy, and since petrolatum is easier to work with in terms of stability and practicality, it was preferred.[30]

Isaksson and colleagues[31] tried to improve on our ability to identify corticosteroid allergy by using mixes and lower concentrations of three corticoids: budesonide, tixocortol pivalate, and hydrocortisone-17-butyrate. Although they found merit in the lower concentration, of more significance was the fact that all tests regardless of concentration were positive when readings were taken at day 10 rather than day 7. The value of late readings in corticosteroids appears to be confirmed. The value of taking patch test reading on corticosteroids beyond day 4 was questioned in a study from the Mayo Clinic. Only 2 patients out of 135 tested developed a reaction at day 7 or beyond that would not have been detected earlier.[32]

In response to the uncertainty of optimal vehicle, concentration, route of exposure (patch test vs intradermal), and proper screening substances, Chang and colleagues[33] recommended testing the commercial formulas of corticosteroids in question for the patient by provocative use tests or repeated open application tests as they did in their patient who was sensitive to 23 different corticosteroids.

CORTICOSTEROID ALLERGEN CLASSES

Four classes of corticosteroids (Coopman classification) have been suggested based on the frequency of

Table 15-4 Four Classes of Corticosteroids Based on Frequency of Crossreactivity

Class A	Class C
Hydrocortisone type	Betamethasone type (not valerate)
Hydrocortisone with C17 and/or C21-acetate ester	Betamethasone and disodium phosphate
Tixocortol pivalate	Dexamethasone and disodium phosphate
Prednisone+/- acetate	Flucortolone
Methylprednisolone+/-acetate	Desoximetasone
Cloprednol	Clocortolone pivalate
Fludrocortisone acetate	Rimexolon
Class B	**Class D1**
Triamcinolone type	Less labile
Triamcinolone acetonide or alcohol	Clobetasol propionate and butyrate
Amcinonide	Betamethasone valerate and dipropionate
Fluocinolone acetonide	Fluocortolone hexanoate and pivalate
Budesonide	Aclometasone dipropionate
Halcinonide	Diflorasone diacetate
Flucinonide	Fluticasone propionate
Desonide	Memetasone furoate
Flunisolide	Beclomethasone dipropionate
Procinonide	**Class D2**
Flucloronide	More labile
Flucloronide acetonide	Hydrocortisone-17-butyrate and 17-aceponate and 17-buteprate
	Prednicarbate

corticosteroid crossreactivity (Table 15.4). Goosens has subclassified Group D corticosteroids into D1 which are halogenated with a C16 substitution and D2 which arelabile prodrug esters without the characteristics found in D1.[34] Although these classes can be used as a guide,[20] many exceptions occur, and nothing can fully substitute for testing the corticosteroid preparation directly on the patient. Sasaki,[19] in a review of 18 cases of corticosteroid allergy and cross-sensitivity, found that betamethasone (Class C) types of allergy rarely crossreact with triamcinolone (Class B). An example of crossreactivity within a class may be seen in the case of Gamboa and colleagues,[35] who reported facial edema, nasal edema, and dermatitis from a budesonide nasal spray confirmed by a 0.2% petrolatum patch test. A crossreaction with amcinonide was observed (both Class B). However, allergic contact dermatitis was reported from prednicarbate (a Class D corticosteroid), and the patch test was positive at the use concentration.[36] This patient crossreacted only to 1% budesonide (Class B) but not to others, including other Class D corticosteroids (Figure 15-5).

The somewhat unpredictable nature of crossreactions among these four classes has given rise to various recommendations for simplified corticosteroid screening. Lauerma[37] found that Classes A, B, and D crossreacted most frequently, and he proposed tixocortol pivalate and hydrocortisone-17-butyrate as a good screening

combination.[37] He also found that Class C (betamethasone type) was the least common corticosteroid allergen in Finland.[37] Although hydrocortisone-17-butyrate (Locoid) is available in the United States, tixocortol is not. Screening with the corticosteroids used by a patient in the commercial formula along with hydrocortisone-17-butyrate would be the reasonable alternative in the United States in the absence of tixocortol availability.

Tixocortol pivalate used as a nasal spray has produced sensitization in as little as 11 days.[38] This would suggest that the greatest use of tixocortol pivalate may be in screening for contact dermatitis rather than in treatment for inflammatory disorders. An example of that use can be seen in the report of a lymphoma patient who received methylprednisolone as part of a chemotherapy program and developed a generalized rash from prednisolone hemisuccinate detected by patch testing with tixocortol.[39] A 5% prednisolone hemisuccinate patch test in 50/50 ethanol/DMSO was also positive.

Challenges to the Coopman classification of corticosteroids into four groups have arisen. In one study of 12 patients who were allergic to budesonide, crossreactivity was not adequately evaluated with patch test results, but rather necessitated intradermal testing. This study did not identify reactions to the Group D corticoids alclomethasone, betamethasone-17-valerate, clobetasol, or hydrocortisone-17-butyrate, or to Group C dexamethasone. Instead,

7 of the 12 patients reacted to hydrocortisone-21-sodium phosphate (Group A) and 1 to methyl-prednisolone (Group A). Another 6 patients reacted to triamcinolone, which would be predicted by the Coopman classification as both triamcinolone and budesonide are in Group B (Figure 15-6).[40]

NARROW VERSUS BROAD CORTICOSTEROID ALLERGY

The four classes of corticosteroids that are based on allergen crossreaction patterns may give the impression that crossreactions are expected and always predictable. This is not the case. Some patients have very narrow allergy and react only to one or two corticosteroids. An example of this is found in the case of Corazza and Virgili,[41] who tested a 26-year-old nurse and found her allergic to 6-alpha-methylprednisolone aceponate, which is allergen Class D. A positive reaction to budesonide 0.1% in petrolatum was found, and this is a known marker for Class B and D allergy. However, no other reactions were noted to members of Classes A, B, or D. Thus, this patient exhibits narrow allergy rather than broad allergy. In a study of crossreactivity between budesonide and desonide based on patch test results, only 1 of 20 budesonide-sensitive patients reacted to 0.1% and 1% desonide in petrolatum. This suggested that the crossreactions predicted on chemical similarity might not be reliable.[42]

The difficulty of testing for corticosteroid allergy is illustrated by the case reported by Quirce and colleagues.[43] Their patient developed periocular dermatitis after use of a corticosteroid eye product containing hydrocortisone and dexamethasone. Patch tests with tixocortol and budesonide were negative, as was hydrocortisone. The patient had a systemic eczematous dermatitis when treated with prednisone 30 mg per day. A challenge with 30 mg of prednisone again caused a systemic eczema. Patch tests with prednisone powder as is and prednisone 5% in ethanol were positive, yet prednisone 10% in petrolatum was negative.

Contact dermatitis from hydrocortisone aceponate, a group D2 corticoid, led to a widespread eruption where no corticoid had been applied. Crossreactions to budesonide and hydrocortisone-17-butyrate (also D2) were identified.[44]

Newer corticosteroids have also caused dermatitis and produced positive patch test reactions. Prednicarbate is one such molecule, and it fits into allergen Class D2. Although it is nonhalogenated, it is esterified at C17 and C21. Villas Martinez and colleagues[45] reported a patient who had broad corticosteroid sensitivity reacting to corticosteroids of Classes A, B, and D. A study of 19 patients

with corticosteroid allergy found tixocortol-21-pivalate to account for most of the reactions (68%). The most common crossreaction seen was between group A hydrocortisone-type compounds and group D2 labile corticosteroid esters with a long-chain ester at C17 or C21 (hydrocortisone -17-valerate, hydrocortisone-17-butyrate, and prednicarbate).[46]

One case has been reported of contact dermatitis from flucortin butyl, detected with a 0.25% petrolatum patch test that did not crossreact with tixocortol or any of the other four corticosteroid classes.[47] This would represent narrow allergy. A patient with broad sensitivity to group B and D corticosteroids was found also to react to desoximethasone a group C corticoid and mometasone furoate from group D1. This individual did not react to group A corticosteroids.[48] This would be an example of broad allergy.

CLASS C—"HYPOALLERGENIC CORTICOSTEROIDS"

Although there are fewer reports of allergic reactions to Class C corticosteroids, it is unclear if desoximetasone, which is a topical agent in Class C, is truly less reactive. It has been reported most commonly as an allergen in the setting of multiple positive corticosteroids, and it has also been a source of erythema multiforme–like eruption.[49]

Paramethasone acetate is a 6-alpha-methylprednisolone 21-acetate, which is in allergen Class C. A Spanish patient with alopecia areata reacted to injections of paramethasone into the balding areas of the scalp.[50] No other Class C corticosteroids reacted, but tixocortol pivalate (Class A) and hydrocortisone-17-butyrate (Class D) reacted. Paramethasone is used primarily for intralesional injections. It has also been reported to cause systemic reactions of an urticarial type.

Mometasone furoate and fluticasone propionate, which are in Class D, were found to produce fewer reactions than other tested corticosteroids in a series by Wilkinson and Beck.[51] Novel substitutions at the C17 position make mometasone less likely to crossreact with other corticosteroids. In the case of fluticasone, fluorine at C6 and C9 rather than the ester at C17 are thought to be responsible for lesser crossreactivity.

INHALED CORTICOSTEROIDS

Contact allergy to budesonide has been reported from nasal sprays as well as oral inhalers.[52] Corticosteroids are administered by inhalation to treat asthma. Reactions may be seen 3 to 4 hours after such treatment. This time-course might suggest immediate sensitivity, as would symptoms such as angioedema of the oral pharynx accompanied by sore throat and dysphagia, but in such a case, Pirker and colleagues found that immediate tests were negative and delayed hypersensitivity was demonstrated by patch testing. In their case, the allergen was budesonide and allergy was established about 2 weeks after therapy was instituted. They did not find allergy to other group A, B, C, or D corticosteroids and their patient was able to safely inhale beclomethasone dipropionate (group D), fluticasone-17-propionate (also D), and dexamethasone-21-isonicotinate (group C).[53] A study of 30 patients on inhaled or intranasal corticosteroids found that 2 patients were sensitized to budesonide.[54]

Fluticasone propionate inhalant, used to treat an asthmatic woman, led to development of immediate type hypersensitivity with cross reactions to deflazacort drops and betamethasone tablets. The patient tolerated oral prednisone.[55] Sultanol and Aldecin both have beclomethasone dipropionate as a common ingredient, and both produced positive patch tests in a patient who inhaled these agents for asthma but developed dermatitis around his tracheostoma. There was no evidence of inflammation of the trachea.[56]

CORTICOSTEROIDS AND ACUTE GENERALIZED EXANTHEMATOUS PUSTULOSIS (AGEP)

Oral prednisolone led to 2 cases of AGEP complete with fever and neutrophilia. Treatment was successful with group D1 (betamethasone dipropionate) and D2 (hydrocortisone-17-butyrate) used topically. Patch tests and lymphocyte transformation tests were confirmatory.[57] While acute generalized exanthematous pustulosis (AGEP) is most commonly a drug eruption, AGEP was the clinical presentation of allergy to topical Class D corticosteroids. The histology showed spongiform pustules within the superficial layers of the epidermis and beneath the stratum corneum.[58]

DEFLAZACORT

Deflazacort is a corticosteroid sold in Spain. Several cases of systemic dermatitis from oral ingestion have been reported, including a case of toxic epidermal necrolysis. An additional case presented with the baboon syndrome and histology of erythema multiforme, and after patch testing, this individual experienced a widespread eruption. Crossreaction with other corticosteroids was not observed or predicted based on the unique chemical structure of deflazacort.[59]

TACROLIMUS AND PIMECROLIMUS

Alternatives to corticosteroids would include topical tacrolimus and pimecrolimus. Allergic contact dermatitis

to both have been reported by Shaw and colleagues. Provocative use testing with tacrolimus produced a reaction on the face in 1 week, but took 7 weeks on the antecubital fossae. A 2.5% concentration in ethanol was required for patch testing.[60] The patient whom Shaw and colleagues[61] reported allergic to tacrolimus was challenged with pimecrolimus, and reacted weakly to the commercial product on patch testing with a negative test to the vehicle. The use test was positive on the face at 1 week and on the wrist at 2 weeks.

Pimecrolimus contact dermatitis was also reported from use on stasis dermatitis with positive patch test results to the commercial product and negative results to the vehicle control.[62] Allergy to the vehicle in pimecrolimus has also been reported and traced to oleyl alcohol tested 10% in petrolatum.[63]

ENDOGENOUS STEROIDS

Glucocorticoid allergy may be a clue to reactivity to other endogenous substances. Infusion of adrenocorticotrophic hormone (ACTH) in patients with corticosteroid allergy has been shown to cause systemic dermatitis.[64] This concept was carried even further in a study of 19 corticosteroid-allergic patients, 11 of whom reacted to 11-deoxycortisol and 5 of whom reacted to 17-alpha-OH-progesterone.[65] This latter group of progesterone-allergic patients could express autoimmune progesterone dermatitis.

An investigation of 5 women with autoimmune progesterone dermatitis and 1 with estrogen-sensitive dermatitis was conducted to examine the relationship of sex steroid allergy to corticosteroid allergy.[66] An extensive patch test evaluation failed to confirm a linkage between the two conditions; furthermore, patch testing with 17-alpha-OH-progesterone was not helpful. Autoimmune progesterone dermatitis has traditionally been diagnosed with intradermal testing. In another such patient, patch tests were investigated as an alternative diagnostic tool but the results were negative.[67]

Systematic patch testing with 17-hydroxyprogesterone hexanoate 1% in ethanol revealed that 19.4% of corticosteroid-sensitive patients also reacted to this progesterone.[68] It had previously been reported that 26.3% of corticosteroid patients react to progesterone. This is an adrenal hormone in men and women but also has ovarian sources in women. This was felt to be a crossreaction and was seen more commonly in the setting of allergy to multiple corticosteroid as opposed to solitary corticosteroid sensitivity. The broader the allergy, the more likely the crossreaction to the sex steroids. Lamb and Wilkinson[69] reported a patient with contact allergies to multiple topical corticosteroids, estradiol, and several progesterone compounds. They recommended that evaluation for sex steroid hormone allergy include patch testing with hydroxyprogesterone 1.0% in ethanol, medroxyprogesterone 1.0% in acetone, progesterone 1.0% in ethanol, estradiol 1.0% in ethanol, and testosterone 1.0% in ethanol.

Sensitizers in Vehicles of Topical Corticosteroids

Table 15.5 lists the ingredients of topical corticosteroid preparations that have caused allergic contact dermatitis from their presence in the base. Use of commercial corticosteroid preparations for patch test screening leaves open the possibility that a vehicle ingredient is at fault, but testing both the ointment and the cream formulas of the positive preparations can sometimes quickly resolve this issue. At other times, only patch tests with individual ingredients may be able to answer the academic and practical questions regarding corticosteroid allergy.

Ethylenediamine hydrochloride was undoubtedly the most common cause of topical corticosteroid sensitivity from its presence in original Mycolog cream, in which it was used as a stabilizer. This ingredient, the parent substance of several antihistamines, is present in aminophylline. It should be noted that original Mycolog ointment was free of ethylenediamine hydrochloride. Currently, only generic formulations of the original Mycolog formula are available. This compound has been reformulated without ethylenediamine and has replaced the original formula from Squibb as Mycolog II cream. When a corticosteroid cream contains an ingredient such as formaldehyde, the use of such products on formaldehyde-allergic patients will not exhibit the normal therapeutic activity that would be expected of the corticoid. A study of 7 such formaldehyde sensitive patients who were treated for experimentally induced nickel dermatitis found only 29% healed, compared to a control group of 17 nickel-allergic (but not formaldehyde-sensitive) patients in whom 71% healed with the corticoid product that was preserved with a formaldehyde-releasing preservative.[70]

The paraben preservatives produce allergic hypersensitivity, particularly in over-the-counter preparations, which may contain this preservative. Fisher[71] saw three patients who became allergic to Cortaid Cream, an over-the-counter preparation that contains paraben.

Lazzarini[72] described a patient allergic to triamcinolone, benzyl alcohol, and isopropyl palmitate, ingredients of certain topical corticosteroids. Black[73] reported contact dermatitis from stearyl alcohol in a fluocinonide cream. Oleffe and colleagues[74] described allergic reactions to chlorocresol and propylene glycol in a steroid cream.

Maibach and Conant[75] described contact urticaria from polysorbate 60, which is present in 1% hydrocortisone cream. It should be noted that polysorbate, an emulsifier, is not related chemically to sorbic acid.

Nonallergic Complications of Topical Corticosteroids

NONSPECIFIC IRRITATION FOR SORBIC ACID

Table 15.6 lists topical corticosteroids that contain sorbic acid. Sorbic acid is a rare sensitizer, but much more commonly it is a primary urticariogenic agent that produces temporary erythema and a stinging sensation from use of the corticosteroid creams shown in Table 15.6. Unless the stinging reaction is marked, this is not a contraindication for the use of these corticosteroid creams. Stinging and erythema are more marked on the face than elsewhere on the body.[10]

Table 15-5 Excipients in Topical Corticosteroids That Have Caused Contact Dermatitis
Benzyl alcohol
Chlorocresol
Ethylenediamine hydrochloride
Isopropyl palmitate
Parabens
Polysorbate 60
Propylene glycol
Stearyl alcohol
Dioctyl sodium sulfosuccinate
Sodium metabisulfite
1,2,6-hexanetriol

Table 15-6 Topical Corticosteroids Containing Sorbic Acid
Aristocort Cream (Lederle)[a]
Fluorone Cream (Upjohn)
Hytone Cream (Dermik)
Kenalog Cream (Squibb)
Maxiflor Cream (Herbert)
Pramosone Cream (Ferndale)[a]

[a]Contains both sorbic acid and potassium sorbate. Aristocort A cream is free of these preservatives.
Note: Sorbitol solution, sorbitan, and polysorbate are emulsifying agents unrelated to sorbic acid.

LONG-TERM COMPLICATIONS FROM THE USE OF TOPICAL CORTICOSTEROIDS

These complications are listed in Table 15.7. Robertson and Maibach[76] noted transient vasodilation rather than vasoconstriction occasionally when patch testing with fluorinated corticosteroids. They also observed persistent erythema of the eyelids with repeated application of fluorinated corticosteroids.

Corticosteroid Creams vs. Ointments

Most topical corticosteroid ointments are free of preservatives because they do not contain water as do most creams; therefore, topical ointments are unlikely to be contaminated with mold and bacteria.

POLYETHYLENE GLYCOLS

These chemicals are solvent vehicles, emollients, and emulsion stabilizers. Halog Ointment, Halog Cream, and Cortaid Cream contain low-numbered polyethylene glycol sensitizers.

The lower molecular weight liquid polyethylene glycols (PEGs) varying from 200 to 700 are used extensively as solvent vehicles in topical medicaments. Fisher[77,78] reported four patients who had allergic reactions to these PEGs in topical medications.

Two patients had immediate urticarial reactions to PEG 400. Two other patients had delayed allergic eczematous reactions, one to PEG 200 and one to PEG 300. Cross-reactions occurred among PEG 200, 300, and 400 but not between these liquid polyethylenes and the higher molecular weight solid polyethylenes from 1,000 to 6,000.

Maibach[79] stressed that PEGs of varying molecular weights are used extensively as vehicles in topical medicaments but are not listed as sensitizers in standard reference books.

Braun[80] studied 40 patients who had delayed allergic contact sensitivity to a medication containing nitrofural, a Furacin-like product. In 3 of 40 cases, the active ingredient, nitrofuran, was not the cause of the dermatitis, and the solvent polyethylene glycol 300 was the culprit.

Benzyl Alcohol

Benzyl alcohol, also known as alpha-hydroxytoluene, phenylmethanol, and phenylcarbinol, is used in topical corticosteroids as a solvent and a preservative and is also used in perfumes.

Fisher[81] found that two patients who had contact dermatitis, one from a perfume and the other from an aftershave lotion, were sensitized by benzyl alcohol. Both patients had positive patch tests to benzyl alcohol 1% in petrolatum. Neither patient had evidence of immediate-type hypersensitivity.

Schultheiss[82] reported a patient who contacted dermatitis from various flavors for drinks. The patient reacted on patch testing to benzyl alcohol 0.5% in olive oil. He had been sensitized previously to balsam of Peru. Lagerholm[83] reported benzyl-alcohol sensitivity from a vitamin B_{12} injection that had been preserved with benzyl alcohol.

Table 15.8 lists topical corticosteroid preparations that contain benzyl alcohol.

Menthol

This antipruritic agent is used in Cordran Lotion. It should be noted that menthol used over a wide area of the body, particularly in elderly persons, may produce a marked chilling effect. Menthol is a rare sensitizer.[84,85]

Urea

This compound is present in Alphaderm HC and in Carmol HC. Although urea does not cause contact allergies, it often produces irritation. Thus, Hannuksela[86] stated that burning and itching sensations are the most usual untoward effects of urea creams. The burning and itching disappear usually within 1 hour. Cramers and Thormann[87] stated that under occlusion, urea cream may cause irritation and that patch testing with urea cream often produces an irritant reaction, frequently in intertriginous areas.

Table 15-7 Nonallergic Complications of Topical Corticosteroids
Atrophy
Granuloma of the diaper area
Hypertrichosis
Hypopigmentation
Masking of cutaneous infections
Perioral dermatitis
Sorbic acid, erythema, and stinging
Steroid acne
Steroid rosacea

Table 15-8 Topical Corticosteroids Containing Benzyl Alcohol
Aristocort A Cream
Cordran Cream
Cyclocort Cream
Original Mycolog Cream (in the perfume)

Perfumes

It is likely that many corticosteroid creams contain fragrances. These, however, may be so-called masking fragrances that are not listed in the ingredients of the vehicles. They are usually of such low concentration that they are unlikely to produce allergic contact dermatitis.

Sodium Bisulfite

This antioxidant, reducing agent is present in Carmol HC Cream. Epstein[88] described a patient who was allergic to the ingredients of Veg-White powder, which contains sodium bisulfite. Patch tests were positive to 5% and to 10% of sodium bisulfite in petrolatum. Sodium bisulfite is also used to prevent discoloration of fruits and vegetables, particularly of foods used in salads. The presence of this antioxidant in foods has been implicated as the cause of toxicity in some persons. Several controls should be tested with this substance for comparison, because patch testing with sodium bisulfite often leads to irritant patch test reactions.

Sodium Metabisulfite

Sodium metabisulfite was also a cause of contact dermatitis in an experimental corticosteroid cream evaluated by Vestergaard and Andersen.[89] They tested 1% sodium metabisulfite in petrolatum in 54 patients and found 3 doubtful positive reactions. However, their patient had a 2+ reaction to 1% and a delayed 2+ reaction to 0.2% sodium metabisulfite. No reaction was seen to sodium sulfite. Tucker and colleagues[90] reported contact dermatitis from sodium metabisulfate found in Trimovate cream.

Cumulative irritancy testing of over-the-counter hydrocortisone preparations led to 2 of 50 subjects becoming sensitized to sodium metabisulfite.[91] A 1% sodium metabisulfite patch test was positive in these two individuals. Higher concentrations in the range of 5% can produce transient day 2 patch test responses. Ketoconazole cream also contains this agent, as do some injectable forms of lidocaine, along with Veg-White, which is used to preserve salad ingredients. Contact dermatitis due to sodium metabisulfite has been reported to all of these exposures.[91]

Sometimes a patient will become sensitized to both the corticoid and a vehicle ingredient. This proved to be the case in a woman who used Trimovate (GlaxoSmithKline) for vulval soreness. She reacted to 0.5% clobetasone butyrate and 0.1% sodium metabisulfite, both of which are present in the product.[92]

Dioctyl Sodium Sulfosuccinate

Excipients in corticosteroids that have been a cause of contact dermatitis include benzyl alcohol, chlorocresol, ethylenediamine hydrochloride, isopropyl palmitate, parabens, polysorbate 60, propylene glycol, stearyl alcohol, and dioctyl sodium sulfosuccinate.[93]

1,2,6-Hexanetriol

Miura and colleagues[94] added 1,2,6-hexanetriol in fluocinonide cream to the list of excipients found in corticosteroids. This agent is used as a humectant and viscosity regulating agent. Patch tests were positive down to 0.5% in petrolatum.

Injectable Depo-Medrol contains miripirium chloride 0.2 mg/mL as a preservative, and this caused finger eczema after intra-articular injection in a patient with rheumatoid arthritis. A patch test with 0.1% was strongly positive at the day 7 reading as well as 0.03%. This allergen is also known as myristyl-gamma-picolinium chloride.[95]

Local Anesthetics

Pramasone Lotion (Ferndale) contains hydrocortisone and the local anesthetic pramoxine hydrochloride. There is only one report in the literature of sensitization to this local anesthetic.[96,97]

Corticaine Cream contains the local anesthetic dibucaine hydrochloride, which has an amide structure and does not crossreact with benzocaine.

References

1. Gonul M, Gul U. Detection of contact hypersensitivity to corticosteroids in allergic contact dermatitis patients who do not respond to topical corticosteroids. Contact Dermatitis 2005;53:67.

2. Foti C, Bonifazi E, Casulli C, et al. Contact allergy to topical corticosteroids in children with atopic dermatitis. Contact Dermatitis 2005;52:162.

3. Sommer S, Wilkinson SM, Sheehan-Dare R. Persistent telangiectasia following patch testing with topical corticosteroids. Contact Dermatitis 2000;43:306.

4. Sams WM, Smith GJ. Contact dermatitis due to hydrocortisone ointment. JAMA 1957;164:1212.

5. Kooij R. Hypersensitivity to hydrocortisone. Br J Dermatol 1959;71:392.

6. Burckhardt W. Contact eczema caused by hydrocortisone. Hautarzt 1959;10:42.

7. Wilkinson RD, McGarry EM, Solomon S. Allergic contact dermatitis to hydrocortisone. J Invest Dermatol 1967;43:295.

8. Fisher AA. Paraben dermatitis due to a new medicated bandage: the "paraben paradox." Contact Dermatitis 1979;5:273.

9. Fisher AA. The management of propylene glycol–sensitive patients. Cutis 1980;25:24.

10. Fisher AA. Cutaneous reactions to sorbic acid and potassium sorbate. Cutis 1980;25:350.

11. Alani MD, Alani SD. Allergic contact dermatitis to corticosteroids. Ann Allergy 1972;30:181.

12. Coskey RJ. Contact dermatitis due to multiple corticosteroid creams. Arch Dermatol 1978;114:115.

13. Zina G, Bonu G. Contact sensitivity to corticosteroids. Contact Dermatitis Newsletter 1967;2:26.

14. Brandao FM, Camarasa JM. Contact allergy to hydrocortisone-17-butyrate. Contact Dermatitis 1979;5:354.

15. Soesman-van Waadenoden Kernekamp A, van Ketel WG. Contact allergy to hydrocortisone-17-butyrate. Contact Dermatitis 1979;5:268.

16. Brown R. Allergy to hydrocortisone-17-butyrate—two more cases. Contact Dermatitis 1980;6:504.

17. Dooms-Goosens A, Morren M. Results of routine patch testing with corticosteroid series in 2073 patients. Contact Dermatitis 1992;26:182.

18. Boffa MJ, Wilkinson SM, Beck MH. Screening for corticosteroid contact hypersensitivity. Contact Dermatitis 1995;33:149.

19. Sasaki E. Corticosteroid sensitivity and cross-sensitivity—a review of 18 cases, 1967–1988 (published erratum appears in Contact Dermatitis 1991 Jul;25(1):79). Contact Dermatitis 1990;23:306.

20. Dunkel FG, Elsner P, Burg G. Contact allergies to topical corticosteroids: 10 cases of contact dermatitis. Contact Dermatitis 1991;25:97.

21. Freeman S. Corticosteroid allergy. Contact Dermatitis 1995;33:240.

22. Wilkinson SM, English JS. Hydrocortisone sensitivity: a prospective study of the value of tixocortol pivalate and hydrocortisone acetate as patch test markers. Contact Dermatitis 1991;25:132.

23. Wilkinson SM, English JSC. Hydrocortisone sensitivity: an investigation into the nature of the allergen. Contact Dermatitis 1991;25:178.

24. Seukeran DC, Wilkinson SM, Beck MH. Patch testing to detect corticosteroid allergy: is it adequate? Contact Dermatitis 1997;36:127.

25. Matura M, Lepoittevin JP, Arbez-Gindre C, Goossens A. Testing with corticosteroid aldehydes in corticosteroid-sensitive patients (preliminary results). Contact Dermatitis 1998;38:106.

26. Isaksson M, Bruze M, Matura M, Goossens A. Patch testing with low concentrations of budesonide detects contact allergy. Contact Dermatitis 1997;37:241.

27. Chowdhury MMU, Statham BN, Sansom JE, et al. Patch testing for corticosteroid allergy with low and high concentrations of tixocortol pivalate and budesonide. Contact Dermatitis 2002;46:311.

28. Isaksson M, Bruze M, Goossens A, Lepoittevin JP. Patch testing with budesonide in serial dilutions: the significance of dose, occlusion time and reading time. Contact Dermatitis 1999;40:24.

29. Isaksson M, Bruze M, Lepoittevin J-P, et al Patch testing with serial dilutions of Budesonide, its R and S diastereomers, and potentially cross-reacting substances. Am J Contact Dermat 2001;12:170.

30. Isaksson M, Beck MH, Wilkinson SM. Comparative testing with budesonide in petrolatum and ethanol in a standard series. Contact Dermatitis 2002;47:123.

31. Isaksson M, Bruze M, Bjorkner B, et al. The benefit of patch testing with a corticosteroid at a low concentration. Am J Contact Dermat 1999;10:31.

32. Davis MDP, Richardson DM, Farmer SA. Low yield for extended reading of patch tests with topical corticosteroids. Dermatitis 2005;16:124.

33. Chang YC, Clarke GF, Maibach IH. Provocative use test (PUT) [repeated open application test (ROAT)] in topical corticosteroid allergic contact dermatitis. Contact Dermatitis 1997;37:309.

34. Goossens A, Matura M, Degreef H. Reactions to corticosteroids: some new aspects regarding cross-sensitivity. Cutis 2000;65:43.

35. Gamboa PM, Jauregui I, Antépara I. Contact dermatitis from budesonide in a nasal spray without cross-reactivity to amcinonide. Contact Dermatitis 1991;24:227.

36. Dunkel FG, Elsner P, Burg G. Allergic contact dermatitis from prednicarbate. Contact Dermatitis 1991;24:59.

37. Lauerma AI. Screening for corticosteroid contact sensitivity: comparison of tixocortol pivalate, hydrocortisone-17-butyrate and hydrocortisone. Contact Dermatitis 1991;24:123.

38. Bircher AJ. Short induction phase of contact allergy to tixocortol pivalate in a nasal spray. Contact Dermatitis 1990;22:237.

39. Fernandez de Corres L, Bernaola G, Urrutia I, Munoz D. Allergic dermatitis from systemic treatment with corticosteroids. Contact Dermatitis 1990;22:104.

40. Ferguson AD, Emerson RM, English JSC. Cross-reactivity patterns to budesonide. Contact Dermatitis 2002;47:337.

41. Corazza M, Virgili A. Allergic contact dermatitis from 6-alpha-methylprednisolone aceponate and budesonide. Contact Dermatitis 1998;38:356.

42. Foti C, Cassano N, Vena GA. Evaluation of cross-reactivity between budesonide and desonide. Contact Dermatitis 2002;47:109.

43. Quirce S, Alvarez MJ, Olaguibel JM, Tabar AI. Systemic contact dermatitis from oral prednisone. Contact Dermatitis 1994;30:53.

44. El Sayed F, Ammoury A, Launais F, et al. Contact dermatitis to hydrocortisone aceponate in Efficort® cream inducing widespread reaction. Contact Dermatitis 2005;53:242.

45. Villas Martinez F, Navarro Echeverria JA, Joral Badas A, Garmendia Goitia FJ. Prednicarbate contact allergy. Contact Dermatitis 1997;37:299.

46. Mimesh S, Pratt M. Allergic contact dermatitis from corticosteroids: reproducibility of patch testing and correlation with intradermal testing Dermatitis 2006;17:137.

47. Aguirre Martinez-Falero A, Calderon Gutierrez MJ, Zubizaretta Salvador J, Diaz-Perez JL. Allergic contact dermatitis from fluocortin butyl. Contact Dermatitis 1990;22:241.

48. Donovan JCH, DeKoven JG. Cross-reactions to desoximetasone and mometasone foroate in a patient with multiple topical corticosteroid allergies. Dermatitis 2006;17:147.

49. Stingeni L, Hansel K, Lisi P. Morbilliform erythema-multiforme-like eruption from desoxymethasone. Contact Dermatitis 1996;35:363.

50. Miranda-Romero A, Bajo-del Pozo C, Sanchez-Sambucety P, et al. Delayed local allergic reaction to intralesional paramethasone acetate. Contact Dermatitis 1998;39:31.

51. Wilkinson SM, Beck MH. Fluticasone propionate and mometasone furoate have a low risk of contact sensitization. Contact Dermatitis 1996;34:365.

52. O'Hagan AH, Corbett JR. Contact allergy to budesonide in a breath-actuated inhaler. Contact Dermatitis 1999;41:53.

53. Pirker C, Kisic A, Frosch PJ. Angioedema and dysphagia caused by contact allergy to inhaled budesonide. Contact Dermatitis 2004;49:77.

54. Bennet ML, Fountain JM, McCarty MA, et al. Contact allergy to corticosteroids in patients using inhaled or intranasal corticosteroids for allergic rhinitis or asthma. Am J Contact Dermat 2001;12:193.

55. Ventura MT, Calogiuri GF, Buquicchio R, et al. Cutaneous adverse drug reactions to fluticasone propionate and Deflazacort in an asthmatic patient. Contact Dermatitis 2005;53:118.

56. Tsuruta D, Sowa J, Kobayashi H, et al Contact dermatitis around a tracheostoma due to salbutamol sulfate and Aldecin®. Contact Dermatitis 2006;54:121.

57. Buettiker U, Keller M, Pichler WJ, et al. Oral prednisolone induced acute generalized exanthematous pustulosis due to corticosteroids of group A confirmed by epicutaneous testing and lymphocyte transformation tests. Dermatology 2006;213:40.

58. Chavarria Mur E, Ballesteros M G-C, Fernandez RS, et al Generalized exanthematous reaction with pustulosis induced by topical corticosteroids. Contact Dermatitis 2005;52:114.

59. Garcia-Bravo B, Repiso JB, Camach F. Systemic contact dermatitis due to deflazacort. Contact Dermatitis 2000;43:359.

60. Shaw DW, Eichenfield LF, Shainhouse T, et al. Allergic contact dermatitis from tacrolimus. J Am Acad Dermatol 2004;50:962.

61. Shaw DW, Eichenfield LF, Shainhouse T, et al. J Am Acad Dermatol 2007;56:342.

62. Saitta P, Brancaccio R. Allergic contact dermatitis to pimecrolimus. Contact Dermatitis 2007;56:43.

63. Andersen KE, Broesby-Olsen S. Allergic contact dermatitis from oleyl alcohol in Elidel cream. Contact Dermatitis 2006;55:354.

64. Lauerma A, Reitamo S, Maibach HI. Systemic hydrocortisone/cortisol induces allergic skin reactions in presensitized subjects. J Am Acad Dermatol 1991;24:182.

65. Schoenmakers A, Vermorken A, Degreef H, Dooms-Goossens A. Corticosteroid or steroid allergy? Contact Dermatitis 1992;26:159.

66. Stephens CJM, McFadden JP, Black MM, Rycroft RJ. Autoimmune progesterone dermatitis: absence of contact sensitivity to glucocorticoids, oestrogen and 17-alpha-OH-progesterone. Contact Dermatitis 1994;31:108.

67. Stranahan D, Rausch D, Deng A, et al. The role of intradermal skin testing and patch testing in the diagnosis of autoimmune progesterone dermatitis. Dermatitis 2006;17:39.

68. Wilkinson SM, Beck MH. The significance of positive patch tests to 17-hydroxyprogesterone. Contact Dermatitis 1994;30:302.

69. Lamb SR, Wilkinson SM. Contact allergy to progesterone and estradiol in a patient with multiple corticosteroid allergies. Dermatitis 2004;15:78.

70. Isaksson M, Gruvberger B, Goon AT, et al. Can an imidazolidinyl urea-preserved corticosteroid cream be safely used in individuals hypersensitive to formaldehyde? Contact Dermatitis 2006;54:29.

71. Fisher AA, Cortaid cream dermatitis and the "paraben paradox." J Am Acad Dermatol 1982;6:116–7.

72. Lazzarini S. Contact allergy to benzyl alcohol and isopropyl palmitate, ingredients of topical corticosteroids. Contact Dermatitis 1982;8:349.

73. Black H. Contact dermatitis from stearyl alcohol in Metosyn (fluocinonide) Cream. Contact Dermatitis 1975;1:125.

74. Oleffe JA, Blondeel A, DeConinch A. Allergy to chlorocresol and propylene glycol in a steroid cream. Contact Dermatitis 1979;5:53.

75. Maibach H, Conant M. Contact urticaria to a corticosteroid cream: Polysorbate 60. Contact Dermatitis 1977;3:350.

76. Robertson DK, Maibach HI. Topical corticosteroids. Int J Dermatol 1982;21:59.

77. Fisher AA. Contact urticaria to polyethylene glycol. Cutis 1977;19:409.

78. Fisher AA. Immediate and delayed allergic contact reactions to polyethylene glycol. Contact Dermatitis 1978;4:135.

79. Maibach HI. Polyethylene glycol: allergic contact dermatitis potential. Contact Dermatitis 1975;1:247.

80. Braun W. Contact allergies to polyethylene glycols. Zeitschrift Fuer Haut-Und Geschlechtskrankheiten 1969;44:385.

81. Fisher AA. Allergic paraben and benzyl alcohol hypersensitivity relationship of the "delayed" and "immediate" varieties. Contact Dermatitis 1975;1:281.

82. Schultheiss E. Benzyl alcohol sensitivity. Dermatologica Wochenschr 1957;135:629.

83. Lagerholm B. Hypersensitivity to phenyl-carbinol preservative in Vitamin B_{12} for injection. Acta Allerg 1958;23:295.

84. Papa GM, Shelley MB. Menthol hypersensitivity. JAMA 1964;189:546.

85. Camarasa G, Alomar A. Menthol dermatitis from cigarettes. Contact Dermatitis 1978;4:169.

86. Hannuksela M. Allergic and toxic reactions caused by cream bases in dermatological patients. Int J Cosmetic Sci 1979;1:257.

87. Cramers M, Thormann J. Skin reactions to a urea-containing cream. Contact Dermatitis 1981;7:189.

88. Epstein E. Sodium bisulfite. Contact Dermatitis Newsletter 1970;7:155.

89. Vestergaard L, Andersen KE. Allergic contact dermatitis from sodium metabisulfite in a topical preparation. Am J Contact Dermat 1995;6:174.

90. Tucker SC, Yell JA, Beck MH. Allergic contact dermatitis from sodium metabisulfite in Trimovate cream. Contact Dermatitis 1999;40:164.

91. Heshmati S, Maibach HI. Active sensitization to sodium metabisulfite in hydrocortisone cream. Contact Dermatitis 1999;41:166.

92. Harrison DA, Smith AG. Concomitant sensivity to sodium metabisulfite and clobetasone butyrate in Trimovate® cream. Contact Dermatitis 2002;46:310.

93. Lee AY, Lee KH. Allergic contact dermatitis from dioctyl sodium sulfosuccinate in a topical corticosteroid. Contact Dermatitis 1998;38:355.

94. Miura Y, Hata M, Yuge M, et al. Allergic contact dermatitis from 1,2,6-hexanetriol in fluocinonide cream. Contact Dermatitis 1999;41:118.

95. Farm G, Erikssohn I. Contact allergy to miripirium chloride in Depo-Medrol. Contact Dermatitis 2001;44:127.

96. Van Ketel WG. Allergy to pramoxine (Pramocaine). Contact Dermatitis 1981;7:49.

97. Fisher AA. Allergic reactions to topical (surface) anesthetics with reference to the safety of tronothane (pramoxine hydrochloride). Cutis 1980;25:584.

PRESERVATIVES AND VEHICLES IN COSMETICS AND TOILETRIES

EXECUTIVE SUMMARY

There are many allergens in topical products such as cosmetics and toiletries. Although we focus on the common allergens, it should be remembered that there will likely have been a report somewhere of an allergy to virtually *any* ingredient in topical products. As a group, the preservatives are the most common allergens, closely followed by fragrances.[1] Many of the other ingredients, called excipients, can also cause allergic contact dermatitis (ACD). This chapter considers the preservatives and other excipients found in cosmetics, skin, and hair care products, recognizing that the same chemicals may be found in industrial settings in coolant fluids, lubricants, and so on. Fragrance allergy is discussed in Chapter 20. In addition, some comments on the cosmetic products themselves are given. This chapter is organized into the following subsections:

- Common Preservative Allergens (Formaldehyde; the Parabens, MCI/MI, MDGN/PE, and IPBC)
- Allergy to Other Preservatives and Antioxidants
- Antioxidants in Topical Products
- Allergy to Other Additives in Topical Products
- Allergy to Vehicles in Topical Products
- Cutaneous Reactions to Cosmetics
- Cosmetics and Toiletries: Reactions and Patch Testing

Virtually all topical products, unless they are totally free of any water, require preservation to retard spoilage and rancidity caused by microbial activity and decomposition of the ingredients. Formaldehyde and the formaldehyde-releasing preservatives (FRPs) are common allergens. Formaldehyde itself and Quaternium-15 have ranked in the top 10 of all allergens tested by the North American Contact Dermatitis Group (NACDG) for the last 20 years at least. Other FRPs and other preservatives are routinely employed on patch test screening panels, since allergy to most of them is common. While fragrance type varies widely around the world, generally the same preservatives are used by manufacturers in most countries. Parabens are perhaps the most commonly used preservatives, but reports of allergy to them are relatively low. Most, if not all, other ingredients in topical products have been reported to cause allergic contact dermatitis (ACD). These include vehicles, surfactants, humectants, emollients,

emulsifiers, sunscreens, and others. The more common ones are useful on screening series, while others should be employed when ACD to specific types of products is suspected. Some "active" components of products are common allergens. These include para-phenylenediamine in hair dye and acrylates in artificial nail products. These and others may cause more allergy in occupationally exposed persons than in the general population.

Patch testing with products may be useful. Generally, products intended to be left on the skin, such as cosmetics, moisturizers, and sunscreens can be tested "as is" on a closed patch. There will be some cases of irritancy and also some false-negative results. The latter occurs when the concentration of an allergen is too low to react on normal skin of the back, but enough to react on sensitive or dermatitic skin. Items that are usually rinsed off, such as cleansing products that contain surfactants, and others with volatile solvents often cause irritant reactions, so they should be tested in an open test or after dilution with an appropriate diluent.

Many potential irritants are also found in topical products. Some are meant to be therapeutic such as retinoids and alpha-hydroxy acids. Others, like propylene glycol, cause non-allergic stinging or burning in persons with "sensitive skin." A few, including sorbic acid and some fragrances, are non-immunologic contact urticants, capable of producing a response in the absence of allergic sensitivity. Patients often confuse these types of reactions and present with a complaint of "being allergic to everything." Although objective measurement capabilities are lacking, it seems that these people make up a small subset of persons with normal-appearing skin and an abnormally heightened sensory perception of irritancy. In addition to those whose skin appears normal, patients with obvious underlying skin diseases, including rosacea, seborrheic dermatitis, and atopic dermatitis, usually complain of increased skin sensitivity, especially on the face.

Common Preservative Allergens

Formaldehyde and the formaldehyde releasers, methyldibromoglutaronitrile, methylisochlorothiazolinone/methylisothiazolinone, parabens, and iodopropynl butylcarbamate are most commonly tested on large patch test series. Many other preservatives are found to be allergens in occasional situations. Preservatives are found in most personal care products and, along with fragrances, are among the most common allergens. In addition, preservatives may be found in industrial fluids, adhesives, paints, and lubricants. Flyvholm has published an extensive listing of such products available in Denmark and the preservatives used in them.[2] Although such a list is not available for US products, it is likely that usage patterns would be similar. An example of the data shows that in 2005, over 5,300 products including 2,900 paints, 260 cleaning products, and 400 printing inks contained formaldehyde.

Formaldehyde

Formaldehyde is one of the simplest organic chemicals with the formula $O=C-H_2$. Perhaps the fact that it is so small allows it to penetrate the stratum corneum to become an effective hapten. Formaldehyde is a common allergen and is a widely used chemical substance found in a variety of applications. A partial listing of formaldehyde-containing products is given in Table 16.1. Apart from specific occupational exposures, the most frequent sources of potential exposure include many skin and hair care products and cosmetics, along with permanent press textiles. Extremely sensitive individuals may react to formaldehyde in paper or smoke. Certain cleaning products and disinfectants may contain formaldehyde, especially those used in medical or food service settings.

The most recent data from the NACDG[1] showed that formaldehyde was positive in 8.7% of 5,130 patients, ranking sixth of all 65 allergens tested.

In addition to causing ACD, formaldehyde vapors may irritate the conjunctiva and nasal mucosa. Formaldehyde may cause cutaneous irritation and contact urticaria.[3]

FORMALDEHYDE IN SKIN CARE PRODUCTS

Formaldehyde itself is rarely listed on ingredient labels as a component of cosmetics and toiletries. In fact, its direct use is forbidden in many countries.[4] However, several preservatives degrade gradually to release formaldehyde as a partial mode of action (Table 16.2). Formaldehyde may be present in some other ingredients as an impurity, and in such cases it will be impossible to identify from reading product labeling.

FORMALDEHYDE IN VINYL AND RUBBER GLOVES

After a flare of hand dermatitis in a formaldehyde-allergic patient when wearing vinyl gloves, it was suspected that formaldehyde might be present.[5] Tests revealed that 4 polyvinyl chloride (PVC), one nitrile, and one natural rubber latex (NRL) glove had significant formaldehyde release. One NRL and two nitrile gloves were negative.

FORMALDEHYDE RELEASE FROM PLASTIC CONTAINERS

Some plastic tubes intended for cosmetics and hand lotions were coated on the outside with melamine or carbamide-formaldehyde resin. Examination revealed that formaldehyde was present in 39 of 113 tubes. The tubes coated with the formaldehyde resins were filled with formaldehyde-free oil in water and water in oil preparations, water, and peanut oil. After 1 or 2 months, the analysis revealed that the contents contained formaldehyde.[6]

PERSISTENCE OF FORMALDEHYDE ALLERGY

Formaldehyde allergy is common, and formaldehyde is present in many products encountered on a daily basis. Patients with formaldehyde allergy must be instructed that time and persistent treatment are necessary for clearing to occur. Perhaps more than with any other allergen, the dermatologist must remind the patient that slow resolution is expected even if the patient attempts careful allergen avoidance. To illustrate this, Agner and colleagues[7]

Table 16-1 Formaldehyde Uses and Exposure

1. Clothing: wash and wear, antiwrinkle, sizing, antishrink, alkali stabilization, stabilization of casein, and mordant for dyes (occurs free or in combination with urea)

   a. wearing apparel that may contain formaldehyde resins and some free formaldehyde:

   Permanent press

   Anticling finishes

   Antistatic finishes

   Chlorine-resistant finishes

   Stiffening on lightweight nylon knits

   Anticurl or lightweight knits

   Waterproof finishes

   Perspiration-proof finishes

   Mothproof finishes

   Mildew-resistant fabrics

   Screen-printed fabrics

   Suede and chamois

   b. formaldehyde-sensitive individuals can usually wear without difficulty clothing made from a single fiber, such as 100% polyester, nylon, or acrylic. Silk is not finished with formaldehyde resins. (see chapter 19)

2. Some glues, papers, and pastes.
3. Embalming fluid and fixatives
4. Some photographic plates, papers, and solutions
5. Cosmetics and personal care products containing formaldehyde releasing preservatives
6. Fumigators—formaldehyde, para-formaldehyde
7. Some household cleaners
8. Some polishes—automobile, cement floor, shoe, and suede shoe
9. Certain medications:
   a. some wart remedies
   b. anhidrotics
   c. methenamine USP (urinary antiseptic)
   d. denatured alcohol
   e. renal dialysis unit disinfectants
   f. root canal preparation disinfectant (Formo-Cresol)
10. Cellulose esters
11. Products used in the manufacture of explosives
12. Mildew preventative in some fruits and vegetables
13. Disinfectants used in some dairy equipment
14. Preservative and coagulant of natural rubber latex- present in some latex and vinyl gloves
15. Some paints and paint-stripping agents
16. Some leather tanning agents (see chapter 19)
17. Printing-etching materials, inks (marking), sealers for cylinder die rolls, "autoprime" used in offset printing machines
18. Some vinyl gloves
19. Reducing agent for recovery of silver and gold
20. Some dry-cleaning spotting agents
21. Coatings and adhesives—phenol, melamine, urea, sulfonamide, and cashew nutshell–type resins
22. Smoke contact and inhalation: formaldehyde is a component of smoke from burning wood, coal, charcoal, cigarettes, and cigars
23. Some papers and cardboards
24. Adhesives in plywood and processed wood
25. Some foam-based building insulation

reported a follow-up study of 57 patients diagnosed with ACD to formaldehyde several years previously. Twenty-eight were clear or nearly so, but 29 (51%) still had frequent or constant dermatitis. Of 709 products analyzed for formaldehyde, 25% were positive. These included cosmetics, toiletries, household cleaners, and paper.

FORMALDEHYDE-RELEASING PRESERVATIVES

The five commonly used formaldehyde-releasing preservatives (FRPs) are listed in Table 16.2. These substances are antibacterial and antifungal in their own right, in addition to offering antimicrobial effects by partly decomposing into free formaldehyde. They may be used alone or in combination with other agents, such as parabens. Generally, the concentration in a commercial product varies between 0.1% and 0.2%. The free formaldehyde concentrations, therefore, would be even lower. Unfortunately, the threshold level that can cause ACD to these agents is unknown.

Presumably, even low concentrations of an allergen applied repeatedly to irritated or abnormal skin may induce sensitization and expression of ACD. For the chemically inclined, Danish workers have written an extensive analysis of the chemical structure and breakdown products of two FRPs, imidazolidinyl urea (IU) and diazolidinyl urea (DU).[8] They showed that the compounds contain polymers of allantoin-formaldehyde condensation products, allantoin, and two hydroxymethyl urea compounds and give the chemical structures.

If a patient is allergic to formaldehyde, but not to the releasers, he may possibly react to the low levels of

Table 16-2 Formaldehyde-Releasing Preservatives and Most Recent Prevalence of Patch-Test Reactions in North America

Bronopol (1%pet)	2.3%
Diazolidinyl urea (2%pet)	3.5%
DMDM hydantoin (1%pet)	2.3%
Imidazolidinyl urea (2%pet)	2.9%
Quaternium-15 (1%pet)	8.9%

formaldehyde liberated from the FRPs in a product. Accordingly, patients allergic to formaldehyde, especially those with strongly positive patch test results, should consider avoiding all the formaldehyde releasers. In doing this, they may avoid some agents to which they are not truly allergic, but may also have the greatest chance of staying free from formaldehyde-induced ACD. Some experts, however, feel that if patch tests are negative to the actual FRP, even in the presence of a positive reaction to formaldehyde, patients need not avoid the preservatives to which they test negative.[9]

Quaternium-15

Quaternium-15 (Q-15) is one of the most widely used topical preservatives. Older names and trade names (which are no longer used in labeling in the United States) include Dowicil 75, 100, or 200; *N*-(3-chlorallyl)-hexaminium chloride; and chlorallyl methenamine chloride. Q-15 is highly soluble in water, and is odorless and colorless. Its antimicrobial activity is independent of the pH of the product.

Most, but not all, individuals allergic to Q-15 are also allergic to formaldehyde. Some cross- or co-reactivity occurs between Q-15 and other FRPs as well.[3] Q-15 was the fifth most common allergen in a report by the NACDG between 2002 and 2004.[1] Of 5,130 patients tested, 8.9% had positive reactions to Q-15 (2% pet). This is very consistent with the levels of allergy noted in North America over the last 15 years. It is a more common allergen in the United States than any of the other topical preservatives.[1,2] However, studies in Europe have shown a lower prevalence rate of positive tests between 1% and 3%.[10] This discrepancy is likely due to different usage rates in various regions and countries.

Q-15 may be an occupational allergen, but the frequency is no greater than for the general patch test clinic population. Health care workers, hair stylists, and machine tool workers may be exposed to Q-15 in hand cleansers and lotions, hair care products, and cutting fluids.[11]

Parker and Taylor[12] studied 89 patients allergic to Q-15 over a 5-year period. They found that neither atopy nor gender had any bearing on Q-15 allergy. However, there were significantly more black (10.4%) than white (5.7%) patients with Q-15 allergy. No reason for this was given, which may reflect referral patterns or product usage patterns at that site. Moisturizers were by far the leading source of Q-15 exposure, occurring in 79% of the patients. Noncoloring hair care products accounted for exposure in one-third of the patients, whereas makeup accounted for about 12%. Fifty-five percent of patients

were also allergic to formaldehyde, whereas reactions to other FRPs occurred in 3% to 6%.

It should be noted that other quaternium compounds are used in some cosmetics, cleaning agents, and industrial products. Quaternium-18 bentonite is the active agent in IvyBlock Lotion. These other quaterniums do *not* crossreact with Q-15, and need not be avoided. Quaternium-15 is the only formaldehyde releaser, and the major sensitizer (Figure 16-1).

Diazolidinyl Urea

Diazolidinyl urea (DU) is the newest of the FRPs. It was introduced in 1982 as Germall II. As with quaternium-15, it is effective at various pH levels, is soluble in water, and has a broad spectrum of activity. It is a superior biocide to imidazolidinyl urea (IU) but is usually combined with another agent for antifungal efficacy.

Jordan[13] found DU to be a stronger sensitizer than IU in human volunteers. In guinea pigs it was found to be a "mild sensitizer."[14] Data compiled by the NACDG from 2002 to 2004 showed a prevalence of positive reactions to DiU of 3.5%.[1] This was slightly higher than the prevalence rate for ImU, DMDM hydantoin, or bronopol but much lower than for Q-15. Cross-sensitivity between DU and IU is common but does not always occur.

Imidazolidinyl Urea

Imidazolidinyl urea (IU), also known as Germall 115, is one of the most commonly used cosmetic preservatives after the parabens. It is reported to be nontoxic and nonirritating.[15] This preservative is compatible with almost all cosmetic ingredients. Its water solubility is high and its oil solubility low. It is colorless, odorless, and tasteless, and is not pH-dependent. IU is more active against bacteria than against yeast and molds. It is active against both gram-positive and gram-negative organisms. Against yeast and molds it is selectively effective.[16]

A key property of IU is its ability to act synergistically with other preservatives, particularly with the parabens, which results in a preservative system that gives not only a wider range of protection against microbial insult but also a greater preservative capacity. Rosen and colleagues[17] reported that a model cosmetic lotion containing 0.2% methyl paraben and 0.1% propylparaben was shown previously to be unsatisfactorily preserved, because it failed to kill *Pseudomonas aeruginosa*. The addition of 0.3% IU to the lotion gave an imidazolidinyl urea–paraben preservative system, which was effective against both an initial challenge of *P. aeruginosa* and two rechallenges.

Theoretically, IU releases about one-eighth as much formaldehyde as Q-15.[18] In one report, only 6 of 15 ImU-sensitive patients also reacted to formaldehyde.[19]

Although guinea pig sensitization testing has given equivocal results, clinical patch test studies suggest that IU is a less frequent sensitizer than formaldehyde or Q-15 and slightly less frequent than DU.[1,20] Fisher[21] studied 30 formaldehyde-allergic patients and found that only 1 reacted to IU, whereas 9 reacted to Q-15.

IU released enough formaldehyde to complicate ACD in a study of 7 patients allergic to both formaldehyde and nickel.[22] Experimentally-induced nickel allergy was treated with a corticosteroid cream containing IU. Compared to controls not allergic to formaldehyde, the allergic patients' dermatitis cleared less completely and more slowly. Formaldehyde concentration in the product was high. Apparently even the corticosteroid could not fully blunt the formaldehyde allergy reaction from the cream.

Bronopol

Invented by the Boots Company in England in the early 1960s, Bronopol (BNPD; 2-bromo-2-nitropropane-1,3-diol) has been used as a preservative, most commonly in cosmetic product formulations and in industrial fluids such as those found in use in paper mills and water cooling towers.[23] It is an odorless, colorless, crystalline solid that is soluble in water, alcohols, glycols, and, to a lesser extent, oils.[23] BNPD has a wide range of antimicrobial properties and is active against gram-positive and gram-negative bacteria, fungi, and yeasts.[23–25] It is particularly effective against *P. aeruginosa.*[26]

Current production is estimated at about 5,000 tons. Most often, products contain bronopol in concentrations of less than 0.1%. The largest group consists of makeup bases, followed by hair conditioners, blushers, cleansing preparations, and eyebrow pencils. Although BNPD is usually encountered in cosmetics, it has also been used as a preservative for milk samples.[27]

Peters and colleagues[24] reported that an analysis of patch tests performed on their patients revealed an incidence of 12.5% relevant positive results to 0.5% or 0.25% BNPD. This result reflects a history of prolonged use of BNPD-containing lubricants in their referral population of patients with different types of severe, extensive dermatitis. Contact sensitization to BNPD in this population is probably facilitated by abnormal cutaneous barrier function.

Storrs and Bell[28] described 7 patients who developed acute ACD after using Eucerin cream on previously dermatitic skin from 5 weeks to 2 years. In 1978, Eucerin was preserved with BNPD to assist in controlling a problem with *P. aeruginosa* contamination. All of the patients were BNPD and Eucerin patch test positive.

In the United States, the rate of positivity in patch test clinic patients has remained stable at about 2% to 3% since the late 1970s (Table 16.2).[1] In other countries, a range of 0.5% to 1.5% positivity is common. Possibly this discrepancy is due to different usage patterns, because test concentration in Europe was equal to or greater than the concentrations used in the United States (0.5% pet).

Microbicidal activity of BNPD is excellent. However, degradation to formaldehyde may limit the shelf life of products containing BNPD. Also, BNPD is a cutaneous irritant in concentrations as low as 0.5% to 1.0%. For these or other reasons, the use of BNPD by the cosmetics industry is on the decline. Because BNPD may be an irritant, patch tests should not be done at a concentration of more than 0.5% in petrolatum.

DMDM Hydantoin

DMDM hydantoin (DMDMH) is a colorless liquid marketed under the name Glydant. It contains 0.5% to 2% free formaldehyde and over 17% combined formaldehyde.[29] Accordingly, formaldehyde-allergic patients would usually be expected to react to DMDMH both in patch testing and from clinical use. Fransway and Schmitz[11] estimate that over 200 ppm formaldehyde would be present in cosmetics preserved with DMDMH. This exceeds recommended threshold levels. DeGroot and colleagues[30] tested formaldehyde-allergic persons to DMDMH along with two related compounds: DMH, which does not contain formaldehyde, and MDMH, a chemical intermediate. None of the patients reacted to DMH. Seven of 21 (33%) reacted to MDMH, and 8 of 15 (57%) reacted to DMDMH.

The NACDG testing with 1% aqueous and 1% petrolatum found 1.4% and 2.3% positive, respectively.[1] Testing at 3% aqueous, deGroot[31] found 1.2% of patients positive. The amount of formaldehyde present, along with the degree of usage of DMDMH, suggests that this allergen should be included on patch test screening series.

FORMALDEHYDE AND RELATED AGENTS USED IN MEDICATIONS

Paraformaldehyde has been used in deodorant and fumigating preparations. Hexamethylenetetramine (methenamine), which decomposes into formaldehyde, is used as a urinary antiseptic. These are covered in Chapter 9.

FORMALDEHYDE IN ASPARTAME?

Belsito reported on a patient with eyelid dermatitis and allergy to formaldehyde whose symptoms improved with topical avoidance but did not fully clear until she stopped ingesting the artificial sweetener aspartame.[32] He states that aspartame is partly degraded into formaldehyde by enzymes present in high levels in the eye. Others have not confirmed this hypothesis.

FRPS IN METALWORKING FLUIDS

All the FRPs used in topical products may be used as biocides to retard bacterial and fungal contamination of coolant and cutting oils. Machinists allergic to these may also react to formaldehyde and FRPs in skin care products. This is discussed in Chapter 24.

Other FRPs occasionally reported to cause ACD in metalworking fluids include dimethylolurea and methylene-bis-morpholine.[33]

FORMALDEHYDE IN CLOTHING

Individuals may react to either formaldehyde or formaldehyde-based textile resins present in permanent-press clothing. Crossreaction with FRPs may confuse the clinical pattern and complicate therapy (see Chapter 19).

OCCUPATIONAL FORMALDEHYDE ALLERGY

Sterilizing agents and fumigants have caused ACD in brewery workers,[34] farmers,[35] workers making binders for paints and glues,[36] newsprint workers,[37] woodworkers,[38] and lithoprinters.[39] Formaldehyde may occur in photography-developing chemicals and steel foundry molds.[40] Formaldehyde may cause ACD in funeral workers and in medical workers who contact histologic specimens.

CONTACT URTICARIA TO FORMALDEHYDE

Formaldehyde has been reported as a rare cause of contact urticaria (see Chapter 31). Three dental patients experienced anaphylactoid reactions after receiving treatment with a paraformaldehyde/cresol mix.[3] Skin prick tests were negative, but serum radioallergosorbent testing (RAST) was positive to formaldehyde 1% aqueous.

TESTS FOR THE PRESENCE OF FORMALDEHYDE

There is no simple and practical chemical test for the presence of formaldehyde in textiles or personal-care products. For the chemically inclined, the following has been reported in prior editions of this text.

The chromotropic acid test, which has been used since the 1930s for the detection of formaldehyde, is limited in its usefulness by the occurrence of frequent false-positive reactions. Fregert and colleagues[41] in 1984 popularized the acetylacetone method, which follows:

Reagent: ammonium acetate 15 g; acetylacetone 0.2 ml; acetic acid (Glacial) 0.3 ml; distilled water to 100 mL.

Procedure: Add 2.5 ml of the reagent to the sample in a clean glass container. Sample size is about 0.5 g. Solids and liquids are tested as is. Ointments, oils, or greasy products are mixed with a few drops of Triton X-100 (Merck), an emulsifying agent. Heat the mixture for 10 minutes at 140°F (60°C). A yellow color develops if formaldehyde is present. This is due to the formation of 3.5 diacetyl-1,4-dihydrolutidine. Positive controls (0.025% to 0.1% formaldehyde) and a negative control (distilled water) should be tested for comparison.

A comparison of this method with high-performance liquid chromatography (HPLC) showed that the acetylacetone test was positive down to about 4 ppm.[42] The chromotropic acid method was not as sensitive and frequently produced a nonspecific discoloration, which obscured the test results.

EXTENT OF EXPOSURE IN FORMALDEHYDE-SENSITIVE PATIENTS

Flyvholm and Menné[43] performed an extensive evaluation of 11 patients with formaldehyde allergy. By using computer records, contacting manufacturers, chemically analyzing products, and so on, they studied not only skin care products but also cleaning products and other household and occupational items suspected of containing formaldehyde. The list of products containing formaldehyde is shown in Table 16.3.

Cronin[44] described 62 women with hand eczema who were allergic to formaldehyde. In 23 of the women, extensive investigations were conducted looking at personal care and household cleaning products. Twenty of the 23 had been using formaldehyde-containing products. Household products containing formaldehyde included dishwashing liquids, furniture polishes, and a window cleaner.

Table 16-3 Types of Formaldehyde-Containing Products in a Danish Study of 11 Patients

Skin and hair care products
Cosmetics
Deodorants
Dishwashing liquid
Liquid soap
Photographic developer
Water-based paint
Laundry detergent (liquid)
Plastic bags
Paper products
Foam rubber

Source: Flyvholm and Menné[43]

These studies illustrate the ubiquitous occurrence of formaldehyde in everyday usage.

FORMALDEHYDE REACTIONS TO MEDICAMENTS AND MEDICAL DEVICES

Logan and Perry[45] reported three patients with ACD due to exposure to orthopedic casts. In each instance, the causative agent was considered to be free formaldehyde derived from the melamine formaldehyde resin incorporated into certain casts. All patients had positive patch tests to formaldehyde, and free formaldehyde was demonstrated in the cast material. Patch tests to the plaster itself were negative when fresh plaster was used but were positive with the use of aged plaster.

RENAL DIALYSIS UNITS

In some renal dialysis units, 2% to 4% formaldehyde solutions are used for sterilization and for home kidney machines. Sneddon[46] reported that in one such unit, 6 of 13 staff members developed dermatitis of the eyelids, face, and hands. Patch tests showed that four people were sensitive to formaldehyde.

Abdel-Aziz and Hodgson[47] reported a man who used formaldehyde to sterilize his wife's kidney machine and who presented with extensive eczema of his hands and arms; patch testing confirmed his sensitivity to formaldehyde. Three cases of formaldehyde dermatitis occurred in the hospital's dialysis unit.

Some individuals exposed to formaldehyde to sterilize artificial kidney machines may develop asthma.[48]

ONE FORMALDEHYDE-SENSITIVE PATIENT'S EXPERIENCE

A 26-year-old woman was referred to Dr. Fisher for the management of a marked formaldehyde sensitivity confirmed by a strongly positive, spreading, pruritic, vesiculopapular patch test reaction to 1% aqueous solution of formaldehyde. The patient, a textile designer and freelance artist, may have acquired her formaldehyde sensitivity in a high school biology class while dissecting animals preserved in formaldehyde.

The patient is a member of the American Association of Textile Chemists and Colorists, and by persistent inquiries and correspondence she has acquired an encyclopedic knowledge of products containing formaldehyde that must be avoided in order to control her dermatitis.

Fisher reports:

To my chagrin, after lying on the table paper of my office examining table for a short while on her initial visit, [the patient] complained of itching on her back and arms, areas which at the time were free of dermatitis. Within an hour a diffuse, erythematous maculopapular eruption developed on the dorsal aspect of her shoulders, arms, and entire back. It was ascertained subsequently that the glossy table paper contained a formaldehyde resin and free formaldehyde. The shiny, heavy, more expensive table paper is much more likely to contain formaldehyde than is the thinner, less expensive, duller, more fragile type of paper. To be on the safe side, formaldehyde-sensitive patients should be protected from table paper with an all-cotton sheet.

The handling of most newspapers, magazines, and both hardcover and paperback books produces dermatitis in this patient. Handling glossy paper readily produced dermatitis.

This patient also acquires dermatitis from many types of paper tissues, paper towels, and paper plates and cups except Marcal brand products. It is of interest to note that, although formaldehyde is not present in the actual ingredients of Dixie brand plates and cups, there is a minute quantity of formaldehyde in the lubricants used to keep the paperboard from wrinkling during their manufacture.

The patient found that she could not tolerate any art paper used for acrylic paint or water colors, except paper with the Grumbacher label. Incidentally, she tolerates Boncour brand acrylic paint, but not Liquitex.[49]

The following excerpts are from a letter recently obtained from Fisher's patient describing some of her trials and tribulations due to formaldehyde sensitivity:

Avoiding formaldehyde completely is next to impossible. There is always one more product or item of clothing which is suspect. While I am free of major dermatitis at present, it is a constant battle to keep exposure to a minimum. The troublesome items and situations to avoid are books, newspapers, and magazines, formaldehyde fumes from a gas stove (confirmed by the Gas Company), and smoke from cigarettes. Most typewriter ribbons give me trouble.

I have had some difficulty with permanent press upholstery in furniture and in automobiles. I find a cotton towel handy to put on chairs and in cars. I recently acquired a contact dermatitis by leaning on a neighbor's plastic tablecloth. A pollution face mask to filter dust while cleaning produced a dermatitis on my face. One must be careful that an ironing board cover does not contain any formaldehyde because ironing formaldehyde-free fabrics on such a board will contaminate the fabrics. Also, I'm having trouble with clotheslines, and

I can't use electric curlers because the heat must be vaporizing formaldehyde from the plastic.

FORMALDEHYDE IN PAPER PRODUCTS AND NEWSPRINT

There are several reports describing the presence of free formaldehyde in various paper products.[44,50] Simpson[51] reported formaldehyde dermatitis from an offset printing machine. The "autoprime" used in the machine contained formaldehyde.

In connection with paper dermatitis, Black[52] reported a formaldehyde-sensitive individual who was allergic to blank newsprint. The estimation of free formaldehyde content of the newsprint showed it to be 0.02%. A similar estimation done on paper towels used in his hospital was 0.03%.

EFFECT OF FORMALDEHYDE ON FOOD

Thomsen[53] described a housewife who complained to the Association of Danish Cooperative Societies that the gelatin she bought was impossible to melt, even by prolonged boiling. The gelatin had been exposed to formaldehyde from an air cleaner. Aldehydes even in such minute concentrations can make gelatin "insoluble." Other similar complaints could be traced to formaldehyde vapor from varnish from kitchen cupboards.

Gluten flour is made to deteriorate by formaldehyde. Dough made from such formaldehyde-contaminated flour will not "rise" and becomes unsuitable for consumption.

Presence of Formaldehyde in Some SLS Preparations

This narrative from Dr. Fisher illustrates the difficulty in avoiding formaldehyde in topical products:

A 37-year-old woman who had atopic dermatitis was informed that she was "allergic" to sodium lauryl sulfate (SLS) and would have to avoid the numerous cosmetics and topical agents containing this surfactant. The patient apparently had not been patch tested with formaldehyde.

Patch testing with a "screening" tray revealed a strongly positive patch test reaction to formaldehyde. Then, patch testing was performed with three batches of SLS (5% aq.) from three different sources. The patient had a positive reaction to two of the SLS preparations but not to the third.[54]

The three solutions of SLS that had been used for patch testing this formaldehyde-sensitive patient were sent for qualitative chemical analyses to determine if formaldehyde was present. The two SLS solutions to which the patient had had a positive reaction were proven by qualitative chemical analyses to contain formaldehyde, whereas the SLS solution to which the patient

had had a negative reaction was proven not to contain formaldehyde.

We then corresponded with the three manufacturers of the different SLS solutions and received the following replies: (a) "This is to inform you that some of our SLS products do contain formalin at a 0.1% level as a preservative"; (b) "The use of formalin as a preservative in SLS is a function of consumer demand. Shampoo manufacturers usually request preserved SLS. Certain other users request nonpreserved SLS," and (c) "We add formalin to our SLS (liquid) on customer request."

It was learned subsequently that many major suppliers of SLS routinely add approximately 0.1% formalin (formalin is 37% wt/wt formaldehyde in water) to their bulk SLS surfactant to preserve it, and that many pharmaceutical manufacturers are not aware of this fact.

WHERE THERE'S SMOKE, THERE MAY BE FORMALDEHYDE

Formaldehyde is a component of smoke from burning wood, coal, charcoal, cigarettes, and cigars. According to the Office of the Surgeon General of the US, cigarette smoke contains 30 parts of formaldehyde per million, which is six times the safe level for industrial exposure.

One patient of Fisher's stated that her gas company has confirmed the fact that fumes from a gas stove may contain free formaldehyde. In a follow-up letter, she wrote: "Parties where a number of people are smoking and there is a wood fire burning are particularly hazardous to me. I learned to be careful of exposure time and ask for ventilation to prevent a formaldehyde 'hangover' of dermatitis, burning eyes, lethargy, and depression."

PATCH TESTING WITH FORMALDEHYDE AND FRPS

Most centers recommend patch testing with formaldehyde 1% in water. Fowler has noted occasional patients who react only to 2% in water. Trattner and colleagues,[55] however, recommend testing at 1% because of increased irritation from the 2% solution. About half of 121 patients were positive to both concentrations, with 32% positive only to 2% and 19% positive only to 1%. The experienced patch-tester, while being alert to potential irritant reactions, may find using a 2% solution of formaldehyde of great help in making the diagnosis of formaldehyde allergy.

Imidazolidinyl Urea and Diazolidinyl Urea

For years, the NACDG has reported higher rates of positivity to these allergens in petrolatum as opposed to water. A sample of the current imidazolidinyl urea test material from one site was analyzed by Dr. Magnus Bruze (Malmo,

Sweden) using HPLC.[56] He found that the petrolatum preparation had 3.1% while the aqueous preparation had 2%. This might help explain the difference. However, the manufacturer performed further tests using the Fourier Transformation Infrared (FTIR) method and stated the sample had only 1.4% imidurea.[57] The discrepancy may be explained by separation of the petrolatum vehicle and allergen in transport. Since the NACDG has not seen a problem with irritant reactions with the petrolatum allergen, perhaps testing with a 3% concentration would be useful.

Allergy to Other Common Preservatives: Parabens, MCI/MI, MDGN/PE, and IPBC

PARABENS

The propyl- and methylparaben esters are popular preservatives incorporated into many cosmetics and topical therapeutic agents to prevent bacterial and fungal contamination. The other paraben esters commonly used are ethyl-, butyl-, and benzylparabens. In addition, some parenterally administered medications, especially those in multidose packages, contain parabens as preservatives. These paraben-containing parenterals include antibiotics, corticosteroids, local anesthetics, radiopharmaceuticals, vitamins, antihypertensives, diuretics, insulin, heparin, and chemotherapeutic agents. Cashman and Warshaw have recently published a review of paraben usage and allergy.[58]

The parabens are rated second only to water as the ingredient most commonly used in cosmetic formulations.[59] The parabens are more active against gram-positive than against gram-negative organisms; as such, they react poorly against Pseudomonas. Generally, parabens are less active against bacteria than against yeast and molds, although the properties of the individual parabens differ in this regard. The parabens are often used in combination with other preservatives. They are colorless, odorless, and nonvolatile. Relative insolubility in water may help explain their poor activity against *P. aeruginosa*. Lorenzetti & Weet[59] state that the parabens meet several of the criteria of an ideal preservative in that they have a broad spectrum of antimicrobial activity, are safe to use (i.e., are relatively nonirritating, nonsensitizing, and nonpoisonous), and are stable over the pH range encountered in cosmetics. In the United States, the paraben concentration in cosmetics is generally less than 0.3%, and a typical paraben preservative system contains 0.2% methyl- and 0.1% propylparaben. Parabens are inactivated by nonionic surfactants. Propylene glycol potentiates paraben activity.

Considering their volume of use, incidence of allergy to the parabens is relatively low compared to the other common preservatives. For example, the NACDG reported allergy to the paraben mix (12% pet) in only 1.1% of 5,130 patients1. Similarly, Schnuch and colleagues[60] reported that parabens were positive in 1.6% of over 28,000 patients tested with a screening series, the lowest of the common preservatives.

The concept that parabens are not as significant as formaldehyde-releasing preservatives is confirmed by several prevalence studies. The NACDG in 1985 reported on 713 patients with presumed reactions to cosmetic or skin care products. There were 19 reactions to parabens, ranking third on the list of preservatives behind quaternium-15 and imidazolidinyl urea. In comparison, 161 reactions to fragrances were seen.[61] More recently, the NACDG found that eyelid dermatitis was associated with paraben allergy in very few cases.[62] Menné and Hjorth[63] found that about 1% of 8,020 patients tested between 1971 and 1986 were positive to parabens. It has been reported that parabens are enzymatically hydrolyzed to parahydroxybenzoic acid (PHBA) in the skin.[64] Because PHBA is apparently a minimal sensitizer, this transformation may account for the relatively low level of paraben allergy.

"Paraben Paradox"

Several puzzling aspects to the use of paraben preservatives have been described by Dr. Fisher as "paradoxes."[65]

Why do the parabens in topical therapeutic agents sensitize about 1.5% of the population, whereas these identical parabens are "safe" in cosmetics so widely used by millions of individuals?

Various investigators have found so many instances of sensitization to the parabens in various topical therapeutic agents that many pharmaceutical manufacturers have removed the parabens from topical therapeutic agents and have replaced them with other preservatives.[66,67] No similar attempt to remove the parabens from cosmetics has been done or seems necessary. Indeed, for example, most mascara preparations on the market, including the so-called hypoallergenic variety, still contain the parabens. Why is it, then, usually safe to use paraben-containing cosmetics without repercussions, even on the thin skin of the eyelids?

The answer to this seeming paradox is that mascara and other cosmetics are usually applied to normal skin, whereas therapeutic agents are applied to inflamed, eczematous, excoriated, or otherwise damaged skin, which is much more readily sensitized than even the thinnest skin. Indeed, some women who are allergic to the parabens can nevertheless apply paraben-containing cosmetics, providing the cosmetic is applied to skin that is normal at the time of application and has not been subjected to a dermatitis in the past. It appears that sites of healed dermatitis sometimes flare when a sensitizer is applied, whereas skin that has never been the site of dermatitis does not react in the sensitized individual. This may be due to local populations of sensitized T lymphocytes residing in the area.

Brauer[68] stated that "[i]t is generally recognized by the food, drug, and cosmetic industries, by worldwide health ministries, as well as by dermatologists who have extensive experience in contact dermatitis with consumer products, that the parabens are representative of the best preservative agents. The consumer population would be ill-served were the parabens to be deleted from commercial use."

Marzulli and Maibach[69] reviewed the literature and concluded that "[t]he clinical impression reported by Fisher and colleagues[70] was that whereas occasional cases of paraben sensitivity occur and are important to the stricken patient's welfare, sensitization is low when the extensive use of the material is considered."

The benefit/risk ratio for the use of parabens in cosmetics is high. The cosmetic microbiologist recognizes that preservatives must be used to ensure product stability and safety and that the parabens are among the most innocuous preservatives. The parabens, therefore, are the preservatives of choice, from an allergenic standpoint, for most formulations.

As with any low-level allergen, false-negative patch test reactions may occur with parabens. This situation is not unique for the parabens, because it is known that a topical medication may sometimes give a false-negative patch test reaction in a sensitized individual even though it contains chemicals to which the patient is allergic.

Such false reactions may have the following causes: (a) A patch test is performed on normal skin. The dermatitis-producing medication, of course, is used on inflamed, eczematous, or ulcerated skin; (b) the concentration in a product of the ingredient that is producing the allergic reaction is too low to produce a positive patch test reaction. For example, the parabens are used in a concentration of less than 0.5% as preservatives in vehicles, but a concentration of at least 3% is necessary to produce a positive patch test reaction on the normal skin in the sensitized individual where the patch test is applied.

Crossreactivity between the parabens and the so-called para group chemicals

The "para" groups include para-aminobenzoic acid (PABA), whose esters form local anesthetics, and para-phenylenediamine (PPDA), used in hair dyes. Rudzki and Kleniewska[71] point out that some authorities (e.g., Paschoud) include the parabens (esters of para-hydroxybenzene acid) in the "para" group, whereas others do not. In their study, Rudzki and Kleniewska found that of 144 PPDA-sensitive patients, 20 were also allergic to parabens, and that of 63 benzocaine-sensitive individuals, 20 were allergic to the parabens.

As regards the parabens, in his material Fisher has not noted crossreactions of parahydroxybenzoic acid esters with the other "para" compounds or with benzoic acid itself. However, Fowler (unpublished observation) has seen several cases with positive patch tests to parabens, PABA, and para-phenylenediamine that appeared to be true crossreactions.

A report from Canada found that only 6 of 253 (2.4%) PPDA also reacted to parabens.[72] Benzocaine was positive in 23 (9%). Of over 4,300 patients tested, only 0.7% reacted to parabens.

Paraben Allergy in Unna Boots

In further support of the concept that paraben allergy is most common when exposure occurs on damaged skin, one report from Cleveland found three cases of paraben allergy from Unna boots used to treat stasis ulcers.[73]

Systemic Allergic Contact Dermatitis to Parabens

Veien and colleagues[74] challenged 14 paraben-sensitive patients with 160 mg each of methyl- and propylparaben and a placebo control. None reacted to placebo. Two of the 14 reacted with a recurrence of vesicular hand eczema to the parabens, and 1 flared at the patch test site. Parabens may be found in some foods, oral medications, and dentifrices.

"Immediate" Urticarial Reactions to the Parabens

Henry and colleagues[75] reported cases of contact urticaria from parabens in cosmetics. The contact urticaria developed in a patient after topical application of several paraben-containing compounds. Positive results of an open patch test and a passive transfer (Prausnitz-Küstner reaction) test demonstrated an immunologic mechanism for the patient's skin reaction.

Nagel and colleagues[76] stated that a hydrocortisone preparation containing methylparaben and propylparaben provoked bronchospasm and pruritus when given intravenously to an asthmatic patient, whereas another hydrocortisone preparation without a paraben preservative did not.

ISOTHIAZOLINONES

Methylchloroisothiazolinone/ Methylisothiazolinone (MCI/MI)

MCI/MI (trade names Kathon CG and Euxyl K100, among others) is a preservative first marketed in 1980.

Over time, its use has increased significantly. Along with this increasing usage has come increasing controversy surrounding the safety of the substance.[77]

However, there is no controversy as to its effectiveness as a preservative. It has a broad spectrum of activity against fungi and gram-positive, and gram-negative bacteria. As such, it is comparable to both FRPs and non-formaldehyde-releasing preservatives. The commercial product Kathon CG is a mixture of MCI and MI in a 3:1 ratio. Other related isothiazolinone biocides are available, under trade names such as Kathon WT, Kathon 893, and Proxel GXL. These others, along with Kathon CG, are used as biocides in a variety of industrial products and systems, such as metalworking fluids, water-cooling towers, and latex emulsions.

The controversy over this preservative began when reports from several European centers identified it as a common allergen, with prevalence of positive reactions as high as 8% to 8.5%.[78,79] Other centers reported lower rates, as did the NACDG.[80] Governmental regulations in some instances limited the use of MCI/MI. In Japan, for example, it may be used in "rinse-off" products only at a concentration of 15 ppm or less. Fransway[77] estimated that over 80 research articles were written in a 7-year period regarding the "pros and cons" of MCI/MI (see Table 16.4).

Guinea-pig maximization testing revealed MCI/MI to be a strong sensitizer.[81] In addition, primary sensitization by patch testing with MCI/MI 300 ppm aqueous occurred in 0.8% of 976 patients, a very high rate.[82] These data establish the fact that MCI/MI has a high allergenic potential. This may not translate directly into a clinical danger, however. If the levels of MCI/MI are kept to below the recommended maximum (15 ppm), sensitization and even elicitation of ACD in those with positive patch tests is limited. Only 5 of 10 patients with a positive patch test to MCI/MI 100 ppm aqueous reacted to repeated application of a lotion containing 15 ppm MCI/MI.[83]

A Danish study confirmed the usefulness of testing MCI/MI at 100 ppm (0.01%) in water.[84]

There are several reasons for the international variations in patch test reactions. The preservative was not released in the United States until after several years of use in Europe. European countries did not require ingredient labeling. Many products in Europe are made by small manufacturers and there may be less strict quality controls among smaller manufacturers. Apparently some cosmetics and skin care products contained levels of MCI/MI well over the 15 ppm limit. Also, some centers tested with concentrations as high as 200 to 300 ppm, which may have generated false-positive readings as well as active sensitization. In the United States, where testing has been done at 100 ppm, prevalence rates have been stable at about 2% to 3% positive. Most recent NACDG data show a prevalence rate of 2.3%.[1] Presumably,

American manufacturers benefited from the European knowledge and limited the concentration of MCI/MI in products to recommended ranges. The Cosmetic Ingredient Review panel has recommended a maximum level of 15 ppm in rinse-off products, such as soaps and shampoos, and 7.5 ppm in leave-on products. A European study, however, suggested that the elicitation threshold is in the range of 0.025 $\mu g/cm^2$, which is obtained by applying a 2 ppm solution to a 9 cm^2 patch. Seven of 25 patients reacted to this level in a repeated open application test (ROAT) at an average time of 17 days, while 14 reacted to a 7.5 ppm solution after an average of 12 days.[85]

Occupational exposure to MCI/MI can cause a caustic burn on direct exposure to the undiluted product. Fowler (unpublished observation) has seen several patients with allergy to MCI/MI after accidental exposure to the chemical in industrial spills. Similar cases have been reported elsewhere.[86,87] Gruvberger and Bruze[88] have reported that both sodium bisulfite and glutathione can inactivate MCI/MI rapidly. These agents, therefore, could be useful in preventing ICD and subsequent ACD after an industrial spill.

A report from Sweden found a high rate of allergy to MCI/MI in workers making paints and glues. Allergy was more common to MCI/MI than to formaldehyde or acrylates in the products.[36] Metalworkers are also at risk for allergy to MCI/MI.[89]

In summary, several statements can be made regarding MCI/MI at this time:

1. In the United States, the prevalence of allergy to MCI/MI is less than allergy to formaldehyde and to most FRPs but somewhat greater than to parabens.
2. The high rate of allergy in some countries is probably due to excessive usage concentrations of M.CI/MI in cosmetics and skin care products.
3. Patch testing with 100 ppm aqueous is adequate and should be included on routine screening series
4. Concentrations of MCI/MI of 15 ppm in rinse-off products and 7.5 ppm in leave-on preparations are apparently unlikely to produce excessive sensitization.

Other Isothiazolinones

The various isothiazolinones usually do NOT cross react.[90] The non-chlorinated isothiazolinones are apparently less allergenic than MCI, as noted in a review of preclinical testing.[91] However, as noted below, cases of ACD do occur.

1,2-benzisothiazolinon-3-one (BIT), which has the trade name Proxel, has been reported to cause allergy, primarily from occupational exposure. Muhn and Sasseville[92] reported cases in several chemical workers, where BIT was used as a microbicide in dyes, adhesives, etc. They state that those at risk include printers, paper

Table 16-4 MCI/MI Allergy Prevalences: 1985–1998[a]

Country	Test conditions	Year(s)	Tested	No. positive	% Positive	Comment
Netherlands	NS	1985	501	7	1.4	Compared to 2% formaldehyde allergy
Sweden	100–150 ppm	1984–1985	658	4	0.6	Most cases occupational, 2+ reaction strength required
Italy	100 ppm	1985–1987	620	52	8.3	All relevant, all PUT (+), all from leave-on product(s)
Denmark	100 ppm	1985–1988	1,396	18	1.3	25% relevant
Netherlands	100 ppm	1986–1987	3,114	155	5.0	70% relevant
Multiple	100 ppm	1984–1986	14,694	165	1.1	Multicenter prevalence range: 0.4%–2.6%
Portugal	NS	1984–1989	4,171	7	0.2	
Switzerland	15 ppm	1984–1986	625	11	1.8	High prevalence at low test concentration
Switzerland	100 ppm	1986–1987	1,320	47	3.6	Multicenter prevalence range: 0.7%–7.5%
North America	100 ppm	1984–1985	495	13	2.6	50% relevant
North America	100 ppm	1985–1987	1,152	20	1.7	
North America	100 ppm	1996–1998	4,083	119	2.9	21st most common allergen
Spain	200 ppm	1989	626	22	3.5	30% relevant
France	100 ppm	1986–1988	540	6	1.1	5/6 relevant
Austria	1.35 ppm	1985–1989	6,202	12	0.2	Claim erroneous test concentration supplied (1.35 ppm)
Austria	100 ppm	1990	400	28	7.0	None reacted at 1.35 ppm
Czechoslovakia	100 ppm	1988–1989	718	6	0.8	All PUT (+)
North America	100 ppm	1988–1989	949	18	1.9	50% PUT (+)
North America	100 ppm	2002–2004	5137	NA	2.2	
Multiple	100 ppm	1988–1989	4,173	141	3.0	Multicenter prevalence range: 0.4–11.1% "Important new allergen"
France	100 ppm	1987–1989	977	35	3.6	Recommended removal from both rinse-off, leave-on product

[a] PUT, provocative use test
NS, not specified
Adapted from reference [64].

hangers, metal workers, painters, paper mill workers, pottery workers, laboratory technicians, and along with makers of adhesives, paints, and air fresheners and those who use these products.

BIT has also been reported to cause allergy in 8 patients due to its presence in vinyl (PVC) gloves as a preservative.[93] Levels in the gloves were from 9 to 32 ppm. These authors saw a total of 20 patients with BIT allergy, with 4 reacting to MCI/MI. They recommend testing with 0.05% in petrolatum, as higher concentrations cause irritancy.

2-N-octyl-4-isothiazolin-3-one caused occupational ACD in 8 Finns.[94] This included 2 machinists, 2 paint workers, 1 textile worker and 3 farmers. The authors of the study could not find a source of exposure in the farmers.

Methyldibromoglutaronitrile/Phenoxyethanol
Marketed under the trade name Euxyl K400, this pre-servative system is a 1:4 mix of the above chemicals. Methyldibromoglutaronitrile (MDGN) is also known as dibromodicyanobutane.[95,96] Use of Euxyl K400 in personal care products began in Europe in the mid-1980s and in the US in the 1990s. Euxyl K400 is effective at low concentration against both bacteria and fungi.81 The manufacturer (Schulke & Mayr, Hamburg, Germany) recommends a use concentration between 0.05% and 0.02%, depending on the product to be preserved.[96] Despite the finding that neither component of Euxyl K400 was capable of sensitizing guinea pigs in the guinea pig maximization test, multiple case reports of allergy to Euxyl K400 have been published.

Due to rising allergy rates, the use of MDGN/PE has been banned in Europe for leave-on products.[97] It has been shown, however, that even in rinse-off products, allergy can develop to MDGN. Seven of 19 allergic individuals reacted to ROAT with a soap containing 0.1% MDGN.[98]

Many cases of allergy to MDGN have been reported. DeGroot and colleagues[99] found six cases caused by moist toilet paper. Tosti and colleagues[100] reported that 24 of 2,057 (1.2%) patients reacted to Euxyl K400 (2% pet). In some of these cases, patch tests were positive at very low dilutions, such as 0.001%. This is below the product concentration recommended.

The NACDG has been testing routinely with MDGN/PE since 1994. For the period 1994 to 1996, 2.0% of 3,074 patients were positive to MDGN/PE (1% pet), and none were positive to PE alone (1% pet).[101] Subsequently, from 2002 to 2004, MDGN/PE (at 2.5% pet) was positive in 6.1% of 5,130 patients, whereas MDGN/PE (at 1% pet) was positive in only 2.7%.[1] This raises concern about patch testing concentrations.

Jackson and Fowler[102] found a positive allergic reaction to 19 of 163 (11.7%) patients tested with 2.5% MDGN/PE (this is equal to 0.5% MDGN). Another 23 patients had mild irritant patch test reactions. Of the 19 with presumed true allergen positives, 7 of 8 with definite relevance were negative to MDGN/PE 1% in petrolatum. This suggests that the optimum patch test concentration for MDGN/PE is closer to 2.5% (or 0.5% for plain MDGN). Most other authors[100–103] also feel the higher concentration is more useful.

A European review found ACD to MDGN/PE in 4.9% of 766 patients.[104] In contrast, a report from Australia noted only 20 cases out of 2,837 patients (0.7%).[105] This may partly be explained because they tested to only 1.5 % MDGN/PE.

It should be noted that Euxyl K100 is an isothiazolinone chemically unrelated to Euxyl K400.

Phenoxyethanol

Phenoxyethanol (PE) had been used previously alone in cosmetics, and still is Only rare cases could be found at this writing of allergy to phenoxyethanol.[106] Contact urticaria has also very rarely been reported to PE.[107]

Iodopropynyl Butyl Carbamate

The preservative iodopropynyl butyl carbamate (IPBC) is an off-white, crystalline powder of molecular weight 281 and CAS # 55406-53-6.[108] It is moderately water soluble and highly soluble in acetone and benzyl alcohol. It was approved for use in the US by the Cosmetic Ingredient Review at levels up to 0.1% in topical products in 1996. At that time, 122 products that were reported to the Food and Drug Administration (FDA), mostly shampoos and hair care products, contained it, but its use seems to be much greater now.[108] It is also used in paints, wallpapers, metalworking fluids, wood preservatives, and canvas as a biocide. It is particularly active against fungi, but also works against *Staphylococcus aureus* and various gram-negative bacilli.

The NACDG began testing with IPBC (0.1% pet) in 1998. More recently, the NACDG has been testing at 0.2% in petrolatum. Current results show a low level of reactivity at 0.5% of 5,130 patients.(1) In Denmark, testing was started in 1996, with 3 of 311 consecutive patients positive.[109] The German group IVDK tested 4,883 patients (0.1% pet), with 16 (0.3%) allergic positive results.[110] They had twice as many reactions that were considered doubtful, and stated that some of these may have been allergic but that the test concentration may have been too low to be sure. These investigators later suggested that testing with IPBC 0.2% gave the best results and minimized false positivity.[111]

Two major questions regarding this potential allergen are unanswered: (a) What is the optimum patch test concentration and (b) Does crossreactivity occur that can be detected with the carbamate mix?

Allergy to Other Preservatives and Antioxidants

BENZALKONIUM CHLORIDE (BAK)

Benzalkonium chloride (BAK), a mixture of alkyl dimethyl benzyl ammonium chlorides, is a quaternary ammonium cationic detergent. It is used widely as a preoperative skin disinfectant, for disinfection of surgical instruments, and in the treatment of burns, ulcers, wounds, and infected dermatoses. It has more recently been added to "antibacterial" soaps and hand-cleaners. It is also present in some cosmetics, deodorants, mouthwashes, dentifrices, lozenges, and ophthalmic preparations. It is used industrially in the fabrication of textiles and dyes and in metallurgy and agriculture. BAK inhibits a wide variety of bacteria but not *Pseudomonas*. It is less active against fungi.[77] Since BAK is a notorious irritant on patch testing, positive reactions must be evaluated critically for relevance. The use of ROAT is especially valuable with this allergen.[112]

Benzalkonium chloride, present in disinfectants such as Zephiran Chloride, has produced ACD in medical personnel from exposure to instruments soaked in it and from its use in the treatment of ulcers, burns, and cutaneous infections.[113] In addition to ACD, irritant dermatitis from BAK may occur.

A bizarre ichthyosis type of dermatitis was reported in Japan to be caused by an ointment containing alkyl benzyl trimethyl-ammonium chloride,[114] which differs from BAK only by an additional methyl group.

Fisher and Stillman[115] reported that one of the authors (M.A. Stillman) developed a conjunctivitis from acquired hypersensitivity to BAK in an ophthalmic medicament, which was then made worse when an unsuspecting ophthalmologist prescribed another preparation containing BAK. Allergy to BAK has been seen from plaster of Paris and where it was used as a denaturent for ethanol.[116,117]

BENZETHONIUM CHLORIDE

This quaternary ammonium compound, which may show crossreactions with benzalkonium chloride, is also a rare sensitizer.[115] Its presence in a roll-on deodorant has produced an allergic axillary dermatitis.[118]

BENZOPHENONES (BZPS)

The benzophenones are used commonly in sunscreens. However, they also may be found in many other skin and hair care products not usually thought of as useful for sun protection. They may have some antimicrobial properties as well. NACDG data showed a rate of positive patch tests to BZP-3, also called oxybenzone, of 0.7% of 5,144 patients.[1]

British authors tested 553 patients to a facial/cosmetic series that included various sunscreen agents. BZP-3 was positive in only 3, BZP-10 was positive in one, but BZP-4 (10% pet) reacted in 13 (2.3%).[119] Ten of the 13 were atopic.

At least a dozen different benzophenones exist with widely different uses. Benzophenones are often incorporated in textiles and plastics to impart protection from and colorfastness to ultraviolet radiation. They are put into transparent shades to protect window displays, plastic lens filters for color photography, aerosol sprays to protect color prints, and many polystyrene, acrylic, and rubber products to prevent darkening and loss of strength. They are often included in paints, varnishes, and fluorescent lacquers to inhibit degradation of colors.

BENZYL ALCOHOL

Benzyl alcohol is used as a preservative in some injectable medications, allergenic extracts, and vaccines, and is also used in topical products and ophthalmologic preparations. Other terms for benzyl alcohol include benzene methanol, phenyl methanol, and phenylcarbanol. It has good activity against gram-positive bacteria but is relatively inactive against gram-negative fungi. Like the parabens, benzyl alcohol is deactivated by nonionic surfactants. It appears that the frequency of positive patch tests to benzyl alcohol in most series is less than 1%.[77]

Benzyl alcohol is unique in that it is not only a preservative but also has local anesthetic and fragrance properties. It is used extensively in perfumes and has also been used increasingly in hair dyes, primarily in connection with direct acid dyes rather than the oxidation colors. Benzyl alcohol, soluble only up to about 5% in aqueous systems, tends to adhere to keratin surfaces from such solutions as a result of solubility partition ratios. The use of benzyl alcohol results in deeper shades in dye concentrations at no extra cost (an important commercial feature). It is a component of MP and a variety of essential oils and foods including cocoa. Curry and Warshaw report a patient who contacted benzyl alcohol from 7 skin-care products, with a 10 year history of ACD.[120] Although an uncommon allergen, its presence in so many over-the-counter and prescription topicals makes it an important one.

Cross-sensitization to benzyl alcohol has been reported in subjects sensitized to Myroxylon Pereirae. Benzyl alcohol was the cause of long-standing vulvar dermatitis due to its presence in various topical agents.[121] Fisher and Stillman[115] reported two patients who had eczematous contact dermatitis owing to benzyl alcohol, the one from perfume and the other from aftershave lotion. Although both patients had strongly positive patch test reactions to benzyl alcohol, neither showed positive reactions to scratch and intradermal testing. Benzyl alcohol can cause non-immunologic contact urticaria as well.

CAPTAN (N-TRICHLOROMETHYLTHIO-4-CYCLOHEXENE-1,2-DICARBOXIMIDE)

Captan (an abbreviation of "mercaptan"), which is used primarily as a fungicide, may also be found as a bacteriostat in cosmetic formulations, particularly for the hair. In barber shops and beauty salons, it may be employed in Dangard.

This fungicide may be used on fruit, vegetables, and plants of all types. Its sensitizing potential was assessed in 205 human subjects by Marzulli and Maibach.[122] They sensitized nine (4.4%) human subjects using a concentration of 1%, both for induction and for challenge. Captan 1% in petrolatum was tested on 509 patients by members of the International Contact Dermatitis Research Group. Sixteen (3%) of these patients reacted, but in none was it considered to be clinically relevant, and the reactions were thought to be mild, irritant responses.

After 3 weeks' exposure to captan, a fruit farmer developed dermatitis of his hands and face. Patch tests with captan 1% in Vaseline and with the related chemical phaltan 1% in petrolatum were both positive.[123]

Epstein[124] reported an instance of photoallergic contact dermatitis owing to Dangard. Dangard is a recrystallized form of N-trichloromethyl-mercapto-4-cyclohexene-1,2-dicarboximide. Another trade name for captan is Vancide

89 RE, which is used in cosmetic and pharmaceutical preparations.

In 1992, captan was deleted from the study series of the NACDG due to an inability to find relevance in most positive reactions. Although it may be useful to retain this allergen for use in agricultural or hairdresser trays, the frequent rate of apparent false positivity makes captan unsuitable for use on a screening series.

CHLORACETAMIDE

Chloracetamide (CAA) is a water-soluble preservative useful especially against yeasts and fungi. In addition, in occasional reports of allergy from cosmetic products, CAA has caused allergy to paints, shoes, adhesives, and cutting oils.[77] One report from Australia caused axillary dermatitis from a deodorant.[125] It is used in some pesticides.

Possibly because of the fairly low frequency of use in cosmetics, prevalence rates of CAA allergy are low. In Belgium, 1 of 156 patients thought to be allergic to cosmetics was positive, whereas 0.3% of more than 5,000 total patients reacted. Fransway[77] reported a similar frequency. Currently, testing is performed with chloracetamide 0.2% in petrolatum. A report from the Swiss Contact Dermatitis Research Group found allergy to CAA in 1.5% of 2,295 patients.[10]

CHLORHEXIDINE

Chlorhexidine is used as a disinfectant and bactericide in cleansing products, especially those used in health care facilities. As such, it may be considered an "active" agent (see Chapter 11). It also may be used occasionally as a preservative in topical products. In addition to ACD, anaphylactic reactions have been reported from topical contact with chlorhexidine.[126] A report from the UK described 5 cases of chlorhexidine allergy seen over a 20-year period.[127] Testing was performed at 0.5% aqueous. One case in a nurse was occupationally related. The remainder were due to disinfectant products used on eczema, wounds, or perioperatively. French workers reported 14 cases of chlorhexidine allergy among 75 patients who were allergic to topical antiseptics.[128]

Chlorhexidine can cause contact urticaria and anaphylaxis.[129]

GLYOXAL

Glyoxal is a disinfectant used primarily in medical and dental facilities, and in metal-working industries. Aalto-Korte and colleagues have reviewed this allergen.[130] They found 20 cases over a 6-year period. Nine were in machinists and 5 were dental workers. They tested with both 1% and 10% aqueous and note that irritant false-positive results were quite frequent with the higher concentration. In one well-documented patient, a machinist with facial dermatitis, they found glyoxal in cutting fluid and air samples, although it was unlisted in any product labeling. Nine of their patients also were allergic to formaldehyde or glutaral.

HEXAMIDINE ISETHIONATE

This agent has been rarely noted to produce ACD. It is occasionally used as an antiseptic and preservative. Patch testing with 0.15% (pet) is recommended.[131]

IODINE

Lee and colleagues have reviewed the difficulties of patch testing with iodine preparations. Irritant reactions are common.[132]

Parachlorometaxylenol (PCMX) and Parachlorometacresol (PCMC)

PCMX, also known as chloroxylenol, is a halogenated phenol used as an additive (preservative) and as an active agent (disinfectant). PCMC, or chlorocresol, is identical to PCMX except for the absence of a methyl group on the basic benzene ring. It is used more commonly in industrial products, such as paints and cutting oils, and less so in topical products than PCMX.[77] Both are soluble in oil and water and have activity against both gram-positive and gram-negative bacteria. PCMX may be less initiating than PCMC.

Both of these agents occasionally cause ACD. The two major sources of exposure seem to be occupational products, especially hand cleaners used in health-care facilities and also found in metalworking fluids, and medical topical products, such as electrode pastes and topical medicaments.[133–135] PCMX is the active agent in carbolated Vaseline. Storrs[135] reported seven cases of ACD from electrocardiograph paste or carbolated petrolatum more than 20 years ago. Industrial and medical hand soaps often contain one or the other agent.[136] Fowler[137] reported two cases related to medical and industrial hand cleaners.

Crossreaction between the two agents is common but not absolute. Burry[138] reported ACD in 13 patients related to use of corticosteroid creams. All reacted to PCMX, and eight also reacted to PCMC. Currently, both PCMX and PCMC are tested at 1% in petrolatum. Most authors in large studies have reported prevalence rates of positive patch tests in the neighborhood of 1%. PCMX appears to react somewhat more often than PCMC. Current NACDG statistics for PCMX show a rate of 0.7% of 5,141 patients tested.[1]

A severe hand and foot dermatitis was traced to PCMC in sorbolene cream used by an Australian mechanic as a "barrier cream."[139] Fatal exfoliative dermatitis occurred in a patient who was allergic to PCMC and received insulin preserved with it.[140]

POLYHEXAMETHYLENE BIGUANIDE (PHMB)

This biocide has been used as a disinfectant in swimming pools and hot tubs, and as a preservative in a variety of topical products. In a German report from 2005, 1975 patients were patch tested with both a 2.5% and 5% (aq) concentration.[141] Ten and 16 patients, respectively, had reactions. Some of these were felt to be irritant reactions, but topical drugs were felt to be causative of dermatitis in 4 and an industrial grease in 1.

THIMEROSAL

This organic mercurial is used as an antiseptic (Merthiolate) and as a preservative, principally in eye medications and cosmetics, contact lens solutions, and injectables such as vaccines.

Frequent positive patch tests are seen to thimerosal 0.1% in petrolatum. The most recent NACDG data gives a 10.2% prevalence rate in more than 4,900 patients, with an equal distribution between men and women. Other studies have ranged from a low of 1% to 6% in the Netherlands to a high of 9.5% in Japan, with most reports in the 4% to 5% range.[77] Because of the frequency of non-relevant reactions, the NACDG stopped testing with this agent in 2003.[1] In Kansas, for example, of 50 positive reactions, relevance could be found in only 4.[142]

This may not be the case worldwide, however. In Israel, 19 of 508 patients (3.7%) were positive. Definite relevance was found in 6 and probable relevance in 8. The explanation for this high rate of relevance may be that many of these patients were from the military and thus may have had exposure from oils and coolants.[143]

Origin of Thimerosal Sensitivity: Vaccinations

Although many positive, morphologically allergic reactions to thimerosal are seen on patch testing, very few are deemed currently relevant. What, then, is the source of sensitization?

The answer to this question, confirmed by several epidemiologic studies, is that injected vaccinations and allergy immunotherapy led to frequent development of thimerosal allergy.[144,145] Thimerosal is often the preservative used in vaccines and "allergy shots," although its use is declining. One study that serves as an example of the evidence implicating vaccination as a source of thimerosal allergy was published by Osawa and colleagues.[146] No reactions were seen in infants who were not yet vaccinated, whereas 25% of 32 persons age 5 to 19

years had positive reactions. Furthermore, over half of a group of guinea pigs given a DPT vaccine containing 0.01% thimerosal became sensitized to thimerosal. Tosti and colleagues[147] documented that patients who had undergone desensitization injections for allergies had a greater rate of thimerosal sensitivity than other patch test clinic patients. As a natural follow-up to these findings, the question of direct reactions to thimerosal in injections has been studied.

Reactions to Thimerosal in Injectables

Forstrom and colleagues[145] found that 13 of 45 thimerosal-allergic patients had a local reaction to a subcutaneous injection of thimerosal. One patient developed a generalized dermatitis. Other studies, however, have shown a much lower rate of actual reactions to vaccine injections. For example, Cox and Forsythe[148] found 4 vaccination reactions in 31 individuals allergic to thimerosal but did not prove thimerosal to be the allergen by intracutaneous testing. Other agents, such as aluminum and neomycin, may also cause localized or generalized reactions to injections.

In a Spanish study, of 125 patients with mercury allergy by patch testing, only 24 had a positive intradermal reaction. Only 5 had a mild local inflammatory reaction to IM thimerosal, and none had any serious reactions.[149]

The conclusion is that, although thimerosal in injectables can cause local or systemic reactions, significant occurrences are uncommon.

Life-Threatening Reaction to Thimerosal

Maibach[150] reported a patient who had a marked reaction to thimerosal, after treating his slight sore throat with a thimerosal first-aid spray. The next day, because of continued discomfort, he repeated its use. Laryngeal obstruction followed within hours. Emergency tracheostomy produced prompt improvement. Patch testing revealed an extreme spreading reaction to thimerosal. It was believed that acute laryngeal obstruction developed as a delayed hypersensitivity reaction to this first-aid spray.

Nature of Thimerosal Allergy

Thimerosal is composed of a thiosalicylate and an organic mercurial. It was once thought that the thiosalicylate fraction is responsible for most of the cases of thimerosal allergy.[151] Many years ago a Japanese report showed that almost all 23 tested patients were allergic to the thiosalicylate. More recent studies, however, have suggested about 20% of thimerosal-allergic patients react to thiosalicylate.[77]

Patients sensitive to thimerosal (Merthiolate) can be divided into three groups: (a) positive to thimerosal but negative to other mercurials and to thiosalicylic acid; (b) positive to thimerosal and to some other mercurials but negative to thiosalicylic acid; and (c) positive to thimerosal and to thiosalicylic acid but negative to other mercurials.

Allergy to Thimerosal and Photosensitivity to Piroxicam

Piroxicam (Feldane) is a nonsteroidal anti-inflammatory agent that can cause photosensitivity.[152] Of 16 patients with a positive thimerosal patch test, 8 had a positive photopatch test to piroxicam.[152] The same authors studied 19 thimerosal patients.[153] None gave positive regular tests to piroxicam. However, 11 were positive on photopatch testing to 1% piroxicam. Of these, 8 were tested to thiosalicylic acid, 0.1%, and all were positive. All who were piroxicam negative were also thiosalicylic acid negative. Cirne DeCastro and colleagues[153] further found that patch tests with a mix of piroxicam and L-cysteine, which was irradiated with UVA *in vitro,* gave positive results in only the piroxicam-photosensitive patients. This implies that piroxicam must combine with cutaneous amino acids to create a photosensitizing product.

Thimerosal as an Allergen in Eye Preparations

There are numerous reports of ACD to thimerosal (Merthiolate) in various eye preparations and contact-lens solutions (Figure 16-2). The allergic reaction may produce conjunctivitis alone, or a combination of conjunctivitis and eyelid dermatitis. In one instance, a sensitized person had a dermatitis of the hands without conjunctivitis (Figure 16-2).

Fregert and Hjorth[154] stated that allergic reactions to eyedrops often produce both conjunctivitis and eyelid dermatitis, whereas van Ketel and Melzer-van Riemsduk[155] pointed out that thimerosal, present as a preservative in many soft lens solutions, produced allergic conjunctivitis, but no eyelid dermatitis, in three of their patients.

Sertoli and colleagues[156] reported that a patient who had allergic thimerosal sensitization developed ACD on the fingers and palms; however, when this same solution was applied to the eyes, it did not produce conjunctivitis or eyelid dermatitis. The patient, a 20-year-old woman, had two small patches of dyshidrosiform vesicles. She had worn soft contact lenses for 1 month before the eruption began. When not worn, the lenses were kept in a lens container with a preserving liquid. They were taken out for use individually with the tip of the left index finger, put onto the right palm, and there washed with a liquid using the tip of the left index finger before being put into the eyes.

Rietschel and Wilson[157] reported that soft contact lenses cleaned and stored in thimerosal-containing solutions may produce an ocular inflammatory process and, if untreated, corneal neovascularization. They examined 38 patients who were using soft contact lenses and found that 31 had positive ocular provocation test results to a thimerosal-preserved, artificial tears solution. Delayed hypersensitivity to thimerosal was demonstrated by positive patch tests in 27 patients.

Contact urticaria from thimerosal may also cause ocular reaction and contact lens intolerance.[158]

TRICLOSAN

Used as an antibacterial agent and preservative, especially in shampoos, soaps, and deodorants, triclosan is also known as Irgasan DP-300. It has some effectiveness against fungi and bacteria but is not active against *Pseudomonas.* In addition to skin care products, triclosan may be incorporated in footwear to retard odors.[77] Its primary use is probably in disinfectant hand cleaners for health-care providers, and for household use.[159]

Apparently triclosan does not crossreact with the photosensitizing halogenated salicylanilides. Allergy to Triclosan is unusual. Prevalence rates of less than 0.5% are commonly reported.[77]

At one time, a few feminine hygiene sprays contained triclosan.

SORBIC ACID AND THE SORBATES

Sorbic acid is known chemically as 2,4-hexadienoic acid and 2-propenyl-acrylic acid. It is a naturally occurring plant substance obtained from the berries of the mountain ash, *Sorbus aucuparia,* L. *rosaceae,* in which it is present as the lactone (parasorbic acid). It is present in cranberries, strawberries, and currants and is used as a preservative in many foods. For commercial purposes, sorbic acid may be made synthetically by the condensation of crotonaldehyde with malonic acid.

Sorbic acid is a white, practically odorless, crystalline powder with a faintly acid taste. Potassium sorbate (popularly used salt form) is also a white, almost odorless powder. It is soluble in water, alcohol, and propylene glycol. It is an excellent fungistatic agent but has little antibacterial activity. It acts by inhibition of microbial enzyme systems. In addition to use in topical products and foodstuffs, sorbic acid may be used in oral medications.

Sorbic acid 0.2% is considered an antimicrobial agent of choice for topically applied vehicles and cosmetics containing fatty acids and polyoxyethylene esters. The sensitizing index of this preservative appears to be low—estimated at 0.3% by Hjorth and Trolle-Lassen.[160] It appears to compare favorably with the parabens from the standpoint of allergenicity.

Sorbic Acid as a Rare Cause of Allergic Contact Dermatitis

Fisher and Pascher[70] found one patient who had allergic hypersensitivity to sorbic acid among 100 patients who were suspected of having allergic reactions to preservatives in topical agents.

Brown[161] reported that a 75-year-old woman who had a long history of varicose eczema experienced a generalized spread of eczema due to sorbic acid in Unguentum Merck. Gorannson and Liden[162] also reported allergy to sorbic acid in Unguentum Merck.

In the US, sorbic acid has shown a patch test prevalence rate of less than 1%. At the Mayo Clinic, 0.9% of 3,759 patients reacted to sorbic acid (2% pet).[77] The rate has been constant, with a report of 0.8% in 1985 and 0.7% in 1993 (unpublished observation) by the NACDG. Slightly higher rates have been reported in Europe. The NACDG has not tested with sorbic acid in its screening series since 1994.

In Denmark, 10 of 718 (1.4%) patients reacted to sorbic acid. Six of these were apparently sensitized through the use of a moisturizing cream (Decubal), which contains 0.15% sorbic acid.[163] None of these patients were known to react to sorbic acid in food, by history, but oral provocation tests were not conducted.

Use of Sorbic Acid in Foods

Sodium and potassium sorbate are recognized as safe for use in foods under regulations of the Food and Drug Administration. At low concentrations these food additives are effective preservatives for the control of mold and yeast in cheese products, baked goods, fruit juices, fresh fruits and vegetables, wines, soft drinks, pickles, sauerkraut, and certain meat and fish products.

Fisher observed one patient who had a 4+ patch test reaction to sorbic acid and who had no flare-up after ingestion of berries. In a report from France, a patient was definitely reactive to sorbic acid present in foods.[164] The dermatitis was on the buttocks and perineal area, reminiscent of the "baboon syndrome." It would seem prudent, therefore, that sorbic acid-sensitive patients at least consider the possibility that oral intake might produce dermatitis.

Effect of Sorbic Acid on the Buccal Mucosa

Clemmensen and Schiødt[165] concluded that "[o]ur findings are in accordance with the clinical impression that sorbic acid in the relevant concentrations, when used as a preservative, is not urticariogenic or otherwise harmful to the oral mucosa."

Sorbic Acid as a Common Cause of Nonspecific Erythema and Nonimmunologic Contact Urticaria

In 1958, Fryklof[166] reported an experiment with ointments and creams in which sorbic acid, used as a preservative, was applied to 20 patients in his laboratory. In half of the patients, the application of these products to the face caused a more or less obvious erythema and slight itching, sometimes even slight edema. The reaction appeared 5 to 15 minutes after the application and disappeared completely 1 to 2 hours later.

Hjorth and Trolle-Lassen[160] tested sorbic acid in various bases and reported that in 18 of 26 persons, ointments containing sorbic acid provoked an erythema persisting after 30 minutes. In a controlled experiment performed simultaneously on the same patients, benzoic acid in identical concentrations and vehicles provoked the same type of response.

In 50 consecutive patients that Fisher studied, he found that in more than half of them, a brisk erythema could be produced on the forearms with 5% sorbic acid in petrolatum within a half hour. In most instances, the erythema was not accompanied by any burning sensation or itching. A stinging sensation, however, developed in a certain group of persons who had "status cosmeticus."

Rietschel[167] reported on a patient who had contact urticaria from cassia oil and sorbic acid limited to the face.

Sorbic acid is one of a group of substances that can produce an immediate nonspecific erythema in most individuals.[168] Other topical agents that may produce immediate nonspecific erythema include benzoic acid, sodium benzoate, MP, cinnamic aldehyde, cinnamic alcohol, and ethyl vanillin.

Potassium Sorbate and Sorbic Acid

Potassium sorbate, because of its high water solubility, is often used to incorporate sorbic acid. The potassium salt of sorbic acid is a weaker preservative than sorbic acid. Like sorbic acid, potassium sorbate is used as a mold and yeast inhibitor, particularly when greater solubility in water is desirable. It should be noted that, depending

Table 16-5 Relation of pH to Sorbic Acid/Sorbate Concentrations

pH	Sorbic acid (%)	Potassium sorbate (%)
4	86	14
5	37	63
6	6	94
7	0.6	99.4
9	0	100

on the pH, most potassium sorbate-containing products have a certain amount of sorbic acid (see Table 16.5).

Fisher observed one sorbic acid patient who acquired an allergic reaction to Clinique's Blended Face Powder, which contains potassium sorbate as a preservative. This appears to be the first instance of a patient with sorbic acid hypersensitivity who acquired ACD from exposure to potassium sorbate in a topically applied agent.

Incidentally, polysorbate 60, an emulsifying agent, is not related to potassium sorbate.

ZINC PYRITHIONE

Muston and colleagues[169] stated that zinc pyrithione (ZPT) has bactericidal and fungicidal properties and is of value in the treatment of dandruff. Only a few cases of sensitivity have been reported.

Pereira and colleagues[170] reported ACD from ZPT in a shampoo. They were able to identify seven cases from the literature. Nielsen and Menné[171] reported allergy to ZPT in a shampoo that triggered an eruption of pustular psoriasis.

Zinc pyrithione may crossreact with piperazine and ethylenediamine hydrochloride derivatives (see Chapter 13).

Antioxidants in Topical Products

Antioxidants in topical products protect from oxidation of lipid components, which leads to a rancid odor. These agents are also useful in the protection of fatty foods, such as mayonnaise, oils, and lard. Also, some foods and topical products may discolor on exposure to oxygen. The darkening of fruits and vegetables, for example, is known as "enzymatic browning." A common example of this is the darkening of sliced apples after several minutes of exposure to the air. Antioxidants retard this oxidation-based discoloration. Generally, the antioxidants are lipid-soluble phenolic substances.[77,172]

BUTYLATED HYDROXYANISOLE, BUTYLATED HYDROXYTOLUENE, AND TERTIARY BUTYLHYDROQUINONE (BHA, BHT, TBHQ)

BHA and BHT are two of the most commonly used antioxidants in both foods and topical preparations. Other names for these agents are butyl methoxyphenol and dibutyl paracresol, respectively. BHA and BHT are also used in the production of petroleum-based products such as plastic, rubber, and fuels, as well as in animal feeds.

In addition to their antioxidant properties, BHA and BHT have some antibacterial effects, particularly against *Corynebacterium* sp. BHA may have a somewhat broader spectrum of action and also is used in topical products somewhat more frequently than BHT.[77]

In general, the prevalence of reactions to BHA or BHT is low. Fisher[172] in 1976 mentioned cases of allergy to antioxidants. Meneghini and colleagues[173] noted only one reaction in 360 patients tested for both BHA and BHT (5% pet). Fransway[77] reported positive rates of 0.7% and 0.5%, respectively, in more than 900 patients. Prevalence of positivity in NACDG studies to BHA was only 0.2% of 4,096 patients.[1] The currently used test concentration is 2% in petrolatum. Most but not all who react to BHT are also allergic to BHA.

White and colleagues[174] specifically looked at reactions to BHA and tertiary butylhydroquinone in 1,096 patients with facial eczema. Seven patients (0.7%) were positive to BHA. All five of the patients tested to TBHQ (a related antioxidant) were also positive.

In Denmark, 1,336 patients were tested with BHT, with no positive reactions.[175] A computerized database of consumer and industrial products indicated that BHT was present in 31 Danish toiletry items out of 440 products overall, mostly coatings, resins, and adhesives.

NORHYDROGUAIARETIC ACID (NDGA)

This agent is not used extensively in the United States. In the 1970s, six patients in Europe were reported allergic to NDGA. Three had been sensitized by one brand of skin cream.[176]

GALLATE ESTERS

These agents have little, if any, preservative action in the sense of being antimicrobial. Propyl gallate is the subject of most ACD reports and is used most frequently. Octyl and dodecyl (lauryl) gallate are also used. Various case reports of ACD to gallate in topical products have been reported.[77,177–179] Causative agents include antibiotic creams, lipsticks, moisturizers, topical corticosteroids, and eye cosmetics. Propyl gallate was a cause of hand dermatitis in a baker who contacted it in cake icings (J. Mark Jackson MD, unpublished observation, 1999). Heine[180] noted six cases from patients using the same body lotion.

Using guinea pig maximization testing, all of eight gallates tested were at least moderate sensitizers. Dodecyl gallate was the strongest.[181] In general, those with a longer side chain showed the strongest sensitizing capacity.

The hypothesis that allergenicity of propyl gallate is enhanced by attachment to liposomes has been presented.[182] Liposomes, phospholipid spheres, are now becoming popular in moisturizers and are marketed as enhancing smoothing and antiwrinkle capability. Marston[182] noted a dramatic increase of ACD to propyl gallate with positive patch tests in 13 of 245 women (5.3%) and no men. In 10 of these women, liposomal moisturizers containing propyl gallate were wholly or partly responsible. In 4 of the 10, propyl gallate was the only allergen.

Perhaps the manufacturers of these "night creams" and "antiwrinkle" creams have inadvertently discovered a method to increase contact allergy instead of decreasing the effects of sun and aging.

VITAMIN E (ALPHA-TOCOPHEROL)

Vitamin E, used as an antioxidant in foods, is used for the same purpose in some skin care products. In addition, it has become a popular agent used as a marketing device to appeal to consumers wanting to use "natural" products. Reports of vitamin E allergy are rare. The NACDG found that 2 of 626 patients suspected of cosmetic allergy reacted to vitamin E but in the late 1990s dropped vitamin E from the screening tray due to a lack of response.[183] However, the NACDG is now testing with di-alpha tocopherol 100% and their most recent publication found 1.1% of 5,130 patients positive.[1] It may well be that the previously used allergen was not the best for identifying allergy.

DeGroot and colleagues[184] found four cases of allergy to tocopheryl acetate (10% pet). The products involved were a face cream, a cream to treat striae distensae, and a product for cellulitis. These four patients were seen in several practices over a 5-year period, suggesting a low incidence of allergy.

Allergy to Other Additives in Topical Products

COPOLYMERS

These large molecular weight molecules include polyvinylpyrrolidone (PVP)/hexadecene copolymer, PVP/

eicosene, polyethylene glycol polymers, and various others. PVP/hexadecene has been reported to cause allergy in several cases from a bath oil, lipstick, and a cosmetic product (Figure 16-3).[185,186] Quartier and colleagues have reviewed the recent literature on copolymers and allergy, noting that although they are used extensively, few cases of ACD have been reported. This is at least partly due to the fact that testing for them is rarely done.[187]

ETHYLENEDIAMINE TETRA-ACETATE (EDTA)

Marketed as the calcium disodium salt of ethylenediamine tetra-acetic acid and as Edathamil calcium, or calcium edetate, EDTA is a chelating agent with a strong affinity for metals such as calcium, lead, and magnesium. It is classed as a sequestering agent. A sequestering agent, such as EDTA, is used frequently as a clarifying agent, because it prevents the formation of calcium, magnesium, and iron soaps, which may cause turbidity.

EDTA prevents discoloration due to traces of metals in antibiotics, antihistaminics, and local anesthetics. It prevents oxidation by trace metals in cosmetic creams and lotions and is used as a stabilizer. It is also used systemically for the treatment of lead poisoning. In ophthalmic solutions, it enhances the antibacterial activity of benzalkonium chloride, chlorobutanol, and thimerosal by disrupting the lipid-protein complexes of cell walls. In addition, EDTA has limited antibacterial properties of its own, especially against gram-negative organisms.

EDTA has rarely caused contact allergy. Raymond and Cross[188] reported it in 1969. A case report of allergy to EDTA in an injected local anesthetic suggests testing with EDTA 1% petrolatum.[189] The patient had facial erythema and edema after a dental injection. Crossreaction with ethylenediamine did not occur. One well-documented case report of allergy to EDTA occurred in a patient with a leg ulcer who was positive to EDTA 1% (aq and pet) but not to ethylenediamine.[190]

Relation of EDTA to Ethylenediamine HCl

Raymond and Cross[188] stated that two of their patients showed crossreactions. Eriksen[191] reported patients with crossreactions, but Fisher[192] could not show any crossreactions.

Dr. C.V. Denehl of Union Carbide (personal communication) wrote: "We have made a few observations in past years that may offer an explanation for your observation on the lack of cross-sensitization between ethylenediamine hydrochloride and ethylenediamine tetra-acetate. We know that the sensitizing properties of ethylenediamine are reduced each time one of the hydrogens of the amine is replaced. The fact that the NH$_2$ group is the active sensitizing part of a compound is supported by the fact that most amines have some sensitizing properties and the property becomes less as hydrogens are substituted."

With these facts in mind it becomes reasonable to conclude that the tetra-acetate that binds each of the hydrogens attached to the nitrogen reduces the sensitizing properties of ethylenediamine. For several years, the NACDG included EDTA in the North American screening tray. There was not a single positive reaction in hundreds of patients who were tested. Furthermore, Fisher[192] tested 100 patients with ethylenediamine hydrochloride sensitivity to EDTA, and in no instance was any crossreaction evident. Likewise, Balato and colleagues[193] found no reactions to EDTA in 32 ethylenediamine-allergic patients. We no longer routinely test with EDTA because it is our conviction that EDTA is a minimal sensitizer.

SURFACTANTS

Sodium laurel sulfate (SLS) has been long used as a surfactant in skin care preparations. In the last decade, nonionic surfactants have become popular substitutes for SLS. These agents, such as cocamidopropyl betaine (CAPB), seem to be less irritating than SLS. They are most often used in shampoos and soapless cleansers.

Sodium Laurel Sulfate (SLS)

Sodium laurel sulfate has the following chemical formula: $CH_3(CH_2)_{10}CH_2OSO_3Na$. SLS is an anionic surface active agent used as an emulsifier in many pharmaceutical vehicles, cosmetics, foaming dentifrices, and even foods.[194]

SLS as an Irritant SLS is well known as a standard skin irritant. Its action on surface tension is the cause of its irritancy, and its great capacity for penetration makes it useful to enhance penetration of other substances in patch tests and in animal assay.[195]

Dahl and Trancik[196] reported that irritant reactions were induced on the forearms of ten normal subjects with 19% aqueous SLS under patch test occlusion for 24 hours.

In general, irritant patch test responses tend to diminish after the patch is removed, whereas allergic responses often increase in size and intensity. Dahl and Trancik, however, found that with SLS, the inflammatory response may initially accelerate after patch test removal and remain intense for at least 48 hours. This does not refute the usefulness of a delayed (96-hour) reading, because the irritant inflammation from SLS had decreased significantly by this time, whereas an allergic reaction would usually not be significantly decreased at the end of 96 hours.

Bergstresser and Eagelstein[197] showed that hydrophilic ointment and a similar vehicle containing 1% SLS invariably produce contact irritant dermatitis when they are occluded 16 hours a day for more than 3 days and that SLS is the provocative irritant agent. Previous experimental work on SLS suggested that denaturation of epidermal proteins and subsequent loss of the epidermal barrier are likely mechanisms.

These investigators concluded that less irritating emulsifiers, or concentrations of SLS less than 1%, should be used in topical products, especially those that might be used under occlusion.

Krook[198] reported that a 74-year-old man who had stasis dermatitis had an allergic reaction to Ficortril, a Swedish hydrocortisone ointment containing 0.9% SLS. Krook deplored the fact that an ointment used for the treatment of eczema should contain an irritant, such as SLS, in such high concentration, and surmises that the irritating effect of SLS in the vehicle had promoted the sensitization to hydrocortisone.

SLS as a Comedogenic Agent Fulton and colleagues[199] reported that the need for a comedogenic-free cosmetic for acne patients led to a study using the rabbit's ear as a model. They found that hydrophilic ointment USP was comedogenic due to the detergent, 1% SLS, in the formula. They declared that SLS was as comedogenic as certain modifications of lanolin and such emulsifiers as butyl stearate and isopropyl myristate, which had proved to be potent acnegens.

SLS as a "Contact Allergen" Kligman[200] stated that no sensitization to SLS was seen in the 100 cases in which SLS was used in "provocative" patch test procedures.

Sams and Smith[201] presumed a specific contact sensitization to SLS when used as an emulsifier in a hydrocortisone cream.

Prater and colleagues,[202] using a "lymphocyte transformation test" in 10 of 12 patients who had an eczematous reaction to an SLS wetting test, found an increased incorporation of H-thymidine and claimed that these results are an almost certain sign of sensitization. Patch tests with SLS 0.1% aqueous solution were positive in 2 of 12 subjects with a positive eczematous reaction.

Foussereau and colleagues[203] reported that in a series of 20 patients treated by "maximization" with a preparation combining hair dyes with SLS, one case of "allergy" to SLS was observed.

There is little if any evidence, then, that SLS acts as an allergen.

Cocamidopropyl Betaine

Cocamidopropyl betaine (CAPB) is a surfactant used in shampoos and cosmetics. Since its introduction in the 1970s, it has increasingly replaced SLS and other anionic surfactants because of its lower irritancy potential. In addition to shampoos for humans, CAPB may be used in bath gels, body washes, liquid detergents, and pet shampoos. CAPB is valued as a viscosity builder and foam booster. It is formed by linking different fatty acids (variable length) with aminopropyl betaine. Coconut oil forms the source of the commercial product and therefore may contribute contaminants such as free fatty acids and sterols.[204]

According to the Cosmetic Ingredient Review, in 1994, 605 of 9,707 (6.23%) of personal care products that were voluntarily reported to the FDA contained CAPB. This product list includes hair shampoo and other hair care products, bath products, and other skin care products.[204]

The majority of cases of ACD to CAPB have been caused by shampoos.[205,206] Sites of dermatitis are usually the scalp and face. The NACDG documented that 59% of patients who were positive to CAPB and/or amidoamine presented with dermatitis on the face, scalp, or neck.[207] Hand dermatitis was present in 12.7%. Hand dermatitis was caused by CAPB in three hairdressers reported by Korting et al. (206) and in one health care worker by Fowler.[208]

Patch testing with CAPB should be performed at a concentration of 1% aqueous. Because the substance is a surfactant, mild false-positive irritant reactions are not unusual. Therefore, caution is advised in interpreting patch test readings, and clinical correlation is essential to determine relevance. Out of 12 patients with positive patch tests to CAPB seen in a 15-month period, we were able to document relevance in 6 by examining shampoo ingredient labeling. In a follow-up study, Fowler and colleagues[209] could reproduce dermatitis under controlled conditions in a use test study in seven of ten patients positive to CAPB on patch testing. These patients reacted to shampoo and/or bath products with CAPB but not to products lacking CAPB but otherwise identical (Figure 16-4).

Six of the subjects also reacted to amidoamine (0.1% aq) on patch testing. Amidoamine is a contaminant found in the manufacture of CAPB, at levels of 3,000 to 30,000 ppm. Specially prepared CAPB that was free of amidoamine caused minimal reactivity, suggesting that the true allergen may be amidoamine in most cases.

In a retrospective analysis, Brey and Fowler[210] identified 49 patients over a period of 1 year with reactions to CAPB (1% aq), amidoamine (0.1% aq), or both (out of 957 patients tested). Fifteen reacted only to CAPB, 12 only to amidoamine, and 8 reacted to both. Thirty five patients were available for follow-up. Of these, 29 (83%) identified CAPB exposure, with 19 considered of "definite" relevance and the rest of "probable" relevance. Interestingly, 23% were positive to formaldehyde (1% aq), which is about twice the level seen in the overall study population.

European investigators have suggested that another contaminant, dimethylaminopropylamine (DMAPA), may be an allergen as well.[211] An English report found that 3 of 4 patients reacting to CAPB reacted to cocamidopropylamine (0.1% aq).[212] This mirrors the results seen by Fowler and colleagues. Only 1 of 6 reacted to DMAPA and only at 10,000 ppm (1%) on normal skin. They emphasize that this level of DMAPA contact is much higher than one would expect to see in the clinical setting. More subjects reacted to DMAPA on tape-stripped skin or when SLS or CAPB were added to the test mixture. However, Foti and colleagues[213] hypothesize that amidoamine may undergo hydrolysis on the skin to form DMAPA, and that therefore DMAPA ends up being present whenever amidoamine or CAPB are tested. They found that of 10 subjects positive on patch testing with CAPB 1% aq from one source (FIRMA, Italy), none reacted to the allergen from another supplier (Chemotechnique, Sweden). All reacted to DMAPA (1% aq) and to amidoamine at 0. 5 and 0.25% aqueous They did not report testing of controls with the DMAPA.

Depending on the source of test materials and supplies for skin-care products, any of the above may be important. In the US, testing with CAPB and amidoamine are recommended.

Cocamide DEA/Lauramide DEA

These nonionic surfactants are also known as coconut diethanolamide and lauric acid diethanolamide. DeGroot and colleagues[214] reported a case of allergy to this in shampoos. Fowler[215] reported three cases of allergy to cocamide DEA (0.5% pet). Other allergens were typically present, but none were allergic to CAPB. In two cases, exposure was expected but unproven (due to lack of cooperation from the employer) to be from hydraulic lubricating oils used in heavy vehicles. In a larger survey, Brey and Fowler[210] found that only 2 of 49 (5.7%) patients who were allergic to CAPB also reacted to CDEA, confirming the lack of crossreactivity.

For the last several years, the NACDG has been testing with CDEA at 0.5% in petrolatum. Most recently, 1.8% of 5,137 patients were positive.[1]

Possible exposure sources include personal care products, lubricating oils, and plastics manufacturing where cocamide DEA may be used in lubricants.

Another related surfactant, undecylenamide DEA (UDEA), was shown to cause ACD in one patient. A liquid soap was the source of exposure.[216]

Oleamidopropyl and Stearamidopropyl Dimethylamine

Oleamidopropyl dimethylamine (OPD) is a surfactant and emulsifier that has been the cause of occasional reports of allergy. Cosmetics, baby lotions, and body lotions have been held responsible for ACD to OPD.[217] However, some older data may need to be revised, as it has been shown that OPD has a propensity to produce irritant patch test reactions.[218] It is now recommended that patch testing be done with 0.1% aq OPD. Even this may irritate, however. Many crossreactions to related amide-amine-type surfactants have been noted.[219] Again, irritant reactions are difficult to separate from allergy with these substances. One report of concomitant reactions in one patient to CAPB, OPD, DMAPA, and amidoamine suggested that in fact the presence of DMAPA as an impurity in the test substances caused all the reactions.[220]

The related chemical stearamidoethyl diethylamine was held responsible for four cases of ACD, three from a skin lotion and one from a deodorant.[221] Testing was done at 0.4% aqueous. All four were believed to be relevant.

Sodium Cocoamphoacetate/Sodium Lauroamphoacetate

Cocoamphoacetate in an eye makeup remover caused ACD in an atopic woman. Testing was positive at both 1% and 2% aqueous.[222] Lauroamphoacetate was found to cause ACD in 4 patients, all from various skin cleansers.[223] Patch tests were positive down to 1% aq, and were also positive to aminoethanolamine (AEE) down to 0.1% aqueous. AEE, a relative of ethylenediamine, is an impurity in lauroamphoacetate.

Nonoxynol-9

This is a nonionic surfactant used in spermicides, disinfectants, cleansers, and cosmetics. Fisher[224] reported ACD of the penis from nonoxynol-9 in a condom. Dooms-Goossens and colleagues[225] found 12 cases of ACD to nonoxynol-9 from various topical antiseptics.

Dihydroxyacetone

This is the principal active agent of self-tanning lotions. The coloration is formed in the superficial epidermal keratin layer. Morren and colleagues[226] reported two cases of ACD due to the dihydroxyacetone acetone in sunless tanning lotions, confirmed by patch testing with the lotion, as well as dihydroxyacetone 10% (aq).

Allergy to Vehicles in Topical Products

ISOPROPYL ALCOHOL

This agent, often used in disinfectant swabs, may rarely cause allergy.[227]

PROPYLENE GLYCOL

Propylene glycol (PG) is a dihydric alcohol, CH_3CHOH-CH_2OH, that is an odorless, viscous liquid, readily miscible with water, acetone, chloroform, and essential oils. It is stable under ordinary conditions. It is very hygroscopic, with an isotonic concentration of 2% in water.

PG is used widely as a vehicle for topical therapeutics, cosmetics, and various hand and body lotions. In recent years, new vehicles based on fatty alcohols and PG have been developed for corticosteroids. In certain preparations, the amount of propylene glycol may be as high as 70%. Moreover, PG has been used as the only base for some antiperspirants. It is particularly useful because it has some antimicrobial properties and enhances penetration of topical pharmacologic agents. Above a 25% concentration, PG is somewhat antibacterial and antifungal and may be considered as a "preservative" in topical medications.

Antimicrobial activity has been shown against *Escherichia coli, Pseudomonas,* and other bacteria, as well as *Candida albicans, Bityrosporum orbiculare,* and some dermatophyte fungi. In vitro, a 30% concentration has been shown to kill *Candida, E. coli,* and *S. aureus* after 20 hours of exposure. Tinea versicolor and seborrheic dermatitis are both somewhat responsive to treatment with high concentrations of propylene glycol.[77]

Fulton and colleagues[228] have found that PG does not produce follicular hyperkeratosis and is therefore non-comedogenic.

Industrial uses of PG include automotive brake fluid and antifreeze formulations, alkyd resin manufacture, as a plasticizer for some resin systems, and as a humectant for tobacco formulations.

PG is used widely in the food-chemical industry as a solvent, humectant, inhibitor of fermentation, preservative (particularly against molds), softening agent, lubricant for food machinery, and heat-transfer fluid for the processing of foods. It is an excellent solvent for food colors and flavoring agents and is added to foods to obtain desirable aesthetic properties.[229]

Review of the Literature Pertaining to Propylene Glycol Patch Testing

Warshaw and Herrmann,[230] over 50 years ago, subjected 84 persons to simultaneous testing with several samples of PG from different sources. These authors concluded that it was often difficult to decide whether a positive reaction was due to specific sensitization or to irritation. Apparently little has changed regarding PG testing. Lessmann and colleagues[231] in Germany used 20% PG aqueous for testing over 45,000 patients. They found 2.3% with positive, 2.4% with "doubtful," and 0.6% with definite irritant reactions.

Meneghini and colleagues[171] performed patch tests with 20% PG in petrolatum in a series of 50 "healthy" persons. They found that this concentration and vehicle were "nonirritating."

Undiluted PG, especially under occlusion, can be a skin irritant. Fifty percent and 10% aqueous solutions of propylene glycol may also be primary irritants in some patients. Atopic patients and those who have eczematous dermatitis may be more sensitive to the irritant effects of PG, thus, topical agents containing it must be used cautiously in these patients. Irritant reactions to PG may be more frequent in winter, and it is speculated that the degree of epidermal hydration may affect the irritant response to propylene glycol.

Trancik and Maibach[232] conducted irritation and sensitization patch test studies using PG in an attempt to ascertain the nature of the cutaneous response to this common excipient. A total of 10 and 203 subjects completed standard irritation and sensitization protocols, respectively. A provocative use test was conducted on subjects reacting to a patch test. Results indicated that propylene glycol is at least a minimal irritant. Fleeting evidence suggestive of sensitization was observed during patch testing but was not substantiated on provocative use testing.

Braun[233] judged that approximately 3 of 78 patients were sensitive to propylene glycol on the basis of positive reactions to 10% propylene glycol solution. Crossreactions between propylene glycol and polyethylene glycol were not observed in this group.

The NACDG reported a rate of positive patch tests to propylene glycol 10% petrolatum of 1% to 2% through the 1980s and early 1990s. Several European studies have shown similar results.[77] As is true of many allergens, higher concentrations of propylene glycol used for patch testing produce larger numbers of positive results. However, at concentrations above 10% irritant reactions are more likely and may be misinterpreted as allergic reactions by less experienced testers. In contrast, testing at less than 10% will probably miss some cases of true positive reactions. Currently, the NACDG tests with 30% propylene glycol in water, with few irritant results. The most recent rate of positivity is 3.3%.[1] Fowler tests all patients with 100% PG and occasionally sees apparent allergic reactions that are not present at 30%, but with a higher number of presumed irritant reactions.

Claverie and colleagues[234] described three patients with allergy to propylene glycol in Zovirax cream. Patch tests were negative with propylene glycol 5% but positive at 10% or 20% only.

Illustrative Case of Propylene Glycol Allergy

A 29-year-old nursing mother of a 4-month-old baby had had vulvitis since the birth of her child, for which she had been treated by her gynecologist with Mycolog cream, Lotrimin solution, Neo-Synalar cream, and Kenalog lotion. With the exception of Lotrimin solution, which was ineffective, all of these medications not only afforded no relief but also resulted in more marked vulvitis.

With the approval of the gynecologist and pediatrician, the patient was given systemic corticosteroids and instructed to apply Xylocaine ointment for the marked pruritus. To their astonishment, the vulvitis became worse.

Preliminary patch tests revealed strongly positive results to Mycolog cream, ethylenediamine hydrochloride, Neo-Synalar cream, neomycin, Xylocaine ointment, and Kenalog lotion. Further testing with the vehicle screening tray showed a strongly positive patch test reaction to 10% propylene glycol. To rule out an irritant reaction, the patient was tested with 5% and 2% propylene glycol. She showed strongly positive reactions to both 5% and 2% propylene glycol. Thus, this patient was allergic to three individual sensitizers in Mycolog cream: ethylenediamine hydrochloride, neomycin, and propylene glycol.

After delving further into the patient's history, it was revealed that during the middle of her pregnancy she had applied Triple Lanolin Cocoa Cream (which contains propylene glycol) to "prevent" formation of abdominal striae. Not only did striae form, but severe abdominal dermatitis was also produced.

This patient also found that eating foods containing propylene glycol produced systemic contact dermatitis with flares of her healed dermatitis and flares of her previous patch test sites of propylene glycol (see Chapter 34).

Propylene Glycol Dermatitis from Corticosteroid Creams and Gels

Many topical steroid preparations contain PG to enhance the penetration and thus the efficacy of the corticosteroid. Fowler[235] found that propylene glycol was present in 48 of 82 corticosteroid creams, gels, ointments, and lotions sold in the United States in 1993. The data are similar today. Because propylene glycol is used so widely in topical corticosteroids, it should be suspected whenever a patient complains of "worsening" after use of such a product. Of course, other excipients and the steroid itself may cause allergy. The clinical picture may be confusing because the benefits of the steroid will moderate somewhat the allergic symptoms.

Propylene Glycol Dermatitis from Deodorants

Propylene glycol is commonly found in deodorants, especially clear gel deodorants. In addition to fragrances and preservatives, it should be considered in all cases of presumed deodorant allergy.

Propylene Glycol Dermatitis from Otic Preparations

Fisher, in a prior edition of this text, noted 5 patients in whom a superimposed ACD developed from corticosteroid preparations used in the treatment of otitis externa. It should be noted that those otic preparations, which contain sensitizers such as PG, neomycin, and others, are not uncommon as causes of secondary ACD in patients who have inflamed ear canals. (Note: The use of a carbol-fuchsin paint [diluted 1:6 with water] may be effective when all else fails in the treatment of otitis externa.)

Propylene Glycol Dermatitis from K-Y Jelly

Propylene glycol was formerly an ingredient of K-Y Jelly that caused occasional allergic reactions.[229]

Propylene Glycol Dermatitis from ECG and TENS Gels

Cases of allergy to propylene glycol in conductive gels used in electrocardiography monitoring and transcutaneous electrical nerve stimulator (TENS) units have been reported[236] (see Chapter 19).

"Systemic" Contact Dermatitis Due to Injectable Valium in a Propylene Glycol–Sensitive Individual

A patient who received a preoperative injection of Valium acquired an eczematous reaction at the sites where she had previously had an allergic contact dermatitis from the application of a steroid gel containing propylene glycol. It had previously been ascertained that she was allergic to propylene glycol in the gel. Propylene glycol was an ingredient in the medication at a concentration of 40%.

Propylene Glycol Intoxication in an Infant

A premature infant became comatose after treatment for burns with dressings containing propylene glycol. Urine levels of propylene glycol were high. Complete recovery ensued after topical treatment was stopped.[237]

OTHER GLYCOLS

1,3 Butylene Glycol

Among the qualities associated with butylene glycol (BG) are the following: (a) It is the humectant most resistant to high humidity; (b) it is particularly valuable in hair sprays and setting lotions; (c) it has a marked ability to retard loss of aromas; (d) it preserves cosmetics against spoilage by microorganisms; and (e) it is a superior solvent for benzoates.[238] It is claimed that 1,3 BG is as efficient a humectant and preservative potentiator as is PG.

Several chemists that Fisher consulted stated that from a theoretical chemical viewpoint, they believed that BG would crossreact with PG. In two patients with PG sensitivity, Fisher found that patch test reactions to 1,3 butylene glycol gave negative results.

A report from Japan identified BG as an allergen in 1 patient who used multiple cosmetic creams.[239] She was not allergic to propylene glycol. Another report detailed facial ACD from BG (1% aqueous), with reactivity also to glycerol, but not to PG.[240] Previous reported cases are referenced in this paper.

Hexylene Glycol

This glycol is less hygroscopic than PG or butylene glycol. However, a 10% hexylene glycol (HG) solution showed antibacterial and anticandidal effects in vitro equal to a 30% solution of PG or butylene glycol.[241]

Hexylene glycol is used at concentrations of 0.1% to 25% in skin care products, soaps, hair care products, and eye cosmetics. In a patch test study comparing HG and propylene glycol, 2.8% of over 800 patients tested with 30% or 50% HG in water developed erythema and edema (+ or ++ reactions).[242] However, only 3 of 22 were still positive to patch tests at 1% or 2% HG aqueous, and they did not react to a use test of a solution of 30% HG. Only one patient with a positive patch test to HG could be identified as definitely clinically relevant. Propylene glycol was shown to have a greater effect on transepidermal water loss than HG in both atopic and nonatopic individuals. The authors concluded that hexylene glycol is an irritant in high concentration, but less so than PG, and that HG is a rare cause of contact allergy.

Polyethylene Glycol

Polyethylene glycol, $HO(CH_2CH_2)_x OH$, is a mixture of glycols. The lower molecular weights from 200 to 700 are liquids, whereas the higher weights of 1,000 to 6,000 are solids. Polyethylene glycols (PEGs) of varying molecular weights are used extensively as vehicles in topical medicaments, suppositories, shampoos, detergents, hair dressings, insect repellents, cosmetics, toothpastes, and contraceptives.[243] They may be used as vehicles for systemic medicaments as well.

In industry, the PEGs are used as solvents for nitrocellulose, as plasticizers for glue and casein, and as wetting agents in epoxy hardeners.

PEG ointment (USP) is made up of solid PEG 4000 (USP) and liquid PEG 300. Carbowax is a solid waxy PEG. Carbowax 1500 is a synthetic soft wax, used as a softener and lubricant sizing agent for textiles. Carbowax 4000, a hard, translucent solid, is a binder for pigments and a lubricant in sizing.

Patch Testing with Polyethylene Glycol Maibach[244] stressed that the PEGs of varying molecular weights are used extensively as vehicles in topical medicaments. In an experimental study, Marzulli and Maibach[245] used as a screen an experimental bar soap for allergic contact sensitization. The soap was tested at 3% in water with the challenge concentration reduced to 1%. One subject (of 200) had a strong spreading reaction at the final elicitation. This was repeated three times at biweekly intervals with similar results. Breakdown testing of the soap components revealed a strong reaction only to 3% PEG 300 in petrolatum. Additional challenges with 3% PEG 100, 1000, 4000, and 6000 were all positive. The same subject also reacted to these at 1% in petrolatum.

Braun[246] studied 40 patients who showed ACD to a medication containing nitrofural, which is a Furacin-like product. In 3 of 40 cases, the active ingredient nitrofural was not the cause of the dermatitis, but the solvent PEG 300 proved to be the culprit. Routine tests in 92 dermatologic patients who had contact allergies gave 4% positive reactions with PEG 300. Group sensitization in the PEG series appeared to occur only with polymers of the same molecular weights. Thus, of 12 subjects sensitized with PEG 300, 5 also reacted to PEG 400 and only 1 of them to PEG 1500 and 6000 as well. No cross-sensitivity could be demonstrated between PG and the PEG derivatives.

Four patients studied by Fisher[243] showed allergic reactions to these liquid PEGs in topical medications. Two had immediate urticarial reactions to PEG 400 in the antifungal agents Lotrimin and Tinactin Solutions. Two other patients had delayed allergic eczematous reactions—1 to PEG 200 and 1 to PEG 300 in an ear solution and a topical liquid anesthetic. Crossreactions occurred between PEG 200, 300, and 400, but not between these liquid polyethylenes and the higher molecular weight solid polyethylenes from 1000 to 6000.

In a study from India, Bajaj and colleagues[247] found 8 of 180 patients with suspected allergy to medicaments reacted to various PEGs. Concentration of the test substances was not given. Four patients reacted only to PEG 400, three to PEG 400 plus either PEG 1500 or 3000, and one to PEG 1500, 3000, and 6000. Relevance was not determined.

In contrast, the NACDG found no reactions to PEG 400 ("as is") in 148 subjects tested. Perhaps the difference in sensitization reflects different patterns of medicament usage in India as compared to the United States. The NACDG no longer recommends testing routinely with PEG, but it still may be useful in suspected cases of cosmetic allergy.

GLYCERIN

Nonirritating Qualities and Rare Sensitization

Among the qualities associated with glycerin are the following: (a) it is stable, nontoxic, nonirritating, and hypoallergenic; (b) it has good water absorption —it is an effective humectant or hygroscopic agent; (c) it is an effective plasticizer; (d) it is an excellent lubricant; and (e) it imparts "smoothness" to cosmetics.

Allergic reactions to glycerin are rare. Hannuksela and Forstrom[248] described one patient who was allergic to glycerol (glycerin). This patient, on the staff of the allergy laboratory of the dermatologic clinic in Helsinki, noticed eczema on both hands. According to her own observations, a mixture of glycerol (1 part) and 70% ethanol (9 parts) applied on the hands after washing them with soap and water was the apparent cause of her eczema. Glycerol tested at 10%, 5%, and 1% aqueous and the glycerol-ethanol mixture already mentioned gave 3+ reactions at 48- and 72-hour readings. The reactions were considered to be allergic. The patient stopped using the glycerol-ethanol mixture, and the eczema disappeared within a couple of days.

Glycerin versus Propylene Glycol

Generally, it is agreed that glycerin is much less active than PG in producing primary irritant and allergic reactions. It is claimed, however, that glycerin is a less desirable solvent than PG. Also, PG has better permeation through the stratum corneum, probably because it has different solvent properties (i.e., propylene glycol is more lipid soluble than glycerin). Because of these superior solubility properties, PG is preferred over glycerin in many pharmaceutical and cosmetic preparations. In addition, propylene glycol is less expensive.

Both glycerin and PG are biodegradable under dilute conditions. Glycerin exhibits antimicrobial properties as a concentrated solution. Thus, glycerin at sufficient concentrations can provide a preservative function in products. Whether or not a product containing glycerin needs a preservative depends on various factors, such as the level of glycerin, other components, and the available water. For example, a dilute solution of glycerin, which contains 10% ethanol, does not need any special preservative because the ethanol will suffice as the preservative.

PETROLATUM

Petrolatum is considered one of the most inert of all topical agents. Nevertheless, there are several case reports of petrolatum allergy. Dooms-Goossens and DeGreef commented on three such cases,[249] and Maibach[250] published the first such case in 1978. Grin and Maibach[251] recently reported a patient with both delayed and immediate allergy to petrolatum. On patch testing, all sites of petrolatum allergens were positive at both day 2 and day 4 with urticarial and eczematous patterns. An open test on the forearms produced urticaria at 30 minutes.

Schnuch and colleagues, [252] in 80,000 patients, saw 29 cases with "positive" patch tests, mostly weak, to petrolatum. However, in all cases, there was no concordance with reactions to the other allergens in petrolatum, leading them to a conclusion that the results represented false positives.

EMULSIFIERS

Emulsifiers are common constituents of skin care products, cosmetics, and topical medications. These agents enhance the miscibility of aqueous and fatty compo-

nents. Generally they are rare sensitizers but mild irritants, especially if applied to damaged skin. Also, irritant patch tests may occur, so delayed readings and clinical correlation are advisable (see Table 16.6).

Cetyl, Stearyl, and Myristyl Alcohols

The first two alcohols have the formula $CH_3 (CH_2)_{14} CH_2OH$ and $CH_3 (CH_2)_{16} CH_2OH$, respectively. They are often used together under the name cetostearyl alcohol (CSA) as an emulsifier and stabilizer. As such, they may be considered preservatives. Only rare cases of allergy to either or both agents occur. Usually there is a predisposing factor that enhances the patient's sensitivity. For example, DeBerker and colleagues[253] reported a patient allergic to stearyl alcohol in 5-fluorouracil cream. The irritant effect of the 5-FU probably predisposed to ACD development. Likewise, cases of allergy in leg ulcer patients have been reported.[254]

A British study found that of 11 patients previously positive to CSA, only 2 reacted on later testing.[255] None reacted to CSA-containing creams in ROAT. The reasons for this apparent "loss of reactivity" are unclear.

Closely related to cetyl and stearyl alcohols, myristyl alcohol has the formula $CH_3(CH_2)_{12} CH_2OH$. It is also known as tetradecanol. There are occasional case reports of allergy to this agent, which may be found in some

Table 16-6 Common Emulsifiers with Selected Patch Test Results

Emulsifier	Other names	Positive Patch Text Percentages			
		Hannuksela et al. (376)		Tosti et al.(380)	
		N= 1,200		N = 739	
		% Pos.	P.T. Conc.	% Pos.	P.T. Conc.
Cetyl alcohol			NT	NT	
Stearyl alcohol			NT	NT	
Cetosteryl alcohol	Lanette O		NT	0.8%	20 pet
Myristyl alcohol			NT	NT	
Stearic acid			NT	NT	
Glyceryl stearate		0	20 pet	NT	
Isopropyl palmitate			NT	NT	
Isopropyl myristate			NT	NT	
Sorbitan sesquioleate	Arlacel 83	0.5%	20 pet	0.9%	20 pet
Polyoxyediylene	Polysorbate 40				
Sorbitan monopalmitate	Tween 40t	0.2%	5 pet	0.7%	10 pet
Polyoxyethylene	Polysorbate 80				
Sorbitan monooleate	Tween 80	0.2%	5 pet	0.5%	10 pet
Sorbitan stearate	Span 60	0.4%	5 pet	NT	
Sorbitan oleate	Span 80	0.4%	5 pet	NT	
Triethanolamine		0.4%	5 pet	2.7%	2.5 pet

P.T. = patch test;
NT = not tested;
Pos. = positive;
pet = petrolatum.

cosmetics and moisturizing creams.[256] It has caused allergy in metal workers, but testing with 10% petrolatum gave 4 positive reactions and 20 probable irritant reactions.[257]

Diethyl Sebacate

This widely used emulsifier has been reported to cause allergy in rare cases. It is especially used in topical medicaments as a penetration enhancer. Patch testing at 5% petrolatum seems appropriate.[258]

Isopropyl Myristate

This emulsifier is a very rare cause of contact allergy. German investigators suggest using a concentration of 10% petrolatum for patch testing, as they found many irritant reactions when using 20%.[259] They found only 16 allergic patients out of over 12,000 (0.13%).

Octylododecanol

This aliphatic alcohol is an emulsifier used in various cleansing and other topical products. Three reports of allergy have been noted.[260]

Oleyl Alcohol

This fatty alcohol has been reported to cause allergy from lipstick and other skin care products. Crossreactions with castor oil have been observed.[261] It has also caused ACD from Elidel cream and from a metalworking fluid.[257,262]

Sorbitan Sesquioleate

Sorbitan sesquioleate is an emulsifier that has been added to our fragrance mix allergens to enhance stability. It is commonly found in skin-care products. Occasional cases of presumed fragrance allergy have in fact been due to this additive in the mix.[263]

Stearic Acid and Glyceryl Stearate

Stearic acid is closely related to stearyl alcohol, containing an extra oxygen atom in place of two hydrogen atoms. Glyceryl stearate is a larger molecule formed by the attachment of glycerin to stearic acid. Both of these agents have been shown to be rare contact sensitizers, although they are used fairly widely in skin care products.[264] Crossreaction between stearic acid, stearyl alcohol, and glyceryl stearate has been studied, but due to the similarities in chemical structure, these might be expected. Hayakawa[265] studied one patient who had a recurrent cheilitis due to lipsticks. She reacted positively to glyceryl stearate, glyceryl disostearate and tri-isostearate, diisostearyl malate, and stearyl alcohol. Testing to stearic acid was negative.

Triethanolamine

Triethanolamine, also known as trolamine or TEA, a mixture of three alkanolamines, is employed frequently as an excipient in hand and body lotions, shaving creams, soaps, shampoos, bath powders, and occasionally pharmaceutical preparations. (An excipient is a presumably "inert" substance that gives a topical agent proper consistency through its action as a dispersant).

Castelain[266] reported ACD due to sensitization to triethanolamine. Suurmond[267] showed crossreactions between triethanolamine and other tertiary amines, such as Phenergan (promethazine). Schwartz[268] cautioned: "These chemicals are combined in the form of an innocuous substance, triethanolamine stearate. On the other hand, in some instances the combined irritant action of chemicals in a cosmetic may be greater than the irritant action of the individual substances."

TEA may be a more common sensitizer in industrial products than in cosmetic agents. A case of allergy to TEA, along with mono- and diethanolamine, in a metal worker has been reported.[269] Fowler (unpublished observation) has seen several such cases. A fluorescent marking pen used in patch testing caused allergy from TEA in one patient.[270]

EMOLLIENTS

Castor Oil

Castor oil is commonly used in lipsticks because of its superior emollient characteristics. Sporadic case reports of allergy to it have implicated ricinoleic acid as the causative agent. Other than one report of allergy to a makeup remover,[271] lipsticks have been the source of exposure. An individual who reacts to "all" lipsticks should be tested with castor oil ("as is").[271,272]

Propolis (Bee Glue) and Beeswax

Propolis (bee glue) is a dark yellow-brown adhesive resin that bees mix with wax to form a cementing substance in their hives. Propolis allergy is discussed also in the chapter on fragrances (Chapter 20). The purified wax from the honeycomb, beeswax, is used widely in cosmetics. Beeswax may be used as cera alba (bleached) or as cera flava (unbleached).

Propolis (bee glue), derived mainly from poplar and other tree resins, contains, among other things, well-known sensitizers such as cinnamic acid and vanillin and may crossreact with MP. ACD from propolis is an occupational hazard for beekeepers.[273] In rare instances a beekeeper may be allergic to beeswax.

Propolis is sold in many health food stores in many forms to be ingested as a cure-all for many diseases, and as a topical agent in the form of various ointments, powders, and cosmetic creams. Solid propolis, which can be chewed, may produce a perioral dermatitis and stomatitis. Thus, Wanscher[274] described two patients who had contact dermatitis from chewing so-called natural propolis products. Petersen[275] predicted that with the increasing employment of propolis for self-medication, an increasing incidence of allergic contact eczema to this preparation must be anticipated.

Hausen and colleagues[276] extensively studied various constituents of propolis and found that several caffeates and benzyl isoferulate are strong sensitizers in guinea pigs. A number of these substances are also found in MP. From 1988 to 1990, 10 of 137 (0.9%) men and 28 of 2,036 (1.4%) women reacted to propolis on patch testing. One report from Prague, where apparently propolis is used commonly, reported allergy in 25 of 605 patients (4.1%). Thirteen of these also reacted to MP.[277]

Beeswax is secreted by bees. Camasara[278] reported a woman who was employed in molding art objects from beeswax and who developed chronic palmar dermatitis. A strongly positive patch test to natural beeswax was obtained.

A beekeeper described by Rothenborg[273] reacted to raw, unpurified beeswax but not to purified beeswax. The raw wax was considered contaminated by poplar tree resins to which the beekeeper was sensitive.

Lanolin

Lanolin (wool fat, wool grease, wool wax, wool alcohol, and adeps lanae anhydrous) and its various esters, fatty acids, and aliphatic alcohols are used in many topical medicaments and cosmetics. Lanolin is a natural product obtained from the sebaceous glands of sheep, and its constituents vary from time to time and place to place.

Lanolin contains sterols, fatty alcohols, and fatty acids. The lanolin sterols (lanolin alcohols or wood alcohols) include principally cholesterol, lanosterol, and agnesterol and are built from one or more benzene rings. Cholesterol is the major ingredient of lanolin alcohol. Oleffe and colleagues[279] emphasized that lanolin is a complex mixture of esters and polyesters of 33 alcohols with high molecular weights and 36 fatty acids.

The fatty alcohols are long-chained and include the closely related stearyl and cetyl alcohols, and are likely to be the main sensitizers.[280] Acetylated lanolin (Modulan), according to Cronin,[281] is less of a sensitizer than is plain lanolin. Dewaxed lanolin (Lantrol), formed by a solvent crystallization process, is also claimed to cause less sensitization than lanolin. Another modification is

hydrogenated lanolin. Vollum[282] reported that it is used frequently in the pharmaceutical and cosmetic industry because it is colorless, odorless, free from tackiness, and more hydrophilic than lanolin. Hydrogenation is carried out by heating lanolin with a catalyst to 330°C at a pressure of 180 atmospheres. The resulting hydrogenated lanolin contains dihydrocholesterol, other hydrogenated steroids, and some saturated alcohol. It was hoped originally that hydrogenated lanolin, or a modification, could be used in cases of lanolin sensitivity, but some patients show a marked sensitivity to hydrogenated lanolin and not to the plain lanolin.

A "purified" anhydrous lanolin product gave a positive patch test in only 1 of 33 subjects previously positive to lanolin.[283] Presumably, the removal of fatty alcohols rendered the "purified" product less allergenic. The development of new derivatives and further purification may contribute to lowering the incidence of skin reactions to this emollient.[284] The results of Giorgini and colleagues[285] confirm the sensitizing action of lanolin alcohols and the fact that acetylation, ethylenation, and transesterification eliminate the allergenic activity of lanolin.

Patch Tests for Lanolin Sensitivity Most investigators routinely test with 30% wool alcohol in petrolatum, but testing is also often carried out with the hydrogenated lanolin, Amerchol L101 (50% pet). Fowler has seen reactions to this with no reaction to the "standard" allergen, so both are probably useful for aimed testing. Wakelin and colleagues agree.[286] They found a rate of 1.7% positive to lanolin from 24,449 patients. A lesser, but important number reacted only to Amerchol L101. Most recent NACDG data show that positive lanolin patch test rates are in the range of 2.2%.[1]

Lanolin derivatives Amerchol L101 and Amerchol CAB are composed of lanolin (wool wax) alcohols. They are useful in cosmetic products as emulsifiers and emollients. A study by Bojs and colleagues[287] showed an identical reaction pattern to Amerchol CAB and Amerchol L101 in lanolin-sensitive patients. Amerchol CAB was present in a corticosteroid ointment made in Denmark.

Matthies and Dockx[288] found a great discrepancy in the frequency of positive reactions to lanolin as opposed to Amerchol L101. Twelve of 323 patients reacted to both lanolin 30% and Amerchol L101 100%, but 32 more reacted to the Amerchol L101 alone. The concern is that some of these may have been irritant reactions. Even so, Amerchol L101 may be a more reliable patch test agent than "standard" wool wax alcohol.

Sensitizing Potential of Lanolin Breit and Bandmann[289] found that 13.2% of 326 cases of leg eczema

Table 16-7 Exposure Data for Personal Care Products	
Median Usage/ Application	Mean Usage/day
Spray Perfume: 0.23gm	0.34 gm
Hairspray (aerosol): 1.83 gm	2.71 gm
Hairspray (pump): 2.66 gm	3.74 gm
Liquid foundation: 0.36 gm	0.45 gm
Shampoo: 9.6 gm	10.75 gm
Body Wash: 9.5 gm	12.9 gm
Antiperspirant (solid): 0.45 gm	0.59 gm

From: Estrin NF, Crosley OA, Haynes CR, eds. CTFA Dictionary, 3e.Washington, DC: Cosmetic, Toiletry, and Fragrance Association, 1982.

Table 16-8 Cosmetic Categories Reported Frequently by Consumers as Causing Adverse Reactions	
Bath soaps and detergents	Mainly irritation
Deodorants (underarm) and antiperspirants	Usually irritation; occasional ACD
Eye shadow	Mainly irritation
Hair dyes	ACD
Mascara	Mainly irritation
Moisturizers	Irritation and ACD
Permanent waves	Irritation and ACD
Shampoos	Irritation and ACD

ACD = allergic contact dermatitis.

were sensitive to wool alcohols. Of the 43 Eucerin-positive patients of Bandmann and Reichenberger,[290] about 70% had stasis eczemas. Thus, stasis dermatitis patients are at unusually high risk. The British report noted above also noted a high rate of lanolin allergy in those with lower-leg dermatitis. In addition, they saw the anogenital area to be frequently involved.[287]

Cronin and colleagues[291] showed that the proportion of atopic patients reacting to wool alcohols was comparable to that of other eczematous patients, except those patients who had stasis eczema.

Cutaneous Reactions to Cosmetics

The cosmetics industry, with the support of the USFDA, in 1976 established an expert panel to review the toxicology of the more than 4,000 ingredients used in cosmetics. The deliberations of this Cosmetic Ingredient Review (CIR) Panel are published in the *International Journal of Toxicology*. Up to this time, about 1,200 cosmetic ingredient have been reviewed, with almost 110 certified as safe for cosmetic use, about 100 with insufficient data, and 9 deemed unsafe.[292] This panel reviews items not only for skin concerns but also for concerns of systemic toxicity.

Knowledge of exposure patterns to cosmetics and personal care products is useful to predict the level of contact with an ingredient and the likelihood of a problem with a product. The Cosmetic, Toiletry, and Fragrance Association (CTFA) surveyed 360 women's usage of products, with assessment of product weights over a 2-week period of use.[293] This information is given in Table 16.7.

ALLERGIC REACTIONS TO COSMETICS

Allergy to cosmetics constitutes a significant portion of the cases of contact dermatitis seen by dermatologists in the United States. In a 64-month study, 11 dermatologists belonging to the NACDG patch tested 13,216

patients; 713 (5.4%) were identified as having reactions caused by cosmetics.[61] It is notable that these contact dermatitis experts and their patients did not initially suspect a cosmetic in half the cases later proven to evoke reactions to cosmetics. Patients who experience reactions to newly purchased cosmetics seldom consult a physician and merely discard or discontinue using the suspected item. These circumstances hinder our ability to learn the true incidence of reactions to cosmetics and their ingredients. Nevertheless, this study provides data to alert physicians to suspect cosmetic contact reactions and notes likely offenders. Fifty percent of the reactions occurred on the face, and 79% were in females.[61]

Fragrances and preservatives constituted the majority of reactions, followed by "active ingredients" such as hair coloring or permanent wave chemicals, sunscreens, and nail care products.

A similar study from the Netherlands identified 119 patients with contact allergy to cosmetic products.[294] In this study, hair cosmetics, except shampoo and conditioners, were not included in the evaluation. Again, the majority of reactions were due to preservatives (32%) and fragrances (27%). A Belgian report of almost 300 patients with cosmetic ingredient allergy found positive patch tests to fragrances in 54%, preservatives in 32% and excipients in 39%.[295] One-third had eyelid dermatitis and almost one-half had facial involvement.

The majority of cosmetic reactions are not due to allergy, however, but are results of irritation of sensitive skin or urticaria, either immunologic or nonimmunologic (see Table 16.8).

METHODS OF TESTING

Closed patch testing can be used safely with many cosmetic preparations in the same way that prepared allergens are tested. When using whole products, however, both false-negative and false-positive reactions may occur.

False-Negative Reactions

The concentration of an allergen in a cosmetic product may be great enough to produce dermatitis after repeated application on sensitive skin but may be too low to produce a positive patch test on the back. This is especially true of fragrances and preservatives. A negative reaction to a cosmetic, therefore, does not rule out allergy to a component of the product.

False-Positive Reactions

Some cosmetic products are inherently irritating on a closed patch. Cleansing products, hair perms, and artificial nail products are particularly problematic. Volatile solvents, as are present in some mascaras, may also irritate and therefore should be allowed to evaporate for 10 to 15 minutes before the patch is applied. However, a positive reaction to a nonirritating product such as a makeup or skin lotion virtually confirms contact allergy.

Recommendations for Cosmetic Testing

Table 16.9 gives guidelines for cosmetic product patch testing. As a general rule, "leave-on" products such as moisturizers and makeup are safe for closed patch testing, whereas "rinse-off" products may frequently irritate. A large German survey confirms this strategy.[296]

Open testing can be done to irritating substances but is much less reliable than properly performed closed patch testing. Often cosmetic manufacturers will supply patch test kits on request with a breakdown of the ingredients in a suspected product. The patch tester should request that materials be provided at proper patch test concentration, not at product use concentrations, to avoid erroneous results. Usually, the proper patch test concentration is higher, but sometimes, in the case of a surfactant or detergent, for example, it may be lower than in the actual product.

Immediate testing for contact urticaria may be helpful if clinically indicated and/or if regular patch testing is unrevealing. The allergen or product is applied to the volar forearm for about 15 minutes. Readings are taken at intervals over the next 2 hours. Very rarely a "delayed" contact urticaria may occur at a later time (see Table 16.10).

The provocative use test (PUT) or ROAT may identify a reaction if patch testing is equivocal. The suspected product is rubbed into the antecubital skin twice daily for up to 1 week. An absence of erythema, pruritus, or other reaction usually confirms absence of allergy.

Finally, a PUT or ROAT may need to be performed on the face or other affected areas. Occasionally, a positive, reproducible reaction will occur only under such testing, especially in the case of contact urticaria.

Photoallergy must also be considered in facial dermatitis in the absence of other positive findings (see Chapter 22).

Fisher has suggested an elimination routine that may be helpful in the diagnosis of reactions to cosmetics. All cosmetics are stopped except lipstick, which is allowed if the lips are problem-free. Unscented shampoo and unscented soap are used to cleanse the scalp and the skin. All cosmetics and cosmetic applicators are brought in for the physician to examine and patch test. When the dermatitis has cleared, a program of beginning systematically to use each cosmetic one at a time is initiated. If a reaction recurs, the cosmetic begun most recently is eliminated. The program is begun again, and the suspected cosmetic is used last.

INGREDIENT LABELING

The diagnosis and treatment of reactions to cosmetics has been facilitated by the FDA regulation requiring the ingredient labeling of all retailed cosmetics. The ingredients are listed in order of descending concentration, although listing them in alphabetical order has been discussed. Because of the complexity of the composition of fragrances and trade secrecy concerns, their compositions are not given but are listed simply as "fragrance." This regulation, besides identifying ingredients, is helpful to dermatologists because it mandated a uniform nomenclature for cosmetic ingredients. The CTFA Ingredient Dictionary, published by the Cosmetic, Toiletry, and Fragrance Association, is the source for the official names. This dictionary provides a brief description of the chemical, alternative names, and names of suppliers.

When the clinical history, appearance of the reaction, or patch test results lead the clinician to conclude that a cosmetic has caused an adverse reaction, it is important to obtain the ingredients for patch testing. The Cosmetic, Toiletry, and Fragrance Association publishes a pamphlet called Cosmetic Industry on Call. This pamphlet lists the names of members of the industry (with addresses, email addresses, and telephone numbers) who are willing to answer questions about their products.

On occasion, "fractionated" samples will be sent for patch testing. Because irritant concentrations of ingredients may be present in these samples, they are often unsuitable to use for closed patch testing. Some manufacturers will supply individual ingredients in the concentration that they appear in the product, as noted earlier. These are often unsatisfactory for patch testing because the nonstandardized concentrations may be too low to provoke an allergic response or may be high enough to elicit irritation under occlusion. See Appendix A in this chapter for contact information for the CTFA.

TYPES OF REACTIONS

Reactions to cosmetics can have a varied appearance; this variety of presentation can challenge the clinician's ability to make the correct diagnosis. Duarte found 176 (87% female) patients in her private practice with complaints of "reactions" to cosmetics.[297] Twenty-eight percent had contact dermatitis (ACD and/or ICD). She felt that just over half of the patients had conditions not caused by cosmetic use including melasma (11%) acne (6%), and other ACD not caused by cosmetics (7.5%).

Table 16-9 Patch Testing Cosmetic Products

Product	Conc.	Vehicle	Comments
Baby products			
Baby shampoo	1[a]	Aq	Test individual ingredients; detergents may require opentest and provocative use tests for confirmation
Baby lotion	as is[b]		
Baby oil	as is		
Baby powder	as is		
Baby cream	as is[b]		
Bath preparation			
Bath oil			
Nonfoaming	as is[b]		Nonfoaming—emulsifiers may irritate.[a]
Foaming			Foaming—treat as detergent; perform open tests and provocative use test[b]
Bubble bath	1[a]	Aq	Test individual ingredients.
Bath capsule			If it contains detergent, dilute 1:100[a]
Other bath preparations			If primarily fragrance, patch test 10% in petrolatum closed and photopatch test. If positive, verify with controls
Eye makeup			
Eyebrow pencil	as is[b]		If positive, verify with controls
Eyeliner	as is[b]		Usually not irritant; if suspected check with open and provocative use test
Eye shadow cream	as is[b]		Rare, irritant reactions. Repeat weak positives with open and provocative use tests
Eye shadow powder	as is		
Eye lotion	as is		
Eye makeup remover	as is[b]		Occasional irritant reaction may contain amphoteric surfactant. Check with open and provocative use tests
Mascara	as is[b]	Dry	Dry 20 minutes to remove volatile solvents. Open and provocative use tests may clarify type of reaction
Fragrance preparations			
Cologne and toilet water	as is	Dry	Dry for 5 minutes. Photopatch test also
Perfume	as is	Dry	Dry for 5 minutes. Photopatch test also
Powder	as is		
Sachet	as is[b]		Photopatch test also
Hair preparations (noncoloring)			
Conditioners	as is[b]		Quaternary ammonium compounds may be irritating under occlusion[c]
Aerosol spray	as is	Dry	
Straightener			Never test except with diluted ingredients
Permanent wave			Never test except with diluted ingredients.
Rinse	2	Aq	
Shampoo	1[a]	Aq	Doubtful value. Test ingredients
Tonic	as is[b]	Dry	Test open and photopatch test. Patch test ingredients. May contain preservatives and fragrance allergens
Hair coloring preparations			
Hair dyes	2	Aq	Prefer: 5 drops dye + 5 drops oxidizer test open and read in 24 hours. Test 1% paraphenylenediamine in petrolatum closed. If negative, test other ingredients
Hair tint			See above: hair dyes
Hair rinse (coloring)			Open test read in 24 hours
Shampoo (coloring)	1[a]	Aq	Irritant due to detergent. If semipermanent dye, test open antecubital area
Bleach			Ammonium persulfate 1 to 2.5% in petrolatum test open (see contact urticaria and text on bleaching)

Table 16-9 (Cont.) Patch Testing Cosmetic Products

Product	Conc.	Vehicle	Comments
Makeup preparation			
Blushers	as is		
Face powder	as is		
Foundation	as is[b]		
Leg and body paint	as is		May be an irritant
Lipstick	as is		Phototest also
Makeup base	as is[b]		
Rouge	as is		
Manicuring preparations			
Basecoat/undercoat	as is[b]	Dry	May test open
Cuticle softener			Do not patch test as is. Test diluted ingredients only
Nail cream	as is[b]		
Nail extender			Patch test ingredients only
Nail polish and enamel	as is	Dry	May test open
Nail polish remover			Do not patch test as is. Test diluted ingredients only
Oral hygiene			
Dentifrice liquid, paste, powder	2[a]	Aq	Detergents may require open and provocative use tests. If positive, verify with controls
Personal cleanliness			
Bath soaps	1[a]	Aq	Alternatively 5% aq open. Both of doubtful value
Detergents			
Deodorant (underarm)	as is[b]		May be mild irritant. Repeat weak positives open inside forearm twice daily for 1 week. Test diluted ingredients also
Antiperspirants			Test ingredients
Douches			
Feminine deodorant sprays	as is[b]		Usually irritant reactions from being applied too close
Shaving preparations			
Aftershave lotion	as is	Dry	Photopatch test. Provocative use test in small area on beard region beard region
Beard softener			
Men's talc	as is		
Preshave lotion			
Shaving cream aerosol			
brushless lather	2[a]	Aq	
Shaving soap	1[a]	Aq	
Skin care preparations			
Cleansing lotion, or pads	as is[b]		Likely to be weak irritants
Depilatory			Test diluted ingredients only
Face, body, or hand cream or lotion	as is		
Foot powder or spray			
Hormone cream or lotion	as is		
Moisturizing cream or lotion	as is		
Night cream or lotion	as is[b]		May be weak irritant
Skin lightener			Test ingredients only
Skin freshener	20	Aq	May be irritant. Provocative use test if in doubt
Suntan and sunscreen preparations			
Sunscreen gel, cream or lotion	as is[b]		
Photopatch test also			
Indoor tanning preparations	as is[b]		

[a]Detergents require provocative use tests.
[b]This category may rarely prodice irritancy with occlusive patch test.
[c]Contact manufacturer requesting irritancy controls.

Table 16-10 Test Procedure for Evaluation of Immediate-Type Reactions in Recommended Order

1. Open application
   Nonaffected normal skin
      Negative

   ↓

   Slightly affected (or previously affected)
      skin
   Negative

   ↓

2. Occlusive application   DIAGNOSIS
   (infrequently needed)   IF   OF
   Nonaffected normal skin   POSITIVE =   CONTACT
      Negative   URTICARIA

   ↓

   Slightly affected (or previously affected)
      skin
   Negative

   ↓

3. Invasive (inhalant, prick, scratch,
   or intradermal injection)[a]

[a]When invasive methods are employed (especially scratch and inhalant testing), adequate controls are required

Adapted from Krogh, G von, Maibach, HI. The contact urticaria syndrome—1982. Semin Dermatol 1982;1:59. (301)

Subjective Irritation

When the application of a cosmetic causes burning, stinging, or itching without detectable visible or microscopic changes, this is designated as subjective irritation. This reaction is common in certain susceptible individuals occurring usually on the face. Some of the ingredients that cause this reaction are not generally considered irritants and will not cause abnormal responses in nonsusceptible individuals.[298] The burning or stinging lasts usually less than 10 minutes. The clinician is dependent on the patient's subjective responses to the use of a product to identify this type of reaction. This is probably the most common cause of dissatisfaction with cosmetics and skin care products.

Objective Irritation

Predictive testing in human beings and rabbits can reliably detect strong or moderate irritants as ingredients in cosmetics or the products themselves.[299] This allows manufacturers to test thoroughly to eliminate these potential hazards before marketing a cosmetic. Mild irritants, however, are more difficult to detect. Because the stratum corneum of the facial skin is penetrated easily, more irritant reactions occur there. Many supposedly nonirritating moisturizers or emollient creams contain surfactants and emulsifiers that may be mild irritants. These cosmetics are applied frequently to facial or inflamed skin, resulting in irritant reactions. In use testing, reproducing an irritant reaction is difficult because penetrability of the stratum corneum varies with environmental conditions such as humidity and temperature. If testing is negative on the back or forearm, provocative use testing may be carried out at the original site of the reactions. This diagnosis rests on the exclusion of contact allergy with patch testing and known exposure to potential irritants.

Examples of irritants in topical products include propylene glycol, PABA, SLS, other surfactants, alphahydroxy acids, and retinoids.

Contact Urticaria

A contact urticarial reaction is a wheal-and-flare response to a topically applied chemical that may be immunologic or nonimmunologic. In practice, patients may present with varied complaints: itching, burning, stinging, chronic dermatitis, generalized urticaria, or systemic anaphylactoid reactions. A careful history alerts a physician to perform the tests that are necessary to observe short-term reactions. A flow sheet designed by von Krogh and Maibach[300] can be used to approach testing in suspected cases (see Table 16.10).

The details of testing can be studied in this review. The testing should be carried out where emergency resuscitation facilities are available, because anaphylactic reactions have rarely been reported even when chemicals have been applied to intact skin in sensitive individuals.

The cosmetic ingredients and products cited in Table 16.11 have been implicated in the contact urticarial syndrome.

Allergic Contact Dermatitis

Although ACD is the most frequently diagnosed reaction to cosmetics, it is suspected initially in less than half the proven cases.

Pigmentation

Pigmentary irregularities are discussed in Chapter 23.

Hyperpigmentation of the face caused by contact dermatitis to ingredients in cosmetics occurs more frequently in dark-complexioned individuals. An epidemic of facial pigmentation reported in Japanese women was attributed to "coal tar" dyes (principally Sudan I, a contaminant of D&C Red No. 31).[301,302] The following fragrance ingredients have also been implicated: benzyl salicylate, ylang-ylang oil, cananga oil, jasmine absolute, hydroxycitronellal, methoxycitronellal, sandalwood oil, benzyl alcohol, cinnamic alcohol, lavender oil, geraniol, and geranium oil.[303] Histologic examination shows hydropic degeneration of the basal layer and pigment incontinence. There may be little other evidence of inflammation. Mathias[304] reported pigmented cosmetic contact dermatitis due to contact allergy to chromium hydroxide used as a dye in toilet soap, and Maibach[250] reported

Table 16-11 Some Cosmetics and Ingredients That Have Been Reported to Cause Contact Urticaria

Type of Reaction	Chemical	Product
Nonimmunologic	Acetic acid	
	Alcohols	
	Balsam of Peru	Perfumes
	Benzoic acid	
	Cinnamic acid	
	Cinnamic aldehyde	
	Formaldehyde[a]	
	Sodium benzoate	
	Sorbic acid	Shampoo
Immunologic	Acrylic monomer	
	Alcohols	
	Ammonia	
	Benzoic acid	
	Benzophenone	
	Diethyltoluamide	
	Formaldehyde[b]	
	Henna	
	Menthol	
	Parabens	
	Polyethylene glycol (PEG-8)	
	Polysorbate 60	
	Salicylic acid	
	Sodium sulfide	
Uncertain	Ammonium persulfate	Hair bleaches
	Paraphenylenediamine	Hair dyes
		Hair spray
		Nail polish
		Rouge
		Toothpaste

[a]Multiple applications may be required for testing.
[b]Single application for testing. Adapted from Krogh, G von, Maibach, HI. The contact urticaria syndrome—1982. *Semin Dermatol* 1982;1:59 (301).

hyperpigmentation in a black man sensitive to petrolatum. These cases are instructive because they alert the dermatologist to search scrupulously for a causative agent; its elimination results frequently in gradual fading of the pigment. Patients require constant encouragement during this slow depigmentation phase; otherwise, they doubt the accuracy of the diagnosis.

Ironically, hydroquinone, used as a bleaching agent, has caused postinflammatory hyperpigmentation. In 1975, Findlay and colleagues[305] from South Africa reported a long-term complication of the use of hydroquinone—deposits of ochronotic pigment in the skin, along with colloid milia. Black patients had no chemical evidence of alkaptonuria. The melanocyte, despite intense hydroquinone use, escaped destruction, and the site of the injury shifted to the dermis and the fibroblast. Polymeric pig-

ment adhered to thickened, abnormal collagen bundles. Since then, reports of exogenous ochronosis have come from other areas, including the United States. A biopsy must be performed to establish this diagnosis.

In addition, a few cases of persistent hypopigmentation have incriminated topical hydroquinone.[306]

Cinnamic aldehyde, which was present in a toothpaste, caused perioral leukoderma.[307]

Paronychia, and Nail Abnormalities

The physician should obtain a detailed description of the nail-grooming habits of patients who have paronychia, onycholysis, nail destruction, or nail discoloration, since any of these problems may be caused by nail cosmetic usage. Nail discoloration has been reported with the use of hydroquinone bleaching creams and hair dyes containing henna.[308] Chronic use of nail polishes may lead to temporary nail staining. Permanent paresthesia and nail loss following usage of acrylic nails has been reported. Fungal infection with dermatophytes or *Candida, Pseudomonas* bacterial infection, and trauma must also be among the considerations in the diagnoses of nail problems.

Hair Breakage

"Perms" and hair straighteners are intended to break the disulfide bonds that give hair keratin its strength. Improper usage or incomplete neutralization of these cosmetics causes hair breakage. Hair that has been damaged by previous applications of permanent waves, straighteners, oxidation-type dyes, bleaches, or excessive exposure to sunlight and chlorine is more susceptible to this damage. Careful examination of the hair shafts is essential to detect any pre-existing abnormalities.

Acneiform Reactions

Acne and folliculitis can be precipitated or aggravated by cosmetic usage. Since 1972, when Kligman and Mills[309] proposed the rabbit's ear model to test cosmetics and their ingredients for comedogenicity, screening programs have been conducted.

Classes of ingredients, such as isopropyl myristate and its analogues, lanolin and its derivatives, detergents, and D&C red dyes, have been incriminated by the rabbit's ear test.[310] In addition, oils such as mineral oil and petrolatum in topical products may cause occlusive folliculitis and formation of comedones. Bronaugh and Maibach[299] reported that results of the rabbit's ear test correlate well with pustule formation noted in use tests of cosmetics performed on women's faces. They noted instances of skin and hair cosmetics that produce papulopustules after 3 to 7 days of use that are strongly positive in the rabbit's ear model.

Frank[311] accurately pointed out inconsistencies in the results reported from the rabbit's ear test. Many questions remain unanswered: Does the mere presence of a comedogenic ingredient in a cosmetic incriminate the product? Are the effects of multiple comedogenic ingredients cumulative?

From a practical standpoint, even cosmetics touted as noncomedogenic may cause acneiform lesions in some patients. Usually "water-based" or "oil-free" cosmetics will be less likely to do so than those containing oils. Although allergen avoidance is fairly easy by reading labels, acnegenicity in a given individual may have to be determined through the "trial and error" method.

Cosmetics and Toiletries: Reactions and Patch Testing

BABY PRODUCTS

These products are marketed primarily for use on the skin and scalps of infants. Some experimental data suggest that infants are less easily sensitized than adults. In clinical practice, ACD is diagnosed relatively infrequently in young children.[312] Partly this may be due to lack of presentation for patch testing and partly it may be due to an inherent low rate of sensitization capability. Patch test results in children mirror frequency of positive reactions in adults, with allergens such as nickel and rubber chemicals often found. Because the diaper area is a frequent site of irritant contact dermatitis, careful attention should be paid to the products used in this area. Often, baby products are fragranced. Baby oil, talc, and cornstarch have simple compositions with little sensitizing potential beside the fragrances. Baby lotions or creams may contain fragrance, preservatives, lanolin, or propylene glycol, and other components that are sensitizers.[1] In the treatment of infants with diaper rash, it is important to examine the ingredients of the cosmetics used on the diaper area and to consider in particular their irritant potential.

BATH PREPARATIONS

Adverse reactions to bubble bath reported to the FDA include skin eruptions, irritation of the genitourinary tract, eye irritation, and respiratory disorders.[313,314] The genitourinary tract reactions in children have been the most serious; some children have been subjected to extensive urologic evaluation before the cause was established. The skin eruptions are assumed usually to be irritant reactions due to the detergent content of this product.

Cocamidopropyl betaine is now present in many bath preparations. Although less irritating than previous surfactants, it is more allergenic. Physicians should warn parents not to allow children to use a bubble bath unsupervised or not to take prolonged bubble baths. Because of their detergent content, these cosmetics may cause or aggravate dryness and inflammation of the skin and are especially unsuitable for atopic individuals.

EYE MAKEUP PREPARATIONS

Mascara, eyeliner, eye shadow, and eyebrow pencil or powders are the most commonly used eye-area makeups. Soft pencils used for shadowing and lining have become popular in recent years, and false eyelashes have become less fashionable. Usually, these cosmetics are unfragranced but do contain one or more preservatives. The parabens are found in almost all eye shadows. Fortunately, these agents are relatively rare sensitizers and may even be tolerated on noninflamed skin in those who are allergic to them (see "The Paraben Paradox" above). Other preservatives, however, may be present and may be more likely causes of allergy. Often overlooked as causes of ACD of the eyelids are the metals nickel, cobalt, and chromate. Nickel is not intentionally present in eye cosmetics but has been found as a contaminant. Both cobalt and chromate may be present in coloring agents.

Eyelid Dermatitis

Most cases of eyelid dermatitis, in the absence of obvious photosensitivity or primary ophthalmologic disease, can be traced to contact dermatitis, seborrheic dermatitis, or atopic dermatitis. Only rarely is contact urticaria or collagen vascular disease the cause. All but ACD and contact urticaria can usually be diagnosed by history and other physical or laboratory findings.

Because the eyelid skin is thin and sensitive, eyelid ACD may be caused not only by directly applied agents but also by allergens transferred by touch and even airborne contact allergens. In addition to cosmetics, allergens in contact lens solutions or eye medications may directly contact the eyelids. Toluene sulfonamide formaldehyde resin in nail polish is a classic cause of eyelid allergy. Acrylates in artificial nails can cause eyelid dermatitis. Rubber in makeup sponges and eyelash curlers may affect the eyelids. Eyelid dermatitis from chromate in airborne cement dust or from allergens in wood dust may occur.

Guin reviewed his extensive experience with eyelid dermatitis.[315] ACD was present in 165 of 215. Thirty seven were atopic but most had relevant contact allergies. Personal care products were positive in 25%, with reactions to metals, rubber, and others also occurring.

Nethercott and colleagues[316] reported on 79 cases of eyelid dermatitis, mostly in women. Forty-six percent had ACD, 15% had ICD, and 23% were atopic. Formaldehyde, formaldehyde-releasing preservatives, fragrances, nickel, and neomycin were among the most commonly positive allergens.

Ingredients of shampoos and other hair care products must also be suspected in cases of eyelid dermatitis. Cocamidopropyl betaine and methyldibromoglutaronitrile are two "newer" shampoo components that may cause eyelid ACD.

Shellac may be a more common cause of eyelid ACD than has been recognized. Several cases have been reported.[317] Testing can be performed with shellac 20% in ethanol.

Although eye cosmetics may be used "as is" for patch testing, the allergen concentration is often too low to give a positive result. Mascaras may cause an irritant reaction on patch testing unless volatile hydrocarbons are allowed to evaporate for 20 minutes or so before applying the patch.[318]

Metals in Eyelid Dermatitis Sainia and colleagues[319] tested 88 colors of 25 brands of eye shadow for levels of cobalt, nickel, chromate, lead, and arsenic. Lead and arsenic values were below toxic levels. Over 10 ppm of cobalt were found in 21 (24%) samples, of nickel in 37 (42%) samples, and of chromium in 33 (37%) samples. The highest levels of nickel and cobalt were 41 and 49 ppm, respectively. Chromium levels in three samples were very high, with over 2,000 ppm. This is particularly significant because usually nickel and cobalt are not listed on ingredient labeling. These levels are significant enough to cause reactivity in some sensitive persons.

More recently, gold has been shown to be a not uncommon cause of eyelid dermatitis, even in the absence of hand dermatitis.[320] Presumably, just as has been seen with nail polish, handling and wearing jewelry and then touching the sensitive eyelids allows for allergen transfer. In a report from the NACDG, gold was the single most common allergen in patients with only eyelid dermatitis.[62] Fragrance was next, followed by nickel and neomycin.

Both black iron oxide (magnetite) and yellow iron oxide (brown limonite) have caused a case of eyelid ACD.[321]

Other Reasons for Eyelid Dermatitis When allergic, seborrheic, and atopic forms of dermatitis are not found, cumulative irritant dermatitis may be present. Dryness, friction, and irritant ingredients of topicals may all contribute to this. Each of these factors must be corrected if treatment is to be successful.

Other than the metals mentioned above, coloring agents are rare sensitizers. In the United States, the pigments used in eye-area cosmetics are restricted. No coaltar derivatives may be incorporated; only purified natural colors or inorganic pigment or lakes of low allergic potential are used.

Eye infections, of either the cornea or the lids, may be due to abrasions from mascara wands when the mascara is not properly preserved.[322] Patients should be urged to use eye cosmetics hygienically and advised not to use eye cosmetics inside the lash line.

HAIR PREPARATIONS (NONCOLORING)

Permanents

Permanent waves are cosmetics that alter the disulfide bonds of hair keratin so that hair fiber configuration can be changed. The disulfide bonds of cystine are broken in the first step when the waving solution is applied to the hair wound around mandrels. In the second step, with neutralization, new disulfide bonds are formed by locking in the curl configuration of the hair.

The waving solutions contain reducing agents that can cause irritant reactions when allowed to run incautiously on the skin surrounding the scalp. Irritant reactions range from erythema to bullous dermatitis. Hair breakage and loss may result when permanent waves are used improperly—in too concentrated a form, for too long a time, or on hair previously damaged by dyes, straighteners, or permanent waves. Old-fashioned hot waves occasionally caused chemical burns, which scarred the scalp, producing permanent alopecia, but modern permanents can cause breakage, which results in temporary loss.

Currently, the majority of salon perms use glyceryl thioglycolate (GTG). These are called "acid" or "heat" perms. GTG has become a major allergen in hairdressers and somewhat less so in their clients. Two factors regarding GTG have been elucidated and doubtless contribute to the chronicity of hand eczema in hairdressers.[323,324]

GTG persists on permed hair for weeks or months. A hairdresser, when cutting hair that has been permed previously, may still react to the GTG. It penetrates intact rubber gloves. The only glove shown to be protective against GTG is a plastic laminate glove (4H glove). Avoidance of this allergen therefore is difficult if not impossible for some hairdressers and may lead to a change in career.

The older type of "cold waves" used for home perms and salon perms contain thioglycolic acid combined with ammonia or another alkali to raise the pH (ammonium thioglycolate). The concentration of the thioglycolic acid and alkali can be varied to change the products' speed of action or to suit the type of hair to be waved (i.e., difficult to wave, normal, or easy to wave). The neutralizer contains hydrogen peroxide or sodium bromate. These perms rarely cause allergic reactions. If a truly allergic reaction is suspected, all the ingredients of the permanent (gums, fragrance, etc.) must be tested as well as the ingredients of the other products used at the same time, such as shampoos, conditioners, and hair sprays. Ammonium thioglycolate can be patch tested at 2.5% aqueous. Allergy to these perms is often assumed but rarely, if ever, proven.

Crossreactions between GTG and ammonium thioglycolate rarely occur.

Another type of perm used primarily at home is the sulfite wave. Although the sulfite wave produces less strong curls and is slower, the odor is more pleasant. Neutralization is done usually with bromates. Occasional allergic reactions are seen with these perms. Use 1% sodium bisulfite in water to patch test.[325]

Cysteamine HCl may be used in some permanent-wave products as a replacement for GTG. Isaksson has reported that 16 of 1,347 hairdressers (1.2%) from the Netherlands had clinically relevant patch test reactions to CHC (0.5% pet).[326] She states that the allergen does not penetrate through latex gloves and that treated hair is not allergenic.

Straighteners

Mme C.J. Walker, in 1901, developed a process to straighten black hair using a heated comb with petrolatum or a mixture of petrolatum, oils, and waxes. The petrolatum or "pressing" oils act as a heat-modifying conductor, which reduces friction when the comb travels down the hair fibers. Mechanical and heat damage can cause hair breakage. Over the years, the heated oils can injure the hair follicles, leading to scarring alopecia ("hot-comb alopecia").

Chemical straighteners containing sodium hydroxide, or "lye," cleave the disulfide bonds of keratin thoroughly and straighten hair permanently.[327] Experience and caution in applying these straighteners are important to avoid hair breakage and chemical burns. Similar products that contain guanidine carbonate mixed with calcium hydroxide are reputed to be milder. It is necessary to straighten new growth every few months. Some manufacturers advise against using permanent hair colors that require peroxide on chemically straightened hair to avoid damage.

Sulfite straighteners, chemically similar to sulfite permanents, are best suited for relaxing curly white hair.

"Soft curls" are a way of styling the hair of some persons with curly hair. Ammonium thioglycolate and a bromate or peroxide neutralizer are used to achieve restructuring of the hair.

Follow-up care is elaborate and includes successive applications of products called moisturizers, curl activators, and oil sheens that saturate the hair and scalp. A plastic cap is worn to bed each night. These cosmetics may contain oils, quaternium compounds, glycerin, propylene glycol, and collagen, as well as fragrance and preservatives.

Shampoos

Shampoos generally have a short contact time with the scalp and are diluted and rinsed off quickly. (Some residues, inadequately quantitated, remain.) These factors reduce their sensitizing potential. Consumers' complaints are commonly directed at their eye stinging and irritating qualities. The importance of eye safety testing for these products became apparent 30 years ago when shampoos based on blends of cationic and nonionic detergents caused blindness in some users.[328]

Shampoos today generally are detergent-based, with a few containing small amounts of soap for conditioning. Anionic detergents and amphoteric detergents are occasional sensitizers.[329] The nonionic surfactant cocamidopropyl betaine, discussed earlier in this chapter, may cause hand dermatitis in hairdressers and facial dermatitis in users. Fatty acid amides used in shampoos as thickeners and foam stabilizers have caused ACD in other products, as well as in shampoos.[330] Individual ingredient patch testing is necessary to incriminate allergens in shampoos because testing with the actual product will usually cause an irritant reaction.

Hair Coloring Preparations

Millions of persons color their hair, using five different types of dyes:

Type 1: Permanent hair dyes, mixtures of colorless, aromatic compounds that act as primary intermediates and couplers. The primary intermediates, principally p-phenylenediamine (PPDA), toluene-2,5-diamine (p-toluenediamine), and p-aminophenol, are oxidized by hydrogen peroxide in the presence of ammonia, polymerize, and combine with couplers to form a variety of colors that blend to give the desired shade. These reactions take place inside the hair shaft, accounting for the fastness of these dyes. Permanent dyes are the most popular because of the variety of natural colors they can achieve, as well as their persistence.

Type 2: Semipermanent hair dyes, containing low-molecular-weight nitrophenylenediamine and anthroquinone dyes, which penetrate the hair cortex to some extent. Their color lasts through approximately five shampoos.

Type 3: Temporary rinses, mixtures of mild organic acids and certified dyes that coat the hair shaft. These rub and shampoo off easily.

Type 4: Vegetable dyes, which in the US contain henna, which only colors hair red.

Type 5: Metallic dyes, containing lead acetate and sulfur. When they are combed through the hair daily, they deposit insoluble lead oxides and sulfides that impart colors that range from yellow-brown to dark gray.

The vast majority of cases of allergy to hair dyes are caused by PPDA. It was introduced in the 1880s and has been problematic ever since.[331,332] In 2006, the American Contact Dermatitis Society called it their "allergen of the year."[332] DeLeo states that "2 out of 5 American women color their hair."[332] Crossreaction may occur to other related amines found in the permanent and semipermanent dyes, and also to "black-rubber" chemicals, benzocaine, PABA, and various medications. Independent sensitization to toluene-2,5-diamine or 2-nitro-p-phenylenediamine dyes or resorcinol occurs rarely, but positive patch tests to toluene-2,5-diamine or 2-nitro-p-phenylenediamine dyes result generally from cross-sensitization to PPDA.

Types 1 and 2, in the United States, bear a label warning about adverse reactions. Instructions for open patch testing are given. In practice, this is seldom carried out in homes or salons. PPDA type dyes are added occasionally to temporary rinses. These rinses must also bear a warning label and patch test instructions.

The severity of PPDA reactions ranges from mild erythema at the hairline or ears to swelling of the eyelids and face, accompanied by an acute vesicular eruption in the scalp that requires prompt medical attention.

One percent PPDA in petrolatum is used in the standard closed patch test. The most recent NACDG data show a positive patch test rate of 4.7%, with almost all being relevant,[1] Broeckx[333] in Belgium reported similar results, with 7.2% of more than 5,000 patients reactive to PPDA. Ortho-nitro PPDA and para-toluenediamine were positive in 1.8% and 1.6%, respectively. Occasional case reports have appeared that suggested that contact reactions occurred to another person's dyed hair.[334,335]

Patients sensitive to PPDA should be warned about possible crossreactions with local anesthetics (procaine and benzocaine), sulfonamides, and para-aminobenzoic acid sunscreens. Also, some persons allergic to PPDA may react to disperse or "azo" textile dyes. It is estimated that 25% of patients who are PPDA-sensitive will react to semipermanent hair dyes. Patients who wish to try these as a substitute should do an open patch test with the dye first.

Several patients have been reported who experienced immediate hypersensitivity reactions to PPDA, and this spectrum of reactions to hair dyes should now be considered as a diagnostic possibility in appropriate patients.[336] Some patients complain of scalp irritation after dyeing their hair, but we are unaware of published data that study the potential of these dyes for irritation. Some hair dye reactions occur most prominently in light-exposed areas, but the phototoxic and photoallergic potential of coal-tar dyes has not been investigated.

PPDA allergy can be a significant occupational problem for hairdressers. One report showed an astounding 58% incidence of allergy in 300 hairdressers.[337]

A relatively new and serious problem with PPDA allergy is arising from "henna" tattoos. These temporary tattoos, popular with youngsters, are often adulterated with very high levels of PPDA. The presence of PPDA is not disclosed.[338]

Henna has not been reported to cause ACD when used as a hair dye, but cases have been reported from coloring the skin with henna.[339,340] Cronin[341] described a hairdresser who noted wheezing and coryza when she handled henna; this patient had a positive prick test to henna.

A single case of contact dermatitis due to lead acetate in the metallic dyes has been reported.[342]

A potential, "hypoallergenic" alternative hair dye called "Elumen Hair Color" is available from Goldwell Cosmetics (Linthicum Heights, MD).[343] These dyes have very low crossreactivity with PPDA.

When hair is bleached, ammonium persulfate, a booster, is added to hydrogen peroxide to obtain the lightest shades. Ammonium persulfate has several industrial uses as well, and it is known to cause irritant reactions and ACD occasionally.[343] One percent aqueous solution of ammonium persulfate can be used in closed patch tests. In addition, observation for immediate reactions should be made at the time of patch testing.

Ammonium persulfate can cause immediate hypersensitivity reactions, including urticaria, facial edema, asthma, and syncope. These reactions are histamine mediated, but at present it is not clear whether or not immunologic mechanisms are involved.[344]

Hairdressers should be instructed that clients who develop hives, generalized itching, facial swelling, or asthma when the hair is bleached should not have the process repeated using persulfate. Clients experiencing such reactions should receive immediate medical attention.

Rastogi and colleagues have noted that after dyeing procedures, significant amounts of unconsumed allergenic components remain.[345]

FACIAL MAKEUP PREPARATIONS

Eleven percent of the reactions to cosmetics in an NACDG study in 1985 were to this group of products, which includes lipstick, rouge, makeup bases, and facial powders.[61]

Before 1960, allergic reactions to lipsticks were common. Most were caused by D&C Red No. 21 (eosin), an indelible dye used in long-lasting deeply colored lipsticks. The sensitizer in eosin proved to be a contaminant; improved methods of purification have reduced its sensitizing potential. Because eosin is strongly bound to keratin, patch tests are performed with 50% eosin in petrolatum.

Other dyes occasionally have been reported as sensitizers.[346,347] Other sensitizers have been reported in lipsticks—castor oil acting as a pigment solvent,[348] antioxidants propyl gallate and monotertiary-butylhydroquinone,[349,350] sunscreens,[351,352] lanolin, preservatives, propylene glycol, and fragrance. Para-tertiary-butylphenol in lipstick caused cheilitis in a patient and depigmentation at the patch test site.[353]

Although allergic reactions to lipstick are uncommon, dermatologists should consider this diagnosis even when the eruption has spread beyond the lips, because the sensitizing chemical may be present in cosmetics other than the lipstick. Each lipstick and lip balm that the patient uses should be tested "closed" as well by photopatch tests, since some of the dyes used may be photoallergens.

Rouge or "blush" is manufactured in various forms—powder, cream, liquid, stick, or gel. It is designed to highlight the cheeks with color. The composition is not unique: Powders are similar to face powder, and creams and liquids are similar to foundation. To achieve bright shades, organic colors are added to rouges as they are to lipsticks. Preservatives and fragrances are common allergens. D&C Yellow No. 11 caused allergic reactions to rouges as well as lipsticks.[346] Some women may use lipstick to color their cheeks in place of rouge, or rouge may be used all over the face to achieve a "healthy glow." Powder blush is less likely to cause allergy than liquid or cream blush, probably because it contains fewer preservatives and other sensitizing ingredients. It may also be better for those patients prone to acne.

Facial makeups or foundations are applied to the skin to give an appearance of uniform color and texture and to disguise blemishes or imperfections. Produced in a variety of forms—emulsions of water and oil, oil-free lotions, anhydrous sticks, poured powders, and pancake makeups—the amount of coverage given is determined by the titanium dioxide (TiO_2) content. Because TiO_2 reflects light, some ordinary makeups achieve significant sun protection factor (SPF) values. Sunscreening agents may be added to some foundations to increase these SPF values. These products with sunscreens may be marketed as "antiaging." PABA derivatives, fragrances, emulsifiers, preservatives, propylene glycol, and lanolin are chemicals with significant sensitizing potential used in makeups. Synthetic esters, such as isopropyl myristate and lanolin derivatives added to these makeups, have been implicated as causes of acne by the rabbit's ear test.[301]

The pattern of dermatitis seen with allergy to facial makeups may be surprisingly irregular, with skipped areas of normal skin interspersed with areas of dermatitis. This raises an interesting question about the existence of resident clones of antigen-presenting cells or T lymphocytes that remain in one area of skin only.

NAIL COSMETICS

In the past, adverse reactions have been reported to numerous nail cosmetics, which have been removed sub-sequently from the market. Nail hardeners containing formaldehyde are in this category.[354] In the United States, this type of hardener is permitted for use only on the free edge of the nail when the skin is protected from contact with the hardener. Some manufacturers sell products called "hardeners," but they have merely increased the resin content of ordinary nail enamel.

Nail enamels, including base coats and top coats, have a similar composition.

1. Film former—nitrocellulose
2. Resins—tosylamide formaldehyde resin, alkyd resins, acrylates, vinyls, or polyesters
3. Plasticizers—camphor, dibutyl phthalate, dioctyl phthalate, and tricresyl phosphate
4. Solvents—alcohol, toluene, ethyl acetate, and butyl acetate
5. Colorants
6. Pearlizers—guanine and bismuth oxychloride

The concentration of each of these chemicals depends on the quality to be achieved in the final product. The base coat will have increased amounts of resin to improve adhesion to the nail plate, but the top coat has increased nitrocellulose and plasticizers to enhance gloss and abrasion resistance.

Patients allergic to nail polish often develop dermatitis at sites distant from the fingers, commonly eyelids, around the mouth and chin, sides of the neck, on the genitalia, and rarely a generalized eruption. Tosylamide formaldehyde resin (TSFR) is responsible for almost all the allergic reactions. In the NACDG study, this resin was the seventh most common ingredient causing allergic contact dermatitis in patients with a cosmetic allergy.[61] In a study from the Netherlands, it accounted for 10% of reactions in 119 cosmetic allergy patients, ranking behind only preservatives, fragrances, and emulsifiers.[294] A small amount of free formaldehyde may be in the resin, but most who react to TSFR are not also allergic to formaldehyde. Patch testing is performed with the resin at 10% petrolatum.[1] The NACDG reports a prevalence of 1.7% from 5,137 patients. "Hypoallergenic" brands of nail polish, which substitute alkyd or other resins, are available for those allergic to TSFR. The durability and abrasion resistance of these other resins is said to be inferior to TSFR. Although onycholysis has been attributed to reactions to TSFR, no published data firmly support this.[355]

Fowler has seen one case of allergy to butyl acetate. The patient was unable to find any brand of nail polish she could tolerate. Dermatitis occurred not only on the face but also on the paronychial areas.

Liden and colleagues[356] show how serious the consequences of ACD to nail polish may be. In a 2-year period, 18 women with nail polish allergy were seen. Eight women had taken 1 or more months of sick leave for a presumed occupational problem before diagnosis. Four were hospitalized and two lost their jobs.

Yellow discoloration of the nail plate, darkest at the distal end, occurs commonly in women who wear colored nail polish. Samman[308] reproduced this staining with the following colors: D&C Red No. 7, D&C Red No. 34, D&C Red No. 6, and FD&C Yellow No. 5 lake. This discoloration will fade over time only if use of nail polish is discontinued.

Nail enamel removers are mixtures of solvents such as acetone and amyl, butyl, or ethyl acetate to which fatty materials and fragrance may be added.[357] ICD is more likely to occur than ACD.

Cuticle removers contain alkaline chemicals, frequently sodium or potassium hydroxide, to break the disulfide bonds of keratin. They should not be left on for prolonged periods or be used by people who are susceptible to paronychia. Cuticle removers are irritants that should not be used for closed patch testing.

Artificial Nails

"Sculptured nails" are popular because they build an attractive artificial nail on the nail plate. Persons who could not grow nails previously can now have the appearance of long nails.

Sculptured nails are applied by a manicurist, or kits may be purchased for home use. The kits consist of a powdered methacrylate polymer, with benzoyl peroxide as an initiator, and a liquid methacrylate ester or mixture of these esters. Polymerization begins when the liquid and the powder are mixed and painted on the nail, which is surrounded by a template that protects the surrounding skin and allows the formation of an artificial extension.

Unfortunately, irritant and allergic reactions to the liquid monomers, as well as secondary infections, may be painful and long-lasting. Paronychia, onycholysis, onychia, and dermatitis of the finger and distant sites may occur. As early as 1957, Fisher and colleagues[358] reported allergic sensitization to the methyl methacrylate monomers in sculptured nails. Acting rapidly, in 1974 the FDA banned the use of methyl methacrylate in these cosmetics.[359] However, analysis of 31 products sold between 1975 and 1981 revealed that this monomer was present in nine of them,[360] and this is probably still true today. Regardless of this, sensitization has also been reported to other monomers, and crossreactions between acrylate monomers are common.[361,362]

Patch testing is essential to determine if an observed reaction is due to acrylate allergy or whether an irritant reaction or allergy to some other component is occurring. A variety of acrylates may be found in artificial nail products. It appears that 2-hydroxymethacrylate, ethyl cyanoacrylate, and possibly methyl methacrylate are sufficient for testing for nail acrylate allergy.[363]

Other sensitizers may be present in artificial nail preparations. Benzoyl peroxide is used as a catalyst and hydroquinone as an inhibitor of polymerization. Both of these are occasional allergens.

Two rare but very serious reactions to acrylates in artificial nails are the development of paresthesias and nail loss. Fisher[364] reported a case of acrylate allergy that resulted in nail loss. After 16 years there was no regrowth. Paresthesia has been caused by acrylate glues not only from nail preparations but also in dentists and orthopedists using acrylate tissue glues.[365] Paresthesias may occur with or without allergic sensitization.[366]

Photobonding of acrylate nail extenders using UV light is a newer method of application. Reactions to this process occur just as with non-UV required products.

Cyanoacrylate, or "Krazy Glue," initially thought to be nonsensitizing, has now been shown to be able to sensitize and cause paronychia, onychia, and ACD.[367,368]

Preformed plastic nails may be designed to cover the nail plate or extended tips. Their prolonged use causes mechanical damage to the nail, and those covering the entire nail plate may cause injury by occlusion. Sensitization to p-tertiary butylphenol formaldehyde resin in the nail adhesive and tricresyl ethyl phthalate of the artificial nail has been reported.[369]

ORAL HYGIENE PRODUCTS

These are fully described in Chapter 33.

DEODORANTS AND ANTIPERSPIRANTS

The action of bacteria on sterile apocrine secretions produces a characteristic odor. Work done by Labows and colleagues[370] incriminated lipophilic diphtheroids as the organisms that produce unique axillary odors. Simple deodorants reduce the number of bacteria in the axilla.

Although deodorants are considered cosmetics, antiperspirants are regulated as over-the-counter drugs as well as cosmetics. Many of these products have been reformulated over the years in response to health concerns. Hexachlorophene was banned because of its neurotoxicity and halogenated salicylanilides because of their photoallergic nature. Chlorofluorocarbon propellants were removed from aerosols because of their proposed role in depleting the stratosphere of ozone. The chlorofluorocarbons have been replaced by hydrocarbon propellants—isobutane, butane, and propane—which are flammable. The FDA OTC Antiperspirant Review Panel recommended the removal of zirconium-containing chemicals from aerosol antiperspirants because of the potential for formation of granulomata in the lung and skin.

Irritant reactions to aluminum salts in antiperspirants are common because of the environmental heat, moisture, and friction and the inflammation caused by shaving in the axilla. Occasional ACD to aluminum in antiperspirants has been reported. Allergic reactions are usually due to the other chemicals in the antiperspirants, most frequently the fragrance ingredients.

Feminine hygiene sprays are primarily fragrance products that cause irritant reactions when sprayed at too close a range. Allergy from fragrances, preservatives, and antimicrobials may occur.

SHAVING PREPARATIONS

Preshave toiletries may contain soaps or detergents in their lather. Reactions to aftershaves and colognes, however, account for most of the contact dermatitis that men experience from shaving cosmetics. The reactions, due to fragrance, may or may not be triggered by light.[371,372] Because these toiletries are applied directly to freshly shaved skin, penetration of the fragrance is enhanced.

In the past, musk ambrette has been reported as a notable photoallergen in aftershaves.[363,364] See Chapter 20 for instructions for patch testing fragrance ingredients. When performing a provocative use test with an aftershave, it is preferable to apply the product repeatedly on a quarter-sized area of the skin that is shaved rather than using the antecubital fossa.

MOISTURIZERS

This category of cosmetics accounted for 28% of all the cosmetic-related contact dermatitis reported by the NACDG.[61] Many of these cosmetic products are creams that contain fragrances, preservatives, emulsifiers, and lanolin, which are responsible for a significant number of adverse reactions.

From 1987 to 1990, the FDA received 12.44 complaints per million units sold of skin moisturizers.[373] Because most adverse reactions are not reported to either the FDA or the manufacturers, this number grossly under-represents the true frequency of such reactions.

Hannuksela and colleagues[374] patch tested over 1,200 eczematous patients with common emulsifiers, with results shown in Table 16.6.

ANTI-AGING PRODUCTS

Retinoids and alpha-hydroxy acids are added to skin care products for putative anti-aging effects. These agents very frequently cause irritant reactions, which usually subside over several weeks as the patient continues using them. Rare cases of allergy have been reported. Kojic acid has been reported to cause several cases of ACD. Testing was done with 0.5% in petrolatum.[375]

DEPILATORIES

Most depilatories contain mercaptans such as calcium thioglycolate 2.5% to 4.0% in conjunction with an alkali to bring the pH to between 10 and 12.5.[376] The keratin of the cortex is more vulnerable before it emerges from the follicle, and depilatories attack it there, leaving a soft rather than sharp end. For this reason, the use of depilatories in place of shaving can prevent pseudofolliculitis barbae in some cases. Irritant dermatitis from the keratolytic action on skin is common. Powdered facial depilatories, produced for beard removal, contain barium or strontium sulfide because these chemicals are quicker acting. Unfortunately, these chemicals cause more irritation and produce an unpleasant odor.[376] To use the less malodorous thioglycolate depilatories for coarser beard removal, hair accelerators such as thiourea, melamine, and sodium metasilicate are added. Depilatories cannot be patch tested directly, and these thioglycolates are seldom sensitizers.

EPILATING WAXES

Epilating waxes are usually warmed to soften, and they harden and enmesh the hair after application. When the wax is pulled off, the hair is removed by the root. Some modified waxes do not have to be warmed and can be applied with a backing material. These cosmetics may contain beeswax, rosin (colophony), fragrance, or rarely benzocaine as potential sensitizers. The problems usually seen with these epilating cosmetics are due to mechanical irritation.

COSMETIC INTOLERANCE SYNDROME

Dermatologists treating reactions to cosmetics will be confronted occasionally by patients who complain bitterly of facial burning and discomfort. This group seriously challenges our diagnostic skills as well as our ability to be empathetic when the severity of patients' symptoms does not match objective signs of disease (see Table 16.12). These patients may have not only subjective symptoms, but also objective inflammation. Fisher[377] coined the term "status cosmeticus" for the condition in which a patient is no longer able to tolerate the use of any cosmetic. Indeed, some of these patients seem to experience irritation (subjective and/or objective) from cosmetics, but during the evolution of this disorder, they become intolerant of many if not all topical agents. Some patients have occult allergic contact dermatitis, allergic photocontact dermatitis, or contact urticarial reactions, and the causal agents

Table 16-12 The Face Intolerant to Cosmetics and Skin Care Agents: Profile of Intolerant Skin Syndrome

Exogenous	
Subjective irritation	Common but difficult for patients to figure out
Objective irritation	Common but often difficult morphology to observe on face
Allergic contact dermatitis	
Photoallergic contact	Less common; discerned dermatitis retrospectively by testing
Contact urticaria	
Endogenous	
Seborrheic dermatitis	Common; a small percentage of patients have an atypical morphology
Rosacea diathesis	
Atopic dermatitis	May be only residual of childhood atopic dermatitis
Status eczematus[a]	Some patients may have no other definable endogenous or exogenous factors
(Status cosmeticus)	
Dysmorphobia[a]	Rare diagnosis made by exclusion

[a]These patients are the most difficult to treat successfully.

are documented by careful clinical review and patch testing.

Others who have a seborrheic/rosacea diathesis with or without inflammation seem to have caused this condition to flare by abandoning the use of soap and water and by overusing cleansing creams and emollients. Both of these conditions may be accompanied by facial erythema or scaling. Some patients require anti-inflammatory therapy, as do a few atopic patients who develop this state.

Prolonged use of the proposed elimination program seems to aid some women who, after 6 to 12 months or more, are able to gradually return to the use of other cosmetics (see Table 16.13). Additions to their regimens of skin care should be made one at a time—no more frequently than every 2 weeks. The final program should be simple and limited in the number and frequency of cosmetics used.

There is a group of patients who experience continuous facial burning without objective signs, whom Cotterill[378] describes as having dermatologic nondisease. Many of these patients have a disturbed body image, dysmorphobia, and complain of physical defects without objective evidence. Frequently these patients are depressed, and in Cotterill's group of 28 patients, several were suicidal. They demand time-consuming care. It is often difficult for these depressed patients to seek the skilled psychiatric care they require.

Table 16-13 Management of Patients Who Are Intolerant to Cosmetic Usage

1. Examine every cosmetic and skin care agent
2. Patch and photopatch test to rule out occult allergic and photoallergic contact dermatitis, or contact urticaria
3. Limit skin care to:
   a. Water washing without soap or detergent
   b. Lip cosmetics—ad libitum
   c. Eye cosmetics—ad libitum—if the eyelids are not symptomatic
   d. Face powder—ad libitum
   e. Glycerin and rose water as moisturizer only if needed
   f. 6 to 12 months of avoidance of other skin care agents and cosmetics
4. Watch for and test, if necessary, depression and other neuropsychiatric aspects

References

1. Warshaw E, Belsito D, DeLeo V, Fowler J, et al. NACDG patch-test results 2003–2004 period. Dermatitis 2007, in press.

2. Flyvholm M. Preservatives in registered chemical products. Contact Dermatitis 2005;53:27.

3. Ebner H, Kraft D. Formaldehyde induced anaphylaxis after dental treatment? Contact Dermatitis 1991;24:307.

4. Fisher AA. Formaldehyde: some recent experiences. Cutis 1976;17:665.

5. Ponten A. Formaldehyde in reusable protective gloves. Contact Dermatitis 2006;54:268.

6. Tegner E, Fregert S. Contamination of cosmetics with formaldehyde from tubes. Cont Derm Newsletter 1973;13:353.

7. Agner T, Flyvholm MA, Menne T. Formaldehyde allergy: a follow-up study. Amer J Contact Dermatitis 1999;10:12–17.

8. Lehmann S, Hoeck U, Breinholt J, et al. Characterization and chemistry of imidazolidinyl urea and diazolidinyl urea. Contact Dermatitis 2006;54:50.

9. Herbert C, Rietschel. Formaldehyde and formaldehyde relaeasers: How much avoidance of cross-reacting agents is required. Contact Dermatitis 2004;50:371.

10. Perrenoud D, Bircher A, Hunziker T, et al. Frequency of sensitization to 13 common preservatives in Switzerland; Swiss Contact Dermatitis Research Group. Contact Dermatitis 1994;30:276.

11. Fransway AF, Schmitz NA. The problem of preservation in the 1990s: 2. Formaldehyde and formaldehyde-releasing biocides: incidences of cross-reactivity and the significance of the positive response to formaldehyde. Am J Contact Dermat 1991;2:78.

12. Parker LU, Taylor JS. A 5-year study of contact allergy to quaternium-15. Am J Contact Dermat 1991;2:231.

13. Jordan WP. Human studies that determine the sensitizing potential of haptens: experimental allergic contact dermatitis. Dermatol Clin 1984;2:533.

14. Stephens TJ, Drake KD, Drotman RB. Experimental delayed contact sensitization to diazolidinyl urea (Germall II) in guinea pigs. Contact Dermatitis 1987;16:164.

15. Berke PA, Rosen WE. Germall, a new family of antimicrobial preservatives for cosmetics. Am Perfum Cosmet 1970;85:55.

16. Rosen WE, Berke PA. Modern concepts of cosmetic preservation. J Soc Cosmet Chem 1973;24:663.

17. Rosen WE, Berke PA, Matzin T, et al. Preservation of cosmetic lotions with imidazolidinyl urea plus parabens. J Soc Cosmet Chem 1977;28:83.

18. Ford GP, Beck MH. Reactions to quaternium 15, Bronopol, and Germall 115 in a standard series. Cont Derm 1986;14:271.

19. Ziegler V, Ziegler B, Kipping D. Dose-response sensitization experiments with imidazolidinyl urea. Contact Dermatitis 1988;19:236.

20. Andersen KE, Boman A, Hamann K, Wahlberg JE. Guinea pig maximization tests with formaldehyde releasers: results from two laboratories. Contact Dermatitis 1984;10:257.

21. Fisher AA. Dermatitis due to formaldehyde-releasing agents in cosmetics and medicaments. Cutis 1978;22:655.

22. Isakkson M, Gruvberger B, Goon A, et al. Can an imidazolidinyl urea preserved corticosteroid cream be safely used in individuals hypersensitive to formaldehyde? Contact Dermatitis 2006;54:29.

23. http://en.wikipedia.org/wiki/bronopol, accessed May 25, 2007

24. Peters MS, Connolly SM, Schroeter AL. Bronopol allergic contact dermatitis. Contact Dermatitis 1983;9:397.

25. Croshaw B. Preservatives for cosmetics and toiletries. J Soc Cosmet Chem 1977;28:3.

26. Preservative properties of bronopol. Cosmet Toiletr 1977;92:87.

27. Ardo Y. Bronopol as a preservative in milk samples. Milchwissenschaft 1979;34:14.

28. Storrs FJ, Bell DE. Allergic contact dermatitis to 2-bromo-2-nitropane-1,3-diol in a hydrophilic ointment. J Am Acad Dermatol 1983;8:157.

29. Rosen M. Glydant and MDMH as cosmetic preservatives. In Kabara JJ, ed. Cosmetic and drug preservation: principles and practice, Vol 1. New York: Dekker, 1984.

30. DeGroot AC, van Joost T, Bos JD, et al. Patch test reactivity to DMDM hydantoins. Relationship to formaldehyde allergy. Contact Dermatitis 1988;18:197.

31. DeGroot AC, Bos JD, Jagtman BA, et al. Contact allergy to preservatives-II. Contact Dermatitis 1986;15:218.

32. Hill A, Belsito D. Systemic contact dermatitis of the eyelids caused by aspartame. Contact Dermatitis 2003;49:259.

33. Rycroft R. Is Grotan BK a contact sensitizer? Br J Dermatol 1978;99:346.

34. Bandmann HJ, Breit R, Mutzeck E. Allergic contact dermatitis from formaldehyde in a brewer. Contact Dermatitis Newsletter 1974;15:452.

35. Fisher AA. Contact dermatitis. 3rd ed. Philadelphia: Lea & Febiger, 1986.

36. Gruvberger B, Bruze M, Almgren G. Occupational dermatoses in a plant producing binders for paints and glues. Contact Dermatitis 1998;38:71.

37. Sanchez I, Rodriguez F, Quinones D, et al. Occupational dermatitis due to formaldehyde in newspaper. Contact Dermatitis 1997;37:131.

38. Meding B, Ahman M, Karlberg AT. Skin symptoms and contact allergy in woodwork teachers. Contact Dermatitis 1996;34:185.

39. Cooke MA, Wilkinson JF. Formalin sensitivity in gum arabic. Contact Dermatitis Newsletter 1973;13:379.

40. Fabry H. Formaldehyde sensitivity. Contact Dermatitis Newsletter 1969;5:56.

41. Fregert S, Dahlquist I, Gruvberger B. A simple method for the detection of formaldehyde. Contact Dermatitis 1984;10:132.

42. Gryllaki-Berger M, Muqny C, Perrenoud D, et al. A comparative study of formaldehyde detection using chromotropic acid, acetylacetone and HPLC in cosmetics and household cleaning products. Contact Dermatitis 1992;27:149.

43. Flyvholm M-A, Menné T. Allergic contact dermatitis from formaldehyde (a case study focusing on sources of formaldehyde exposure). Contact Dermatitis 1992;27:27.

44. Cronin E. Formaldehyde is a significant allergen in women with hand eczema. Contact Dermatitis 1991;25:276.

45. Logan WS, Perry HO. Case dermatitis due to formaldehyde sensitivity. Arch Dermatol 1972;106:717.

46. Sneddon IB. Formalin dermatitis in a renal dialysis unit. Contact Dermatitis Newsletter 1968;3:47.

47. Abdel-Aziz AHM, Hodgson C. Formalin dermatitis in a renal dialysis unit. Contact Dermatitis Newsletter 1974;15:441.

48. Hendrick DJ, Lane DJ. Occupational formalin asthma. Br J Industr Med 1977;34:11.

49. Fisher AA, Kanof NB, Biondi EM. Free formaldehyde in textiles and paper. Arch Dermatol 1962;86:753.

50. Fregert S. Allergic contact dermatitis from formaldehyde in paper. Contact Dermatitis Newsletter 1974;15:459.

51. Simpson J. Formalin sensitivity—offset printing machines. Contact Dermatitis Newsletter 1969;6:133.

52. Black H. Contact dermatitis from formaldehyde in newsprint. Contact Dermatitis Newsletter 1971;10:162.

53. Thomsen HF. Hidden sources of formaldehyde. Contact Dermatitis Newsletter 1973;13:380.

54. Fisher AA. Dermatitis due to the presence of formaldehyde in certain sodium lauryl sulfate (SLS) solutions. Cutis 1981;27:360.

55. Trattner A, Johansen JD, Menné T. Formaldehyde concentration in diagnostic patch testing: comparison of 1% with 2%. Contact Dermatitis 1998;38:71.

56. Rietschel R, Bruze M, Zug K, et al. The relationship of vehicle and concentration of imidazolidinyl urea, with attention to formaldehyde status. Dermatitis 2006;17:48.

57. Niklasson B. The relationship of vehicle and concentration of imidazolidinyl urea, with attention to formaldehyde status-reply Dermatitis 2006;17:93.

58. Cashman R, Warshaw E. Parabens: A review. Dermatitis 2005;16:57.

59. Lorenzetti OJ, Weet TC. Topical parabens: benefits and risks. Dermatologica 1977;154:244.

60. Schnuch A, Geier J, Uter W, Frosch PJ. Patch testing with preservatives, antimicrobials and industrial biocides: results from a multicentre study. Br J Dermatol 1998;138:467.

61. Adams RM, Maibach HI. A five-year study of cosmetic reactions. J Am Acad Dermatol 1985;13:1062.

62. Warshaw E, Rietschel R, Sasseville D, et al. Common allergens found in eyelid dermatitis. Contact Dermatitis 2007, accepted for publication

63. Menné T, Hjorth N. Routine patch testing with paraben esters. Contact Dermatitis 1988;19:189.

64. Hansen J, Mollgaard B, Avnstorp C, Menne T. Paraben contact allergy: patch testing and in vitro absorption/metabolism. Am J Contact Dermat 1993;4:78.

65. Fisher AA. The paraben paradox. Cutis 1973;1:830.

66. Schorr WF. Paraben allergy—a cause of intractable dermatitis. JAMA 1968;204:859.

67. Evans S. Epidermal sensitivity to lanolin and parabens—occurrence in pharmaceutical and cosmetic products. Br J Dermatol 1970;82:625.

68. Brauer EW. Parabens in cosmetic creams. Contact Dermatitis 1979; 5:265.

69. Marzulli FN, Maibach HI. Status of topical parabens: skin hypersensitivity. Int J Dermato1974;13:3197.

70. Fisher AA, Pascher F, Kanof NB. Allergic contact dermatitis due to ingredients of vehicles. Arch Dermatol 1971;104:286.

71. Rudzki E, Kleniewska D. Cross reactions between parabens and the para group. Br J Dermatol 1970;83:543.

72. Turchin I, Moreau L, Warshaw E, et al. Cross-reactions among parabens, para-phenylenediamine, and benzocaine. Dermatitis 2006;17:192.

73. Praditsuwan P, Taylor JS, Rownigk HH Jr. Allergy to Unna boots in four patients. J Amer Acad Dermatol 1995;33:906.

74. Veien NK, Hattel T, Laurberg G. Oral challenge with parabens in paraben-sensitive patients. Contact Dermatitis 1996;34:433.

75. Henry JC, Tschen EH, Becker LE. Contact urticaria to parabens. Arch Dermatol 1979;115:1231.

76. Nagel JE, Fuscaldo JT, Fireman P. Paraben allergy. JAMA 1977;237:1594.

77. Fransway AF. The problem of preservation in the 1990s: 3. Agents with preservation function independent of formaldehyde release. Am J Contact Dermat 1991;2:145.

78. DeGroot AC. Methylisothiazolinone/methylchloroisothiazolinone (Kathon CG) allergy: an updated review. Am J Contact Dermat 1990;1:151.

79. Tosti A. Prevalence and sources of Kathon CG sensitization in Italy. Contact Dermatitis 1988;18:173.

80. Rietschel RL, JR Nethercott, EA Emmett, HI Maibach. Methylchloroisothiazolinone-methylisothiazolinone reactions in patients screened for vehicle and preservative hypersensitivity. J Am Acad Dermatol 1990;22:734.

81. Chan PK, Baldwin RC, Parsons RD, et al. Kathon biocide: manifestation of delayed contact dermatitis in guinea pigs is dependent on the concentration formulation and challenge. J Invest Dermatol 1983;81:409.

82. Bjorkner B, Bruzw M, Dahlquist I, et al. Contact allergy to the preservative Kathon® CG. Contact Dermatitis 1986;14:85.

83. Marks J, Moss JN, Parno JR, et al. Methylchloroisothiazolinone/methylisothiazolinone (Kathon CG) biocide—United States multicenter study of human skin sensitization. Am J Contact Dermat 1990;1:157.

84. Fewings J, Menne T. The patch test concentration for methylchloroisothiazolinone/methylisothiazolinone. Contact Dermatitis 1998;39:320.

85. Zachariae C, Lerbaek A, McNamee P, et al. An evaluation of dose/unit area and time as key factors influencing the elicitation capacity of MCI/MI in MCI/MI allergic patients. Contact Dermatitis 2006.55:160.

86. Kanerva L, Tarvainen K, Pinola A, et al. A single accidental exposure may result in a chemical burn, primary sensitization and allergic contact dermatitis. Contact Dermatitis 1994;31:229.

87. Primka EJ III, Taylor JS. Three cases of contact allergy after chemical burns from methylchloroisothiazolinone/methylisothiazolinone: one with concomitant allergy to

methyldibromoglutaronitrile/phenoxyethanol. Am J Contact Dermatitis 1997;8:43.

88. Gruvberger B, Bruze M. Can chemical burns and allergic contact dermatitis from higher concentrations of methyl-chloroisothiazolinone/methylisothiazolinone be prevented? Am J Contact Dermat 1998;9:11.

89. Madden SD, Thiboutot DM, Marks JG Jr. Occupationally induced allergic contact dermatitis to methylchloroisothiazolinone/ methylisothiazolinone among machinists. J Amer Acad Dermatol 1994;30:272.

90. Geier J, Schnuch A. No cross sensitization between MCI/MI, benzisothiazolinone, and octylisothiazolinone. Contact Dermatitis 1996;34:148.

91. Alexander BR. An assessment of the comparitive sensitization potential of some common isothiazolinones. Contact Dermatitis 2002;46:191.

92. Muhn C, Sasseville D. Occupational contact dermatitis from 1,2-benzisothiazolinon-3-one. Contact Dermatitis 2005; 52:129.

93. Aalto-Korte K, Alanko K, Henricks-Eckerman H, et al. Antimicrobial allergy from polyvinyl chloride gloves. Arch Dermatol 206;142:1326.

94. Aalto-Korte K, Alanko K, Henricks-Eckerman M, et al. Occupational allergic contact dermatitis from 2-N-octyl-4-isothiazolin-3-one. Contact Dermatitis 2007; 56:160.

95. Torres V, Soares AP. Contact allergy to dibromodicyanobutane in a cosmetic cream. Contact Dermatitis 1992;27:114.

96. DeGroot AC, Weyland JW. Contact allergy to methyldibromoglutaronitrile in the cosmetics preservative Euxyl K400. Am J Contact Dermat 1991;2:31.

97. European commission. Opinion of the scientific committee on cosmetic products and non-food products intended for consumers. Methyldibromo glutaronitrile. COLIPA No:P77;2002.

98. Jensen C, Johansen J, Menne T, et al. Methyldibromoglutaronitrile in rinse off products causes contact dermatitis. Br J Dermatol 2004;150:90.

99. DeGroot AC, DP Bruynzeel, PJ Coenraads, et al. Frequency of allergic reactions to methyldibromoglutaronitrile (1,2-dibromo-2,4-dicyanobutane) in the Netherlands. Contact Dermatitis 1991;25:270.

100. Tosti A, Vincenzi C, Trevisi P, Guerra L. Euxyl K400: incidence of sensitization, patch test concentration and vehicle. Contact Dermatitis 1995;33:193.

101. Marks JG, Belsito DV, DeLeo VA, et al. North American Contact Dermatitis Group patch test results for the detection of delayed-type hypersensitivity to topical allergens. J Amer Acad Dermatol 1998; 38:911.

102. Jackson JM, Fowler JF. Methyldibromoglutarolnitrile (Euxyl K400): a new and important sensitizer in the United States? J Amer Acad Dermatol 1998;38:934.

103. Gruvberger B, Andersen K, Brandao F, et al. ROAT with MDGN, a multicentre syudy. Contact Dermatitis 2005;52:19.

104. Zachariae C, Johansen J, Rastogi S, et al. Allergic contact dermatitis from methyldibromoglutaronitrile. Contact Dermatitis 2005;52:6.

105. Williams J, Frowen K, Nixon R. Allergic contact dermatitis from methyldibromoglutaronitrile. Contact Dermatitis 2007;56:164.

106. Lovell CR, White IR, Boyle J. Contact dermatitis from phenoxyethanol in aqueous cream BP. Contact Dermatitis 1984;11:187.

107. Birnie A, English J. 2-phenoxyethanol induced contact urticaria. Contact Dermatitis 2006;54:349.

108. Bergfeld WF, Belsito DV, Carlton WW, et al. A final report approved by the Expert Panel of the Cosmetic Ingredient Review: iodopropynyl butylcarbamate (IPBC). Washington, DC, 1996.

109. Bryld LE, Agner T, Rastogi SC, Menne T. Iodopropynyl butylcarbamate: a new contact allergen. Contact Dermatitis 1997;36:156.

110. Schnuch A, Geier J, Brasch J, Uter W. The preservative IPBC: frequency of allergic reactions and cosmetic considerations. Contact Dermatitis 2002; 46:153.

111. Brasch J, Schnuch A, Geier J, eta l: IPBC 0.2% is suggested for patch testing. Br J Dermatol 2004;151:608.

112. Basketter D, Marriott M, Gilmour N, et al. Strong irritants masquerading as skin allergens: the case of baenzalkonium chloride. Contact Dermatitis 2004;50:213.

113. Wahlberg JE. Two cases of hypersensitivity to quaternary ammonium compounds. Acta Dermatol Venereol (Stockh.) 1962;42:239.

114. Seiji M, Mizuno F. Unusual cornification in ichthyosis-like dermatitis. Acta Dermatol 1970;50:338.

115. Fisher AA, Stillman MA. Allergic contact sensitivity to benzalkonium chloride (BAK): cutaneous, ophthalmic and general medical implications. Arch Dermatol 1972;106:169.

116. Stanford D, Georgouras K. Allergic contact dermatitis from benzalkonium chloride in plaster of Paris. Contact Dermatitis 1996;35:371.

117. Ortiz-Frutos FJ, Argila D, Rivera R, et al. Allergic contact dermatitis from benzalkonium chloride used as a denaturant of ethanol. Contact Dermatitis 1996;35:302.

118. Shmunes E, Levy EJ. Quaternary ammonium compound contact dermatitis from a deodorant. Arch Dermatol 1972;105:91.

119. Hughes T, Stone N. Benzophenone 4: an emerging allergen in cosmetic and toiletries? Contact Dermatitis 2007;56:153.

120. Curry E, Warshaw E. Benzyl alcohol allergy. Dermatitis 2005;16:203–08.

121. Li M, Gow E. Benzyl alcohol allergy. Australas J Dermatol. 1995;36:219.

122. Marzulli FN, Maibach HI. Antimicrobials: experimental contact sensitization in man. J Soc Cosmet Chem 1973;24:399.

123. Fregert S. Allergic contact dermatitis from the pesticides captan and phaltan. Contact Dermatitis Newsletter 1967;2:28.

124. Epstein S. Photoallergic contact dermatitis. Cutis 1968;4:856.

125. Taran J, Delaney T. Contact allergy to chloroacetamide. Australas J Dermatol 1997;38:95.

126. Thune P. Two patients with chlorh95exidine allergy—anaphylactic reactions and eczema. Tidsskr Nor Laegeforen 1998;118:3290.

127. Goon A, White I, Rycroft R, et al. Allergic contact dermatitis from chlorhexidine Dermatitis 2004;15:45.

128. Barbaud A, Vigan M, Delrous J, et al. Conatct allergy to antiseptics. Ann Dermatol Venereol 2005; 132:962.

129. Ebo D, Bridts C, Stevens W. IgE mediated anaphylaxis from chlorhexidine. Contact Dermatitis 2006;55:301.

130. Aalto-Korte K, Makela E, Huttunen M, et al. Occupational contact allergy to glyoxal. Contact Dermatitis 2005; 52:276.

131. Dooms-Goossens A, Vandaele M, Bedert R, Marien K. Hexamidine isethionate: a sensitizer in topical pharmaceutical products and cosmetics. Contact Dermatitis 1989;21:270.

132. Lee S, Zhai H, Maibach H. Allergic contact dermatitis from iodine preparations: a conundrum. Contact Dermatitis 2005;52:184.

133. Goncalo M, Goncalo S, Moreno A. Immediate and delayed sensitivity to chlorocresol. Contact Dermatitis 1987;17:46.

134. Adams RM. P-chloro-m-xylenol in cutting fluids: two cases of allergic contact dermatitis in machinists. Contact Dermatitis 1981;7:341.

135. Storrs FJ. Para-chloro-meta-xylenol allergic contact dermatitis in seven individuals. Contact Dermatitis 1975;1:211.

136. Libow LF, Ruskowski AM, DeLeo VA. Allergic contact dermatitis from paracloro-meta-xylenol in hurosep soap. Contact Dermatitis 1989;20:67.

137. Fowler JF. Para-chloro-meta-xylenol allergy and hand eczema. Am J Contact Dermat 1993;4:53.

138. Burry JN, Kirk J, Reid J, Turner T. Chlorocresol sensitivity. Contact Dermatitis 1975;1:41.

139. Mackenzie-Wood A, Freeman S. Severe allergy to sorbolene cream. Australas J Dermatol 1997;38:33.

140. Rajpar S, Foulds I, Abdullah A, et al. Severe adverse cutaneous reaction to insulin due to cresol sensitivity. Contact Dermatitis 2006;55:119.

141. Schnuch A, Geier J, Uter W, et al. The biocide polyhexamethylene biguanide remains an uncommon contact allergen. Contact Dermatitis 2007; 56:235.

142. Suneja T, Belsito D. Thimerosal in the detection of clinically relevant allergic reactions. J Am Acad Dermatol 2001;45:23.

143. Slodownik D, Ingber A. Thimerosal - is it really irrelevant? Contact Dermatitis 2005;53:324.

144. Moller H. Merthiolate allergy: a nationwide iatrogenic sensitization. Acta Derm Venereol 1977;57:509.

145. Forstrom L, M Hannuksela, M Kousa, E Lehmuskallio. Merthiolate hypersensitivity and vaccination. Contact Dermatitis 1980;6:241.

146. Osawa J, Kitamura K, Ikezawa Z, Nakajima H. A probable role for vaccines containing thimerosal in thimerosal hypersensitivity. Contact Dermatitis 1991;24:178.

147. Tosti A, Guerra L, Bardazzi F. Hyposensitizing therapy with standard antigenic extracts: an important source of thimerosal sensitization. Contact Dermatitis 1989;20:173.

148. Cox NH, Forsythe A. Thimerosal allergy and vaccination reactions. Contact Dermatitis 1988;18:229.

149. Audicana M, Munoz D, del Pozo M, et al. Allergic contact dermatitis from mercury antiseptics and derivatives. Am J Contact Dermat 2002;13:3.

150. Maibach HI. Acute laryngeal obstruction presumed secondary to thimerosal (Merthiolate) delayed hypersensitivity. Contact Dermatitis 1975;1:221.

151. Takino C. Thimerosal contact dermatitis (Japanese). Jap J Clin Dermatol 1971;25:1175.

152. Cirne DeCastro JL, Vale E, Martins M. Mechanism of photosensitive reactions induced by piroxicam. J Am Acad Dermatol 1989;20:706.

153. Cirne DeCastro JL, Freitas JP, Menezes Brandao F, Themiido R.. Sensitivity to thimerosal and photosensitivity to piroxicam. Contact Dermatitis 1991;24:187.

154. Fregert S, Hjorth H. In: Rook AJ, Wilkinson DS, Ebling JFG, eds. Textbook of dermatology. Oxford: 1972.

155. Van Ketel WG, Melzer-van Riemsduk FA. Conjunctivitis due to soft lens solutions. Contact Dermatitis 1980;6:321.

156. Sertoli A, E Di Fonzo, P Spallanzani, E Panconesi. Allergic contact dermatitis from thimerosal in a soft contact lens wearer. Contact Dermatitis 1980;6:292.

157. Rietschel RL, Wilson LA. Ocular inflammation in patients using soft contact lenses. Arch Dermatol 1982;118:147.

158. Podmore P, Storrs FJ. Contact lens intolerance: allergic conjunctivitis? Contact Dermatitis 1989;20:98.

159. Campbell L, Zirwas M. Triclosan. Dermatitis 2006;17:204.

160. Hjorth N, Trolle-Lassen C. Skin reactions to preservatives in creams with special regard to paraben esters and sorbic acid. Am Perfumer 1962;77:43.

161. Brown R. Another case of sorbic acid sensitivity. Contact Dermatitis 1979;3:268.

162. Gorannson K, Liden S. Contact allergy to sorbic acid and Unguentum Merck. Contact Dermatitis 1981;7:277.

163. Ramsing DW, Menné T. Contact sensitivity to sorbic acid. Contact Dermatitis 1993;28:124.

164. Giordano-Labadie F, Pech-Ormieres C, Bazex J. Systemic contact dermatitis from sorbic acid. Contact Dermatitis 1996;34:61.

165. Clemmensen OJ, Shiødt M. Patch test reaction of the buccal mucosa to sorbic acid. Contact Dermatitis 1982;8:341.

166. Fryklof LE. A note on the irritant properties of sorbic acid in ointments and creams. Stockholm: Apotekens Kontrol-laboratorium, 1958.

167. Rietschel RL. Contact urticaria from synthetic cassia oil and sorbic acid limited to the face. Contact Dermatitis 1978;4:347.

168. Lahti A. Skin reactions to some antimicrobial agents. Contact Dermatitis 1978;4:302.

169. Muston HL, Messenger AG, Byrne JPH. Contact dermatitis from zinc pyrithione, an antidandruff agent. Contact Dermatitis 1979;5:276.

170. Pereira F, Fernandes C, Dias M, Lacerda MH. Allergic contact dermatitis from zinc pyrithione. Contact Dermatitis 1995;33:131.

171. Nielsen NH, Menné T. Allergic contact dermatitis caused by zinc pyrithione associated with pustular psoriasis. Amer J Contact Dermatitis 1997;8:170.

172. Fisher AA. Reactions to antioxidants in cosmetics and foods. Cutis 1976;17:21.

173. Meneghini CL, Rantuccio F, Lomuto M. Additives, vehicles and active drugs of topical medicaments as causes of delayed-type allergic dermatitis. Dermatologica 1971;143:137.

174. White IR, Lovell CR, Cronin E. Antioxidants in cosmetics. Contact Dermatitis 1984;11:265.

175. Flyvholm M, Menné T. Sensitizing risk of butylated hydroxytoluene based on exposure and effect data. Contact Dermatitis 1990;23:341.

176. Roed-Petersen J, Hjorth N. Contact dermatitis from antioxidants: hidden sensitizers in topical medications and foods. Br J Dermatol 1976;94:233.

177. Bojs G, Nicklasson B, Svensson A. Allergic contact dermatitis to propyl gallate. Contact Dermatitis 1987;17:294.

178. Raccagni AA, Frattagli M, Baldari U, Righini MG. Lauryl gallate hand dermatitis in a cheese counter assistant. Contact Dermatitis 1997;37:182.

179. Hernandez N, Assier -Bonnet H, Terki N, Revuz J. Allergic contact dermatitis from propyl gallate in desonide cream (Locapred). Contact Dermatitis 1997;36:111.

180. Heine A. Contact dermatitis from propyl gallate. Contact Dermatitis 1988;18:313.

181. Hausen BM, Beyer W. The sensitizing capacity of the antioxidants propyl, octyl and dodecyl gallate and some related gallic acid esters. Contact Dermatitis 1992;26:253.

182. Marston S. Propyl gallate on liposomes. Contact Dermatitis 1992;27:74.

183. Storrs FJ, Rosenthal LE, Adams RM, et al. Prevalence and relevance of allergic reactions in patients patch tested in North America—1984 to 1985. J Am Acad Dermatol 1989;20:1038.

184. DeGroot AC, Berretty PJM, van Ginkel CJW, et al. Allergic contact dermatitis from tocopheryl acetate in cosmetic creams. Contact Dermatitis 1991;25:302.

185. Fowler JF. Allergic contact dermatitis to polyvinylpyrrolidone/hexadecene copolymer. Amer J Contact Dermatitis 1995;6:243.

186. DeGroot AC, Brunynzeel DP, Bos JD, et al. The allergens in cosmetics. Arch Dermatol 1988;124:1525.

187. Quartier S, Garmyn M, Becart S, et al. Allergic contact dermatitis to copolymers in cosmetics. Contact Dermatitis 2006;55:257–67.

188. Raymond JZ, Cross PR. EDTA: preservative dermatitis. Arch Dermatol 1969;100:436.

189. Bhushan M, Beck MH. Allergic contact dermatitis from disodium ethylenediamie tetra-acetic acid (EDTA) in a local anaesthetic. Contact Dermatitis 1998;38:183.

190. DeGroot AC. Contact allergy to EDTA in a topical corticosteroid preparation. Contact Dermatitis 1986;15:250.

191. Eriksen KE. Allergy to ethylenediamine. Arch Dermatol 1975;111:791.

192. Fisher AA. Does ethylenediamine hydrochloride cross-react with ethylenediamine tetraacetate? Contact Dermatitis 1975;1:267.

193. Balato N, Cusano F, Lembo G, Ayala F. Ethylenediamine dermatitis. Contact Dermatitis 1986;15:263.

194. CTFA Cosmetic ingredient dictionary. 3rd ed. Washington, DC: Cosmetic Toiletry and Fragrance Association, 1982.

195. Nilzen A, Wikstrom K. The influence of sodium lauryl sulfate on the sensitization of guinea pigs to chrome and nickel. Acta Derm Venereol 1955;35:292.

196. Dahl MV, Trancik RJ. Sodium lauryl sulfate irritant patch tests: degree of inflammation at various times. Contact Dermatitis 1977;3:263.

197. Bergstresser PR, Eagelstein WH. Irritation by hydrophilic ointment under occlusion. Arch Dermatol 1973;108:218.

198. Krook G. Contact dermatitis due to Ficortril (hydrocortisone 1 percent ointment, Pfizer). Contact Dermatitis Newsletter 1974;15:460.

199. Fulton JE, Bradley S, Aqundex A, et al. Non-comedogenic cosmetics. Cutis 1976;17:344.

200. Kligman AM. The SLS provocative patch test in allergic contact sensitization. J Invest Dermatol 1966;36:573.

201. Sams WM, Smith G. Contact dermatitis due to hydrocortisone ointment: report of a case of sensitivity to emulsifying agents in a hydrophilic ointment base. JAMA 1957;164:1212.

202. Prater E, Goring HD, Schubert H. Sodium lauryl sulphate—a contact allergen. Contact Dermatitis 1978;4:242.

203. Foussereau J, Petitjean J, Lants JP. Sodium lauryl sulphate. Contact Dermatitis Newsletter 1974;15:460.

204. Expert Panel of the American College of Toxicology. Final report on the safety assessment of cocamidopropyl betaine. J Am Coll Toxicol 1991;10:33.

205. VanHoute N, Dooms-Goossens A. Shampoo dermatitis due to cocobetaine and sodium lauryl ether sulphate. Contact Dermatitis 1983;9:169.

206. Korting HC, Parsch EM, Enders F, Przybilla B. Allergic contact dermatitis to cocamidopropyl betaine in shampoo. J Am Acad Dermatol 1992;27:1013.

207. Fowler J, Zug K, Taylor J, et al. Allergy to cocamidoprepyl betaine and amidoamine in North America. Dermatitis 2004;15:5.

208. Fowler JF. Cocamidopropyl betaine: the significance of positive patch tests in 12 patients. Cutis 1993;52:281–284.

209. Fowler JF, Fowler LM, Hunter JE. Allergy to cocamidopropyl betaine may be due to amidoamine: a patch test and product use test study. Contact Dermatitis 1997;37:276.

210. Brey N, Fowler JF. Relevance of positive patch-test reactions to Cocamidopropyl betaine and amidoamine Dermatitis 2004;15:7.

211. Angelini G, Rigano L, Foti C, et al. 3-dimethylaminopropylamine: a key substance in contact allergy to cocamidopropyl betaine? Contact Dermatitis 1995;32:96.

212. McFadden J, Ross J, White I, Basketter D. Clinical allergy to CAPB: reactivity to cocamidopropylamine and lack of reactivity to 3-DMAPA. Contact Dermatitis 2001; 45:72.

213. Foti C, Bonamonte D, Mascolo G, et al. The role of 3-DMAPA and amidoamine in contact allergy to cocamidpropyl betaine. Contact Dermatitis 2003; 48:194.

214. DeGroot AC, De Wit FS, Bos JD, Weyland JE. Contact allergy to cocamide DEA and lauramide DEA in shampoos. Contact Dermatitis 1987;16:117.

215. Fowler J. Allergy to Cocamide DEA. Am J Contact Dermat 1998;9:40.

216. Christersson S, Wrangsjo K. Contact allergy to undecylenamide diethanolamide in a liquid soap. Contact Dermatitis 1992;27:191.

217. DeGroot AC, Liem DH. Contact allergy to oleamidopropyl dimethylamine. Contact Dermatitis 1984;11:298.

218. Bruynzeel DP, Niklasson B. The patch test dilution of oleamidopropyl dimethylamine. Contact Dermatitis 1992;27:190.

219. DeGroot AC, Jagtman BA, van der Meeren HL, et al. Cross-reaction pattern of the cationic emulsifier oleamidopropyl dimethylamine. Contact Dermatitis 1988;19:284.

220. Moreau L, Sasseville D. Allergic contact dermatitis from cocamidopropyl betaine, cocamidoamine, DMAPA, and oleamidopropyl dimethylamine. Dermatitis 2004;15:146.

221. Taylor JS, Jordan WP, Maibach HI. Allergic contact dermatitis from stearamidoethyl diethylamine phosphate: a cosmetic emulsifier. Contact Dermatitis 1984;10:74.

222. Goosens A, Bruze M, Gruvberger B, et al. Contact allergy to sodium cocoamphoacetate present in an eye makeup remover. Contact Dermatitis 2006;55:302.

223. Foti C, Bonamonte D, Mascolo G, et al. Aminoethylethanolamine: a new allergen in cosmetics? Contact Dermatitis 2001;45:129.

224. Fisher AA. Allergic contact dermatitis to nonoxynol-9 in a condom. Cutis 1994;53:110–111.

225. Dooms-Goossens A, Deveylder H, D-Alam H, et al. Sensitivity to nonoxynols as a cause of intolerance to antiseptic preparations. J Am Acad Dermatol 1989;21:723.

226. Morren M. Contact allergy to dihydroxyacetone. Contact Dermatitis 1991;25:326.

227. Vujevich J, Zirwas M. Delayed hypersensitivity to isopropyl alcohol. Contact Dermatitis 2007;56:287.

228. Fulton JE Jr, Bradley S, Agundez A, et al. Non-comedogenic cosmetics. Cutis 1976;17:344.

229. Fisher AA. Propylene glycol dermatitis. Cutis 1978;21:166.

230. Warshaw TG, Herrmann F. Studies of skin reaction of propylene glycol. J Invest Dermatol 1952;19:423.

231. Lessmann H, Schnuch A, Geier J, et al. Skin sensitizing and irritant properties of propylene glycol. Contact Dermatitis 2005;53:247.

232. Trancik RG, Maibach HI. Propylene glycol: irritation or sensitization? Contact Dermatitis 1982;8:185.

233. Braun W. Contact allergies against polyethylene glycols. Z Hautkr Geschlechtskr 1969;44:385.

234. Claverie F, Giordano-Labadia F, Bazex J. Eczema de contact au propylene glycol. Ann Dermatol-Venereol 1997;124:315.

235. Fowler JF. Contact allergy to propylene glycol in topical corticosteroids. Am J Contact Dermat 1993;4:37.

236. Fisher AA. Dermatologic hazards of electrocardiography. Cutis 1977;20:686.

237. Peleg O, Bar-Oz B, Arad I. Coma in a premature infant associated with the transdermal absorption of propylene glycol. Acta Paedatr 1998;87:1195.

238. Hibbot HW, Monks J. Butylene glycol. J Soc Cosmet Chem 1961;12:2.

239. Sugiura M, Hayakawa R. Contact dermatitis due to 1,3-butylene glycol. Contact Dermatitis 1997;37:90.

240. Tamagawa-Mineoka R, Katoh N, Kishimoto S: Allergic contact dermatitis due to 1.3 butylene glycol and glycerol. Contact Dermatitis 2007;56:295.

241. Kinnunen T, Koskela M. Antibacterial and antifungal properties of propylene glycol, hexylene glycol, and 1,3-butylene glycol in vitro. Acta Dermatol 1991;71:148.

242. Kinnunen T, Hannuksela M. Skin reactions to hexylene glycol. Contact Dermatitis 1989;21:154.

243. Fisher AA. Immediate and delayed allergic contact reactions to polyethylene glycol. Contact Dermatitis 1978;4:135.

244. Maibach HI. Polyethylene glycol: allergic contact dermatitis potential. Contact Dermatitis 1975;1:247.

245. Marzulli F, Maibach H. Use of graded concentration in studying skin sensitizers: experimental contact sensitization in man. Food Cosmetic Toxicol 1974;12:219.

246. Braun W. Contact allergies to polyethylene glycols. Z Haut-Geschlechtskrankheiten 1969;44:385.

247. Bajaj AK. Contact sensitivity of polyethylene glycols. Contact Dermatitis 1990;22:291.

248. Hannuksela M, Forstrom L. Contact hypersensitivity to glycerol. Contact Dermatitis 1976;2:291.1992;27:1013.

249. Dooms-Goossens A, DeGreef H. Sensitization to yellow petrolatum used as a vehicle for patch testing. Contact Dermatitis 1980;6:146.

250. Maibach H. Chronic dermatitis and hyperpigmentation from petrolatum. Contact Dermatitis 1978;4:62.

251. Grin R, Maibach H. Long lasting contact urticaria from petrolatum mimicking dermatitis. Contact Dermatitis 1999;40:110.

252. Schnuch A, Leesman H, Geier J, et al. White petrolatum is virtually non-sensitizing. Contact Dermatitis 2006;54:338.

253. DeBerker D. Contact sensitivity to the stearyl alcohol in Efudex cream. Contact Dermatitis 1992;26:138.

254. Martinez-Falero AA, Martinez-Falero A, Calderon Gutierrez MJ, et al. Allergic contact dermatitis from fluocortin butyl. Contact Dermatitis 1990;22:241.

255. von-der-Werth JM, English JS, Dalziel KL. Loss of patch test positivity to cetylstearyl alcohol. Contact Dermatitis 1998;38:109–110.

256. DeGroot AC, Bruynzeel DP, van Joost T. Weyland JW. Cosmetic allergy from myristyl alcohol. Contact Dermatitis 1988;19:76.

257. Andersen K, Broesby-Olsen S. Allergic contact dermatitis from oleyl alcohol in Elidel Cream. Contact Dermatitis 2006;55:354.

258. Narita T, Oiso N, Ota T, et al. Allergic contact dermatitis to diethyl sebacate in a hand cream. Contact Dermatitis 2006;55:117.

259. Uter W, Schnuch A, Geier J, et al. Isopropyl myristate recommended for aimed rather than routine testing. Contact Dermatitis 2005;50:242.

260. Singh M, Winhoven S, Beck H. Contact sensitivity to octylodecanol and trometamol in an anti-itch cream. Contact Dermatitis 2007;56:288.

261. Tan BB, Noble AL, Roberts ME, et al. Allergic contact dermatitis from oleyl alcohol in lipstick cross-reacting with ricinoleic acid in castor oil and lanolin. Contact Dermatitis 1997;37:41–42,

262. Geier J, Lessmann H, Becker D, et al. Patch testing with components of a water based metal working fluid. Contact Dermatitis 2006;55:322–29.

263. Orton D, Shaw S. Sorbitan sesquioleate as an allergen. Contact Dermatitis 2001;44:190–1.

264. DeGroot AC, van der Meeren HL, Weyland JW. Cosmetic allergy from stearic acid and glyceryl stearate. Contact Dermatitis 1988;19:77.

265. Hayakawa R. Lipstick dermatitis due to C18 aliphatic compounds. Contact Dermatitis 1987;16:215.

266. Castelain P. Generalized diffuse eczema due to sensitization to triethanolamine. Bull Soc Franc Derm Syph 1967;74:562.

267. Suurmond D. Patch test reactions to Phenergan cream: promethazine and triethanolamine. Dermatologica 1966;133:503.

268. Schwartz L. Sensitivity testing in cosmetics: science and technology. New York: Interscience Publishers, 1967.

269. Blum A, Lischka G. Allergic contact dermatitis from mono-, di- and triethanolamine. Contact Dermatitis 1997;36:166.

270. Hamilton TK, Zug KA. Triethanolamine allergy inadvertently discovered from a fluorescent marking pen. Amer J Contact Dermatology 1996;7:164.

271. Brandle I. Allergy to castor oil. Contact Dermatitis 1983;9:424.

272. Fisher AA. Allergic cheilitis due to castor oil in lipsticks. Cutis 1991;47:389.

273. Rothenborg HW. Occupational dermatitis in a beekeeper due to poplar resins in beeswax. Arch Dermatol 1967;95:381.

274. Wanscher B. Contact dermatitis from propolis. Br J Dermatol 1976;94:451.

275. Petersen HO. Allergy to propolis (bee glue) in patients with eczema. Ugeskr Laeg 1977;139:2331.

276. Hausen BM, Evers P, Stüwe H-T, et al. Propolis allergy (IV). Contact Dermatitis 1992;26:34.

277. Machackova J. The incidence of allergy to propolis in 605 consecutive patients patch tested in Prague. Contact Dermatitis 1988;18:210.

278. Camasara G. Occupational dermatitis from beeswax. Contact Dermatitis 1975;1:124.

279. Oleffe JD, Blondeel A, Boschmans L. Patch testing with lanolin. Contact Dermatitis 1978;4:233.

280. Fregert S, Dahlquist I, Trulsson L. An attempt to isolate and identify allergens in lanolin. Contact Dermatitis 1984;10:16–9.

281. Cronin E. Lanolin dermatitis. Br J Dermatol 1966;78:617.

282. Vollum DI. Sensitivity to hydrogenated lanolin. Arch Dermatol 1969;100:774.

283. Edman B, Moller H. Testing a purified lanolin preparation by a randomized procedure. Contact Dermatitis 1989;20:287.

284. Peter C, Schropl F, Franzwa H. Experimental investigation regarding allergenic effects of wool wax alcohols. Hautarzt 1969;20:450.

285. Giorgini S, Melli MC, Sertoli A. Comments on the allergenic activity of lanolin. Contact Dermatitis 1983;9:425.

286. Wakelin S, Smith H, White I, et al. A retrospective analysis of contact allergy to lanolin. Br J Dermatol 2001;145:28.

287. Bojs G, Bruze M, Svensson A. Contact allergy to the lanolin derivative amerchol CAB. Am J Contact Dermat 1992;3:83.

288. Matthies L, Dockx P. Discrepancy in patch test results with wool wax alcohols and Amerchol L-101. Contact Dermatitis 1997;36:150.

289. Breit R, Bandmann H-J. Dermatitis from lanolin. Br J Dermatol 1973;88:414.

290. Bandmann H-J, Reichenberger M. Beobachtungen and Untersuchungen zur Frage der durch Eucerin Bedingten seltenen Allergies. Hautarzt 1957;8:11.

291. Cronin E, Bandmann HJ, Calnan CD, et al. Contact dermatitis in the atopic. Acta Derm Venereol (Stockh.) 1970;50:183.

292. Bergfeld W, Belsito D, Marks J, et al. Safety of ingredients used in cosmetics. J Am Acad Dermatol 2005;52:125.

293. Loretz L, Api A, Barraj L, et al. Exposure data for personal care products. Food Chem Toxicol 2006;12:2008.

294. de Groot A, Bruynzeel DP, Bos JD, et al. The allergens in cosmetics. Arch Dermatol 1988; 124:1525.

295. Kohl L, Blondeel A, Song M. Allergic contact dermatitis from cosmetics. Dermatology 2002;204:334.

296. Uter W, Balzer C, Geier J, et al. Patch testing with patients own cosmetics and toiletries. Contact Dermatitis 2005;53:226.

297. Duarte I, Campos-Lage A. Frequency of dermatoses associated with cosmetics. Contact Dermatitis 2007; 56:211.

298. Frosch PJ, Kligman AM. A method for appraising the stinging capacity of topically applied substances. J Soc Cosmet Chem 1977;28:197.

299. Bronaugh RL, Maibach HI. Primary irritant, allergic contact, phototoxic, and photoallergic reactions to cosmetics and tests to identify problem products. In: Frost P, Horwitz SN, eds. Principles of cosmetics for the dermatologist. St Louis: Mosby, 1982.

300. Krogh G von, Maibach HI. The contact urticaria syndrome—1982. Semin Dermatol 1982;1:59.

301. Sugai T, Takahashi Y, Takagi T. Pigmented cosmetic dermatitis and coal tar dyes. Contact Dermatitis 1977;3:249.

302. Kozuka T, Tashiro M, Sano S, et al. Pigmented contact dermatitis from azo dyes: 1. Cross-sensitivity in humans. Contact Dermatitis 1980;6:330.

303. Nakayama H, Harada R, Toda M. Pigmented cosmetic dermatitis. Int J Dermatol 1976;15:673.

304. Mathias CG. Pigmented cosmetic dermatitis from contact allergy to a toilet soap containing chromium. Contact Dermatitis 1982;8:29.

305. Findlay GH, Morrison JGL, Simson IW. Exogenous ochronosis and pigmented colloid millium from hydroquinone bleaching creams. Br J Dermatol 1975;93:612.

306. Fisher AA. Hydroquinone uses and abnormal reactions. Cutis 1983;31:240.

307. Mathias CG, Maibach HI, Conant MA. Perioral leukoderma simulating vitiligo from use of a toothpaste containing cinnamic aldehyde. Arch Dermatol 1980;116:1172.

308. Samman PD. Nail disorders caused by external influences. J Soc Cosmet Chem 1977;28:351.

309. Kligman AM, Mills OH. Acne cosmetica. Arch Dermatol 1972; 106:843.

310. Fulton JE, Pay SR, Fulton JE, III. Comedogenicity of current therapeutic products, cosmetics and ingredients in the rabbit ear. J Am Acad Dermatol 1984;10:96.

311. Frank SB. Is the rabbit ear model, in its present state, prophetic of acnegenicity? J Am Acad Dermatol 1982;6:373.

312. Hjorth N. Contact dermatitis in children. Acta Derm Venereol (Stockh.) 1981;95:36.

313. Marshall S. The effect of bubble bath on the urinary tract. J Urol 1965;93:112.

314. Roberts HJ. Bubble bath cystitis and cosmetic vulvitis neglected hazards. J Fla Med Assoc 1973;60:31

315. Guin JD. Eyelid dermatitis: a report of 215 patients. Contact Dermatitis 2004;50:87.

316. Nethercott J, Nield G, Holness DL. A review of 79 cases of eyelid dermatitis. J Am Acad Dermatol 1989;21:223.

317. Gallo R, Maro I, Pavesi A. Allergic contact dermatitis from shellac in mascara. Contact Dermatitis 2005;53:238.

318. Epstein E. Misleading mascara patch tests. Arch Dermatol 1965;91:615.

319. Sainia E, Jolanki R, Hakalde, Kanerva L. Metals and arsenic in eye shadows. Contact Dermatitis 2000;42:5.

320. Fowler J. Gold. Am J Contact Dermat 2001;12:1.

321. Saxena M, Warshaw E, Ahmed D. Eyelid allergic contact dermatitis to black iron oxide. Am J Contact Dermat 2001;12:38.

322. Wilson LA, Ahearn DG. Pseudomonas-induced ulcers associated with contaminated eye mascaras. Am J Ophthalmol 1977;84:112.

323. Warshawshki L, Mitchell JC, Storrs FJ. Allergic contact dermatitis from glyceryl monothioglycolate in hair dressers. Contact Dermatitis 1981;7:351.

324. Rapaport M. Irritant contact dermatitis to glyceryl mono-thioglycolate. J Am Acad Dermatol 1983;9:739.

325. Schorr WF. Multiple injuries from permanents: cosmetic symposium. Am Acad Dermatol, Dec. 3, 1983.

326. Isaksson M, van der Walle H. Occupational contact allergy to cysteamine hydrochloride in permanent-wave solutions. Contact Dermatitis 2007;56:295.

327. Harris RT. Hair relaxing. Cosmet Toiletr 1979;94:51.

328. Henkin H. Technical history of shampoos. Cosmet Toiletr 1981;96:39.

329. Haute N Van, Dooms-Goossens A. A shampoo dermatitis due to cocobetaine and sodium lauryl ether sulphate. Contact Dermatitis 1983;9:169.

330. Nurse DS. Sensitivity to coconut diethanolamine. Contact Dermatitis 1980;6:502.

331. Corbett J. An historical review of the use of dye precursors in the formulation of commercial oxidation hair dyes. Dyes and Pigments 1999;41:127.

332. DeLeo V. Para-phenylenediamine. Dermatitis 2006;17:53.

333. Broeckx W. Cosmetic intolerance. Contact Dermatitis 1987;16:189.

334. Foussereau J, Reuter G, Petitjean J. Is hair dyed with PPD-like dyes allergenic? Contact Dermatitis 1980;6:143.

335. Warin AP. Contact dermatitis to partner's hair dye. Clin Exp Dermatol 1976;1:283.

336. Engasser PG, Maibach HI. Cosmetics and dermatology: hair dye toxicology. In: Rook AJ, Maibach HI, eds. Recent advances in dermatology, vol. 6. New York: Churchill Livingstone, 1985.

337. Valks R, Conde-Salazar L, Malfeito J. Contact dermatitis in hairdressers. Dermatitis 2005;16:28–31.

338. Brancaccio R, Brown L, Chang Y, et al. Identification and quantification of PPDA in a temporary black henna tat-too. Am J Contact Dermat 2002;13:15.

339. Pasricha, JS, Gupta R, Panjwani S. Contact dermatitis to henna (Lawsonia). Contact Dermatitis 1980;6:288.

340. Garcia-Ortiz J, Terron M, Bellido J. Contact allergy to henna. Int Arch Allergy Immunol 1997;114:298.

341. Cronin E. Immediate-type hypersensitivity to henna. Contact Dermatitis 1979;5:198.

342. Edwards EK, Jr, Edwards EK. Allergic contact dermatitis to lead acetate in a hair dye. Cutis 1982;30:629.

343. White IR, Catchpole HE, Rycroft RJG. Rashes among persulfate workers. Contact Dermatitis 1982;8:168.

344. Fisher AA, Dooms-Goossens A. Persulfate hair bleach reactions. Arch Dermatol 1976;112:1407.

345. Rastogi S, Sosted H, Johansen J, etal. Unconsumed pre-cursors and couplers after formation of oxidative hair dyes. Contact Dermatitis 2006;55:95.

346. Calnan CD. Quinazoline yellow dermatitis D&C Yellow 11 in eye cream. Contact Dermatitis 1981;7:271.

347. Weaver JE. Disparate skin allergenicity of 2 quinoline dyes. Contact Dermatitis 1983;9:526.

348. Andersen KE, Nielsen R. Lipstick dermatitis related to castor oil. Contact Dermatitis 1984;11:253.

349. Cronin E. Lipstick dermatitis due to propyl gallate. Contact Dermatitis 1980;6:213.

350. Joost T van, Liem DH, Stolz E. Allergic contact dermatitis to monotertiary-butylhydroquinone in lip gloss. Contact Dermatitis 1984;10:189.

351. Calnan CD, Cronin E, Rycroft RJG. Allergy to phenyl salicylate. Contact Dermatitis 1981;7:208.

352. Calnan CD. Amyldimethyl aminobenzoic acid causing lipstick dermatitis. Contact Dermatitis 1980;6:233.

353. Angelini E, Marinaro CeCarrozzo AM, et al. Allergic contact dermatitis of the lip margins from para-tertiary-butylphenol in a lip liner. Contact Dermatitis 1993;28:146.

354. Mitchell JC. Non-inflammatory onycholysis from formalde-hyde-containing nail hardener. Contact Dermatitis 1981;7:173.

355. Paltzik RL, Enscoe I. Onycholysis secondary to toluene sulfonamide formal dehyde resin used in a nail hardener mimicking onychomycosis. Cutis 1980;25:647.

356. Liden C, Berg M, Farm G, Wransjo K. Nail varnish allergy with far-reaching consequences. Br J Dermatol 1993;128:57.

357. Wilkinson JB, Moore RJ. Harry's cosmeticology. New York: Chemical Publishing, 1982.

358. Fisher AA, Franks A, Glick H. Allergic sensitization to acrylic nails. J Allergy 1957;28:84.

359. Food and Drug Administration seizure actions. FDA Consumer 1974;8:37.

360. Fuller M. Analysis of paint-on artificial nails. J Soc Cosmet Chem 1982;33:51.

361. Marks JG, Bishop ME, Willis, WP. Allergic contact dermatitis to sculptured nails. Arch Dermatol 1979;115:100.

362. Fisher AA. Cross reactions between methyl methacrylate monomer and acrylic monomers presently used in acrylic nail preparations. Contact Dermatitis 1980;6:345.

363. Constant L, Hecke E, Naeyaert J, Goosens A. Screening for contact allergy to artificial nails. Contact Dermatitis 2005;52:73.

364. Fisher A. Permanent loss of fingernails due to allergic reaction to an acrylic nail preparation: a sixteen year follow-up study. Cutis 1989;43:404.

365. Fisher A. Paresthesia of the fingers accompanying dermatitis due to methyl methacrylate bone cement. Contact Dermatitis 1979;5:56.

366. Baran R, Schibli H. Permanent paresthesia to sculptured nails. Derm Clin 1990;8:139.

367. Pigatto P, Giachetti A, Altomare GF. Unusual sensitization to cyanoacrylate ester. Contact Dermatitis 1986;14:193.

368. Belsito D. Contact dermatitis to ethyl cyanoacrylate containing glue. Contact Dermatitis 1987;17:234.

369. Burrows D, Rycroft, RJG. Contact dermatitis from PTBP resin and tricresyl ethyl phthalate in a plastic nail adhesive. Contact Dermatitis 1981;7:336.

370. Labows JN, McGinley KJ, Kligman AM. Axillary odor: current status. In: Frost P, Horwitz SN, eds. Principles of cosmetics for the dermatologist. St Louis: Mosby, 1982.

371. deGroot AC, Liem DH. Facial psoriasis caused by contact allergy to linalool and hydroxycitronellal in an after-shave. Contact Dermatitis 1983;9:230.

372. Raugi GJ, Stoors FJ, Larsen WG. Photoallergic contact dermatitis to men's perfumes. Contact Dermatitis 1979;5:251.

373. Jackson E. Moisturizers: what's in them? How do they work? Am J Contact Dermat 1992;3:162.

374. Hannuksela M, Kousa M, Pirila V. Contact sensitivity to emulsifiers. Contact Dermatitis 1976;2:201.

375. Mata T, Sanchez J. Allergic contact dermatitis to kojic acid. Dermatitis 2005;16:89.

376. Rieger MM. Depilatories: 1979 update. Cosmet Toiletr 1979;94:71.

377. Fisher AA. Current contact news (cosmetic actions and reactions: therapeutic, irritant, and allergic). Cutis 1980;26:22.

378. Cotterill JG. Dermatological nondisease: a common and potentially fatal disturbance of body image. Br J Dermatol 1981;104:611.

HAND DERMATITIS DUE TO CONTACTANTS: SPECIAL CONSIDERATIONS

EXECUTIVE SUMMARY

Occupational exposures may result in irritant contact dermatitis that 5 years after diagnosis may still be active to a moderate degree in half of the cases and severe in another third. Preventative measures are frequently disappointing.

Patch tests are necessary to distinguish irritant from allergic contact dermatitis of the hands. Population studies have found that hand dermatitis is experienced by approximately 10% of women and 5% of men over periods of time ranging from 1 to 3 years.

Allergens found to play a prominent role in contact dermatitis of the hands include nickel, potassium dichromate, ethylenediamine, rubber, paraphenylenediamine, and preservatives. Oral ingestion of nickel and chromium has been linked to pompholyx.

Handling foods can cause hand dermatitis by either delayed hypersensitivity or contact urticaria. Immediate sensitivity can present with a mixed morphologic picture of urticaria and vesiculation. Food additives that have caused hand problems include butylated hydroxyanisole, butylated hydroxytoluene, sodium bisulfite, lauryl gallate, propyl gallate, potassium and ammonium persulfate, and benzoyl peroxide. Additional additives that can cause dermatitis include waxes, gums, color additives, spices, and flavoring agents.

Studies of the role of soaps and detergents in hand dermatitis have produced some counterintuitive findings, suggesting that such exposures help rather than hurt hand dermatitis. However, "wet work" has been repeatedly linked to hand dermatitis, and decreasing an individual's exposure to wet work is beneficial.

Barrier creams in general are of limited use in preventing hand dermatitis, but frequent moisturizing does seem beneficial. Gloves may help but must be chosen to match the nature of the exposure. Latex-based gloves are not protective against acrylic bone cement, nickel, and hair dyes. Alcohol-based hand disinfectants may be less irritating than frequent handwashing.

There are several varieties of allergic contact dermatitis (ACD) of the hands. Table 17.1 lists these varieties, together with the type of skin testing that may help determine the etiology of the different kinds of hand dermatitis owing to various contactants.

Irritant Contact Dermatitis

Irritant contact dermatitis (ICD) due to a nonspecific reaction can occur in all individuals, provided the irritants are in contact with the skin for a sufficient length of time and are in sufficiently high concentrations. This dermatitis is usually characterized by dryness, some fissuring, and thickening of the skin. It differs from allergic dermatitis in that vesicles are usually rare. Defatting, degreasing agents, such as detergents and solvents, are the main causes of "gradual" irritant dermatitis. Strong acids and alkalis may produce an acute "severe" irritant dermatitis. In general, irritants damage the skin by direct, cytotoxic action. The diagnosis of irritant dermatitis is one of exclusion, because "proof" cannot be obtained by "skin tests."

Table 17-1 Hand Eczema–Skin Test Correlations	
Type	Test
Irritant	No specific test
Allergic	
Contact (delayed)	Patch test
Contact (systemic)	Patch test
Contact (immediate)	Immediate patch, prick, scratch test
Endogenous	No specific tests

One form of ICD was formerly called "housewife's eczema" or "dishpan hands." Medical and dental workers, food preparation and service workers, janitors, housekeepers, and anyone who frequently washes his or her hands or is exposed to cleaners may develop this type of eczema. Irritant contact dermatitis of the hands due to occupational exposures is not easily resolved. A questionnaire 5 years after such a diagnosis was answered by 124 patients. In 50%, a moderate amount of hand dermatitis persisted, and 32% still reported severe hand dermatitis. More than half the patients reported changing jobs, but the preventive measures failed to improve most cases. Glove use was found to be low and most exposures to skin irritants were by unprotected skin.[1]

Patch tests, however, may reveal a superimposed allergic dermatitis. The trapping of soaps and detergents under a ring often initiates an irritant hand dermatitis. It has been estimated that 65% of atopic individuals who do wet work in hospitals develop dermatitis of the hands.[2]

PATCH TEST REACTIVITY IN PATIENTS WITH HAND ECZEMA

Bjornberg[3] analyzed the skin reactions to 11 primary irritants in patients who had eczema and in normal persons. It has been assumed generally that an irritant reaction observed after a 24-hour patch test subsides rapidly. This assumption, which has been used to differentiate allergic from irritant patch test reactions, has often been incorrect. Severe irritant patch test reactions in particular often increase over the first 72 hours.[4]

The average concentration of an irritant causing a faint erythema can be taken as a measure of the skin irritancy of a compound. Only 0.2% of croton oil in petrolatum was necessary to evoke this erythema, whereas 0.9% of sodium lauryl sulfate and the surprisingly high figure of 17.5% of potassium soap were necessary. No marked difference was present between patients and controls. Many authors have described the irritant reaction as an "all or none" response, but phenol was the only substance that conformed to this pattern. With all other substances, the intensity of reaction increased in proportion to concentration and exposure time. All age groups react similarly to sodium lauryl sulfate.

The increased skin susceptibility to irritants in remote body regions was an important finding in patients who had hand eczema. This is the first proof of the validity of the commonly used term "status eczematicus" and must be taken into account in establishing the concentration of substances used for patch testing and in assessing the reaction to substances that are at the same time allergens and irritants. This increased reactivity may cause nonspecific patch test reactions, may add to the risk of accidental patch test sensitization, and may cause unexpected side effects from therapeutic agents.

Patients who had healed (in contrast to active) hand eczema showed a normal reactivity to most irritants, but both groups gave stronger reactions to soap, sodium lauryl sulfate, and benzalkonium chloride than did the controls.

Agner[5] used various objective determinations of patch test reactions to sodium lauryl sulfate, including measurements on an evaporimeter, an ultrasound A-scan, a laser-Doppler flowmeter, and a chromameter. He verified the fact that patch test results in hand eczema patients differ from those of controls only when the hand eczema is active.

Allergic Contact Dermatitis of Hands

It is often impossible to distinguish between irritant and allergic contact dermatitis of the hands without performing patch tests. Patch testing is the only scientific "proof" that a contactant is a dermatitis-producing allergen in a particular case. It has been found valuable to patch test patients who have a chronic hand dermatitis with the "standard" patch test series. Jordan[6] reported 220 cases of hand eczema that were evaluated for uncomplicated allergic contact dermatitis. In 12% of the 220 patients, the diagnosis was established with the aid of a standard screening tray. Another 5% of the cases were diagnosed as a result of testing with additional allergens. The hand eczema in these patients (17%) changed dramatically as a result of allergic contact investigation. Wilkinson and colleagues[7,8] agree that patch testing is of great value in the management of hand dermatitis.

Epidemiology of Hand Eczema

Several studies of large groups of individuals have been conducted to analyze the prevalence of hand eczema.

Lantinga and colleagues[9] studied over 1,900 people in the city of Vlagtweddle in the Netherlands twice over a 3-year period. At the last point in the study, 10% of women and 4.5% of men, age 30 to 60, had hand eczema of some type. Irritant contact dermatitis alone accounted for about half the cases and ACD alone for 15%, with the remainder being a combination of these or other diagnoses such as atopic or nummular dermatitis. Of 141 patients patch tested, 20% tested positive for nickel (26% women, 7% men). Other allergens were not particularly remarkable.

At about the same time, Kavli and Førde[10] studied hand eczema in northern Norway. This was done by questionnaire, not by patient examination. Five percent of men and 13% of women claimed they had had hand eczema over the preceding 12 months. Of the total sample of 14,667, 49 men (0.7%) and 105 women (1.4%) had taken sick leave for hand eczema during the preceding 3 years.

In a more recent work, Meding and Swanbeck[11] studied hand eczema in Goteborg, Sweden. Twenty thousand persons age 20 to 65 were surveyed by mail, resulting in examination of 1,238 persons with confirmed hand eczema. The 1-year period prevalence was 11.8%. Patch testing of 1,071 patients with 26 standard allergens showed that 15% were allergic to nickel. Other frequent allergens were cobalt (6.7%), fragrance mix (5.8%), balsam of Peru (4.9%), and rosin (3.2%).

Two-thirds of the 1,238 had sought medical help, and 21% had taken sick leave because of eczema. Those with ACD had more serious consequences than those with other forms of eczema.[12] A 15-year follow-up study of patients with hand eczema found that 66% of patients continued to experience hand eczema and 44% reported that they had had symptoms in the previous year. However, 74% felt that their hand eczema had improved. Out of 868 patients who responded to the survey, 20 had changed jobs due to hand eczema and 15 reported improvement with the job change.[13]

Rystedt[14–16] has extensively studied hand eczema in patients with atopy. She found that those with childhood atopic dermatitis of either moderate or severe degree (44% and 55%, respectively) developed hand eczema even without irritant work exposure, whereas 68% to 81% who worked as housecleaners, nurses, food handlers, or hairdressers developed hand eczema. Those atopic individuals who changed jobs because of hand eczema were less likely to see improvement than those who were not atopic, and were also less likely to have ACD than nonatopics (22% vs 45%). Although women, those with a family history of atopic dermatitis, and those with respiratory atopy were somewhat more likely to have hand eczema, these factors are of much less significance than a personal history of atopic dermatitis.

Hand dermatitis among nurses is related to wet work, and prevention that focused on a reduction of wet-work exposure was investigated with questionnaires and direct observation. Observation found that the actual amount of wet-work exposure was approximately double what was reported on questionnaires. Exposure to irritant was found to relate more to the frequency of wet hand exposure than to the duration of wet hands. In order to improve outcomes it was recommended that nurses should be encouraged to wear gloves, not just to prevent infection but also to protect against hand dermatitis.[17]

Three major factors were found to pose significant risks for the development of hand eczema in metalworkers. Atopic diathesis, mechanical forces, and limited time for the skin to recover from an insult were key. Disruption of the epidermal barrier with limited time for the barrier to reconstitute itself were the newer findings.[18]

Role of Certain Allergens in the Standard Patch Test Series in Hand Dermatitis

Allergic reactions to nickel, dichromate, ethylenediamine hydrochloride, rubber compounds, paraphenylenediamine, and topical preservatives play a significant role in the production and maintenance of hand dermatitis.

NICKEL

As a rule, dermatitis to nickel-plated objects is not confined to the hands, because other sites also are usually exposed to nickel-containing jewelry, clips, and zippers. External hand dermatitis occurs principally as a reaction to handles, knobs, pencils, scissors, surgical instruments, knitting needles, thimbles, and coins. Traces of nickel in detergents are probably not significant in the US, although in some countries the nickel content may be high enough to cause dermatitis.

Clemensen and colleagues[19] studied the nickel content of water specimens from consecutive stages during the cleaning process in a Danish hospital. Statistically significant increases of the nickel concentrations were found from step to step of the cleaning, eventually exceeding the theoretical sensitizing safety limit. The dimethylglyoxime test indicates the presence of nickel.

Among hospital cleaners, rubber gloves are used widely. An investigation has shown that nickel penetrates rubber but not vinyl.[20]

Pompholyx of Hands Due to "Ingestion" of Nickel (Positive Patch Test)

Allergic contact eczema and hand pompholyx may flare following ingestion of nickel in patients sensitized to this metal, according to several investigators.[21–24] It has been reported that the oral administration of nickel in a double-blind test provoked an aggravation of hand eczema in 9 of 12 patients, and in 7 of the patients this was accompanied by secondary eruptions, including outbreaks of earlier, healed eczema.

Nickel excretion in urine in 4 female patients sensitive to nickel with an intermittent dyshidrotic eruption was measured with flameless atomic absorption. Excretion of nickel increased in association with outbreaks of vesicles. The results would support the idea that the chronic hand condition was maintained by ingestion of nickel in food. Jensen and colleagues[25] conducted a modified meta-analysis of oral exposure to nickel and concluded that oral exposures in the range of 0.22 to 0.53 mg of dietary nickel will provoke a reaction in 1% of nickel-sensitive individuals. Exposure to 0.55–1.33 mg of dietary nickel will make 10% of nickel-sensitive individuals respond.

Christensen,[26] after studying female patients who had nickel allergy and hand eczema and who were reinvestigated 6 years after the primary investigation, found that 30% of the patients had healed. Patients who had the pompholyx-type eczema had the worst prognosis. Because the control of pompholyx in nickel-sensitive individuals with diet is difficult, a chelating agent such as disulfiram (Antabuse) has been employed.

Thus, Christensen and Kristensen[27] reported 11 patients who had nickel allergy and hand eczema of the pompholyx type who were treated with disulfiram (Antabuse) at 200 mg daily for 8 weeks. Two patients healed, and 8 patients improved considerably. Mild relapses were observed in all patients within 2 to 16 weeks after discontinuation of treatment.

Fowler[28] showed that of nine patients with nickel allergy and hand eczema, eight improved while taking disulfiram 250 mg daily, and none improved and five worsened on placebo. The study was a double-blind, placebo-controlled-crossover evaluation. Some patients were maintained on periodic doses of disulfiram after the study period with continued good results.

Patients receiving disulfiram (Antabuse) must avoid drinking alcohol, and their liver enzymes should be monitored during such therapy. Before using disulfiram, a preliminary patch test with the "thiram mix" should be done to rule out sensitivity to this compound.[29]

Ragweed and Pompholyx

A study that compared contact allergy from ragweed (*Ambrosia artemisiifolia*) of American and Swedish origin found that patients in Sweden reacted to both sources. Pompholyx was the clinical presentation of this allergy in 16 of 17 cases, and most patients' hands flared when patch tested with ragweed. A sesquiterpene lactone mix patch test identified this group of patients.[30]

POTASSIUM DICHROMATE

Aside from many industrial exposures, particularly cement, individuals sensitized to potassium dichromate may acquire dermatitis of the hands from leather gloves, shoes, and other leather objects. In addition, matches, bleaches, antirust compounds, varnishes, yellow paints, spackling compounds, and certain glues that contain dichromates may cause dermatitis of the hands in sensitized individuals (see Chapter 32).

Role of Dichromate Sensitivity in "Housewife's Eczema"

From Israel, Spain, and Yugoslavia have come reports that the dichromates play an important role in the production of "housewife's eczema."[31–34] In the US, chromates have not been implicated in "housewife's eczema." Spot tests for chromates may be positive in American soaps and detergents, but the quantity is apparently not sufficient to produce dermatitis. Chromates are part of the earth's crust, and traces of chromates are present in practically all raw materials. Phosphate-containing soaps and detergents have a higher concentration of chromates than do those that are free of this chemical.

In Fisher's series of 50 women who had severe "housewife's eczema," only one showed a positive reaction to potassium dichromate.

Pompholyx from Chromate Ingestion

Cronin[35] reported that the experimental ingestion of 10 drops of a 0.001% solution of $K_2CR_2O_7$ equaling about 0.5 mg $K_2CR_2O_7$ daily for several days can produce vesicular eruption of the palms and flares of dermatitis in chromate-sensitive individuals. Schleif[36] also found that the ingestion of chromates can produce pompholyx-like eruptions and flares of chromate dermatitis in chromate-sensitive individuals. These authors speculated that chromium may be released by cooking acid or salty food in stainless-steel cooking utensils.

Kaaber and Veien[37] also reported that the dermatitis of 11 of 31 patients who had chronic chromate dermatitis was aggravated following the ingestion of an amount of chromate comparable to that found in a normal daily food intake, and that those patients who had pompholyx were the ones most affected by ingestion of chromates.

As Burrows[38] pointed out, however, most chromium is changed in the acid medium of the stomach to trivalent chrome, which is not absorbed. Also, in view of the small quantity of chromium that exists in the diet, it would be difficult to reduce intake much further apart from the avoidance of cloves, thyme, and pepper. Dermatitis of the hands in professional gamblers and card players may be caused by exposure to chromium salts used for dyeing green felt or baize, which covers gambling tables.[39]

PROGNOSIS OF HAND DERMATITIS DUE TO CHROMATES

Several investigators state that the prognosis is poor for workers who have hand dermatitis owing to exposure to chromates. The term "chrome cripples" has been applied to such workers.[40,41]

Fregert,[42] however, was more optimistic. He stated that cement chromium hand eczema is often chronic but not as severe as nickel hand eczema, although the change of work does not guarantee healing of the eczema. Fregert advised that chrome-sensitive men should work as carefully as possible and should avoid other chromium sources (e.g., matches). Many people are able to continue their jobs for years with proper topical treatment.

PREVENTION AND MANAGEMENT OF CEMENT CHROMATE HAND DERMATITIS

Because one cannot depend on "hardening" or hyposensitization to occur, early diagnosis of chromate dermatitis and avoidance of chromates is imperative if prolonged disability is to be avoided. Once acquired, chromate dermatitis has a great tendency to become chronic.

The following prophylactic measures have been advocated: (a) Replace the chromates in circulatory water cooling systems with tannins and benzoates. (b) Reduce the sensitizing water-soluble chromates in Portland cement by the addition of 0.2% ferrous sulfate. (c) Replace zinc chromate and lead chromate in primer paints and in rust-preventing agents used on iron sheets with molybdates. (d) Use only disposable towels; hand towels used by workers in the chromate industry, even after washing, contain enough chromate to give a positive "spot test" for chromium.

ETHYLENEDIAMINE HYDROCHLORIDE

A positive patch test to ethylenediamine hydrochloride in a patient who had hand dermatitis probably means that the patient was sensitized to this compound through the use of Mycolog cream (Squibb) or generics. Such patients may need to avoid hydroxyzine and aminophylline. Mycolog II cream is free of ethylenediamine (see Chapter 16). In addition, it must be remembered that

certain epoxy amine hardeners crossreact with ethylenediamine hydrochloride. Such patients must also be patch tested with epoxy amine hardeners, particularly if they have handled epoxy resins.

Rudzki and Krajewska[43] reported that a consecutive series of 1,544 patients and 137 patients in occupational contact with epoxy resins were tested with ethylenediamine or triethylenetetramine; some were tested with diethylenetriamine. Guinea pigs sensitized to triethylenetetramine were tested with ethylenediamine and diethylenetriamine. The results showed that crossreactions may occur between triethylenetetramine and ethylenediamine, although most patients were sensitized to only one of the compounds.

RUBBER

Mercaptobenzothiazole and thiram (tetramethylthiuram disulfide) are the most common causes of allergic rubber dermatitis in the general population. Rubber finger cots, rubber gloves, rubber bands, rubber hoses, tubing, adhesive tape, and adhesive bandages cause allergic rubber dermatitis of the hands, which may also complicate other types of hand dermatoses.

Patients who have hand dermatitis often become sensitized to rubber gloves used to "protect" their hands. Dermatitis owing to rubber gloves should be suspected when a hand dermatitis stops abruptly at the wrists. Patch tests may be performed with a half-inch square cut from the rubber gloves, and those tests may be supplemented by testing with mercaptobenzothiazole and thiram.

Rubber may cause allergic contact dermatitis even when completely "cured." It appears that not all antioxidants and accelerators take part in the final crystallization of rubber and that some are released imperceptibly over many years. Release is enhanced by sweating and heat; this provides the opportunity for sensitization and may even cause occupational depigmentation.

More recently, rubber gloves have been found to cause urticaria, eczema, and even anaphylaxis due to allergy to natural latex proteins. Health care workers are at risk for these reactions. Testing for rubber accelerators is negative. Patch, prick, or scratch tests with latex rubber glove extracts are positive within 10 to 30 minutes (see Chapter 29).

PARAPHENYLENEDIAMINE

Dermatitis of the hands owing to allergic sensitization to paraphenylenediamine (PPDA) occurs mainly in hairdressers and furriers. Hair dyeing, however, may be done occasionally at home by nonprofessionals who may develop allergic contact dermatitis of the hands from the procedure.

If the patient has a positive patch test reaction to PPDA and apparently has not handled the dye, patch tests should be performed with other "para-amino" compounds such as benzocaine, procaine, and para-aminobenzoic acid, with which PPDA may crossreact.

In addition, PPDA-sensitive individuals who handle certified azo dyes incorporated into foods, drugs, and cosmetics should be tested with such dyes, as crossreactions may rarely occur. Allergic dermatitis of the hands from ballpoint pens containing azo dyes may occur in patients sensitized to PPDA.

TOPICAL PRESERVATIVES

Hand eczema, whether it begins as ICD, ACD, or endogenous dermatitis, may become worse because of allergy to preservatives or other agents in topical medicaments and skin care products. The formaldehyde releasers, such as quaternium-15, imidazolidinyl urea, and diazolidinyl urea, are particularly common as causes of ACD. Other preservatives, fragrances, and vehicles may also be a problem in selected individuals. Whenever a hand eczema seems to spread or worsen after using a topical product, all of the ingredients in that product must be held suspect as allergens until proven otherwise.

FRAGRANCES

It might seem obvious that when a fragrance-sensitive patient places the hands in a solution of their allergen, a dermatitis will most certainly develop. However, the relationship between allergen and real-life exposure turned out to be more complex when carefully studied. Heydorn and colleagues[44] exposed fragrance-sensitive patients with a history of hand eczema to solutions of their allergens for 10 minutes daily for 2 weeks. The concentrations of the fragrance allergens were 10 ppm and 250 ppm, which mimic the concentrations of diluted and undiluted liquid soap products that contain fragrance. A control immersion of the opposite hand to a solution without the allergen was also done. There was no difference in the 15 patients between exposure and non-exposure to allergens. Three of the patients developed changes on the allergens finger, 3 on the control finger, and 3 on both.[44]

Dermatitis of Hands Due to Contact with Foods

Homemakers, chefs, bakers, and others who handle food may acquire contact dermatitis of the hands.[45–47] Such contact dermatitis is of five varieties: (a) an irritant dermatitis, (b) a "delayed" allergic eczematous contact dermatitis, (c) an immediate urticarial type of dermatitis, (d) an immediate vesicular eruption, and (e) a phototoxic dermatitis.

A study of 52 bakers with hand eczema found both immediate and delayed allergens unique to bakers. Of 45 bakers who had reactions to contact allergens, there were four reactions to benzoyl peroxide, two to 2-tert-butyl-4-methoxyphenol (BHA), and one each to alpha-amylase, d-limonene, cinnamic aldehyde, isoeugenol, and rye flour. Contact urticaria evaluation by prick testing found 19 (42%) of 45 bakers to react to wheat, rye, barley, oats, soy flours, alpha-amylase, or storage mite (*L. destructor*).[48]

IRRITANT CONTACT DERMATITIS

The juices of many foods can produce a nonspecific irritant dermatitis of the hands that may be similar to dermatitis from any wet work. This type of irritant hand dermatitis is often accompanied by paronychia, particularly of the monilial variety. Irritant dermatitis owing to food is characterized usually by edema, erythema, and fissuring rather than the vesiculation and severe pruritus that occur in allergic contact dermatitis. At times, only patch tests will distinguish between the irritant and allergic dermatitis of the hands owing to food. Two recognized irritant hand dermatitides are due to corn and pineapple. Corn dermatitis (corn itch or corn poisoning) is an irritant occupational eruption of the hands similar to the contact dermatitis seen in other vegetable processing and in wet work in food plants. Excoriations and secondary infections often complicate the dermatitis.[49] Pineapple dermatitis is due to pineapple juice, which contains bromelain, a proteolytic enzyme that can readily produce an irritant dermatitis.[50]

ALLERGIC ECZEMATOUS CONTACT DERMATITIS FROM FOODS

In sensitized individuals, contact with certain foods may produce a classic "delayed" allergic contact dermatitis with a positive patch test reaction. This type of reaction is seen most often with the oleoresins of fruits and vegetables or with spices such as cinnamon. Orange and lemon peel contain oil of limonene and other sensitizing terpenes that may crossreact with turpentine. Limonene is found not only in lemons and oranges, but also in dill, caraway oil, and celery seed oil. In addition, the peel of lime may produce not only allergic contact dermatitis but also photodermatitis.

Patch tests for citrus peel contact sensitivity may be done with either 1% oil of limonene in alcohol or orange, lemon, and lime peel, "as is." Should positive reactions be obtained, the test should be performed on three normal controls, because occasionally the oil of these citrus peels may be irritants. In addition, the peel

Table 17-2 Vegetables: "Delayed" Eczematous Dermatitis

Positive Patch Test

Artichoke	Cucumber
Asparagus	Endive
Carrot	Garlic
Celery	Horseradish
Chicory	Leek
Chives	Lettuce
Corn	Onion

of limes should be tested by both closed and open methods with exposure to sunlight, because certain limes are photosensitizers.

The mango can produce allergic contact dermatitis owing to the oleoresin present in the mango tree sap or the skin of the fruit, which crossreacts with poison ivy oleoresin.

Allergic eczematous contact dermatitis from vegetables (see Table 17.2) may be due to the essential oils of edible vegetables including carrots, parsnips, parsley, and celery. Pinene, terpineol, and eucalyptol are probably the actual sensitizers. In addition, onions and garlic may cause a contact dermatitis that may show crossreactions with tulips and hyacinths.

If prepared oleoresins of vegetables are not available, patch tests may be performed with the fresh vegetables and the results compared with three controls.

Celery, parsnips, and parsley may produce a phototoxic reaction in the presence of moisture and sunlight. Patch tests with celery, parsnip, and parsley should be performed with the vegetable moistened with water and exposed to sunlight or artificial ultraviolet radiation to "prove" phytophoto dermatitis.

Mustard oil (allyl isothiocyanate) is an irritant and a sensitizing chemical found in horseradish, cabbage, broccoli, and Brussels sprouts.[51]

Allergic dermatitis owing to spices (see Table 17.3) occurs in the United States, principally from five spices: capsicum, cinnamon, cloves, nutmeg, and vanilla.[52] Blends of mace and nutmeg are used extensively for flavoring foods. Bakers in particular may acquire allergic dermatitis of the hands from handling these spices. Oil of cloves is rich in eugenol, which may be a sensitizer, and is used widely as an ingredient in perfumes, soaps, toothpastes, and mouthwashes.

Table 17-3 Spices: "Delayed" Eczematous Dermatitis

Positive Patch Test

Capsicum	Laurel
Cayenne pepper	Mace
Cinnamon	Nutmeg
Cloves	Vanilla

Dermatitis due to vanilla occurs in individuals employed in the cultivation, trade, or industrial use of vanilla. Vanillism, an allergic contact dermatitis acquired by workers who handle the vanilla plant, produces marked edema and erythema. Rhinitis, asthma, and vertigo may accompany the eruption.

Spencer and Fowler[53] reported a case of hand eczema in a Girl Scout cookie maker due to vanilla.

Nethercott and Holness[47] studied 20 bakers and food service workers in Toronto. Half were felt to have ICD and half ACD. Rubber allergens and fragrance/flavorings such as cinnamic aldehyde and balsam of Peru were most common. Contact urticaria due to shellfish was present in one patient.

Sinha and colleagues[54] studied 53 patients who had a fissured contact dermatitis on the fingertips and who showed positive patch tests to several vegetables, the most common being garlic, onion, tomato, and carrot, in that order of frequency. Of several preparations (made from garlic, onion, tomato, and carrot), the juices used as such gave the maximum number of positive patch test reactions.

IMMEDIATE CONTACT URTICARIA OF HANDS FROM FOODS

Foods that can cause contact urticaria with resulting hand dermatitis are listed in Table 17.4[55–60] (see also Chapter 31). Sensitivity to potatoes may be so severe that a wheal may form merely by rubbing the unabraded skin with a raw potato. More often, a strongly positive scratch test reaction

Table 17-4 Foods Producing Immediate Urticaria

Seafood
- Codfish
- Lobster
- Prawns
- Shrimp

Vegetables
- Bean
- Carrot
- Lettuce
- Onion
- Parsley
- Parsnip
- Potato
- Rice
- Tomato

Meat
- Beef
- Calves' liver
- Lamb
- Pork
- Turkey meat
- Turkey skin

to the raw potato consisting of a large wheal and flare is obtained. No reaction occurs in controls. Scratch tests with cooked potatoes usually produce negative results. Potato sensitivity can cause "housewife's" hand eczema and can be classified as an "occupational" allergy.

Sensitized patients also may show positive scratch test results to uncooked fish, shellfish, shrimp, and cheese. Allergic hand dermatitis of the "immediate" variety can be produced by handling these foods, probably because of some proteinaceous substance, particularly in those persons with damaged skin due to an irritant or an allergic contact dermatitis from other causes.

It should be stressed that in these cases of "immediate" food contact dermatitis, the patch tests are negative and therefore scratch tests may be necessary to prove the cause of this variety of contact food dermatitis.

Maibach[59] stressed that the handling of certain foods can produce a burning and stinging sensation in the chronically eczematous skin but not in otherwise normal skin and that tests on intact skin may be negative. Scratch tests with certain foods produced positive results only on intact skin. Intradermal tests with commercial antigens were negative.

When performing scratch tests with whole foods, at least three control subjects also should be tested. A positive reaction in the patient that is not duplicated in the controls makes it likely that the reaction is allergic. At present, it appears that patients who have allergic contact hand dermatitis owing to food handling can eat such foods without experiencing a flare of the dermatitis. It is most likely that either cooking the foods or the action of digestive juices renders the foods hypoallergenic for these patients.

At present, it is not clear whether the food antigens that allergists use in testing for allergic rhinitis, asthma, and gastrointestinal allergy are also the antigens responsible for the immediate allergic contact dermatitis of the hand from handling certain foods.[59] Hannuksela and Lahti[60] found that scratch tests with apple, carrot, parsnip, parsley, potato, tomato, and onion revealed positive reactions in patients who had various disorders. These patients had itching and tingling sensations with or without edema of the lips, mouth, and tongue after eating raw fruits and vegetables. In addition, laryngeal and abdominal disturbances, rhinitis, and hand dermatitis were recorded.

IMMEDIATE VESICULAR HAND DERMATITIS

Lettuce, endive, and tomatoes may produce immediate, vesicular, and intensively pruritic eruptions within a few minutes of contact with these vegetables in previously sensitized skin (see Table 17.5). Some-

Table 17-5 Foods Causing Immediate Vesicular Eruptions When Applied to Damaged Skin
Fruits and Vegetables
Chicory
Endive
Apples
Kiwi fruit
Peaches
Strawberry
Lettuce
Tomato
Miscellaneous foods
Beer
Cheese
Egg
Flour
Milk
Mayonnaise (sorbic acid)

times a combined urticarial and vesicular eruption arises as a reaction to these vegetables.[61] A prerequisite, then, for the appearance of the immediate, vesicular reaction observed in some cases seems to be that the allergen may come into contact with previously damaged skin, even if the skin appears normal to the naked eye.

Parsnip, parsley, and limes are capable of producing phototoxic reactions. They can be tested with ultraviolet light or sunlight.[62]

Dermatitis of Hands Due to Food Additives

Table 17.6 lists the preservatives added to foods, and Table 17.7 lists miscellaneous food additives and their uses (see also Chapter 28). Other food additives, aside from the preservatives, include antioxidants, dyes, flavoring agents, "spoilage retarders," "dough conditioners," "flavor protectors," and "cloudiness preventatives." Some of these chemicals, which may produce contact dermatitis of the hands in certain sensitized individuals, particularly homemakers, food handlers, bakers, and cooks, are often the same agents that have proved to be sensitizers in topical medications and cosmetics.[63,64]

Table 17-6 Preservatives Added to Foods	
Benzoic acid	Polysorbate
Calcium propionate	Guaiac gum
Citric acid	Sodium benzoate
Monoglycerol citrate	Sodium bisulfite
Parabens	Sorbic acid

Table 17-7 Miscellaneous Food Additives and Their Uses

Additive	Use
Calcium disodium EDTA	Stabilizer—chelating agent
Chlorophyll	Color for pastry
Dyes, certified	Coloring agents
Gum arabic (acacia)	Cream and cheese additive
Karaya	Pastry filler
Lanolin	Chewing gum additive
Propylene glycol aginate	Filler—many salad dressings
Sodium silicon aluminate	Lump preventor in cake mix
Tragacanth	Vegetable gum filler

ANTIOXIDANTS IN FOODS

One of the most common types of food spoilage is an undesirable change in color or flavor caused by oxygen in the air. Thus, sliced, fresh apples and peaches turn brown when exposed to air for any length of time, and foods such as mayonnaise and lard turn rancid and become inedible if kept unprotected too long. Both of these conditions are caused by oxidation and can be retarded by using antioxidants.

The darkening of some fruits and vegetables is a type of oxidation known as "enzymatic browning." If foods containing certain enzymes are cut or bruised or are overmature and exposed to air, the tissues darken and turn brown. Apples, apricots, bananas, cherries, peaches, pears, and potatoes contain such enzymes. Antioxidants prevent or delay this enzymatic browning. Table 17.8 lists the antioxidants that are used in foods.

Oxidation can also cause the rancid taste and odor that sometimes develop in fats, oil, mayonnaise, and lard. Accordingly, processed foods that contain these fatty materials must be protected from possible oxidation in order to maintain their best flavor during storage.

At present, such antioxidants as butylated hydroxyanisole (BHA) and butylated hydroxytoluene (BHT) are largely replacing gum benzoin. These antioxidants, which

Table 17-8 Antioxidant Food Additives

Ammonium persulfate (flour color improver—some European countries)
Benzoyl peroxide (flour color "improver")
Butylated hydroxyanisole
Butylated hydroxytoluene
Dodecyl gallate
Gum benzoin
Lauryl and propyl gallate
Sodium bisulfite
Vitamin E (tocopherols)

may also be present in cosmetics, may be tested 2% in petrolatum.

Butylated Hydroxyanisole

This antioxidant is used in many products, including beverages, chewing gum, ice cream, candy, baked goods, gelatin, desserts, soup bases, potatoes, glacéed fruits, potato flakes, sweet potato flakes, dry breakfast cereals, dry yeast, dry mixes for desserts and beverages, lard, shortening, and unsmoked dry sausage, and in emulsions for stabilizers for shortenings. Roed-Petersen and Hjorth[65] reported that in two patients who had allergic dermatitis owing to BHA or BHT, acute flares of vesicular dermatitis on the fingers appeared after the experimental oral administration of these antioxidants.

Butylated Hydroxytoluene

This antioxidant has uses similar to those of BHA.

Sodium Bisulfite in Salads

Epstein[66] described hand eczema in a salad maker owing to "Veg-White," an antioxidant used to prevent discoloration of fruit and vegetables used in salads. The specific sensitizer in this preparation was sodium bisulfite. Patch tests can be performed with a 10% aqueous solution of sodium bisulfite. Sulfites in foods can also cause immediate anaphylactic reactions in very sensitive individuals.

Lauryl Gallate

Brun[67] reported contact dermatitis in a baker from lauryl gallate added to margarine as an antioxidant.

Propyl Gallate

Liden[68] reported a patient who had allergic hypersensitivity from this preservative in Alphosyl and pointed out that bakers are also exposed to this antioxidant, which is chemically closely related to the parabens.

Potassium and Ammonium Persulfate

These have been used as boosters with hydrogen peroxide to produce "platinum bleached" hair. When they have been used in the past in certain European countries as flour "improvers" to render flour whiter, they have caused dermatitis of the hands in bakers.[69]

Benzoyl Peroxide

This is used as an antiacne agent and for the treatment of stasis ulcers. It is also used occasionally as a "flour improver" and can cause hand dermatitis in bakers.[70]

WAXES AND GUMS ADDED TO FOODS

These agents include some known skin sensitizers, namely, guaiac, guar, karaya, acacia (gum arabic), tragacanth, benzoin spermaceti, carnauba, and beeswax (the last four being used for glazing confectionery). Acacia (gum arabic) is permitted in chocolate drinks, creams, French dressing, malt liquors, milk, mustard, pickles, cheese, ice cream, and sherbet. Guaiac gum is used as a preservative for fats and oils, and guar gum is used in milk products. Guar gum is also used as a stabilizer; as a thickening and film-forming agent for cheese, salad dressings, ice cream, and soups; and as a binding and disintegrating agent in tablet formulations, suspensions, emulsions, lotions, creams, and toothpastes. Some of these waxes and gums crossreact with balsam of Peru.

COLORS ADDED TO FOODS

Several "natural" approved colors can be added to foods. In addition, ten synthetic organic dyes are permitted. Citrus Red 2 and Sunset Yellow have formulas that indicate possible crossreactions with paraphenylenediamine and sulfanilamide.

SPICES AND FLAVORING AGENTS

Many spices and flavoring agents have been implicated in the production of contact dermatitis owing to foods. These flavoring agents include oil of almond, anise seed, bergamot, capsicum, chamomile, caraway, cinnamon, clove, coconut, ginger, laurel, mace, menthol, minonene, mustard, nutmeg, palm, peppermint, and sesame.[71,72]

POTATO CHIP DERMATITIS

Inman[73] traced three cases of contact dermatitis occurring in a potato chip factory that were due, respectively, to cheese powder, wheat filler, and onion powder.

METALS IN FOODS

Most foods contain traces of various metals, including nickel and chromium. Ethylenediamine tetra-acetate (EDTA) is added to many foods to chelate such metals. It must be emphasized that EDTA is not a sensitizer and does not crossreact with ethylenediamine hydrochloride, which is a notorious sensitizer.

It is interesting to note that the addition of nickel is permitted as a catalyst for hydrogenated fats and that aluminum sulfate may be added to canned fish, pickles, relishes, and starch. Table 17.9 lists metals that may be present in food.

Table 17-9 Metals in Foods*
Aluminum
Chromium
Cobalt
Nickel (may also be added to hydrogenated fats)

*Ethylenediamine tetra-acetate is often added to chelate these metals.

SULFATES IN FOODS

Sodium lauryl sulfate is permitted in egg whites. Sodium sulfate can be added to biscuits, and sodium thiosulfate can be added to table salt (see Table 17.10).

"Housewife's Eczema"

"Housewife's eczema" is probably the most common type of contact dermatitis of the hands encountered in clinical practice. This type of eruption occurs principally on the fingers and the webs and dorsa of the hands of women who do house and laundry work that entails more or less regular exposure to soaps, detergents, and other household cleansers. "Housewife's eczema," however, may affect not only homemakers but also those whose profession or other activities involve excessive exposure to soaps and detergents. Included in this group are surgeons, medical personnel, dentists, bartenders, dishwashers, kitchen workers, canners, and individuals employed in those occupations necessitating frequent washing and immersion of the hands in various detergent solutions. The eruption of "housewife's eczema" begins usually with mild dryness, redness, and scaling. As the condition becomes more severe under continued exposure to soap and water, fissuring, crusting, and eventually chronic eczema are produced.[74,75]

Hand eczema often begins in cold weather with "chapping" of the hands. A young mother's hands remain frequently in fairly good condition until 3 to 6 months after childbirth. At this time, the increased exposure of the hands to soaps and water in the bathing and care of the infant causes a "breakdown" of the skin. Such eczema may be intensified by any one of many common household irritants such as bleaches, waxes, polishes, and turpentine. The patient not infrequently excoriates the itchy skin, causing secondary infection and lichenifications. Atopic individuals are particularly prone to develop "housewife's eczema."[76,77]

Table 17-10 Sulfates in Foods
Sodium bisulfite (biscuits)
Sodium lauryl sulfate (egg white)
Sodium thiosulfate (table salt)

HAND ECZEMA PATTERNS

Cronin[78] performed an exhaustive study of hand eczema patterns in 263 women. She found that 44% had primary palmar involvement, 15% dorsal, 19% fingers only, and 22% generalized hand eczema. Of those with palmar involvement, only 42% had ICD, whereas 75% of dorsal eczema patients had significant contact with irritants. Those with dorsal or finger involvement were more often atopic than those with palmar predominance. Nickel was the most significant allergen, with about 30% of the women positive. Fragrances and rubber allergens were also common.

Role of Rings in Hand Dermatitis

Allergic reactions to nickel-plated rings may occur in nickel-sensitive individuals. Gold and palladium occasionally cause allergy. Platinum and silver almost never cause ACD. The dermatitis under a ring may be produced in several ways:

1. Soaps, detergents, waxes, polishes, or even cosmetic creams may accumulate under the ring and may cause a primary, irritant type of dermatitis. Therefore, whenever possible, rings should be removed when washing the hands with soaps or exposing them to detergents. Rings must be cleaned at regular intervals to remove such accumulated material.
2. Certain rings, especially alloys of copper and silver, can corrode readily on the skin and form a primary irritant in the presence of an adequate concentration of salt.
3. Industrial smog contains fumes thick with sulfides from the burning of low-grade, sulfur-laden coal and fuel oil, or other corrosive metals such as phosphates. These air pollutants can attack gold alloys directly, even when jewelry is not being worn. When a tarnished ring slips back on the finger, or a bracelet onto the arm, the thin film of tarnish rubs off in a black smudge and may irritate the skin.
4. Simon and Harly[79] reported that radiodermatitis of the fingers is produced by gold rings contaminated with gold seeds containing decayed radon. Leone[80] found that a radioactive gold ring made from improperly salvaged gold radon seeds caused a long-standing radiodermatitis.

Thus, hand eczema begins frequently under a ring. In many instances, when a dermatitis begins on a left fourth finger, the patient changes the ring to the right side and so produces a dermatitis on both hands. If a dermatitis owing to rings is not treated properly, the eruption may spread from the finger onto the hand and to other fingers. The irritated skin produced by a recurring ring dermatitis is subject to secondary infection and sensitization to other chemicals.[81]

REMOVAL OF A RING FROM A SWOLLEN FINGER

It is not uncommon for a finger to become swollen suddenly from a contusion, an edematous dermatosis, or some other transient cause.

Leider[82] has described in detail how to remove a ring from a swollen finger without damage to the ring. The procedure is as follows:

- Lubricate the finger with oil or petrolatum.
- Take a longish piece of soft string of moderate caliber and good strength and start winding it from the beginning of the first interphalangeal joint up to the ring, being careful to make every turn comfortably snug and touching close to the preceding one. Such winding progressively reduces the bulk of the tissue and drives edema toward, under, and beyond the ring.
- When the ring is reached by as many successive turns as it takes to encase completely the swollen digit to that point, feed the advancing end of the string under the ring and beyond it with a slender blunt instrument, such as one prong of a tweezer. This can always be done; there is always enough space to accommodate the girth of a string of loose enough and compressible enough cotton.
- When the maneuver is accomplished to the point at which the ring is caught by the string (now passed under and beyond it and made taut), start to unwind the turns of the string off the finger gently and slowly, all the while keeping the string taut and almost perpendicular to the finger. In most cases, the ring will move forward gradually with every unwind, as it is caught by the string which is always behind it.
- As soon as the second interphalangeal joint is passed, the job is largely done and the ring readily slips off the rest of the finger, to the great relief of both patient and operator.

This procedure works almost every time and in all but the most severely swollen fingers. In average cases, the amount of discomfort is moderate and it is almost always endurable.

Several precautions must be observed: (a) If the finger is swollen from pyogenic infection, has a cut, or is badly abraded, the procedures should not be done. (b) If the unwinding is done roughly or too rapidly, the skin may be too severely crushed, lacerated, or abraded by the moving ring and string as it is unwound. Some slight damage may be done to the epidermis even when this procedure is done gently and slowly, but it is of no great consequence. Such skinning heals readily. (c) If the ring has an impediment such as an expander or a massive setting in the form of a large, bezeled stone or other raised, broad ornament in its position on the dorsal surface of the finger, the string must be depressed parallel to the finger every time the setting is reached and until it is passed each time. The maneuver is gratifyingly successful if it is done skillfully. The string removes the ring as it unwinds, and the patient's praises ring in the operator's ear.

Exner[83] has also removed rings successfully from swollen fingers.

Differential Diagnosis of Contact Dermatitis of Hands

Dermatitides of the hands from entirely different causes may resemble each other so closely that the cause of the dermatitis can often be discerned only after prolonged observation and special diagnostic tests. Thus, allergic and irritant contact dermatitis of the hands may be difficult to distinguish from atopic eczema, tinea infections, psoriasis, nummular eczema, a blistering eruption called pompholyx (dyshidrotic eczema), or a pustular eruption called pustular bacterid or pustular psoriasis (see Table 17.11).

The original condition of the hand dermatitis often becomes changed radically by secondary infection or by a superimposed contact dermatitis resulting from

Table 17-11 Differential Diagnosis of Contact Dermatitis of Hands

Dermatophytosis
  KOH, culture
  Examine finger—toenails, soles, and interweb areas
  Rule out dermatophytid of hands (trichophyton test)
Psoriasis
  Examine nails, elbows, knees, scalp, and intergluteal area
Pustular psoriasis
  In psoriatic, discrete pustules in normal or in eczematized skin
Dyshidrosis
Discrete vesicles on sides of fingers, palms, and soles
Atopic dermatitis
  History of asthma, allergic rhinitis, infantile eczema, or presence of eczema—popliteal, antecubital, dorsal aspect of toes and nuchal areas
Pustular bacterid
  Leukocytosis 12,000–19,000 may respond to oral antibiotics focus of infection
Nummular eczema
  Discrete discoid (coin-shaped) lesions on back of hand
Chronic acral dermatitis[87]
  A pruritic, papulovesicular, and keratotic dermatitis of the hands, feet, and extremities had marked elevated serum IgE levels up to 100,000 ng/ml

reactions to topical medications and irritating soaps and detergents.

A listing by the physician of all previously used medications, hand creams, and lotions is necessary to evaluate the role of these preparations in alleviating or exacerbating the dermatitis. A detailed history of contactants encountered not only in the workplace but also in various hobbies is important.

EXAMINATION OF PATIENT

Always examine the patient's feet. The patient often protests such a procedure, saying, "I don't have anything on my feet." The physician who believes such a statement is often misled, because the patient may not realize that thickening and yellowish discoloration of the toenails or slight scaling of the soles may mean that he or she has psoriasis or a fungus infection that also affects the hands. Scaling between the toes may indicate an active fungal infection that can cause tiny blisters on the palms, which, in turn, can become "eczematized" and can result in a full-blown hand dermatitis.

Examine the soles and heels for blisters or pustules. The presence of a vesicular or pustular eruption on the feet often means that the eruption of the hands is not a "simple" contact dermatitis. Thus, many patients are being treated for contact dermatitis from external or occupational causes when, in reality, they have pompholyx, pustular bacterid, pustular psoriasis, or nummular eczema, which are of endogenic origin.[84,85]

Examine the patient's knees, elbows, scalp, and intergluteal area for the dry, scaly evidence of psoriasis. Particularly in dentists and surgeons, psoriasis frequently may localize on the hands because of trauma and may be mistaken for an occupational contact dermatitis (Koebner's phenomenon).

Find out if the patient is atopic. Does the patient have asthma or allergic rhinitis? Does he or she remember having eczema as a child? Examine the antecubital and popliteal areas and the back of the neck for evidence of atopic eczema. Atopic eczema of the hands is often localized on the dorsal surfaces of the joints. Irritants and housework often cause the dermatitis to localize on the hands in an individual who has an atopic constitution.

Examine the dorsal aspect of the extremities for the coin-shaped lesions of nummular eczema, particularly if the hand dermatitis is predominantly on the dorsal aspect. Nummular eczema of unknown origin is often confused with contact dermatitis.

Chronic paronychia, particularly of the monilial variety, is usually evidence that the hands are wet much of the time. Paronychia may be due occasionally to wax, hair, bristles, threads, and scales that enter the parony-chial tissues as foreign bodies.

Abnormalities of the nails (Figure 17-1) should be noted, particularly for evidence of fungal infections and psoriasis. The role of such dermatoses in hand dermatitis must be evaluated. Subungual hemorrhages may be caused by excessive exposure to a combination of water, detergents, and trauma, as in the case of professional dishwashers.

Study the distribution of the eruption. A recurrent, pruritic, vesicular eruption on the palms and sides of the fingers that is symmetrical and bilateral will more prob-ably be pompholyx (dyshidrotic eczema) than will one caused by external contactants. The cause of pompholyx is unknown, but in some nickel-sensitive individuals the ingestion of nickel in foods has been implicated as a cause of the eruption. Rarely, penicillin will produce a symmetrical, vesicular eruption of the hands, resembling pompholyx.

Examine the eruption for discrete pustules of varying sizes. In the absence of any crusting or itching, such an eruption will most probably be a so-called pustular psor-iasis or bacterid rather than an instance of infected contact dermatitis. The etiology of such eruptions is obscure. Some cases respond to antibiotic therapy and removal of foci of infection or to intralesional injection of corticosteroids.

Keratoderma climactericum is a disorder of the palms and soles occurring in menopausal women. The disorder is characterized by discrete oval patches of mild kerato-derma. The lesions progress slowly to reach a size and shape that remain almost unchanged in appearance for a long time. The hyperkeratosis is generally quite mild. Vesiculation is not a feature. Both palms and soles may be involved, but usually only the palms are affected. The lesions improve ultimately but are generally unrespon-sive to therapy.

These dermatoses, which must be distinguished from contact dermatitis, are often complicated by a superim-posed, irritant contact dermatitis resulting from the use of soaps, detergents, or chemicals encountered in various occupations. A superimposed allergic contact dermatitis resulting from the use of topical medications or occupa-tional sensitizers is not uncommon. It is, therefore, necessary to find out what medication the patient has used in the past that seemed to make the hand dermatitis worse. In addition, find out the patient's occupation and whether he or she is handling irritants or allergens. The role of irritants is determined by taking a careful history. The role of allergens is proved by patch tests.

Hand dermatitis often becomes secondarily infected. Sensitization to bacteria may produce an infectious, ecze-matoid dermatitis with dissemination to the forearms and more distant areas.

CHRONIC ACRAL DERMATITIS WITH HIGH IGE

Some patients who have a pruritic, papulovesicular der-matitis of the hands, feet, and extremities have sharply elevated IgE serum levels of up to 100,000 ng/mL. There is no personal or family history of atopic disease. A variety of immunologic, physiologic, and pharmacologic studies of the skin have normal results. The course of this unique dermatitis is chronic, lasting many years, and it is resistant to all treatments except the administration of systemic corticosteroid drugs. Winkelmann and Gleich[86] have labeled this condition "chronic acral dermatitis."

Role of Soaps and Detergents in Hand Dermatitis

The role of soaps and detergents in hand eczema is controversial. Wechsler[75] suggested that the term "deter-gent hands" is a misnomer because of the limited role of soaps and detergents as irritants. Indeed, Suskind[87] found that immersion of hands in solutions of soaps or synthetic detergents in the concentrations recommended by the suppliers actually improves hand dermatitis. In a study of dishwashing liquids with pH adjusted to 7.4, 10.0, or 10.8 in 30 persons with normal hands, repeated exposure did not show a difference among the three exposures in skin changes or hydration. Increasing the pH to 10.8 did not worsen overall hand appearance.[88]

Kligman and Wooding[89] pointed out that hand eczema in homemakers was once attributed to soap, but since World War II, synthetic detergents have been incriminated. Their introduction, however, has not led to any notable increase in "housewife's eczema," and wide-spread use of dishwashers and washing machines over the last 10 years has not led to any conspicuous decline.

All investigative methods distinguish between detergents causing a low and a high degree of irritancy. The results, however, show unexplained discrepancies, which suggest that detergents are by no means homogeneous and that the damage may be produced by different mechanisms.

Wood and Bettley,[90] who studied the denaturing action of detergents on keratin and irritancy in human skin, also found considerable differences among deter-gents. Glickman and Silvers[91] found that 82% of patients who have hand eczema have a history of atopy.

The incidence of "housewife's eczema," "dishpan hands," and "detergent hands" is low compared to the number of people exposed. Cleaning personnel, laun-derers, dishwashers, and others who earn their living by having their hands immersed in solutions of these deter-gents, however, do frequently develop dermatitis. In many instances, the inflamed skin does not tolerate soap and detergents well, and contact with these compounds should be avoided, at least until the acute phase has subsided.

Hand eczema from wet work is related to frequent exposure to water and surfactants. Ethoxylated surfactants oxidize with normal use over time and the oxidation products have been found to be sensitizers in guinea pigs. But in a human study, formaldehyde and acetaldehyde were the unexpected exposures that could cause allergic reactions in patients engaged in wet work and the use of ethoxylated surfactants.[92]

Under appropriate circumstances, excessive exposure to water, soap, and detergents leads to changes in the skin. The amount of damage depends on traumatic and environmental influences, such as cold weather, low humidity, impairment in alkali neutralization capacity, emotional stress, hyperhidrosis, exposure to other contactants (e.g., vegetables, fruits, meat juices, and other foods), and contact with cleansing and polishing products containing bleaches, abrasives, alkalis, and solvents.

Soaps and detergents probably damage skin by the following mechanisms:

1. Alkali-induced damage of the keratin layer of the epidermis that increases the permeability of the horny layer
2. Irritative effects of certain fatty acids
3. Removal of lipids and the protective mantle of the skin and prevention of re-establishment of the mantle and its normal acidity
4. Alteration of the buffering capacity of the skin
5. Removal of amino acids with damage to the water-holding capacity of the horny layer; this is particularly likely with synthetic detergents

Often irritation by soaps and detergents is heightened by concentration of the detergent solution on the skin, such as when cleansers become trapped under rings or when, during dishwashing, dishes are held tightly for a period of time in the detergent-moistened hand. Soaps for fine fabrics are probably the least irritating of the detergent cleansers.

"BUILDERS"

Practically all laundry soaps contain "builders," or other ingredients used to build a finished product—additives, such as sodium carbonate, sodium phosphate, ash, borax, or sodium silicate, that may irritate but not sensitize.

ABRASIVE AGENTS

Many powdered, industrial hand cleansers have ingredients to increase the mechanical, cleansing action. The inorganic scrubbers include pumice, talc, sand, and borax; the organic agents include ground nut shells, cornmeal, and wood flours. These agents are effective in removing heavy oil, greases, tar, and other stubborn dirt from the hands, but the inorganic variety is particularly rough on the skin.

PATCH TESTING WITH SOAPS AND DETERGENTS

Patch testing with soaps and detergents is performed usually with a 1% to 2% aqueous solution. The test site occasionally becomes slightly red, desquamates, wrinkles, or appears glazed. These reactions are not indicative of allergic sensitization but are merely owing to the irritant effect of soap or detergent solutions under the covered patch. Patch test reactions with these agents should always be checked on at least three control subjects.

The irritant reactions under a covered patch may interfere with the interpretation of allergic reactions. Whenever possible, therefore, patch tests should be performed with the suspected ingredients. Occasionally, however, photosensitivity reactions owing to antiseptics in soaps are clear, even when the testing is done with soap solutions.

The alkalis and fatty acids of soaps are rare sensitizers. Any white, unscented soap that is free of antiseptics, other medication, or lanolin is hypoallergenic, and patch testing except for investigative purposes is usually unrewarding. Similarly, the synthetic detergents without additives are rarely sensitizing and do not usually yield patch test results of clinical significance.

Numerous methods have been devised for testing new soaps and detergents before they are introduced for general use. Such testing may be of value in detecting unusual irritant qualities of new products.

The following additives to soaps may be allergens:

1. Lanolin
2. Perfumes
3. Rosin
4. Antiseptics
5. Deodorants
6. Vitamin E
7. Antiperspirants
8. Turpentine (special industry soap)
9. Dyes
10. Surfactants and emulsifiers (rarely)

ROSIN (COLOPHONY)

Yellow (soft) laundry bars owe their properties to the presence of rosin, which is the solid resin residue remaining after the distillation of spirits of turpentine derived from the crude oleoresin of certain species of pine. Rosin consists of a mixture of complex abietic acids and esters. It makes laundry bars more soluble and hastens sudsing in cool water. Some toilet soaps also contain a small percentage of this agent.

PERFUMES

It should be noted that some soaps with the label "Contains no perfume," may contain small amounts of "masking" perfumes to disguise the odor of certain fats. The concentration of such perfumes is not usually a hazard for perfume-sensitive patients.

ENZYMES IN DETERGENTS

Currently 70% to 75% of laundry detergents sold in the US contain enzymes. Depending on the brand and type, these products contain as much as 0.1% active enzymes, which are prepared by fermentation with the widely distributed nonpathogenic soil organism *Bacillus subtilis*.

The Food and Drug Administration made public a study in which the average enzyme detergent laundry product in normal use by consumers did not produce more primary irritation of the skin than did similar products containing no enzymes.[93] Ducksbury and Dave,[94] however, reported that 12 women in the home-help service in Nottingham developed an irritant dermatitis after using enzyme detergents. A survey based on a questionnaire showed an incidence of 5% among people using these products. Onychia may result from their use.

Allergic Reactions to Enzyme Detergents

Exposure to the concentrated enzyme in industry has caused dermatitis, allergic rhinitis, and asthma.[95]

Belin and colleagues[96] stated that sensitization to enzyme detergents can also occur in consumers of enzyme-containing detergents and in every situation in which these enzymes are dust particles. These investigators obtained positive scratch tests in sensitized patients.

Patch test can be done with a 0.25% aqueous solution of the commercial product. The "pure subtilisms" can be patch tested with a 0.1% solution in water.

BARRIER CREAMS FOR PREVENTION OF HAND ECZEMA

In general, barrier creams have not been proven to be helpful in combating hand eczema. Perhaps this is because the very factors that aggravate hand eczema (friction, solvent and detergent exposure, wet work, etc.) also serve to remove the barrier cream from the skin.

In a study of four "barrier creams," Loden[97] found that three had no effect on absorption of formaldehyde, whereas the other reduced absorption by about 40% only. None had any blocking effect on the solvent benzene.

Some barrier creams may in fact aggravate skin irritation. Frosch and colleagues[98,99] found that two barrier creams actually increased irritancy from sodium hydroxide in guinea pigs. One other cream did, however, suppress irritation from sodium lauryl sulfate and toluene. These guinea pig studies, of course, cannot duplicate the aggravating factors of actual job performance, so results in actual use would likely be much poorer.

Boman and Mellstrom[100] also found that several barrier creams were of no use in blocking organic solvent absorption in guinea pigs.

The exception to this may be in the use of a barrier cream for prevention of urushiol dermatitis from poison ivy, oak, and sumac. Epstein[101] showed that an organoclay compound may be helpful, and Orchard and colleagues[102] also found a linoleic acid containing preparation was efficacious. Smith,[103] however, found no benefit from a popularly marketed poison ivy shielding preparation.

Hand dermatitis in manufacturing was found to derive significant benefit from a program of care that included skin moisturizers as compared to care without moisturizer. This was demonstrated in the workplace using a randomized trial design and both bioengineering and visual assessments.[104] An emollient that contained skin lipids which are thought to contribute to restoration of a more normal stratum corneum barrier (Locobase Repair) was found useful in an acute barrier disruption model of tape stripping. A significant acceleration of repair of barrier damage was observed. However, in a study of chronic hand dermatitis, management with the ceramide-containing emollient was no better than with petrolatum-based emollient, although both were deemed beneficial.[105]

Role of Gloves in Management of Hand Dermatitis

There are several types of gloves available for hand protection. Those used most commonly are either natural latex rubber or synthetic rubber. Vinyl gloves are available for both home and occupational use. The 4-H glove is a polyethylene laminate glove with good barrier properties for organic chemicals and others.

Latex rubber gloves are most commonly used in health care settings because they are inexpensive and easily distensible, allowing for maximum comfort. However, individuals may become sensitive to latex or to the various additives used in glove manufacture, especially when gloves are worn over already dermatitic skin. Vinyl gloves are available for both home and medical use. Vinyl gloves are by nature hypoallergenic, because no rubber accelerators or latex are present. However, vinyl gloves do not fit closely and, therefore, are not good in settings where fine touch is important. This is not so much of a problem for household use. One benefit of vinyl gloves is that they are somewhat more protective than latex gloves for certain allergens, including nickel. Vinyl gloves are more subject to developing microcracks from stretching and, therefore, after being worn for a period of time may decrease in their protective abilities, not only against chemicals but also against microbial agents.

Irritant contact dermatitis manifest by bilateral dry skin was studied in 30 female assembly line workers. They were given one aloe vera gel coated glove to wear on one hand for an 8 hour work day. The study was a 30-day use followed by a 30-day rest period and then 10 more days of use. No improvement was seen in the non-gloved hand, but good to marked improvement was seen in the gloved hand by several grading methods. Improvement was noted in as little as 3 days and was marked by 10 days of glove use.[106]

ALCOHOL-BASED HAND DISINFECTANTS

The use of alcohol-based hand disinfectants was compared to the use of detergent. The 17 healthy volunteers in the study used the products every 10 minutes for an hour twice daily. After 4 weeks it was concluded that alcohol-based disinfectant had caused less visible skin irritation and less skin barrier disruption, on the basis of transepidermal water loss measurements. Alternating detergent with alcohol-based disinfectant was also less irritating than use of detergent alone.[107]

PROBLEM OF PROTECTING THE HANDS OF ORTHOPEDIC SURGEONS FROM ACRYLIC BONE CEMENT

Acrylic bone cement is a mixture of polymethyl methacrylate and methyl methacrylate (acrylic monomer). It is used for fixation of prostheses to bone in surgical procedures on the hip joint. The brochure describing the bone cement contains the following statement: "The liquid component (methyl methacrylate monomer) is a powerful, lipid solvent. It should not be allowed to come into direct contact with sensitive tissues or be absorbed by the body. Also, it should not be permitted to come in contact with rubber, including rubber gloves."

Ironically, a surgeon can in no way prevent the cement from coming into contact with rubber gloves, because rubber gloves are the only type used regularly in the operating room. The manufacturer of the bone cement recommends: "The surgeon should wear two pairs of rubber gloves when handling the cement directly and discard these for a fresh pair immediately after he [or she] has finished putting the cement in place." This method is thought to provide sufficient protection for an operator unless he or she is sensitive to the methyl methacrylate monomer. In that case, the stratagem may not work.

There are many reports of allergic contact dermatitis from acrylic bone cement, which readily penetrates rubber gloves.[108–111]

Some surgeons who have become sensitized to bone cement sometimes allow an assistant to perform that part of the operation requiring the handling of bone cement; the sensitized surgeon then completes the operation.

A unique feature of allergic contact dermatitis caused by acrylic monomer is that it is accompanied by a distressing paresthesia of the fingertips in the form of a burning and tingling sensation and a slight numbness. The paresthesia may persist for several weeks after the dermatitis has subsided. The prolonged paresthesia accompanying sensitization to acrylic monomer may occur because the acrylic monomer is a powerful solvent that readily penetrates damaged skin and thus produces an inflammation of the nerve endings in the fingers.

The only currently available glove protective against acrylates is the 4-H plastic polymer glove (Safety 4 Company, Lyngby, Denmark). This glove is thin but has no elasticity and so does not fit snugly against the fingers. A rubber glove, however, can be worn over the 4-H glove to increase fine touch.[112]

NICKEL

Moursiden and Faber[113] showed that positive patch tests to nickel sulfate (2.5%) could be obtained even when the allergen was separated from nickel-sensitive skin by a segment of rubber glove material. Similar tests, using polyvinyl chloride material instead of rubber, proved negative (Figure 17-2).

Wall[20] reported that during an investigation of an outbreak of nickel dermatitis in an electrode factory, it was found that the inside lining of the fingertips of the rubber gloves used by the operators was dimethylglyoxime positive, proving that the nickel penetrated rubber gloves.

HAIR DYES

Moursiden and Faber[113] described a case of allergic, occupational dermatitis in a hairdresser who was sensitive to toluenediamine and aminoazobenzene, which progressed in spite of careful use of rubber gloves. These authors felt that vinyl gloves offer more protection than the rubber variety against hair dyes and most other allergens. Hand dermatitis is a common problem among hairdressers. A study of 2,352 hairdressing apprentices found that unprotected wet work of greater than 2 hours per day and low ambient absolute humidity were the main risk factors. The risk of hand dermatitis decreased as age increased. Improving work conditions and providing skin protection proved beneficial, regardless of whether the workers were atopic or not.[114]

The 4-H glove is also useful in protecting hairdressers from dye and perm chemicals, probably to a greater degree than vinyl gloves.[115]

SOAPS AND DETERGENTS

Homemakers and others who are exposed to soaps and detergents often acquire a dermatitis from the rubber gloves that they use to protect their hands.[116] Vinyl gloves adequately protect the hands from soaps and detergents without causing rubber dermatitis.

NITROGEN MUSTARD

Thomsen and Mikkelsen[117] reported that patients who have early stages of mycosis fungoides are often treated with topical nitrogen mustard (HN_2). HN_2, however, is a potent sensitizer, and 13 of 23 patients who had mycosis fungoides were sensitized.

The only glove that protected the patients against penetration of HN_2 was the one made of polyvinyl chloride. Rubber gloves did not give protection, and a polyethylene glove also permitted penetration of HN_2.

SOLVENTS

Sansone and Tewari[118] have shown that various solvents penetrate most types of gloves. Polyvinyl chloride provided the least protection, and neoprene and nitriles were the most effective.

A study by the National Institute for Occupational Safety and Health revealed that most of the gloves that were tested did not give any protection at all.[119] In many cases, they were worse than not wearing anything at all. The study tested the permeation rates of various gloves when immersed in 1,2-dichloroethane; 1,1,1-trichloroethane; 1,1,2-trichloroethane; and a polychlorinated biphenyl mixture. The glove and garment materials tested included butyl rubber, neoprene rubber latex, nitrile rubber latex, polyethylene (medium-density), surgical rubber latex, DuPont's Teflon and Viton, and butylcoated nylon. Normalized times for breakthrough ranged widely, with Viton in all cases resisting permeation the longest.

Viton is a fluorinated elastomer (made by DuPont) that the Norton Company (Charleston Safety Products Division, Charleston, SC) makes into an unsupported, liquid-proof glove.

SURGICAL GLOVE DERMATITIS

Many surgeons become sensitized to the accelerators or antioxidants used in surgical rubber gloves. In a study of 11 surgeons who acquired an allergic contact dermatitis of their hands from surgical gloves, patch testing revealed that 7 had positive patch tests to mercaptobenzothiazole, a common cause of allergic rubber dermatitis. The other 4 were allergic to various other rubber chemicals. Such surgeons must use "hypoallergenic" rubber gloves free of mercaptobenzothiazole and other rubber sensitizers in order to avoid hand dermatitis.

Blue nitrite gloves, made of acrylic nitrite and butadiene, have no latex and generally low levels of accelerators.

MECHANICAL FACTORS

Gloves provide the most effective protection when they can be used, but there are many jobs in the engineering industry in which gloves are dangerously liable to get caught in the moving parts of the machine or in which the components being handled are so small that the wearing of gloves is impossible.

Often, however, patients in certain occupations, such as hairdressing, claim they are unable to do their work properly when they are wearing gloves. When it is pointed out that surgeons must wear gloves when they have to do microsurgery or other delicate operations, such patients sometimes consent to wear gloves.

References

1. Jungbauer FHW, van der Vleuten P, Groothoff JW, et al. Irritant hand dermatitis: severity of disease, occupational exposure to skin irritant and preventive measures 5 years after initial diagnosis. Contact Dermatitis 2004;50:245.

2. Lammintausta K, Kalimo K. Atopy and hand dermatitis in hospital wet work. Contact Dermatitis 1981;7:301.

3. Bjornberg A. Skin reactions to primary irritants in patients with hand eczema. Goteborg, Sweden: Oscar Isacson, 1968.

4. Coenraads PJ, Bleumink E, Nater JP. Susceptibility to primary irritants: age dependence and relation to contact allergic reactions. Contact Dermatitis 1975;1:377.

5. Agner T. Skin susceptibility in uninvolved skin of hand eczema patients and healthy controls. Br J Dermatol 1991;125:140.

6. Jordan WP. Allergic contact dermatitis in hand eczema. Arch Dermatol 1974;110:567.

7. Wilkinson DS. Contact dermatitis of the hands. Trans St Johns Hosp Dermatol Soc 1972;58:163.

8. Wilkinson DS, Bandmann HJ, Calnan CD, et al. The role of contact allergy in hand eczema. Trans St Johns Hosp Dermatol Soc 1970;56:19.

9. Lantinga H, Nater JP, Coenraads PJ. Prevalence, incidence and course of eczema on the hands and forearms in a sample of the general population. Contact Dermatitis 1984;10:135.

10. Kavli G, Førde OH. Hand dermatoses in Tromsø. Contact Dermatitis 1984;10:174.

11. Meding B, Swanbeck G. Occupational hand eczema in an industrial city. Contact Dermatitis 1990;22:13.

12. Meding B, Swanbeck G. Consequences of having hand eczema. Contact Dermatitis 1991;23:6.

13. Meding B, Wrangsjo K, Jarvholm B. Fifteen-year follow-up hand eczema: persistence and consequences. Brit J Dermatol 2005;152:975.

14. Rystedt I. Work related hand eczema in atopics. Contact Dermatitis 1985;12:164.

15. Rystedt I. Factors influencing the occurrence of hand eczema in adults with a history of atopic dermatitis in childhood. Contact Dermatitis 1985;12:185.

16. Rystedt I. Atopic background in patients with occupational hand eczema. Contact Dermatitis 1985;12:247.

17. Jungbauer FHW, Lensen GJ, Groothoff JW, et al. Exposure of the hands to wet work in nurses. Contact Dermatitis 2004;50:225.

18. Berndt U, Hinnen U, Iliev D, et al. Hand eczema in metalworker trainees – an analysis of risk factors. Contact Dermatitis 2000;43:327.

19. Clemensen OJ, Menne T, Kaaber K, Solgaard P. Exposure of nickel and the relevance of nickel sensitivity among hospital cleaners. Contact Dermatitis 1981;7:14.

20. Wall LM. Nickel penetration through rubber gloves. Contact Dermatitis 1980;6:461.

21. Fisher AA. Possible role of diet in pompholyx and nickel dermatitis—a critical survey. Cutis 1978;22:412.

22. Christensen OB, Moler H. External and internal exposure to the antigen in the hand eczema of nickel allergy. Contact Dermatitis 1975;1:136.

23. Menné T, Thorboe A. Nickel dermatitis—nickel excretion. Contact Dermatitis 1976;2:353.

24. Hjorth N. Nickel vasculitis. Contact Dermatitis 1976;2:356.

25. Jensen CS, Menne T, Johansen JD. Systemic contact dermatitis after oral exposure to nickel: a review with a modified meta-analysis. Contact Dermatitis 2006;54:79.

26. Christensen OB. Prognosis in nickel allergy and hand eczema. Contact Dermatitis 1982;8:7.

27. Christensen OB, Kristensen M. Treatment with disulfiram in chronic nickel hand dermatitis. Contact Dermatitis 1982;8:59.

28. Fowler JF. Disulfiram is effective for nickel allergic hand eczema. Am J Contact Dermat 1992;3:175.

29. Christensen JD. Disulfiram treatment of three patients with nickel dermatitis. Contact Dermatitis 1982;8:105.

30. Moller H, Spiren A, Svensson A, et al. Contact allergy to Asteraceae plant Ambrosia artemisiifolia L. (ragweed) in sesquiterpene lactone-sensitive patients in southern Sweden. Contact Dermatitis 2002;47:157.

31. Feuerman EJ. Contact dermatitis in housewives. Br J Dermatol 1979;82:205.

32. Wahba A, Cohen T. Chrome sensitivity in Israel. Contact Dermatitis 1979;5:101.

33. Garcia-Perez A, Martin-Pascual A, Sanchez-Misiega A. Chrome content in bleaches and detergents: its relationship to hand dermatitis in women. Acta Derm Venereol (Stockh) 1973;53:353.

34. Perisic S, Jovovic D. Allergic contact sensitivity to chromates in housewives. Dermatovenerol Jugoslav 1977;4:15.

35. Cronin E. Contact dermatitis XVII: reactions to contact allergens given orally or systemically. Br J Dermatol 1972;86:104.

36. Schleif P. Provokation des Chromatekzems zu Testzwecken durch interne chromzufuhr. Hautarzt 1968;19:209.

37. Kaaber K, Veien NK. Chromate ingestion in chronic chromate dermatitis. Contact Dermatitis 1978;4:119.

38. Burrows D. Chromium and the skin. Br J Dermatol 1978;99:587.

39. Fisher AA. "Blackjack disease" and other chromate puzzles. Cutis 1976;18:21.

40. Burry JN, Kirk J. Environmental dermatitis: chrome cripples. Med J Aust 1975;2:720.

41. Briet R, Turk RMB. The medical and social fate of the dichromate allergic patient. Br J Dermatol 1976;94:349.

42. Fregert S. Chromium valencies and cement dermatitis. Br J Dermatol 1981;105:7.

43. Rudzki E, Krajewska D. Cross-reactions between ethylenediamine, diethylenetriamine and triethylenetetramine. Contact Dermatitis 1976;2:311.

44. Heydorn S, Menne T, Andersen KE, et al. The fragrance hand immersion study – an experimental model simulating real-life exposure for allergic contact dermatitis. Contact Dermatitis 2003;48:324.

45. Hjorth N. Battery for testing of chefs and other kitchen workers. Contact Dermatitis 1975;1:63.

46. Fisher AA. Allergic eczematous contact dermatitis due to foods. Cutis 1975;16:603.

47. Nethercott JR, Holness DL. Occupational dermatitis in food handlers and bakers. J Am Acad Dermatol 1989;21:485.

48. Meding B, Wrangsjo K, Brisman J, et al. Hand eczema in 45 bakers- a clinical study. Contact Dermatitis 2003;48:7.

49. Seligman EJ, Key MM. Corn dermatitis. Arch Dermatol 1968;97:664.

50. Polunin I. Pineapple dermatoses. Br J Dermatol 1951;63:441.

51. Mitchell JC, Jordan WP. Allergic contact dermatitis from radish. Raphanus sativus. Br J Dermatol 1974;91:183.

52. Fisher AA. Dermatitis due to cinnamon and cinnamic aldehyde. Cutis 1975;16:383.

53. Spencer LV, Fowler JF. "Thin mint" cookie dermatitis. Contact Dermatitis 1988;18:185.

54. Sinha SM, Pasricha JS, Sharma RC, Kandhari KC. Vegetable responsible for contact dermatitis of the hands. Arch Dermatol 1977;113:776.

55. Rostenberg A, Jr. Contact urticaria from food. Arch Dermatol 1970;101:491.

56. Fisher AA. Allergic "protein" contact dermatitis due to foods. Cutis 1975;16:793.

57. Fisher AA, Stengel F. Allergic occupational hand dermatitis to calves' liver: an urticarial "immediate" type hypersensitivity. Cutis 1977;19:561.

58. Hjorth N. Occupational dermatitis in the catering industry. Br J Dermatol 1981;105:37.

59. Maibach H. Immediate hypersensitivity in hand dermatitis. Arch Dermatol 1976;112:1289.

60. Hannuksela M, Lahti A. Immediate reactions to fruits and vegetables. Contact Dermatitis 1977;3:79.

61. Krook G. Occupational dermatitis from Lactuca sativa (lettuce) and Cichorium (endive). Contact Dermatitis 1977;3:27.

62. Sommer RG, Jillson OF. Phytophotodermatitis (solar dermatitis from plants) gas plant and wild parsnip. N Engl J Med 1967;276:1484.

63. Fisher AA. Contact dermatitis due to food additives. Cutis 1975;16:961.

64. Mitchell JC. The skin and food additives. (letter to the editor) Arch Dermatol 1971;104:329.

65. Roed-Petersen H, Hjorth N. Contact dermatitis from antioxidants. Br J Dermatol 1976;94:233.

66. Epstein E. Sodium bisulfite. Contact Dermatitis Newsletter 1970;7:115.

67. Brun R. Eczema de contact à un antioxydant de la margarine (gallate) et changement de métier. Dermatologica 1970;140:390.

68. Liden S. Alphosyl sensitivity. International Symposium on Contact Dermatitis. Gentofte, Denmark, 1974.

69. Fisher AA. Persulfate hair bleach reactions. Arch Dermatol 1976;112:1407.

70. Fisher AA. Hand dermatitis—a "baker's dozen." Cutis 1982;29:214.

71. Fisher AA. Contact dermatitis due to cinnamon and cinnamic aldehyde. Cutis 1975;16:383.

72. Neering H, van Ketel WG. Allergy from spices used in Indonesian cooking. International Symposium on Contact Dermatitis. Gentofte, Denmark, 1974.

73. Inman PM. Dermatitis in a crisp factory. Acta Derm Venereol (Stockh) 1965;45:295.

74. Glickman FS, Silvers SH. Hand eczema and atopy in housewives. Arch Dermatol 1967;95:487.

75. Wechsler AL. Soaps, detergents and hand eruptions. Cutis 1970;6:525.

76. Blohm SG, Lodin A. Eczema of the hands in women: "housewives' eczema." Acta Derm Venereol (Stockh) 1968;48:7.

77. Calnan CD, Bandmann HJ, Cronin E, et al. Hand dermatitis in housewives. Br J Dermatol 1970;82:543.

78. Cronin E. Clinical patterns of hand eczema in women. Contact Dermatitis 1985;13:153.

79. Simon W, Harly J. Skin reactions from gold jewelry contaminated with radon deposit. JAMA 1967;200:254.

80. Leone RA. Radiodermatitis caused by a radioactive gold ring. JAMA 1968;206:2113.

81. Gaul EG. Ring dermatitis. Arch Dermatol Syphilol 1958;77:526.

82. Leider M. Removal of ring from a swollen finger without injuring the ring. J Dermatol Surg Oncol 1980;6:298.

83. Exner FB. Removal of ring from swollen finger. JAMA 1969;210:558.

84. Epstein E. Therapy of recalcitrant hand dermatitis. Cutis 1975;15:347.

85. Osmet LS. Recurrent and recalcitrant vesiculopustular eruptions of the hands. Cutis 1973;11:601.

86. Winkelmann RK, Gleich GJ. Chronic acral dermatitis. JAMA 1973;225:378.

87. Suskind RR. Cutaneous effects of soaps and synthetic detergents. JAMA 1957;163:943.

88. Park KS, Kim YS, Cho YH, et al. Effects of alkalinity of household dishwashing liquids on hand skin. Contact Dermatitis 2001;45:95.

89. Kligman AM, Wooding WM. A method for the measurement and evaluation of irritants on human skin. J Invest Dermatol 1967;49:78.

90. Wood DC, Bettley L. The effect of various detergents on human epidermis. Br J Dermatol 1971;84:320.

91. Glickman FS, Silvers SH. Hand eczema and atopy in housewives. Arch Dermatol 1967;95:487.

92. Matura M, Bodin A, Skare L, et al. Multicentre patch test study of air-oxidized ethoxylated surfactants. Contact Dermatitis 2004;51:180.

93. National Academy of Sciences. Enzyme-containing laundering compounds and consumer health. Washington, DC, 1971:15, 23.

94. Ducksbury CFL, Dave VK. Contact dermatitis in home help following the use of enzyme detergents. Br Med J 1970;1:537.

95. Weill H, Waddell LC, Ziskind M. A study of workers exposed to detergent enzymes. JAMA 1971;217:425.

96. Belin L, Falsen E, Hoborn J, Andre J. Enzyme sensitization in consumers of enzyme-containing washing powders. Lancet 1970;2:1153.

97. Loden M. The effect of four barrier creams on the absorption of water, benzene and formaldehyde into excised human skin. Contact Dermatitis 1986;14:292.

98. Frosch PJ, Schulze-Dirks A, Hoffmann M, et al. Efficacy of skin barrier creams (I). The repetitive irritation test (RIT) in the guinea pig. Contact Dermatitis 1993;28:94.

99. Frosch PJ, Schulze-Dirks A, Hoffmann M, Axthelm I.. Efficacy of skin barrier creams (II). Ineffectiveness of a popular "skin protector" against various irritants in the repetitive irritation test in the guinea pig. Contact Dermatitis 1993;29:74.

100. Boman A, Mellstrom G. Percutaneous absorption of 3 organic solvents in the guinea pig (III): effect of barrier creams. Contact Dermatitis 1989;21:134.

101. Epstein WL. Topical prevention of poison ivy/oak dermatitis. Arch Dermatol 1989;125:499.

102. Orchard S, Fellman JA, Storrs FJ. Poison ivy/oak dermatitis: use of polyamine salts of a linoleic acid dimer for topical prophylaxis. Arch Dermatol 1986;122:783.

103. Smith WB. Lack of efficacy of a barrier cream in preventing Rhus dermatitis. Arch Dermatol 1993;129:787.

104. Arbogast JW, Fendler EJ, Hammond BS, et al. Effectiveness of a hand care regimen with moisturizer in manufacturing facilities where workers are prone to occupational irritant dermatitis. Dermatitis 2004;15:10.

105. Kucharekov M, Van De Kerkhof PCM, Van Der Valk PGM. A randomized comparison of an emollient containing skin-related lipids with a petrolatum-based emollient as adjunct in the treatment of chronic hand dermatitis. Contact Dermatitis 2003;48:293.

106. West DP, Zhu YF. Evaluation of aloe vera gel gloves in the treatment of dry skin associated with occupational exposure. Am J Infect Control 2003;31:40.

107. Pedersen LK, Held E, Johansen JD, et al. Less skin irritation from alcohol-based disinfectant than from detergent used for hand disinfection. Brit J Dermatol 2005;153:1142.

108. Fisher AA. "Hypoallergenic" surgical gloves and gloves for special situations. Cutis 1975;15:797.

109. Pegum JS, Medhurst EA. Contact dermatitis from penetration of rubber gloves by acrylic monomer. Br Med J 1971;2:141.

110. Fisher AA. Contact dermatitis in surgeons. J Dermatol Surg Oncol 1975;1:63.

111. Fries IB, Fisher AA, Salvati EA. Contact dermatitis in surgeons from methylmethacrylate bone cement. J Bone Joint Surg Am 1975;57:547.

112. Tobler M, Freiburghaus AV. A glove with exceptional protective features minimizes the risks of working with hazardous chemicals. Contact Dermatitis 1992;26:299.

113. Moursiden HT, Faber O. Penetration of protective gloves by allergens and irritants. Trans St John's Hosp Dermatol Soc 1973;9:230.

114. Uter W, Pfahlberg A, Gefeller O, et al. Hand dermatitis in a prospectively-followed cohort of hairdressing apprentices: final results of the POSH study. Contact Dermatitis 1999;41:280.

115. McClain TC, Storrs FJ. Protective effect of both a barrier cream and a polyethylene laminate glove against epoxy resin, glyceryl monothioglycolate, frullania, and tansy. Am J Contact Dermat 1992;3:201.

116. Epstein E. Therapy of recalcitrant hand dermatitis. Cutis 1975;15:346.

117. Thomsen K, Mikkelsen HI. Protective capacity of gloves used for handling nitrogen mustard. Contact Dermatitis 1975;1:268.

118. Sansone EB, Tewari YB. The permeability of laboratory gloves to selected solvents. Am Hygiene Assoc J 1978;39:169.

119. Protective gear flunks permeation tests (Editorial). Chemical Week 1981 Feb 25:20.

TEXTILES AND SHOES

EXECUTIVE SUMMARY

A variety of allergens is present in shoes and textiles. Dyes and formaldehyde-related textile finishing resins are of major importance in clothing. Dyes of the "azo" type, used on synthetic fabrics, tend to cause a more acute, florid dermatitis, while textile resins more often account for a smoldering, chronic reaction. Other fabric components such as metal fasteners, elastic, and decorations cause allergy occasionally. Textile allergy often presents as dermatitis predominantly in areas where clothing fits snugly. If formaldehyde is involved, however, allergy to related preservatives in topical products may complicate the picture. Some reports have suggested that the elderly are at greater risk for textile resin sensitization.

Major causes of shoe allergy include rubber, glues, dyes, and leather (usually chromate). There is an interesting variability in frequency of allergy to these components based on geographic location in the world and prevalence of footwear types. Important allergens used to screen for dermatitis to shoes and textiles include formaldehyde, formaldehyde textile resins, disperse dyes, basic dyes, chromate, the rubber allergens, para-tertiary butyl phenol formaldehyde resin (shoe glues), and nickel.

Beyond allergic contact dermatitis (ACD), skin changes from occlusion and friction may occur. Irritant contact dermatitis (ICD) is fairly common with rough fibers like wool and burlap. In textile workers, frictional ICD from repeated rubbing of garments against the hands and arms is not unusual. Folliculitis may result under areas of occlusion, especially in humid climates.

Textile Dermatitis

A variety of allergens may cause ACD from textiles, but the fabrics themselves are very rarely to blame. The "natural" fabrics include vegetable-based fibers such as cotton, linen (flax), hemp, and bamboo, and animal-derived fibers such as silk, fine animal hairs, and wool. Swerev has written an excellent overview of textile fabrics that should be read by any dermatologist with a special interest in the topic.[1]

The vegetable-based fibers may come from the seed (cotton), stalk, leaf, or fruit. Animal fibers include sheep's wool, silk from the silk worm, and fine hairs from many species such as goats (cashmere), camels (alpaca), and rabbit (angora). Animal-derived fibers, like human skin and hair, are composed of keratin. Silk consists of fibroin. The vegetable fibers are composed primarily of cellulose. Manmade or synthetic fibers include regenerated cellulose-based fibers such as acetate and viscose, and chemical-based fibers like polyester, polyamide, acrylic, polypropylene, polyethylene, and others. The chemical-based fibers are generated by polymerization of monomers such as amines, ethylene glycol, and acrylonitrile. Mineral fibers may occasionally be used in textiles such as asbestos, glass, or metals.

Yarns are produced from individual fibers to make woven or knitted fabrics. Nonwoven fabrics are produced by using mechanical, thermal, or chemical bonding procedures. Various chemical and mechanical finishing processes may be performed on the fabrics in order to enhance such qualities as durability, tactile smoothness, and water repellency. The chemicals and dyes used in these processes are usually the cause of ACD to textiles. Synthetic fabrics, such as nylon, rayon, acrylics, and acetates are more commonly are implicated in ACD, not in and of themselves but because of the dyes and finishes often used on them.

Irritant reactions from textiles are not unusual. Wool, of course, may cause irritation with pruritus and a prickly sensation, especially in atopic individuals, but this is unrelated to allergic mechanisms. In addition to ACD and ICD, petechial and urticarial lesions may occur in both textile workers and consumers.

CLINICAL PICTURE OF CLOTHING DERMATITIS

The distribution of the eruption generally conforms to a pattern that coincides with the places on the skin where the garment fits most snugly. Variation in styling of men's and women's clothing explains some differences in distribution. Men might be more likely to have a neck dermatitis from a stiffened dress shirt collar, for example. Dermatitis on the anterior and posterior axillary folds from dress or shirt fabrics is typical for both men and women. Dermatitis on the inner and anterior thighs, as well as on the popliteal fossae, would implicate allergy to pants. Any location where the clothing is held more tightly against the skin is a likely spot for textile dermatitis to occur (Figure 18-1). Patients may often mistake allergy to textile dyes or finishes for allergy to rubber in elastic if dermatitis occurs around the waistline.

Allergy to finishes on bedlinens or furniture fabrics may produce a worsening of dermatitis on the back, posterior legs, or other locations of prominent contact. Warmth and moisture tend to increase the appearance of textile ACD. Because of wearing heavier clothing, textile dermatitis is worse in the winter in some persons. Sparing of parts of the skin protected by underclothing is a distinctive feature of fabric finish and dye-related ACD, but spreading into these areas may occur. Cross-reaction with formaldehyde-based preservatives may complicate the picture by causing dermatitis on the face and hands.[2]

Allergy to rubber additives or natural rubber latex may produce dermatitis around the waist and brassiere straps at sites of elastic contact (Figure 18-2). Belt buckles and metal buttons produce dermatitis at expected contact sites in the nickel-allergic individual.

In general, dermatitis from dyes tends to be acute and rapid in onset.[3] Permanent-press finishes based on formaldehyde resins more commonly produce a smoldering chronic dermatitis. Generalized erythroderma may also result from formaldehyde allergy. Older patients may have a more widespread eruption than younger individuals.[2] Purpuric dermatitis has been reported from allergy to a rubber antiozonant, N-isopropyl-N-phenyl-paraphenylenediamine (IPPD).[4]

Irritant dermatitis (ICD) can occur from frictional irritation or because of the material itself, e.g., wool. In addition, tight clothing may produce follicular irritation with resulting miliaria or folliculitis. Ramam and colleagues from India[5] have reported cases of "frictional sweat dermatitis" occurring in hot summer months, limited to areas of tight clothing. Clinical features include mild stinging or burning and a glazed, wrinkled skin surface with sharp margins. Recovery is spontaneous.

CLOTHING DERMATITIS FROM DETERGENTS AND CONTAMINANTS

In evaluating possible clothing-related dermatitis, it should be remembered that clothing may trap and hold allergens from the environment or workplace. This can be seen in individuals exposed to airborne dusts or oils, for example.

Patients frequently complain that a laundry detergent has caused skin irritation. Often the first item that is changed in the household when someone develops a dermatitis is the laundry detergent. True rates of allergic or irritant reactions, however, have rarely been studied. A report from Great Britain discussed 98 patients with a facial rash that occurred while staying at a holiday resort.[6] The "attack rate" was 7.0 to 14.2 per 1,000 visitors, depending on the site of the accommodations. Replacement of washed bed linens with new ones resulted in total clearing with no new cases. The author concluded that the "rash" was due to irritation from detergent retained in poorly rinsed linens. Enzymes derived from Bacillus subtilis are used in detergents. Although they cause irritant dermatitis and respiratory problems in manufacturers, neither irritant nor allergic reactions attributed to the wearing of clothing washed in these products has been proved with certainty.[7,8]

Fragrances in laundry products are often thought by patients to be a problem, but documentation is difficult. Corea and colleagues point out that an extremely low level of fragrance is likely to be retained on clothing after laundering.[9] They considered the theoretical deposition of fragrance allergens on clothing from laundry products such as fabric softeners and compared this to a calculated level where elicitation of ACD would be likely to occur. For 24 fragrance allergens discussed, they calculated a "margin of safety" of 55 to 17,000 times the expected exposure.

Belsito and members of the NACDG evaluated potential allergy from clothing detergents.[10] Patients (n=738) were tested to a granular and liquid detergent, each at 0.1% aq. Five (0.7%) reacted to the granular detergent and 3 of these to the liquid. All were felt to have current or past relevance. One was allergic to fragrance and none were allergic to nickel or chromate. Two were available for further testing. One showed no reaction to dilutional testing while the other reacted to laundered clothing as well as unlaundered controls, suggesting a nonspecific irritant response. The rate of 0.7% then may actually be too high.

SOFTENERS

Anionic, cationic, and nonionic softeners are used to modify fabric stiffness. Sulfated natural oils and fatty esters (anionic); fatty acid–diethanolamine condensates, quaternary ammonium salts, and cetyl trimethyl bromide (cationic); ethylene oxide condensates (poly-oxyethylene derivatives); and oleic-acid alcohols and esters (nonionic) all exemplify such softeners. Occasionally, these softeners may contain preservatives, probably at levels too low to cause dermatitis. The softener is added to a finishing bath, and modern fabric finishing does not employ after-washes. Any un-cross-linked formaldehyde preservative remaining in the cloth would be eliminated in the first home wash.

Fabric softeners can also be added to apparel in the home. This is often done during a rinse cycle or in the dryer. Patients frequently believe that they are "allergic" to fabric softeners, but this has not been substantiated experimentally. It seems possible, however, that a highly fragrance-allergic patient could react to the perfume left on clothing from a fabric softener.

Poison ivy oleoresin (urushiol) may cling to clothing and retain its dermatitis-producing potential for weeks. In India, ACD (*dhobi* itch) may be produced by laundry markings made with the oleoresin of the India marking nut tree.

Hosiery can be contaminated by chemicals and dyes leached out of shoes. Hosiery dermatitis may, therefore, actually be due to the chemicals in shoes. Fowler has seen cases of ACD in flexural areas especially from allergy to wood dusts that become trapped in clothing and held against the skin.

FIBERS USED IN CLOTHING

In addition to the basic fibers used in textiles, various other components may be added. Elastic fibers are made from either natural rubber or synthetic "snap-back" fibers known as elastomers (spandex). Synthetic elastomers are polyurethanes. Fibers used in some drapery materials and in some industrial cloths can be made of spun glass (fiberglass). Metal fibers used in clothing usually consist of aluminum filaments covered with plastics.[11]

A condensed description of fibers used in clothing is found in Table 18.1.

Current US labeling regulations require that clothing be marked with the content of the various fabrics. Garments are often made from yarns that are formed by combining natural and synthetic fibers into "blends." These blends, as well as the 100% synthetic and natural fibers that are their parents, have many brand names and manufacturers (Table 18.2).

DERMATITIS FROM NATURAL FIBERS

Cotton

Cotton is made from untreated cotton cellulose. Pure cotton has not been reported to cause ACD. One can presume that any cotton fiber that claims crease resistance is treated with a durable or permanent-press finish,

Table 18-1 Fibers Used in Clothing

Type	Generic name	Raw materials
Natural fibers		
Cotton	Cotton	Cellulose
Linen	Linen	Cellulose
Silk	Silk	Protein
Wool	Wool	Protein
Hemp	Hemp	Cellulose
Bamboo	Bamboo	Cellulose
Synthetic fibers		
A. From natural polymers		
Cellulose (1900s)		Wood cellulose
Viscose rayon	Rayon	
Cellulose acetate	Acetate	
Cellulose triacetate	Triacetate	
B. From synthetic polymers		
Condensation polymers		
Polymides (1930s)	Nylon	Petroleum or oat hulls and corncobs
Polyesters (1950s)	Polyester	Petroleum
Polyamide aramid	Nomex	
Vinyl-type addition polymers(1950s) (polyacrylonitriles)		
Vinyl chloride	Modacrylic (35%–85% petroleum acrylonitrile)	
Vinyl cyanide	Acrylic (85% Petroleum acrylonitrile)	
Elastomers		
Polyurethanes	Spandex	Petroleum
Vinylidene chloride	Saran	Petroleum
Polyvinyl alcohol	Vinylon	Petroleum and coke

Table 18-2 Permanent-Press Finishing

Unlikely to be finished with formaldehyde resins

Fabric made totally (100%) of any synthetic (except rayon): nylon, polyester, acrylic, etc.

Silk

Wool

Linen

Cotton denim

100% cotton T-shirts

Any 100% cotton that easily wrinkles

Likely to be finished with formaldehyde resins

Rayon

Polyester/cotton blends

Other synthetic/natural fiber blends

Cotton garments labeled "wash and wear", "no-ironing needed", "wrinkle resistant", etc.

Wrinkle resistant linen

as are many cotton synthetic fiber blends (see section on durable-press finishes). It is impossible to identify with absolute certainty whether a 100% cotton fabric is finish free. Price is not a determinant, although easily wrinkled or shrinkable cottons are less likely to have been treated (Table 18.2).

Genetically enhanced cotton that is less prone to wrinkling is now available, although it does not hold its stiffness as well as fabrics treated with formaldehyde resins.

Cotton "breathes" but does not dissipate perspiration as well as either silk or nylon.[12]

Various chemical and mechanical processes may be applied to cotton. These include sanforizing, mercerizing, and sizing.

1. Sanforizing. This is a controlled-shrinkage process. The yarns are rearranged mechanically and are shortened by the amount they would be if they were laundered. No chemicals are used, and no skin hazard exists. Linen is rarely sanforized.
2. Mercerization. In this finishing process, the cotton is impregnated with a cold, strong (about 25%) sodium hydroxide solution (caustic soda). The process increases the penetrability of finishing resins and dyes and, when done under tension, enhances the fabric's luster. The sodium hydroxide is removed so that no hazard exists to the wearer. Only cotton is mercerized.
3. Sizing. Starch, glues, vegetable gums, rosins, or shellac may be applied to the cotton to impart a stiff, polished, or glazed surface. Organdy, piqué, sheeting, and mosquito netting may be sized. Traces of glues and rosins in sized cotton cloth may produce dermatitis in sensitized individuals.[13] Sizing processes may be used on many fabrics other than cottons.

Linen

This fiber is made from the inner bark of the flax plant. It is treated occasionally with durable-press finishes to combat its tendency to wrinkle. In its unfinished state, it should not cause allergic reactions.

Wool

The warmth, softness, extensibility, ability to felt, and ability to take up a third of its own weight in water without feeling damp are all qualities of wool that have not been duplicated in any synthetic fiber.[11] Fibers derived from natural proteins (Table 18.1) approximate the "handle" of wool but fail to reproduce all of its other merits. These synthetic wools are largely obsolete now. Pure woolen garments are not usually treated with durable-press finishes, but some old patents and

processes do describe the use of formaldehyde on wool to prevent shrinkage and bacterial degradation.[14] Modern wool processing tends to avoid such finishing because it alters the natural handle of wool. Woolen blends may be finished, however.

Allergic dermatitis to natural wool has been very rarely documented.[15] Wool is often included in lists of substances that cause contact urticaria and has been documented to do this at least once.[15–16]

Irritant dermatitis related to wool, particularly in people who have atopic dermatitis, is common.[17] Atopic dermatitis may be aggravated at sites on the body at which wool touches the skin. Smooth and soft fabrics worn between the atopic skin and wool can minimize this aggravation.

Hellier[18] in 1960, and Romaguera and colleagues[19] in 1981 suggested the possibility that purpuric eruptions associated with wool could be related to allergy from a urea or melamine-formaldehyde resin finish. Chromium can be used as a mordant in wool-dyeing processes. Allergic dermatitis in association with the wearing of green woolen military textiles with chrome allergy has been reported.[20]

Silk

Silk is the least extensively used natural fiber.[11] Silk, like other fabrics, may be sold under several names, including crepe, satin, chiffon, taffeta, and jersey.

Contact urticaria caused by silk has been reported.[21] In a case from Japan, with allergy to silk undergarments, scratch tests were positive to sericin 5% aqueous, raw silk, and silkworm cocoon. Lymphocyte stimulation tests to sericin was positive.[22] Allergic reactions to silk are rare, however, and the nature of the allergen is disputed.[23] The proteinaceous silk fiber (fibroin), the gum or glue (sericin) in raw silk, and the silkworm protein are the antigen candidates. Silk used as a filter for biological products may cause anaphylaxis.[24]

Hemp and Bamboo

Hemp and bamboo fibers may be extracted from the stems of the plants and woven into clothing.[25] To our knowledge, ACD to these fibers has not been reported.

DERMATITIS FROM SYNTHETIC FIBERS (RAYON, NYLON, POLYESTER, AND ACRYLICS)

Until 1971, nylon led the synthetic fiber market, but since then the polyesters and polyacrylonitrites have surpassed nylon.[11] Nylon, Dacron, and Orlon have been the backbone of the synthetic fiber industry for 50 years.[11] One would expect that as oil reserves decrease, more cellulose-based fibers would be made. Cellulose-based Rayon constitutes a minority of synthetic fiber production, however.

Despite the prevalence of synthetic fibers, allergic reactions to untreated synthetic fibers are rare. Allergic contact dermatitis to virgin nylon has been reliably reported once in the United States and twice in Europe.[26,27] One case of allergy to nylon-6 from Japan gave a positive patch test to the nylon monomer epsilon-aminocaproic acid (3% pet).[28] A similar case has been reported from Spain. A textile factory worker was allergic to epsilon-caprolactin (5% pet) used in the synthesis of nylon-6.[29]

Nylon is not very absorbent, and thus a freely perspiring individual may complain of pruritus and dermatitis from the maceration and irritation of unabsorbed sweat when he or she wears nylon garments. Pure rayons and polyester are not known as allergens. One report has been made of an allergy related to an acrylonitrile used in a finger splint.[30] Five workers in a factory producing acrylonitrile (CH_2CHCN) for use in synthetic fibers developed ACD. All gave 3+ reactions to acrylonitrile 0.1% petrolatum. The guinea pig maximization test (GPMT) showed that acrylonitrile has strong allergenic potential.[31]

The vinylidene chloride polymers (saran) are used occasionally in belts, suspenders, and raincoats. Dermatitis has been reported in association with Saran Wrap.[32] Other vinyl plastics such as polyvinyl chloride may find occasional use in swimwear or as identification armbands. Unexplained irritant dermatitis was reported in seven children wearing such armbands.[33] Plasticizers added to the vinyl chlorides (dibutyltin maleate, dibutyl sebacate, dibutyl phthalate, dioctyl phthalate, and epoxy resins) are usually the explanation for both irritant and allergic reactions attributed to the plastic fabrics[34] (see Chapter 27).

Contact Urticaria from Nylon

A 21-year-old woman reported urticaria with pruritus within 15 minutes of putting on nylon panties or stockings. Immediate patch tests was repeatedly positive to dye-free nylon.[35]

DERMATITIS FROM RUBBER AND ELASTOMERS IN CLOTHING

Spandex (an anagram of "expands") is a polyurethane-based synthetic polymer that substitutes for rubber. The major tradename is Lycra. Pure spandex fibers have not been proven to cause dermatitis. In the past, spandex fibers were treated with mercaptobenzothiazole (MBT). Allergy to this accelerator explained some ACD associated with elastic undergarments.[36] More recently, a benzotriazole

chemical (Tinuvin P) used in spandex in underwear caused one case of ACD (personal communication, FJ Storrs, MD, 1984). Spandex is lighter and whiter than rubber, and its advantages suit its use in underclothes and swimsuits. It is an excellent rubber substitute for people who are sensitive to rubber additives. Antioxidants such as butylated hydroxytoluene also may be used on spandex to prevent deterioration.

Clothing containing rubber, including elastic, can cause dermatitis in rubber-allergic people. Usually this is due to allergy to thiurams, carbamates, mercaptos or possibly thioureas. Thioureas are used increasingly in the production of neoprene rubber and in elastic in underwear (see Chapter 29).

Several rarer explanations have arisen for rubber-related clothing contact dermatitis. IPPD (also called 4-isopropylaminodiphenylamine or isopropylphenyl p-phenylenediamine [PPD]) is an antiozonant and antioxidant used in the rubber industry. Allergy to IPPD explained a purpuric eczematous dermatitis in 23 patients caused by the elastic in their undergarments.[37] IPPD can cross-react with PPD, and patch test reactions to both of these chemicals can be petechial or purpuric.[4,38] IPPD imparts a black or gray color to rubber treated with it, although this color can be masked by weaving the elastic fibers into other material.[38] Fisher[39] has noted reactions to IPPD used in a rubber diving suit, in elasticized shorts, and in a rubberized leg support bandage. IPPD can also cross-react with some azo dyes used in textiles.

Elasticized clothing may also cause skin eruptions as a consequence of mechanical pressure. Pressure urticaria, acneiform eruptions, exaggeration of preexisting dermatoses, and nondescript erythematous changes may develop at skin sites at which clothing fits too snugly.[40] Pressure dermatographism may be persistent.

Wearing underclothing made of spandex usually prevents ACD in individuals sensitive to rubber accelerators and antioxidants. Pure cotton French-cut boxer shorts, which button and contain no elastic, are sold by retail stores and in catalogs.

Jordan and Bourlas[41] reported ACD to underwear elastic that resulted only when the undergarment was bleached. The rubber accelerator, zinc dibenzyldithio-carbamate, present in the elastic, formed eight reaction products in the presence of sodium hypochlorite (bleach). One of these reaction products, N,N-dibenzylcarbamyl chloride, was the sensitizer. Sensitized individuals who wore unbleached underwear avoided the dermatitis.

FIBERGLASS DERMATITIS

Glass can be spun into a fiber and woven into a fabric. It has not been used in garments, fortunately. Glass cloth is used as a fireproof material in curtains, lampshades, furniture covers, and awnings. It has some use in construction as well as for wrapping wires and in insulation.

Fiberglass is an irritant. It has caused a pseudoclothing dermatitis when fabrics made of fiberglass were washed in an automatic washing machine with a family's clothes.[42] The glass fibers can become embedded in the nonglass garments and subsequently cause a papular, pruritic dermatitis that can resemble scabies. This dermatitis is most likely to be caused by large glass fibers. Small fibers may contact the skin and cause no difficulty. When the lesions are biopsied, glass particles may be seen in foreign body granulomas.[43] It is sometimes possible to see fiberglass fragments in a potassium hydroxide preparation taken from scrapings of the involved skin.[44]

Although the fiberglass itself does not cause ACD, it can be finished with formaldehyde resins like other synthetic fibers. An allergic reaction to such a finish used on fiberglass wool has been noted.[45] Fisher[46] has reviewed the similarities and differences between rockwool (mineral wool) dermatitis and fiberglass dermatitis (see Chapter 27).

DERMATITIS FROM PERMANENT-PRESS TEXTILE RESINS

Fabric treatment with formaldehyde was first discussed about 100 years ago.[14] In the 1930s, N-methylol (formaldehyde) compounds derived from urea and melamine formaldehyde polycondensation products were polymerized within the interstices of cellulose fibers. The desired property of wrinkle resistance was offset by a tendency of the resins to absorb chlorine from bleaches. The resultant chloramides produced yellowing, breakdown with heat (ironing), and eventual weakening of the fabric. An undesirable amount of formaldehyde was released from the resins during manufacture, storage, and wear.[47]

In the 1950s and 1960s, escalation in the development of synthetic fibers (Table 18.1) and then mixing (blending) with cellulose (cotton and rayon) was accompanied by the introduction of the cyclic ethylene and propylene urea compounds (Table 18.3). These resins represented an improvement over the condensation resins in that they combine directly with the cellulose fiber. They release less formaldehyde, and are more wash and chlorine fast. Etherified glyoxal reactant modifications of these cyclic ureas (Table 18.3) are used today and have further decreased formaldehyde release from fabric-finishing resins.

Alteration in the handle of cellulose (cotton, rayon) or cellulose synthetic fiber blends is the result of the development of covalent cross-linkages that develop between the cellulose and the N-methylol (formaldehyde) finishing compounds. Synthetic fibers that are 100% noncellulose (i.e., synthetics) do not require finishing

Table 18-3 Cross-Linking Fabric Finishing Agents (Permanent Press)
Polycondensation polymers (1930s)
Urea formaldehyde (dimethylol urea) (DMU)
Melamine (MF)
Linear reactants
Dimethylol carbamates
Cyclic ureas
N-methylol propyl ene urea derivatives:
-dimethylolpropylene urea (DMPU)
-dimethylolethylene urea (DMEU)
Dimethyloldihydroxyethylene urea (DMDHEU)
Dimethoxymethyl dihydroxyethylene urea (1980s) (methylated DMDHEU)
Uron formaldehyde
N,N-bis-(methoxymethyl) uron (UF)
N,N-dimethyl-4,5 dihydroxyethylene (DHDMI)

with formaldehyde resins. The resins are incapable of chemically cross-linking 100% synthetic fibers. Wool can be treated with N-methylol resin to prevent shrinkage. Because the treatment alters the desired natural handle of wool, it is seldom done. Silk is not treated, because the process can actually injure the fibers.[11]

The reaction is driven by heat during curing. If some acid catalyst remains in the fabric and if no washing or formaldehyde scavenging is done after curing, then hydrolysis can occur under warm, humid conditions. The finishing reaction is reversed and formaldehyde is released. An even more important reason for formaldehyde release from fabric is the failure of some resin to fully cross-link.

By 1981, the textile industry was able to claim that levels of formaldehyde release had decreased to the point that 100 to 200 ppm rather than 200 ppm was the rule.[48] This would provide a level of 0.1 ppm in the air of a textile factory, which is well within NIOSH's (National Institute of Occupational Safety & Health) recommended level of 1 ppm.[49] Most of this decrease is probably due to preparation of purer resins and use of less of them. Additionally, the use of methylated dimethyloldihydroxyethylene urea (DMDHEU) (see Table 18.3) eliminates or decreases the NCH_2OH groups in the finish and, thus, the main source of formaldehyde release.[49]

In 1975, the Japanese Department of Health and Welfare restricted the content of formaldehyde in underclothes to less than 75 ppm for adults and to less than 15 ppm for babies.[50] Before the restriction, some Japanese textiles contained more than 10,000 ppm formaldehyde. Formaldehyde and formaldehyde donor release are also restricted in Japanese cosmetics.

The textile resins now in use in the United States are listed in Table 18.3.

CLINICAL AND PATCH-TEST FINDINGS IN TEXTILE RESIN ALLERGY

The most recent NACDG data indicate a rate of positive patch tests to formaldehyde (1% aq) of 8.7% of 5,142 patients. Ethyleneurea melamine formaldehyde resin (ETUMFR) was positive in 2.0% and DMDHEU was positive in 0.8%.[51]

Marcussen,[52] in Denmark, saw 26 patients with formaldehyde textile allergy between 1934 and 1958. He tested formaldehyde at a concentration of 4%, which may have produced some false-positive irritant reactions. In Norway, Hovding[53] found free formaldehyde between 5,000 and 12,000 ppm in 227 of the 256 rayon and cotton samples he analyzed in 1959. Hovding[54] reported 45 patients whom he saw between 1953 and 1958 among 2,110 routinely patch-tested patients who were formaldehyde sensitive and who had a dermatitis in a clothing distribution.

Cronin,[55] in England, saw 30 patients who had a textile dermatitis not caused by dyes between 1953 and 1961. She saw an additional 33 patients from 1970 to 1976. Patch tests to pieces of suspect clothing were often negative, but these same pieces of clothing gave positive chemical reactions for formalin.[55] In 1964, Berrens and colleagues[56] also noted that patients in the Netherlands who were sensitive to formaldehyde (even to concentrations as low as 0.3% to 0.03%) would usually not react to pieces of suspect clothing, even when it was shown to contain formaldehyde. Avoidance of the formaldehyde-containing clothing, however, resulted in resolution of their dermatitis.

Further, Fisher and colleagues,[57] in 1962, could not make formaldehyde-positive patients in the United States react to pieces of fabric known to contain formaldehyde. The U.S. patients did not have dermatitis in a clothing pattern, and these authors concluded that American fabrics contained too little formaldehyde release to cause dermatitis. Fisher's patients were chosen, however, for their formaldehyde sensitivity rather than for their clothing distribution. Fisher and colleagues[57] believed that the few U.S. cases could be explained by the fact that after-washing was more common in the finishing process in the United States than it was in Europe.

In 1964, Malten[58] in the Netherlands tested 66 patients who had a suspected textile-finish hypersensitivity dermatitis. Of these 66 patients, 27 reacted to at least one of the 37 substances that were being used in textile finishing. Only seven of the patients reacted to formaldehyde.

A most interesting group of formaldehyde-negative, resin-finish-positive patients appeared in Canada in 1973.[59,60] These 11 patients developed an extensive pruritic, follicular eczema after sleeping in colored Wabasso polyester/cotton bedsheets. None of the 11 patients were positive to formaldehyde, nor were 39 additional patients reported from London in 1976 after similar offending sheets were distributed in England.[61] Six of the Canadian patients had positive patch tests to white pieces of their own sheets.[59] Five of the six reacted to the raw permapress resin (*N,N*-dimethylol-4-methoxy-5,5-dimethyl propylene urea).[60] Allergens useful for patch testing for textile-resin allergy are noted in Table 18.4.

A dramatic change in this trend was reported by Fowler and colleagues.[2] In a period of 28 months, 17 cases of formaldehyde resin allergy were diagnosed from among 1,022 patients tested in Louisville, Kentucky, and New York City. Clinical data are given in Table 18.5. Five had occupationally related disease. The others tended to be older and to have widespread dermatitis. Only 12 reacted to formaldehyde (1% aq). Twelve also reacted to formaldehyde-related preservatives. Ethylene urea melamine formaldehyde resin (EUMFR) (Fixopret AC) (10% pet) was the best screening agent, with 14 positives (82%). The authors theorized that a trend toward using imported textiles, even if the finished garment is made in the United States, may account for this upsurge in cases. Alternatively, cases of generalized dermatitis may have previously gone unrecognized as being caused by textile resins. A lack of suspicion of textile allergy may lead to inappropriate withholding of patch testing. Even if patch testing is done, some patients who are formaldehyde negative may be missed on limited screening.

Sherertz[62] reported that 10 of 11 patients with clothing allergy to formaldehyde compounds reacted to urea

Table 18-4 Patch Testing for Textile Resin Allergy

Allergen	Concentration	Brial	Chemo technique	Hermal
Formaldehyde*	1% aq	X	X	X
Dimethylol dihydroxyethylene urea	4.5% aq	X	X	
Dimethyl dihydroxy thyleneurea	4.5% aq		X	
Dimethylol dihydroxyethyle neurea, modified	5% aq		X	
Ethyleneurea, melamine for maldehyde*	5% pet	X	X	
Urea formaldehyde	10% pet		X	
Melamine formaldehyde	7% pet		X	

* Most important for screening

Table 18-5 Clinical Patterns of Textile Resin ACD

Patients tend to be older, with no gender predilection

Face, hand, feet usually spared unless allergic also to formaldehyde-releasing preservatives (FRPs)

Frequent reaction to FRPs (especially quaternium-15)

About 30% negative to formaldehyde alone

Areas of tight clothing (e.g., waist, shoulders, thighs) usually the worst

May go misdiagnosed as scabies, neurodermatitis, etc., for months or years

Itching generally severe

Clinical pattern is that of a chronic, lichenified dermatitis, sometimes nummular dermatitis

formaldehyde resin, but only 8 reacted to formaldehyde 1% aqueous.

From the hot and humid climes of New Orleans, 24 cases of formaldehyde textile resin allergy were identified.[63] Seven were negative and 1 doubtful to formaldehyde (1% aq). All reacted to DMPU (5% aq).

A more recent report from Cleveland shows that the problem of ACD to textile resins is not decreasing.[64] The authors found that 7.2% of 852 patients tested over a 4.5 year period were positive to formaldehyde (1% aq). ETUMFR was positive in 2.0% and DMDHEU was positive in 2.3%, including several who were negative to formaldehyde. The authors contacted clothing manufacturers and give a list of clothing makers who claim their products are very low in formaldehyde and therefore may be less likely to cause ACD in formaldehyde-sensitive patients.

In addition to dermatitis, formaldehyde can cause urticaria.[65] One case of severe contact urticaria associated with formaldehyde used in leather dresses has been reported from Finland.[66]

Jordan and colleagues[67] identified patients who gave allergic responses to aqueous formaldehyde patch tests in concentrations as low as 30 ppm (0.003%). One of their patients could predictably identify (by the development of itching without an observable skin reaction) solutions sprayed into his axilla containing 30 ppm of formaldehyde. No lower concentrations were tested, but Jordan has theorized that sensitive formaldehyde-allergic people might itch without urtication or eczematization from even lower concentrations (WP Jordan, personal communication, 1984). This suggests that for some of our patients, even brief contact with garments containing formaldehyde can reactivate ACD.

CONSEQUENCES OF DURABLE-PRESS ALLERGIC CONTACT DERMATITIS

If a person is sensitized to FTRs and not to formaldehyde itself, simple avoidance of the relevant fabrics should bring relief.[59–61] When formaldehyde allergy is at the root of the

problem, however, the consequences can be more far-reaching. Formaldehyde-sensitive people, for example, can react to a series of formaldehyde related preservatives (FRPs) that are used as biocides both in cosmetics and in industry.[68]

The decrease in the incidence of formaldehyde allergy in Japan coincident with restrictions on its use has been noted. The NACDG has noted an increase in formaldehyde allergy from 3.4% in 1974 to 6.7% in 1980 to 9.3 % in 1998[51,69,70] and 8.7% in 2004. Most of this increase was attributed to formaldehyde releasers in cosmetics. A review of the incidence of positive reactors to various allergens around the world gives formaldehyde ratings from 1.3% (Spain) to 7.0% (Japan in 1976).[69] Most Western countries show reaction rates between 4% and 5% for formaldehyde.[69–71]

PATCH TESTING FOR DURABLE-PRESS ALLERGY

Although formaldehyde identifies about 60 to 70% of people who are allergic to fabric-finishing *N*-methylol resins, it is obvious from the foregoing discussion that some people will be missed if the resins are not tested as well. The fabric is often negative on testing. Soaking the fabric in water for 10 minutes before it is applied may produce more positive reactions.

Patch testing with the substances identified in Table 18.4 should detect most ACD caused by permanent-press finishes. Currently, the NACDG uses ETUMFR (5% pet) and DMDHEU (4.5% pet) as screening agents for textile allergy. Scheman and colleagues[72] recommend the latter.

In most centers, formaldehyde is tested at 1% aqueous. Fowler has not infrequently seen cases of negative reactions to 1% but definite, relevant positives to 2% aqueous. Therefore, if formaldehyde allergy is strongly suspected, testing should be done with both 1% and 2% concentrations. Conversely, the physician must remember that 2% and occasionally 1% formaldehyde may give a mild irritant reaction. This usually appears as a "glazed" appearance at the site with very mild erythema but without induration or papules. This irritant reaction is not indicative of allergy.

METHODS FOR DETECTING FORMALDEHYDE IN TEXTILES

Various methods have been used in the past to determine free formaldehyde release from fabrics, but there are no practical testing methods for physicians or their patients known to the authors. The reader is referred to previous editions of this text if more information on testing is desired.

Such analyses done in 1960 showed 3,900 to 6,200 ppm of formaldehyde released from various resin-treated fabrics. This could be reduced to 1,500 to 3,500 ppm by an afterwash.[47] Schorr and colleagues[73] looked at 112 randomly selected American fabrics in 1974. The treating resin used was not determined, but in general the authors verified that finished cellulose and blends could release up to 3,600 ppm of formaldehyde by the chromotropic acid method. One hundred percent synthetics released 1 to 2 ppm of formaldehyde, which could well have been from biocides in the softeners used on their surfaces.

MANAGEMENT OF CLOTHING DERMATITIS ASSOCIATED WITH PERMANENT-PRESS FINISHES LIKELY TO RELEASE FORMALDEHYDE

These patients are some of the most miserable contact allergy sufferers because of ubiquitous exposure to the allergens. Often systemic corticosteroids are required for temporary relief. Even after good efforts at allergen avoidance, some individuals may require several months to completely clear. Counseling and encouragement are especially critical at this stage. Other systemic therapy such as psoralen plus ultraviolet light A (PUVA) or immunosuppressive agents may be necessary in some cases of formaldehyde dermatitis.

Table 18.6 lists several instructions for formaldehyde- or textile resin-allergic patients.

Wearing an undergarment made of cotton or silk may allow formaldehyde and formaldehyde-resin-sensitive people to wear treated clothing temporarily. Fowler found silk to be better for this purpose. Cool weather also allows sensitive people to wear treated clothing that

Table 18-6 Instructions for Formaldehyde Resin Patients

1. Avoid permanent-press, wrinkle-resistant clothing and bed linens as much as possible. If necessary to wear such garments, wear only cool, loose-fitting items for short time periods. Perspiration and heat make the problem worse.
2. Wash *all* new textile products, permanent-press or not, at least twice before using.
3. Soft, easily wrinkled fabrics are safest. Avoid heavy, stiff fabrics.
4. Most blended fabrics (e.g., polyester-cotton) are likely to be treated with resins and should generally be avoided.
5. Silk, linen, wool, denim, and pure 100% synthetics such as nylon or acrylics or polyester are unlikely to be treated and are almost always safe.
6. Rayon blends, corduroy, and "shrink-proof" wool should be avoided.
7. Cotton that is mercerized or sanforized is safe because these finishes do not use formaldehyde.

they cannot tolerate when they are sweating in hot weather.

DERMATITIS FROM TEXTILE ADDITIVES OTHER THAN DURABLE-PRESS FINISHES

Numerous chemicals other than cross-linking durable-press finishes are applied to textiles to alter the fabrics' "hand" and to impart special characteristics. These include softeners, weighters, acrylic and vinyl hand modifiers, water repellents, biocides, antistats, soil retardants, mothproofers, antislip finishes, and fire retardants. Once clothing is manufactured, it may be treated with spot removers and drycleaning agents.

Isophoronediamine (IPDA), used as an epoxy resin hardener, caused occupational ACD in a worker using it to manufacture water-resistant fabric.[74] The cloth was intended for use in hospital garments and drapes where blood and water resistance was needed.

Oilcloth

Foussereau and colleagues[75] found that allergy to alpha-phenyl-indole explained a dermatitis to American oilcloth in 11 of 18 patients whom they studied. Twenty patients reacted to the entire cloth. This report highlights the fact that although they are most unusual, chemicals other than formaldehyde-releasing fabric finishes are used on fabrics and should, on occasion, be considered when evaluating a baffling case of clothing-related dermatitis.

Biocides

Biocides are used to inhibit mildew growth and thus prevent the rotting of fabrics likely to be used outdoors. Tributyl tin, copper-8-quinolate, zinc naphthenate, organomercury compounds, quaternary ammonium compounds, phenols and chlorophenols, zinc dimethyl dithiocarbamate, zinc-2-mercaptobenzothiazole, and even neomycin have all been used as biocides on textiles in the United States. Fabrics used by the military and canvas fabrics likely to be used for outdoor recreational use may contain biocides. Molin and Wahlberg[76] reported 70 soldiers who developed an irritant dermatitis on their feet when tribrityltin oxide was used in excess to disinfect their socks.

Spin Finishes

Biocides can also be used in spin finishes, which are complex aqueous emulsions of oils, waxes, surfactants, and biocides used on synthetic fibers to reduce friction and static. Savage[77] suggested but did not prove that methylol chloracetamide (Grotan HD) caused an allergic hand dermatitis in seven nylon yarn workers who used a nylon spin finish. Burrows and Campbell[78] felt that the ten dermatitis patients whom they saw who developed problems after polyester spin finish exposure had an irritant rather than an allergic contact dermatitis. Their patients' patch test reactions were equivocal. Methylene bisthiocyanate, mixed halogenated amides, N-methylolchloraretamide, and dimethoxane were the biocides used in the spin finishes that they studied. An isothiazolone biocide (Kathon 930) caused hand dermatitis in eight textile workers. The substance was used in a finishing rinse. Interestingly, the patients did not cross-react to Kathon CG.[79] In most instances, biocides are added to fabric-finishing compounds in concentrations so low that even patients who are sensitive to a particular chemical have no problem with fabrics so treated.[80]

An English textile worker developed ACD from the biocide N,N-methylene bis-5-methyloxazolidine, used in a nylon spin finish. Testing was positive at 1% aq. This is a formaldehyde-releaser also known as Grotan OX. This patient was not allergic to formaldehyde.[29]

Soil Retardants and Stain Repellents

Antistatic compounds help reduce soiling. Colloidal alumina, titanium alkylates, methyl and ethyl silica, and fatty alcohol–ethylene oxide condensates also assist in the removal of stains. One patient has been described who had an apparent allergic reaction to Scotchgard, which contained a fluorocarbon, acrylates, and rubber materials. The sensitizer was not identified.[81]

Antipill Finish

The tendency of some fabric to produce tiny balls on the surface with friction or wear is called "pilling." An antipill finish, Evafanol-AS-1, containing 1,6-diisocyanatohexane, caused dermatitis in 11 workers at two factories making dresses. This constituted 10% of the workforce. Testing was done at 1% aqueous strength. Another name for this agent is hexamethylene diisocyanate.[82]

MISCELLANEOUS SOURCES OF POTENTIAL ALLERGY AND IRRITATION IN CLOTHING

Epoxies

Taylor and colleagues[83] described three boys who developed ACD on their knees that was caused by an epoxy resin (Epon 825) used as a knee-patch adhesive constituent. Epoxies are seldom if ever used now as part of the durable-press finishing of fabrics, although they had some use in the past. Fowler has seen cases of epoxy allergy in workers handling canvas tent fabric, with documentation of the presence of epoxy resin in the fabric.

Flame Retardants

Some fabrics such as brushed nylon and wool have an innate flame resistance.[11] Polyvinyl chloride fiber and to some extent the modacrylics are flameproof as well.[11] Melamineformaldehyde resins also enhance the flame resistance of polyester blends.

Nomex is a synthetic polyamide aramid made by DuPont. Nomex 111A is a blend of Nomex, Kevlar, and carbon core nylon with inherent flame resistance. It is said to be unaffected by most bleaches, solvents, and acids. Vinex is another inherently flame-resistant fabric made of Vinal (a polyvinylalcohol-treated polymer).[84]

Flame-retardant chemicals are used in textiles, carpets, home furnishings, plastics, paints, adhesives, and construction materials. A flame retardant composed of 23-bromocresylglycidyl ether caused severe ACD in a worker after an accidental exposure. It is uncertain whether this is used on textiles.[85]

Durable flame-retardant chemicals contain phosphorus, nitrogen, chlorine, or bromine. Flame retardants decrease flammability by favoring charring as well as by facilitating the snuffing of a flame in their volatile phase.

A flame retardant that has been indicted as a relevant contact allergen is Proban, a polymer produced by cross-linking the condensate of tetrakis (hydroxymethyl) phosphonium chloride (THPCL) and urea with ammonia followed by oxidation.[86]. Proban-induced dermatitis and urticaria were suspected by Martin-Scott[86] in two children who gave positive patch test reactions to Proban-treated fabric. They were not tested to Proban itself.

The International Contact Dermatitis Research Group included Firemaster LVT 23P in 5% petrolatum in its standard series of patch tests for a limited period of time to determine the incidence of sensitization against Firemaster. Of 1,103 individuals tested, 2 showed a positive response (Maibach H, personal communication, 1986).

Belsito[87] reported 12 patients with ACD from diammonium hydrogen phosphate (DAP) used as a flame retardant in hospital surgical caps. The 100% rayon caps apparently had excessive levels of DAP. Patch testing was done with DAP (0.5% aq).

If the tetrakis phosphonium compounds are applied to cotton or rayon fabrics in their hydroxide form, they react within cellulose to form firm covalent cross-links with themselves. Commercial THPCL has been reported to contain free formaldehyde, and formaldehyde can be recovered from extracts of fabrics that have been cross-linked with THPCL.[88,89] One of Martin-Scott's[86] two fabric-positive patients were also formaldehyde patch test positive.

Manufacturers of flame-retardant fabrics indicate that free formaldehyde may be found on the surface of such textiles in concentrations of up to 500 ppm. This is especially true of tetrakis compounds but may occur with other treated fabrics as well. This formaldehyde is not cross-linked within the cellulosics, and the flame-retardant industry feels that it washes out readily.

Dry-Cleaning Preparations

The chemicals used in dry cleaning are irritants but are probably only rare allergens. Perchloroethylene (PCE, tetrachloroethylene) is used for most closed-machine dry cleaning and also for metal degreasing.[90] TCE is a central nervous system depressant. Six cases of textile dermatitis were reported in a semiconductor manufacturing facility. The problem was traced to high residual levels of perchloroethylene in dry-cleaned uniform coats. The dermatitis produced was probably irritant rather than allergic contact.[91] Other commonly used dry-cleaning compounds include trifluorotrichloroethane (Arklone and Valclene) and trichloroethylene (Trilene). All of these dry-cleaning compounds are irritating and volatile. If garments are properly aired before being worn, they should cause no difficulty.

A Japanese report described three patients with bullous dermatitis, presumed to be irritant, from dry-cleaned clothing. The cleaning agent was not perchloroethylene but rather a "petrolatum solvent" composed of paraffins or paraffin plus naphtens.[92]

Spot Removers

Powerful skin irritants such as hydrofluoric acid, glacial acetic acid, carbolic acid, nitrobenzene, and strong alkalis can also find occasional use as spot removers. Van Ketel[93] described two women employees in the clothing industry who developed hand dermatitis while working with stain removers containing hydrazine. They both had positive patch test reactions to hydrazine sulfate 1% in H_2O. They were of special interest in that they showed crossreactivity to other hydrazine derivatives such as apresoline, phenylhydrazine-HCl, and isoniazid.

DYES

Textile fibers have been dyed by people for thousands of years. Natural indigo was known in several parts of the world by 2000 B.C.[94]

As more synthetic fibers were developed in the 1930s and 1950s (Table 18.1), dye technology became more complex in an effort to meet new fiber requirements. Nylon stockings were introduced into the United States in 1939, and shortly thereafter contact dermatitis caused by nylon stocking dyes was reported. Although this problem is much less prevalent now, even at its height its incidence was estimated to be no more than one case of dermatitis for every 13,309,000 pairs of nylon stockings sold.[95]

Textile dye chemistry classification is complex. Different types of fabrics can be dyed with different chemical entities, so knowledge of the fiber type in a textile is critical. A list of many allergenic dyes is given in Table 18.7.

Disperse Dyes (Plastosoluble Dyes)

In 2004, the worldwide production of disperse dyes was listed as 180,000 tons.[96] These are used to dye synthetics, especially polyesters and acetates; also used on triacetate polyamides and polyacrylonitriles, in printing, and on some plastics. Disperse dyes present as colloidal dispersions; the dye dissolves into the fabric. They come from azoic anthraquinone and nitroarylamine chemical classes. This dye class is the principal source of ACD.

Hatch and Maibach[97,98] in 1995 and again in 1999 reviewed textile dye allergy. It is clear from these reviews that almost all of the sensitizing dyes belong to the disperse group and that the azo and anthraquinone dyes in this group sensitize more often. Although disperse dyes were developed for use on synthetic fibers, it is difficult to make them fast to the fiber, which may well relate to their tendency to sensitize.

Among Cronin's[3] 16 original patients, a disperse dye was identified as the sensitizer in 14. Four patients were allergic only to anthraquinone dyes, three only to azo dyes, two to both anthraquinone dyes and azo dyes, and three to dyes of different groups. Cross-reactions to paraphenylenediamine (PPDA) were found in 85% of Cronin's azo dye-positive patients, whereas such crossreactivity was all but nonexistent in the other groups. Other authors have since shown, however, that PPDA alone is not a good screen for dye allergy. Seidenari and colleagues[99] found only 20 PPDA reactors in 100 patients. Many of his patients were allergic to azo dyes, which theoretically may cross-react with PPDA but apparently did not do so clinically. Likewise, Pratt reported that only 8 of 40 patients with textile dye allergy reacted to PPDA.[100] These findings highlight the inadvisability of relying on a PPDA patch test reaction to identify clothing dye contact dermatitis. Cronin's initial series also made it clear that the color of the culprit dye often bears no relationship to the color of the offending garment. Thus, a purple suit caused a dermatitis from a disperse yellow dye used as one component of the final purple color.

Cronin[101] also described 21 women and 26 men who had one or more relevant positive reactions to one of a series of routinely tested clothing dyes. Disperse Blue 124

Table 18-7 Some Fabric Dyes Known to Be Potentially Allergenic

Textile class (generic number)	Color index (C.I.) number	Color index chemical class
Disperse Yellow 1	10345	Nitro
Disperse Yellow 3	11855	Azo
Disperse Yellow 4	12770	Azo
Disperse Yellow 9	10375	Nitro
Disperse Yellow 39	—	Indo lindigo
Disperse Yellow 49	—	Methine
Disperse Yellow 54	—	Quinoline
Disperse Yellow 64	47023	Quinoline
Disperse Orange 1	11080	Azo
Disperse Orange 3	11005	Azo
Disperse Orange 13	—	—
Disperse Orange 76	—	Monoazo
Disperse Red 1	11110	Monoazo
Disperse Red 11	62015	Aq
Disperse Red 15	60710	Aq
Disperse Red 17	11210	Monoazo
Disperse Red 55	—	Aq
Disperse Blue 1	64500	Aq
Disperse Blue 3	61505	Aq
Disperse Blue 7	62500	Aq
Disperse Blue 26	63305	Aq
Disperse Blue 35	—	Aq
Disperse Blue 85	11370	Azo
Disperse Blue 106	—	Azo
Disperse Blue 124	—	Monoazo
Disperse Black 1	11365	Azo
Disperse Black 2	11255	Azo
Disperse Brown 1	—	—
Acid Black 48	65005	Aq
Acid Yellow 23	19140	Azo
Acid Yellow 159	—	Disazo
Acid Yellow 198	—	Disazo
Acid Red 151	26900	Disazo
Acid Blue 40	62125	Aq
Acid Violet 17	42650	—
Basic Red 46	—	—
Vat Green 1	59825	Aq
Wool Red B	—	—
Solvent Yellow 1	11000	Azo
Foron Blue	—	Aq
Black Base 1	—	—
Acid Yellow 61	18968	Azo
Acid Red 118	—	Azo
Direct Orange 34	40215	Azo
Acid Red 359	—	Azo
Reactive Red 238	—	—
Reactive Violet 5	—	—
Reactive Blue 122	—	—
Reactive Black 5	20505	—
Reactive Yellow 17	18852	—

(azo dye) was the most frequent sensitizer among the women and Disperse Orange 76 (azo dye) among the men. Pratt's article gives detailed results on textile dye ACD.[100] Of 271 patients for which she had some suspicion of textile ACD, 40 were positive to dyes. Disperse blue 106 was positive in 33 (82.5%) and Disperse Blue 124 in 32. Disperse Red 1 and 17 each gave reactions in 10 (25%) patients. Thirty-five of her patients were female. Ten of 11 reacted to clothing pieces, nine to dark colored acetate or polyester clothing liners, and one to an acetate/cotton blend. Eighteen (45%) reacted to "para" group allergens such as PPDA, IPPD, benzocaine, or para-aminophenol. All of her patients had moderate to severe acute or subacute eczema.

In 1972, Sim-Davies[102] reported 15 men, age 21 to 73, who were all allergic to disperse dyes used in coloring trousers or pajamas made of 100% polyester or Terylene (polyethylene) and polyester wool fabric blends. All of the men were patch test positive to pieces of the guilty fabric. Several men reacted to dyes in more than one chemical class. None of the patients reacted to formaldehyde. Disperse Yellow 39, a methine dye, was the most common sensitizer (6 of 15 patients).

A report from Israel found that 22 of 55 (40%) patients tested with the same textile series reacted to dyes. The researchers found Disperse Blue 124, Blue 85, Red 17, and Blue 106 most common.[103] The editors of the *American Journal of Contact Dermatitis* called Disperse Blue dyes the "allergens of the year" in 2000.[104]

Seidenari and colleagues[105] studied cross-reactivity in 437 patients with reactions to at least 1 azo textile dye. Overall 437 (6.7%) of 6,478 subjects reacted to at least one dye. Of these, 196 reacted to Disperse Blue 106, 193 to DB 124, 143 to disperse orange 3, 109 to para-aminoazobenzene (PAAB), 95 to Disperse Yellow 3 and 92 to Disperse Red 1. Those reacting to Disperse Orange 3 reacted to PPDA about 63% of the time, but those allergic to the other allergens reacted only 7% of the time. Goon and colleagues[106] performed a recall study with disperse dyes on 128 PPDA positive patients. Disperse orange 3 was positive in 46 %, Disperse Yellow 3 and Black 1 were positive in about 21%, and many others showed lower levels of crossreactivity. Reactivity to Disperse Blue 106 and 124 was not reported. The authors note that the dyes with a high degree of crossreactivity are structurally very similar to PPDA and that they may be degraded by skin enzymes to PPDA.

A German report found 86 (4.3%) of 1986 patients positive to a Disperse Blue 106 and or 124 with good concordance and high relevance.[107]

Interesting case reports of dye allergy include one patient with hand and textile dermatitis allergic to multiple disperse dyes.[108] The hand dermatitis was due to handling dyed maggots while fishing. In another case, Disperse Blue 85 caused allergy to a knee brace.[109] Thioureas are more frequent causes of neoprene knee brace allergy.

The local lymph node assay has been used in Europe as a tool to estimate the potential for chemicals to cause allergic sensitization. Dinitrochlorobenzene (DNCB) is a potent allergen in this assay. One study showed that DB 106 was as potent as DNCB as a contact allergen.[6]

Disperse Dye Allergy from Non-Textile Sources
A patient with dermatitis to his plastic eyeglass frames was allergic to PPDA, PAAB, and many disperse dyes. The supplier indicated that Disperse dyes were probably present in the plastic, but since the product came from "far-Eastern sources," the exact nature could not be confirmed.[110]

Allergy to Non-Disperse Dyes It must be emphasized that allergy to all other textile dyes is reported much less frequently than is allergy to disperse dyes.

Acid Dyes

Acid dyes may be used on proteinaceous fibers such as wool, silk, and animal hair. As is implied by the name, these dyes are applied to fabrics in an acidic solution. Chemical types of acid dyes include the anthraquinone type (blue shades), azo type (reds), and triphenylmethane type (yellow and green).[7]

Acid dyes have been indicted several times in cases of textile dermatitis. Hatch's review found seven cases of allergy to acid black 48 and isolated cases of allergy to other acid dye colors, mainly res and yellows.[97] Cronin[3,101] identified Acid Violet 17 (C.I. 42650) as a cause of underwear dermatitis and Acid Black 48 (C.I. 65005) in an instance of clothing dermatitis in a man. Pedersen8 reported Acid Red 85 (C.I. 22245) as an explanation for a hand dermatitis in a dyehouse worker. In an Italian study,[111] five nondisperse azo dyes were tested in 1,814 patients. Eight reactions were noted to Acid Dyes: Acid Yellow 61 (5), Acid Red 359 (2), and Acid Red 118 (1).[101]

Aniline Dyes

In India, the tie-and-dye industry involves much manual labor and handling of dyestuffs. Mathur and colleagues[112] found that 20% of 250 workers developed a severe dermatitis. Fourteen of 26 that were patch tested were positive. Red RC salt (C.I. 37120) (0.2% aq) was positive in all 14. Other common reactors were Orange GC (C.I. 37005) in seven and Bordeaux GP (C.I. 37135) in three.

Basic (Cationic) Dyes

These are used in dyed fur, leather, wool, silk, cotton, and some modified acrylics.[113] They may be used to color paper. Chemically, they are primarily anilines. Some azo and anthraquinone dyes are also used (some as medications, e.g., crystal violet, methylene blue). Fluorescent textile dyes are in this group. Pratt reported 2 patients reactive to Basic Red 46 amongst 40 dye-allergic patients.[100] Both of theses patients reacted to Disperse Dyes. Other rare reports of allergy to these dyes have been noted.[97] Scheman[114] found a patient allergic to Basic Red 46 in a flame-retardant Nomex fabric. Nixon found a number of cases from Australian socks.[115]

Although basic (cationic) dyes have rarely been implicated in clothing allergy, they have caused ACD when used in medicaments (gentian violet, brilliant green, and malachite green), especially on the legs.[116]

Direct Dyes

Direct dyes are used on the natural fibers as well as rayon, nylon, paper, and leather. They are easy and convenient to apply, but lack "washfastness" and so may "bleed" continually. Chemically direct dyes are mostly azoics, with a sulfonate moiety. They adhere to fibers through hydrogen bonding and Van der Waals forces.[117]

In an Italian study,[111] five nondisperse azo dyes were tested in 1,814 patients. Eight reactions were noted to Direct Orange 34. Five of these eight also reacted to PPDA and/or disperse dyes. All dyes were tested at 5% petrolatum. Hatch's review noted a number of cases of allergy to Direct Black 38 from one report.[97]

Insoluble Azoics and Naphthol AS

Dermatitis associated with both the diazonium salts and the coupling agents used to form these dyes within a fabric have been described.

Malten[118] described diazonium salt allergy (diazotized ice red color TR) among workers in a Dutch cotton printing mill. Foussereau and colleagues[119] described the chemistry of this problem in some detail. Ancona-Alayon and colleagues[120] studied 24 Mexican workers who developed ACD and 32 who developed hyperpigmentation while working with the coupling agent Naphthol AS (3,hydroxide-2,naphthanilide), coupling component 2 (C.I. 37505), which was being used with an azo dye in a textile mill. The allergic patients had positive reactions to Naphthol AS 5% in water. Kiec-Swierczynska[121] described similar textile workers in Poland who developed hyperpigmentation or allergic dermatitis and who had positive patch test reactions to both "Texas" textiles and to 1% aqueous Naphthol AS used in the dyes.

A Danish report, using Naphthol AS (1% pet) in a general screening series, detected six cases of allergy.[122] One of these was work related, and the rest were clinically typical of textile allergy.

Mordant Dyes

A mordant is an organic or inorganic molecule which combines with a dye to deposit and fix an insoluble color on a fiber. Various acids, such as tannic acid and metal salts including chromium are used as mordants.[123] Chemically, mordant dyes are mostly anionic and hence can be considered a subset of acid dyes. Examples of mordant dyes include Alizarin Red S and hematein (natural black 1).

Allergic dermatitis attributed to chrome has occurred in a woolen blanket factory and in association with the wearing of green woolen military textiles.[20]

Reactive Dyes

Reactive dyes form a covalent bond between the fiber and the dye molecule. Thus the dye is bound tightly to the fabric, is the most permanent of all dyes, and is therefore perhaps less likely to cause ACD than disperse dyes. They are primarily used on cellulosic, proteinaceous, and polyamide fibers. They are sometimes used for wool and nylon.[124]

Manzini and colleagues[125] in Italy studied allergy to reactive dyes. Eighteen of 1,813 (0.99%) consecutive patients reacted to one or more of 12 dyes tested. Reactive Red 238 (Red Cibacron CR) and Reactive Violet 5 (Violet Remizol 5R) gave eight and five positives, respectively. Other reactors included Reactive Blue 122, Reactive Black 5, and Reactive Yellow 17. Testing concentration was at 5% petrolatum. Of the 18 patients, 1 had occupational exposure and 6 were felt to have relevant exposure to these dyes in clothing. Two reacted to disperse dyes. In a separate article, the authors tested 312 patients to five or more reactive dyes, with no positive results.[126]

A dark-colored cotton T-shirt was the cause of a case of reactive dye ACD. The patient reacted to 6 different dyes on patch testing, but not to other dyes.[127]

Sulphur Dyes

The first sulphur dye, Videl black, was discovered in 1873.[128] Insoluble in water, they are applied to fabrics in a sodium sulfide solution. They offer only a few shades of brown, navy, and black colors and may be used on cellulosics. Many navy and khaki overalls are dyed with sulphur dyes. Allergy to sulfur dyes is unreported.

Vat Dyes

Vat dyes are applied to fibers in a reduced, soluble form and then oxidized to the insoluble dye while on the item. They are commonly anthraquinones and indigo derivatives. Natural fibers are the substrate for vat dyes. Vat dyes rarely cause dermatitis. In fact, Levi Strauss's 501 "Shrink to Fit" jeans, which are dyed with Vat Blue 1 (C.I. 73000), can be a reliable and safe trouser substitute for disperse dye-sensitive people.

Foussereau and colleagues[119] described a group of cases of ACD among workers in a factory in which Vat Red 1 (C.I. 73360) was synthesized. A complicated and common green anthraquinone dye, Vat Green 1 (C.I. 59825) was reported by Wilson and Cronin[129] to explain five cases of dermatitis from blue uniforms in nurses. Each nurse was patch test positive to both a piece of her uniform and the dye, 1% in soft paraffin.

Miscellaneous Dyes

When leather is used as clothing, dyes incorporated into it can cause problems. Disperse Black 1 and Bismarck Brown in a leather watch strap and orthodichlorobenzene in a belt resulted in dermatitis.[130,131]

A report from Italy in 1991 implicated several "new" dyes as occasional allergens.[132] Unfortunately, dye type and C.I. numbers were not given. Brilliant green (2% pet), said to be used on wool, and Supramine Red (2% pet) for wool and polyamide were each positive in 2 of 569 patch test clinic patients. Supramine Yellow and Red, Turquoise Reactive (cotton), and Neutrichrome Red (wool and polyamide) each reacted once.

Phosgene (2,5-dichlorophenyl) hydrazone from yellow sweaters caused ACD in 12 men in Japan. The chemical was formed by the action of bleach on Pigment Yellow 16 in the garments.[133]

SCREENING FOR TEXTILE DYE ALLERGY

On the basis of current reports, the disperse dyes are exponentially more likely to cause ACD than all the other types of textile dyes. However, since the other dyes are rarely employed for patch testing, it is possible that allergy to these entities may be overlooked. Currently either Disperse Blue 106 or DB 124 seem to be the most common dye allergens. Using these two dyes individually or in a mix together makes sense for screening purposes. In cases where there is a strong clinical suspicion of textile allergy, other disperse dyes, as well as several acid, basic, reactive, and direct dyes may be useful (Table 18.8).

In addition to the dyes themselves, several dye intermediaries are positive on patch testing in some cases. Para-aminoazobenzene, also called Solvent Yellow 1 or Anidine Yellow (C.I. 11000), may react at times but was positive in only 27% in one study. PPDA reacts in about one-fifth to one-third of patients. Occasional reactions are seen to the "black-rubber mix" of substituted PPDA derivatives.[101]

An Italian group employed a textile-dye mix in retesting 67 patients with known disperse dye allergy. The mix consisted of Disperse Yellow 3, Red 1, and Orange 3, each at 0.25%, and Blue 124 at 0.1% in petrolatum. Sixty of the 67 reacted to the mix[134] (Figure 18-3).

Other Reports of Dye-Related Healh Effects

PHOTOTOXIC TEXTILE DERMATITIS

The phototoxic potential of Disperse Blue 35, an anthraquinone-based dye, was elaborately studied by Gardiner and colleagues.[135] They studied 16 employees in a dye-manufacturing factory in which over 130 workers had been seen over a 10-year period for acute redness and swelling of their light-exposed skin. Visible light in the 400-to-700-nm region caused phototoxic skin reactions with the whole dye in individuals whether they had been exposed to the dye in their work or not, verifying a phototoxic as opposed to a photoallergic explanation for the workers' complaints.

Hjorth and Moller[136] described two women who developed phototoxic textile dermatitis and hyperpigmentation on skin covered by bikini bathing suits. Disperse Blue 35 was not absolutely proved to cause this problem, but an extract of the bathing suit dye contained two fractions also found in Disperse Blue 35.

ALLERGIC DERMATITIS AND RESPIRATORY DISEASE

Estlander[137] reported five persons who were occupationally sensitized to reactive dyes. Two had only skin disease, but three also had respiratory symptoms. None were atopic. All reacted on patch testing and the latter three also on scratch testing. Involved dyes were in both the azo and anthraquinone families. None of the patients cross-reacted to PPDA or disperse dyes.

DERMATITIS FROM WOMEN'S AND MEN'S HOSIERY

Nylon stockings were introduced in the United States in 1939 and was first made in Britain in 1947.[95] By 1940, dermatitis caused either by nylon stocking dyes or finishes was being reported in the United States.[138] By 1956, nylon stocking dye dermatitis was being described in Britain.[139]

In 1947, Dobkevitch and Baer[140] studied 13 patients who had nylon stocking dermatitis caused by azo dyes used in stockings. None of the patients reacted to anthraquinone dyes used in the hosiery. All of them reacted to a piece of the suspected hosiery, to paraphenylenediamine, and to one or more of the suspect azo dyes.

Allergen	Concentration	Brial	Chemo technique	Hermal
Acid Yellow 36	1% pet			X
Acid Yellow 61	5% pet		X	
Acid Red 118	5% pet		X	
Acid Red 359	5% pet		X	
Basic Red 46	1% pet		X	
Bismarck Brown R	0.5% pet			X
4-aminoazobenzene	1% pet	X	X	X
4-aminophenol	1% pet	X	X	X
Aniline	1% pet	X		
Direct Orange 34	5% pet		X	
Disperse Blue Mix (124/106)*	1% pet	X	X	
Disperse Blue-1	1% pet	X		
Disperse Blue-3	1% pet	X	X	X
Disperse Blue-35	1% pet		X	
Disperse Blue-85	1% pet		X	
Disperse Blue-124*	1% pet		X	
Disperse Blue-153	1% pet		X	
Disperse Blue-106*	1% pet	X	X	
Disperse Orange 3	1% pet	X	X	X
Disperse Red-1	1% pet	X	X	X
Disperse Red-11	1% pet	X		X
Disperse Red-17	1% pet	X	X	X
Disperse Yellow 3	1% pet	X	X	X
Disperse Yellow 9	1% pet	X	X	X
Eosin	5% pet		X	
Erythrosine-B	0.25% pet	X		
Metanil Yellow	1% pet	X		
Methyl Violet	0.5% pet	X		
Naphthol-AS	1% pet	X		X
p-aminodiphenylamine	0.25%	X		
Phenolphthalein	0.5% pet	X		
Reactive Black 5	1% pet		X	
Reactive Blue 21	1% pet		X	
Reactive Blue 238	1% pet		X	
Reactive Orange 107	1% pet		X	
Reactive Red 123	1% pet		X	
Reactive Red 238	1% pet		X	
Reactive Red 228	1% pet		X	
Reactive Violet 5	1% pet		X	
Sudan III	1% pet	X		
Vesuvine brown	0.5% pet	X		

Table 18-8 Textile Dye Allergens for Patch Testing

* Most important for screening

When Calnan and Wilson[139] described six women who had nylon stocking dermatitis in 1956, all British hosiery manufacturers were using azo dyes. The patients reacted to pieces of stocking and to one or more dyes. Only one patient had a paraphenylenediamine reaction. None of the patients reacted to melamine or urea formaldehyde resins, which at that time were used to provide an antisnag finish.

Fourteen patients in Finland became allergic to a brown stocking dye mixture (Synten Brown), which consisted of nitro- and aminodiazobenzene and aminoanthraquinone dyes.[141] Nine of these patients reacted to para-aminoazobenzene, nine to Disperse Orange 3 (C.I. 11005), and four to Disperse Yellow 3 (C.I. 11855). Three of these patients had previously worked with textiles and had hand eczemas. Efforts to flare six of these patients with peroral azo food dyes (tartrazine and amaranth) failed.

Men's nylon or acrylic socks have been described as sources of ACD in France, Britain, Australia, and many years ago in the United States.[95,101,142] This seems to be a rare event today, although patients still report intolerance to colored, as opposed to white, socks. Perhaps this lack of recognition of intolerance to colored socks is due to inadequate patch testing. Nixon and colleagues noted 20 cases of allergy to Basic Red 46 in patients with foot dermatitis. Chemical analysis found the dye in dark colored acrylic blend "loop knit" socks.[115]

OPTICAL WHITENERS

"Whiter than white" fabrics are created by the application of colorless dyes, which absorb incidental and invisible ultraviolet light and reflect it as visible bluish light. The resultant reflected light tends to mask off-whites or yellowish tinges and produces radiant whites.[11]

The dyes are applied directly to textile fibers, plastics, and papers and can be incorporated into detergents. They tend to concentrate in textile fibers with increasing numbers of washes.

Allergic contact dermatitis has been reported from Denmark and Spain. In 1971, Osmundsen and Alani[143] described 167 patients in Copenhagen who developed a reticulate, occasionally hyperpigmented, long-lasting dermatitis in a clothing distribution. These patients washed their clothing in a detergent that contained 0.02% to 0.2% Tinopal CH 3566 (CPY) as an optical whitener. This compound was a mixture of 1-(3-chlorphenyl)-3-phenyl pyrazoline and 1-(3-chlorphenyl)-3-(4-chlorphenyl)-pyrazoline. All of the affected patients had positive patch tests with the brightener at 0.1% to 1% in petrolatum. Half of the patients who were patch tested to "nylon" pieces washed in the

suspect detergent had positive reactions, and 16 of 88 patients tested to benzyl salicylate reacted positively. Benzyl salicylate is a common perfume ingredient in detergents, and this may have represented a cosensitization.[144] A special feature of the Danish subjects who had dermatitis was the development of hyperpigmentation in a clothing distribution in nine of them without obvious antecedent dermatitis.[140] This pigmentation was reproduced on patch testing. Tinopal CH 3566 (CPY) was shown to be a strong sensitizer in a guinea pig maximization test: CPY was never used in the United States and was withdrawn in Denmark.

The 103 Spanish patients were also associated with CPY and had clinical features like the Danish patients'.[145] The Spanish study also had 12 patients who were stilbene sensitive.

Manufacturers of optical whiteners have tried to screen these agents for their sensitizing potential. One such study examined 31 agents and found three sensitizers.[146] Two of these chemicals were pyrazolines (one was CPY and the other 1-phenyl-2-(naphtho(2,1-d)oxazol-2-yl) ethylene). This compound was positive in some of Osmundsen's[147] CPY-positive patients.

No recent patients who have textile-distributed dermatitis attributed to optical whiteners have been described in the United States or Europe. The Danish and Spanish epidemics of subtle, long-lasting, elusive dermatitis are, however, a fine example of the value of alertness in examining the sensitizing potential of clothing and its numerous and almost countless additives.

PATCH TESTING IN CLOTHING DERMATITIS

A list of allergens that can be used to evaluate a suspect case of clothing dermatitis is presented in Table 18.9. It should be remembered, that neither formaldehyde nor especially paraphenylenediamine is an absolute indicator of fabric finish or dye allergy.

Patch testing with a piece of the suspect fabric is most useful for a dye allergy, in which case it is usually positive. It is of least help for durable-press finishes, in which it is often negative. Aids for extracting finishes have already been mentioned. We usually simply soak the fabric in water for 10 minutes before applying it. On occasion, more positive reactions are seen with a piece of suspect fabric if it is left in place for longer than 48 hours (e.g., 96 to 120 hours).

DERMATITIS DUE TO MECHANICAL PRESSURE AND FRICTION OF CLOTHING

Tight-fitting clothing may cause irritation and folliculitis from the effects of friction and/or trapping of

Table 18-9 Patch Testing for Textile Dermatitis

I. *Most standard screening trays contain*
   "Black rubber mix"—dyes and rubber accessories
   Chromate—leather
   Epoxy—adhesives, labels
   Formaldehyde—permanent press
   Lanolin—finishes
   MBT, thiuram, thiourea, carbamate—rubber, adhesives
   Nickel—metal accessories
   PTBFR—adhesive
   PPDA—some azo dyes
II. *Formaldehyde resins: see Table 18.4*
III. *Dyes: see Table 18.8*
IV. *Others*
   p-aminozobenzene (0.25% pet)—dye marker
   Perchloroethylene (25% olive oil)—dry cleaning
   Triclosan (0.5% pet)—fungicide
   Naphthol AS (5% aq)—dye coupler
V. *Piece of suspect clothing:* Soak in water for 15 minutes for formaldehyde resins or warmed ethanol for 60 minutes for dyes. Leave on 48 hours. If no reaction, leave another 24 to 48 hours (see text).

MBT = mercaptobenzothiazole; PPDA = paraphenylenediamine; PTBFR = paratertiary butylphenol formaldehyde resin

perspiration. Folliculitis may be compounded by either bacterial or yeast colonization. Underlying ACD, whether it is from the clothing itself or other allergens, may be exacerbated by pressure under bras, underwear, etc. and may cause the patient to suspect allergy to elastic. The isomorphic response of Koebner may occur under areas of clothing occlusion.

Systemic urticaria is commonly exacerbated by pressure in areas of tight clothing.

Blousing Garter Dermatitis

This is a syndrome of pigmentation of the ankles and dorsa of the feet in soldiers who wear either blousing garters or bootlaces around their legs to keep fatigues neatly in place. The resultant mild edema and subsequent deposition of hemosiderin and melanin resemble changes of the lower extremities in patients with stasis dermatitis secondary to varicose veins. If the constriction is prolonged, one would assume hemosiderin deposits would occur, as in the pigmented purpuric eruptions. The cutaneous changes occur distal to the site of constriction.

CLOTHING ACCESSORY DERMATITIS

The many accessories used on clothing, particularly nickel-plated or rubber objects, may produce areas of dermatitis around sites of contact. Nickel-plated zippers, clips, buckles, and pins, therefore, may produce dermatitis in nickel-sensitive individuals. It is common to see ACD to nickel on the abdomen from blue-jean buttons and/or belt buckles. Rubber shoulder pads, dress shields, collars, and the rubber portion of girdles and bras can produce dermatitis in sensitized individuals. Other accessories such as studs and buttons, dyed dress labels, clothing marked with inks, and articles carried in pockets may produce dermatitis. Coins, keys, wallets, and plastic cards routinely carried in the same pocket are not unusual causes of localized ACD.

Some garments contain inlaid patches of different colors and materials, such as gloves with leather inlays and socks with stripes of different colors, which may produce circumscribed areas of dermatitis.

FACTORS AFFECTING CLOTHING DERMATITIS

Friction, heat, humidity, and particularly excessive perspiration play important roles in the production of clothing dermatitis. Tight-fitting clothing can produce dermatitis, which may not recur when the patient wears a larger garment or loses weight. The patient may acquire dermatitis from a particular article in the summer, but not in cooler weather or in drier climes. Hyperhidrosis, particularly when clothing is nonabsorbent, readily produces miliaria. The change of pH in sweat when evaporation is hindered may be a factor in producing dermatitis. Sweat also leaches dyes and finishes from clothing, which may produce dermatitis in sensitized patients. Control of excessive perspiration enables some patients to wear clothing that would otherwise produce dermatitis.

Occupational Textile ACD and ICD

Soni and Sherertz[148] evaluated 72 textile workers over a 5-year period with possible occupational contact dermatitis. Almost three-fourths had work-related ICD, ACD, or a combination, with 38% felt to be ICD. Frictional irritation was prominent. Allergens included textile dyes in 12 cases, formaldehyde finishes in 11, and rubber allergens in 10. The hands were the primary site of involvement, with hand dermatitis found in 82% of those with work-related dermatitis.

Thiourea derivatives have caused allergy in workers handling diazo paper used for patterns.[149] An interesting papergiving an overview of textile finishing practices and occupational allergy came from South Africa recently.[150]

Bio-Functional Textiles

A new category of clothing materials has been termed "bio-functional" textiles. This concept concerns modification of textiles to be useful for supporting therapy and prevention of dermatologic disease.[151] The major focus at this time appears to be providing textiles with active antimicrobial properties due to treatment with bacteriostatic agents. Such fabrics could potentially be useful in atopic individuals who suffer from frequent skin colonization with bacteria. Silver and quaternary-ammonium compounds seem to be particularly popular.[152,153] Contact dermatitis specialists would not be surprised to find significant irritant and allergic contact dermatitis problems with these fabrics, although the field is too new to have any reports so far.

Shoe Contact Dermatitis

The hot, humid environment within a shoe, combined with exposure to a variety of dyes, rubber allergens, glues, chromium, and other materials, creates an ideal situation for the development of allergic or irritant contact dermatitis.

CLINICAL PICTURE

The pattern of dermatitis on the foot of a person allergic to a footwear constituent may mimic the location of the offending chemical or material in the shoe (Figures 18-4 and 18-5), but spreading of a reaction is common. Of course, since most patients wear a variety of shoes, the localization of dermatitis is not always especially helpful. One exception is that ACD is rarely localized between the toes. Instead, this pattern should suggest fungal infection. In addition, a secondary fungal infection of the foot is not uncommon, especially when the patient has been treating ACD with topical corticosteroids. The elderly, diabetics, and patients with stasis changes are at greater risk for fungal infections of the feet and nails.

The patterns of foot dermatitis also reflect the changing vogue in shoe manufacture. Thus, when rubber was being added to the thermoplastic inner box toes of oxfords, shoe dermatitis classically began on the dorsal surfaces of the toes, especially the big toe. Dorsal toe allergic shoe dermatitis is still reported and may well relate to the rubber that covers the outer toe surface of some tennis shoes. Many athletic shoes now contain uppers and tongues made of foam-rubber, with resultant dorsal foot dermatitis in those allergic to rubber components.

Plantar dermatitis may be seen when the patient is allergic to rubber, adhesives, or leather components of insoles. The most typical sole involvement spares the instep and the toes' flexural creases. According to Cronin, when the instep only is involved with small vesicles or pustules, a shoe dermatitis is unlikely.[101] The anterior portion of the sole may be involved exclusively. The dermatitis may be unilateral. Symmetry is more common, however, as is a history of increased sweating.

A secondary vesicular dermatitis on the hands may occur with shoe dermatitis. This "id" reaction or autosensitization was well studied by Gaul and Underwood,[154] who observed hand involvement in over half of their 140 patients. The pattern of hand dermatitis tended to mimic the foot's distribution. Hand involvement was most likely when the shoe dermatitis began on the soles and disappeared when the guilty shoes were discarded. Calnan and Sarkany[155] and Fisher[156] have all reported similar "id"-like reactions with shoe dermatitis. In addition to these hand eruptions, a generalized dermatitis that begins as a shoe allergy has been described.[154] Storrs has seen this happen with mercaptobenzothiazole allergy from a rubber insole (FJ Storrs, MD, personal communication, 1996).

People of all ages may develop shoe allergy. Virtually all reports have included children in the first decade of life, as well as adults in their sixties.[155] Over half of Adam's patients were under 20 years old, and most of Gaul and Underwood's[154] patients were 40 years old or under. Weston and colleagues[157] studied three children age 1 or under among their nine children who were under 6 years of age and who had proven relevant shoe allergens. One Italian study of 17 children with foot dermatitis found nine positive patch tests. Two reacted to chromate, two to dodecyl mercaptan in rubber, and six to thimerosal.[158] Those with only thimerosal allergy did improve after avoiding certain leather shoes, suggesting the allergen may have been present in the leather.

In a British study, 15 of 29 children and 26 of 57 adults with foot dermatitis had relevant allergies.[159] Rubber allergens predominated in both groups, with only one child and three adults allergic to chromate in leather. Somewhat less commonly seen in both groups were allergies to fragrances, preservatives, and topical medication. Similarly, in a small French study all 8 children seen with footwear allergy reacted to various rubber allergens.[160]

Leukoderma may be seen as a late sequela of some phenols used in rubber. Bajaj and colleagues[161] described 19 cases of depigmentation of the feet, some of which were felt to be due to hydroquinones and/or phenols. In six, dermatitis preceded the depigmentation but patch tests were negative. Even petechial and purpuric eruptions can occur when problems are traced to black rubber boots.[4]

DIFFERENTIAL DIAGNOSIS

The differential diagnosis of shoe allergy includes other allergies, mechanical irritant dermatitis, juvenile plantar dermatosis (JPD), atopic dermatitis, tinea pedis, endogenous dermatitis, pustular psoriasis, lichen planus, and mycosis fungoides.

Ill-fitting shoes and anatomic foot deformities may cause excessive friction and wearing away of protective linings and may thus allow more intimate contact of shoe sensitizers with the skin. New shoes or orthopedic shoes can correct this problem.[156] Shoes soaked by perspiration may overdry and become brittle. Ridges may form in the shoes' linings that irritate the skin of the feet. Slow drying of the shoe on wooden shoe trees helps alleviate this problem.[162]

Atopic dermatitis may be a special differential diagnostic problem in that irritation can precipitate an attack of dermatitis, especially in areas of greatest friction. Almost half of Freeman's[163] 55 patients were atopics.

JPD tends to occur on the toes and distal foot. Although its distribution, with instep sparing, can be exactly that of a shoe dermatitis, the absence of vesicles or signs of a more acute dermatitis is a distinguishing feature. The clinical pattern in most cases consists of chronic, scaling, mildly erythematous dermatitis, with minimal symptoms. Repeated cycles of wetting by sweat or environmental moisture followed by drying may predispose to JPD. Consequently, treatment must be focused on eliminating that situation.

In a study by Mackie, 42% of the 269 reported patients had a personal or family history of atopy.[164] Some authors have reported some histologic features of JPD suggesting chronic eczema; thus, these patients have often been patch tested. Ten percent of Mackie's[164] series of patients had positive patch tests to shoewear constituents, but changes of footwear did not always resolve the dermatitis. Romaguera and colleagues[165] found relevant shoe allergens in 4 of 15 children whom they initially diagnosed as having JPD. Weston and colleagues[157] found no positive relevant allergens in any of the 15 children they saw with plantar involvement and called these cases "JPD by default."

OVERVIEW OF SHOE CONTACT DERMATITIS

Allergy to shoe components is quite variable in different regions of the world.

The NACDG has compiled an extensive review of their data on shoe dermatitis compiled over the first 4 years of this millenium.[166] Of 10,061 patients, 109 had foot dermatitis and were listed as having footwear as the cause. The adhesive PTBFR was causative in 25% of these. Next were chromate (17.5%), and carbamate (12%). As a group, however, the rubber allergens were most common at 40%. Nineteen of the 109 were allergic to allergens not in the 65 NACDG standard allergens.

Freeman[163] studied 55 patients with shoe dermatitis and was able to follow up with 48 at a later time. Most patients had hyperhidrosis and 43% were atopic. Allergens were rubber (43.1%), chromate (23.6%), *p*-tert-butylphenol

formaldehyde resin (PTBFR) (20.0%), rosin (9.0%), and PPDA (3.6%). Positive reactions to shoe pieces with negative reactions to individual chemicals occurred in 14.5%. At mean follow-up of almost 3 years, 87.5% were clear or better (over half clear), 10% the same, and one patient worse.

Holden and Gawkrodger[167] saw 230 patients with foot dermatitis over a 10-year period. Forty-four patients (19%) showed relevant reactions to the British standard series, led by chromate (9 patients), neomycin (7), MBT (8), thiuram (6) and so on. Only one was allergic to PTBFR. Their shoe series gave positive reactions to several other rubber chemicals, dyes, and biocides. They did not test to Basic Red 46.

In Pakistan, 109 patients with suspected shoe dermatitis were patch tested, with 87 showing positive results.[168] Adhesives (34%) were the most common allergens, with PTBFR accounting for 27% of the positives. Chromate accounted for 16%, rubber allergens for 8%, and dyes for 8%.

An Israeli report noted that 58 of 140 patients with presumed shoe allergy had positive results on patch testing.[169] Chromate was positive in 27% and only 9% were positive to PTBFR.

Jordan[170] estimated that he saw one new patient with dermatitis related to shoes every 6 weeks in 1972. From 1977 to 1980, Lynde and colleagues,[171] in Vancouver, Canada, suspected shoe dermatitis enough to apply a shoewear screening tray to 119 of 2,910 patients with eczema whom they patch tested in that period (prevalence of 4.1%). In Italy, Angelini and colleagues[172] estimated a shoe contact dermatitis prevalence of 6.3% among patients who had dermatitis whom they evaluated for 4½ years up to 1980.

COMPONENTS OF FOOTWEAR

In order to evaluate a patient who has a shoe allergy and to assist that patient in finding shoes that he or she can wear without difficulty, it is important that the physician know how shoes are constructed as well as which chemicals used in shoe manufacture are most likely to cause problems. This is easier said than done.

Gaul and Underwood[154] noted that their efforts to learn about shoe adhesives were met by a "decided reluctance [of the manufacturing companies] to divulge their ingredients." Hack[173] contacted manufacturers who allegedly made "hypoallergenic" shoes and found that his inquiries "elicited amazed replies in some cases and amazing replies in others." It must be remembered that a modern shoe is composed of many parts and that the final assembler may not be aware of all of the chemicals that have been used to prepare each of them, because they may have come from all over the world to finally come together in a finished piece of footwear. (Storrs F, personal communication, May, 2007).

In addition to "classical" materials like leather and rubber, shoes may be constructed of plastics, woods, or metals and glued together with different adhesives.

DIFFICULTY IN IDENTIFYING SHOE ALLERGENS

The difficulty in finding out components of specific shoes may be appreciated by reviewing US government data on shoe imports. In 2006, over 2 billion pairs of non-rubber footwear and 340 million pairs of rubber and plastic footwear were imported into the USA.[174] China was the leading supplier with over 1.6 billion and 300,000 pairs respectively. It is no wonder then that consumers and physicians are forced to make educated guesses about shoe components.

Although groups of chemicals can be collected that are useful for the diagnosis of the cause of shoe allergy (Table 18.10), it has long been the experience of dermatologists who make such investigations that they often fail to find a precise explanation for their patients' obvious shoe dermatitis. Dahl[175] suspected shoe allergy in 59 patients but confirmed specific relevant allergens in only 33 patients, although shoes were positive in 42 patients. Angelini and colleagues[172] found positive patch tests in only 108 of 165 patients who had clinically suspect shoe allergies, and in many instances these were to medicaments. Only 32 of the 119 suspect patients of Lynde[171] had possibly relevant positive reactions to their shoewear screening tray.

In Spain, Grimalt and Romaguera[176] collected 45 unexplained patients who had shoe dermatitis. They were able to explain all but 17 of them by testing with neoprene and polyurethane resins and their constituents (see the following section on adhesives).

Constituents of rubber, adhesives, and leather are the most common causes of shoe ACD. Substances in natural and synthetic fabrics, as well as biocides or dyes added to the finished or refinished shoe, are also suspect but seldom reported. It must be remembered that what is common in one country (e.g., rubber in North America) may be rare in another (e.g., chrome and dyes in Italy).[171,172]

LEATHER

Leather is created by tanning animal hides, principally cattlehide. Chrome tanning was invented in 1858. It produces leather that is more pliable and water-resistant than vegetable tanned leather and is more able to take-up a variety of colors. It accounts for about 90% of US

Table 18-10 Patch-Test Allergens for Shoe Dermatitis
From typical screening series
Adhesives
PTBFR
Rosin (colophony)
Epoxy resin
Dyes
PPDA
Disperse Blue 106 or 124
Rubber Allergens
Black rubber mix (or IPPD)
Carbamate Mix
MBT and mix
Thiourea mix
Thiuram mix
Tanning agents
Chromate
Glutaral
Formaldehyde (rarely)
Miscellaneous
Metals: nickel and cobalt- grommets, decorations
Additional allergens
Adhesives
PTBP
Dodecylmercaptan
PTBC
Benzoyl peroxide
Dimethylaminoethyl ether
Biocides
Thimerosal
Chloracetamide
Phenylmercuric nitrate
Isothiazolinones
Dyes
Para-aminoazobenzene
Disperse Dyes
Bismarck Brown
Plastics
Isophorone diisocyante
Rubber
Dithiodimorpholine
Monobenzyl ether of hydroquinone
Shoe pieces

leather production.[177] Hausen[178] has summarized what is known of wood-derived tannins.

Vegetable tanned leather (mostly from tree-bark tannins) is more susceptible to shrinkage. Aldehyde-tanned leather is usually white or cream-colored. Glutaraldehyde is principally used, although occasionally formaldehyde may still be used. Chamois leather is an example of this type. Synthetic resins (e.g., melamine formaldehyde resin) were used to tan leather in past times. White leather was produced and free formaldehyde can be detected from these leathers. Aluminum salts are occasionally used, but are not waterproof. Rawhide is untanned, but is soaked in lime and dried, producing a brittle product. Bonded leather or "reconstituted leather" is made of leather scraps with epoxy, urethane, or other resins as binding agents.

Tanning agents and dyes are most likely to explain shoe allergy caused by leather. Reviews of shoe dermatitis have noted that early reports of allergy in the 1930s and 1940s were concerned mostly with leather and dyes. By the 1950s and 1960s, leather had slipped to second place behind rubber constituents in the United States and England.[98] In the United States, there are regional differences: Storrs (personal communication, 2000) in Oregon frequently sees shoe allergy due to leather but Fowler rarely sees it. Perhaps this is due to greater use of leather sandals without socks by the Oregonian-type individual. In Italy, leather allergy was still more common than rubber allergy.[172]

Chrome Tanned Leather

Chromium allergy is detected by patch testing with potassium dichromate 0.25% petrolatum in the United States and 0.5% petrolatum in some other countries. Although trivalent chrome salts, such as chromic acid, chromic sulfate, and chrome trichloride, are the usual tanning agents, patch testing with trivalent chrome salts is much less reliable than using the hexavent potassium dichromate.

Although chrome allergy explains some shoe dermatitis, in many areas it is less important than rubber and adhesive allergy.[158] In 1959 in Britain, Calnan and Sarkany[155] found that 62% of their 102 patients who had shoe dermatitis reacted to leather, but only 9 of these leather-sensitive patients reacted to chromate. Twelve of these chrome-negative patients were shown subsequently to react to East Indian vegetable-tanned leather.[155] In Canada, only 3 of the 32 patients of Lynde and colleagues[171] who had positive reactions to shoewear reacted to chromate, whereas 49 (30%) of the patients of Angelini and colleagues[172] had positive and probably relevant reactions in Italy. It is likely that better fixation of chrome to leather, coupled with the cooler climate of North America, explains the decreasing prevalence of chrome allergy. It is known, for example, that individuals sensitized to chrome from other sources can wear chrome-tanned shoes without difficulty.[101] Fisher[156] found that only 18 of 68 (26%) dichromate-sensitized persons had shoe dermatitis.

In "ideal" circumstances, leather shoe dermatitis caused by chromates can reach epidemic proportions. Scutt[179] saw 86 cases in 3½ years among sailors in the British navy who were assigned to the Far East. These "foreign service invalids" wore unlined chrome-tanned sandals next to their skin. The severe and chronic foot eczema that they developed resulted in "invaliding" to a temperate climate (Britain) at no small cost to the British taxpayer. Once shoe chrome dermatitis develops, it can become chronic, although like other shoe allergies, it may minimize with time.

Vegetable-Tanned Leather

Vegetable tanning is very time consuming. Chrome tanning requires 6 to 14 hours, whereas vegetable tanning can take up to 6 months.162 Vegetable-tanned leathers are more expensive and more easily scuffed. It should be remembered that, on occasion, leather is both chrome- and vegetable-tanned. Usually only black and brown leathers are available in vegetable tanning.

British authors have long suspected and documented that vegetable-tanned leather was responsible for many of their unexplained shoe leather–positive patients.[155] The precise sensitizer was never identified, however. Calnan and Cronin[180] did find one patient in 1978 who reacted to a leather watch strap and to myrabolam extract powder and quebracho extract powder, as well as to potassium dichromate. Lewis,[181] however, reported a remarkable case of a man who appeared to have an authentic ACD to "tannic acid," which he was using as a wet compress. He was patch test positive to tannic acid 0.25% aqueous.

A group of patients felt to be allergic to vegetable tannins was first reported by Lynch.[182] Patients developed a vigorous dermatitis under the sandal straps of their Indian leather sandals. Subsequently, reports of this problem came from around the United States and Denmark.[183,184] Sumac sap was indicted as the allergen, but patients known to be allergic to poison ivy did not react to the leather,[183] nor was it possible to extract a catechol-like substance from the Indian sandal leather.[184] In fact, Spoor[184] hypothesized that an oil added to the leather as a softening agent and not a vegetable tannin was the actual sensitizer. Some of his patients developed both a generalized and a foot dermatitis.

Formaldehyde and Glutaraldehyde

Although formaldehyde patch test reactions are seen in patients who have shoe dermatitis, their relevance is suspected but is seldom fully explained.[171,175] Hack[173] saw a formaldehyde-allergic woman whose shoe dermatitis coincided perfectly with the skin covered by the white leather of her pumps.

Glutaraldehyde has been used to tan upper-shoe leather.[185] It may be used to retan chrome-tanned leather. It finds occasional use, as well, in preparing leather for vegetable tanning. It provides great water resistance and reduces shrinkage. Although glutaraldehyde is thought to be irreversibly bound to leather, the researchers were able to obtain positive patch test reactions to glutaraldehyde-tanned leather in five patients who had been sensitized to glutaraldehyde in disinfectants. None of these patients had a shoe dermatitis. It is doubtful that glutaraldehyde in leather causes much sensitization.

Dyes

Dyes used to color leather are unusual causes of leather dermatitis. Cronin[101] reported no cases of shoe dermatitis owing to a dye at St. John's Hospital in London. Fisher[156] had seen no problems from the manufacturer's original shoe dye. However, he had seen problems from shoes that were redyed. He noted that leather dyes are usually azo-aniline group dyes that fix firmly to the leather. Redyed shoes do not fix these dyes as firmly. Para-aminoazobenzene accounted for 5 of 35 reactions in foot dermatitis patients in one Indian study.[112]

Dahl[175] did not list which dyes his five dye-allergic patients who had shoe dermatitis reacted to. Some of Dahl's patients also reacted to paraphenylenediamine, which is not uncommon in azo-dye allergy. A proven case of ACD caused by Acid Yellow 36 (C.I. 13065), which was used to dye the inners and stiffeners of an industrial leather protective shoe, was reported by Ancona and colleagues.[186]

Angelini and colleagues[172] found that 24.8% of their patients with shoe dermatitis reacted to paraphenylenediamine. Paraphenylenediamine is not used to dye shoe leather, and the researchers felt that patients' reactions represented cross-reactions with some rubber additives (see the following section), or with dyes used in fabric or plastic shoes or in stockings. They did not mention any specific guilty dyes. Allergic reactions attributed to dyes used to color leather used as clothing have already been discussed.[130] Dyes are also used in plastic materials in shoes but have not yet been indicted in a case of shoe dermatitis.

Shoe polishes are also rarely or never the cause of allergic dermatitis. Gaul and Underwood[154] listed irritant and questionably allergic reactions to some shoe polishes but did not describe them in any detail.

RUBBER

Rubber allergy is a common manifestation of shoe contact dermatitis (Figure 18-6). The rubber accelerator mercaptobenzothiazole (MBT) usually leads the list of culprits. The thiurams and carbamates have also been responsible for some problems. The antioxidant IPPD has been a problem in rubber boots.[4] In the past, monobenzyl ether of hydroquinone (MBH) and an assortment of other rubber additives have been causative.[187] MBH

was responsible for three positive reactions in the series of shoe dermatitis patients of Lynde and colleagues.[171]

Rubber may be used on the outer sole of shoes, and in the case of some sports shoes it may wrap over the outer upper toe of the shoe. It may also be used as a component of the shoe's midsole. Insoles, tongues, and uppers in athletic shoes may be made of foam or latex-based rubber. At one time, rubber (thermoplastic) box toes were the most common cause of shoe contact dermatitis in the United States,[156] but they are now essentially obsolete.

No matter where the rubber is in the shoe, it is important to remember that when the shoe becomes wet after being worn, the suspect chemicals can migrate to distant parts of the shoe. The importance of patch testing individuals with shoe dermatitis on their soles to pieces of the outer sole of their shoes should be remembered. Marcussen[188] showed that MBT can diffuse out of rubber. A piece of canvas became reactive in an MBT-allergic person if it sat for 24 hours in a solution with a piece of rubber that contained MBT.

Mercaptobenzothiazole, Carbamates, and Thiurams

Mercaptobenzothiazole (MBT) has been identified as the most frequent rubber allergen as well as the most frequent shoe allergen in various series.[157,171,176] MBT accounted for 20% and TMTD for 11% of positive reactions among the shoe-sensitive patients of Lynde and colleagues.[171] Together, they were the most common positives. In a general population of 4,190 eczema patients tested by this same group in Vancouver, between 1972 and 1981, MBT was positive in 3.2% of the patients and the thiuram mix in 5.4%.[66] In some countries, rubber allergy is still a less common cause of shoe dermatitis than leather.

As noted above, the rubber allergens as a whole, led by MBT, were the most common allergens in a report from the NACDG.[48]

Belsito, however, in a small series, found dithiodimorpholine allergy in 6 of 23 patients.[189] It was more common than other rubber allergens, although MBT and thiuram were each positive in 5 patients. Carbamate was positive in 3 patients.

In Newfoundland, none of the 30 patients sensitive to rubber boots were found to react to paraphenylenediamine (PPD).[190] IPPD itself was not tested and often does not crossreact with PPD.[4] The Newfoundland patients were interesting, nonetheless, in that although some of them reacted to MBT, they also reacted to chemicals used in rubber that are only rarely reported as sensitizers in footwear, such as zinc diethyldithiocarbamate, diphenylguanidine, and trimethylquinoline.[190] All of these patients reacted to a piece of boot rubber, but only 13 of them had positive reactions to specific chemicals.

Disulfiram (tetraethylthiuram disulfide, Antabuse) is used in the treatment of alcohol abuse. At least one patient with TMT-based rubber allergy from footwear has developed a generalized (systemic) dermatitis after using disulfiram.[191]

N-Isopropyl-N-Phenyl-Paraphenylenediamine

N-isopropyl-*N*-phenyl-*p*-phenylenediamine (also called isopropylphenyl-*p*-phenylenediamine or 4-isopropylamino diphenylamine, or IPPD) has caused ACD in rubber boot wearers.[4] One epidemic of 109 patients in Prague is summarized by Cronin.[101] Of special interest is the purpuric nature of the eczema that can be reproduced on patch testing.[4] Allergy to IPPD has also been indicted as an explanation for shoe contact dermatitis from Maleki shoes in Iran. The soles of these shoes are made from recycled rubber tires.[192]

Neoprene Rubber Allergens

Roberts and Hanifin[193] reported allergy to ethylbutyl thiourea used as an accelerator in a polychloroprene (neoprene) adhesive used in running shoes. They noted, however, that thioureas may find their way into other neoprene products, such as orthopedic supports and sporting goods.

PLASTIC ALLERGENS IN SHOES

Synthetic materials are used commonly in shoe manufacture. Problems with these synthetic materials have mostly to do with adhesives. Some of the same chemicals used in adhesives, however, are also used in solid shoe materials.

Polyurethanes are also used in both solid shoe materials and adhesives. Polyurethanes are polyaddition products resulting from the reaction between diisocyanates and polyhydroxy compounds (polyalcohols, polyesters) with free OH groups.[119] Grimalt and Romaguera[176] reported allergy to the polyurethane constituents Desmocoll 400, Desmodur R, and Desmodur RF in 13 patients who had shoe dermatitis in Spain. They also identified 15 patients who were allergic to dodecyl mercaptan, which is used to arrest polymerization in some neoprenes. The Spanish authors confirmed the presence of dodecyl mercaptan in DuPont's Neoprene ACM resin, which is used as glue in the Spanish shoe industry. Such arresters can also be found, however, in solid neoprenes.[176]

Belsito reported allergy to a urethane monomer, isophorone diisocyanate in 3 of 23 patients and to an epoxy hardener, dimethylaminoethyl ether in another 3.[189]

Cronin[101] described several patients who were sensitized to polyvinyl chloride (PVC) shoe linings, but the allergen was not identified. Neither Foussereau and colleagues[119] nor Adams[194] mentions polyurethanes as potential allergens in shoemakers, despite excellent discussions of their chemistry. Bisphenol A, an epoxy resin component, has caused shoe dermatitis from plastic shoes in India.[195]

In the past, an occlusive plastic shoe made in Japan caused an irritant sort of dermatitis that came to be known as the "Japanese hot foot."[196] The dermatitis, which replicated the ripple sole, was attributed to occlusion.

ADHESIVES

Shoe cements came into use in 1910.[154] Most shoe adhesives were rubber based for many years. In the 1950s and 1960s, neoprene- and urethane-based adhesives became more popular.

Rubber Adhesives and Rosin

The first reports of shoe dermatitis attributed to rubber adhesives were vague. Gaul and Underwood[154] and Fisher[156] noted that their patients who reacted to shoe adhesives or rubber parts were often also allergic to adhesive tape ("plaster"). Although they suspected the same chemicals were used in both the glue and the adhesive tape, the precise chemicals were not named. Fisher, Shatin, and Reisch all felt that rubber cements were only rarely the cause of shoe allergy.

In her 1980 textbook, Cronin[101] stated that thiurams and MBT were used to formulate some latex glues used for shoe linings. She relied on the work of Jordan[171] and Dahl,[175] who assumed, but did not verify, that some of their MBT- and TMTD-positive patients were troubled by the presence of these chemicals in latex adhesives.

Modern rubber cements are used usually for sole attaching or for sticking layers below the insole. They help decrease the squeak of leather shoes. They are not as permanent as neoprene or urethane glues and need not be, especially if the sole is sewn. Most of them rely on rosin esters that are present as tackifiers, for example, glyceryl ester of rosin or various esterified wood rosins.

Neoprene Adhesives and Paratertiary Butylphenol Formaldehyde Resin (PTBFR)

Neoprene glues are usually used for the sole attachment but may find use anywhere below the shoe insole.[197]

Occasionally, thiurams are added to neoprene glues to control polymerization.[192] Dodecyl mercaptan (or mercapthane), also used to arrest polymerization in neoprene adhesives (e.g., Neoprene ACM by DuPont), has caused allergic reactions. Allergy to ethyl butyl thiourea, used as an accelerator in a neoprene adhesive, has already been mentioned.[193]

PTBFR allergy can explain 10% to 20% of patients allergic to footwear. Four of Jordan's[171] 25 patients, and 8 of Dahl's[175] 42 patients were allergic to phenolic resins.

The first cases of allergy to PTBFR in neoprene shoe adhesives were reported by Malten.[198] in 1958. None of his ten patients, who were shoemakers, reacted to neoprene AC, but all of them reacted to PTBFR and to PTBP itself. Two patients also reacted to formaldehyde, but it was uncertain whether this was related to formaldehyde's presence in the resin or to a fungicide in the shoe.[199]

By the mid- to late 1960s, more patients with shoe allergy attributed to PTBFR were being reported (1990). These later PTBFR-positive patients were not always positive to PTBP, which suggested that less free PTBP was present in the newer glues. Although sensitization can occur to either PTBP or PTBFR alone, group sensitization reactions between the two can also occur.

Other compounds besides PTBFR itself may be sensitizers in PTBFR adhesives. Rycroft[200] suggested 2-monomethylol phenol (tested 10% in petrolatum) as the sensitizing molecule in phenol formaldehyde resin allergy. He stressed the importance of testing with a patient's exact resin, because the screening phenol formaldehyde resin may be negative.

In a study from the Netherlands, 30 of 1,966 (1.5%) patients patch tested reacted to PTBP/PTBFR.[201] Of these, six had shoe dermatitis and five were allergic to watchbands.

In 1976, Foussereau and colleagues[202] collected 106 cases of PTBFR allergy. Thirty-one (29%) of the patients had footwear allergies, and the remaining cases were occupational. They affirmed that formaldehyde plays only a minor role in PTBFR allergies.

PTBFR adhesives find use in clothing items such as belts, watch straps, and hats. They are used widely in automobile upholstery and for hobby purposes. Individuals have been reported in whom allergic dermatitis was caused by PTBFR present in their amputation prostheses.[203]

Urethane Adhesives

Urethanes find wide use as adhesives because of their lightness and durability, and many of them require little curing. Although urethanes are commonly used as shoe adhesives, allergy caused by them is rarely reported. The nature of polyurethanes and the presence of allergy to their isocyanate component in shoe-allergic patients has already been mentioned.[171,185,192] It is unclear whether these patients reacted to urethane adhesives or to solid urethane materials such as might be used in the foamy

insole material. Tertiary amines such as triethylenediamine, cyclic amines such as diaminodiphenylmethane, plasticizers such as dibutyl tin or tin dilaurate, and the various diisocyanates themselves should all be kept in mind as possible causes of shoe dermatitis associated with modern synthetic shoes that are not explained with standard shoe allergens.

Patch Testing to Shoes

Patch testing with a standard screening series including chromate, rubber allergens, and PTBFR should detect most cases of foot dermatitis caused by shoe allergy. Adding the special "shoe" allergens listed in Table 18.10 will increase that yield. However, as the previous pages have documented, some patients with reactions to shoe pieces do not react to these allergens. It may be helpful to patch test directly with pieces of the suspect shoe. Because different parts of the shoe (uppers, lowers, soles, insoles, etc.) contain different allergens, one should attempt to obtain pieces of suspect shoe from an area in contact with the affected skin location. The piece should be thin to avoid pressure effects. Use of an adhesive bandage or plain Scanpor tape is recommended because the Finn chamber may cause pressure effects, leading to a false-positive result. The sample can be collected with a biopsy punch, curette, or scissors. It should be remembered that allergens in shoes may migrate under the moist conditions of chronic wearing. An insole, for example, may contain chemicals originally found in the outer sole.

It is difficult in patch testing to replicate the conditions of shoe wearing. For this reason, Jordan[171] has suggested soaking shoe-piece patches in water for 15 minutes before testing. It may be helpful to leave the pieces of shoe in place on the back for 4 or 5 days rather than for the traditional 48 hours.

When a patch test to a piece of shoe is positive but standard allergens are negative, there may be two explanations. Most likely, the allergen is an unusual chemical added to some shoe component such as a biocide in leather or other rarely used additive. However, positive patch tests to shoe pieces have at times been due to uptake by the shoe material of patient applied agents. For example, Storrs[204] has reported a case of allergy to topical steroids that had been absorbed into the shoe material. The patient had not bought any new shoes for several years and was, therefore, re-exposing himself to the offending allergens accidentally by wearing his old, "contaminated" shoes.

An equally interesting observation is that two patients with MBT allergy from their shoes gave positive reactions to pieces of white socks that had been soaked in dilute solutions of MBT (0.1% to 1%) for 24 hours and then washed and boiled. Rietschel[205] suggested that shoe allergens may concentrate in stockings and play an additional role in chronicity.

Stocking dermatitis can simulate shoe dermatitis. Thus, patch testing to stockings themselves or to the textile allergens listed in Table 18.8 will occasionally identify a cause in a patient with foot dermatitis.

MANAGEMENT OF SHOE DERMATITIS

Once the source of allergy in a shoe is identified, a patient can be guided to a shoe least likely to cause further problems. Because so many American shoes are imported, such guidance is not always easy. The patient can, however, be told what materials to avoid or seek.

While the physician sorts out the shoe allergens, or if a trial away from potentially allergenic shoes seems warranted, wooden or plastic shoes may be used as temporary substitutes. Plastic or wooden shoes should not be purchased with glued insoles.

For Rubber Allergy

Wear all leather shoes such as sewn leather moccasins with no insole and no attached outer sole. Injection-molded 100% plastic shoes with no insole should be fine. Some tennis shoes are rubber free. These shoes are made of polyolefins, urethanes, and ethylene vinyl acetate. Check the shoe's label for materials. Replace insoles with cork, felt, or gel insoles. Wooden shoes are also good substitutes.

For Leather Allergy

Wear wooden, plastic, or all-fabric shoes. Vinyl shoes and boots are also acceptable. Remove leather insoles because these may be chrome tanned. Specially made vegetable-tanned leather shoes are usually tolerated.

For PTBFR Adhesive Allergy

It may be necessary to contact individual manufacturers. One hundred percent leather, plastic (if not neoprene), or wooden shoes should be tolerated. Urethane-glued shoes are desired. Liners can be removed and replaced with gel, cork, or felt insoles glued in place with acrylic (e.g. Super Glue) adhesives or Elmer's type glue.

GENERAL TREATMENT OF SHOE DERMATITIS

Many locales have local manufacturers of special orthopedic or corrective shoes. Occasionally, these small companies will take enough interest to provide specially made products to avoid specific allergens. The cost for this may be prohibitive, however.

Topical therapy with wet dressings and corticosteroids or calcineurin inhibitors, as well as the occasional use of systemic corticosteroids, will assist in resolving acute eruptions. Despite these topical measures and even with shoe substitution, chronic foot dermatitis may be a problem. Minimizing shoe friction, using lubricants and occasionally topical corticosteroids, and discarding socks worn in the relevant shoes will all assist in hastening the resolution of a chronic shoe dermatitis.

It is possible that a patient may have a unique allergy to an unusual dye, fungicide, vegetable tannin, or adhesive ingredient that is present in only one pair of shoes. After the dermatitis has been cleared with medical measures and the patient has worn one pair of all-leather, all-wood, or all-plastic shoes (depending on the physician's suspicions), the suspect shoes can be slowly reintroduced. This should be done one pair at a time and no more often than weekly. Such a procedure can be used to apprehend the shoes in question.

TREATMENT OF HYPERHIDROSIS

People who have hyperhidrosis are especially prone to the development of shoe dermatitis. On occasion, controlling hyperhidrosis will allow a patient with a minimal problem to wear the "incriminated" shoes for short periods of time.

Zeasorb powder (Stiefel) dusted into shoes and hosiery may lessen perspiration. Drysol (Person & Covey), which is 20% aluminum chloride in ethyl alcohol, can also be used to treat hyperhidrosis. The Drionic device (General Medical Corp.) is an iontophoretic device that passes a slight electric current through the skin. Repeated treatments inactivate eccrine sweat glands for periods of up to several weeks. Intradermal injection of botulinum toxin can control hyperhidrosis for up to 6 months.

Tea foot baths are another way to help decrease foot sweating. They also assist in calming an acute dermatitis, but have the side effect of staining the feet and toenails.

Instructions for Tea Foot Baths

1. Boil six to eight tea bags in 1 quart of water for 10 minutes.
2. Place in basin and allow to cool to lukewarm temperature.
3. Soak feet for 30 minutes once or twice daily.
4. After 1 to 2 weeks, frequency of treatments can usually be reduced.

Formaldehyde and glutaraldehyde soaks have in the past been used to treat hyperhidrosis. Because of their allergenic potential, however, this cannot be recommended.

GENERAL MEASURES FOR MANAGEMENT OF CLOTHING DERMATITIS

When clothing is suspected of producing or aggravating an existing dermatitis, the following procedures may be helpful.

Washing of Clothes

Whenever washable garments are suspected of causing dermatitis, such clothes, particularly socks, stockings, shirts, and undergarments, should be washed to remove irritants and sensitizers before being worn again. All undergarments should be carefully washed and rinsed to remove all detergents, sebum, and sweat.

Handling of Dry-Cleaned Clothes

Clothing that has been dry cleaned should be removed from the plastic bag and thoroughly aired before being worn to allow complete evaporation of solvents and irritants used in the dry-cleaning process.

Control of Hyperhidrosis

Attempts to control hyperhidrosis with antiperspirants may aid in the prevention of clothing dermatitis. Botulinum toxin is effective at reducing axillary hyperhidrosis.

Use of Protective Undergarments

White cotton or silk undergarments may protect hypersensitive skin from irritation of rough woolen and tweed garments. Scarves are useful to protect the neck from the friction of furs and of collars of coats or blouses. Fowler feels that silk is more protective than cotton.

Management of Dermatitis from Linings

Removal of an allergenic clothing liner and replacement with undyed cotton or silk may allow continued use of an expensive garment.

Use of Skin Protectants

Several products are marketed as "skin protectants." Their efficacy in preventing textile dermatitis is unproven, but they may be worth trying.

MANAGEMENT OF ACD CAUSED BY DYES

Although textile dye chemistry is complex, the management of dye allergy is simple: **avoid synthetic fabrics** (Table 18.11). Since the vast majority of dye allergy is due to disperse dyes, which are not used on the natural fibers, cotton, linen, wool, silk, etc., of any color should be safe for most dye-allergic patients. White, or very light-colored synthetics may also be safe for these patients. If for

Table 18-11 Suggestions for Disperse Dye Allergic Patients
Wear any 100% "natural fabric" (cotton, silk, linen, wool, hemp, bamboo, etc.) of ANY color
For synthetics wear only white or very light colors
Wash new clothing once or twice before wearing
Darker synthetics may be tolerated if 1) they are worn for a short time only, 2) they are loose fitting, 3) the environment is cool
Cotton, or even better, silk, undergarments may block dye allergy reactions for a short time

some reason, substitution with non-synthetic garments is impossible, wearing undergarments between the clothing and the skin may reduce ACD, but usually is not sufficient to totally block a reaction. Silk may be more useful than cotton for this purpose (Fowler J, personal observation). Also, loose-fitting clothing is less likely to cause a problem than tighter garments.

Acknowledgement

Portions of this chapter are revisions of material written for the 3rd and 4th editions by Frances J. Storrs, MD, Portland, Oregon. Her contribution is greatly appreciated.

References

1. Swerev M. What dermatologists should know about textiles. In: Elsner P, Hatch K, Wigger-Alberti W. Textiles and the skin. Karger Basel, Switzerland, 2003, pp 1–23.

2. Fowler J, Skinner S, Belsito D. Allergic contact dermatitis from formaldehyde resin in permanent press clothing. J Am Acad Dermatol 1992;27:962.

3. Cronin E. Clothing and textiles. In: Ronin E, ed. Contact dermatitis. Edinburgh: Churchill Livingstone, 1980:36.

4. Calnan CD, Peachey RDG. Allergic contact purpura. Clin Allergy 1971;1:287.

5. Ramam M, Khaitan B, Singh M, Gupta S. Frictional sweat dermatitis. Contact Dermatitis 1998;38:49.

6. Betts C, Dearman R, Kimber, et al. Potency and risk assessment of a skin-sensitizing disperse dye using the local lymph node assay. Contact Dermatitis 205;52.268.

7. www.en.wikipedia.org/wiki/acid_dye, accessed May 8, 2007.

8. Pedersen NB. Occupational contact dermatitis from C.I. Acid Red 85 (C.I. 22245). Contact Dermatitis 1982;8:142.

9. Corea N, Basketter D, Clapp C, et al. Fragrance allergy: assessing the risk from washed fabrics. Contact Dermatitis 2006;55:48.

10. Belsito D, Fransway A, Fowler J, et al. Allergic contact dermatitis to detergents. J Am Acad Dermatol 2002;46:200.

11. Moncrieff RW. Man-made fibers. Toronto: John Wiley & Sons, 1975;1.

12. Otomasu K, Yamauchi M, Ohwatari N, et al. Analysis of sweat evaporation from clothing materials by the ventilated sweat capsule method. European J Appl Physiol 1997;76:1.

13. Braitman M. Dermatitis and fabrics. J Med Soc NJ 1955;52:757.

14. Walker JF. Formaldehyde. American Chemical Society Monograph Series, no. 159. New York: Robert E. Krieger Publishing Co., 1964:1.

15. Lord LW. Cutaneous sensitization to wool. Arch Dermatol 1932; 26:707.

16. Davies JH, Barker AN. Textile dermatitis. Br J Dermatol Syphilol 1944;56:33.

17. Osborne ED, Murray PF. Atopic dermatitis: study of its natural course and of wool as dominant allergenic factor. Arch Dermatol 1953;68:619.

18. Hellier FF. Dermatitis purpurica nach Kontakt mit Textilgeweben. Hautarzt 1960;11:173.

19. Romaguera C, et al. Occupational purpuric textile dermatitis from formaldehyde resins. Contact Dermatitis 1981;7:152.

20. Fregert S, et al. Allergic contact dermatitis from chromate in military textiles. Contact Dermatitis 1978;4:223.

21. Rudzki E. Contact urticaria from silk. Contact Dermatitis 1977;3:52.

22. Inoue A, Ishido I, Shoji A, Yamada H. Textile dermatitis from silk. Contact Dermatitis 1997;37:185.

23. Urbach E, Gottlieb PM. Allergy. New York: Grune & Stratton, 1946:245.

24. Brown SE, Coleman M. Severe immediate reactions to biologicals caused by silk allergy. JAMA 1957;165:2178.

25. http://www.shirtsof bamboo.com.

26. Morris GE. Nylon dermatitis. N Engl J Med 1960;263:30.

27. Prassa MN. Bullous dermatitis of feet caused by pure nylon. Bull Soc Trans Dermatol Syphilol 1955;62:508.

28. Tanaka M, et al. Contact dermatitis from nylon-6 in Japan. Contact Dermatitis 1993;28:250.

29. Batten K, et al. Occupational ACD from N,N methylen bis-5-methyloxazolidine in a nylon spin finish. Contact Dermatitis 1999;41:165.

30. Balda B. Allergic contact dermatitis due to acrylonitrile. Contact Dermatitis Newsletter 1971;9:219.

31. Bakker J, et al. Occupational contact dermatitis due to acrylonitrile. Contact Dermatitis 1991;24:50.

32. Osbourn RA. Contact dermatitis caused by Saran Wrap. JAMA 1964;188:1159.

33. Schulsinger C, Mollgaard K. Polyvinyl chloride dermatitis not caused by phthalates. Contact Dermatitis 1980;6:477.

34. Fregert S, Rorsman H. Hypersensitivity to epoxy resins used as plasticizers and stabilizers in polyvinyl chloride resins. Acta Derm Venereol (Stockh) 1963;43:10.

35. Dooms-Goossens A, Duron C, Loncke J, et al. Contact urticaria due to nylon. Contact Dermatitis 1986;14:63.

36. Porter PS, Sommer RG. Contact dermatitis due to spandex. Arch Dermatol 1967;95:43.

37. Batschvarow B, Minkow DM. Dermatitis and purpura from rubber in clothing. Trans St Johns Hosp Dermatol Soc 1968;54:178.

38. Shmunes E. Purpuric allergic contact dermatitis to paraphenylenediamine. Contact Dermatitis 1978;4:225.

39. Fisher A. Allergic petechial and purpuric rubber dermatitis: the PPP syndrome. Cutis 1974;14:25.

40. Mihan R, Ayres S. Stretch garment dermatitis. Calif Med 1968;108:109.

41. Jordan WP, Bourlas MC. Allergic contact dermatitis to underwear elastic. Arch Dermatol 1975;111:593.

42. Abel RR. Fiber glass: washing machine and fiberglass. Arch Dermatol 1966;93:78.

43. Kalimo K, Saarni H, Kytta J. Immediate and delayed type reactions to formaldehyde resin in glass wool. Contact Dermatitis 1980;6:496.

44. Fisher BK, Warkentin JD. Fiberglass dermatitis. Arch Dermatol 1969;99:717.

45. Bjornberg A, Lowhagen G. Patch test reactions to rockwool. Contact Dermatitis 1975;1:242.

46. Fisher AA. Fiber glass vs mineral wool (rockwool) dermatitis. Cutis 1982;29:412.

47. Reid JD, Arceneaux RL, Reinhardt RM, Harris JA. Studies of wrinkle resistance finishes for cotton textiles: release of formaldehyde vapors on storage of wrinkle-resistant cotton fabrics. Am Dyestuff Reporter 1960;49:29.

48. Vail SL, Reinhardt RM. What do formaldehyde tests measure? Text Chem Colorist 1981;13:13.

49. Formaldehyde. Current Intelligence Bulletin 34, NIOSH, April 15, 1981.

50. Sugai T, Yamanoto S. Decrease in the incidence of contact sensitivity to formaldehyde. Contact Dermatitis 1980;6:154.

51. 48. Pratt M, Belsito D, DeLeo V, Fowler J, et al. NACDG patch test results 2003–2004. Dermatitis 207, in press.

52. Marcussen PV. Contact dermatitis due to formaldehyde in textiles 1934–1958. Acta Derm Venereol (Stockh) 1959;39:348.

53. Hovding G. Free formaldehyde in textiles. Acta Derm Venereol (Stockh) 1959;39:357.

54. Hovding G. Contact eczema due to formaldehyde in resin finished textiles. Acta Derm Venereol (Stockh) 1961;41:194.

55. Cronin E. Formalin textile dermatitis. Br J Dermatol 1963;75:267.

56. Berrens L, Young E, Jansen LH. Free formaldehyde in textiles in relation to formalin contact sensitivity. Br J Dermatol 1964;76:110.

57. Fisher AA, Kanof NB, Biondi E. Free formaldehyde in textiles and paper. Arch Dermatol 1962;86:97.

58. Malten KE. Textile finish contact hypersensitivity. Arch Dermatol 1964;89:102.

59. Pannaccio F, Montgomery DC, Adam JE. Follicular contact dermatitis due to coloured permanent-pressed sheets. Can Med Assoc J 1973;109:23.

60. Wilkinson RD. Sheet dermatitis. Can Med Assoc J 1973;109:14.

61. Rycroft RJG, Cronin E, Calnan CD. Canadian sheet dermatitis. Br Med J 1976;2:1175.

62. Sherertz E. Clothing dermatitis: practical aspects for the clinician. Am J Contact Dermat 1992;3:55.

63. Metzler-Brenckle L, Rietschel R: Patch-testing for permanent–press allergic contact dermatitis Contact Dermatitis 2002;46:33.

64. Carlson R, Smith M, Nedorost S. Diagnosis and treatment of dermatitis due to formaldehyde resins in clothing. Dermatitis 2004;15:169.

65. Schwartz L. Dermatitis from synthetic resins. J Invest Dermatol 1945;6:239.

66. Helander I. Contact urticaria from leather containing formaldehyde. Arch Dermatol 1977;113:1443.

67. Jordan WP, Sherman WJ, Kins S. Threshold responses in formaldehyde-sensitive subjects. J Am Acad Dermatol 1979;1:44.

68. Dahl M. Formaldehyde sensitivity in patients allergic to formaldehyde-releasing biocides. Br J Dermatol 1982;106:119.

69. Lynde CW, Warshawski L, Mitchell JC. Screening patch tests in 4190 eczema patients 1972–1981. Contact Dermatitis 1982;8:417.

70. Marks J, Belsito D, DeLeo V, Fowler J, et al. North American Contact Dermatitis Group patch-test results, 1996–1998. Arch Dermatol 2000;136:272.

71. Agathos M. Formaldehyde contact allergy. Contact Dermatitis 1982;8:79.

72. Scheman A, Carroll P, Brown K, Osburn A. Formaldehyde related textile allergy: an update. Contact Dermatitis 1998;38:332.

73. Schorr WF, Keran E, Plotka E. Formaldehyde allergy. Arch Dermatol 1974;110:73.

74. Tarvainen K, Jolanki R, Henriks-Eckerman ML, Estlander T. Occupational allergic contact dermatitis from isophoronediamine (IPDA) in operative-clothing manufacture. Contact Dermatitis 1998;39:46.

75. Foussereau PJ, Meynadier J, Reuter G, et al. L'Eczema allergique aux toiles cirées. Dermatosen Beruf Umwelt 1980;28:46.

76. Molin L, Wahlberg JE. Toxic skin reactions caused by tributyltin oxide (TBTO) in socks. Berufs-dermatosen 4;138.

77. Savage J. Chloracetamide in nylon spin finish. Contact Dermatitis 1978;4:179.

78. Burrows D, Campbell HS. Contact dermatitis to polyester spin-finishes. Contact Dermatitis 1980;6:362.

79. Kawai K, et al. Occupational contact dermatitis from Kathon 930. Contact Dermatitis 1993;28:117.

80. Weaver JE, Maibach HI. Dose response relationships in allergic contact dermatitis: glutaraldehyde-containing liquid fabric softener. Contact Dermatitis 1977;3:65.

81. Eskelson YD, Goodman LS. Contact dermatitis from "Scotchgard," a stain repellent for fabrics. JAMA 1963;183:136.

82. Wilkinson S, et al. Allergic contact dermatitis from 1,6-diisocyanatohexane in an anti-pill finish. Contact Dermatitis 1991;25:94.

83. Taylor JS, Bergfeld WF, Guin JD. Contact dermatitis to knee patch adhesive in boy's jeans: a non-occupational cause of epoxy resin sensitivity. Cleve Clin Q 1983;50:123.

84. Baltinger, W. Westex Inc. technical bulletin. Chicago, 1997.

85. Parlew R, King CM, Evans S. Primary sensitization to a single accidental exposure to a flame retardant and subsequent allergic contact dermatitis. Contact Dermatitis, 1995;33:286.

86. Martin-Scott I. Contact textile dermatitis. Br J Dermatol 1966;78:632.

87. Belsito D. Contact dermatitis from diammonium hydrogen phosphate in surgical garb (Abstract). Contact Dermatitis 1990;23:267.

88. Ulsamer AG, Osterberg RE, McLaughlin J. Flame-retardant chemicals in textiles. Clin Toxicol 1980;17:101.

89. Blum A, Ames BN. Flame-retardant additives as possible cancer hazards. Science 1977;195:17.

90. http://en.wikipedia.org/wiki/tetrachlorethylene, accessed June 2, 2007.

91. Redmond S, Schappert K. Occupational dermatitis associated with garments. J Occup Med 1987;29:243.

92. Aoki T, Kageyama R. Three cases of dry cleaning dermatitis. Nippon-Hifuka-Gakkai-Zasshi 1989;99:1035.

93. Van Ketel WG. Contact dermatitis from a hydrazine-derivative in a stain remover; cross sensitization to

apresoline and isoniazid. Acta Derm Venereol (Stockh) 1964;44:49.

94. Jenkins CL. Textile dyes are potential hazards. J Environ Health 1978;40:279.

95. Fleming AJ. The provocative test for assaying the dermatitis hazards of dyes and finishes used on nylon. J Invest Dermatol 1948;10:281.

96. www.pubs.acs.org/cen/coverstory/8241/8241process3.html, accessed May 8, 2007.

97. Hatch KL, Maibach HI. Textile dye dermatitis. J Am Acad Dermatol 1995;32:631.

98. Hatch K, Maibach H. Dyes as contact allergens. Text Chem Colorist 1999;1:53.

99. Seidenari S, et al. Contact sensitization to textile dyes: description of 100 subjects. Contact Dermatitis 1991;24:253.

100. Pratt M, Taraska V. Disperse Blue Dyes 106 and 124 are common causes of textile dermatitis and should serve as screening allergens for this condition. Am J Contact Dermatitis 2000;1:30.

101. Cronin E. Studies in contact dermatitis XVIII: dyes in clothing. Trans St Johns Hosp Dermatol Soc 1968;54:156.

102. Sim-Davies D. Studies in contact dermatitis XXIV: dyes in trousers. Trans St Johns Hosp Dermatol Soc 1972;58:251.

103. Lazarov A, Trattner A, David M, Ingber A. Textile dermatitis in Israel: a retrospective study. Am J Contact Dermatitis 2000;1:26.

104. Storrs, F. Disperse Blue Dyes. Am J Contact Dermatitis 2000;1:1.

105. Seidenari S, Giusti F, Massone F, et al. Sensitization to disperse dyes in a patch test population over a five year period. Am J Contact Dermat 2002;13:101.

106. Goon A, Gilmour N, Basketter D, et al. High frequency of simultaneous sensitivity to disperse orange 3 in patients with positive patch tests to PPDA. Contact Dermatitis 2003;48:248.

107. Uter W, Geier J, Lessmann H. Contact allergy to disperse blue 106 and disperse blue 124 in German and Austrian patients. Contact Dermatitis 2001;44:173.

108. Warren L, Marren P. Textile dermatitis and dyed maggot exposure. Contact Dermatitis 1997;36:106.

109. Lazarov A, Ingber A. Textile dermatitis from Disperse Blue 85 in a knee brace. Contact Dermatitis 1998;38:357.

110. Batchelor R, Wilkinson S. Contact allergy to disperse dyes in plastic spectacle frames. Contact Dermatitis 2006;54:66.

111. Seidenari S, Manzini B, Schiavi M, Motolese A. Prevalence of contact allergy to non-disperse azo dyes for natural fibers: a study in 1814 consecutive patients. Contact Dermatitis 1995;33:118.

112. Mathur N, Mathur A, Benerjee K. Contact dermatitis in tie and dye industry workers. Contact Dermatitis 1985;12:38.

113. www.greatvistachemicals.com/dyes_ and_pigments, accessed May 8, 2007.

114. Scheman A. Allergic contact dermatitis from Basic Red 46 in a flame-retardant work clothing. Contact Dermatitis 1998;38:340.

115. Nixon R, Opie J, Frowen K. Basic Red 46: an important allergen in foot dermatitis? (abstr) Dermatitis 2004; 15:99.

116. Bielicky T, Novak M. Contact-group sensitization to triphenylmethane dyes: gentian violet, brilliant green and malachite green. Arch Dermatol 1969;100:540.

117. http://www.greatvistachemicals.com/dyes_and_pigments/direct_dye.html, accessed May 8,2007.

118. Malten K. Eczema in a cotton-printing mill (Proceedings of the XI International Congress of Dermatology). Acta Derm Venereol (Stockh) 1957;2:353.

119. Foussereau J, Benezra C, Maibach H. Occupational contact dermatitis: clinical and chemical aspects. 1st ed. Philadelphia: WB Saunders, 1982:1.

120. Ancona-Alayon A, et al. Occupational pigmented contact dermatitis from Naphthol AS. Contact Dermatitis 1976;2:129.

121. Kiec-Swierczynska M. Occupational contact dermatitis in the workers employed in production of Texas textiles. Dermatosen Beruf Umwelt 1982;39:41.

122. Roed-Petersen J, Batsberg W, Larsen E. Contact dermatitis from naphthol-AS. Contact Dermatitis 1990;22:161.

123. http://www.greatvistachemicals.com/dyes_and_pigments/direct_dye.html

124. www.greatvistachemicals.com/dyes_and_pigments accessed May 8, 2007.

125. Manzini B, Motolese A, Conti A, et al. Sensitization to reactive textile dyes in patients with contact dermatitis. Contact Dermatitis 1996;34:419.

126. Manzini B, Donini M, Motolese A, Seidenari S. A study of 5 newly patch tested reactive textile dyes. Contact Dermatitis 1996;35:313.

127. Moreau L, Goossens A: Allergic contact dermatitis associated with reactive dyes in a dark garment. Contact Dermatitis 2005;53:150.

128. www.greatvistachemicals.com/dyes_and_pigments/sulfur

129. Wilson H, Cronin E. Dermatitis from dyed uniform. Br J Dermatol 1971;87:67.

130. Calnan CD, Woods B. Dermatitis from dye in a leather watchstrap. Contact Dermatitis 1978;4:179.

131. Wright RC. Dermatitis from orthodichlorobenzene in a leather dye. Contact Dermatitis 1979;5:124.

132. Manzini B, et al. Contact sensitization to newly patch-tested non-disperse textile dyes. Contact Dermatitis 1991;25:331.

133. Kojima S, et al. Phosgene (chlorophenyl) hydrazones, strong sensitizers found in yellow sweaters bleached with sodium hypochlorite. Contact Dermatitis 1990;23:129.

134. Francalanci S, Angelini G, Balato N, et al. Effectiveness of disperse dyes mix in detection of contact allergy to textile dyes: an Italian multicentre study. Contact Dermatitis 1995;33:351.

135. Gardiner JS, Dickson A, Macleod TM, Frain-Bell W. The investigation of photocontact dermatitis is a dye manufacturing process. Br J Dermatol 1971;85:264.

136. Hjorth N, Moller H. Phototoxic textile dermatitis ("bikini dermatitis"). Arch Dermatol 1976;112:1445.

137. Estlander T. Allergic dermatoses and respiratory diseases from reactive dyes. Contact Dermatitis 1988;18:290.

138. Fanburg SJ. Dermatitis following the wearing of nylon stockings. JAMA 1940;115:354.

139. Calnan CD, Wilson HTH. Nylon stocking dermatitis. Br Med J 1956;1:147.

140. Dobkevitch S, Baer RL. Eczematous cross-hypersensitivity to azo dyes in nylon stockings and to paraphenylenediamine. J Invest Dermatol 1947;9:203.

141. Kousa M, Soini M. Contact allergy to a stocking dye. Contact Dermatitis 1980;6:472.

142. Foussereau J, Tanahaski Y, Grosshans E, et al. Allergic eczema from Disperse Yellow 3 in nylon stockings and socks. Trans St Johns Hosp Dermatol Soc 1975;58:75.

143. Osmundsen PE, Alani MD. Contact allergy to an optical whitener, "CPY," in washing powders. Br J Dermatol 1971;85:61.

144. Rothenborg HW, Hjorth N. Allergy to perfumes from toilet soaps and detergents in patients with dermatitis. Arch Dermatol 1968; 97:417.

145. Rinol Aguade J, et al. Dermatitis por blanqueradores opticas. Medicina Cutanea 1971;5:249.

146. Griffith JF. Fluorescent whitening agents. Arch Dermatol 1973; 107:728.

147. Osmundsen PE. Contact dermatitis from an optical whitener in washing powders. Cutis 1972;10:59.

148. Soni BP, Sherertz EF. Contact dermatitis in the textile industry: a review of 72 patients. Am J Contact Dermatitis 1996;7:226.

149. Dooms-Goossens A, Boyden B, Ceuterick A, Degruf H. Dimethylthiourea, an unexpected hazard for textile workers. Contact Dermatitis 1979;5:367.

150. Maiphetlho L. Contact dermatitis in the textile industry. Curr Allergy Clin Immunol 2007;20:28.

151. Elsner P, in: Biofunctional textiles and the skin. Hipler U and Elsner P, eds. Karger, Basel, Switzerland, 2006, pp: X.

152. Ricci G, Patrizi A, Mandrioli P, et al: Evaluation of the antibacterial activity of a special silk textile in the treatment of atopic dermatitis. Dermatology 2006;213:224.

153. Hofer D: Antimicrobial textiles in Biofunctional Textiles and the Skin. Hipler U and Elsner P, eds. Karger, Basel, Switzerland, 2006, pp. 42–51.

154. Gaul LE, Underwood GB. Primary irritants and sensitizers used in fabrication of footwear. Arch Dermatol 1949;60:649.

155. Calnan C, Sarkany I. Studies in Contact dermatitis IX. Trans St Johns Hosp Dermatol Soc 1959;43:8.

156. Fisher A: Some practical aspects of the diagnosis and management of shoe dermatitis Arch Dermatol 1959;79:267.

157. Weston JA, Hawkins K, Weston WL. Foot dermatitis in children. Pediatrics 1983;72:824.

158. Trevisan G, Kokelj F. Allergic contact dermatitis due to shoes in children: a 5-year follow-up. Contact Dermatitis 1992;26:45.

159. Cockayne SE, Shah M, Messenger AG, Gawkrodger DJ. Foot dermatitis in children: causative allergens and follow-up. Contact Dermatitis 1998;38:203.

160. Raoul S, Ducombs G, Leaute-Labreze C, et al. Footwear contact dermatitis in children. Contact Dermatitis 1996;35:334.

161. Bajaj A, et al. Footwear depigmentation. Contact Dermatitis 1996; 35:117.

162. Hack M. Chemical and mechanical etiology of shoe dermatitis Cutis 1970;6:259.

163. Freeman S. Shoe dermatitis. Contact Dermatitis 1997;36:247.

164. Mackie R. Juvenile plantar dermatosis Semin Dermatol 1982;1:67.

165. Romaguera C, Grimalt F, Ferrando J. Dry feet syndrome or juvenile plantar dermatosis. Contact Dermatitis 1982;8:219.

166. Warshaw E, Schram S, Belsito D, et al. Shoe allergens: review of the literature and retrospective analysis of cross-sectional data from the NACDG 2001–2004. submitted for publication 2007.

167. Holden C, Gawkrodger D. 10 years' experience of patch testing with a shoe series in 230 patients. Contact Dermatitis 2005;53:37–39.

168. Rani Z, Hussain I, Haroon T. Common allergens in shoe dermatitis: our experience in Lahore, Pakistan. Int J Dermatol 2003;42:605–7.

169. Trattner A, Farchi Y, David M. Shoe-contact dermatitis in Israel. Am J Contact Dermat 2003;14:12.

170. Jordan WP. Clothing and shoe dermatitis. Postgrad Med 1972;52:143.

171. Lynde CW, Warshawski L, Mitchell JC. Patch test results with a shoewear screening tray in 119 patients, 1977–80. Contact Dermatitis 1982;8:423.

172. Angelini G, Vena GA, Meneghini CL. Shoe contact dermatitis. Contact Dermatitis 1980;6:279.

173. Hack M. The shoe in contact dermatitis. J Am Podiatr Assoc 1976;66:408.

174. www.ita.doc.gov/td/ocg/imp316212–9q.htm accessed May 9, 2007.

175. Dahl MV. Allergic contact dermatitis from footwear. Minn Med 1975;58:871.

176. Grimalt F, Romaguera C. New resin allergens in shoe contact dermatitis. Contact Dermatitis 1975;1:169.

177. www.en.wikipedia.org/wiki/leather (accessed

178. Hausen BM. Woods injurious to human health: a manual. Berlin: Walter deGruyter, 1981.

179. Scutt RWB. Chrome sensitivity associated with tropical footwear in the royal navy. Br J Dermatol 1966;78:337.

180. Calnan CD, Cronin E. Vegetable tans in leather. Contact Dermatitis 1978;4:295.

181. Lewis GM. Dermatitis venenata due to tannins. Arch Dermatol 1944;50:138.

182. Lynch PJ. Indian sandal strap dermatitis. JAMA 1969;209:1906.

183. Minkin W, Cohen HJ, Frank S. Contact dermatitis to East Indian leather. Arch Dermatol 1971;103:523.

184. Spoor HJ. Indian leather dermatitis. Cutis 1973;11:805.

185. Jordan WP, Dahl MV, Albert HL. Contact dermatitis from glutaraldehyde. Arch Dermatol 1972;105:94.

186. Ancona A, Serviere L, Trejo A, Monroy F. Dermatitis from an azo dye in industrial leather protective shoes. Contact Dermatitis 1982;8:220.

187. Gaul LE. Results of patch testing with rubber antioxidants and accelerators. J Invest Dermatol 1957;29:105.

188. Marcussen PV. Rubber footwear as a cause of foot eczema. Acta Derm Venereol (Stockh) 1943;23:331.

189. Belsito D: Common shoe allergens undetected by commercial patch testing kits. Am J Contact Dermat 2003;14:95.

190. Robb JB. Rubber boot dermatitis in Newfoundland: a survey of 30 patients. Can Med Assoc J 1969;100:13.

191. Webb PK, Gibbs SC, Mathias CT, et al. Disulfiram hypersensitivity and rubber contact dermatitis. JAMA 1979;241:2061.

192. Leppard BJ, Parhizgar B. Contact dermatitis to PPD rubber in Maleki shoes. Contact Dermatitis 1977;3:91.

193. Roberts JL, Hanifin JM. Athletic shoe dermatitis: allergy to ethyl butyl thiourea. JAMA 1979;241:275.

194. Adams RM. Occupational skin disease. San Francisco: Grune & Stratton, 1983.

195. Srinivas C, et al. Footwear dermatitis due to Bisphenol-A. Contact Dermatitis 1989;20:150.

196. Shellow H. Dermatitis from Japanese rubber thong slippers. Fam Phys 1961;1:44.

197. Malten KE, Rath R, Pastors PHM. *p*-tert-butylphenol formaldehyde and other causes of shoe dermatitis. Dermatosen Beruf Umwelt 1983;31:149.

198. Malten KE. Contact sensitization caused by *p*-tert-butylphenol and certain phenol-formaldehyde-containing glues. Dermatologica 1967;135:54.

199. Malten K. Occupational eczema due to PTBFR in a shoe adhesive. Dermatologica 1958;135:54.

200. Rycroft RG. Contact sensitization to 2-monomethylol phenol in phenol formaldehyde resin as an example of the recognition and prevention of industrial dermatoses. Clin Exp Dermatol 1982;7:285.

201. Geldof B, et al. Clinical aspects of para-tertiary butylphenol-formaldehyde resin (PTBP-FR) allergy. Contact Dermatitis 1989;21:312.

202. Foussereau J, Cavelier C, Selig D. Occupational eczema from para-tertiary-butylphenol formaldehyde resins: a review of the sensitizing resins. Contact Dermatitis 1976;2:254.

203. Correcher BL, Perez AG. Dermatitis from shoes and an amputation prosthesis due to mercaptobenzothiazole and paratertiary butyl formaldehyde resin. Contact Dermatitis 1981;7:275.

204. Storrs FJ. Shoe dermatitis. Presented at American Contact Dermatitis Society Meeting, July 1993, New Orleans, LA.

205. Rietschel RL. Role of socks in shoe dermatitis. Arch Dermatol 1984;120:398.

MEDICAL DEVICES, IMPLANTS, AND EQUIPMENT

EXECUTIVE SUMMARY

Patients who receive artificial internal parts are at risk for allergy to components of these implants. Nowadays our patients may be treated with cardiovascular devices including pacemakers, valves, stents, umbrellas, and plugs, artificial orthopedic joints, genitourinary stents and supports, gastrointestinal bands and staples, and so on. Allergy to these implants is rare, but can cause dermatitis and/or failure of the implant. This is one of the areas in contact dermatitis that has been the subject of intense interest in the new millennium. Metals have been most commonly implicated in the rare cases of allergy, but other components such as acrylates and resins may cause allergy as well. In addition, evidence has begun to be presented that patients with endovascular stents have higher rates of metal allergy than controls. The currently unproven concern is that allergy to metals in a stent may increase the risk of restenosis. Gold, especially, has been implicated in this problem.

Many more cases of allergic contact dermatitis (ACD) and irritant contact dermatitis (ICD) occur from medical devices, dressings, and equipment that contact the skin. Examples include ostomy appliances, prosthetic limbs, hearing aids, eyeglasses, transcutaneous electrical nerve stimulation (TENS) units, and catheters.

Fortunately, in most cases of externally induced ACD or ICD from these medical items, the cause is suspected because of the location and history of the dermatitis. Metals, rubber allergens, adhesives, disinfectants, and plastics chemicals are the usual culprits. Many of these can be detected with a standard screening series of patch test allergens, and the rest are usually identifiable by aimed testing.

Reactions and Dermatitis Due to Metals Used in Orthopedic Surgery

COMMON PROSTHETIC METALS

Vitallium, stainless steel, and titanium are used widely for prosthetic devices. These metals are resistant to corrosion by physiologic fluids and can be left in the body indefinitely.[1]

Vitallium, a cobalt-based alloy designed for casting, contains about 30% chromium (Cr) and about 5% molybdenum (Mo). Since 1937, vitallium has been used successfully for orthopedic implants. Being a cast alloy, however, vitallium cannot be drawn into suture wire or worked into other complex shapes.

"Stainless steel" is a generic term covering several dozen iron-chromium alloys. The metallurgical definition of stainless steel requires a minimum of 10% chromium in an iron-based alloy.[2] Oxidation protects steel from degradation, while chloride exposure leads to pitting and potential breakage.[3] Addition of tantalum, niobium, or titanium aid in making steel amenable to welding. Two alloys, AISI Type 302 and AISI Type 316 steels, have found uses in orthopedic surgery. Shortly before World War II, however, it was recognized that Type 316 steel (17% Cr, 13% nickel [Ni], 2.5% Mo) was more inert to physiologic fluids than was Type 302 steel. The addition of molybdenum helps to prevent pitting by body chlorides. Widespread use of AISI Type 316 steel came about during World War II. Type 316 steel has some desirable features that vitallium lacks: greater strength, greater fatigue resistance, the ability to be easily worked into useful forms, and relatively low cost (Table 19.1). Most stainless steel contains nickel,

Table 19-1 Common Metals Used in Orthopedic Implants
Vitallium—cobalt, chromium steel
Type 316 stainless steels- chromium, molybdenum, cobalt, nickel
Titanium alloys
Nitinol-nickel titanium alloy

molybdenum, chromium and sometimes small amounts of other metals,

Titanium is one of the newer metals to be used in prosthetic applications. Although it lacks the strength of Type 316 stainless steel or vitallium, it is apparently inert to physiologic fluids. In fact, bone has a tendency to grow in contact with titanium and becomes very adherent to it. Titanium has been used successfully in various reconstructions. In cases of known or strongly suspected allergy to nickel, cobalt, or chromate, titanium prosthesis may be preferable.

NEWER ORTHOPEDIC ALLOYS

Nitinol is an alloy composed of about 55% nickel and 45% titanium. It is called a "metal with a memory" because it returns to its initial shape when heated. It may be used in some suture fixation devices and in spinal rods.[1] Other titanium alloys containing zirconium and niobium may be stronger than titanium alone.

Reactions to Implanted Metal Prostheses

Orthopedic implants may be either static, such as rods and screws, or dynamic, such as an artificial hip or knee joint. Most joint implants now have a metal-to-plastic interface. In patients who have old metal-to-metal prostheses, elevated concentrations of chromium and cobalt occur in blood and urine as well as in the tissue adjacent to the joint prostheses. In patients with metal-to-plastic prostheses, the metal concentrations in blood and urine are usually normal, and only slightly elevated in the tissues when compared with controls.[4,5]

Nickel is released from stainless steel prostheses by the action of sweat, blood, and physiologic saline solution.[6] In laboratory animals, solubilized nickel is localized in the tissue near the implant.[7]

The sensitization potential of implanted metal alloys has been evaluated in retrospective and prospective clinical studies. The significance of these studies is difficult to interpret, because metal allergy is a common phenomenon in the general population.

In retrospective studies concerning patients with metal-to-metal prostheses (cobalt and chromium), a high incidence of metal sensitivity has been found. In 14 patients who had loose prostheses, 9 were sensitive to either cobalt or chromium. Of 24 patients who had normally functioning prostheses, none was metal sensitive.[5] Elves and colleagues[8] studied 50 patients with metal-to-metal prostheses. Of the 50 patients, 23 had a nontraumatic failure of the prosthesis. Fifteen of these were sensitive to metals, 7 were cobalt-sensitive, 3 were sensitive to cobalt and nickel, 2 to nickel, 2 to chromium, and 1 to both nickel and vanadium. In the other 27 patients who had stable prostheses or who had a traumatic failure, only 4 were metal sensitive. Benson and colleagues[9] found an incidence of 28% metal sensitivity in patients with metal-to-metal prostheses. Among 34 patients with pain and loosening of the prostheses, Munro-Ashman and Miller[10] found 16 patients with metal sensitivity. Thirteen were sensitive to cobalt, 4 to nickel, and 2 to chromium. The results of these studies are similar and, although retrospective, they suggest that at least cobalt sensitization occurs as a consequence of systematic exposure to the metal when released from an implanted metal alloy.

Lodi and colleagues[11] patch tested 66 patients an average of 8 years after implantation with a large battery of metal allergens. There was one positive test each to nickel, cobalt, and chromate, but seven to vanadium trichloride (5% pet). Many irritant responses were also seen to the vanadium, so the significance of this data is uncertain. There was no comment regarding the type of prosthesis—metal to metal or metal to plastic.

In older prospective studies concerning similar patients in whom the preoperative status has been evaluated by patch testing, no evidence was found of sensitization to the implanted metal alloys when retested months to years after the operation.[12–15] In the retrospective part of the study by Carlsson and colleagues,[12] a statistically significant increase in the number of metal-sensitive patients was found among those with loose prostheses. Among the patients studied prospectively, only a few had complications with pain and loosening of the prostheses. Rooker and Wilkinson[15] studied 69 patients prospectively. Before the operation, six patients were metal sensitive, but only one remained so afterward. The authors suggested that the minimal systemic exposure to the hapten led to immunologic tolerance. The safety of the metal-to-plastic prostheses from the point of sensitization is in agreement with the small amounts of metal released from this type of prosthesis.[4,5]

Sensitization from metal prostheses has been reported mostly in patients with loosening of the prostheses. This does not prove that the allergy is the cause of the loosening. The alternative explanation is that the loosening causes the allergy. The present evidence supports the latter hypothesis.[16,17]

Skin symptoms in patients who have undergone implantation of metal prostheses are rare. They occur in two forms: either as a dermatitis localized to the skin that covers the area of the metal prostheses[10,18] or as a generalized dermatitis.[19–22] Those who develop rashes from osteosynthesis screws have a more persistent disease, and removal of the screws has been followed by a rapid clearing of the dermatitis.[18,19,21,23]

In a literature review, Dujardin and colleagues[23] found 54 cases of dermatitis due to various implants. None were caused by titanium. The difficulties of making a firm diagnosis without removal of the prosthesis are discussed.

CASE REPORT ILLUSTRATING POTENTIAL PROBLEMS WITH A METAL IMPLANT

Thomas and colleagues gave an extensive report on a patient with impaired healing of a hand fracture, along with dermatitis in the area.[24] The eczema began within a few weeks after a titanium plate and screws were placed. Patch tests were negative, but lymphocyte transformation tests were positive to titanium dioxide. Fifty controls were negative. Removal of the titanium resulted in prompt healing of both the fracture site and the skin lesions.

REACTION TO ACRYLATES IN ORTHOPEDIC SURGERY

Occasionally, allergic reactions have been seen to methyl methacrylate in orthopedic bone cements (Figure 19-1). More often, the surgeon may suffer a hand dermatitis from these agents. Joint loosening apparently occurs rarely, if at all.[24]

ROLE OF PREOPERATIVE PATCH TESTING

The utility of preoperative patch testing is unclear. Fowler has noted an increase in patients and orthopedic surgeons requesting such tests over the last few years. Some of this may be driven by a greater understanding of the potential problems associated with metal allergy and joint implants, while some is undoubtedly related to concern over potential litigation if a poor surgical result occurs. Concern over degradation of polyethylene sockets may be leading orthopedists to return to the use of more metal-on-metal prostheses. A 10% failure rate is expected.[25] Carlsson and colleagues[12] recommended that a patient who had a history of metal allergy should be examined

by a dermatologist and should be patch tested. If a metal allergy is found, an implant should be used that does not contain the metal in question. Only long-term prospective studies, which are currently unavailable, can determine whether it is necessary to take these precautions.

SUMMARY

Gawkrodger[25] reviewed the subject and agreed that modern prostheses of the metal to plastic variety rarely cause metal allergy. Occasionally, eczema, either localized or generalized, may be seen with static implants, but even this is rare.

An important concern in the debate about preoperative patch testing is medicolegal liability. If any adverse event occurs in a metal-sensitive patient after implantation of that metal, the surgeon may be held liable, rightly or wrongly. Therefore, even though cutaneous and other reactions to implanted metals are rare, knowledge of the patient's allergic status should be taken into consideration when determining implant usage.

The following summarizes our current state of knowledge regarding orthopedic implants and metal allergy:

1. Even if a patient has a proven metal allergy, any reaction to an orthopedic implant is rare.
2. The most likely reaction to occur seems to be dermatitis. This may be limited to the site of the implant, may affect a distant site especially the hands, or may become generalized.
3. Failure of the implant or poor wound healing has been documented in a very few cases.
4. Pre-operative patch testing can usually identify pre-existing metal allergies.
5. Documented allergy to titanium is exceedingly rare, so if tests to other metals are positive titanium is as safe an alternative as possible.
6. In cases of known metal allergy, legal concerns may outweigh medical concerns, since an implant allergy may be blamed by a litigious patient for post-operative problems even if the allergy is not the cause.

Allergy to Endovascular Stents

Several years ago, a report suggested that metal allergy may be implicated in restenosis of cardiac artery stents.[26] In this paper, patients were patch tested with several metals and their stent status was evaluated some time after surgery. Although many who were not allergic to metals had restenosis, the percentage with metal allergy and restenosis was significantly greater. Subsequent reports suggested that gold plated stents had higher restenosis rates than identical types without gold.[27]

Swedish dermatologists and cardiologists evaluated 22 patients 18 months after gold stent placement.[28] Ten of 22 (45.5%) were allergic to gold, as compared to 20.5% of a matched control group. Three of the ten gold-allergic patients (30%) had restenosis as compared to 2 of 12 in the non-allergic group (17%). The difference was suggestive but not statistically significant. The small number of patients may have mitigated against detecting significance.

There is evidence then, of an increased rate of metal allergy in patients who have received endovascular stents. The current limited data suggests that the presence of allergy increases the risk of stent restenosis, but this must be considered speculative at this time. Cause and effect is unknown; does allergy cause inflammation and stent occlusion or does inflammation and occlusion lead to the development of allergy?

Ostomy Dermatitis

Ostomies are artificial openings to the gastrointestinal (GI) or urinary tracts. They are used widely in the treatment of a variety of inflammatory, neoplastic, and posttraumatic processes. The proper care of the operative stoma and of the appliance fitted to it is crucial to proper functioning of the surgical diversion and to the complete rehabilitation of the patient. Fortunately, specially trained ostomy nurses or technicians are available to most ostomy patients to provide optimum routine management. The dermatologist rarely needs to become involved unless intractable dermatitis develops.

The peristomal skin is prone to irritation and development of ACD partly because of the continuous exposure to GI or urinary fluids and moisture, and partly because of the occlusion necessary around the stoma to prevent leakage.

Rothstein[29–32] has written extensively on the care and management of the ostomy site. He states that several factors relating to the stomal surgery itself are important in providing an optimal stoma result. These include gentle handling of the skin to avoid scarring and proper anatomic placement of the stomal stump to avoid surface irregularities that allow for leakage. Also, the length of the stump is critical so that excess irritation from friction or secretions will not occur. Depending on the stoma location, discharge may be more fluid or more solid. Obviously, fluid drainage is more likely to cause irritation because of the presence of fecal enzymes and an alkaline pH.

PERISTOMAL ALLERGIC AND IRRITANT CONTACT DERMATITIS

Allergic contact dermatitis (ACD) may be caused by a variety of allergens in the peristomal area. It has been well documented that ACD is more likely to develop in areas where skin breakdown from other causes occurs, and this situation may be present around a stoma. Pruritus and spread of dermatitis around the affected site are typical of ACD.

Martin and colleagues have recently reviewed reports of peristomal ACD.[33] They identified 23 cases from the English language literature. The most commonly reported cause is the stoma bag, with epoxy resin the usual allergen. Allergy to Gantrez, a PMV/methacrylate copolymer, has been reported[34] several times. Gantrez is a patented polymer with an ability to adhere to moist areas. It is N-butylmonoester of polymethyl vinyl ether maleic acid.[34] Contact sensitivity has been reported to Hollister adhesive, Stomahesive, and rubber.[31–34]

Table 19.2 lists some of the reported causes of peristomal ACD. Patch testing is essential to determine the allergen(s) responsible. On screening patch test series, the rubber allergens, rosin, epoxy resin, neomycin, fragrance, and preservatives are all candidates to cause peristomal ACD. Other potential allergens include topical antimicrobials, disinfectants, acrylates, corticosteroids, and plasticizers.

Irritant dermatitis is common and must be expected to occur in almost any ostomy patient occasionally. Chemical irritation may occur from excreted fluids, from solvents, cleansing materials, or disinfectants used when changing the device, or from pressure and friction from the sealing ring and ostomy pouch. Gentle changing of the ostomy pouch, without the use of solvents, if possible, may be necessary if irritation develops. It has been suggested that the use of a karaya ring instead of common adhesive rings may be useful if irritation develops.[35] The pouch can be held in place

Table 19-2 Reported Allergens in Stomal Dermatitis

Adhesive tapes (rubber, acrylates, rosin)
Adhesive remover solvents
Deodorizers e.g. d-limonene
Disinfectants
Epoxy resin components
Gantrez
Myroxylon Pereirae, fragrances
Rosin
Rubber additives
Stomahesive paste
Topical medications (corticoids, excipients)

with hypoallergenic tape or a belt temporarily. The bag itself may cause an irritant reaction owing to friction or a prickly, heatlike eruption owing to sweat retention.[35] Secondary yeast infection is also common at ostomy sites and may be treated with topical or systemic antifungal agents.

Karaya is a polysaccharide gum made from the sterculia tree.[32] It is available as a powder, which is good for absorbing moisture, a paste, or as an ostomy ring. Rothstein suggests mixing karaya with milk of magnesia or an antacid such as aluminum hydroxide, which may inhibit fecal enzyme activity.[30] Burt-McAliley and colleagues,[36] however, prospectively studied 112 patients given either a karaya-based or a pectin-based barrier. They found that irritation was more likely to develop in those using a karaya-based product.

DEODORANT DERMATITIS

Davies and colleagues[37] reported that an ostomy deodorant sensitized two patients and was due to oil of citronella.

UROSTOMY DERMATITIS

Urostomies are subject to encrustations. These are verrucous, gray-white excrescences that seem to grow on the stomal mucosa or on improperly cleaned reusable pouches. They are crystallized alkaline salts, mainly amorphous ammonium phosphates. Because of their gritty texture, they may excoriate the skin if they are allowed to seep beneath the pouch. Prolonged exposure of the skin to moisture may create pseudoepitheliomatous hyperplasia—a condition of epidermal thickening characterized histologically by acanthosis and increased mitoses but without atypia.[38]

Mann and colleagues[39] reported sensitivity to a urostomy pouch plastic in a patient with epoxy resin sensitivity. The patient's eczema cleared completely on subsequently changing the system to another pouch. Van Ketel and colleagues[40] also reported epoxy resin dermatitis from a Squibb ileostomy bag, which was made of polyvinyl chloride, in which epoxy resin was used as a plasticizer.

TRACHEOSTOMY ALLERGIC CONTACT DERMATITIS

ACD to rubber and in another case to the medications salbutamol and Aldecin, which contains betamethasone, have been reported.[41,42]

MANAGEMENT OF OSTOMY DERMATITIS

Rothstein[31,32] reviewed important considerations in ostomy management. Obviously, avoidance of further irritation and identification of allergens is a critical first step. Temporary ostomy appliances may be tolerated for several days to allow the skin to heal before reapplying permanent devices. A topical or oral anti-*Candida* agent will reduce yeast infections and colonization. Low- to medium-strength topical corticosteroids may be needed, but care must be taken so as not to allow development of steroid atrophy or secondary infections. Systemic corticosteroids may be needed for a short time for severe cases.

Covering the pouch with a commercial cloth bag or even flannel or gauze may reduce frictional irritation.

Two "skin protective" products may offer some benefit at reducing irritation or allergen penetration, but have not been studied for this use. These include Pro-Q foam (Ponsus Pharma, Stockholm, Sweden) and Ivy-Block Lotion (Hyland Inc., Chicago, Il.). To be effective, such products would need to be applied to the skin before the appliance is seated and also applied under tape and the pouch.

Contraceptive Dermatitis

The most common contraceptives in use at present—the condom, the diaphragm, chemical contraceptives, female pouches, the intrauterine device, and "the Pill"—may all occasionally produce allergic or other reactions[43] (Table 19.3).

CONDOMS

Condoms are popularly called "sheaths," "French letters," prophylactics," "rubbers," "skins," or "safes" and are made mostly of rubber. Allergic reactions to condoms may produce itching and edema of the

Table 19-3 Contraceptive Dermatitis Patch Test Series	
Patch Test Substance	Concentration[a]
Chemical contraceptive used	As is
Thiuram Mix	
Carbamate Mix	
Mercapto Mix	
Mercaptobenzothiazole	
Mixed thioureas	
Hexylresorcinol	1% pet
Nonoxynol-9	0.05% aq
Oxyquinoline sulfate	1% pet
Phenoxypolyetoxy ethanol	0.5% pet
Phenyl mercuric acetate	0.01% pet
Quinine hydrochloride	1% aq
Rubber condom	As is

prepuce or distal part of the shaft of the penis, which may initiate an eczematous dermatitis and spread to the entire shaft, the scrotum, and the inguinal and suprapubic areas. The eruption may spread to other areas of the body.

The rubber condom may also produce an acute dermatitis of the vulva and inner thighs in a rubber-sensitive female sexual partner.

Rubber condom dermatitis is usually due to sensitivity to one or more rubber antioxidants or accelerators or to latex itself.[44] (Rubber allergy is discussed more specifically in Chapter 29.) Occasionally, a preservative powder which has been dusted onto the condom or a lubricant is the cause of the dermatitis rather than the rubber itself. In one instance, the powder contained 10% monobenzylether of hydroquinone (agerite alba), which is a sensitizer and depigmenting agent.

Patch tests may be performed with the condom suspected of producing the reaction. If a powder or lubricant is present with the condom, tests should also be performed with these substances. Patch tests should also be performed with the usual rubber allergens.

Immediate hypersensitivity (contact urticaria) to latex may cause localized urticaria in either partner. More severe reactions, including anaphylaxis, have occasionally been reported (see Chapter 29). Such reactions are especially surprising and unpleasant during times when condoms are in use.

Some have found by trial and error that only certain brands of rubber condoms produce allergic reactions, but in general, individuals with rubber sensitivity should use nonrubber condoms.

A rubber-sensitive woman can acquire an acute diffuse dermatitis of the vulva and inner thighs from contact with a rubber condom worn by a man.

Nonrubber Condoms

Condoms made of processed lamb cecum are available for individuals who cannot tolerate rubber condoms. Such preparations are popularly called "fishskins." Because these condoms may not be as effective in preventing the spread of sexually transmitted diseases, a rubber condom may be worn over the natural condom if the man is sensitive or under the natural condom if the woman is sensitive to rubber.

Lubricants Used with Condoms

Many condoms are lubricated with aqueous gums containing preservatives. Some of these preservatives, particularly the parabens, have been shown to be sensitizers.

Oils and petrolatum should be avoided as lubricants, because they cause rubber to deteriorate.

ALLERGIC OR IRRITANT CONTRACEPTIVE DERMATITIS IN WOMEN

Allergic or irritant mucosal reactions can occur from chemical contraceptives. Often, in mild cases, the patient complains of pruritus vulvae or a burning vaginal sensation, and little is noted on examination. This may indicate either an irritant dermatitis or mild ACD. In more severe degrees of allergic reactions, redness and edema of the vulva occurs, and the adjacent skin shows an eczematous reaction.

CHEMICAL CONTRACEPTIVES

Many chemical contraceptives are available. They consist essentially of a foaming agent or surfactant to emulsify the ejaculate and a spermicide to act upon it. They are produced as creams, jellies, pastes, gelatin vagatories, waxy vagatories, and foaming tablets. These chemical contraceptives are all intended for vaginal insertion before coitus.

These preparations may contain monophenoxypolyetoxy ethanol derivatives (nonoxynol-9), hexylresorcinol, and chloramine predominantly. Nonoxynol-9 is a very rare allergen but a common cause of temporary, low-grade irritation in either partner. German manufacturers also commonly use quinine and ammonium thiocyanate. Hungarian "state-manufactured" preparations contain cetylpyridium bromide. In Sweden, sodium dioctylsulfosuccinate and sodium lauryl sulfate are combined commonly in a contraceptive cream. In Russia, quinine pessaries have been used widely for contraception.

Sensitizers in Vaginal Spermicides

These chemicals include phenylmercuric acetate, oxyquinoline sulfate, quinine hydrochloride, and hexylresorcinol.

Patch tests with chemical contraceptives must be interpreted with care because some contraceptives contain surfactants that may show nonspecific irritant reactions under a closed patch. A positive patch test reaction to a chemical contraceptive should be followed by testing in controls and if possible, with the individual ingredients of the product. Testing with a screening series, such as the North American Contact Dermatitis Group (NACDG) series, will cover the most common causes of contraceptive ACD including rubber allergens, preservatives, fragrances, lanolin, and propylene glycol. Individual allergens in spermicides should be determined by contacting the manufacturer and tested when possible.

Sensitivity to quinine hydrochloride may manifest itself as an allergic purpuric dermatitis medicamentosa.

Intrauterine Devices (IUDs)

An IUD made of a copper ring and a polyethylene carrier of metallic copper is available. Several cases of dermatitis due to the IUD in copper-sensitive individuals have been reported.[45–47]

Hemodialysis (Renal) Dermatitis

Formaldehyde, glutaral, other disinfectants, epoxy resin, and thiurams have produced ACD in individuals servicing hemodialysis machines or in patients receiving dialysis.

FORMALDEHYDE DERMATITIS

Sneddon[48] reported that formaldehyde solutions 2% to 4% are used for sterilization in some renal dialysis units and for home kidney machines. In one such unit, 6 of 13 staff members developed dermatitis of the eyelids, face, and hands. Four staff members were sensitive to formaldehyde. The dermatitis ceased when formaldehyde was replaced by another disinfectant. Abdel-Aziz and Hodgson[49] treated a man who used formaldehyde to sterilize a kidney machine and who subsequently developed an extensive eczema on his hands and arms. Patch testing confirmed the patient's sensitivity to formaldehyde. Three cases of formaldehyde dermatitis occurred in the hospital's dialysis unit.

Hendrick and Lane[50] stated that formaldehyde used to sterilize artificial kidney machines caused asthma and productive coughs among the staff of a hemodialysis unit. Glutaraldehyde may also be used on dialysis equipment and can cause ACD in staff and patients.

A prospective double-blind study documented that five of ten patients with anaphylactoid symptoms on dialysis reproduced their symptoms when exposed to formaldehyde sterilized equipment but not when the equipment was gas sterilized.[51]

EPOXY RESIN DERMATITIS

Mork[52] described contact sensitivity from epoxy resin in a hemodialysis set at the site where an adhesive strip containing epoxy resin fixed the needle. Brandao and Pinto[53] studied two patients on hemodialysis who developed dermatitis at the site of needle puncture. Patch tests were positive to epoxy resin and to the glue that binds the needle to the plastic butterfly. Filter paper test and thin layer chromatography confirmed that the glue was a low-molecular-weight epoxy resin of the bisphenol A

type. (See also Chapter 27). Both patients changed needles and had no more trouble.

THIURAM DERMATITIS

Another cause of dermatitis in hemodialysis units has been described by Penneys and colleagues.[54] An outbreak of dermatitis among patients in such a unit was traced to various thiuram compounds, probably leaching out of the rubber components of the hemodialysis apparatus.

PRURITUS WITH EXCORIATIONS

Many patients with severe renal dysfunction, whether or not they are on dialysis, develop severe itching, for reasons totally unrelated to allergy, which induces scratching and excoriations.

Dermatitis of Amputation Stumps

The skin of an amputee who wears a prosthesis is subject to many abuses, even though the devices have improved greatly in recent years. The artificial limb now weighs about 1 lb compared to 10 to 12 lbs a decade ago.[55]

With the conventional prosthesis for the leg amputee, the stump fits into the hollow of the socket and the device is held on with a pelvic band.

Suction suspension is used more frequently. As the amputee places his weight on the prosthesis, air is forced out through the valve in the socket; then, as the amputee shifts his or her weight to the normal leg, the artificial limb is held to the stump by negative pressure. Uneven loading on the socket, which provides for weight bearing, may cause stress on areas of the stump skin. Common disorders are cysts developed under friction and pressure, dermatitis, and edema at the end of the stump.

Therapy by the dermatologist requires close cooperation with the orthopedic surgeon and prosthetist, which will include eliminating all mechanical factors contributing to edema. These factors can include poor fit and alignment and excessive negative pressure in a suction-socket prosthesis. As with ostomies, the modern prosthesis technician is usually well equipped to handle routine problems. Cases of persistent dermatitis, especially ACD, may require dermatologic intervention and evaluation.

SUCTION-SOCKET PROSTHETIC DERMATITIS

An amputee can expect edema, hyperemia, and pigmentation resulting from capillary hemorrhage, and other relatively innocuous conditions to occur when starting to wear a suction-socket prosthesis. These changes, which usually do not require therapy, are the result of altered conditions forced on the skin and subcutaneous tissues. They can be partially prevented, however, by gradual compression of the stump tissues with an elastic bandage or "shrinker" sock prior to use of the prosthesis.

NONSPECIFIC ECZEMATIZATION OF AMPUTEE SKIN

Nonspecific eczematization of the stump skin has been seen in several instances. In one case, the amputee presented a weeping, itching, nonhealing plaque of dermatitis over the distal portion of the stump. The lesion, at first dry and scaly, suddenly and without an apparent reason, became moist. It waxed and waned over a period of months to years. In some instances a significant history of recurrent allergic eczema or active eczematous lesions on other portions of the body was found to account for the eruption on the stump. In other instances, the eczema was secondary to edema and congestion of the terminal portion of the stump, so that only with the alleviation of these problems did the condition clear.

EPIDERMAL CYSTS IN AMPUTEES

Allende and colleagues[56] reported the following:

1. Epidermoid cysts appearing in the stumps of amputees have been studied from clinical, bacteriologic, and histopathologic points of view.
2. These cysts occur as the result of mechanical shearing forces produced by the socket on the skin, which result in invagination and implantation of keratin plugs and epidermal fragments into the dermis. These plugs become separated from the epidermis and are surrounded by a foreign-body reaction; the cyst that forms may become liquefied and rupture to the surface, producing a sinus.
3. Many therapeutic measures, including surgical incision and drainage, excision and grafting, topical therapy, injection of hydrocortisone and triamcinolone, antibiotic therapy, and griseofulvin therapy, have been only palliative.
4. Improvement in prosthetic fit, with reduction of shearing forces, seems to be the most promising approach to the problem.

VERRUCOUS HYPERPLASIA

Hyperplasia appeared to be secondary to an underlying vascular disorder, poor prosthetic fit and alignment, and possibly bacterial infection. Working with the orthopedic surgeon and the engineering department permits successful treatment. Levy[55] reported a patient with longstanding verrucous hyperplasia and an ulceration who developed a squamous cell carcinoma of the stump.

External compression combined with adequate control of bacterial infection proved, through trial and error, to be the best method of treatment. When support of the stump end was provided in the socket by building up a temporary platform with foam rubber, the verrucose condition was reduced. The greater the compression on the distal stump, the more immediate and lasting was the improvement.

ROLE OF HYGIENE IN PREVENTION OF AMPUTEE DERMATITIS

Amputees must be instructed carefully in the hygienic care of their stumps. The primary requirement is that the stump should be kept clean. Washing should not be done in the morning or just before the prosthesis is put on, because damp skin may swell, stick to the socket, and be irritated by rubbing. The socket itself should be cleansed frequently—every day in warm weather—also after the prosthesis is removed and not just before it is put on. The stump sock should be changed daily.

Des Groseilliers and colleagues[57] stated that of 50 amputees seen in 1 year, 17 amputees were affected. The most common lesions were due to badly fitting prostheses or to poor hygiene, which caused callus formation or breakdown of the skin with or without ulceration in 12 patients.

Van Ketel[58] reported that the friction and pressure of prostheses, in addition to close and prolonged contact with the skin, are important factors responsible for the skin becoming easily damaged. Trophic changes in the stumps are mainly the result of these factors.

ALLERGIC CONTACT DERMATITIS OF THE STUMP

1. *Plastics.* The sockets of leg prostheses are commonly finished with an inside application of varnish or lacquer and an outside coating of plastics and resins. These substances are capable of causing ACD. The epoxy resins, if cured incompletely in their manufacture, may serve as specific allergic sensitizers or may produce primary-irritant dermatitis. These resins are used frequently to improve the appearance of a socket and to render it impervious to external agents.[59] Paratertiary butyl catechol and paratertiary butylphenol formaldehyde resin have caused cases of dermatitis in amputees.[60,61] Unsaturated polyester resin caused allergy in a child with an arm prosthesis.[62] Curing agents, known as catalysts or hardeners, are added to solidify the plastic material. These agents are organic amines of various types and, when left in excess by incomplete baking or curing at high

temperatures, are able to produce a dermatitis. Benzoyl peroxide, used as a catalyst in plastic manufacture, caused allergy in one case.[63] There are at least two reports of ACD to methyl methacrylate in leg prosthesis wearers. Other acrylates may also be involved.[64,65]

2. *Rubber allergens.* Allergy to thiurams and/or mercaptobenzothiazoles can cause ACD when the stump contains a rubber portion or suction device.[66] Thioureas are especially common cause of ACD to neoprene rubber.

3. *Topical medications, cleansers, and antibacterial agents.* In seven patients with amputation stumps of the thighs, allergic contact eczema could be confirmed by positive patch tests by Fisher. Two patients were allergic to hexomedine, an antibacterial that is often used because it penetrates easily into the skin.

4. *Leather and metals.* Of five patients wearing leather prostheses, one was sensitized to paraphenylenediamine and other para dyes. Two patients showed positive patch tests to potassium dichromate. Because most leathers are tanned with chromium compounds, these reactions could be considered relevant. Another patient reacted to paratertiarybutylphenol and paratertiarybutylphenol formaldehyde resin. These compounds were probably used in a glue in the manufacture of prostheses. One patient showed a positive patch test to chamois leather, which was used for patch testing. In this prosthesis, pieces of chamois leather were used to protect the skin from pressure.

Manneschi and colleagues[67] reported two patients allergic to nickel from metal components of arm prostheses. One also reacted to cobalt, paraphenylenediamine, and a formaldehyde resin.

Dermatologic Hazards of Electrocardiography

GELS AND PASTES USED IN ELECTROCARDIOGRAPHY

In the very early days of electrocardiography (ECG), a patient's hands and left foot were placed in three large pots of saline solution. In 1910, with the introduction of contact electrodes, this method of partial immersion in saline solution was replaced by bandaging the limbs with saline pads and malleable metal electrodes. The saline-soaked bedclothes of bedridden patients often produced not only maceration of the skin but also short-circuiting of the equipment. In the 1930s, commercial electrode jellies and pastes consisting principally of sodium chloride and an abrasive became available and are now widely used.

Dermatitis Due to Parabens in a "Nonirritating" Jelly (Natrosol) Used for Long-Term Electrocardiographic Monitoring

An 8-year-old boy with mild atopic dermatitis required long-term ECG monitoring. He began to complain of marked itching under the electrodes. Upon examination, the areas where the electrodes had been applied revealed a sharply demarcated erythematous oozing dermatitis. It was learned that electrode jelly (Natrosol) had been used. A positive patch test to this jelly was obtained. The electrode jelly consisted of hydroxycellulose, polyvinyl pyrrolidone, sodium, potassium, and calcium chlorides in deionized water, and parabens. Patch tests with the various ingredients gave negative results except for the parabens.[68]

Various ECG gels and pastes and metal and rubber electrodes may produce irritant and allergic contact dermatitis.

Dermatitis Due to FD&C Yellow No. 5 in Camcreme ECG Paste (Cambridge)

A 40-year-old woman acquired dermatitis at sites where Camcreme ECG paste had been applied. Camcreme is a complex mixture containing sodium sulfate, lanosterol, cholesterol, mineral oil, cetyl alcohol, polyethylene glycol 40 (PEG-40), stearate, stearamide, MEA stearate, glyceryl stearate, stearyl sapamine, laureth-4, preservatives (propylparaben, methylparaben, phosphoric acid, and ethoxydiglycol), and fragrances, and colored with FD&C Yellow No. 5 and No. 6. The patient showed a positive patch test reaction to the FD&C Yellow No. 5 and to paraphenylenediamine. FD&C Yellow No. 5 is tartrazine, which has been implicated as a cause of chronic urticaria.[69]

Dermatitis Due to Propylene Glycol in Spectra 360 Electro Gel (Parka Lab)

A 62-year-old man acquired dermatitis following the use of this ECG gel, which contains propylene glycol, organic "polymers," and cellulose. Patch test results were positive only to 5% aqueous solution of propylene glycol and negative to the other ingredients.[70] Many other brands of electrode gels and pads contain propylene glycol.

ACD Due to Parachlorometaxylenol (PCMX) in Redux ECG Paste

A 70-year-old woman acquired a sharply defined erythematous vesicular dermatitis at the site where Redux ECG paste had been applied. Positive results were obtained with the paste and with the PCMX, which is used widely as a preservative in numerous topical medications and cosmetics. Storrs[71] documented allergic dermatitis due to PCMX in three men and four women whose dermatitis was precipitated by exposure either to Vaseline First Aid Carbolated Petroleum Jelly or to Redux ECG paste.

Other cases of ACD to ECG Electrode Jelly

A 57-year-old man proved to be allergic to this ECG jelly and to pine oil, which is one of its ingredients. Although the pine oil is present in only a 1:10,000 concentration, it was apparently sufficient to produce dermatitis. Pine oil is also present in various disinfectants and deodorants and certain liquid scrub soaps.

Coskey[72] reported a patient with allergic hypersensitivity to this ECG jelly and incriminated the gum tragacanth as the cause of the allergic dermatitis.

RUBBER STRAPS USED TO FASTEN ECG ELECTRODES

Two patients were studied who acquired bandlike, erythematous, vesicular dermatitis at the sites of contact with the rubber straps used to fasten the ECG electrodes. Both patients showed a positive reaction to a piece of the rubber strap and to mercaptobenzothiazole.[73]

NICKEL-PLATED ECG ELECTRODES

Fisher reported that a 26-year-old nurse acquired dermatitis at the sites where electrodes had been applied. It was at first suspected that she was allergic to the ECG pastes, but patch testing with the paste, which was performed elsewhere, gave negative results. The history revealed that she could not wear costume jewelry without acquiring dermatitis. A strongly positive patch test reaction to nickel sulfate was obtained, and the metal electrodes gave a strongly positive reaction to dimethylglyoxime, indicating the presence of "available" nickel in the metal electrode.

ALCOHOL IN A PREPACKAGED GAUZE PAD USED AS A SUBSTITUTE FOR ECG PASTE

A 38-year-old man had a sharply localized rectangular patch of vesicular dermatitis corresponding to the sites of the ECG electrodes. In this patient, alcohol-impregnated cotton sponges were used as conductors instead of ECG paste. This patient was found allergic, on patch testing, to the isopropyl alcohol used in the gauze pad and to ethyl alcohol. Thankfully, no systemic reaction, however, was produced from drinking alcoholic beverages.[74]

There are several reports in the literature of various types of topically applied alcohol capable of producing ACD.[75] In some of the patients with delayed-type allergic hypersensitivity to alcohol, an eruption may also develop after the ingestion of alcohol.

Table 19-4 Causes of Pacemaker Dermatitis
Epoxy resin
Metals
Mercury
Titanium
Nickel
Chromate
Cobalt
Gold
Polychloroparaxylene (parylene)
Rubber allergens

Cardiac Pacemaker Dermatitis

Contact dermatitis due to a cardiac pacemaker is a very rare event that may occur over the site of the pacemaker or may be widespread and may resemble a nummular eczema. Table 19.4 lists the reported causes of pacemaker dermatitis; Table 19.5 lists the composition of a popular pacemaker.

Epoxy resin allergy is one of the more common causes of the rare occurrence of pacemaker dermatitis. Andersen[76] reported that a pacemaker with an epoxy resin coating produced a dermatitis in a patient who later tolerated a pacemaker in a titanium capsule. Romaguera and Grimalt[77] studied a man with a generalized dermatitis due to epoxy resin cement in a pacemaker that was presumably incompletely polymerized after nearly a year.

Raque and Goldschmidt[78] described a patient with circumscribed eczematous dermatitis occurring over the site of a pacemaker within 3 weeks of implantation. Later, widespread nummular eczema developed. The authors discussed whether it was an irritant dermatitis due to a medical-grade silicone elastomer or nummular eczema provoked by an irritant dermatitis. Patch tests in a patient and two control subjects with the uncured silicone adhesive gave positive reactions that were thought to be irritant reactions. The patient's dermatitis was not resolved.

Table 19-5 Composition of a Popular Pacemaker	
Battery:	Lithium
Casing:	Epoxy resin
	Silicone
	Titanium
Insertion tip:	Iridium (10%)
	Platinum (90%)

Polychloroparaxylene, also called parylene, is a coating for pacemakers and has been reported to cause allergy in one patient.[79] Polyurethane and titanium patch tests were both positive in one patient with pacemaker sensitivity.[80]

Pacemakers caused a localized dermatitis over the sites of implant in two patients investigated by Brun and Hunziker.[81] Allergy to mercury accounted for the first patient, but sensitization to titanium was considered the most likely cause in the second case, despite negative patch tests to metallic titanium and titanium tetrachloride. These tests were interpreted as false-negative reactions because compounds for patch testing were yet to be determined.

Peters and colleagues[82] did find a positive patch test to titanium in one patient with pacemaker dermatitis. A granulomatous reaction to a pacemaker with titanium found on electron probe microanalysis but with negative patch tests has been reported. The eruption resolved spontaneously over several years.[83] Other reports have implicated metals including nickel, chromate, cobalt, and cadmium, as reviewed by Buchet and colleagues.[84] A pompholyx eruption from a nickel-containing pacemaker has been reported.[85] Some reports have failed to identify an allergen but suggest allergy because the dermatitis resolved upon removal of the implant.

At the Seventh International Symposium on Contact Dermatitis, held in East Germany in June 1983, Dr. B. Bandemir, of Neubrandenburg, reported:

A 76-year-old patient, who had a cardiac infarction in 1978, had a pacemaker with a casing of chromium, nickel, and steel implanted into the left thorax. Some weeks later signs of inflammation as well as an eczematous reaction of the skin appeared in the area of the implanted pacemaker. In the area of the hypogastrium as well as the thighs, small papulous and badly itching efflorescences were seen.

Micro-organisms could not be found in the bed of the pacemaker case. Patch tests with the standard series were positive to potassium dichromate after 1 day and 2+ positive after 2 and 3 days with a focal reaction in the area of the implanted pacemaker, the hypogastrium, and the thighs as well as itching on the whole integument. Patch tests with epoxy resin and triethanolamine were completely negative.

In December 1981, a subpectoral implantation of an Axios pacemaker with a pure titanium casing was carried out. Since that time. no reactions of the integument have occurred.

DERMATITIS FROM SUBCUTANEOUS PRESSURE?

Wilkerson and Jordan[86] studied a man with localized dermatitis that began 2 years after a pacemaker was inserted over the left upper abdomen. Patch tests were negative. When the pacemaker migrated to a different location, the original dermatitis cleared and the new location became dermatitic. Eventually the unit perforated through the skin and had to be replaced. The authors concluded the dermatitis was caused by an isomorphic response to pressure, as no evidence of allergic contact dermatitis was ever detected. However, the possibility must be considered that an allergy to an unidentified allergen was the true cause.

Ferringer and Mowad reported a 76 year-old man with reticulate erythema over the site of an implanted defibrillator with negative patch tests.[87] Histology was benign and infection was absent. The etiology of the reaction is uncertain, but pressure, warmth, and electromagnetism have been speculated as culprits.

Dermatitis Associated with Transcutaneous Electrical Nerve Stimulation

Transcutaneous electrical nerve stimulation (TENS) is being used increasingly to relieve postoperative pain and chronic pain from such diverse causes as cancer, bursitis, fractures, causalgia, and postherpetic neuralgia.

TENS uses the passage of small electrical currents through the skin, which are presumed to effect "depolarization" of the affected sensory nerve endings and nerves themselves by the conduction of impulses along them, resulting in the inhibition (of awareness or perception) of paresthesias and particularly pain.[88] The "system" generally used in TENS is a battery-operated "pulse generator" that contains the power source and the electronics of the system. The electrical impulses are transmitted through cables attached to electrodes, which in turn are fastened to the skin by straps, adhesive, or tapes. In most systems, an electrolyte gel is interposed between the electrode and the skin.

ELECTRICAL BURNS FROM TENS

Skin burns occur if the patient uses excessive stimulation with small-area electrodes (such as ECG electrodes) or if the interface between skin and electrode is dry. Shealy and Maurer[89] stated that the electrode surface area must be greater than 4 cm2 for a 500 msec 85 mA pulse, 185 pps stimulus. The heat produced must be less than 250 mcal/cm2/sec in order to avoid localized burns.

Burton[90] described another type of injury, which he termed "micropunctate burns," due to poor electrical contact between skin and electrode. The explanation is that current flow is not distributed over a wide surface area but is concentrated in small punctate areas (usually hair follicles). Because of the concentration of a large volume of current in small areas, current density is high and skin burns result. These micropunctate skin burns represent true thermal damage to the skin, but Burton felt that they are of little clinical significance in themselves, and, as with allergic reactions, simple discontinuation of use of the electrodes will allow recovery.

SKIN IRRITATION FROM TENS

Even with adequately sized electrodes, skin irritation may occur with the prolonged use of TENS, particularly with a high output. It is advisable in instances of prolonged use to periodically move the electrodes to adjacent positions to prevent such irritation. Loeser and colleagues[91] noted that if the patient did not heed their warnings about changing the stimulation sites and washing the electrode sponges, areas of erythema might occur after 24 to 48 hours of continuous stimulation. This is easily controlled by discontinuation of stimulation at the inflamed sites.

Zugerman[92] stated that multiple irritant follicular papules and erosions may be caused by electrochemical reactions at the electrode-tissue interface. For example, carbon-containing silicone rubber or polyolefin plastic electrodes generate acids at the positive electrode and bases at the negative electrode as electrons are respectively accepted and repelled by the electrode surface during direct current stimulation.

These pH changes are most pronounced at sites of high current density and are associated with the formation of punctate erythema degenerating to bullous lesions, if stimulation is prolonged or intense (current density >10 mA/cm^2).

In the laboratory, it was found that by placing a 1- to 2-mm pad of fabric, thoroughly moistened with physiologic saline or weak buffer solution, between the electrode and the skin, these lesions are prevented by distributing the current uniformly over the entire electrode area and by providing a reservoir of liquid or buffer, which dilutes or minimizes the pH changes. This liquid also serves to hydrate the stratum corneum, the principal barrier to the passage of direct current through the skin.

An alternative way to minimize skin damage associated with these electrochemical reactions is to use a bidirectional pulse or alternating pulse train of opposing polarity, so that the electrochemical effects of each pulse or pulse train are canceled by those of the succeeding one. This would achieve the same neural stimulation effect, while minimizing cumulative electrochemical by-products at the electrode-tissue interface.

IRRITANT DERMATITIS FROM TENS GELS

Two patients were encountered who acquired an irritant dermatitis from Sanborn "Redux" Gel. Patch test results did not indicate an allergic reaction but did reveal an irritant, follicular reaction. This type of gel is said to contain silicon oxide, which can produce irritation similar to that of "ground glass" on thin, delicate skin. This patient was able to tolerate EC-Z Cream (Grass Instruments) without difficulty.

ALLERGIC REACTIONS TO TENS ELECTRODES

Several types of electrodes are in use. As with ECG electrodes, rubber allergens and metals may cause contact allergy. Theoretically, there should be more chance of reactivity to TENS devices because of prolonged contact with the skin.

ACD FROM TENS GELS CONTAINING PROPYLENE GLYCOL

Fisher[88] cited three cases of ACD due to propylene glycol in an electrolyte jelly. One of these patients is reported on through the courtesy of Dr. W. Clendenning of the Hitchcock Clinic in Hanover, New Hampshire. One other patient, seen in consultation with Dr. Mary T. Hunsicker of East Stroudsbourg, Pennsylvania, also proved to have propylene glycol hypersensitivity. The third patient was a New York woman who was allergic to propylene glycol in this TENS gel and in certain of her cosmetics. He also reported a case of ACD to propylene glycol in a sterile lubricant (K-Y lubricating jelly) used by a patient undergoing TENS who had previously developed contact sensitivity to propylene glycol in a conductive material.[93]

Zugerman[92] reported a patient who developed ACD to propylene glycol in a conductive jelly (Neuromod TENS gel). In an attempt to continue therapy, the patient changed to a poorly conductive surgical lubricant jelly, which caused irritation and micropunctate burns. Electrodes not utilizing conductive jelly were applied subsequently, with excellent results.

Dermatitis from Antabuse Implants

Because some alcoholic patients discontinue the use of oral Antabuse, the subcutaneous implantation of disulfiram pellets has been used to overcome the problems of vacillating motivation.[94] Lachapelle[95] described two cases of ACD to implanted Antabuse pellets. He further stated, "It is also interesting to compare the evolution of both patients. Whereas, one of them was able to take oral disulfiram without any further skin reaction, the other patient developed a severe systemic, eczematous, contact-type dermatitis in the 24 hours following the oral absorption of one tablet of disulfiram.."

Alcohol can exacerbate ACD from Antabuse. The explanation of this interaction is probably quite different from the aldehyde syndrome. Similarly unexplained is the fact that some patients who have been implanted with Antabuse pellets experience itching, burning, and redness at the site of the implantation when they drink alcohol.[96]

Acupuncture Needle Dermatitis

Romaguera and Grimalt[97] reported that a 48-year-old woman presented with a papulovesicular dermatitis of the neck, elbows, and wrists. She had also been suffering from a vesicular eruption on the forearms, upper part of the back, and face for the previous 8 days. All the lesions were accompanied by marked itching. The patient was receiving treatment with acupuncture for cervical arthritis. She denied any previous reaction to nickel exposures.

Patch tests with the metal series showed a positive reaction to nickel sulfate. An acupuncture needle was introduced experimentally into the forearm; after 8 hours, the needle was removed. Around the site of the puncture a vesicular, edematous plaque with pseudopodia and marked itching was seen. With conventional treatment and termination of the acupuncture sessions, all the lesions disappeared in 18 days. The composition of the metal needles was unknown.

These same authors reported ACD in a nickel-sensitive individual from a permanent acupuncture needle inserted into the helix of the patient's right ear.[98] A severe contact dermatitis appeared at this site around and near the acupuncture needle. Composition of the acupuncture needle, which originated in China, was unknown to the authors.

Eun[99] reported that the earliest needles used were fish bones, bamboo splinters, and pointed stones, which were superseded by needles made of such metals as iron and copper. At present, most needles are made of silver, gold, or stainless steel. Some Korean acupuncture needles are stainless steel composed of iron with 13.3% chromium

and 6.7% nickel. The Chinese and French acupuncture needles, however, were found to be different. Data from Lee's analysis are given in Table 19.6.

Eun[99] tested some of the Korean stainless steel needles presently in use. All samples were dimethylglyoxime spot test negative. Thin, fiber-shaped gold needles, which are inserted into the body until broken into thin segments and retained permanently as part of a special technique, were also found to be negative to the dimethylglyoxime test.

Table 19-6 Quantitative Analysis (% Weight) of Various Acupuncture Needle Materials

	Iron	Chromium	Nickel	Silver	Copper	Tungsten
Korean	+++	13.3%	6.7%			
Chinese (A)	+++	12.5%	8.5%			
Chinese (B)	+++	10.4%	6.6%			
Handle of needle (A)				+++	1.0%	
Handle of needle (B)					+++	
French						+++

+++ = present, majority component of needle.
From: Fisher A. Allergic dermatitis from acupuncture needles. Cutis 1986;38:226–228.

Table 19-7 Sensitizers in Eyeglass Frames

Azo dyes
Beeswax-turpentine mixture
Plastic materials (see chapter 27)
  Butyl acrylate
  Ethyl acrylate
  2-hydroxyethyl methacrylate
  Methyl methacrylate
  Cellulose acetate
  Cellulose propionate
  Epoxy resin
  Ethyl acetate
  Ethylene glycol
  p-tert-butylphenol
  Phenyl salicylate
  Resorcinol monobenzoate
  Tricresyl phosphate
  Triphenyl phosphate
Metals
  Chromate
  Cobalt
  Gold
  Nickel
  Palladium
  Platinum
  Titanium

Eyeglass Frame Dermatitis

Most eyeglass frames are usually made of metal or plastic. Wood and tortoiseshell are now rarely used. Table 19.7 shows many possible sensitizers in eyeglass frames.

CELLULOSE PLASTIC FRAMES

Contact dermatitis from cellulose plastics is infrequent and due usually to cellulose acetate or cellulose propionate. The plastic itself is nonallergenic, but some of the additives used in its manufacture can sensitize. Eyeglass frames are the most common cause of dermatitis from cellulose acetate, but it has also been attributed to ballpoint pens, hearing aids, patch test films, and steering wheels.[100]

In addition to the plastic base itself, other ingredients of the finished plastic may include plasticizers, stabilizers, and coloring agents. Any of these may be sensitizers. Coloring agents include either pigments, which are normally inert, or dyes, frequently amino compounds, which can sensitize. Solvents and formaldehyde resins, used in the processing of some plastics, are not usually used here. (See chapter 27)

The manufacturing process used in these products is known as "injection molding." In this process, the cellulose (obtained usually from nature in the form of wood fibers), after being esterified, is simply mixed with a plasticizer, a stabilizer, and a coloring agent. The entire mass is then heated to increase mixing of the components and decrease viscosity, but no chemical reaction occurs (i.e., these plastics are not "cured"). Hence, the individual components are not bound chemically to one another and remain more or less available to be leached out. As a final step, the hot mixture is injected into molds of desired shape and is allowed to cool.

Vail[101] reported instances of ACD from Cool-Ray sunglass frames made of cellulose propionate plastic, due probably to an unknown additive.

Tritolyl Phosphate (Tricresyl Phosphate) and Triphenyl Phosphate

Pegum's[102] patient was sensitive to tritolyl phosphate in polyvinyl chloride (PVC), and she also had dermatitis from triphenyl phosphate in her cellulose acetate eyeglass frames. She reacted to triphenyl phosphate (1% in both peanut oil and acetone), tritolyl phosphate (5% in peanut oil), the eyeglass frames, and PVC from various articles.

Andersen of Denmark (Andersen K, personal communication, 1982) observed a 46-year-old woman with eyeglass frame dermatitis. She had positive patch test results to the dyed plastic frame but not to the sidebars. Supplementary patch tests showed positive reactions to

tricresyl phosphate, phenolformaldehyde resin, and a phosphate ester used in Firemaster flame-retardant compounds from Michigan Chemical Corporation consisting of halogenated phosphate esters. Liquid Firemaster caused delayed hypersensitivity maximization test results in human subjects and is classified as a weak to mild sensitizer. Sensitized persons could have reactions to fabrics containing this flame retardant.

The International Contact Dermatitis Research Group included Firemaster LVT 23P in 5% pet in their standard series of patch tests for a limited period of time to determine the incidence of sensitization against Firemaster. Of 1,103 individuals tested, only 2 showed a positive response (Maibach H, personal communication, 1986).

"Optyl" Epoxy Frames

Fisher[103] reported a patient with epoxy resin sensitivity acquired from wearing eyeglass frames from Hong Kong made of Optyl, a plastic material of the epoxy series. This epoxy plastic is covered with a polyurethane lacquer. Positive patch tests were obtained to scrapings from the eyeglass frames but not in three controls. Negative tests were obtained with polyurethane resin monomers. In this instance, an apparently "cured" epoxy resin was capable of producing ACD in a sensitized individual.

Turpentine

Jordan[104] reported that a man known to be sensitive to turpentine developed eyeglass frame dermatitis. It was traced to a turpentine-beeswax mixture used in the final polishing. Patch testing revealed that the patient was positive to the turpentine-beeswax polish and a piece of buffed plastic but was negative to beeswax and unbuffed plastic.

ULTRAVIOLET INHIBITORS OR STABILIZERS IN EYEGLASS FRAMES

Resorcinol Monobenzoate

Resorcinol monobenzoate is a colorless, ultraviolet light absorber that is added to plastics to prevent deterioration by sunlight. This compound was the sensitizer in two cases of dermatitis from sunglasses reported by Jordan and Dahl.[100] In patch tests, both patients reacted to resorcinol monobenzoate (1% pet) but not to resorcinol. Two of three patients sensitive to resorcinol monobenzoate were also allergic to *Myroxylon pereirae* (MP). Calnan[105] also reported ACD to resorcinol monobenzoate in eyeglass frames.

Phenyl Salicylate

Rycroft[106] reported three cases of contact dermatitis behind the ears from wearing the same brand of industrial safety spectacles. In each case a positive patch test was obtained with scrapings of the plastic. In both cases positive patch tests were obtained with phenyl salicylate. Phenyl salicylate is used as an ultraviolet inhibitor in some cellulose acetate butyrate and cellulose acetate propionate formulas. It has been reported previously as a contact sensitizer from its use as a sunscreen in a lip salve. Positive patch test reactions were also obtained variously in these cases with MP, resorcinol monobenzoate, and epoxy resin.

METAL IN EYEGLASSES

Jirasek and colleagues[107] reported that a celluloid eyeglass frame was reinforced with metal struts made of an alloy containing 30% nickel, 1% to 3% manganese, and 65% to 68% copper. As the plastic aged, the nickel was leached out and caused a retroauricular dermatitis. Nickel, cobalt, chromium, gold, palladium, and titanium all potentially could cause ACD from eyeglasses, but titanium allergy is very rare.

NOSE-PAD DERMATITIS

Hambly and Wilkinson[108] studied a woman with dermatitis from the plastic nose pads of her eyeglass frames. In a patch test she reacted to butyl acrylate 1% (olive oil) but not to ethyl or methyl acrylate. An eyeglass manufacturer confirmed that such acrylates might be present in acrylic frames.

Jordan and Dahl[109] found that eyeglass dermatitis limited to the nose occurred in one patient. Patch testing revealed the offending agent to be a common solvent, ethylene glycol monomethyl ether acetate, used to chemically weld the nose pads to the eyeglass frame. The patient also had an unrevealed allergy to ethyl acetate.

Trichloroethane

Fowler[110] reported a case of contact urticaria in a worker polishing and grinding eyeglass lenses due to trichloroethane.

Reactions in Contact Lens Wearers

Contact allergy to ophthalmic drugs and contact lens solutions has been reviewed in detail by Herbst and Maibach.[111] They give a suggested patch test tray based on their review. Preservatives (e.g., thimerosal) and antibiotics, especially neomycin, were the most frequent allergens. Other active ingredients and excipients were occasional allergens.

Tosti and Tosti[112] reported multiple cases of ACD and conjunctivitis to thimerosal in contact lens solutions.

Virtually all such solutions now marketed in the United States are free of thimerosal.

Nickel and cobalt were found in a contact lens solution in Spain that caused intense periorbital dermatitis in a metal-sensitive individual.[113]

The surfactants cocamidopropyl betaine and disodium cocoamphodipropionate in contact lens solutions have caused allergy.[114,115]

Two workers manufacturing soft, disposable contact lenses became sensitized to 2-hydroxyethyl acrylate and developed hand dermatitis.[116]

Hearing-Aid Dermatitis

A 64-year-old patient who had acquired a new hearing aid soon developed a dermatitis of the ear that was in direct contact with the hearing aid. It was ascertained that this hearing aid was composed of a vinyl plastic. The patient was patch tested with various available types of plastics used in hearing aids and was found to have a strongly positive reaction to the vinyl variety but not to silicone, acrylic, and polyethylene.

A patient described by Guill and Odom[117] developed dermatitis from a new "in the ear" hearing aid made of cold-cured methyl methacrylate, whereas a replacement with a heat-cured aid was comfortable. Upon patch testing, the patient reacted to 10% methyl methacrylate in olive oil and to pieces of a cold-cured plastic but not to the heat-cured one.

Jordan and Dahl's[100] patient developed a dermatitis from a cellulose ester plastic used in a hearing aid. In this patient the specific sensitizer was resorcinol used as an ultraviolet stabilizer in the plastic. Diethyl phthalate has caused allergy from both hearing aids and eyeglass frames.[118] Paratertiary butylphenol formaldehyde resin (PTBFR) may be used to bond plastic parts in hearing aids and has been reported to cause allergy.[119]

Hearing aids may contain resorcinol monobenzoate as an ultraviolet stabilizer or as an inhibitor and may produce ACD in MP-sensitive individuals.[120]

In two separate studies from Scandinavia, methacrylates were found to be common sensitizers in hearing aids or the molds for them. In the first study, three laboratory technicians and four patients were allergic to methacrylates.[121] In the second, 6 of 22 patients with chronic dermatitis of the ear canal reacted to methylmethacrylate or related acrylates. Ingredients of topical medications also caused allergy in some cases.[122]

Because previous allergic reactions have been reported to acrylic and polyethylene plastics used in hearing aids and none have ever been reported from silicone, it was decided to use silicone hearing aid material. The silicone hearing aid was well tolerated.

In addition to ACD, the differential diagnosis of dermatitis in the area of a hearing aid should include seborrhea, irritant contact dermatitis, psoriasis, and yeast and bacterial infection.

Nasal Cannula Dermatitis

Wright and Fregert[123] reported two patients who each had dermatitis of their upper lips from the use of an oxygen nasal cannula. In the first patient, scrapings from the oxygen cannula showed a positive patch test. The manufacturer of the cannula indicated that vanilla and epoxidized soybean oil were added to polyvinyl chloride in the production of the nasal cannula. A second series of patch tests revealed the following results: vanilla 10% (w/v) in acetone, negative; repeat scrapings from suspect nasal cannula, 2+; scrapings from another nasal cannula made from pure polyvinyl chloride, negative; epoxy resin 1% pet, 2+. A cannula made from pure vinyl chloride was prescribed, and the dermatitis resolved.

The second patient was a 54-year-old woman who had been on continuous oxygen therapy for 10 years and during that period of time had used a plastic oxygen cannula. She had experienced no difficulty until 3 weeks prior to being seen in a dermatologic consultation. She had developed some irritation after using a cannula from a different supplier. On physical examination, dermatitis was present on the upper lip and the cheeks in the area of contact with the cannula. Because of the prior experience with the first patient, a patch test to epoxy resin (1% pet) was carried out and showed a 2+ reaction.

Toome[124] reported a similar case also allergic to epoxy resin. A PVC cannula without epoxy resin was obtained from a different manufacturer.

Irritant dermatitis from the drying effects of the oxygen flow is much more common than ACD.

Stethoscope Dermatitis

Nickel-sensitive physicians and nurses may acquire a bilateral, bandlike, linear dermatitis at the sides of their necks whereon the nickel-plated, metallic portion of the stethoscopes rests. Rubber or plastic components of the stethoscope may also cause allergy in the wearer.

Infusion Pumps

Acrylates and epoxy resins in glues in insulin infusion pumps have caused ACD in diabetics.[125,126] Van den Hoveand colleagues[126] suggested that a pump called Pureline Basic or Disetronic Plus has no glue and therefore may be safe for use in these cases.

Medical Adhesive Tapes

Medical adhesive bandages (tapes) consist of a pressure-sensitive adhesive and a backing, which is a carrier for the adhesive. Depending on its intended use, the bandage's backing may be made of plastic, cloth, paper, or foam. There are two types of medical adhesive tape: older tapes, based on rubber and rosin; and newer, "hypoallergenic" tapes, composed of acrylic resins. (See Chapters 29 and 30.)

RUBBER, ROSIN-BASED ADHESIVES

The rubber-based adhesives contain rubbers, tackifiers, plasticizers, antioxidants, and other stabilizers. Tackifiers provide stickiness and are usually resins derived from terpenes, rosin (colophony), and petroleum. Plasticizers soften and facilitate the conformability of the adhesives. Antioxidants provide resistance to oxygen and thermal deterioration. Abietic acid, a major component in rosin, dihydroabietyl alcohol, plasticizers, and antioxidants have all been shown to cause ACD.[127] Most such adhesive tapes also contained zinc oxide and substances derived from coniferous resins, such as turpentine, balsams, and rosin. In addition, antioxidants, to provide resistance to deterioration, and plasticizers, to facilitate spreading of the adhesive mass on cloth, are the ingredients in many adhesive tapes and plasters.

In a European report, diphenylthiourea was found as a cause of allergy to adhesive tape in eight patients.[128] Zinc diethyldithiocarbamate, a rubber accelerator, was reported as a cause of rubber adhesive dermatitis.[129] Murphy and colleagues[130] identified diamylhydroquinone as the allergen in both Scotch tape and an adhesive tape. Allergy to PTBFR was found to cause severe dermatitis in four patients. A particular athletic tape containing PTBFR was the culprit, and one patient also reacted to her athletic shoes.[131]

Factitial dermatitis was caused by rosin in adhesive tape in a case from Australia.[132]

ADHESIVE TAPE REACTIONS FROM TENS UNITS

Seven patients were either allergic to or irritated by the ordinary adhesive used to fasten the electrodes to the skin. These patients were able to use an acrylate type of adhesive such as Dermicel (Johnson & Johnson) and Micropore (3M). One patient was studied who was allergic to these acrylate adhesive tapes and also could not tolerate ordinary adhesive.[133] Special straps had to be used in this instance.

ACRYLATE-RESIN-BASED ADHESIVE TAPES

These single-component adhesives were developed to avoid the allergic reactions and instability associated with rubber-based adhesives. These so-called hypoallergenic adhesives are formed by the combination of an acrylic ester monomer with a polar monomer. On occasion, the acrylic ester monomer is replaced with an acrylic monomer combined with another type of monomer, such as vinyl acetate.

Ethylhexyl Acrylate

Jordan[134] reported that during predictive testing he found seven volunteers who reacted to Curad adhesive but not to Dermicel. All reacted to ethylhexyl acrylate and three to N-tert-butyl maleamic acid. No crossreactions were present between the acrylates and the methacrylates.

Heskel and colleagues[135] stated that the major components of Curad adhesive are 2-ethylhexyl acrylate and alkyl maleamic acid (a polar monomer). He reported two patients who proved to be allergic to N-dodecyl maleamic acid. The alkyl group in the maleamic acid is derived from tertiary amines whose alkyl groups range from C_8 to C_{16}, with an average of C_{12} (dodecyl maleamic acid). No tackifiers or plasticizers are used. The resultant polymer is polar and of high molecular weight. During the reaction, approximately 98% of the monomers are converted to a polymer. The polymer is washed, dissolved in solvent, coated on a vinyl film, and heated in order to remove solvents and residual monomers, which are capable of producing sensitization.

The tendency of acrylic ester monomers to cause an allergic reaction has been shown to decrease as the size of the acrylic ester group increases. Methacrylates are less allergenic than the corresponding acrylic esters. Jordan[134] found that allergy to acrylates does not necessarily mean allergy to methacrylates. The di- and triacrylate esters are potent allergens, whose frequency of sensitization increases as the number of unsaturated groups in the monomer increases.[136,137]

TRAUMATIC, IRRITANT, AND DERMATOGRAPHIC ADHESIVE TAPE DERMATITIS

Most skin reactions related to adhesive tape are mechanical. One type of traumatic adhesive tape reaction results from the shearing stresses at the tape-skin interface and is encountered most frequently when tape is applied with tension that exceeds the physiologic tolerance of skin. Narumi[138] showed that adhesive plaster applied with tension can readily produce erythema and even blistering.

Patch testing is an excellent indirect test for dermatographism. The rare individual with severe dermatographism will develop urticaria in an exact pattern matching the location of the adhesive portion of the patch tests. This may persist until the final reading, and likely gives a clue as to the diagnosis.

The other type of irritant, adhesive tape reaction, involves the mechanical plugging of the follicular and sweat ostia, producing a follicular rash resembling prickly heat. Also, patients with dermatographism commonly develop erythema and even urticaria at sites of tape removal, such as in patch tests. This reaction to friction and pressure usually resolves spontaneously within several hours.

Traumatic or irritant adhesive tape dermatitis remains localized usually to the site of contact, but the allergic reactions tend to spread.

BAND-AID PATCHES

Occasionally, the vinyl film backing of Band-Aids may produce ACD because of plasticizers and stabilizers in the film.

SALICYLIC ACID PLASTER

Rasmussen and Fisher[139] reported two patients who developed ACD while applying 40% salicylic acid plaster to their plantar warts. Patch testing identified the allergen as a dehydroabietic acid, a sensitizer in rosin.

Reactions to Transdermal Drug Delivery Systems

Transdermal drug delivery systems (TDDS), also called transdermal therapeutic systems (TTS), provide a low, continuous dosage of a medication. It is especially useful for drugs with a short half-life that could otherwise require frequent oral dosing or in cases where oral absorption may be impaired. Drugs administered by this route include nitroglycerin, estradiol, scopolamine,

Table 19-8 Patch Test Series for Suspected Allergy to Transdermal Drug Delivery Systems

Clonidine	9% aq
Estrogen	5% aq or pet
Scopolamine	1% aq or pet
Nitroglycerin	2% aq
Nicotine	10% aq
Testosterone	2% aq or pet
Hydropropyl cellulose	70% alc
Ethanol	5% aq
Acrylates	as per screening series
Placebo patch	as is

Aq, aqueous; pet, petrolatum.

nicotine, fentanyl, clonidine, lidocaine, methylphidate and testosterone, among others.

Reaction can occur either to the active drug or to a component of the patch system (Table 19.8). Reaction to the active drug is more common. Musel and Warshaw have reviewed the topic.[142]

NONALLERGIC REACTIONS

Because the patch may be left in place for several days or more, folliculitis and miliaria rubra may develop from occlusion. Yeast or bacterial overgrowth may occur under a path left in place for prolonged periods. Vasodilatation from nicotine may be mistaken for ACD or ICD.[143] In one case, apparently a burn was caused by microwave radiation from a leaky oven.[140]

Irritant contact dermatitis (ICD) may occur due to the adhesive and frictional effects of the patch. TDSs with a drug reservoir, as opposed to having the drug incorporated into the adhesive matrix, may have more irritancy.[142] One of the newest TDSs, the Daytrana patch containing methylphenidate, has shown a fairly high incidence of irritancy.

ALLERGY TO ACTIVE AGENTS

Scopolamine, clonidine, nicotine, lidocaine, testosterone, estradiol, methylphenidate, and nitroglycerin have all caused ACD. Patients allergic to scopolamine have not reacted to atropine.

In one study, 21 of 320 patients (6.5%) developed cutaneous reactions to a TDS containing glyceryl trinitrate used for angina pectoris. About half of these had to discontinue therapy. More irritant than allergic reactions were observed.[144] Not only nitroglycerin TDS but also nitroglycerin pastes can cause allergic contact dermatitis.

The sensitizing capacity of topical antihistamines was illustrated by a report on an experimental triprolidine TDS. Five out of six study subjects exposed twice to this patch in clinical testing developed allergy. Further development of this technique was halted by these investigators.[145]

Clonidine is a fairly common cause of ACD in TDS but not when applied topically in petroaltum. Some studies suggest up to 25% of patients may develop allergy to it.[146] However, almost all patients who react topically can tolerate oral clonidine.[147] Nicotine reacted in several patients in one Swiss study.[148]

Allergy to estrogen in an Estraderm TTS50 patch was followed by generalized dermatitis after oral estrogen administration. Patch test was positive to 17-beta-estradiol.[149] Another report detailed a woman who was allergic to both estradiol and norethisterone acetate from both a patch and a gel.[150]

Testosterone has caused allergy from TDS application.[151]

Nicotine in TDSs has been reported to cause ACD in up to 3% of patients.[152]

REDUCTION OF ALLERGY IN TDS

Silva and Berman[153] suggested that Maalox applied to the skin before applying clonidine patches reduces the appearance of ACD in sensitized individuals. Jordan[154] reported that scrotal testosterone TDS was tolerated much better than a nonscrotal system, with less allergy and irritation. Coadministration of a topical steroid also reduces sensitization in TDS.[155]

ALLERGY TO OTHER PATCH INGREDIENTS

Various components of the patch, although usually inert, may sometimes cause ACD. Hydroxypropyl cellulose, the major component of the drug reservoir, caused ACD in one case.[156] Ethanol has also caused ACD in TDDS.[157] Several other instances of apparent allergic contact dermatitis to patch components have been reported, although the offending ingredients were not identified.[140,141]

In addition to causing ICD, TDS adhesives may occasionally cause ACD. Unfortunately, the exact causative agent in the adhesive is usually unidentified.[158] Methacrylates in the adhesive of patches may cause allergy.[159]

ACD of Legs Due to Bandages and Dressings

A critical fact in diagnosing ACD is that it is more common in areas of underlying dermatitis. Stasis dermatitis leads to secondary allergic sensitization frequently.

A woman used a Dome Paste Bandage on a stasis ulcer that produced a severe superimposed contact dermatitis under the entire bandage. This medicated bandage contains zinc oxide, calamine, and gelatin. The unlisted preservative proved to be the parabens. The patient had strongly positive reactions to a piece of the bandage and to the parabens. Four cases of allergy to preservatives in Unna boots was reported, three to parabens and one to hexachlorophene. Preservative free wraps were tolerated.[160]

Hydrogel dressings gave positive patch tests in 9.5% of 200 patients with venous leg ulcers.[161] Tests were negative in 200 controls. Propylene glycol (PG) was positive in a few of these patients, but the testing was done with only 5 or 10% propylene glycol. This is too low to identify most cases of ACD to PG, so in fact it may have been the cause in many of the patients. The same report listed rubber accelerators as positive in 13.5%. Elastic compression bandages were the likely cause in many of these.

ELASTIC LEG SUPPORT BANDAGES

Malten,[162] who reported ACD from paraphenylenediamine and related dyes and mercaptobenzothiazole in rubberized leg bandages and support hose, advocated the use of undyed fabrics with known rubber auxiliary substances declared on the label.

Patients with dermatitis from support bandages usually tolerated the Lycra spandex variety.

Joint Support Sleeves and C-PAP Straps

Tight-fitting elastic sleeves are used to support joints such as knees, ankles, and elbows during athletic activities. These are usually made of neoprene rubber, sometimes with a layer of cloth. Components may be glued or stitched together. In Fowler's[163] experience, allergy to these support devices has usually been caused by thioureas used in the rubber itself or possibly in the adhesives. Scalf and Fowler[164] have also reported allergy to the rubber straps holding a mask used with a continuous positive airway pressure device (known as a C-PAP) for treating sleep apnea. Thiourea was again the offending agent (Figures 19-2, 19-3, and 19-4).

Allergy to Sutures and Skin Clips

Polypropylene (Prolene) suture gave a positive patch test in one patient.[165] Fisher has reported nylon suture allergy[166] and silk suture sensitivity has been suspected.[167]

Lhotka, et al, analyzed metal surgical clamps and staples and patch tested 184 patients after orthopedic surgery.[168] Patch test were to chromium, cobalt, nickel, molybdenum, and titanium. Chromium and nickel were present in the items at an average concentration of 16% and 11% respectively. The levels of the other metals was < 1.5%. Forty patients (22%) were allergic to nickel and reported that all of them had "clinical reactions". These ranged from a local allergic reaction in 20, delayed wound healing in 17 and generalized dermatitis in 3. Controls were not performed and correlation of allergy to chromate was not mentioned.

References

1. Kasser J, ed. Orthopedic knowledge update-5. Rosemont, IL: American Academy of Orthopedic Surgeons, 1996:41.

2. <www.steel.org> Accessed July 12, 2007.

3. <http://en.wikipedia.org/wiki/stainless_steel> Accessed November 10, 2007.

4. Coleman RF, Harrington J, Scales JT. Concentrations of wear products in hair, blood, and urine after total hip replacement. Br Med J 1973;2:527.

5. Evans EM, Freeman MAR, Miller AJ, Vernon-Roberts B. Metal sensitivity as a cause of bone necrosis and loosening of the prosthesis in total joint replacement. J Bone Joint Surg 1974;56B:626.

6. Haudrechy P, Foussereau J, Mantout B, et al: Nickel release from nickel plated metals and stainless steels. Contact Dermatitis 1994;31:249.

7. Samitz MH, Katz SA. Nickel dermatitis hazards from prostheses. Br J Dermatol 1975;92:287.

8. Elves MW, Wilson JN, Scales JE, Kemp HBS. Incidence of metal sensitivity in patients with total joint replacements. Br Med J 1975;4:376.

9. Benson MK, Goodwin PG, Brostoff J. Metal sensitivity in patients with joint replacement arthroplasties. Br Med J 1975;4:374.

10. Munro-Ashman D, Miller AJ. Rejection of metal prosthesis and skin sensitivity to cobalt. Contact Dermatitis 1976;2:65.

11. Lodi A, Chiarelli G, Mancini LI, et al. Skin sensitivity to endoprosthetic materials in the recipients of hip prostheses. Contact Dermatitis 1995;32:58.

12. Carlsson AS, Magnusson B, Mieller H. Metal sensitivity in patients with metal-to-plastic total hip arthroplasties. Acta Orthop Scand 1980;51:57.

13. Deutman R, Mulder TJ, Brian R, Nater JP. Metal sensitivity before and after total hip arthroplasty. J Bone Joint Surg 1977;49A:862.

14. Nater JP, Brian RG, Deutman R, Mulder TJ. The development of metal hypersensitivity in patients with metal-to-plastic hip arthroplasties. Contact Dermatitis 1976;2:259.

15. Rooker GD, Wilkinson JC. Metal sensitivity in patients undergoing hip replacement. J Bone Joint Surg 1980;62B:502.

16. Metal allergy: a false alarm? Br Med J 1980;281:1303.

17. Can metal sensitivity loosen joint replacements? Lancet 1980;2:1284.

18. Cramers M, Lucht U. Metal sensitivity in patients treated for tibial fractures with plates of stainless steel. Acta Orthop Scand 1977;48:245.

19. Barranco VP, Solomon H. Eczematous dermatitis caused by internal exposure to nickel. South Med J 1973;55:447.

20. Kubba R, Taylor JS, Marks KE. Cutaneous complications of orthopedic implants. Arch Dermatol 1981;117:554.

21. Oleffe J, Wilmet J. Generalized dermatitis from an osteosynthesis screw. Contact Dermatitis 1980;6:365.

22. Balato N, Costa L, Lembo G, et al: Allergic contact dermatitis from orthopedic devices. Contact Dermatitis 1995;32:314.

23. Dujardin F, Fevrier V, Lecorvaisier C, Joly P. Allergic dermatitis caused by metallic implants in orthopedic surgery. Rev-Chir-Orthop-Reparatrice-Appar-Mot 1995;81:473.

24. Thomas P, Bandl W, Maier S, et al: Hypersensitivity to titanium osteosynthesis with impaired fracture healing, eczema, and T-cell hyperresponsiveness in vitro. Contact Dermatitis 2006;55:199.

25. Gawkrodger D: Metal sensitivities and orthopedic implants revisited. Br J Dermatol 2003;148:1089.

26. Koster R, Vieluf D, Kiehn M, et al: Nickel and molybdenum contact allergies in patients with coronary in-stent restenosis. Lancet 2000;356:1895.

27. Park S, Lee C, Hong M, et al: Comparison of gold-plated Nir stents with uncoated Nir stents in patients with coronary artery disease. Am J Cardiol 2002;89:872.

28. Svedman C, Tillman C, Gustavsson C, et al: Contact allergy to gold in patients with gold-plated stents. Contact Dermatitis 2005;52:192.

29. Rothstein MS. Management of peristomal skin: routine care and maintenance. J Dermatol Allergy 1982;5:20.

30. Rothstein MS. Ostomy skin care. Dialog Dermatol 1982;10:6.

31. Rothstein MS. Management of stomal wounds. Clin Dermatol 1994;12:81.

32. Rothstein MS. Dermatologic considerations of stoma care. JAAD 1986;15:411.

33. Martin J, Hughes T, Stone N: Peristomal allergic contact dermatitis. Contact Dermatitis 2005;52:273.

34. Scalf L, Fowler J: Peristomal allergic contact dermatitis due to Gantrez in Stomahesive paste. J Am Acad Dermatol 2000;42:355.

35. Stevenson CJ. Skin problems with surgical stomata. Contact Dermatitis 1975;1:243.

36. Burt-McAliley D, Eberhardt D, van Rijswijk L. Clinical study: peristomal skin irritation in colostomy patients. Ostomy-Wound-Manage 1994;40:28–30, 32–34, 36–37.

37. Davies MG, Hodgson GA, Evans E. Contact dermatitis from an ostomy deodorant. Contact Dermatitis 1979;5:317.

38. Pappas M. Urostomy skin care. Ostomy Q 1979;Fall:50.

39. Mann RJ, Stewart E, Peachey RDG. Sensitivity to urostomy pouch plastic. Contact Dermatitis 1983;9:80.

40. Van Ketel WG, van de Burg CKH, de Haan P. Sensitization to epoxy resin from an ileostomy bag. Contact Dermatitis 1983;9:516.

41. Mitxelena J, Aguirre A, Bilbao I, et al: Contact dermatitis in a tracheotomized patient due to a rubber disc. Contact Dermatitis 1998;32:181.

42. Tsurata D, Sowa J, Kobayashi H, et al: Contact dermatitis around a tracheostoma due to salbutamol and Aldecin. Contact Dermatitis 2006;54:121.

43. Fisher AA. Allergic reactions to contraceptives. Cutis 1974;13:337.

44. Fisher AA. Practical management of allergic contact dermatitis due to rubber in manufactured articles. Dermatol Digest 1963;2:23.

45. Barranco VP. Eczematous dermatitis caused by internal exposure to copper. Arch Dermatol 1972;106:386.

46. Barkoff JR. Urticaria secondary to a copper intrauterine device. Int J Dermatol 1979;15:594.

47. Romaguera C, Grimalt F. Contact dermatitis from a copper-containing intrauterine contraceptive device. Contact Dermatitis 1981;7:77163.

48. Sneddon IB. Formalin dermatitis in a renal dialysis unit. Contact Dermatitis Newsletter 1968;3:47.

49. Abel-Aziz AHM, Hodgson C. Formalin dermatitis in a renal dialysis unit. Contact Dermatitis Newsletter 1974;15:441.

50. Hendrick DJ, Lane DJ. Occupational formalin asthma. Br J Industr Med 1977;34:11.

51. Bousquet J, Rivory J, Maurice F, et al. Allergy in chronic hemodialysis: 1. Double-blind intravenous challenge with formaldehyde. Clin-Allergy 1987;17:499

52. Mork NJ. Contact sensitivity from epoxy resin in a hemodialysis set. Contact Dermatitis 1979;5:331.

53. Brandao FM, Pinto J. Allergic contact dermatitis to epoxy resin in hemodialysis needles. Contact Dermatitis 1980;6:218.

54. Penneys NS, Edwards LS, Katsikas JL. Allergic contact sensitivity to thiuram compounds in a hemodialysis unit. Arch Dermatol 1976; 112:811.

55. Levy SW. Disabling skin reactions associated with stump edema. Int J Dermatol 1977;16:122.

56. Allende MF, Levy SW, Barnes GH. Epidermoid cysts in amputees. Acta Dermato-Venereol 1967;43:56.

57. Des Groseilliers JP, Desjardins JP, Germain JP, Krol AL. Dermatologic problems in amputees. Can Med Assoc J 1978;118:535.

58. van Ketel WG. Allergic contact dermatitis of amputation stumps. Contact Dermatitis 1977;3:50.

59. Requena L, et al. Epoxy dermatitis of an amputation stump. Contact Dermatitis 1986;14:320.

60. Freeman S. Contact dermatitis of a limb stump caused byp-tertiary butyl catechol in the artificial limb. Contact Dermatitis 1986;14:68.

61. Romaguera C, et al. Paratertiary butylphenol formaldehyde resin in prosthesis Contact Dermatitis 1985;12:174.

62. MacFarlane A, Curley R, King C. Contact sensitivity to unsaturated polyester resin in a limb prosthesis. Contact Dermatitis 1986;15:301.

63. Vincenzi C, et al. Allergic contact dermatitis due to benzoyl peroxide in an arm prosthesis. Contact Dermatitis 1991;24:66.

64. Foussereau J, Cavelier C, Protois JP, et al. Contact dermatitis from methyl methacrylate in an above-knee prosthesis. Contact Dermatitis 1989;20:69.

65. Romaguera C, Vilaplana J, Grimalt F, et al. Contact sensitivity to meth (acrylates) in a limb prosthesis. Contact Dermatitis 1989;21:125.

66. Baptista A, Barros M, Azenha A. Allergic contact dermatitis on an amputation stump. Contact Dermatitis 1992;26:140.

67. Manneschi V, Palmerio B, Pauluzzi P, Patrone P. Contact dermatitis from myoelectric prosthesis. Contact Dermatitis 1989;21:116.

68. Fisher AA. Dermatologic hazards of electrocardiography. Cutis 1977;20:686.

69. Lockey SD. Drug reactions and sublingual testing with certified food colors. Ann Allergy 1973;31:423.

70. Hannuksela M, Pirila V, Salo PO. Skin reaction to propylene glycol. Contact Dermatitis 1975;1:112.

71. Storrs FJ. Para-chloro-meta-xylenol allergic contact dermatitis in seven individuals. Contact Dermatitis 1975;1:211.

72. Coskey RJ. Contact dermatitis caused by ECG electrode jelly. Arch Dermatol 1977;113:839.

73. Fisher AA. Allergen replacements in allergic contact dermatitis. Int J Dermatol 1977;16:319.

74. Richardson DR, Caravati CM Jr, Weary PE. Allergic contact dermatitis to "alcohol" swabs. Cutis 1969;5:1115.

75. Lewes D. Electrode jelly in electrocardiography. Br Heart J 1965;27:105.

76. Andersen KE. Cutaneous reactions to an epoxy-coated pacemaker. Arch Dermatol 1979;115;97.

77. Romaguera C, Grimalt F. Pacemaker dermatitis. Contact Dermatitis 1981;7:333.

78. Raque C, Goldschmidt H. Dermatitis associated with an implanted cardiac pacemaker. Arch Dermatol 1970;102:646.

79. Iguchi N, Kasanuki H, Matsuda N, et al. Contact sensitivity to polychloroparaxylene-coated cardiac pacemaker. Pacing-Clin-Electrophysiol 1997;20:372.

80. Abdallah H, Balsara R, O'Riordan A. Pacemaker contact sensitivity: clinical recognition and management. Ann Thorac Surg 1994;57:1017.

81. Brun R, Hunziker N. Pacemaker dermatitis. Contact Dermatitis 1980;6:212.

82. Peters MS, Schroeter AL, Van Hale HM, et al. Pacemaker contact sensitivity. Contact Dermatitis 1984;11:214.

83. Viraben R, Boulinguez S, Alba C. Granulomatous dermatitis after implantation of a titanium pacemaker. Contact Dermatitis 1995; 33:437.

84. Buchet S, Blanc D, Humbert P, et al. Pacemaker dermatitis. Contact Dermatitis 1992;26:46.

85. Landwehr A, van-Ketel W. Pompholyx after implantation of a nickel-containing pacemaker in a nickel-allergic patient. Contact Dermatitis 1983;9:147.

86. Wilkerson PG, Jordan WP. Pressure dermatitis from an implanted pacemaker. Dermatol Clin 1990;8:189.

87. Ferringer T, Mowad C: Telangiectatic erythematous cutaneous reaction to an implantable cardioverter defibrillator. Am J Contact Dermat 2003;14:37.

88. Fisher AA. Dermatitis associated with transcutaneous nerve stimulation for control of pain. Surg Neurol 1974;2:45

89. Shealy CN, Maurer D. Transcutaneous nerve stimulation for control of pain. Surg Neurol 1974;2:45.

90. Burton C. Transcutaneous electrical nerve stimulation to relieve pain. Postgrad Med 1976;59:105.

91. Loeser JD, Black RG, Christman A. Relief of pain by transcutaneous stimulation. J Neurosurg 1975;42:308.

92. Zugerman C. Dermatitis from transcutaneous electric nerve stimulation. J Am Acad Dermatol 1982;6:936.

93. Fisher AA, Brancaccio RR. Allergic contact sensitivity to propylene glycol in a lubricant jelly. Arch Dermatol 1979;115:1451.

94. Fisher AA. Dermatologic aspects of disulfiram (Antabuse) use. Cutis 1982;30:461.

95. Lachapelle JM. Allergic "contact" dermatitis from disulfiram implants. Contact Dermatitis 1975;1:218.

96. Swinson RP. Disulfiram implant. J Alcohol 1970;5:40.

97. Romaguera C, Grimalt F. Nickel dermatitis from acupuncture needles. Contact Dermatitis 1979;5:195.

98. Romaguera C, Grimalt F. Contact dermatitis from a permanent acupuncture needle. Contact Dermatitis 1981;7:156.

99. Eun HC. Nickel in acupuncture needles. Contact Dermatitis 1981;7:334.

100. Jordan WP, Dahl MV. Contact dermatitis from cellulose ester plastics. Arch Dermatol 1972;105:880.

101. Vail JT. Allergic contact dermatitis due to eyeglass frames. Cutis 1972;9:703.

102. Pegum JS. Contact dermatitis from plastics containing tri-aryl phosphates. Br J Dermatol 1966;78:626.

103. Fisher AA. Epoxy resin dermatitis. Cutis 1976;17:1027.

104. Jordan WP. Turpentine in eyeglasses. Contact Dermatitis Newslett 1972;12:309.

105. Calnan CD. Resorcinol monobenzoate. Contact Dermatitis 1975;1:59.

106. Sonnex T, Rycroft R. Dermatitis from phenyl salicylate in safety spectacle frames. Contact Dermatitis 1986;14:268.

107. Jirasek L, Kobikova M, Jiraskova M. Retroauricular eczema caused by the nickel of celluloid-rimmed spectacles. Cesk Dermatol 1976;51:369.

108. Hambly EM, Wilkinson DS. Contact dermatitis to butyl acrylate in spectacle frames. Contact Dermatitis 1978;4:115.

109. Jordan WP, Dahl MV. Contact dermatitis to a plastic solvent in eyeglasses: cross-sensitivity to ethyl acetate. Arch Dermatol 1971;104:524.

110. Fowler J. Contact urticaria to 1,1,1 trichloroethane. Am J Contact Dermat 1991;2:239.

111. Herbst R, Maibach H. Contact dermatitis caused by allergy to ophthalmic drugs and contact lens solutions. Contact Dermatitis 1991; 25:305.

112. Tosti A, Tosti G. Thimerosal: a hidden allergen in ophthalmology. Contact Dermatitis 1988;18:268.

113. Vilaplana J, Romaguera C, Grimalt F. Contact dermatitis from nickel and cobalt in a contact lens cleaning solution. Contact Dermatitis 1991;24:232.

114. Cameli N, Tosti G, et al. Eyelid dermatitis due to cocamidopropyl betaine in a hard contact lens solution. Contact Dermatitis 1991;25:261.

115. De-Groot A, Weijland J. Contact allergy to disodium cocoamphodipropionate. Contact Dermatitis 1996;35:248.

116. Peters K, Andersen K. Allergic hand dermatitis from 2-hydroxyethyl acrylate in contact lenses. Contact Dermatitis 1986;15:188.

117. Guill MA, Odom RB. Hearing aid dermatitis. Arch Dermatol 1972;105:880.

118. Oliwiecki S, Beck M, Chalmers R. Contact dermatitis from spectacle frames and hearing aid containing diethyl phthalate. Contact Dermatitis 1991;25:264.

119. Matrolonardo M, Loconsole F, Conte A, et al. Allergic contact dermatitis to PTBFR in a hearing aid. Contact Dermatitis 1993;28:197.

120. Jordan WP. Resorcinol monobenzoate, balsam of Peru sensitivity. Arch Dermatol 1973;108:278.

121. Koefoed-Nielsen B, Pedersen B. Allergy caused by light cured ear moulds. Scand-Audiol 1993;22:193.

122. Meding B, Ringdahl A. Allergic contact dermatitis from the earmolds of hearing aids. Ear-Hear 1992;13:122.

123. Wright RC, Fregert S. Allergic contact dermatitis from epoxy resin in nasal cannulae. Contact Dermatitis 1983;9:387.

124. Toome BK. Allergic contact dermatitis to a nasal cannula. Arch Dermatol 1989;125:571.

125. Boom B, et al. Allergic contact dermatitis to epoxy resin in infusion sets of an insulin pump. Contact Dermatitis 1985;12:280.

126. Van den Hove J, et al. Allergic contact dermatitis from acrylates in insulin pump infusion sets. Contact Dermatitis 1996;35:108.

127. Cronin E, Calnan CD. Allergy to hydroabietic alcohol in adhesive tape. Contact Dermatitis 1978;4:57.

128. Dooms-Goossens A, et al. Contact and photocontact sensitivity problems associated with thiourea and its derivatives. Br J Dermatol 1987;116:573.

129. Calnan CD. Diethyldithiocarbamate in adhesive tape. Contact Dermatitis 1978;4:61.

130. Murphy JC, Reif AE, January HL. Cutaneous hypersensitivity to adhesive and scotch tapes. J Invest Dermatol 1958;31:45.

131. Shono M, Ezoe K, Kaniwa M, et al. Allergic contact dermatitis from PTBP-FR in athletic tape and leather adhesive. Contact Dermatitis 1991;24:281.

132. Dwyer P, Freeman S. Allergic contact dermatitis to adhesive tape and contrived disease. Australas J Dermatol 1997;38:141.

133. Marron P, DeBerker D, Powell S. Methacrylate sensitivity and transcutaneous electrical nerve stimulation (TENS). Contact Dermatitis 1991;25:190.

134. Jordan WP. Cross sensitization patterns in acrylate allergies. Contact Dermatitis 1975;1:13.

135. Heskel NS, Samour CM, Storrs FJ. Allergic contact dermatitis from dodecyl maleamic acid in Curad adhesive plastic bandages. J Am Acad Dermatol 1982;7:747.

136. Emmett EA. Contact dermatitis from polyfunctional acrylic monomers. Contact Dermatitis 1977;3:245.

137. Nethercott JR. Skin problems associated with multifunctional acrylic monomers in ultraviolet curing inks. Br J Dermatol 1978;98:541.

138. Narumi J. Friction dermatitis due to adhesive plaster. Narumi Dermatology Clinic, Beppu, Japan. Jpn J Clin Dermatol 1970;24:1185.

139. Rasmussen JE, Fisher AA. Allergic contact dermatitis to salicylic acid plaster. Contact Dermatitis 1976;2:237.

140. Hogan DJ, Maibach HI. Adverse dermatologic reactions to transdermal drug delivery systems. J Am Acad Dermatol 1990;22:811.

141. Holdiness MR. A review of contact dermatitis associated with transdermal therapeutic systems. Contact Dermatitis 1989;20:3.

142. Musel A, Warshaw E: Cutaneous reactions to transdermal therapeutic systems. Dermatitis 2006; 17: 109.

143. Von Bahr B, Wahlberg J: Reactivity to nicotine patches wrongly blamed on contact allergy. Contact dermatitis 1997;37:44.

144. Kounis N, Zavras G, Papadaki P, et al. Allergic reactions to local glyceryl trinitrate administration. Br J Clin Pract 1996;50:437.

145. Robinson M, et al. Evaluation of the primary skin irritation and allergic contact sensitization potential of transdermal triprolidine. Fundam-Appl-Toxicol 1991;17:103.

146. Horning J, Zawada E, Simmons J, et al: Efficacy and safety of two-year therapy with transdermal clonidine for essential hypertension. Chest 1998; 93:941.

147. Maibach HI. Oral substitutions in patients sensitized by transdermal clonidine treatment. Contact Dermatitis 1985;19:225.

148. Bircher AJ, Howald H, Rufli T. Adverse skin reactions to nicotine in a transdermal therapeutic system. Contact Dermatitis 1991;25:230.

149. El-Sayed F, Bayl-Lebey P, Marquery M, et al. Sensibilisation systémique au 17 beta-oestradiol induite par la voie transcutanée. Ann-Dermatol-Venereol 1996;123:26.

150. Koch P, Allergic contact dermatitis from estradiol and norethisterone acetate in a transdermal hormonal patch. Contact Dermatitis 2001;44:112.

151. Shouls J, Shum K, Gadour M, et al. Contact allergy to testosterone in an androgen patch. Contact Dermatitis 2001;45:124.

152. Eichelberg D, Stolze P, Block M, et al. Contact allergies induced by TTS treatment. Methods Find Exp Clisn Pharmacol 1989;11:223.

153. Silva SK, Berman B. The effect of topical Maalox on transdermal clonidine induced contact dermatitis. Am J Contact Dermat 1992;3:79.

154. Jordan W. Allergy and topical irritation associated with transdermal testosterone administration: a comparison of scrotal and nonscrotal transdermal systems. Am J Contact Dermat 1997;8:108.

155. Amkraut A, Jordan W, Taskovich L. Effect of coadministrations of corticosteroids on the development of contact sensitization. J Am Acad Dermatol 1996;35:27.

156. Schwarz BK, Clendenning WE. Allergic contact dermatitis from hydroxypropyl cellulose in a transdermal patch. Contact Dermatitis 1988;18:106.

157. Pecquet C, et al. Allergic contact dermatitis from ethanol in a transdermal estradiol patch. Contact Dermatitis 1992;27:275.

158. McBurney E, Noel S, Collins J. Contact dermatitis to transdermal estradiol system. J Am Acad Dermatol 1999;20:508.

159. Dwyer C, Forsyth A. Allergic contact dermatitis from methacrylates in a nicotine transdermal patch. Contact Dermatitis 1994;30:309.

160. Praditsuwan P, Taylor J, Roenigk H. Allergy to Unna boots in four patients. J Am Acad Dermatol 1995;33:906.

161. Tavadia S, Bianchi R, Dawe M, et al: Allergic contact dermatitis in venous leg ulcer patients. Contact Dermatitis 2003 ; 48 : 261.

162. Malten KE. Sensitizers in leg bandages. Contact Dermatitis 1977;3:217.

163. Fowler J. Contact allergy to a rubber knee brace. Am J Contact Dermat 1991;2:211.

164. Scalf L, Fowler J. Allergic contact dermatitis caused by dialkyl thioureas in a patient with sleep apnea. Am J Contact Dermat 1999;10:169.

165. Sanchez-Morillas L, Martos R, Rodriguez-Mosquera M, et al. Delayed sensitivity to Prolene. Contact Dermatitis 2003;48:338.

166. Fisher A. Nylon allergy: nylon suture test. Cutis 1994;53:17.

167. Kurosaki S, Otsuka H, Kunitomo M, et al. Fibroin allergy. Nippon Ika Daigaku Zasshi 1999;66:41.

168. Lhotka C, Szekeres T, Fritzer-Szekeres M, et al. Are allergic reactions to skin clips associated with delayed wound healing? Am J Surg 1998;176:320.

FRAGRANCE ALLERGY

EXECUTIVE SUMMARY

The prevalence of positive patch tests to fragrance allergens is among the highest of all allergens routinely tested. In North America, the North American Contact Dermatitis Group (NACDG) has reported 9.1% of patients positive to the fragrance mix FM-1 and 10.6% to *Myroxylon pereirae* (MP, formerly called balsam of Peru).[1] These two allergens are commonly used to screen patients for fragrance allergy. A second fragrance allergen mix, FM-2, has recently been tested in Europe and is beginning to be used in North America.[2] In addition, it is becoming increasingly recognized that oxidation products of some fragrance substances, eg, linalool, are much more allergenic than the fresh chemical. Therefore, testing may be necessary with these added materials when fragrance is strongly suspected as the culprit.

Reasons for the high rate of fragrance allergy are twofold: many fragrance substances are good allergens, and exposure to fragrances is ubiquitous. In addition to "fine" fragrances used in perfumes and colognes, we are under constant assault from fragrances in skin and hair care products, laundry and cleaning products, room deodorizers, etc. Only one-fourth of the patients with a fragrance allergy in a European study reacted to perfume or cologne.[3] The rate of positive patch tests to fragrance increases with increasing age of patients, presumably a result of lifelong exposures (Figure 20-1).

Beyond the obvious sources, exposure to allergens related or identical to fragrance allergens may occur when a person uses products that contain herbal or "botanical" ingredients. Many, but not all, of these botanical extracts contain allergens that crossreact with the allergens in our screening patch tests. This is an area where testing with patient-supplied materials can be very useful.

Fragrance allergens such as cinnamic and mint derivatives are frequently found in dental care products and can cause stomatitis, cheilitis, and possibly systemic allergic contact dermatitis (ACD) in sensitized persons.[4] Another source of systemic exposure to fragrance-related allergens includes a variety of foods, spices, and flavorings that have been characterized as "balsam-related edible products." Ingestion of these allergens may cause non-specific dermatitis, hand dermatitis, or reactivation of dermatitis at previous sites of topical exposure.[5] Salaam and Fowler[5] reported that almost 50% of a group of patients with positive patch tests to either FM-1 or MP

could identify foods that caused a flare of their dermatitis, after having incomplete clearance with fragrance avoidance alone.

The prevalence of positive patch tests to fragrance allergens varies geographically. This may be due partly to the allergens employed for testing but more to the character of the fragrances preferred by different ethnic and national populations. While positive patch tests to fragrances are common, a few authors believe that true ACD from fragrances is less so. The problem is the difficulty in being certain of the actual chemical composition of a given fragranced product, since such information is almost never released by industry.

In addition to ACD, photodermatitis is seen occasionally, as are contact urticaria, irritation, and depigmentation.

Fragrance allergy generally has been well recognized only since the 1940s. Bonnevie[6] in 1948 reported that balsam of Peru (now called *Myroxylon pereirae*, abbreviated to MP) was a common allergen and identified cinnamic aldehyde as an important allergenic constituent. In 1961, Hjorth[7] extensively described allergy to balsam of Peru, both topically and systemically. Larsen[8] in 1977 developed the fragrance mix and reported on its usefulness as a screening allergen. These pioneers have allowed us to have a much clearer understanding of the diagnosis and prevalence of fragrance allergy.

The approximate concentration of perfume oils used in various products is shown in Table 20.1. More than five thousand fragrance materials are in use today. A typical complete perfume may consist of 10 to 300 separate

Table 20-1 Approximate Concentrations of Perfumes in Various Products

Colognes	4.0%
Cosmetics	0.5%
Masking perfumes	0.1% or less
Perfumes	20.0%
Toilet water	5.0%

components. Defining the specific offending allergens can, therefore, be difficult. Fortunately, there are often chemical similarities among fragrances that lead to crossreactions.

Prevalence of Fragrance Allergy

Thirty years ago, a prospective cosmetic adverse reaction study showed that fragrances are the leading cause of ACD due to cosmetics.[9] A follow-up study by the same investigators found 713 patients over a 6-year period with cosmetic dermatitis.[10] Of 536 positive patch tests, 161 (30%) were to fragrances. Preservatives accounted for 27% of reactions.

The most recent data from the North American Contact Dermatitis Group (NACDG) from 2004, indicate that fragrance mix-1 (FM-1) (8% pet) was positive in 9.1% of 5,140 patients tested, and MP was positive in 10.6%.[1] This compares with 14.0% and 10.4%, respectively, seen in the period 1994 to 1996.[11] Only nickel and neomycin gave more positive reactions.

DeGroot and Frosch[12] summarized fragrance allergy in Europe. Prevalence rates of about 5% to 11% are reported in various studies, with a European multicenter study reporting 8.3% of 1,072 tested patients positive to the fragrance mix.[13] From Finland, of almost 12,000 patients tested between 2000 and 2002, FM was positive in 6.9% and MP in 6.2%.[14] They noted that MP positivity had increased from 4.0% in 1996.

A retrospective analysis of patch tested patients over a 2-year period in Spain found positive reactions to MP (T.R.U.E.-Test) in 5.8% of 863 patients.[15] They speculated that handling citrus fruits may have contributed to allergy in their population.

In the general population, the frequency of fragrance allergy is uncertain. In a study from Denmark, about 1% of unselected subjects were positive to the fragrance mix.[16] Guin and Berry,[17] however, found that 18% of 90 student nurses were positive to the fragrance mix (16% concentration). Positive patch tests to fragrance increases with ageing, at least in Britain.[18] In children (age < 19 years), the NACDG has found a rate of positive patch tests to fragrance mix of 5.1%, in comparison to 9.1% in the entire tested group (Kathryn Zug, MD, personal communication, 2007).

Screening for Fragrance Allergy

Because there are hundreds of individual fragrance chemicals, the use of screening allergens is essential in diagnosing fragrance allergy.

MYROXYLON PEREIRAE (BALSAM OF PERU)

The name "balsam of Peru" has recently been changed to *Myroxylon pereirae* by the International Nomenclature of Cosmetic Ingredients (INCI), the international body charged with naming constituents in skin care products. *Myroxylon pereirae* is generally included in standard screening patch test series as an indicator of fragrance sensitivity. A naturally occurring substance obtained from Central and South American fir trees, MP is composed of many allergens including benzyl acetate, benzyl alcohol, cinnamic acid, cinnamic alcohol, cinnamic aldehyde, eugenol, and isoeugenol.

MP itself is rarely used in fragrances, although distillates are used that may be less allergenic. Some individuals may be sensitized to BP through medicinal exposure. Crossreactions with benzoin and resorcinol have been reported. BP as a marker substance is positive in about 50% of cases of fragrance allergy.

FRAGRANCE MIXES

A second agent used to screen for fragrance allergy is a fragrance mix. Typically, a mixture of eight common individual fragrance allergens (FM-1), listed in Table 20.2, is used. Currently, each allergen is included at a 1% concentration (8% total). This is superior to a 16% mix in terms of reduced irritancy, but may miss some reactions that would be positive at 16%. Santucci and colleagues[19] found a 3.6% to 5.2% range of positive reactions to fragrance mix depending on concentrations.

Based on international work, a second fragrance mix, FM-2, was added in 2007 to the NACDG standard series, and in some other centers. The components are listed in Table 20.2.

An interesting observation by Enders and colleagues[20] has led to the discovery that sorbitan sesquioleate (SS), an emulsifier, can enhance the diagnostic value of patch testing fragrances. They noted that less than half the patients positive to fragrance mix reacted to any of the agents separately. Subsequently, after finding the presence of SS in the mix, but not the individual allergens, they retested patients after adding SS to each single allergen. Ninety-three percent reacted to one or more allergen and none to SS (20% pet). The authors suggest that adding SS or another emulsifier may enhance patch test diagnostic

Table 20-2 Components of Patch Test Fragrance Mixtures-I and II			
Fragrance Mix I (each at 1%)			
1. oak moss absolute	2. cinnamic aldehyde	3. cinnamic alcohol	4. alpha-amyl cinnamic alcohol
5. geraniol	6. hydroxycitronellal	7. isoeugenol	8. eugenol
Fragrance Mix II (14%)			
1. Lyral (2.5%)	2. Citral (1%)	3. Farnesol (2.5%)	4. Citronellol (0.5%)
5. Hexyl Cinnamic Aldehyde (5%)	6. Coumarin (2.5%)		

power.[21] However, SS itself is a rare allergen and must be excluded as a cause of reaction to fragrance patch tests.

If an irritant reaction from fragrance mix is suspected and it is crucial to rule in or rule out fragrance allergy, then retesting at a later time with the individual components with SS is recommended. If a particular product is suspected as the cause, a request to the manufacturer for patch test materials containing a breakdown of the fragrance components is often helpful. Although fragrance formulas in many products are closely guarded, a coded patch test series may be supplied. Without divulging the whole formula, the manufacturer may disclose only the agents causing positive reactions.

The Cosmetics, Toiletry and Fragrance Association (CTFA) and/or the Research Institute for Fragrance Materials (RIFM) can be helpful in supplying information to assist the physician investigating fragrance or other cosmetic problems (see Appendix A).

Testing with BP and fragrance mix will probably detect over 90% of the cases of fragrance allergy. Larsen and colleagues[22] tested known perfume-sensitive patients and found that over 90% reacted to BOP, FM, or both. Three essential oils, sandalwood, narcissus, and ylang-ylang, detected almost all the remaining few patients who did not react to BP or FM.

Testing with Individual Fragrance Agents and Patient-Supplied Materials

Perfumes and colognes usually can be tested as is, although the patch should be allowed to dry before application to avoid irritation from volatile solvents.[23] Individual fragrance should be tested at concentrations listed in Table 20.3.

The NACDG collected data on frequency of positive patch tests to individual fragrance chemicals before 1991. For the years 1989 to 1990, 614 patients were tested with these allergens (Table 20.3). Twenty-two percent had one or more reactions. Twelve of these 135 patients (9%) had occupationally related fragrance allergy. Of the 199 total reactions, 162 (81.4%) were considered relevant to a past or current skin problem. A worldwide, multi-center study re-tested 178

known fragrance-allergic patients with the fragrance mix 1 (FM-1; 8%) and 20 other fragrance chemicals.[22] 79% reacted to FM-1. Other reactions are noted in Table 20.4.

Table 20-3 Positive Patch Tests to Fragrances in 614 Patients	
Allergen (pet)	Positive (%)
Cinnamic alcohol 5%	47 (7.6)
Cinnamic aldehyde 1%	30 (4.9)
Hydroxycitronellal 4%	13 (2.1)
Eugenol 4%	33 (5.4)
Isoeugenol 4%	19 (3.1)
Oak moss %%	11 (1.8)
Benzyl alcohol 5%	8 (1.3)
Geraniol 5%	17 (2.8)
Alpha-amyl cinnamic alcohol 5%	1 (0.2)
Benzyl salicylate 2%	7 (0.2)
Anisyl alcohol 5%	3 (0.5)
Sandalwood oil 2%	10 (1.6)
Coumarin 5%	8 (1.3)
Musk ambrette 5%	3 (0.5)

Source: NACDG. Unpublished data, 1991.

CINNAMIC ALCOHOL, CINNAMIC ACID, AND CINNAMIC ALDEHYDE

These commonly used fragrance materials are well-known allergens. An estimate of worldwide usage in a year 2000 survey was that between 100 and 1000 metric tons of cinnammic aldehyde and alcohol (each) and 1–10 tons of cinnamic acid were produced for the fragrance industry.[24] Cinnamic aldehyde and alcohol and chemically related components are used as flavoring agents, as well as fragrances. They are used in beverages (cola), vermouths, bitters, chewing gums, mouthwashes, soaps, and toothpaste. Sanitary napkin dermatitis due to cinnamic alcohol has been reported.

Because of its sensitizing capacity, the International Fragrance Research Association (IFRA) recommends that cinnamic alcohol should not be used as a fragrance ingredient at a level of more than 4% in fragrance compounds and that cinnamic aldehyde use should be less than half of one

Table 20-4 Allergy to Various Fragrance Materials

Fragrance Material *Total number of patients tested = 178*	# positive	% positive
Fragrance mix 8% pet (FM-1)	140	78.7
Jasmine absolute 10% pet	30	16.9
Geranium oil bourbon 10% pet	15	8.4
1-citronellol 5% pet	10	5.6
Spearmint oil 5% pet	9	5.0
1,3,4,6,7,8-hexahydro-4,6,6,7,8,8-hexamethylcyclopenta-gamma-2-benzopyran 7% pet	6	3.4
Omega-6-hexadecenlactone 5% pet	6	3.4
Dimethyltetrahydrobenzalaldehyde (isomer mixture) 5% pet	4	2.3
α-amylcinnamaldehyde 5% pet	4	2.3
1-(1,2,3,4,5,6,7,8-octahydro-2,3,8,8-tetramethyl-2-napthylenyl)ethanone 5% pet	3	1.7
Cyclopentadecanone 5% pet	3	1.7
2-methyl-5-(2,3-dimethyltricyclo[2.2.1.0 (2,6)]hept-3-yl-2-pentenol(α-form) and 2-methyl-5-(2-methyl-3-methylenebicyclo [2.2.1]hept-3-yl-2-penten-1-ol(beta form) 5% pet	2	1.1

Adapted from reference # 22

percent.[25,26] However, a European multi-center study showed that ACD can be triggered with a much lower concentration of cinnamic aldehyde. In this study, a ROAT was positive in individuals with axillary dermatitis from deodorants. The concentration of cinnamic aldehyde of 0.1% or less gave positive reactions in all subjects tested.[27]

Cinnamic aldehyde has shown stronger sensitization than cinnamic alcohol in guinea pig tests.[28] There is some crossreactivity between the two. The enzyme alcohol dehydrogenase, present in human skin, can readily convert the alcohol to the aldehyde. Cinnamic aldehyde has been shown to cause non-immunologic contact urticaria, with immediate flushing and release of several prostaglandins.[27] This could be blocked by prior administration of aspirin.

GERANIOL

This substance is found in many essential oils, including rose, geraniums, citronella, jasmine, and lavender oils. It is colorless with a scent of roses.[12]

ALPHA-AMYL CINNAMIC ALDEHYDE

This is a synthetic fragrance with a jasmine odor. It is a weak sensitizer, as noted in studies where individual fragrance allergens are tested (Table 20.3).

HYDROXYCITRONELLAL

Hydroxycitronellal is a fragrance used widely in floralizing perfume materials. It may also be found as a fragrance in antiseptics and insecticides. This widely used fragrance material is synthetic and is not found in nature.

ISOEUGENOL AND EUGENOL

Eugenol is a component of essential oils obtained from spices, including cloves and cinnamon leaf, with an odor and taste of cloves. Positive patch tests to eugenol and isoeugenol, respectively, were found in 1.4% and 2.4% of 1,016 patients reported by the NACDG. Of the patients reactive to either substance, 13% reacted to both, indicating a low degree of crossreactivity. The chemical structure of these substances is very similar. Eugenol is found in mouthwashes, toothpaste, dental cements and packing agents, antiseptics, and inhalants, as well as in fragrance mixtures. Eugenol has been shown to have the ability to "quench" nonimmunologic contact urticaria when applied before urticants such as sorbic acid and cinnamic aldehyde.[29] Unfortunately, it does not inhibit ACD in the same situations.[30]

Isoeugenol has a weaker odor than eugenol and may be found in ylang-ylang and nutmeg oil. In 1998, the IFRA suggested reducing the limit of 0.2% in consumer products to 0.02%. White and colleagues[31] reported that isoeugenol acetate (1.2% ethanol), a possible replacement for isoeugenol, gave positive patch tests in most isoeugenol sensitive patients. Isoeugenol in deodorants is a common cause of axillary dermatitis. Bruze and colleagues showed that experimental formulations containing isoeugenol that were applied like deodorants could elicit dermatitis in some patients even with a concentration of 0.0063%.[32] Substitution of isoeugenol with related fragrance chemicals may not achieve much reduction in contact allergy. From 65 to 95% of patients that reacted on patch testing with isoeugenol acetate, isoeugenol benzoate, or isoeugenol phenylacetate also reacted to isoeugenol.[33] A few patients reacted to isoeugenol methyl ether or benzyl ether and did not react to isoeugenol, however.

OAK MOSS ABSOLUTE

Oak moss absolute is a natural product derived from a tree lichen, *Evernia prunastri*. Atranorin and chloroatranorin, along with their degradation products atranol and chloroatranol, are potent sensitizers, present in oak moss.[34,35] In one study, half of 10 subjects reacted to atranol and/or chloroatranol at 1ppm or less.[36] Other allergens include evernic acid and fumarproto-cetaric acid. Consort contact dermatitis has been reported in a woman due to exposure to her husband's aftershave lotion, which contained oak moss.[37] Oak moss absolute is a commonly used fragrance material in aftershave lotions.

BENZYL ALCOHOL

Benzyl alcohol is a fragrance ingredient that is also used as a preservative and antiseptic topically and as a preservative in injectable medications. Allergy to benzyl alcohol as a fragrance ingredient has been reported.[38] However, allergy from other exposure sources, such as preservatives and solvents, is also common. Shaw[39] gives an excellent review of the topic. (See also Chapter 16.)

MUSK AMBRETTE AND MUSK MOSKENE

Musk ambrette is a synthetic chemical that has been used widely for the last 60 years.[40] This nitro-musk compound is used as a fixative in perfume formulations in concentrations from 1% to as high as 15%. In 1978, Larsen[41] reported the first case of photoallergic contact dermatitis to musk ambrette. The patient used a well-known aftershave lotion and broke out with a severe dermatitis on the sun-exposed areas of the face and neck.

Since that time, numerous reports of photosensitivity to musk ambrette have been made.[42] In addition, musk ambrette can cause nonphotoallergic contact dermatitis. It is apparent that putting aftershave lotion on a recently shaved face and going outdoors is analogous to a continuous photomaximization test. Musk ambrette should be a component of any photo patch testing series.

In addition to photoallergy, an apparent case of airborne ACD of the face with hyperpigmentation has been reported. Chronic burning of incense for several years was the source of exposure.[43]

A case of ACD to musk moskene, a related perfume, has been reported from contact in facial cosmetics.[44] Testing at 5% petrolatum was negative in controls. Musk moskene is reported to cause less photosensitivity and allergy than musk ambrette.

The IFRA recommends that musk ambrette should not be used as a fragrance ingredient at a level of more than 4% in fragrance compounds. It recommends further that musk ambrette should not be used at a level of more than 0.5% in fragrance compounds intended for use in aftershave products.

6-METHYLCOUMARIN (6-MC)

The synthetic compound 6-methylcoumarin is related structurally to the furocoumarins. In 1980, an epidemic of photodermatitis occurred in people using a popular sunscreen containing 6-MC.[45] The reaction occurred primarily in women and developed within several hours after they applied suntan lotion and went into the sun.

The U.S. Food and Drug Administration (FDA) received many consumer complaints, and it initiated a shelf recall of all those suntan products containing this ingredient.[46] Subsequent phototesting suggested that 6-MC is indeed a potent photosensitizer, at least under the conditions of this particular application.[47]

The IFRA recommends that 6-methylcoumarin and also 7-methylcoumarin should not be used as a fragrance ingredient.

CITRAL (3,7 DIMETHYL-(2,6)-OCTADIENAL)

Citral is the major component of oil of lemon grass and is also found in oils from verbena, oranges, and lemons. It imparts a lemon-like odor and bittersweet taste. Heydorn and colleagues[48] patch tested 586 dermatitis patients with citral (2% pet). Probable allergic reactions were seen in 28 (5%) and irritant reactions in 82. Of the 28, 12 patients did not react to other fragrance allergens. Women accounted for 71% of the citral- reactors. The high ratio of irritant to allergic patch test responses makes evaluation of this potentially important allergen problematic.

LINALOOL

Linalool (dimethyhl octadienol) occurs naturally in over 200 essential oils from herbs, flowers, etc. and has been called one of the most common fragrances in domestic and occupational products.[49] True, pure, linalool seems to be a very rare sensitizer, but oxidized linalool showed a good ability to sensitize guinea pigs.[50] In humans, 1.3% of 1511 consecutive patients in Europe reacted to oxidized linalool.[51]

R-LIMONENE

R-Limonene is widely in fragrances in both personal and occupational products and also as a solvent, insecticide, and flavoring agent.[52] While the non-oxidized substance is non-allergenic, oxidation is common and rapid and produces several allergens. In a multicenter European study of 2,273 patients, 63 had allergic patch tests to "aged" (10 weeks) limonene (3% pet) and/or "limonene hydroperoxide fraction"(0.5% pet).[53] Only half of these reacted to other screening fragrance allergens.

LICHEN EXTRACTS

Lichens, plantlike organisms often found on tree bark, leaves, and soil, produce various substances with aromatic and biocidal poperties. Allergy to lichen components has been seen mostly in forestry and wood workers, or from perfumes.[54] A lichen acid mix for patch testing contains usnic acid, atranorin, and everinic acid. Storrs and colleagues reported four cases of axillary dermatitis, positive to lichen-acid mix, clearly caused by a "natural" deodorant that contained lichen extracts.[55]

LYRAL

This fragrance allergen, also known as (hydroxy methyl-pentyl)cyclohexene-carboxaldehyde (HMPCC or HICC), has been reported to be an important sensitizer in Europe.[56] In North America, however, of 1,600 patients from 6 centers only 8 reacted to HMPCC (1.5% or 5% pet).[57] Three of these also reacted to either MP or FM-1. An extensive review of Lyral ACD has recently been published.[58] It seems that only about half of those allergic to Lyral will show a positive reaction to MP or FM-1. An evaluation of dose response estimated that 10% of HMPCC-allergic patients will react to 25 ppm. In a ROAT deodorant test, 9 of 14 subjects reacted within 2 weeks to a deodorant with 200 ppm.[59]

JOJOBA (*SIMMONDSIA CHINENSIS*)

Jojoba extacts are used in cosmetic and other skin care products and in folk medicines. Cases of ACD to Jojoba have been reported from Italy and Germany.[60,61]

VERSALIDE (AETT)

Versalide (AETT) is a tetralin musk formerly used widely as a musk fixative in many cosmetics, including soaps, colognes, and antiperspirants. It found wide use as a masking agent in nonscented antiperspirants. In 1979, Avon toxicologists discovered that during routine dermal tests with rats exposed to perfume oil, the skin and internal organs of the rats developed a blue color. The central nervous system was among those organs showing the most intense coloration. The pathologic change found in the nervous tissue was demyelination of nerve tracts.[62] This neurotoxic effect was reported to the RIFM, and the two fragrance companies that made versalide stopped supplying this compound for use in consumer products. The FDA took no action because the compound was no longer available for human use. The IFRA recommends that versalide should not be used in any fragrance compounds.

TEA-TREE OIL

The extract of the *Melaleuca alternifolia* plant, tea-tree oil, is promoted as being useful for a wide spectrum of skin disorders such as scabies, herpes, and micorbial infections, and therefore is found in assorted topical products.[63,64] Crawford and colleagues[63] offer a recent worthwhile review. Systemic neurologic toxicity may occur in animals from overingestion. They comment on a study from Australia that found rates of allergy between 3 and 5% in 219 volunteers, 63% of whom had had known prior contact. This is likely higher than will be

Table 20-5 Allergens Identified in Tea-Tree Oil (in order of frequency)
Terpinolene
Ascaridol
Alpha-terpinene
Trihydroxy menthane
Alpha-phellandrene
Limonene
Myrcene
Viridiflorene
Carvone
Aromadendrene
Sabinene
Terpinen-4-ol

Based on Reference #68

seen in other areas since the tree is indigenous to and very popular in Australia.

Allergy in patients was reported by Rubel and colleagues.[65] Extensive patch testing with tea-tree oil components documented allergy to the sesquiterpenoid fractions. Another report implicated a monoterpene, O-limonene, as responsible for tea-tree oil allergy in six cases.[66] More recently, terpinen-4-ol and 1,8 cineole have been reported to be major constituents of tea tree oil.[67] Hausen has noted allergy to a variety of components listed in Table 20.5.[68] Crossreactivity with MP on patch testing appears to be common. Fowler noted frequent crossreactivity between tea-tree oil and MP and FM (Fowler J, personal communication, 2007).

ROSE OIL

Scheinman[69] reported 9 of 299 (3%) consecutive patients positive to rose oil (2% pet). In an Indonesian study, 7 of 32 patients positive to FM also reacted to rose extract.[70]

Further study of rose oil/extract would seem to be in order.

Unscented Cosmetics and Masking Fragrances

Some cosmetics and skin care products are labeled "unscented" but actually contain a low concentration of a "masking fragrance." The masking fragrance is intended to cover the fatty odor of soap or the "medicinal" smell of some chemicals without giving a recognizable aroma of its own. Ethylene brassylate (Musk T) is often used for this purpose. It is uncertain how often this fragrance crossreacts with other fragrances, but if a patient wishes to completely avoid fragrance exposure, this substance should be looked for in ingredient lists. Generally, products labeled "fragrance-free" have no fragrance chemicals, including a masking fragrance. Therefore, the fragrance-sensitive consumer should look for this designation rather than the label "unscented."

Fragrances Masquerading as "Botanical" or "Herbal" Ingredients

In recent years some personal care products such as skin lotions and soaps have been marketed as being "unscented" or "fragrance-free," yet they contain herbal ingredients or oils from botanicals. Technically, although they import a fragrance, they are classified as "moisturizers" rather than fragrances. Unwitting consumers may be duped by marketing claims stating that a product contains only "natural" ingredients and may not realize that these herbal and botanical extracts can cause allergy in fragrance-sensitive persons.[69,71]

Both Scheinman[69] and Nakayama and colleagues[72] reported cases of ACD from "hidden" fragrances in soaps and other toiletries. Offending allergens included rose oil, vanilla, and sweet almond oil. Kiken and Cohen have reviewed ACD to botanical extracts.[73] They noted that up to that time, allergy had been reported to aloe, Arnica, Centella asiatica, chamomile, cucumber, gingko, lavender, peppermint, rosemary, sage, tea-tree oil, and witch hazel.

Storrs and colleagues[74] tested 140 Oregonians to 47 botanical extracts, including 21 at "high-risk" (known users of botanicals) and the rest without history of use of botanicals. Ten of the high risk group (48%) and 4 (3.4%) of the rest had positive patch tests. Propolis, feverfew (parthenium), spearmint, chamomile, and tea-tree oil gave the most reactions, but many others showed relevant positives. They propose a screening tray for botanical extract allergy (Table 20.6). This is one instance where testing with materials supplied by the patient may be very useful.

Table 20-6 Suggested Botanical Screening Tray

Tea tree oil 5% pet.
Lichen acid mix 0.3% pet.
Geranium oil (Bourbon) 2% pet.
Spearmint oil 5% pet.
Dandelion 2.5% pet.
Neroli oil 4% pet.
Lavender (absolute) 2% pet.
Sandalwood oil 2% pet.
Cananga oil 2% pet.
Rose oil (Bulgarian) 2% pet.
Ylang-ylang oil 2% pet.
Compositae mix 6% pet.

Based on reference # 74.

Fragrance-allergic patients should be counseled to read ingredient labels and avoid products containing covert fragrance allergens such as "herbal," "natural," or "botanical" extracts. As Fisher was fond of saying, the notorious sensitizer poison ivy is a natural substance.

Contact Urticaria

Contact urticaria may be allergic or nonallergic.[75] Myroxylon pereirae and some of its derivatives can cause nonallergic urticaria. The chief agent responsible for this is cinnamic aldehyde, although cinnamic acid, benzoic acid, and benzaldehyde are also active. The mechanism of action is probably a nonallergic histamine-liberating effect that may be more than a purely cutaneous phenomenon, because some individuals suffering from chronic respiratory allergies precipitate symptoms of their condition on exposure to certain fragrance materials. Fowler has observed immediate, presumably nonimmunologic contact urticaria at patch test sites of cinnamic aldehyde and MP. Cancian and colleagues[76] reported generalized urticaria with foci at patch sites of FM and BOP that resolved after 6 hours.

(Further discussion of contact urticaria is found in Chapter 31.)

"Predictive Testing" for Fragrance Sensitization

In humans, most fragrance allergy potential is documented with the maximization method. False-negative assays, however, occur with this method.[77]

Malten and colleagues[78] reported on 22 fragrance substances included by the RIFM in human maximization testing. Some agents showing a high rate of sensitization, such as diethylmaleate, are listed as prohibited in Table 20.7. However, several agents, including eugenol, hydroxycitronellal, and cinnamic alcohol, showed a very low sensitization potential yet are proven to give positive patch tests in certain ACD patients.

The fragrance industry is trying constantly to eliminate those fragrance materials that cause adverse reactions. The IFRA indicates chemicals the use of which is not recommended at all as well as those with limits and concentrations (consult Table 20.7).

The Future

We will not learn about new fragrance allergens unless we look for them by testing patients who are suspected to be allergic to cosmetic and toiletries, and by determining

Table 20-7 Suggested Restrictions in Ingredient Usage

Excluded	Limit on concentration on product use*	Use with quenching agent(s)
AETT (acetyl ethyltetramethyltetralin	5-acetyl-1,1,2,3,3,6-hexamenthyl indan	Carvone oxide
Acetyl isovaleryl	Allyl heptine carbonate	
Allanroot oil (elocampane oil)	Amyl cyclopentenone	Cinnamic aldehyde
Allylisothiocyanate		
Anisylidene acetone	Angelica root	Cinnamic aldehyde methyl anthranilate Schiff base
	cis- and trans- asarone	
Benzylidene acetone	Bergamot oil	Citral
p-tert-butylphenol	Bitter orange oil expressed	
Chenopodium oil	p-tert-butyl-dihydrocinamaldehyde	
Cinnamylidene acetone		
Colophony	Cassia oil	
		Phenylacetaldehyde
Costus root oil, absolute and concrete		
3,7-dimethyl-2-octen-1-ol (6,7-dihydrogeraniol)		
Diethyl maleate	Cinnamic alcohol	
Dihydrocoumarin	Cinnamon bark oil, Ceylon	
2,4-dihydroxy-3-methyl-benzaldehyde	Citrus oils and other furocoumarins containing essential oils	
4,6-dimethyl-8-t-butyl coumarin	Coatus root, essential oil, absolute and concrete	
Dimethylictraconate	Cumin oil	
Diphenylamine	Cyclamen alcohol	
Esters of 2-octynoic acid, except methyl and allyl heptine carbonate	Grapefruit oil expressed trans-2-hexenal	
Esters of 2-nonynoic acid, except methyl octine carbonate	a-hexylidene cyclopentanone	
	Hydroxycitronella	
	Isocyclogeraniol	
	Isoeugenol	
Ethyl acrylate	Lemon oil, cold pressed	
Ethylene glycol monoeathyl ether and its acetate	Lime oil, expressed	
Ethylene glycol monomethyl ether and its acetate	Marigold oil and absolute (tagetes oil and absolute)	
Fig leaf absolute	Menthadienyl formate	
Furfurylideneacetone	Methoxy dicyclopentadiene carboxaldehyde	
	2-methoxy-4-methylphenol	
trans-2-heptenal	Methyl heptadienone	
Hexahydrocoumarin		
trans-2-hexenal diethyl acetal		
trans-2-hexenal dimethyl acetal		
Hydroabietyl alcohol		
Hydroquinone monoethylether		
Hydroquinone monomethylether		
6-isopropyl-2-decalol	Methyl heptine carbonate	
Massoia bark oil	p-methylhydrocinnamic aldehyde	
Massoia lactone		
Melissa oil		
Methyl methacrylate		
7-methoxycoumarin	Methyl N-methyl anthranilate	
	3-methyl-2(3)-nonenenitrile	
	Methyl octine carbonate	
	Oak moss extracts	
	1-octen-2-yl acetate	
N-methyl anisylidene acetone	Opoponax	

Table 20-7 (Cont.) Suggested Restrictions in Ingredient Usage

6-methylcoumarin	Perilla aldehyde
	Balsam of Peru
7-methylcoumarin	
4-methyl-7-ethoxy coumarin	Propylidene phthalide
Methylcrotonate	Rue oil
Musk ambrette	
Nitrobenzene	Safrole, isosafrole, dihydrosafrole
	Styrax
	Tree moss extracts
	1-(trimethylcyclohexenyl/cyclohexadienyl)-
	2-butenn-1-ones (Rose ketones)
Pentylidene cyclohexanone	Verbena absolute
Phenylacetone (methyl benzyl ketone)	
Phenylbenzoate	
Pseudoionones	
Pseudomethylionone	
Thea sinensis absolute	
Verbena oil	

*These items are restricted to various maximum concentrations in the final product. Based on IFRA guidelines, 1999.

the offending allergens. This is done most easily by testing the actual product as is, except when it is irritating, as with shampoos and cleansers. If testing of the final formulation is positive, all the components, including the fragrance, should be obtained wherever possible and should be tested separately. Most major cosmetic and toiletry manufacturers will often assist by sending patch test materials when requested. If the fragrance component is positive, further breakdown of the fragrance to its individual components should be done to discover new fragrance allergens.

Prevention

The avoidance of fragranced cosmetics and toiletries is fairly straightforward if patients read labels and learn to avoid fragrances and, if appropriate, botanical extracts. More cosmetic lines are developing fragrance-free cosmetics, allowing for a wider choice of products by consumers. ROAT testing can be performed by a patient to help identify products with a fragrance that they can safely use, if total fragrance avoidance is unpalatable. Application of a product twice daily to non-dermatitic skin in the antecubital space is recommended.

References

1. Pratt M, Belsito D, DeLeo V, Fowler J, et al. NACDG patch-test results 2003–2004 period. Dermatitis 2007, in press.

2. Frosch P, Pirker C, Rastogi S, et al. Patch testing with a new fragrance mix detects additional patients sensitive to perfumes and missed by the current fragrance mix. Contact Dermatitis 2005;52:207.

3. DeGroot AC, Bruynzeel DP, Bos J, and colleagues The allergens in cosmetics. Arch Dermatol 1988;124:1525.

4. Saino L, Kanerva L: Contact allergens in toothpastes. Contact Dermatitis 1995;33:100.

5. Salaam T, Fowler J: Balsam-related systemic contact dermatitis. J Am Acad Dermatol 2001;45:377.

6. Bonnevie P. Some experiences of war-time dermatoses. Acta Derm Venereol (Stockh) 1948;28:231.

7. Hjorth N. Eczematous allergy to balsams, allied perfumes and flavoring agents with special reference to balsam of Peru. Acta Derm Venereol (Stockh) 1961;41(Suppl 46):1–216.

8. Larsen W. Perfume dermatitis. Arch Dermatol 1977;113:623.

9. Eiermann HJ, Larsen WG, Maibach HI, Taylor JS. Prospective study of cosmetic reactions, 1977–80. J Am Acad Dermatol 1982;6:909.

10. Adams RM, Maibach HI. A five-year study of cosmetic reactions. J Am Acad Dermatol 1985;13:1062.

11. Marks J, Belsito D, DeLeo V. North American Contact Dermatitis Group patch test results, 1996–1998. Arch Dermatol 2000;136:576.

12. DeGroot A, Frosch P:Adverse reactions to fragrances. Contact Dermatitis 1997;36:57.

13. Frosch P, Pilz B, Andersen K, and colleagues Patch testing with fragrances: results of a multicenter study of the EECDRG with 48 frequently used constituents of perfumes. Contact Dermatitis 1995;33:333.

14. Hasan T, Rantanen T, Alanko A, et al. Patch test reactions to cosmeticallergens in 1995–1997 and 2000–2002 in Finland. Contact Dermatitis 2005;53:40.

15. Avalos-Peralta P, Garcia-Bravo B, Camacho F: Sensitivity to Myroxylon pereirae resin (Balsam of Peru). Contact Dermatitis 2005;52:304.

16. Nielsen N, Menne T. Allergic contact sensitization in an unselected Danish population. Acta Derm Venereol (Stockh) 1992;72:456.

17. Guin J, Berry V. Perfume sensitivity in adult females. J Am Acad Dermatol 1984;11:1168.

18. Buckley D, Rycroft R, White I, et al. The frequency of fragrance allergy increases with their age. Br J Dermatol 2003;149:986.

19. Santucci B, and colleagues Contact dermatitis to fragrances. Contact Dermatitis 1987;16;93.

20. Enders F, Przybilla B, Ring J. Patch testing with fragrance mix at 16% and 8%, and its individual constituents. Contact Dermatitis 1989;20:348.

21. Enders F, Przybilla B, Ring J. Patch testing with fragrance-mix and its constituents: discrepancies are largely due to the presence or absence of Sorbitan sequioleate. Contact Dermatitis 1991;24:238.

22. Larsen W, Kakayama H, Fischer T, and colleagues Fragrance contact dermatitis—a worldwide multicenter investigation. Am J Contact Dermat 1996;7:77.

23. Johansen J, Frosch P, Rastogi S, Menne T: Testing with fine fragrances in eczema patients. Contact Dermatitis 2001;44:304.

24. Bickers D, Calow P, Greim H, et al, A toxicological and dermatologic assessment of cinnamyl alcohol, cinnamaldehyde, and cinnamic acid when used as fragrance ingredients. Food and Chem Toxicology 2005; 43: 799.

25. Cocchiara J, Letizia C, Lalko J, and colleagues Fragrance material review on cinnamaldehyde. Food and Chem Tixicology 2005;43: 867.

26. Bruze M, Johansen J, Andersen K, et al, Deodorants: an experimental provocation study with cinnamic aldehyde. J Am Acad Dermatol 2003;48:194.

27. VanderEnde D, Morrow J: Release of markedly increased quantities of prostaglandin D2 from the skin in vivo in humans after the application of cinnamic aldehyde. J Am Acad Dermatol 2001;45:62.

28. Basketter DA. Skin sensitization to cinnamic alcohol: the role of skin metabolism. Acta Derm Venereol (Stockh) 1992;72:264.

29. Safford RJ, et al. Immediate contact reactions to chemicals in the fragrance mix and a study of the quenching action of eugenol. Br J Dermatol 1990;123:595.

30. Basketter DA, Allenby CF. Studies of the quenching phenomenon in delayed contact hypersensitivity reactions. Contact Dermatitis 1991;25:160.

31. White I, Johansen D, Arnau E, et al. Isoeugenol is an important contact allergen: can it be safely replaced with isoeugenol acetate? Contact Dermatitis 1999;41:272.

32. Bruze M, Johansen J, Andersen K, et al. Deodorants: an experimental provocation study with isoeugenol. Contact Dermatitis 2005;52:260.

33. Tanaka S, Royds C, Buckley D, et al. Contact allergy to isoeugenol and its derivatives : problems with allergen substitution. Contact Dermatitis 2004;51:288.

34. Thune P, et al. Perfume allergy due to oak moss and other lichens. Contact Dermatitis 1982;8:396.

35. Bernard G, Gimenez-Arnau E, Rastogi S, et al. Contact allergy to oak moss. Arch Dermatol Res 2003;295:229.

36. Johansen J, Bernard G, Gimenez-Arnau E, et al. Comparison of elicitation potential of chloroatranol and atranol- 2 allergens in oak moss absolute. Contct Dermatitis 2006;54:192.

37. Held JL, Ruszkowski AM, Deleo VA. Consort contact dermatitis due to oak moss. Arch Dermatol 1988;124:261.

38. Corazza M, Mantovani L, Maranini C, et al. Allergic contact dermatitis from benzyl alcohol. Contact Dermatitis 1996;34:74.

39. Shaw D. Allergic contact dermatitis to benzyl alcohol in a hearing aid impression material. Am J Contact Dermat 1999;10:228.

40. Opdyke DL. Musk ambrette: monographs of fragrance raw materials. Food Cosmet Toxicol 1975;13:875.

41. Larsen WG. Photoallergy to musk ambrette found in an aftershave lotion. Presented at the American Academy of Dermatology Meeting, San Francisco, Dec 1978.

42. Kochever IE, et al. Assay of contact photosensitivity to musk ambrette in guinea pigs. J Invest Dermatol 1979;73:144.

43. Hayakawa R, Matsunaga K, Arima Y. Airborne pigmented contact dermatitis due to musk ambrette in incense. Contact Dermatitis 1987;16:96.

44. Hayakawa R, Hirose O, Arima Y. Pigmented contact dermatitis due to musk moskene. J Dermatol 1991;18:420.

45. Jackson RT, Nesbitt LT, Jr, DeLeo VA. 6-methylcoumarin photocontact dermatitis. J Am Acad Dermatol 1980;2:124.

46. Eiermann HJ. Regulatory issues concerning AETT and 6-MC. Contact Dermatitis 1980;6:120.

47. Kaidbey KH, Kligman AM. Identification of topical photosensitizing agents in humans. J Invest Dermatol 1978;70:149.

48. Heydorn S, Menne T, Andersen K, et al. Citral a fragrance allergen and irritant. Contact Dermatitis 2003;19:32.

49. Rastogi S, Heydorn S, Johansen J, et al. Fragrance chemicals in domestic and occupational products. Contact Dermatitis 2001;45:221.

50. Skold M, Borje A, Matura M, et al. Studies on the autoxidatin and sensitizing capacity of the fragrance chemical linalool, identifying a linalool hydroperoxide. Contact Dermatitis. 2002;46:267.

51. Matura M, Skold M, Borje A, et al. Selected oxidized fragrance terpenes are common contact allergens. Contact Dermatitis 2005;52:320.

52. Rastogi S, Heydorn S, Johansen, J, Basketter D: Fragrance chemicals in domestic and occupational products. Contact Dermatitis 2001;45:221.

53. Matura M, Goosens A, Bordalo O, et al, Patch testing with oxidized R-(+)-limonene and its hydroperoxide fraction. Contact Dermatitis 2003; 49:15.

54. Wood B, Rademaker M. Allergic contact dermatitis from lichen acids. Contact Dermatitis 1996;34:370.

55. Sheu M, Simpson E, Law S, Storrs F. Allergic contact dermatitis from a natural deodorant. J Am Acad Dermatol 2006;55:332.

56. Johansen J, Frosch P, Svedman C, et al. Hydroxyisohexyl 3 cyclohexene-carboxaldehyde-known as Lyral. quantitative aspects and risk assessment of an im portent fragrance allergen. Contact Dermatitis 2003; 48:310.

57. Belsito D, Fowler JF, Sasseville D, et al. Delayed-type Hypersensitivity to fragrance materials in a select North American population. Dermatitis 2006;17:23.

58. Militello G, James W: Lyral: a fragrance allergen. Dermatitis 2005;16: 41.

59. Jorgensen P, Jensen C, Rastogi S, et al. Experimental elicitation with hydroxyisohexyl-3-cyclohexene carboxaldehyde containing deodorants. Contact Dermatitis 2007;56:146–50.

60. Wantke F, Hemmer W, Gotz M, Jarisch R: Contact dermatitis from jojoba oil and myristyu lactate/maleated soybean oil. Contact Dermatitis 1996; 34:71–2

61. Di Berardino L, DiBerardino F, Castelli, et al. A case of contact dermatitis from jojoba. Contact Dermatitis 2006;55:57–8

62. Spencer PS, et al. Neurotoxic changes in rats exposed to the fragrance compound acetyl ethyl tetramethyl tetralin. Neurotoxicology 1979;1:221.

63. Crawford G, Sciacca J, James W: Tea Tree Oil: cutaneous effects of the extracted oil of *Melaleuca alternifloria*. Dermatitis 2004;15:59.

64. Walton S, McKinnon M, Pizzutto S, et al. Acaricidal activity of *Melaleuca alternifolia* (tea tree) oil. Arch Dermatol 2004;140:563.

65. Rubel D, Freeman S, Southwell I. Tea-tree oil allergy: what is the offending agent? Aust J Dermatol 1998;39:244.

66. Knight T, Hausen B. Melaleuca oil (tea-tree oil) dermatitis. J Am Acad Dermatol 1994;30:423.

67. Cox S, Mann C, Markham J: Interactions between components of the essential oil *of Melaleuca alternifolia*. J Appl Microbiol 2001;91:492.

68. Hausen B: Evaluation of the main contact allergens in oxidized tea-tree oil. Dermatitis 2004; 15: 213.

69. Scheinman P. Is it really fragrance free? Am J Contact Dermat 1997;8:239.

70. Roesyanto-Mahadi I, Guersen-Reitsma A, vanJoost T, and colleagues Sensitization to fragrance materials in Indonesian cosmetics. Contact Dermatitis 1990;22: 212.

71. Scheinman P. The foul side of fragrance-free products: what every clinician should know about managing patients with fragrance allergy. J Am Acad Dermatol 1999;41:1020.

72. Nakayama H, Nogi N, Kashara N, et al. Allergen control, an indispensable treatment for allergic contact dermatitis. Dermatol Clin 1990;8:197.

73. Kiken D, Cohen D: Contact dermatitis to botanical extracts. Am J Contact Dermat 2002;13:148.

74. Simpson E, Law S, Storrs F: Prevalence of botancal extract allergy in patients with contact dermatitis. Dermatitis 2004;15:67.

75. Von Krogh G, Maibach HI, eds. The contact urticaria syndrome. In: Marzulli FN, Maibach HI, eds. Dermatotoxicology, 2nd ed. New York: Hemisphere Publishing, 1983:301.

76. Cancian M, Fortina A, Peserico A. Contact urticaria syndrome from constituents of balsam of Peru and fragrance mix in a patient with chronic urticaria. Contact Dermatitis 1999;41:300.

77. Marzulli F, Maibach HI. Contact allergy: predictive testing of fragrance ingredients in humans by draizé and maximization methods. J Environ Pathol Toxicol 1980;3:235.

78. Malten KE, et al. Reactions in selected patients to 22 fragrance materials. Contact Dermatitis 1984;11:1.

APPENDIX A

Information Sources For Fragrances

RESEARCH INSTITUTE FOR FRAGRANCE MATERIALS (RIFM)

50 Tice Blvd.
Woodcliff Lake, NJ 07677
Telephone: 201–689–8089
Fax: 201–689–8090
Website: www.rifm.org

INTERNATIONAL FRAGRANCE RESEARCH ASSOCIATION (IFRA)

Avenue des Arts 6
1210 Brussels, Belgium
Telephone: 32-2-214-20-60
Fax: 32-2-214-20-69
E-mail: secretariat@ifraorg.org
Web site: www.ifraorg.org

COSMETICS, TOILETRY, AND FRAGRANCE ASSOCIATION (CTFA)

1101 17th Street, N.W. #300
Washington, DC 20036
Telephone: 202-331-1770
Fax: 202-331-1969
Web site: www.ctfa.org

CHAPTER 21

ALLERGIC SENSITIZATION TO PLANTS

EXECUTIVE SUMMARY

The best-known plant allergens are the Toxicodendrons, which include poison ivy, poison oak, and poison sumac, all of which contain identical allergens. Crossreactions occur between these notorious plant allergens and Japanese lacquer and cashew nut trees, mango, and the Indian marking nut tree.

Sesquiterpene lactones are another plant allergen found in many plants such as ragweed, sagebrush, burdock, chamomile, and chrysanthemum species including tansy, feverfew, and pyrethrum. The water-soluble protein fraction of ragweed causes the respiratory allergy while the oleoresin found in the pollen, stem, and leaf causes dermatitis.

Parthenium dermatitis in India is due to accidental introduction from American wheat contaminated with feverfew. Severe, refractory airborne contact dermatitis has resulted.

While some plants produce irritant contact dermatitis (spurge, cowhage) others produce phytophotodermatitis (limes, parsnip, figs, celery, dill, and fennel).

Many common decorative plants are potential sources of allergic contact dermatitis (English ivy, philodendron, daffodil, bougainvillea, hydrangea, narcissus, verbena, and marigold). Tulip bulbs and Alstroemeria share a common allergen. Primrose is a major source of contact dermatitis in Europe.

Common vegetables, such as carrots, squash, asparagus, and cucumber have been reported to cause contact dermatitis.

A large number of spices cause contact dermatitis, including cinnamon, nutmeg, mace, cloves, vanilla, laurel, cayenne pepper, thyme, and rosemary.

Patch tests done with parts of plants can cause irritant reactions or may be potentially useful with non-irritant plants.

Plant dermatitis may be classified as allergic sensitization, mechanical irritation, chemical irritation, phytophotodermatitis, and pseudophytodermatitis.

The plant substances responsible for dermatitis do not enter directly into the metabolism of the plant and are classified as secondary products. The relative proportion of these secondary products depends on vigor of growth, cultural conditions, and the stage of development of the plant. Thus, the amount of ragweed oleoresin increases tenfold when the plant pollinates and is at the height of growth.

Another factor that may be clinically significant is the distribution of the dermatitis-producing substances in the plant. For example, primin, the antigenic substance of the primrose, is stored in fragile cells in superficial glandular hairs and is released by casual contact. In contrast, the sensitizing substance in some daisies is stored in resin canals and is released only when the plant is bruised or crushed.[1] In some plants, the sensitizers may be in the leaves and stem; in others, they are found, in addition, in the flowers, pollen, and roots.

Pentadecylcatechols in the plant oleoresin, consisting of 1,2-dihydroxy benzenes (catechols) with a 15-atom side chain in the third position, are the sensitizers in the *Toxicodendron* plants. These pentadecylcatechols may show crossreactivity with other phenolic compounds, such as resorcinol, hexylresorcinol, and hydroquinones, but not with phenol.

A 1:10 dilution of the oleoresin in acetone usually equals a 1:1,000 dilution of pentadecylcatechols in antigenicity. Patch testing, except for investigational purposes, is not advisable.

The oleoresin contains unstable, unsaturated compounds that are probably more potent sensitizers than the stable, unsaturated pentadecylcatechols. Members of the Anacardiaceae plant family include common poison ivy *(T. radicans)*, poison oak *(T. toxicodendron, T. diversiloba)*, poison sumac *(T. vernix)*, mango, lacquer tree, cashew nut, Indian marking nut, and rengas tree (black varnish tree). The ginkgo tree fruit contains related allergenic catechols.

Toxicodendron Plants

In the United States, the *Toxicodendron* group of plants is responsible probably for more cases of allergic contact dermatitis than are all other provocatives combined.

In the eastern United States, *Toxicodendron* dermatitis occurs usually in the spring and summer, but in the Southwest, where outdoor living is common all year, poison oak dermatitis appears at any time, regardless of the season. Even in the East, poison ivy may be acquired from the roots of the plant throughout the year.

Poison ivy and poison oak are the principal causes of *Toxicodendron* dermatitis in the United States. Poison oak *(T. toxicodendron, T. diversiloba)* is more prominent on the West Coast than elsewhere, but poison ivy *(T. radicans)* occurs throughout the United States. Poison sumac or poison dogwood *(T. vernix)* is found only in woody, swampy areas. Cross-sensitivity between the *Toxicodendron* plants exists, and the antigens of all of them are essentially the same. Table 21.1 shows some distinctive characteristics of the various *Toxicodendron* plants.

Poison ivy, the most ubiquitous of the *Toxicodendron* group, is a versatile plant that may climb for many feet on a pole, a tree, or a house. On several occasions poison ivy has been discovered being cultivated as an ornamental vine, growing up the side of a house as high as the second story and producing severe, recurrent poison ivy dermatitis on the unsuspecting occupants. The leaflets of the poison ivy and oak plants usually grow in groups of three, giving rise to the warning, "Leaves three, leave them be!"(Figure 21-1)

The allergic contact dermatitis whether produced by poison ivy, poison oak, or poison sumac is the same. Furthermore, because the *Toxicodendron* plants belong to the Anacardiaceae family, crossreactions may occur with the following related plants and substances:

1. A furniture lacquer that may sensitize is obtained from the Japanese lacquer tree.

Table 21-1 Characteristics of Poisonous Toxicodendron Plants[a]

Name	Habitat	Identification aids
Poison ivy *(T. radicans)*	United States (except extreme Southwest) and southern Canada	Groups of three leaflets, the margins of each entire, to toothed, to lobed, flat, or wavy. Leaflets 5 to 15 cm long, apex pointed. Fruits off-white. Stems with or without aerial rootlets, usually clambering or climbing.
Poison oak *(T. toxicodendron, quercifolia)*	Same as above	Groups of three leaflets, the margins of which are more wavy, more lobed, more "oaklike" than *T. radicans,* and the plant appears more shrublike and less vinelike. *Leaflets 5 to 15 cm long,* more apex pointed than rounded. Conservative botanists consider this a variety or form of poison ivy. Fruits off-white.
Poison oak *(T. diversiloba)*	Generally west of the Cascade and Sierra Nevada mountains, from the Puget Sound to Mexico	Group of three to five leaflets, the margins of each wavy to deeply lobed, more "oaklike" than either of the two above. *Leaflets 3 to 7 cm long,* apex rounded. Fruits off-white. Stems smooth to pubescent, usually stiff and shrublike, less commonly vinelike. This is the poison oak variety found in California.
Poison sumac *(T. vernix)*	Damp, swampy places east of the Rocky Mountains, particularly east of the Mississippi River Groups of three leaflets, the margins of each entire, to toothed, to lobed, flat, or wavy. *Leaflets 5 to 15 cm long,* apex pointed. Fruits off-white. Stems with or without aerial rootlets, usually clambering or climbing.	Groups of 7 to 13 leaflets, arranged as pairs along central rib, with single leaflet at the end. Fruits white.

[a]In the United States and Canada, any species of Toxicodendron with white fruits should be avoided until positive identification is made. Red-fruited species generally are safe.

2. The oil from the shell of the cashew nut contains a potent sensitizer, which is destroyed by heat. Imported Haitian voodoo dolls and swizzle sticks made from cashew nuts may produce a reaction resembling poison ivy dermatitis. Cashew oil may be used in the synthesis of phenolformaldehyde resins and in mucilages, varnishes, and printer's ink. Components of the oil of cashew nut shells may crossreact with the fruit pulp of the ginkgo tree. The ginkgo fruit pulp may produce an eruption indistinguishable from that of poison ivy dermatitis.

3. The rind of the mango contains a catechol similar to the catechol of the poison ivy group.

4. The marking nut tree of India produces a black, tarry oleoresin used to mark laundry. Because this black ink is a potent sensitizer unaffected by boiling, it can cause repeated attacks of allergic contact dermatitis (dhobi itch) when used to mark clothing. (A *dhobi* is a laundryman.)

Dark-skinned individuals seem less susceptible than others to *Toxicodendron* dermatitis. It has been estimated that at least 70% of the population of the United States would acquire it if exposed casually to the plants. Prolonged exposure would probably sensitize even more of the population. Although elderly individuals are not usually as susceptible to poison ivy as are younger people, Fisher[2] observed poison ivy dermatitis in several individuals who were in their late 70s. Newborn infants can readily be sensitized by a single application of the oleoresin to a localized area, such as a patch test site. More than 50% of infants thus sensitized showed positive patch test reactions 2 to 3 weeks after the initial sensitizing application.

Table 21.2 has a list of plants that contain urushiols, which are related to the poison ivy group. Tests for the pyrocatechols in these anacardiaceous plants are presented in Table 21.3.

Goldstein[3] pointed out that rengas trees, which grow primarily in Malayan jungles, furnish lumber resembling mahogany that is used for furniture. Unlike mahogany, however, rengas sap crossreacts with other urushiol plants and trees. If rengas wood furniture is varnished before it is dried thoroughly, the sap may come through the varnish and cause reactions in those using it.

Indian sandal strap dermatitis may be due to the urushiol-containing sumac used to tan leather in certain Indian villages.

A contact dermatitis can be caused by the oleoresin of the mango tree sap or the skin of the fruit. Ingestion of the fruit may produce anaphylactic reactions.

JAPANESE LACQUER TREE

Dermatitis from the Japanese lacquer tree is known to be due to urushiol. The lacquer resin of *Melanorrhoea usitata* is used for the same purposes in Thailand. The allergen is closely related to urushiol and is known as thitsiol. In Vietnam, the lacquer contains laccol.[4]

JAPANESE WAX TREES

In Japan, Australia, and New Zealand, *Rhus succedanea* and *R. vernicifua* are sources of poison ivy. Known

---

Table 21-2 Anacardiaceae Plants Related to the Poison Ivy Group

Common names	Scientific names	Distribution	Modes of contact
Brazilian pepper	*Schinus terebinthifolius*	Brazil, Hawaii, France, Florida	Direct—plant to skin
Cashew nut shell oil		India, Africa, Central America, East Indies	Direct—plant to skin Voodoo dolls, swizzle sticks, resins, mucilages, printer's ink, electric insulation
Cashew oil	*Anacardium occidentale*		
El litre tree	*Lithraea caustica*	Chile	
Ginkgo tree	*Ginkgo biloba*	Southeastern United States, China, Japan, Europe	Oriental lacquerware, stepping in seeds
Indian marking nut dhobi (laundryman) itch	*Semecarpus anacardium*	India, Malaya	Laundry marking ink
Lacquer tree	*Rhus vernicifera*	China, India, Japan	Wood boxes, bracelets, bar rails
Mango	*Mangifera indica*	Hawaii, California, Florida, India, Central America, Mediterranean	Direct—plant to skin
Pepeo tree	*Mauria puberula*	Venezuela	Direct—plant to skin Direct—plant to skin
Rengas tree, black varnish tree	*Anacardium melanorrhoea*	Malaya	Furniture, wood carvings

Table 21-3 Tests for Pyrocatechols

Green to black with ferric chloride
Green to brown with alcohol and caustic soda
White with lead acetate

collectively as Japanese wax trees, the fat from the berries is used for candles and the resin for lacquer. These ornamental sumacs are valued for their bright red-orange leaves in the fall.[5]

In South America, the *Lithraea* genus causes allergic contact dermatitis. *Lithraea molleoides, caustica,* and *brasiliensis* are commonly referred to as Aroeira or Aruera, followed by the suffix *brava,* which means "harmful" or "hazardous." These are trees *(L. molleoides)* or shrubs *(L. brasiliensis).* They are members of the Anacardiaceae family and do crossreact with *Toxicodendron.* In a study of 17 *Lithraea*-sensitive patients, all reacted to urushiol. This is not surprising, given that the allergens identified in *Lithraea* include 3-pentadecylcatechol, 3-pentadecenylcatechol, 3-heptadecenylcatechol, and 3-hepta-dec-dienilcatechol.[6]

DERMATITIS-PRODUCING FACTORS OF TOXICODENDRON PLANTS

The leaves, stems, seeds, flowers, berries, and roots of certain plants contain a milky sap that turns into a black substance resembling varnish on exposure to air. Alcohol and other solvents can be used to extract a crude yellow-brown viscous substance from the sap. The residue remaining after evaporation of the solvents is the antigenic oleoresin. The term "urushiol" is often used for the oleoresins of the Anacardiaceae plants, including the *Toxicodendron* group. Urushiol is antigenic even after the plant has died.

The dermatitis-producing principle of the oleoresin is related to the presence of pentadecylcatechols (PDCs), which are 1,2-dihydroxy benzenes (catechols) with a 15-atom side chain in the third position. Some investigators, however, suggest that individuals may be sensitive to another component of the oleoresin. Some people with allergic hypersensitivity to PDCs show crossreactivity to other phenolic compounds, such as resorcinol, hexylresorcinol, and the hydroquinones, but not to phenol.

A 1:10 dilution of the oleoresin in acetone usually equals a 1:1,000 dilution of PDCs in antigenicity. The oleoresin contains unstable, unsaturated compounds, however, which are probably more potent sensitizers than the stable, saturated PDCs.

Aside from phenolic substances, the oleoresins contain variable mixtures of polymers of unknown chemical composition.

Nature of Toxicodendron Dermatitis

The eruption produced by poison ivy is an allergic eczematous contact dermatitis usually characterized by redness, papules, vesicles, and bullae, plus linear streaking (Figure 21-2). Occasionally, urticaria and eruptions, resembling erythema multiforme, measles, or scarlatina, occur from systemic absorption of the poison ivy antigen.

The dermatitis is produced by exposure to some portion of the bruised plant, allowing the oleoresin to contact the skin. The uninjured plant is innocuous. Pure smoke from burning the poison ivy plant is also harmless provided the particulate matter does not contain the oleoresin. Involvement of the mucous membranes, with stomatitis or proctitis, due to chewing of the leaves or overdosage in oral hyposensitization, is not rare.

The fluid content of vesicles and bullae present in poison ivy dermatitis is not antigenic. Patch tests performed with it give negative reactions.

One can acquire poison ivy dermatitis from oleoresin-contaminated animals, clothing, tools, golf clubs, fishing rods, and baseball bats. Fomites contaminated with the oleoresin in a dry atmosphere may remain antigenic for a long time, whereas a warm, moist climate favors loss of potency. The urushiol of the Japanese lacquer tree (*Toxicodendron verniciflua*) polymerizes to a nonallergenic state over 10 to 20 or more years, but heating accelerates this. The reaction seen from urushiol stored at 20°C for 10 years is equal to that seen with urushiol stored at 110°C for 1 week or 150°C for 11 hours.[7] Washing with soap or detergents renders oleoresin-contaminated clothing and objects harmless. The *Toxicodendron* oleoresin may remain under a person's fingernails unless removed deliberately by thorough cleansing. If not removed, for several days after contact with the plants, the antigen may be spread from the fingers to the covered parts of the body and even to other individuals.

After first exposure to the oleoresin, sensitization and dermatitis occur after 7 to 10 days. After a previously sensitized person contacts the oleoresin, the eruption appears usually within 2 days, and delay of onset rarely exceeds 10 days. In a few cases, the skin reaction may occur within 8 hours of exposure. Such temporal differences are due probably to the degree of exposure, individual susceptibility, and regional variation in cutaneous reactivity. In some recent experimental work with urushiol antigen, it was observed that most subjects react between day 4 and 5 after exposure to a moderate antigen dose (RLR, personal observation).

Toxicodendron dermatitis begins usually with itching and redness. Streaks of erythema or papules in linear arrangement soon appear. Complications include eosinophilia, kidney damage, urticaria, dyshidrosis, and marked pigmentation or leukoderma. Impetigo and pyoderma are frequent complications.

In the differential diagnosis, it must be remembered that arthropod bites, particularly those due to bedbugs, often cause a linear eruption. In addition, phytophotodermatitis (dermatitis bullosa striata pratensis) due to the psoralen of plants may produce lesions consisting of bullae that are striate or irregularly linear on exposed portions of the body. The lesions develop 12 to 24 hours after plants, such as celery, parsley, gas plants, limes, and figs, have been crushed on the skin and after subsequent exposure to sunlight. The bullae heal, leaving pigmentation that may persist for many months.

Toxicodendron plants are not photosensitizers, and the dermatitis is distinguished by occurring on both covered and uncovered parts of the body and by not requiring sunlight for its development.

PATCH TESTING FOR POISON IVY SENSITIVITY

The plant oleoresin diluted 1:10 in acetone may be used for patch testing. The pure synthetic antigen, 3-pentadecylcatechol, a stable crystalline material, may also be used in various dilutions, but it is not readily available. There is also some question as to whether it contains all the antigenic materials of the poison ivy oleoresin.

Patch testing reveals that about 50% of the population of the United States has been sensitized to poison ivy. A strong possibility exists that 5% to 10% of nonsensitized individuals may become sensitized by being patch tested with either the synthetic antigen or the natural oleoresin.

The diagnosis of poison ivy dermatitis is usually fairly obvious, and there is not much point in proving the diagnosis by such a procedure. Patch testing with the oleoresin or pentadecylcatechol should be restricted to investigative procedures or to proving hyposensitization by prophylactic treatment.

The only objective proof of successful hyposensitization procedures is a negative or weakly positive patch test reaction to poison ivy in individuals who had previously shown a strongly positive reaction to the oleoresin. The oleoresins may give intense vesicular and even bullous reactions in sensitized individuals.

Urushiol is insoluble in water, as is its component, PDC. This limits some of the *in vitro* investigations that can be carried out. A water-soluble allergen, tetrahydrourushiol glycoside (THUG), gives concordant reactions with urushiol and PDC. Similar intensity of patch test responses was observed with 0.002% urushiol in petrolatum as compared with 0.1% PDC in petrolatum and 0.1% THUG in water.[8]

GENERAL PROPHYLAXIS *OF TOXICODENDRON* DERMATITIS

The best prophylaxis for any type of allergic contact dermatitis is complete avoidance of the allergen. Patients should be taught to recognize and avoid the *Toxicodendron* group. They should carefully observe and search surrounding terrain before choosing a picnic or camping site. When a poison plant is present in the garden or cannot be avoided, its chemical destruction or physical removal is indicated. Farmer's Bulletin No. 2158, *Chemical Control of Brush and Trees*,[9] issued by the U.S. Department of Agriculture, should be consulted for information on specific chemicals for destroying poison ivy or poison oak.

All individuals exposed to these plants should thoroughly wash the entire body with soap and water. One need not use strong soaps for this purpose. Complete change of clothing is also advisable, and, whenever possible, contaminated clothing should be washed with soap and water.

The poison ivy antigen enters the skin so rapidly that the oil must be totally removed within 10 minutes of exposure. When such early washing is not feasible, however, it is worthwhile for the individual to wash at the first opportunity to remove any oleoresin remaining on the skin and thereby prevent its being transferred to other parts of the body.

Topical prophylaxis of poison ivy/oak has been demonstrated with topical linoleic acid dimer.[10]

In a double-blind evaluation of seven different barrier creams, three were deemed significantly more effective in protecting against experimental toxododendron dermatitis. Stokogard, Hollister Moisture Barrier, and Hydropel were helpful, and Stokogard proved most effective, but no product was completely effective.[11]

Experimentally induced poison ivy dermatitis was effectively prevented by application of a 5% quaternium-18 bentonite lotion. About 70% of the 144 urushiol-sensitive subjects had total or near total protection.[12] The product is sold under the brand name Ivy Block, and the active agent has been renamed bentoquantum.

Poison Ivy

SOME UNUSUAL FEATURES OF THE TOXICODENDRON GROUP

"Leaves three, leave them be!" is the common warning. However, as Gillis[13] stated, "Although typical poison ivy and poison oak normally have but three leaflets, occasionally additional leaflets are formed. Added leaflets are common especially in western poison oak, in which nearly every clone studied can be found to have some leaves with *five or more* leaflets. I have seen one population that consistently produced additional leaflets, ranging even up to seventeen!"

LACK OF PROTECTION BY RUBBER GLOVES

The catechols in urushiol are soluble in rubber. Therefore, rubber gloves do not protect the hands from poison ivy. Use heavy-duty vinyl gloves instead.

BLACK LACQUER DEPOSITS DUE TO SELF-BLACKENING OF TOXICODENDRON SAP

Guin[14] demonstrated that a black enamel–like deposit is seen frequently on injured areas of *Toxicodendron* plants. The black deposit can be produced by crushing leaves from the plant onto a sheet of white paper and exposing the paper to the air for a few minutes. When the oleoresin is released by injury to the plant, it darkens and hardens to form a black "lacquer." Mallory and colleagues[15] reported four patients with clinical *Toxicodendron* dermatitis that presented with dramatic black lacquer like deposits on several lesions. This black deposit was also observed at sites of injury on poison ivy plants and was reproduced on volunteers by the application of plant sap on the skin. Histologically, the observed material was identified in the stratum corneum. An example of the characteristic "lacquer dot" is seen in Figure 21-3.

ROLE OF AGE, SEX, COLOR OF SKIN, AND SPECIES

Poison ivy does not spare age, sex, color of skin, or race. Poison ivy dermatitis can occur at any age, although infants are apparently not as easily sensitized as adults. After the age of 3, children become highly susceptible, and by 12 years of age nearly all have become sensitized to poison ivy.[16]

Of all animals, only humans and a few of the higher primates are sensitive to poison ivy. Even rhesus monkeys may be sensitized only with difficulty, and they lose their sensitivity relatively rapidly. A few instances are on record of deliberately sensitizing dogs once the poison was applied directly to the skin with the hair removed.

URUSHIOL

The oleoresin component of poison ivy contains the pentadecylcatechols that produce dermatitis. These catechols are soluble in rubber and in oil and fat solvents.

Urushiol retains its antigenic potential in the dry state indefinitely. Thus, several 100-year-old herbarium specimens containing urushiol have been known to produce dermatitis in a sensitized individual who has handled them.[17]

The reaction of urushiol with the sensitized skin is almost immediate, a complex protein being formed almost at once.

It is known that the sap from *Toxicodendron* plants turns black when touched to surfaces other than skin. The juice from the vine made a satisfactory indelible ink, and some Native American tribes even made a black dye from the vines. This use is similar to that of the Japanese lacquer tree, whose sap, when exposed to the air, forms a black varnish. *Semecarpus anacardium,* the usual cause of dhobi mark dermatitis, is used to make laundry marks in India because of similar properties. Contact urticaria from a dhobi mark has been reported.[18]

Fisher[19] pointed out that urushiol binds with sensitized skin, forming a catechol-protein complex that is not removed by thorough washing. The black deposits could not be removed with soap and water in volunteers after 4 hours, although no attempt was made to remove the deposit with an organic solvent. The oleoresin-protein complex or the oleoresin itself probably accounts for the yellowish, amorphous material observed in the stratum corneum of biopsies.

No amount of washing will remove the already reacted complex of catechol protein. After the dermatitis appears, washing will have no effect. Washing may remove excess ununited urushiol from dry areas of the skin.

Urushiol is nonvolatile and dries quickly on clothing, shoes, and tools, retaining its potency for months or even years on such fomites. Cleaning fluid solvents can effectively remove urushiol from fomites, and for contaminated clothing ordinary laundering is usually effective in removing urushiol.

Epstein and colleagues[20] reported that 21 adults, highly sensitive to urushiol, ingested up to 300 mg of urushiol over 3 to 6 months. A control group received placebo capsules. The study was done double blind to evaluate changes in patch test reactivity to urushiol, altered reactivity to an unrelated contact sensitizer, side effects, and duration of hyposensitization. A significant number of subjects in the experimental group (15 of 21) became hyposensitized. Such hyposensitization was not seen in the control group (2 of 12), and the difference between groups was significant. No change in reactivity to an unrelated contact sensitizer occurred in subjects hyposensitized to urushiol, suggesting antigen specificity. Retesting up to 3 months after completion of the protocol indicated that subjects remained hyposensitized without a "rebound" effect during that time. Side effects, detected by a questionnaire, were limited to vesicular and urticarial rashes and pruritus ani in 18 of 21 test subjects.

GEOGRAPHY

Poison ivy is most abundant along the sandbars off the coast of New Jersey, New York, through the Carolinas, and along the rocky coast of New England.[14] Poison ivy can grow to a rather large size. At least one poison ivy tree is on record from Sanibel Island, Florida, that stands 15 to 20 feet high. Poison ivy vine can grow as high as 30 feet on a telephone pole.

Poison ivy is native to North and South America and eastern Asia. In the lower Mississippi River basin, a form of poison ivy exists that is confined virtually to the cotton-growing areas of rich soils in places such as the Delta region of Arkansas, Louisiana, and Mississippi.[21]

In the Edwards Plateau region of Texas and continuing north to the Arbuckle Mountains of Oklahoma, another subspecies of poison ivy is found with sharply pointed lobes on the leaflets. A species of poison ivy, which is common in Mexico in the Sierra Madre Occidental, extends northward into the southeastern corner of Arizona, and to the southern tip of Baja, California.[22] Reports of poison ivy dermatitis in Europe and Australia involve introduced plants.

COMPLICATIONS

On rare occasions, patients with poison ivy dermatitis may develop immune complex disease with accumulations of IgG in the kidney and skin associated with the appearance of skin sensitive antibodies to urushiol in serum with resulting nephrosis.[23]

Hyperpigmentation is a common complication of poison ivy dermatitis in black skin, but is rare in white skin. Urticaria or erythema multiforme or scarlatiniform eruptions may occur occasionally from systemic absorption of poison ivy antigen.

Oral or injected administration of poison extract can produce an allergic systemic contact dermatitis with a flare of poison ivy dermatitis at previously affected sites.

DIFFERENTIAL DIAGNOSIS

Three dermatoses resembling each other clinically and characterized by linear or striate papules and vesicles, and sometimes urticaria, include poison ivy dermatitis, phytophotodermatitis, and Portuguese man-of-war envenomization. Allergic contact dermatitis from scorpion weed, *Phacelia*, in the southwestern United States closely resembles poison ivy/oak dermatitis.

IMMUNITY AND DESENSITIZATION

The U.S. Food and Drug Administration (FDA) has not approved as yet any desensitizing procedure.[24]

NATURAL DESENSITIZATION OR HARDENING

Immunologists cannot explain why repeated skin exposure to poison oak and poison ivy allergens often reduces patch test reactivity. The phenomenon of "hardening," which occurs presumably with certain industrial chemicals, has been reported in certain settings. Japanese lacquer craftspeople who are new to the job are exposed to 60% to 65% urushiol in raw lacquer. After 1 month on the job, five of eight such individuals became sensitized with patch test verification.[25] After 9 to 10 months, seven of eight showed decreased sensitivity, and the one who did not "harden" was suspected to have had antecedent sensitization.[25] Another study of the Japanese lacquer industry by questionnaire revealed that 81% of 232 craftspeople developed dermatitis, but only 1.3% did not decrease reactivity, and those with more than 2 hours per day exposure "hardened" better than those with less exposure.[26] This usually occurred within 1 month. These observations are similar to those found in the cashew nut shell oil industry, where 9 of 13 workers showed decreased or no reactivity to poison ivy/oak after several months of occupational exposure.[27]

Repeated patch tests with urushiol give unpredictable results, sometimes reducing, sometimes heightening responses. Administration of live, attenuated measles virus vaccine to a small group of subjects resulted in a *temporary* reduction of sensitivity to poison ivy most marked between the third and sixth weeks after immunization.[28]

Some persons appear to be relatively immune to poison ivy. Probably few persons are potentially totally immune, but rather have a high threshold for sensitization or have never been sensitized.

THE "SPREAD" OF POISON IVY

Poison ivy may be spread in the smoke of burning poison ivy because of tiny droplets of the urushiol present on the particles of dust and ash in the smoke. Smoke that does not contain urushiol is not antigenic. Such "airborne" urushiol, however, may produce severe involvement of the eyelids and conjunctivitis. It must be emphasized that urushiol is not volatile even at the usual temperature of bonfires and therefore cannot be spread from burning poison ivy as a gas.

THE "EXOTIC" MEMBERS OF THE ANACARDIACEAE FAMILY

Poison ivy closely related to the East Coast variety is found in China and Japan. The lacquer from the lacquer trees of China and Japan consists of a dried urushiol, and even when dried, the lacquer can still produce dermatitis.

The nuts of the cashew tree contain cardol oil, a urushiol whose sensitizing property is destroyed by roasting. Brake linings, electrical insulations, resins, mucilages, and printer's ink are made from cashew nut shell oil. Swizzle sticks (drink stirrers) and voodoo dolls made from cashew nuts may cause urushiol dermatitis.

The ginkgo fruit pulp contains catechols that may produce cheilitis, stomatitis, proctitis, and pruritus ani when ingested by sensitized individuals.[29] The seeds of the ginkgo tree fruit are free of catechols.[30]

The catechols of the mango are restricted to the stem or pedicle and the exocarp ("skin") of the fruit.[31] Black deposits on the edible mango can also result from contamination by sap from the stem.

POISON IVY AND BRAZILIAN PEPPER ("FLORIDA HOLLY")

Morton[32] reports that the Brazilian pepper tree (*Schinus terebinthifolius,* of the family Anacardiaceae) is closely related to poison ivy and is native to Brazil. It has been commonly cultivated in Florida for more than 50 years as an ornamental, and use of its sprays of showy red fruits for Christmas decoration gave rise to the popular misnomer "Florida holly." Too late, it was found to become a large, spreading tree; aggressive seedlings began springing up near and far. Jungles of *Schinus* have crowded out native vegetation over vast areas of Florida and the Bahamas, as in all the islands of Hawaii.

When in bloom, the tree is a major source of respiratory difficulty and dermatitis. The abundant nectar yields a spicy, commercial honey, and beekeepers are opposed to eradication programs. This plant has produced many cases of severe dermatitis in Florida.

Hurtado and colleagues[33] found that the oleoresin of *Mauria puberula,* a poisonous species of the Anacardiaceae that is indigenous to the Venezuelan Andes, can cause both primary irritant dermatitis and allergic contact dermatitis in guinea pigs and humans. Cross-sensitization reactions were found in persons with known allergy to *Toxicodendron* spp. or *Lithraea caustica* and in guinea pigs sensitized to 3-n-pentadecylcatechol. These results suggest that the active principles of *Mauria* are chemically related to, but not identical to, those of *Toxicodendron.*

ERADICATION OF POISON IVY

The following is reprinted from *Poison Ivy, Poison Oak and Poison Sumac* by Donald M. Crooks and Dayton L. Klingman, Farmer's Bulletin No. 1972, published by the U.S. Department of Agriculture, U.S. Government Printing Office, Washington, D.C., 1976.[22]

Control by Mechanical Means

Poison ivy and poison oak can be grubbed out by hand quite readily early in spring and late in fall, if a few plants are involved. Roots are most easily removed when soil is thoroughly wet. Grubbing when soil is dry and hard is almost futile because the roots break off in the ground,

leaving large pieces that later sprout vigorously. Grubbing is effective if well done.

Poison-ivy vines climbing on trees should be severed at the base, and as much of the vine as possible should be pulled away from the tree. Often the roots of the tree and weed are so intertwined that grubbing is impossible without injury to the tree. Bury or destroy roots and stems removed in grubbing, because the dry material is almost as poisonous as the fresh.

Smoke from burning poison-ivy plants or contaminated articles may carry the poison in a dispersed form. Take extreme caution to avoid inhalation or contact of smoke with the skin or clothing. (Pure smoke from burning poison ivy plants, since it does not contain any particles of the plant, will not cause any dermatitis.)

Old plants of poison ivy produce an abundance of seeds, and these are freely disseminated, especially by birds. A poison-ivy seedling 2 months old usually has a root that one mowing will not kill. Seedling plants at the end of the first year have well-established underground runners that only grubbing or herbicides will kill. Seedlings are a threat as long as old poison ivy is in the neighborhood.

Plowing is of little value in combating poison ivy and poison oak. Mowing with a scythe or a sickle is not an efficient means of controlling poison ivy and poison oak. It has little effect on the roots unless frequently repeated. Weed burners are also inefficient in controlling poison ivy and poison oak.

Control by Herbicides

Poison ivy and poison oak can be destroyed with herbicides without endangering the operator. One usually may stand at a distance from the plants and apply the herbicide without touching them. Most herbicides are applied as a spray solution by sprayers equipped with nozzles on extensions 2 feet or more in length. The greatest danger of poisoning occurs in careless handling of gloves, shoes, and clothing after work is finished.

The most satisfactory herbicides for control of poison ivy, poison oak, and poison sumac are: 1) amitrole (3-amino-s-triazole); 2) silvex [2-(2,4,5-trichlorophenoxyl) propionic acid]; 3) ammonium sulfamate; and 4) 2,4-D [2, 4(dichlorophenoxy) acetic acid]. These herbicides are sold under their common names and under various trade names.

Any field or garden sprayer, or even a sprinkling can, can be used for applying the spray liquid, but a common compressed-air sprayer holding 2 to 3 gallons is convenient and does not waste the spray.

Use moderate pressure giving relatively large spray droplets, rather than high pressure giving a driving mist, because the object is to wet the leaves of the poison ivy and poison oak and avoid wetting the leaves of desirable plants. High pressures cause formation of many fine droplets that may drift to desirable plants.

Follow the manufacturer's recommendations shown on the container label in preparing the spray solution. Cover all foliage, stems, shoots, and bark of poison plants with herbicide spray. Although best results normally are obtained soon after maximum foliage development in the spring, applications may be made up to 3 weeks before fall frost is normally expected under good growing conditions in humid areas.

Many herbicides used on poison ivy and poison oak will injure most broad-leaved plants. Apply them with caution if the surrounding vegetation is valuable. During the early part of the growing season, the leaves of poisonous plants usually tend to stand conspicuously apart from those of adjacent plants, and they can be treated separately if sprayed with care. Later in the season, the leaves become intermingled, and injury to adjacent species is unavoidable. Chemicals other than oil are not injurious to the thick bark of an old tree, and poison ivy clinging to the trunk safely can be sprayed with them. Cutting the vine at the base of the tree and spraying regrowth, however, may be more practical.

Apply sprays when there is little or no air movement. Early morning or late afternoon, when the air is cool and moist, is usually a favorable time. No method of herbicidal eradication can be depended on to kill all plants in a stand of poison ivy and poison oak with one application. Retreatments made as soon as the new leaves are fully expanded are almost always necessary to destroy plants missed the first time, to treat new growth, and to destroy seedlings. Plants believed dead sometimes revive after many months. An area under treatment must be watched closely for at least a year and retreated where necessary.

Dead foliage and stems remaining after the plants have been killed with herbicides are slightly poisonous. Cut off dead stems and bury or burn them, taking care to keep out of the smoke. (The smoke may carry droplets of the catechols that also may cause the dermatitis.)

Precautions

1. Herbicides used improperly may cause injury to [humans] and animals. Use them only when needed and handle them with care. Follow the directions and heed all precautions on the labels.
2. Keep herbicides in closed, well-labeled containers in a dry place. Store them where they will not contaminate food or feed, and where children and animals cannot reach them.
3. When handling a herbicide, wear clean, dry clothing.
4. Avoid repeated or prolonged contact of herbicides with your skin.
5. Wear protective clothing and equipment if specified on the container label. Avoid prolonged inhalation of herbicide mists.
6. Avoid spilling herbicide concentrate on your skin, and keep it out of your eyes, nose, and mouth. If you spill any on your skin, wash it off immediately with soap and water. If you spill it on your clothing, remove clothing immediately and wash contaminated skin. Launder the clothing before wearing it again.
7. After handling a herbicide, do not eat, drink, or smoke until you have washed your hands and face. Wash any exposed skin immediately after applying a herbicide.
8. Avoid drift of herbicide to nearby crops.
9. To protect water resources, fish, and wildlife, do not contaminate lakes, streams, or ponds with herbicide. Do not clean spraying equipment or dump excess spray material near such water.
10. It is difficult to remove all traces of herbicides from equipment. For this reason, do not use the same equipment for applying herbicides that you use for insecticides and fungicides.
11. Dispose of empty herbicide containers at a sanitary land-fill dump, or crush and bury them at least 18 inches deep in a level, isolated place where they will not contaminate water supplies. If you have a trash-collection service, wrap small containers in heavy layers of newspapers and place them in the trash can.

Plants and Spices

Most of the dermatitis-producing plants belong to a limited number of families, and many of the plant sensitizers that have been isolated also appear to belong to closely related chemicals, such as catechols and lactones.

Many cases of plant dermatitis are occupational. The *Toxicodendron* group (poison ivy, oak, and sumac) produces many instances of both occupational and nonoccupational dermatitis. In Europe, *Primula obconica* (primrose) is the principal cause of nonoccupational plant dermatitis.

SEX DISTRIBUTION OF PLANT DERMATITIS

Even among city dwellers, ragweed dermatitis occurs almost exclusively in men. Primula dermatitis occurs principally in women. *Toxicodendron* reactions occur equally in both sexes and at all ages.

PLANT SENSITIZERS

The most recent development in the study of plant dermatitis has been the isolation of specific chemicals that are the sensitizers. It is hoped that these chemicals will become useful in hyposensitizing procedures.

SESQUITERPENE LACTONES

Mitchell and colleagues[34,35] showed that such lactones are the allergens responsible for allergic contact dermatitis caused by ragweed *(Ambrosia)*, sneezeweed *(Helenium)*, sagebrush, wormwood and mugwort *(Artemisia)*, boneset *(Eupatorium)*, poverty weed *(Franseria)*, marsh elder *(Iva)*, cocklebur *(Xanthium)*, burdock *(Arctium)*, chamomile *(Anthemis)*, artichoke *(Cynara)*, gaillardia, and chrysanthemum species (tansy, feverfew, and pyrethrum).

The presence of an alpha-methylene group exocyclic to the gamma-lactone appears to be the immunochemical requisite for such dermatitis. For patch test purposes, Mitchell and Dupuis[34] used alantolactone 0.25% in petrolatum.

A major allergen in airborne and occupational contact dermatitis from Compositae is parthenolide, which is the main sesquiterpene lactone in feverfew and tansy, according to Hausen.[36] Parthenolide is water soluble. In fact, one-third of the allergen extractable with chloroform can actually be removed with water alone. Parthenolide may make up 0.3% to 1% of tansy and feverfew, respectively, and is found in 12 other Compositae and Magnoliaceae species.[36]

Compositae dermatitis presents a pattern on exposed surface mimicking either a photodermatitis or windblown distribution, but when carefully studied, hand eczema was more common than these more widespread patterns.[37]

Because more than 1,350 sesquiterpene lactones have been identified so far, no ideal substance has been found for fool-proof patch testing. A 1% costus oil in petrolatum test was used in a study of 740 patients, and 1.5% of patients (13) were found sensitive.[37] Nine of the 11 patients had hand eczema. Mixtures of sesquiterpene lactones have been evaluated in an attempt to provide an improved screening tool. About 1.5% of patients undergoing diagnostic patch testing were found to be positive to a 0.1% petrolatum mix of equimolar amounts of alantolactone, costunolide, and dihydrocostus lactone.[38] Of the positive reactions, 41% were deemed relevant to the dermatitis evaluation.

A similar study found a Compositae mix to give reactions in 124 of 3,489 patients. About half were sensitive to yarrow, and none were photoaggravated.[39] The airborne nature of the clinical presentation was believed to be caused by an increase in allergen concentration as the plants withered.

Lovell and Rowan[40] concluded that shortcomings of any mix attempting to cover so many possible allergens can be anticipated. The commercial sesquiterpene lactone mix failed to detect five of seven patients sensitive to

Taraxacum officinale, a dandelion in the chrysanthemum family. A 3:1 chloroform/methanol extract in petrolatum at 1% concentration was positive from the leaf, flower, and root.[40] The possibility of crossreactions further confuses some of the investigations of plant contact dermatitis. A crossreaction occurs between marigolds *(Tagetes)* and the Compositae plant *Arnica* and other sesquiterpene-lactone-containing species, even though the genus *Tagetes* is not known to produce sesquiterpene lactone, but rather thiopene compounds.[41]

When patients report summer-exacerbated dermatitis, suspect (a) sensitivity to flowers or plants, (b) sensitivity to pollen (especially in atopic individuals or, (c) photosensitivity, but keep in mind that half of patients sensitive to Compositae plant extracts are not photosensitive.[42]

Similar lactones have been implicated as the sensitizers in *Frullania*, a genus of liverworts. Like ragweed dermatitis, many cases of Frullania dermatitis occur in males. Mitchell[43] also reported that dermatitis may be due to usnic acid, which is derived from lichens. Such dermatitis occurred only during work in forest areas and was worse during wet weather. These cases may represent multiple sensitization to usnic acid, lichen chemicals, and lactones.

Calnan[44] reported two patients who developed allergic contact dermatitis from incense cedar wood *(Libocedrus decurrens)* used in pencils. The allergen was thymoquinone. Calnan stated that there are at least eight different cedar woods belonging to several species, and that the terms "cedar wood dermatitis" and "cedar poisoning" are inaccurate.

Various other plants, including trees, grasses, flowers, vegetables, fruits, and weeds, as well as airborne pollens, can produce contact dermatitis. The term "phytodermatitis" is usually applied in such cases.

Most cases of plant dermatitis are the result of allergic hypersensitivity, which is dependent on immunologic changes induced by previous contact with the same plant or with a closely related species.[45] Certain plants are such potent sensitizers that brief contact is sufficient to produce sensitization in a considerable proportion of those exposed. This is true for poison ivy. Sensitivity may develop within 7 to 10 days of first contact or only after many years of exposure. No plant can be dismissed as a cause of dermatitis solely because the patient has handled it for a long time with impunity.[46]

Other plants that are fairly common sensitizers include the following:

Family Compositae. The members of this family that are sensitizers include chrysanthemums and daisies.
Family Ambrosia. These include both giant and dwarf ragweed.

Family Liliaceae. This group consists of the tulip, hyacinth, and asparagus.[47] *Family Alleaceae.* Garlic and onion.

Family Amaryllidaceae. Includes the daffodil and narcissus.*Family Umbelliferae.* Carrots, celery, and wild parsnips are members of this group.

Family Cannabidaceae. Includes hops.

Family Rutaceae. The sensitizers in this family include the orange, lemon, and grapefruit. *Dictamnus albus* (the gas plant fraxinella, burning bush, or dittany) is a photosensitizer.

Plant Sensitizers

The sensitizing substances of many plants are present mainly in the oleoresin fraction. In a few plants, the allergens are water-soluble glucosides or other aqueous fractions.[48]

OLEORESIN FRACTION

This fraction consists of a mixture of substances, including essential oils, terpenes, resins, phenols, and camphors. The potency and amount of oleoresin increase as the growth of the plant becomes more vigorous. The oleoresin may be present throughout the plant and in the pollen. When the pollen is freely airborne, contact dermatitis occurs without touching the plant. In ragweed dermatitis, the contact is usually from such pollen and from small light fragments of dry dead plant material and detached plant hairs that are blown about as a dust.

ESSENTIAL OIL FRACTION

This fraction of oleoresin contains most of the sensitizing substances identified until now. Essential oils ordinarily occur in localized regions of the plant, for example, predominantly in the flowers (lavender), leaves (eucalyptus), bark (cinnamon), wood (sandalwood), and peel (citrus fruits).

An essential oil is a volatile, nongreasy, nonsaponifying oil with a characteristic odor, which is obtained from plants or plant constituents by distillation. Accidental contact with the oleoresin essential oils may occur when the plant is crushed or bruised. More than five hundred compounds have been identified in essential oils. These compounds may be classified into five main groups:

1. Phenols and aromatic alcohols and aldehydes
2. Terpenes
3. Aliphatic and aromatic esters
4. Substituted benzene hydrocarbons (including the mustard oils)
5. Quinines

Of special interest to the dermatologist are phenols, aromatic alcohols, aldehydes, and terpenes. The phenols include dihydric phenols, plus catechols, resorcinols, and hydroquinones. The catechols and related compounds are the sensitizing substances in the *Toxicodendron* (poison ivy) plants and other members of the Anacardiaceae family, which include the marking nut tree of India, the Japanese lacquer tree, the mango, and the cashew nut.[49]

SUBSTITUTED CATECHOLS

These substances, including eugenol and vanillin, are occasionally sensitizers. Eugenol is used in dentistry and is present in cinnamon oil, oil of cloves, some perfumes and soaps, and bay rum. More complex substituted catechols are now appearing in industry. The *p*-tertiary butyl catechol, for example, is used in duplicating papers, in paint, in rubber manufacture, in the oil industry, and as an oxidation catalyst in the manufacture of polyester and polystyrene resins.

The chemical 2-methoxy-6-*n*-pentyl-*p*-benzoquinone is the major allergen of *Primula* (primrose).[50] Other plants and woods contain allergenic quinones that show cross-sensitivity to primin. This assumption is supported by the finding of a coincidence between positive reaction to *Primula obconica* leaf and Dalbergia wood.

Oranges

This fruit may be treated with ethylene gas and biphenyl, a mold retarder. In addition, the azo dye (Citrus Red No. 2) may be used for the peel of Florida oranges, but not those from California (JC Mitchell, personal communication). This azo dye is a rare sensitizer, which may be tested as 2% in acetone.

The outer layer of orange peel consists of numerous oil-containing cells from which an oil of limonene, other terpenes, linalool, and a resinous residue can be expressed. The natural coloring is mainly hesperidin and carotene. The terpene limonene is probably the principal sensitizer of orange peels.

Patch tests with the orange peel may lead to primary irritant reactions.

Lemons

This fruit may produce dermatitis in sensitized individuals because of lemon oil, which contains terpenes (limonene).[51] Allergic dermatitis may also occur in carpenters from contact with lemon wood and sawdust. In addition, an irritant dermatitis may occur in waiters and bakers from contact with citric acid, which also has been implicated in the production of aphthous ulcers.

Turpentine

Turpentine is extracted from species of pine. The irritant and sensitizing potentials vary from country to country. An individual who is sensitized may show crossreaction with balsam of Peru, benzoin, ragweed oil, chrysanthemum, and pyrethrum. The most commonly used products containing turpentine include varnishes, sealing wax, paint thinners, and dry-cleaning materials. Freshly distilled turpentine is less antigenic than turpentine that has been stored and become oxidized. The principal sensitizer in turpentine is a carene; pinene and limonene (dipentene) may be less potent sensitizers.[52]

TERPENES

These substances are sensitizing agents in dermatitis caused by citrus fruits, celery, and turpentine (Table 21.4). Terpenes or their derivatives are present in other plants, such as chrysanthemums, and plant products, such as resins and balsams.

In discussing the terpenes, D.S. Wilkinson (personal communication) stated that, in addition to carbohydrates, proteins, and glycerides, plants contain oily substances, which are insoluble in water. Many of these essential oils are terpene, but oils of wintergreen, aniseed, and mustard are not.

The true terpenes (e.g., limonene, pinene, and camphene) are hydrocarbons with the molecular formula $C_{10}H_{16}$; their alcohols, aldehydes, ketones, and other related compounds are equally important and widespread (e.g., menthol and camphor).

The function of terpenes in the life of the plant is not known; they may attract or repel insects or may be waste products of metabolism. Their precursors in nature are also unknown, although two possibilities are leucine and certain carbohydrates.

Camphene is solid, but the other true terpenes are liquids, boiling between 155°C and 185°C. They have strong, not unpleasant smells, and are volatile in steam.

Geraniol, $C_{10}H_{17}OH$, is a straight-chain terpene alcohol. It occurs in many Indian grasses and as a glucoside in Pelargonium odorantissimum.

Citral, $C_9H_{15}CHO$, is the aldehyde of lemon grass oil.

Citronellol, $C_{10}H_{19}OH$, is an alcohol in rose oil and geranium oil. It is also a glandular secretion of the alligator.

Linalool, $C_{10}H_{17}OH$, has many botanical sources (e.g., oil of linaloe).

Table 21-4 Sources of Exposure to Turpentine

Polishes: automobile, metal, porcelain and metal, shoe, stove, silver (dip type), wood and furniture

Preservatives: paintbrush, wood

Repellants: bird

Waxes: general purpose, paste

Fertilizers

Cosmetics: liquid soaps, soap powders, bath oils, emollient creams, hair tonics, hand tonics, hand lotions, lilac and lily of the valley perfumes, talcum powders, and suntan preparations

Cleaners: metal, general-purpose industrial soaps

Insecticides: products with pine oil, tree sprays, dairy stock sprays, and preparations for dog and cat fleas and lice, floral garden pests, grubs, mites, moths, thrips, ticks, flies, and aphids

Mange treatment

Deodorizers: cleanser type

Degreasers

Liquid starch

Paints: including anticorrosion paints

Solvents and thinners: for paints, dry cleaners, and waxes

Varnishes, shellacs, and lacquers

Stains and finishes

Terpineol: solvent for resins

Dutch Drops (Haarlem Oil): proprietary remedy for colds and fever

Any cleaning, cosmetic, or painting product having a pine odor

Shoe polish

Eyeglass frames

Substances that may crossreact with turpentine: ragweed, burwood marsh elder, chrysanthemum, and pyrethrum (found in disinfectants, insecticides, fungicides, soil conditioners, wood preservatives, repellents, dog and cat soaps)

Monocyclic terpenes. These compounds always have one ring in the molecular structure.

Myrcene, $C_{10}H_{16}$, is an open-chain hydrocarbon with three double bonds and is found in oil of bay and oil of hops.

(+) *Limonene* is found in lemon oil, oil of neroli, dill and bergamot, oil in orange peel, caraway oil, and celery seed oil.

(2) *Limonene* is found in spearmint and pine needles. Dipentene is a form of limonene.

Cineole occurs in wormseed oil, cajeput oil, eucalyptus oil, and rosemary.

Phellandrene occurs in elemi oil, ginger grass oil, oil of cinnamon, and bitter fennel oil.

(2) *Phellandrene* occurs in eucalyptus oils, pimento oils, Canada balsam oil, and Japanese peppermint oil.

(+) *Phellandrene* occurs in fennel oil, and lemon oil.

Carvone, $C_{10}H_{14}O$, is a constituent of dill and caraway oils.

(2) *Menthone,* $C_{10}H_{18}$, which occurs in oil of peppermint, is a liquid.

(2) *Menthol,* $C_{10}H_{19}OH$, occurs in peppermint oils and Japanese mint oil.

Dicyclic terpenes. These compounds, $C_{10}H_{16}$, always have one six-membered ring, a second closed chain, and one olefinic link.

Alpha-pinene is the principal constituent of oil of turpentine, which is obtained from members of the order Coniferae.

(+) *Camphor,* $C_{10}H_{16}O$, occurs in the camphor laurel and in feverfew oil.

Camphene occurs widely in nature, particularly the (2) form, which is found in the oil of *Abies sibirica.*

Borneol, $C_{10}H_{17}OH$, occurs in many oils, such as pine oil. Wilkinson (personal communication) states that the terpene-free diet shown in Table 21.5 may, on occasion, be useful for trial on patients who are allergic to flavors and perfumes.

Resins and Balsams

Resins and balsams are plant products that may be sensitizers. Balsams are similar to resins but are pathologic secretions after injury to the plant. Resins are acidic substances occurring either as amorphous vitreous solids or as solutions in essential oils. Some are phenolic derivatives, but others are polymerization and oxidation products of terpenes. The residue remaining after distillation of crude oil of turpentine is rosin or colophony, which consists mainly of abietic acid and pimaric acids. Some resins are plant exudations containing mixtures of true gums, oils, and resin.

Table 21-5 Terpene-Free Diet

No oils of:
Lemon, spearmint, rosemary, cinnamon, bitter fennel, pimento, peppermint, camphor, eucalyptus, orange, caraway, dill, and red palm—or any foods or condiments containing them (e.g., fruit drinks, boiled sweets, flavorings, or colorings)

No red or yellow fruits:
Including apples, apricots, bananas, blackberries, cherries, gooseberries, oranges, pears, peaches, plums, pineapples, prunes, raspberries, and strawberries

Fruits allowed:
Currants, damsons, figs, grapefruit, white grapes, white melon, raisins, sultanas, and nuts

No green, leafy vegetables:
Including asparagus, broccoli, cabbage, brussels sprouts, carrots, French beans, runner beans, cauliflower, endive, leeks, lettuce, mint, parsley, peas, spinach, and tomatoes

Vegetables allowed:
Artichokes, broad beans, butter beans, beetroot, celery, cucumber, horse radish, lentils, marrow, onions, parsnips, split dried peas, potatoes, shallots, rutabaga, and radishes

Foods to avoid:
Liver, kidneys, and heart
Fatty fish (e.g., herring, kippers, salmon, sardines, and oysters)
Dairy products, including milk, butter, margarine, cheese, egg yolks, and cream
Avoid any foods containing them (e.g., cakes, sweets, and puddings)

Foods allowed:
Skimmed milk
Egg white
Vegetable oils
Bacon, pork, beef, mutton, and poultry
White fish
All cereals, including wheat, rye, macaroni, rice, and semolina
Sugars, jams, honey, and syrups
Tea, coffee, rose hip syrup, and ribena
Beers, ciders, wines, and spirits

BALSAM OF PERU

The term "balsam of Peru," a viscid fluid with an odor recalling cinnamon and vanilla, is a misnomer. Hjorth[53] in his fine monograph, *Eczematous Allergy to Balsams,* points out that the balsam comes almost exclusively from El Salvador. The balsam is not found preformed in the wood of the tree *(Myroxylon balsamum)* from which it is obtained, but it is produced by inflicting wounds on the tree's bark. The balsam then exudes out as a sort of granulation tissue to heal the bark's lesions and is used subsequently in many ways.

Hjorth[53] stated that approximately two-thirds of Peruvian balsam comprise the volatile oil cinnamein, which contains the following chemicals: cinnamic acid, cinnamic aldehyde, cinnamic alcohol, methyl cinnamate, benzyl cinnamate, vanillin, and eugenol.

The remaining one-third consists of polymers of esters of coniferyl alcohol with benzoic acid and cinnamic acid that may prove to be the major allergens of balsam of Peru.

The following food items and other products may contain balsams (NK Veien, personal communication):

Products that contain the peel of citrus fruits (oranges, lemons, grapefruits, bitter oranges, tangerines, and mandarin oranges), e.g., marmalade, juice, and bakery goods.

Flavoring agents, such as those found in Danish pastries and other bakery goods, candy, and chewing gum

Perfumed products, such as perfumed tea and tobacco
Certain cough medicines and lozenges
Eugenol used by dentists
Suppositories containing balsam of Peru
Ice cream
Cola and other spiced soft drinks

Spices such as cinnamon, cloves, vanilla, and curry. These spices are used in such products as ketchup, chili sauce, chutney, spiced herring, pickled vegetables like beets and cucumbers, highly spiced bakery goods, liver paste, vermouth, and various other bitter, spiced drinks.

The following compounds often show crossreactions with balsam of Peru: cinnamon, clove, orange peel, benzoin, rosin, vanilla, cinnamic aldehyde and alcohol, cinnamates, benzyl benzoate, benzyl salicylate and alcohol, eugenol, and various perfumes.[53]

CHRISM

Chrism is a consecrated oil used by certain churches in various rites, such as baptism. Such aromatic oil may contain or crossreact with balsam of Peru.

Many patients with allergic perfume sensitivity show strong patch test reactions to balsam of Peru.

Many topical medications and sunscreens contain balsam of Peru (see Chapter 10).

ALLERGIC REACTION TO CERTAIN FLAVORING AGENTS

Cinnamon oil is used for flavoring foods, cakes, toothpaste, chewing gum, tobacco, vermouth, aperitifs, bitters, and beverages of the cola type. Cassia is a Chinese cinnamon. The ingestion of cinnamon oil may produce an eczematous contact–type flare-up in individuals previously sensitized by contact with the oil. Fisher[54] observed a balsam of Peru–sensitive patient, sensitized to a cinnamon in a toothpaste, whose dermatitis flared after drinking vermouth containing cinnamon.

Hjorth[55] reported two children who were sensitive to balsam of Peru and orange peel and whose eczema flared after eating fruits and ices. Hjorth also described a man with a severe hand eczema who was allergic to balsam of Peru and whose eczema flared when he ate a jar of

orange marmalade. The patient then avoided perfumes, cola drinks, vermouth, throat tablets, and cinnamon, and his hand eczema cleared up.

Pirila[56] reported that eating vanilla sugar caused a flare of eczema in a patient sensitive to balsam of Peru. Thus, dermatitis due to sensitization to balsam of Peru may flare with ingestion of cinnamon, oranges, and other flavors. A low-balsam diet has produced long-term benefit in 47% of patients, but a positive provocation has not proved to be predictive of those who will derive benefit.[57]

RESORCINOL MONOBENZOATE, STEERING WHEELS, AND BALSAM OF PERU

Jordan[58] reported: "Resorcinol monobenzoate (RMB) has... been described as a cause of allergic contact dermatitis in seven patients who had been in close contact with cellulose ester plastics." A 69-year-old man with an intractable palm eczema was patch test positive to his car steering wheel, RMB, and balsam of Peru. The plastics manufacturer confirmed the existence of RMB in the steering wheel. Steering wheels made of cellulose ester plastic should not contain RMB after 1971.

Jordan and Dahl[59] also reported that plastic sunglasses, hearing aids, and ballpoint pens contain resorcinol monobenzoate as an ultraviolet stabilizer or inhibitor and may produce allergic contact dermatitis in balsam of Peru–sensitive individuals. Thus, resorcinol monobenzoate allergy should be considered when a candidate for plastic dermatitis reacts to balsam of Peru. To date, six RMB-sensitive patients have reacted to balsam of Peru.

COLOPHONY (ROSIN)

The sap tapped from pine trees is referred to as gum rosin, whereas wood rosin refers to rosin extracted from pine stumps or wood. The more liquid tall oil rosin is a by-product of the pulp industry.[60] Gum rosin is mostly abietic acid. Modified rosin is usually treated with maleic anhydride or fumeric acid with the subsequent product used as paper size. The modified rosin esters are used as printing ink, varnish, or adhesives. The major allergen in the modified rosin has been reported to be maleopimaric acid.[60]

Mitchell and Rook[61] found that the constituents of rosin are about 90% resin acids and 10% neutral matter. Of the resin acids, about 90% are isomeric with abietic acid $(C_{20}H_{30}O_2)$; the other 10% is a mixture of dihydroabietic acid $(C_{20}H_{32}O_2)$ and dehydroabietic acid $(C_{20}H_{28}O_2)$. Malten and colleagues[62] found that rosin is a mixture of certain resin acids, namely, abietic acid and its isomers; neoabietic acid, palustric acid, pimaric acid, and levopimaric acid.

Ehrin and Karlberg[63] concur that 90% of colophony is resin and found 30% to 50% of the resin to be abietic acid, which, along with dihydroabietic acid, has been linked to allergy. Pimaric acids in colophony appear to be nonallergenic. The importance of colophony as an allergen is its widespread use, with 1.2 million tons produced in 1988. Of this production, 66% was used for paper, adhesives, and printing inks. The rosin content of most paper is 0.1% to 0.2% of the weight, whereas rosin core solder is 15% to 20% rosin, and tall oil is 2% to 20% rosin. Soluble cutting oils tend to be 15% to 20% tall oil or 0.4% to 4.0% rosin.[63]

Rosin may be combined with glycerin or alcohol to form emulsions of acid ester gums that may be used as fabric finishers and can produce allergic contact dermatitis when sensitized persons come in contact with the clothing.

Exposure to and Dermatitis from Rosin (Colophony)

There are many opportunities for a person to become exposed to rosin and in some cases sensitized to it. The North American Contact Dermatitis Group lists over three hundred products that contain rosin (Table 21.6).

Agrup[64] found that dermatitis due to adhesive tape, furniture polish, and sawdust was often caused by sensitivity to rosin. Kirk[65] reported a case of "colophony collar dermatitis," whereas Fregert[66] found that colophony in cutting oil and in soap water used as cutting fluid produced allergic dermatitis in certain workers. Adams[67] reported that rosin could be an industrial cause of contact dermatitis, and Wilkinson and Calnan[68] cited a patient with allergic reactions to rosin used for a belt-driven machine. Perioral lip lickers–like dermatitis has also been traced to colophony in chewing gum.[69]

Relationship of Abietic Acid to Rosin (Colophony)

Abietic acid is a principal sensitizer in rosin. During a 6-month period, Wahlberg[70] found 15 patients who were allergic to rosin; of these 15, 6 were also allergic to abietic acid.

Cronin and Calnan[71] found a patient who was allergic to hydroabietic alcohol (Abitol) in adhesive tape but not to abietic acid or rosin. Dooms-Goossens and colleagues[72] reported on a woman with mascara dermatitis who was allergic to both dihydroabietyl alcohol (as Abitol is known in Europe), present in mascara, and hypoallergenic adhesive tape containing methyl abietate. Results also indicated that colophony crossreacted with abietic

acid. Because Abitol is produced from abietic acid and other rosin acids, it would be expected that crossreactions could occur readily between Abitol and abietic acid.

Rapaport,[73] reviewing sensitization to Abitol, stated: Abitol is a colorless, tacky balsamic resin. It is a high moleculate primary monohydric alcohol derived from rosin acids that have been hydrogenated to reduce unsaturation. It has a high refractive index, excellent color, low odor, good adhesion, and resistance to oxidation. Typically, Abitol has found wide application with natural and synthetic rubber, nitrocellulose, and other polymers as a plasticizer and with emulsions, solvents, and hot-melt adhesives as a tackifier. Toxicologic data have shown Abitol to be safe. It was tested many years ago by a modified Schwartz technique and showed little irritation. It was interpreted as a nonsensitizer from data at that time (p. 137).

Rasmussen and Fisher[74] described salicylic acid plaster dermatitis from rosin. Fisher[75] reported contact dermatitis in a violinist from rosin. Solder flux, newsprint paper, and sandcores have produced rosin dermatitis.[76–78]

Dermatitis Due to Plant Oleoresins, Including Pollen

Dermatitis from plant pollens, particularly that of ragweed, is a fairly common cause of plant dermatitis. The shell of the pollen grain contains the allergen, a resin-like material. Reactions occur mostly in farmers, gardeners, carpenters, salespeople, harvesters, and others who work outdoors and have prolonged contact with pollen-bearing plants.

The typical seasonal appearance is often masked because of the secondary lichenification and infection, which prolong the duration beyond the pollen seasons. In persons who have the dermatitis throughout the year, however, a careful history reveals that exacerbations occur during the pollen seasons. Often such cases masquerade as neurodermatitis.

The principal sites of pollen dermatitis are the exposed surfaces, namely, the face, neck, V area of the chest, arms, and legs. This pattern is always suggestive of an airborne dermatitis. Pollen dermatitis is usually subacute, but vesiculation may be found on the areas where pollen grains have adhered. The diffuse and even distribution of the eruption is attributed to the coalescing of minute individual papules produced by the grains of pollen.

Aside from the oleoresin, an aqueous protein fraction in pollen may produce asthma, hay fever, and occasionally atopic dermatitis. Rarely is there both an immediate

Table 21-6 Exposure to Rosin (Colophony)

Adhesives, adhesive plasters, and tapes

Asphaltic products, emulsions, and foundry supplies

Caulking compounds

Cements (linoleum, rubber, shoe, thermoplastic tile, lens-coating), cement agents

Chewing gum

Cleaners for leather and office machines, and grease remover for clothes

Corrosion inhibitors (automobile cooling systems, brake-shoe lining)

Cosmetics (brilliantine, depilatories of wax, eyeshadow, mascara, rouge, hair pomade, nail varnish)

Disinfectants and insecticides

Fillers (putty, wood dough)

Fireworks

Glues

Grease and lubricant thickener, axle grease, and greases

Insulating tapes (less frequent)

Jointing tapes

Linoleum, floor coverings, and floor tiles: adhesive bedding, cement

Insulations, electrical and thermal

Match tips

Medicaments (human and veterinary)

Modeling clay

Ostomy appliances

Paints: oleoresinous, anticorrosion, antifouling, house paint and enamel, finishes, varnishes (metallic drier, paint drier, emulsifiers)

Paper: Paper can be coated with rosin size. Rosin is added to paper to increase its water resistance, to prevent feathering or spreading of ink. Protective coating for glossy paper, price labels, plastics, and stickers. Rosin is applied as a finishing film to protect print on paper and as a surface coating for price labels. Ink can contain rosin derivatives (ceramic, marking, mimeograph, printing inks). Water-fast colors in artists' pens. Photographic paper. One of the largest single uses of colophony is in the sizing of paper and paperboard. Small quantities of resin acids can be transferred from paper to articles packed in it (e.g., food substances).

Polish (floor, furniture, metal, shoe, car)

Polythene (polyethylene)

Rosins and derivatives: gum rosin, wood rosin, rosin oil, tall oil (rosinol, retinol abitol), and ester gums. Resins (alkyd, synthetic ester, metals, phenolic resin modifier). Epoxy resins

Sawdust and resin of pine and spruce

Sealants and wood swellers

Shoes and clothing

Soaps: Brown soap, clear (transparent) soap, yellow soap, soap water used with cutting oil, yellow (soft) laundry bar soap. Rosin makes laundry bars more soluble and hastens sudsing in cool water

Soldering fluxes and soldering agents

Solvents

Stains

Surface coatings (lager beer casks, rust-proof coatings, coatings for price labels, can labels), polish for roasted coffee beans

Tacky substances—to prevent slipping

  Athletic grip aids

  Carpentry nails, rosin applied with tar

  Drive belts and clutches in automobile industry and engineering

  Grafting wax for trees

  Machine belts in industry

Table 21-6 (Cont.) Exposure to Rosin (Colophony)

Nonslip applications

Postage stamp glue

Powdered rosin as an application to belts on machinery to prevent slipping

Rosin bag for baseball players

Sticky flypaper

Handles for sports (golf club, tennis racket, etc.)

Rosin applied to bows of stringed musical instruments and to dancers' shoes

Rosin for wrestlers, gymnasts, ballplayers, and bowlers

Mixed with rubber (e.g., in car tires). Rubber-compounding aids, reclaiming agents, and emulsifying agents in producing synthetic rubber

Rosin used on floors to prevent slipping

Rosin is not infrequently used as an adulterant of other resinous products. Traces of turpentine may be present in gum rosin. Evidence for cross-sensitivity between colophony (rosin) and balsam of Peru is scanty

Tall oils, cutting oils, and core oils

Varnishes: Rosin reacts with maleic anhydride to produce adducts known as maleic resins

These are used extensively in oil and spirit varnishes and lacquers

Water-proofing agents (cardboard, walls) and oilcloth

Wax: sealing, shoemaker, tree wax, and grafting wax. Wax modification. Car, floor furniture wax and polish.

Physiotherapy wax (contaminated)

Zein compositions

urticarial sensitivity reaction (due to the protein fraction) and a delayed eczematous sensitivity reaction (due to oleoresin) to the pollen. In some patients, exacerbations of atopic dermatitis in the summer, aside from those due to humidity and sweating, are thought to be caused by inhalation of plant pollens.

Airborne pollen dermatitis with marked involvement of the exposed areas may resemble a photosensitivity dermatitis due to plants, drugs, or topical substances. Lesions on exposed areas due to simple pollen dermatitis, without photosensitivity, are not usually as sharply demarcated from normal skin as in the case of a photosensitizing dermatitis, because the pollen grains often get inside the collar and extend the dermatitis to the upper part of the chest and shoulders. Similarly, pollen grains may get inside trousers and affect the legs and even the inguinal area and genitals. Such involvement under the clothes may help differentiate simple pollen dermatitis from photosensitivity reactions. It must be remembered, however, that certain pollens, particularly ragweed, are photosensitizers as well as causes of dermatitis venenata.

RAGWEED OIL DERMATITIS

The oleoresin that produces ragweed dermatitis is present in the pollen and the stem and leaf of the plant. Ragweed pollen has two chief components: an inner core containing the water-soluble protein fraction, which may

Table 21-7 Compositae Dermatitis Synonyms
Australian bush dermatitis
Chrysanthemum dermatitis
Compositae dermatitis/airborne contact
Parthenium dermatitis
Pollen dermatitis
Ragweed (oil) dermatitis
Sesquiterpene lactone dermatitis
Sesquiterpenoid dermatitis
Weed dermatitis

Table 21-8 Some Plants Known to Contain Sesquiterpene Lactones

Common name	Genus
Arnica	Arnica
Artichoke, globe	Cynara
Artichoke, wild	Olearia
Bitterweed	Helenium
Boneset	Eupatorium
Broomweed	Amphiachyris
Burdock	Arctium
Bursage	Ambrosia
Burrobrush	Hymenoclea
Capeweed	Cryptostemma
Chamomile, German	Matricaria
Chamomile, Roman	Anthemis
Champaca of perfumery	Michelia[a]
Chicory	Cichorium
Chrysanthemum	Chrysanthemum
Cocklebur	Xanthium
Cosmos	Cosmos
Costus of perfumery	Saussurea
Cottonthistle	Onopordon
Encelia	Encelia
Feverfew	Parthenium
Fireweed	Gaillardia
Fleabane	Erigeron
Guayule	Parthenium
Hempweed	Mikania
Ironweed	Veronia
Laurel oil	Laurus
Leafcup	Polymnia
Lettuce	Lactuca
Liverwort	Frullania
Marguerite	Chrysanthemum
Marigold	Calendula
Marsh elder	Iva
Oxeye	Telekia
Pyrethrum	Chrysanthemum
Ragweed	Ambrosia
Sagebrush	Artemisia
Sneezeweed	Helenium
Sowthistle	Sonchus
Starthistle	Centaurea
Stinkwort	Inula
Sunflower	Helianthus
Tansy	Tanacetum
Tulip tree	Liriodendrona
Whitewood of commerce	Liriodendrona
Wormwood	Artemisia
Yarrow	Achillea

[a]Not a member of the Compositae family.

produce allergic rhinitis or asthma, and an outer portion, which is waxy and can produce allergic contact dermatitis in the sensitized individual at the time of ragweed pollination.[79] The sesquiterpene lactone parthenin is oil-soluble and has been detected in the waxy coat of the allergenic plant *Parthenium hysterophorus*. Ragweed oil dermatitis and ragweed hay fever are unrelated entities caused by different antigens of the ragweed plant. Most individuals with ragweed oil dermatitis are *not* atopic and do *not* have ragweed rhinitis or asthma.

Sensitized individuals may acquire dermatitis also by contact with the stem or leaves of the ragweed plant in the spring or summer, even before pollination takes place. In most instances, however, ragweed oil dermatitis is due to contact with airborne pollen when the plant is at maximal growth and its oleoresin is most concentrated.[80,81]

Dermatitis due to airborne pollen is seasonal, lasting initially from August to the first frost. As the patient advances in age and as the seasonal exposures continue, the dermatitis may begin in June and extend to December.

The early, uncomplicated case usually involves the face, particularly the eyelids, the sides of the neck, the sternal area, and the extensor region of the arms. The dermatitis is often sharply limited by a protective undershirt. In chronic cases, it may extend to involve the trunk, groin, and lower extremities and become so widespread that it resembles a generalized erythroderma. Spontaneous remissions of ragweed oil dermatitis are rare, but even the untreated patient may show variations in severity.

The patient who is sensitive to ragweed oil may have associated allergic contact hypersensitivity to pyrethrum, chrysanthemum, and turpentine.[81] Synonyms for Compositae dermatitis are shown in Table 21.7. Some of the numerous members of the Compositae family are shown in Table 21.8.

COMPOSITAE FAMILY

Sesquiterpene lactones present in the oil-soluble plant oleoresin are responsible for allergic dermatitis caused by these plants. The presence of an alpha-methylene group exocylic to the gamma-lactone appears to be the immunochemical requisite for such dermatitis. A screening test for Compositae with 0.1% sesquiterpene lactone mix has been evaluated against individual Compositae oleoresins. The mix identified only 35% of the cases. The mix is considered an inadequate screening tool based on these results.[82]

This family of plants includes ragweed (*Ambrosia*), sneezeweed and bitterweed (*Helenium*), sagebrush, wormwood, mugwort (*Artemisia*), boneset (*Eupatorium*), poverty weed (*Franseria*), marsh elder (*Iva*), cocklebur (*Xanthium*), burdock (*Arctium*), chamomile (*Anthemis*), artichoke (*Cynara*), gaillardia, chrysanthemum, tansy (*Tanacetum*), feverfew (*Chrysanthemum parthenium*), pyrethrum (*Chrysanthemum species*), and broomweed (*Amphiachyris dracunculoides*).

Ragweeds of the plant genus Ambrosia have water-soluble antigens, which release IgE from the basophils and mast cells of the nose, producing hay fever: This is a Type 1 reaction. The same plant, ragweed, may produce contact dermatitis through a Type 4 reaction to one of the several lipid-soluble antigens, among which are the sesquiterpene lactones. Thus, ragweed possesses several different antigens that can cause different types of hypersensitivity responses.

Ragweed and parthenium dermatitis occur almost exclusively in adult men. Children and women seem to be immune. Oral hyposensitization in cases of Compositae allergic contact dermatitis cannot be recommended with complete confidence, but may be somewhat helpful.[80] Airborne contact dermatitis from Compositae oleoresin simulating photodermatitis has been reported from the United States, India, Australia, United Kingdom, and most recently from Scandinavian countries.[34]

Ragweed dermatitis appears initially in the fall and clears after the first frost, but untreated cases may become perennial. Crossreactions between Compositae species are often observed, owing to some 3,500 crossreacting allergenic sesquiterpene lactones distributed in this family.

Airborne contact dermatitis from triangle-leaf bursage (*Ambrosia deltoidea*) is seen in the desert southwest of the United States. Patch test with the leaves was positive, and air samples collected onto Teflon filter from air outside the patient's home in one case proved both the specific source and general environmental exposure responsible for the eruption. Similar air samples from inside the home were negative.[83]

Airborne contact dermatitis to feverfew (*Tanacetum parthenium*) had been considered to be due to airborne release of the plant's sesquiterpene lactones. However, it was learned that the volatile material released is not sesquiterpene lactone but rather monoterpenes. In a study of 17 patients who reacted to feverfew and parthenolide, participants were challenged with monoterpenes, and 13 had positive or doubtful positive reactions to one

or more monterpene. This provides another explanation for airborne dermatitis from feverfew. Dried plant parts might provide another way for the sesquiterpene lactone in the plant to become airborne and cause dermatitis, but direct evidence for this was lacking.[84]

It was thought originally that Compositae dermatitis was not present in Europe. Hjorth and colleagues,[81] however, reported a series of Danish patients who had been treated for 1 to 50 years for photodermatitis (or in one instance of actinic reticuloid), all of whom turned out to be strongly positive to oleoresin from several Compositae species.

CAN RAGWEED DERMATITIS BE AIRBORNE?

After Fisher studied 18 male New Yorkers who were not farmers and had not been exposed to ragweed plants, he became convinced that ragweed dermatitis can be airborne from pollen containing the oleoresin.

Howell[85] stated, however, that he could not produce dermatitis by blowing ragweed onto the moistened skin of patients with ragweed dermatitis.

Grater[86] stated, "Everyone who has made an allergy extract knows that the pollen contains a considerable amount of oleoresins. In the preparation of extracts for pollens, they are defatted with ether, thus the hyposensitization has none of the active principle causing the dermatitis" (p. 159).

Hjorth and colleagues[81] stated flatly that wind-borne plant material is responsible for a true airborne contact etiology. Furthermore, Burry and colleagues,[87] in discussing Compositae dermatitis in Australia, suggested "Australian bush dermatitis" as a suitable name for a chronic dermatitis of exposed areas occurring in men living in the Australian bush. Sensitivity to ragweed revealed by patch testing was common to five patients suffering from the dermatitis, but was thought to be incidental and not clinically relevant. Wind-borne pollens or dust, released during dry summer conditions by other plants of the Compositae family present in the Australian bush, are suggested as probable causes. The incapacitating chronicity of Australian bush dermatitis indicates that dermatologic, botanical, and chemical research into its origins is desirable.

Ragweed dermatitis is not often recognized, usually being misdiagnosed as "photodermatitis" from other causes.[88,89] Coexistence of ultraviolet light sensitivity and Compositae sensitivity does occur, however.[90]

As commercial sesquiterpene lactone patch test mixes have become available, the diagnosis of Compositae dermatitis has been established in 1% to 2% of patients patch tested, with clinical relevance found in about one-half of the positive cases.[38] The trend that has evolved is for hand eczema to be as or more prevalent than photodermatitis or airborne dermatitis. At the European Contact Dermatitis Society meeting in Brussels, October 1992, Ross reported 1.8% of 7,420 patients were allergic to sesquiterpene lactones and about one-third showed an airborne pattern, one-third hand eczema, and one-fifth generalized dermatitis. The remainder had facial dermatitis. Only 22% of the sesquiterpene lactone allergic patients were found photosensitive.[91] At the same meeting, du Peloux Managé reported 9% of these patients who were photosensitive reacted to ultraviolet B (UVB) only, 82% to ultraviolet A (UVA) and UVB, and 8% were sensitive to UVA, UVB, and visible light.[91]

PARTHENIUM DERMATITIS EXPORTED TO INDIA

Parthenium hysterophorus (feverfew, carrot weed), an American weed introduced accidentally to India by a shipment of American wheat, has produced hundreds of cases of severe contact dermatitis in the Poona area, located on the western coast of India near Bombay. In some cases, the dermatitis progressed to a generalized erythroderma with fatal results. The weed has spread to other parts of India and so devastated the countryside that it has been called the "scourge of India."[92]

Parthenium, a member of the Compositae group of plants, which includes tansy and pyrethrum, crossreacts with ragweed *(Ambrosia)*. As in ragweed dermatitis, the contact sensitizer parthenolide is an oil-soluble oleoresin present throughout the plant and pollen. Up to one-third of the oil-soluble fraction can be removed with water alone.[36] In contrast, ragweed and parthenium allergic rhinitis and asthma are due to water-soluble proteins present only in the pollen. Parthenolide makes up 0.3% to 1% of the plant weight and is found in 12 other Compositae species.[36]

The principal source of exposure to parthenium is direct contact with the living plant whose plant hairs (trichomes) contain abundant dermatitis-producing sesquiterpene lactones. The airborne pollen of parthenium, however, also contains the oleoresin, and the resulting contact dermatitis may be entirely "airborne." In addition, the plants crumble during the dry season to a fine dust that is scattered throughout the countryside. This dust is another source of "airborne" contact dermatitis.[93] Because spontaneous cures of parthenium and ragweed dermatitis apparently do not occur, hyposensitization procedures are worthwhile, particularly in those patients who cannot avoid exposure to the plants. An allergenic sesquiterpene lactone, parthenin, has been detected in parthenium pollen.

Features of Parthenium Dermatitis

1. This is the first instance of an "imported" sensitizer causing allergic contact dermatitis in thousands of people.
2. The eruption may become generalized and produce a universal erythroderma that is not amenable to systemic corticosteroids and may be fatal.
3. The only effective treatment presently is to remove the patient from the area in which the weed is growing in India. Because thousands of Indians are affected, such a procedure is not practical.
4. In the southwestern United States, parthenium usually causes only a mild dermatitis, subsiding after the first frost when the plant becomes dormant. Shelmire,[94] however, described a patient in Texas with a generalized parthenium dermatitis who showed a positive patch test reaction to a 1:100,000 parthenium extract. The eruption was recurrent from May to December.
5. In India, parthenium is no longer a rural problem. The weed is extraordinarily prolific and aggressive, growing rapidly all over the city in vacant lots and any open space in cities, on roadsides and paths, and even from crevices in the walls of buildings and houses. In Poona, a city with a population of 1.5 million, a bank manager, an urban physician, and other office workers were affected with dermatitis. The plant in pastureland is harmful to cattle, contaminates milk, and interferes with crops and agricultural food production.
6. The principal sensitizing chemical of parthenium is the sesquiterpene lactone, parthenolide. Patch testing has revealed crossreactions to numerous other plants of the Compositae group and to their sesquiterpene lactones.[36,95]
7. Although Indian authorities claim that no herbicide is effective, Hausen[96] has stated that control of *Parthenium hysterophorus* is possible with Ansar-529, a weed killer containing arsenic.
8. Parthenium dermatitis, like ragweed dermatitis, affects men almost exclusively. The dermatitis is rare in women and does not affect children. About 4% of exposed males acquire parthenium dermatitis.
9. Parthenium dermatitis, like ragweed dermatitis, resembles photodermatitis because skin surfaces not usually covered with clothing are initially involved.

The parthenium oleoresin may contain phototoxic chemicals.[97] Mitchell,[98] in discussing "dermatitis at a distance," states that it is possible that the airborne pollen of parthenium is capable, on phytochemical grounds, of providing allergens for the production of dermatitis. Recently, allergenic oil-soluble sesquiterpene lactones have been detected in the waxy coat of parthenium pollen.

Dr. A. Lonkar (personal communication) wrote:

The treatment of parthenium dermatitis has been frustrating. The systemic as well as topical steroids are of limited value. Prolonged corticosteroid administration has its own hazards. The clue given by the age of the patients, involvements of only postmenopausal women, although rarely, absence of the disease before puberty and activation or increase due to sunlight stimulated me in trying short courses of antimalarials and female hormones. I use Chlorquin 200 mg tid for about 1 week and then taper it off to suit the need. Ethinyl estradiol 0.05 mg at bedtime for about 3 weeks is given to both adult males and females. This combination does seem to modify the course of the disease. I have not advocated this as a standard treatment in parthenium dermatitis, but I feel that it provides a clue in the pathogenesis of the disease.

EFFECT OF PYRETHRIN INSECTICIDES ON RAGWEED-SENSITIVE INDIVIDUALS

Fisher[99] stated that a sharp distinction must be made between pyrethrum and the commercially refined pyrethrin extracts used in insecticides.

It has been known for a long time that insecticidal pyrethrins present in pyrethrum powder are not the cause of respiratory allergy.[100] As far as the dermatitis-producing oleoresin is concerned, Mitchell and colleagues[101] have shown that the oleoresin fraction of ragweed that produces contact dermatitis is a sesquiterpene lactone and that the dermatitis-producing fraction of pyrethrum is pyrethrosin, a sesquiterpene lactone that is not used for insecticidal properties. Furthermore, Head[102] has shown that pyrethrosin is not present in the commercially refined pyrethrin extracts used as insecticides. Hausen and Schulz[103] confirmed Mitchell's observation that the pyrethrins (i.e., constituents with strong insecticidal activity) play no role in chrysanthemum and pyrethrum dermatitis.

In addition, Fisher[2] completed a study of 50 patients with either ragweed dermatitis or ragweed rhinitis or asthma. Twelve of these patients were men with ragweed dermatitis, with a strongly positive patch test reaction to ragweed oleoresin. Thirty-eight patients had ragweed rhinitis or asthma with positive scratch test reactions to the aqueous ragweed fraction. None of these patients showed any patch or scratch test reaction to RID (Pfizer), a pediculicide that contains purified pyrethrins.

One can, therefore, conclude that pyrethrum-derived pyrethrin insecticides are safe for patients with respiratory allergy or dermatitis due to ragweed.

Frullania (Liverworts)

Liverworts of the genus *Frullania* are small, reddish or brownish plants, which frequently grow with mosses and lichens, from which they may be distinguished by their compact ropelike appearance. So-called cedar or hemlock poisoning is a misnomer because the dermatitis is actually caused by liverwort plants growing on the trees and in nearby forests or due to lichens.

Mitchell and colleagues[104] identified *Frullania* (liverwort) as the causative agent of some cases of so-called cedar wood poisoning in the forests of the Pacific Northwest. They demonstrated positive patch tests in addition to several members of the Compositae family or their oleoresin extracts, and deduced that the sesquiterpene lactones were the chemicals common to Compositae and the unrelated *Frullania*. Some of the patients were said to exhibit evidence of photosensitivity. Comparison of the chemical structures of a series of sesquiterpene lactones indicated that the presence of an exocyclic, carbon-to-carbon double bond (methylene) conjugated with the cyclic carbonyl (lactone) was essential for antigenicity.

Storrs and colleagues[105] emphasized the unvarying clinical picture of both Compositae and *Frullania* dermatitis, with the exception that the Frullania reactors by contrast flare in the wet winter in the Pacific Northwest. They suggest that the more water-soluble oleoresin sensitizers may even contaminate rainwater, which might explain slight submental-sparing simulating photodermatitis.

Despite initial clinical impressions, phototesting was negative. The authors drew attention to several positive patch tests to balsam of Peru, turpentine, and colophony, which contain terpenes and might be crossreactive.

Storrs and colleagues[105] stated that many individuals with allergic hypersensitivity to the d-usnic acid in lichens are also allergic to *Frullania*. This is not a true crossreaction, because reactions to d-usnic acid probably represent separate sensitization to lichens rather than a true crossreaction to sesquiterpene lactones. D-usnic acid is not a sesquiterpene lactone, does not occur in *Frullania* or Compositae, and exhibits stereoisomeric specificity in the production of delayed hypersensitivity (only the d- form is active). As a sensitizer, d-usnic acid is not as potent as the sesquiterpenoids. Stereoisomeric specificity was reported for two species of *Frullania*. *F. dilatata* produced the 1 or (-) form of frullanolide, and *F. tamarisci* produced the d- or (+) form. These enantiomers (mirror images) did not crossreact. Routine screening with frullanolide is not recommended, as it may sensitize. It should be used as an "aimed test" when highly likely to be helpful on clinical history.[106]

Allergic contact dermatitis due to *Frullania* and Compositae responds rapidly to withdrawal of the patient from exposure to the causative antigen. Systemic and topical corticosteroids hasten recovery. The only patients who have not had continued problems are those who have changed occupations or retired. In the case of forest workers, this involves total avoidance of tree bark. Fallers, buckers, log truckers, toppers, hook tenders, choker setters, scalers, and timber cruisers are all susceptible. Switching from one to another of these occupations does not benefit the patient; however, because persons who work with debarked trees (sawyers, graders, and finishers) seem to have no difficulty with *Frullania* sensitivity, transfer to one of these jobs can be a suitable alternative to switching industries completely.

Persons sensitive to *Frullania* must also be cautioned to avoid the particular members of the Compositae family to which patch testing has revealed sensitivities. Thus, transfer of a sensitized logger to a ranching position might result in continued dermatitis from tansy or sagebrush. Conversely, a sagebrush-sensitive rancher might have problems as a logger.

Some French investigators[107] have been able to hyposensitize some of their *Frullania*-sensitive patients using repeated biweekly applications of whole *Frullania*. Theoretically, oral hyposensitization with plant extracts could be achieved in a manner similar to that used for the treatment of ragweed or *Toxicodendron* dermatitis. In Oregon, Storrs and colleagues[105] attempted this procedure in four patients, using mixtures of Compositae oleoresins prepared according to the patient's specific sensitivity pattern by Hollister-Stier. Two of these treated patients believed that their summer tansy-related dermatitis was "somewhat better" while taking the oleoresin-filled capsules. An explosive flare of dermatitis occurred in one patient each time he began oral hyposensitization. In the fourth patient, the severe dermatitis never cleared sufficiently to allow therapy without fear of worsening the condition. Oral hyposensitization therapy in cases of Frullania and Compositae allergic contact dermatitis cannot yet be recommended with confidence.

Dermatitis due to Lichens

Lichens, plants composed of fungi living in symbiosis with algae, have caused allergic contact dermatitis in foresters. The specific sensitizing substance is apparently usnic acid, which accumulates in lichenized fungi. It is chemically related to the furocoumarins, but it is apparently not a photosensitizer.

So-called cedar poisoning or wood cutter's eczema may actually be a contact dermatitis due to lichens. The general population may be exposed by burning lichen-infested logs in fireplaces. Lichen mosses used to simulate trees and shrubs are the source of exposure in model railroad operators and architects. Lichens may also be used in making clothing dyes and funeral wreaths. Litmus is derived from lichen pigment. Ointments containing usnic acid are used for treatment of skin infections, particularly in Scandinavia and Germany. Patch tests may be performed with 1% usnic acid in petrolatum.

Salo and colleagues[108] reported the frequency and immunologic background of dermatitis occurring in lichen pickers who were studied in a small community in northern Finland. Thirty of 164 lichen pickers had suffered from dermatitis at least on the fingers and the dorsa of their hands, and many of them also had dermatitis on their forearms and faces. Fifteen were subjected to epicutaneous and photoepicutaneous testing with crushed *Cladonia alpestris* (L.) Rab. and some fractions of it. Allergic contact reactions were seen in nine subjects, three of whom also had positive photoepicutaneous test reactions from lichen allergens. No immediate reactions were seen in scratch or scratch chamber tests with crushed *Cladonia alpestris* or with its alcoholic extract.

Plant Dermatitis due to Mechanical Irritation

Mechanical irritation may be produced by spines, thorns, specialized bristles, and hairs. The large or small wounds produced by such mechanical irritation may be complicated by bacterial or fungal infection, particularly sporotrichosis. Many grasses and cereals, including barley, millet, rice, and bamboo, have sharp trichomes, which may produce urticarial papules in workers handling crops or litter straw. Dogwood has t-shaped hairs, which may produce urticaria when the leaf is rubbed on the skin in the direction of the hairs.

Many European herbs of the borage family are covered with coarse, stiff hairs, which can produce an irritant dermatitis. Certain tropical plants, including palms and cacti, have spicules, which may also produce dermatitis.

The prickly pear cactus has barbs (glochidia), which can enter the skin, producing a dermatitis resembling scabies. Covered parts of the body may be secondarily affected through the transfer of the broken-off barbs from primarily affected sites. In Israel, harvesting the pears of this plant produces an occupational hazard called sabra dermatitis. Mechanical removal of the barbs is difficult. Peeling ointments or salicylic acid plasters may be used to bring about exfoliation of the skin with the embedded barbs.

Primary Irritant Dermatitis due to Plant Chemicals

Chemical irritation may occur from contact with fluids or crystals in specialized hairs or other portions of the plant.

Plants may injure the skin by direct chemical action. No allergic mechanism is involved, and if the degree of exposure is sufficiently great, a reaction is provoked in everyone so exposed. Variation in susceptibility is attributed to anatomic factors, notably, the thickness of the horny layer, and to climatic factors, which favor or impede the penetration of the irritant substances. Primary irritant dermatitis is particularly common in children.

Aside from irritant hairs, many plants contain chemicals that are strong primary irritants. The buttercup is an important irritant plant. It contains an unsaturated lactone, protoanemonin, formed by the breakdown of a glucoside in injured plants. Children chewing the leaves or stems of the injured plants may acquire blisters on the face and around the lips.

Certain members of the daisy family may also produce an irritant bullous eruption when crushed on the skin.

Cactus-like plants (spurges) of South Africa contain a copious milky latex in their stems, which has strong caustic properties. The manchineel tree of the West Indies and certain vegetables, such as tropical gourds and cucumbers, contain a juice that can irritate the skin.

Plants of the mustard and radish family contain the glucoside sinigrin, which is harmless in the dry state, but is converted into the irritant, volatile oil of mustard in the presence of water.

Pineapple juice contains bromelin, a proteolytic enzyme that can cause a primary irritant dermatitis. The enzyme causes separation of the superficial layers of the skin and increases skin and capillary permeability. These effects resemble the mechanical damage produced by needle-shaped calcium oxalate crystals of tulip bulbs. Both the enzyme and the crystals produce itching and increased permeability of capillaries with the formation of wheals, which are suggestive of histamine liberation in the skin.

The tropical plant *Mucuna pruriens* (itch plant) is a member of the bean family. It does not occur in the United States, but it grows wild in all tropical areas. Short, barbed spicules cover its seed pods. The active itch-producing principle of the plant is a proteolytic enzyme named mucunain, which is the principal ingredient of the "itch powder" used by practical jokers.

Sometimes irritant effects give way to more classic delayed reactions. A 9-year-old boy fell into a nettle bush and experienced a 12-hour bout of urticaria, which at 48 hours changed to a vesicular dermatitis.[109]

Table 21.9 summarizes plant irritant dermatitis.

Table 21-9 Irritant Dermatitis Due to Plants

Chemical
1. *Euphorbiaceae*—
   a. *Euphorbia (spurge)*
   b. *Hippomane mancinella* (manchineel tree)
2. *Mucuna pruriens* (cowhage)
   Itch powder
   Proteolytic enzyme
3. Pineapple
   Calcium oxalate and bromelin, a keratolytic enzyme
Mechanical irritant
   a. Opunita family—prickly pear cactus pines (glochidia), produce foreign body granulomas
Pharmacologic
   Nettles (Urticaceae family): 5–hydroxy tryptamine, histamine, acetylcholine

PHYTOPHOTODERMATITIS

Photosensitization contact dermatitis due to plants is caused largely, if not entirely, by photosensitizing compounds related to furocoumarin (psoralens). Some other chemical compounds, such as thiophenes, have so far been reported to induce phototoxicity only in microbial systems.[110] Phytophotodermatitis can be diagnosed usually by the clinical history and characteristic skin lesions that follow exposure to psoralen-containing plants.

Two requisites for the initiation of phytophotodermatitis are contact with a sensitizing furocoumarin in the juice of the plant and subsequent exposure to ultraviolet radiation of wavelengths greater than 320 nm (usually sunlight). All individuals exposed sufficiently to the plant are susceptible, because a phototoxic and not an allergic mechanism is involved.

Table 21.10 shows the differential diagnosis of an allergic contact plant dermatitis (poison ivy) and one due to phytophotodermatitis. Table 21.11 lists plants implicated in causing phytophotodermatitis.

Phytophotodermatitis, evoked by exposure to UVA and a psoralen plant, such as the gas plant or a plant product (such as a bergamot orange oil in perfume), is a cutaneous phototoxic reaction. First exposure can result in redness, burning pain, and blistering of the skin that appears at about 48 hours; the reaction is confined to the initial sites of contact. Hyperpigmentation, which can result, even without obvious dermatitis, often persists for months.

Meadow grass dermatitis (dermatitis bullosa striata pratensis) is a phototoxic eruption produced by contact with wild parsnip and other vegetation and exposure to sunshine. A network of crisscross, striate bullae, resembling poison ivy dermatitis, is produced. The lesions develop 12 to 24 hours after the plants have been crushed

Table 21-10 Clinical Features of Poison Ivy-Oak (Toxicodendron) Dermatitis and of Phytophotodermatitis of Plants with Psoralens

Disorder	Onset	Mechanism	Symptoms	Course
Poison ivy dermatitis	First exposure can result in sensitization and dermatitis after 5 or more days; on reexposure, dermatitis appears within 48 hours, often within 12 hours	Contact allergic	Itching	Fresh disseminated lesions often appear during 1 week after exposure
Phytophotodermatitis	First exposure can result in redness and blistering of the skin, which appears at about 48 hours; on reexposure, the reaction time is about 48 hours	Phototoxic	Burning pain	Reaction is confined to initial sites of contact

on the skin and there has been subsequent exposure to sunlight. If the skin is moist, the photodynamic effect is enhanced. The bullae soon heal, leaving marked pigmentation, which may persist for many months.

Table 21-11 Common Plants Implicated in Causing Phytophotodermatitis

Common name	Botanical name	Family
Angelica	Angelica archangelica	Umbelliferae
Bergamot	Citrus bergamia	Rutaceae
Bitter orange	Citrus aurantium	Rutaceae
Celery	Apium graveolens	Umbelliferae
Citron	Citrus medica (C. acida)	
Cow parsley	Heracleum sphondylium	Umbelliferae
Cow parsley, wild chervil	Anthriscus sylvestris	Umbelliferae
Dill	Anethum graveolens	Umbelliferae
	Peucedanum oreoselinum	Umbelliferae
Fennel	Foeniculum vulgare	Umbelliferae
Figs	Ficus carica	Moraceae
Gas plant, burning bush	Dictamnus albus (D. fraxinella)	Rutaceae
Giant hogweed	Heracleum mantegazzianum	Umbelliferae
	H. maximum	Umbelliferae
	(H. dulce)	
Lemon	Citrus limon	Rutaceae
Lime	Citrus aurantifolia	Rutaceae
Lovage	Levisticum officinale	Umbelliferae
Masterwort	Peucedanum ostruthium	Umbilliferae
	Ammi majus	Umbelliferae
Parsnip (garden variety)	Pastinaca sativa (P. urens)	Umbelliferae
Parsnip (wild parsnip)	Heracleum giganteum	Umbelliferae
Persian lime	Citrus aurantifolia	Rutaceae
(Tahitian)	"Persian"	Rutaceae
Rue	Ruta graveolens	
Wild carrot, garden carrot	Daucus carota	Umbelliferae

Furocoumarins continue to be identified in a variety of plants including lovage, which is an herb that contains 0.64 mg/g of psoralen and caused phytophotodermatitis in a woman harvesting it.[111] Celery that has been rendered most resistant to fungal contamination ironically contains psoralens that caused phytophotodermatitis in grocery store clerks.[107] Celery normally contains psoralen precursors. Under attack by fungus, celery produces psoralen as a defensive mechanism. Fungus-infected celery (pink rot) causes blisters on the hands of harvesters in sunlight. Botanists have produced strains of celery that contain psoralens and are therefore resistant to pink rot. Psoralen-containing strains of celery produce hyperpigmentation of the forearms of produce workers. Picking the leaves and flowers of *Ruta corsica* can produce phytophotodermatitis.[112]

Primula dermatitis is not usually a photodermatitis, but one case has been reported in which 5.9 J of UVA caused a positive patch test to 0.01% primin in petrolatum, whereas the unirradiated test was negative[113] (see also Chapter 22).

Pseudophytodermatitis

Pseudophytodermatitis is an eruption that appears to be due to plants, but in reality is produced by arthropods infesting the plants or by dyes and waxes applied to the skin of citrus fruits and plant insecticides.

PSEUDOPHYTODERMATITIS DUE TO MITES

Grain Itch Mites

Pediculoides ventricosus, the North American itch mite, feeds on various insect larvae that infest wheat, barley, rye, and other grain straw and beans. The mites attack humans, especially persons sleeping on straw mattresses, and may produce a generalized eruption consisting of petechiae, wheals, vesicles, and pustules.

Farmers, harvesters, chaff cutters, handlers of old hay, strawboard factory workers, millers, bakers, packers, unloaders, and persons working in grain elevators or places where grain and straw are handled may become infested with grain itch mites.

Frequent bathing and change of clothing may prevent infestation when there is massive exposure to the mites. The wearing of clothing impregnated with benzyl benzoate may be effective. Prophylactic use of Kwell or Eurax is beneficial.

Food Mites

Tyroglyphus farinae, the flour mite, may infest not only grain stores, mills, and bakeries, but also food in homes. Contact with the food produces a papular dermatitis.

Tyroglyphus siro, the cheese mite, infests not only cheese but also dried fruit, sugar, roots, bulbs, and copra. Grocer's itch, a pruritic papular eruption, is produced in persons handling these infested plant products. Cheese mites do not suck blood, but their migration under superficial scales of the epidermis produces pruritus and an eruption that is difficult to distinguish from that of allergic contact dermatitis.

Cheese mites have been controlled by painting the cheese with paraffin and by wiping or dipping cheese with mineral oil, cotton seed oil, or glycerin. Good packaging to prevent the mites from obtaining entrance to the food is important for prevention of infestation.

Miscellaneous Mites

Barley itch usually occurs in dock workers unloading barley infested with food mites. Baker's itch occurs among workers in granaries, flour mills, and bakeries, particularly in small establishments that do not use mechanical processes and have few sanitary arrangements to destroy mites.

Individuals handling cotton seed in bulk may acquire a mite rash known as cotton seed itch. When the seeds are handled in bags, dermatitis does not occur. The mite in cotton seed is related to *Pediculoides ventricosus.* Bulb mite itch is contracted by individuals who store infested bulbs above their beds on shelves or in attics; these persons, while asleep, are attacked by the mites.

Bakers, workers in sugar refineries or chocolate candy factories, and those who can and pack fruits and syrups may acquire a dermatitis from the sugar mite.

Dried fruits may be infested by the mite *Carpoglyphus passularum.* Sorters, peelers, and packers of infested prunes may acquire a follicular, papular eruption. Women sorting partly damaged dates may also be affected. Dock laborers and workers engaged in shoveling figs for a jam factory have developed dermatitis produced by a fruit mite. A mite found on dried beans can produce dermatitis in workers handling these legumes.

PSEUDOPHYTODERMATITIS DUE TO CONTACT WITH POISON HAIRS OF CATERPILLARS

Outdoors, exposure to caterpillars is not uncommon. In the home, caterpillars may crawl into clothes and bedding. Fomites infested with caterpillars may produce dermatitis for long periods, even in cold storage. Caterpillar dermatitis is an occupational disease in plantation workers.

Dead larvae and cocoons of caterpillars as well as debris from infested pine forests can cause dermatitis. Caterpillar dermatitis, therefore, may occur throughout the entire year. The eruption is caused by microscopic hairs containing a toxin that produces lesions in all individuals exposed. An entire community may suffer from urticaria epidemica due to caterpillars.

This type of dermatitis appears usually as a urticarial, papular eruption, but vesiculation and even necrosis may also occur. Nodular conjunctivitis and severe damage to the eyeball are serious complications.

PSEUDOPHYTODERMATITIS DUE TO DYES

Certified azo dyes applied to the skin of oranges and grapefruits rarely cause dermatitis.

PSEUDOPHYTODERMATITIS DUE TO WAXES

Carnauba wax, from the South American palm, is used to wax oranges and is an ingredient of shoe, furniture, and automobile polishes, cosmetic creams, lipsticks, and solid perfumes. J. C. Mitchell has not encountered allergic contact dermatitis from this wax.

PLANT INSECTICIDES

Various plant insecticides, including arsenical sprays and malathion, can produce contact dermatitis, which may initially be diagnosed as plant dermatitis.

Dermatitis due to Flowers and Decorative Plants

Many varieties of wild and cultivated flowers may cause dermatitis.

Sensitivity occurring in gardeners and florists is confined usually to the hands, forearms, face, and neck; episodic, acute vesicular reactions occur. Dermatitis in commercial flower growers is a known hazard of the trade. Those affected are often seasonal workers who leave the work when dermatitis appears or carry on despite it and do not come to the attention of dermatologists. The growing of chrysanthemums by commercial growers and hobby gardeners involves close contact by "pinching out" the buds of the plants as they mature. Cutting back and pruning many garden plants (e.g., English and Algerian ivy) involve contact with the sap and risk of contact dermatitis.

CHRYSANTHEMUM

Chrysanthemums, asters, and daisies all belong to the same family of plants. Most of these flowers can produce dermatitis under certain conditions. Chrysanthemums are the most common offenders, and the resulting dermatitis appears usually in the late fall and early winter—the blooming season. Because the blooms emit a pollen, the eyelids may be the first areas involved. Many sensitized individuals also have facial involvement. Widespread chrysanthemum dermatitis is not uncommon. The diagnosis may be confirmed by a patch test. Patients who react to one species of chrysanthemum may react to other Compositae plants as well. For example, crossreactions may also take place with arnica and aster.

PHILODENDRON

This plant is widely used for interior and patio decoration. Contact dermatitis from several species, especially *Philodendron cordatum,* has occurred. Hands and arms are usually involved. Exposure takes place when the patient washes, oils, or plucks the leaves. Because the plant grows indoors, there is no relationship of the dermatitis to a particular season. A patient may have numerous attacks of dermatitis, which are not readily diagnosed. Dieffenbachia, a common house plant related closely to the philodendron, may also cause dermatitis.

Contact dermatitis to philodendron (*Philodendron scandens*) is common in Hawaii. The allergen in philodendron is an alkylresorcinol, which is chemically close to the catachols found in *Toxicodendron*. However, a study of patients sensitive to one or the other of these two plants found cross-activity to be rare.[114]

ALGERIAN IVY

This plant may be used as a ground cover. The history reveals usually that the patient cut the ivy a day or so before the onset of the dermatitis.

ENGLISH IVY

A dermatitis may be caused by the leaves, stems, and even the roots of this ornamental plant. The lesion sometimes resembles a *Toxicodendron* eruption.

OLEANDER

Dermatitis results when crushed leaves of this plant come into contact with the skin of persons who have become sensitized by previous exposure. Often children playing near shrubs are affected. Because oleander is not deciduous, it may produce dermatitis at any time of year. Patch testing confirms the diagnosis.

CASTOR BEAN

Dermatitis may occur at any time of year when there is exposure to the juice of the leaves or stems of the plants or to the beans. Castor oil extractors, fertilizer workers, and farmers may acquire occupational dermatitis from handling the plants or the beans. The beans are poisonous when ingested.

DAFFODIL/NARCISSUS

These plants can cause a papular, pruritic eruption with most severe involvement on the face, hands, and forearms. Daffodils and narcissi are members of the Amaryllidaceae family. Those affected are usually engaged in cutting, bunching, or packing daffodils and narcissi. Daffodil pickers characteristically get a papular and excoriated dermatitis on the dorsum of their hands due to the manner in which the flower is harvested. The hand is exposed to the calcium oxalate crystals in the sap, and this produces an irritant contact dermatitis. Paronychia is common in these individuals.[115]

CHINESE RICE PAPER PLANT

This popular ornamental shrub may cause severe dermatitis. The toxic substance is present in a heavy yellow pollen produced in the fall and winter. Irritant contact dermatitis can be caused by the trichomes of the Chinese rice paper tree (*Tetrapanax papyriferum*). This is a member of the Araliaceae family, which contains other plants known for both irritant and allergy, such as *Hedera helix, Fatsia japonica,* and *Schefflera* sp.[116] The allergens in *Dendropanax trifidus* have been found to crossreact with *Fatsia japonica, Hedera helix,* and *Schefflera arboricola,* which are members of the Araliaceae family. Chemically, the allergens are cis-9,17-octadecadiene-12,14-diyne-1,16-diol (comp.I)(+), 16-hydroxy-cis-9,17-octadecadiene-12,14-diynoic acid (comp.II)(+) and cis-9, trans-16-octadecadiene-12,14-diynoic acid (comp.III)(+) tested at 0.05% in petrolatum.[117]

DENDROPANAX

In Japan, the plant commonly known as kakuremino (because it resembles a Japanese straw coat) is *Dendropanax trifidus* Makino. There has been some confusion as to whether this member of the Araliaceae family crossreacts with the Japanese lacquer tree or *Fatsia japonica*. The allergen has been identified as cis-9,17-octadecadiene-12,14-diyne-1,16-diol. This is an analog of falcarinol. The apparent crossreactions to urushiol were considered coincidental. Falcarinol is the allergen found in *Hedera helix* and *Schefflera arboricola*.[118] Falcarinol allergy was detected in a cook. Vegetables that contain flacarinol and caused positive patch tests included carrot, parsley and celery. Falcarinol is present in common ivy (*Hedera helix*) and the patient also reacted to ivy and falcarinol 0.03% in petrolatum.[119]

The allergen identified in Dendropanax has been found to be present in 7 times greater concentration than in *Fatsia japonica*. Two additional allergens have been found in *Dendropanax trifidus*: 16-hydroxy-cis-9,17-ocadecadiene-12,14-diynoic acid and cis-9,trans-16-octadecadiene-12,14-diynoic acid.[120]

PHACELIA CRENULATA

This plant is known as the desert or false heliotrope. It blooms profusely in March and April in the desert areas of southern Utah, New Mexico, Arizona, southeastern California, and the Baja peninsula. The plant produces an eruption similar to that of poison ivy dermatitis.

BOUGAINVILLEA

This popular genus of South American origin is planted both indoors and outdoors. Localized urticaria outbreaks accompanied by some shortness of breath have been reported.[121] A scratch chamber test reproduced the urticarial reaction in 20 to 30 minutes.[121]

COLEUS

Facial dermatitis suspected to be due to airborne contact with dried leaves of coleus has been reported.[122] The allergen coleon O tested at 0.01% has been deemed a strong sensitizer.[122]

GARDENIA FRUIT

A folk remedy known as Sokujikoh in Japan was found to contain 16% powdered gardenia fruit (*Gardenia jas-* *minoides,* member of the Rubiaceae family), which was responsible for contact dermatitis.[123] Extracts with alcohol of the pericarp and seeds were positive.[123]

CENTELLA ASIATICA

This plant is known as the Indian penyworts and is an Umbelliferae. A 2% extract of *Centella asiatica* was included in a vasotonic cream that also contained neomycin, lavender, and geraniol, but the plant extract proved to be the allergen.[124]

HYDRANGEA

Hydrangea allergy is seen mainly in nursery workers and is due to the allergen hydrangenol, which is an isocoumarin. While the concentration in *Hydrangea macrophylla* rarely exceeds 3% and in other species is usually less than 2%, the leaves readily give positive patch tests in those who are sensitive to the plant.[125]

There are 25 species of hydrangea, and the allergen is found in both leaf and flower.[126] Hydrangenol is tested at 0.1% in petrolatum and is extractable with alcohol.[127] Hydrangenol is not uniformly found throughout the 25 species.[126] Generally, rubber gloves are protective.[127]

DAHLIA

There are three patterns of dermatitis reported among 20 patients with dahlia dermatitis. Hand dermatitis was seen in 10, hand and face in 7, and an airborne pattern in 4. The exposure was occupational in 87% of these cases.[128] A 1:10 ethanol extract can be used for patch testing.

ELECAMPANE

Crude extracts of elecampane (*Inula helenium* L.) are potent sensitizers at 1% concentration. Positive reactions to helenin 0.1% and alantolactone 0.1% were found in these cases.[129]

NARCISSUS AND HYACINTHS

Dermatitis from these plants may be allergic, but it is usually an irritant reaction to bundles of needle-shaped crystals of calcium oxalate in the outer layers of the bulbs. These do not occur in tulip bulbs. The outer scales of hyacinth bulbs contain about 6% calcium oxalate, and the dust on worktables has a similar concentration. The crystals penetrate the skin and cause a dermatitis resembling fiberglass dermatitis. Itching can be abolished by washing with dilute acetic acid. Hyacinth itch is thus rarely of allergic origin.

MARIGOLD

Three potential sensitizers have been identified in marigolds (*Tagetes* sp.). Tests in guinea pigs have defined the allergenic potential of these compounds as 5-(3-buten-1-ynyl)-2,29-bithiophene [strong], alpha-terthienyl [less strong], and hydroxytremetone [weak]. Thiophenes abundantly occur in many species of Compositae, and both phototoxic and sensitizing properties have been found.[130]

TRACHELIUM

A plant know as *Trachelium caeruleum* grows in the western Mediterranean region and is used in cut flower bouquets. It is a member of the Campanulaceae (bell-flower) family and has caused allergic contact dermatitis in a male florist who had previously had contact allergy to chrysanthemum. No crossreactivity was suspected, as the plants come from different families, and the patient's allergy developed after about 1 year of exposure to *T. caeruleum*.[131] Florists are increasingly using *Trachelium caeruleum* for floral arrangements. The petal and left can produce positive patch tests. Two cases have been reported.[132]

VERBENA

Anaphylactic symptoms developed in a teenage boy after contact with *Verbena hybrida*. The incident followed retrieving a ball from a garden. A 62000 Dalton allergen caused specific IgE mediated response. *Verbena elegans* 'Cleopatra' has also produced contact urticaria and delayed hypersensitivity.[133]

GERBERA

Contact urticaria, conjunctivitis, and rhinitis would occur in a botanist who studied *Gerbera hybrida*, which is a member of the Asteraceae family (Compositae). Type 1 reactions to this family are rare. Prick tests and RAST were positive. Pollen gave stronger reactions than did petals or leaves.[134] A greenhouse worker developed both type I and type IV reactions to this plant. Patch test with the leaf, petal and stamen/pollen were positive. Scratch tests with the sap were also positive. This plant has more commonly been associated with conjunctivitis and respirator allergy due to type I sensitization.[135]

DITTRICHIA VISCOSA AND OTHERS

Dittrichia viscosa (L.) Greuter is a member of the Compositae (Asteraceae) family, which grows in Portugal. It contains sesquiterpene lactones rather than alantolactone or isoalantolactone.[136]

Jojoba (*Simmondsia chinensis*) in a cosmetic body cream sensitized a women who used the product. The confirmatory patch test was performed with 15% jojoba seed powder in petrolatum.[137]

Aloe vera is a popular folk treatment for a variety of skin conditions. The safety of the plant extracts was evaluated in 702 patients. Patch tests with the oily extract of the leaves, pulverized whole plant, and a concentrated gel were negative in all 702 cases, attesting to the safety of the plant extracts.[138]

Work with *Cannabis* plants in a forensic laboratory led to the development of contact urticaria in a woman whose job involved stripping, grinding, and growing the plants. She did not have recreational exposure.[139]

MISCELLANEOUS FLOWERS AND SHRUBS

Less commonly, dermatitis venenata is produced by dichondra, magnolia, tea roses, greasewood, *Wigandia caracasana*, daffodils, poinsettias, *Ficus repens*, century plants, and Australian silk oak trees.

Dermatitis due to Trees

Colloquial, common, and trade names of commercial woods can be completely misleading; for example, Canadian hemlock is often shipped as Alaska pine. A dictionary of commercial trees lists in several languages the large number of trade names of commercial woods. No reliance can be placed on the trade name of a wood as an indication of the botanical species of the tree from which the wood is derived. Expert identification by a department of botany or by a forest products laboratory is essential for meaningful tests in suspected contact allergy from sawdust.[140]

Forest workers who fell trees and cut them up can be irritated or sensitized by the wood itself, but more common is sensitivity to lichens and *Frullania* (a liverwort resembling a moss) that grows on the bark of the trees. Sensitized workers develop, during work with vegetation in forest areas, occupational allergic contact dermatitis of exposed skin surfaces, which resolves on leaving work in the forests.

Dermatitis from the solid wood of finished articles is much less common, but has followed prolonged contact with musical instruments, bracelets, or knife handles made of the strongly allergenic Dalbergia rosewoods. Furniture made of rengas or obeche can also give trouble.

Hausen[141] listed the main sensitizers in woods (see also Table 21.12). Fisher and Bikowski[142] reported allergic contact dermatitis due to a wooden cross made of *Dalbergia nigra*. A search of the available literature revealed that all previous reports of allergic contact dermatitis due to *Dalbergia nigra* were concerned with occupational exposure to the wood in carpenters,

Table 21-12 Concentrations of Essential Contact Allergens of Wood Species for Epicutaneous Tests

Sensitizer	Timber	Concentration
Anthothecol	*Khaya anthotheca*	1
Chlorophorin	*Chlorophora excelsa*	1–10
Cordiachromes	*Cordia* and *Patagonula* species	0.1
Deoxylapachol	*Tectona grandis; Tabebuia* species	0.01–0.1
R-3,4-dimethoxydalbergione	*Machaerium* species	0.01
S-4,49-dimethoxydalbergione	*Dalbergia* species	1
S-49-hydroxy-4-methoxydal	*Dalbergia* species	1
2,6-dimethoxy-1,4-benzoquinone	Various wood species	10
Lapachol	*Tectona grandis; Bignoniaceae* species	1–10
"Macassar quinone"	Oxidation product of Macassar II from *Diospyros celebica*	1
Mansonone A	Mansonia altissima	0.1
Obtusaquinone	*Dalbergia retusa*	1
Oxyayanin A and B	*Distemonanthus benthamianus*	1
Thymoquinone	*Calocedrus decurrens*	0.1

woodworkers, and cabinetmakers. This is apparently the first report of "nonoccupational" dermatitis from *Dalbergia nigra*. It is of interest to note that this wooden cross produced an erythema type of eruption.

Martin and colleagues[143] reported a case of erythema multiforme–like eruption from Brazilian rosewood in a 35-year-old carpenter who initially developed rhinitis and conjunctivitis, which was succeeded by a generalized erythema multiforme–like eruption. A patch test with the wood dust produced a positive + + + reaction at 48 hours.

Hausen and Rothenborg[144] reported a case of allergic contact dermatitis caused by olive wood jewelry. Chemical analysis revealed that the olive wood contains quinoid compounds similar to sensitizers in teakwood and East Indian rosewood. Exposure to olive wood can take place not only from wood jewelry, but also from napkin rings, knife handles, and musical instruments.

EUCALYPTUS

IgE-mediated contact urticaria to eucalyptus pollen without any systemic symptom has been reported.[145] Eucalyptus oil has been found allergenic also. Tea-tree oil has been used as a topical medicament and produced contact dermatitis, which upon oral ingestion causes a flare of the prior dermatitis and a generalized eruption.[146] Tea-tree oil contains 98.5% eucalyptol, which is 1,8-cincole, and cajapulol. This is the primary ingredient in eucalyptus oil, and as little as 3.5 g of ingested eucalyptol can be fatal.[146] Tea-tree oil comes from *Melaleuca alternifolia*.

Trees may contain irritants or sensitizers in the bark, wood, or pollen.

IRRITATION DERMATITIS

Sawdust and fragments of wood produced by machine tools can cause contact dermatitis. The severity depends on whether the cut fragments are hard or soft, dry or moist.

About 120 commercial woods exist that can cause contact dermatitis in sawyers, carpenters, and those who come in contact with sawdust. The hands and face are affected, together with skin folds in which dust accumulates. Involvement of the face, ears, and scalp can resemble seborrheic dermatitis or an airborne photodermatitis. Table 21.13 lists steps for testing with sawdust.

SENSITIZATION DERMATITIS TO SAWDUST

Sensitizing chemicals are more often found among the extractives of the heartwood and therefore affect sawyers, carpenters, joiners, polishers, and finishers exposed to fine dust. The picture is that of an airborne contact dermatitis, beginning on the dorsa of the hands and forearms, eyelids, face, and neck and rapidly involving the genitals through handling in urination. In bald men,

Table 21-13 Steps Recommended for Patch Testing Workers Suspected of Allergy to Sawdust

1. Obtain botanical identification if possible from the wood (not the dust).
2. Place no reliance on trade (lumber) names.
3. Patch test with dry and then with damp sawdust. (Damp sawdust may release formic acid and other irritants.)
4. It is best to patch test with freshly ground sawdust 10% in petrolatum and test controls.
5. Care must be taken not to actively sensitize workers by using allergens in too strong a concentration.

the scalp is often affected. If the clothing gives poor protection, fine dust may drift inside it and may affect the sweaty area of the axillae, waistband, and groin and sometimes the ankles and dorsa of the feet.

Mild cases have only erythema and slight irritation, but often there is papular or vesicular dermatitis, which may progress to chronic dermatitis, after repeated exposure. Severe fissured lichenification of the palms was described as *mains de crocodile*.

The latent period varies from a week to many years, but is most commonly 10 to 15 days. In successive attacks, the latent period becomes shorter and eczema usually increases in severity, but hardening is not unusual. Crossreactions to other woods, or other sources of related antigens, are common.

ALLERGIC DERMATITIS

In the United States, the native woods that are cutaneous sensitizers include acacia, alder, ash, beech, birch, chestnut, cedar, elm, maple, mesquite, oak, pine, poplar, prune, and spruce. Some patch test concentrations for specific extracts are found in Table 21.12.

The major components of wood, such as cellulose and lignin, are not sensitizers, but the minor components, such as resins, terpenes, oils, phenols, formic acid, and nitrogen-containing substances, may cause allergic contact dermatitis. In addition, certain species of poplar contain a glucoside that may be a primary irritant.

Freshly cut woods are more apt to cause a dermatitis than are older woods, but Rengas wood, used in furniture making, may produce dermatitis only when it is old and begins to disintegrate.

Birch bark contains a fine powder on its inner aspect, which can produce a follicular acneiform eruption by mechanically plugging the follicles of exposed skin.

The bark of aspen trees *(Populus tremula)* was found to contain salicyl alcohol, the source of contact dermatitis in a farmer who developed the dermatitis while pruning using a chain saw.[147] Synonyms for salicyl alcohol include 2-hydroxybenzyl alcohol and 2-methylolphenol. Bruze used the latter term in his work with phenol-formaldehyde resins in which crossreactions occurred between phenol-formaldehyde resins and 2-methylolphenol. Balsam of Peru can also crossreact with this constellation of seemingly diverse allergens. The allergens in aspen bark *(Populus tremula)* have been found to be salicyl alcohol and salicylaldehyde, both of which are present at about 0.9 µg/mg of bark. Lesser amounts of these two allergens can be found in rowan *(Sorbus aucuparia)*, tea-leaved willow *(Salix phylicifolia)*, and goat willow *(Salix caprea)*. Salicyl alcohol is also known as 2-methylolphenol and can be found in phenol-formaldehyde resins.[148]

Tropical Woods

Working with tropical wood may result in inflammations of the oral mucosae and the respiratory system, as well as acute contact dermatitis, especially of the face and extremities. The condition often occurs in persons who are exposed to high concentrations of fine sawdust. Exotic woods seem to be the most sensitizing. Obeche wood may cause contact urticaria. Teak and mansonia contain sensitizing quinones.

Other types of dermatitis that have been mistakenly called wood poisoning include bacterial and fungal infections, seborrheic and atopic dermatitis, and contact dermatitis from common weeds, such as poison oak. In addition, chemicals sprayed onto the wood and agents, such as chloronaphthalenes, impregnated into wood for protection may cause dermatitis.

These woods are used in musical instruments, in boat construction, in furniture, and as handles for kitchen utensils. Cocus wood, known as "green ebony" or "grenadil," is used to make flutes, recorders, and clarinets. Wood shavings can produce positive patch tests, and the allergens Cocus I and II tested at 1% in ethanol. The structure of Cocus II is not fully known, but Cocus I is 7,8-dihydroxy-2,4,5-trimethoxisoflavan.[149] Clarinetists and saxophonists may develop cheilitis from cane reeds used in the instruments.[150,151] A scratch or prick test is sometimes positive when patch tests are negative.[151] A plastic-coated reed (Plasticover, available from Encore Music Co., Woodburn, IN 46797) is a suitable alternative for these patients.[151]

Fig and rubber trees, belonging to the *Ficus* genus of plants, contain a milky sap, which is commonly called latex. Fig tree latex may produce both allergic dermatitis and photodermatitis. Rubber latex rarely sensitizes.

Latex from other trees, such as gutta percha, chicle, and balata gum, rarely cause dermatitis.

The fruit of the female ginkgo tree may produce an allergic dermatitis simulating poison ivy dermatitis. Ginkgo fruit and *Toxicodendron* contain related catechols.

Perupok is a shrub found in Southeast Asia (*Lophopetalum dubium* or *Lophopetalum floribundum)*. Due to a shortage of wood worldwide, it is being increasingly used and wider contact is expected. Contact dermatitis confirmed with a 50% petrolatum patch test to the sawdust identified this plant as the source of dermatitis in a botanist.[152]

Brazilian Box Tree Wood

Sources of dermatitis from this plant include "orange sticks" for manicuring and unvarnished surfaces of organs. Dermatitis appears on hands, fingers, eyelids, and face. Both irritant and allergic reactions to *Aspidosperma* sp. Occur.[153]

Planthymenia

The Brazilian tree *Plathymenia foliosa,* also known as vinhatico, is a member of the Leguminosae family. A carpenter exposed to the dust of this tree developed a pigmented contact dermatitis. This is not surprising, as the tree is thought to contain psoralens.[154]

Tali Wood

The wood of *Erythrophleum guianense* is an irritant to nasal mucosa and can cause bradycardia, vomiting, and vertigo. A patch test to a 10% ethanol extract in petrolatum confirms contact dermatitis. This wood is used for flooring.[155]

Australian Blackwood

There are 125 Australian and 3 African species of *Acacia,* and the *A. melanoxylon* R. Br. is known as the Australian blackwood. The sensitizers are 2,6-dimethoxy-1,4-benzoquinone, acamelin, and melacacidin. The latter substance occurs in all species.[156]

Apuleia Leiocarpa

Carpenters at times are exposed to exotic woods and can develop airborne contact dermatitis to sawdust from these materials. Such was the case for a 42-year-old man who became allergic to *Apuleia leiocarpa* wood. This tree from Brazil is also known as tatajuba, bagasse, and crebianco giono.[157]

Jelutong

Wood from the *Dyera costulata* tree in southeastern Asia is commonly known as jelutong. It is a soft wood used for carving; the sap is used for chewing gum and some medicine. This tree is from the family Apocynaceae. Contact dermatitis was found in 19% of teachers who used the wood in woodworking classes. This finding, plus guinea pig sensitization studies, confirms this material to be a potent sensitizer.[158]

Milo Wood

Thespesia populnea is a tree native to Hawaii. The wood is used for carved bowls and artifacts. The tree is commonly known as milo in Hawaii and portia in California. In the Philippines, it is known as banago. The allergen in this wood is mansonone: 7-hydroxy-2,3,5,6-tetrahydro-3,6,9-triimethylnaphtho [1,8 bc] pyran-4,8-dione. It is a moderate sensitizer.[159]

Sucupira Wood

Bowdichia nitida of the family Papilionaceae or Fabaceae is known as sucupira wood. Because it is very hard, it is used for railroad ties, stakes, floors, and joists. This wood contains benzoquinone, and crossreactions with hydroquinone and primula (which contains benzoquinone) have been reported.[160]

Iroko

Iroko (*Chlorophora excelsa*), also known as African teak, is a member of the Moraceae family. It was used in building a staircase and ship repair by a man who in that setting developed airborne contact dermatitis. The allergen in this wood is chlorophorin, which is an oxystilbene.[161]

Iroko is also known as kambala, rokko, African oak, swamp mahogany, rock elm, West African mulberry, and bush oak. It caused dermatitis in a Swiss carpenter working as a joiner.[162]

Obeche Wood

Obeche wood comes from the African whitewood or African maple (*Triplochiton scleroxylon*). It is very resistant to warping and does not get as hot as other woods; therefore, it is used to make sauna benches. In Finland, occupational asthma has frequently been traced to obeche wood. A carpenter who used obeche wood to make organs developed contact urticaria when sitting on obeche wood in saunas and occupational rhinitis. He did not develop contact urticaria from the wood unless moisture was a part of the exposure.[163]

Tree Pollens

Contact dermatitis may be caused by ether-soluble portions of tree pollen oleoresin. Like ragweed oil dermatitis, tree pollen oil dermatitis is usually confined to a short season during which the pollen is airborne. The history usually reveals that the skin becomes clear after the pollination has ended and remains clear until the next season. Individuals sensitized to the oil fractions of the pollen, which produce allergic contact dermatitis, may not be sensitized to the aqueous protein fraction, which produces allergic rhinitis and asthma.

Airborne contact urticaria manifested as erythema, edema of the hands and neck, and angioedema of the lips and eyes was found to be due to mulberry (*Morus alba*) pollen rather than mulberry leaves. Prick test to the pollen extract was positive, and specific IgE to the pollen was elevated.[164]

Beekeepers can acquire an allergic contact dermatitis from bee glue (propolis) derived mainly from poplar and other tree resins. This glue is also used as a local anesthetic in Russia. In Africa, it is used as a wood and leather varnish and as a base for ointments, cosmetics, and polishes.

A tree surgeon who developed dermatitis while working on poplar trees was found sensitive to a mixture of three caffeic acid pentenyl esters thought to be the major

sensitizers in poplar bud resin. The individual also reacted to propolis, balsam of Peru and Tolu, wood tars, eugenol, and isoeugenol.[165]

Contact Dermatitis Due to Vegetables

The essential oils of the edible umbellifers carrots, parsnips, parsley, squash, asparagus, and celery (including celery salt) may cause allergic eczematous dermatitis in sensitized individuals.[166] Pinene, terpineol, and cineole are probably the sensitizers. Some members of this family are also photosensitizers. Onions and garlic may cause a contact dermatitis that can crossreact with tulips and hyacinths.[167]

Corn dermatitis (corn itch or corn poisoning) is an occupational eruption similar to the contact dermatitis seen in other vegetable processing or wet work with food plants.[168] Excoriations often complicate the dermatitis, and occasionally secondary infection occurs. Protective gloves and barrier creams help reduce exposure. In addition, a photosensitizing dermatitis may appear in workers harvesting celery parasitized by fungi (rusts or smuts).[169]

CARROTS

Klauder and Kimmich[170] described a patient with a sensitivity to carrots who developed a cheilitis and perioral dermatitis when she ate this vegetable raw or cooked.

If the oleoresin of carrots is not available for testing, patch tests may be performed with the external surface of an unpeeled raw carrot or with the surface of a slice of carrot. The reaction is usually stronger to the slice than to the outside portion. The essential oil of carrot contains pinene, terpineol, cineole, and limonene.

CELERY

This plant may cause an ordinary allergic contact reaction and photocontact dermatitis. Crossreaction may occur with the essential oil of orange, lemon, bergamot, caraway, dill, and balsams.

WILD PARSNIPS AND PARSLEY

The dermatitis produced by these vegetables is usually due to photosensitization. Moisture is necessary for the reaction. Some individuals acquire the photocontact dermatitis only when they are perspiring profusely or have become wet from water.[169]

Exposure to sunlight within 48 hours after the moist contact with the plants is necessary for the phototoxic reaction.

Photo patch tests with parsnip and parsley can be performed with the vegetable moistened with water and exposed to sunlight or artificial ultraviolet radiation.

Both contact urticaria and chronic urticaria have occurred from eating *Eruca sativa,* a popular salad garnish in Italy. A positive reaction was found with RAST and scratch tests but not open application to skin.[171]

SQUASH

Butternut squash caused hand dermatitis in a 30-year-old woman who had no antecedent history of atopic dermatitis. Rechallenge with the plant *(Cucurbita moschata)* reproduced the eczematous reaction. Previous reports of squash dermatitis were due to turban or winter squash *(C. maxima).*[172]

ASPARAGUS

Harvesting and canning of asparagus is associated with allergic contact dermatitis. The frequency of reactions is such that the condition has been called "asparagus scabies." The allergen in asparagus *(Asparagus officinalis)* has been identified as 1,2,3-trithiane-5-carboxylic acid. This is a growth inhibitor, which is present in asparagus mainly in the early part of the season.[173]

CUCUMBER

Although not common, contact allergy to cucumber *(Cucumis sativus)* has been reported in a greenhouse worker. Patch tests were found positive to the leaf and stem but not the peel.[174]

Tulip Bulb Dermatitis

Alpha-methylene-gamma-butyro-lactone is the chemical cause of tulip dermatitis. This lactone, which is split off the plant glycoside, is most highly concentrated in the bulbs. Less is found in the stems, and the least in the petals. The lactone, found in members of both *Tulipa* and *Alstroemeria,* is known as Tuliposide A.

Patch tests with the pure allergen in dilutions down to 1:600 may give positive reactions in control subjects, whereas patients suffering from "tulip fingers" usually have positive reactions to a concentration of 1:20,000. Because the pure tulip allergen is not available for clinical use, patch tests can be performed with the moist, fleshy outer layers of the bulb, from which the thin outer skin has been removed. Tests in control subjects are required to exclude irritant reactions.

Tulip bulbs may cause a painful, dry, fissured, and hyperkeratotic eczema, at first underneath the free margin of the nails, then extending to the fingertips and periungual region. Dermatitis of the face, the hands and forearms, and the genital region may also occasionally occur.

Sensitivity to other bulbs, such as hyacinth *(Hyacinthus)* and daffodil *(Narcissus)* are important causes of contact dermatitis in the bulb-growing industry.

ALSTROEMERIACEAE (ALSTROEMERIA)

Alstroemeria (Peruvian lily), which can produce allergic contact dermatitis of the hands in floriculturalists, cross-reacts with *Tulipa;* both contain the allergen Tuliposide A. Alstroemeria dermatitis can be confined to the fingertips of workers who string the flowers on garlands.[175,176]

Although *Alstroemeria* has gotten a good deal of recent attention as a cause of dermatitis among florists, a study of 164 persons working in floral shops found 46% had a rash at some time. The most commonly suspected plant was daffodil stems followed by primula, Christmas tree, and Cupressus for wreaths.[177] Wholesale florists usually are reactive to chrysanthemums, tulips, and alstroemeria.[178]

Dry fissured fingertips have been associated with *Alstroemeria,* garlic, tulip bulbs, and the northern India shrub *Tabernaemontana coronaria,* a member of the Apocynaceae family.[179]

Miscellaneous Plant Families that Produce Dermatitis

ALLIACEAE (ONION FAMILY)

Onion *(Allium cepa)* and garlic *(A. sativum)* can produce irritant and allergic contact dermatitis on cooks' hands. The eruption tends to start on the fingertips and to be unilateral. By patch test, onion and garlic do not always co-react. The allergen may be allyl disulfide.

CAPPARIDACEAE (CAPER FAMILY) AND CRUCIFERAE (MUSTARD FAMILY)

The mustard family and its tropical counterpart, the caper family, characteristically contain thioglucosides.[180,181] These release isothiocyanates, which, by their irritant and vesicant action, provide the counterirritant effect of a traditional mustard plaster. In making the familiar condiment, mustard powder, the ground dry seeds of *Brassica nigra,* is wetted, thus allowing action by the plant enzyme, myrosinase, and release of isothiocyanate from its thioglucoside.

Crushed seeds of mustard have been reported to cause a dermatitis deemed irritant. The dermatitis flared 5 days after oral ingestion of mustard. One month later,

patch tests were negative to commercial mustard 1:10, crushed seeds 1:1 in olive oil, and allylisothiocyanate up to 1% in ethanol. At this point, oral ingestion was asymptomatic.[182]

Familiar members of these families are *Capparis* (the pickled flower buds form capers), horseradish *(Armoracia),* cress *(Lepidium),* cabbage, brussels sprouts, cauliflower and broccoli *(Brassica* species), and nasturtium *(Tropaeolum);* the pickled seeds of the last can form a poor man's caper.

A compress of leaves and fruit of capers *(Capparis spinosa)* resulted in a dermatitis detected by patch tests to the leaf and fruit as is, mustard oil 1% and 0.1% in petrolatum, allyl isothiocyanate 0.1% and 0.05% in petrolatum, and benzyl isothiocyanate 0.1% in petrolatum. Other isothiocyanate plants were negative.[183]

The radish *(Raphanus)* is not only pungent and irritant but also sensitizing, and it is likely that the pronounced irritant effects of isothiocyanates have obscured their allergenic potential.

Allyl and benzyl isothiocyanates present in mustard oils are usually primary irritants that produce vesiculation. Occasionally, however, they may also be sensitizers. These chemicals can be tested at a concentration of 0.05% in petrolatum.

The botanical sources of allyl isothiocyanate and benzyl isothiocyanate are as follows: 1) *Allyl isothiocyanate:* wild garlic, madwort, horseradish, winter cress, mustard greens, black mustard, (root) cabbage, kohlrabi, kale, brussels sprouts, cauliflower, broccoli, sea rocket, shepherd's purse, sea kale, and white wall rocket). *Benzyl isothiocyante:* blister cress, rocket, candytuft, charlock, wild mustard, hedge mustard, penny cress, wild garlic, bitter cress, wart cress, garden cress, cow cress, pepper grass, and mignonette nasturtium of gardens.

PRIMROSE FAMILY

Primin, 2-methoxy-6-*n*-pentyl-*p*-benzoquinone, is the major allergen of primrose dermatitis. A patch test concentration of 0.01% primin in petrolatum was evaluated in 3,075 patients. Of this group, 1.8% were positive, and only two patients were sensitized by the patch test itself. There was an active primin dermatitis present at the time of testing in 41% of those who tested positive.[184] Allergy to primin was rarely found in patients under age 35.[184]

Primrose dermatitis is common in Europe. Although the plant is not supposed to grow in the United States, the late Dr. Neils Hjorth in a personal communication stated that he had seen plenty of primrose in California. The allergen content of the plants varies considerably, depending on the season, the number of hours of sunshine, the method of cultivation, and the horticultural variety. Patch testing with the leaf may be unreliable because of these variations, which result in false-negative patch test reactions, especially during winter. Therefore, an extract of *Primula obconica* is preferable for routine patch testing.[185,186] While primin in *Primula obconica* is a common allergen, other species of Primula have produced allergic contact dermatitis absent allergy to primin. *P. auricula* and *P. denticulata* contain primetin and miconidin, which are other allergens found in some *Primula sp*.[187] Aplin and Lovell[188] went on to demonstrate that allergy to *Primula auricular* is more common than previously recognized and that other species may also be implicated, including *P. vulgaris, P allionii, P. marginata* and *P. forrestii.*

Several other plants and woods containing allergenic quinones show crossreactivity with primin, particularly rosewood extract.[50]

CHENOPODIACEAE (SPINACH FAMILY)

Wild spinach or *Chenopodium album* can be cooked and eaten as a vegetable. An angioedema-like eruption of sun exposed skin can result from ingestion and furocoumarins are thought to be the cause of the phototoxic reaction.[189]

Russian thistle *(Salsola kali)* is a widespread weed native to Russia but a common and troublesome pest in arid regions of the United States, where it can cause "tumbleweed dermatitis." The spines of the plant by mechanical injury produce a papular eruption and contact urticaria.

Powell and Smith[190] reported that Russian thistle *(Salsola kali)*, the most common plant referred to as "tumbleweed" in the western United States, can cause a dermatitis in persons who come into direct contact with it. Tests were conducted to determine the mechanism of this dermatitis. Mechanical contact with plant branches, as well as scratch, patch, and photopatch tests with Russian thistle extract and scratch tests with 1.5% potassium nitrate, a plant constituent, was used. The tests, along with transparent adhesive tape preparations and a skin biopsy, showed that in nonsensitized persons, dermatitis was due only to mechanical irritation of plant floral bracts. In sensitized individuals, Russian thistle floral bracts pierced the skin and stimulated a urticarial reaction.

CANNABIDACEAE (HEMP FAMILY)

Hops *(Humulus lupulus)* are used to flavor beer. Hop pickers' dermatitis is an affliction of seasonal workers who pick the female inflorescence (hop cone), which is aromatic with hop oil and sticky with resin containing humulone and lupulone. These chemicals may be the

sensitizers. The dermatitis affects the dorsa of hands, forearm flexures, and face. Possibly 1 in 30 pickers are affected, but the incidence is difficult to determine because of the casual workforce. The milder cases may clear or become "hardened," but the more severe ones tend to get worse; some quit the casual work without coming to medical attention. Hops can produce allergic contact dermatitis from myrcene in fresh hop oil, "hop rash" which is an irritant dermatitis due to the rough hairs on the stem and hops, and (rarely) occupational asthma and anaphylaxis. Contact urticaria has been documented by positive prick tests and specific IgE.[191]

TOBACCO (NICOTIANA TABACUM)

The green and yellow cured tobacco leaf, but not nicotine or pesticide, caused contact dermatitis in a 40-year-old female seasonal tobacco plantation worker. One percent ether, acetone, and alcohol extracts in petrolatum were all positive.[192]

CACTACEAE (CACTUS FAMILY)

In addition to the obvious and injurious spines of cacti, the hobbyist may encounter tufts of short, fuzzy, barbed bristles, or glochids, five to eight on each of the 25 to 30 areolae per opuntia (cactus) leaf. The glochids have barbs that prevent their ready extraction once in the skin.

The glochids of *Opuntia lingularis* (cholla) cause immediate pain on entering the skin. Erythema and swelling develop in 72 hours and subside after 1 to 3 days, only if the glochids are removed. Retained glochids produce papules and plaques, sometimes like granuloma annulare, with a central punctum and bristle. It may take 3 to 4 months for these changes to resolve once the bristles have been rejected, and during extrusion the epidermis may become warty.

Allergic reactions consisting of flesh-colored, domed papules, 2 to 4 mm in diameter, each with a central black dot, can occur on the limbs, usually in groups of 3 to 6, and last for 2 to 8 months. Skin tests with glochid extracts have given positive responses.

O. ficus indica, prickly pear or sabra of North America, Mexico, and the Mediterranean region, causes dermatitis in workers who pick, distribute, and sell the fruit. Vacationers in the Mediterranean have also been affected. The glochids break off readily, get into the clothes, and cause sabra dermatitis, a pruritic papulovesicular eruption that looks rather like scabies. To remove glochids, depilatory wax or adhesive tape can be applied to the skin and pulled off.

Cactus spines, when embedded in the skin and not readily visible at the surface, can cause deep injuries, such as pseudotumors of bone.

AGAVE AMERICANA

The century plant derives its name from the legend that it flowers only once every 100 years. Although this is not true, the *Agave americana* produces contact dermatitis more often than that. It is highly irritating and contains sapogenins, hecogenins, oxalic acid, and calcium oxalate crystals.[193] Tequila is distilled from *Agave tequilana*, which contains needle-like calcium oxalate crystals that produce an irritant dermatitis in both plantation and distillery workers. The crystals are referred to as raphides, and those longer than 180mm have been found to cause irritation. Raphides from the *Agave tequilana* range from 30 to 500 µm in length.[194]

ARACEAE (ARUM FAMILY)

Plants of the Arum family are grown mainly as houseplants, some as outdoor plants in warm areas for their attractive foliage. The plant tissues contain sharp, stinging calcium oxalate crystals, which are irritant to the lips and tongue. Acute cheilitis, stomatitis, and glossitis can occur inindividuals, usually children, who chew the stems of dieffenbachia and monstera. Some other chemicals besides the crystals, and as yet unidentified, probably play a part. The stem and leaf of dieffenbachia may produce a positive patch test result.[195]

The common houseplant philodendron is a sensitizer for nursery workers and hobbyists; the allergen is an alkyl-resorcinol similar to those of Proteaceae and with phytochemical affinities to the allergenic catechols of Anacardiaceae. Co-reaction of the genus *Philodendron* and *Toxicodendron*, however, has not been reported. Contact may be accidental during watering the plant or result from plucking or polishing the leaves. Hobbyists are exposed far less than nursery workers, as they water the plant with greater care and handle it less. Dermatitis from *P. scandens* and related species resembles mild poison ivy reactions with streaky, blotchy vesicular erythema on the hands and forearms, less often on the abdomen and lower limbs. The eyelids may be affected alone, or as part of widespread dermatitis.

Hammershoy and Verdich[196] reported allergic contact dermatitis due to *P. scadens*. In four patients with dermatitis, allergy to philodendron was found through patch testing with leaves, stems, and ether extracts from eight philodendron species. Although this allergy appears to be rare, it ought to be considered in patients with dermatitis on hands, arms, and face.

Scindapsus aureus is a popular indoor climber in Scandinavia despite its needle-like hairs; biting the stem causes intense irritation, and the plant is also allergenic. Reactions from it as a garden plant are known in Hawaii.[197]

The roots of some Arum contain a starchy material that is edible if boiled or otherwise treated to destroy irritant calcium oxalate crystals. The starch from the tubers of *Arum maculatum* (cuckoo pint, wake robin, and lords-and-ladies) forms arrowroot, which is made into biscuits. In Elizabethan times, the starch of this species used to stiffen ruffs irritated the hands of laundresses. In 1713, Ramazzini, the father of occupational medicine, described gangrene of the genitals of an apothecary who contacted another arum (*A. arisarum*). Many others, perhaps most of the 2,000 species in the plant family, have irritant properties. The clinical history obtained in cases of dermatitis will suggest immediate irritancy rather than a delayed allergic effect. For example, in Venezuela, laborers cutting *Montrichardia arborescens* with a machete develop erythema instantly on contact with the sap. The erythema fades in 24 to 72 hours.

ARALIACEAE (IVY FAMILY)

Hedera (ivy), the best known genus, is popular as a houseplant or as ground cover in the garden. Algerian or Canary Island ivy (*H. canariensis*) causes more dermatitis than English ivy (*H. helix*), possibly because it grows faster and requires more cutting back. Like poison ivy, the plant parts of ivy must be bruised to release the allergenic sap. The clinical picture of Hedera dermatitis resembles that from poison ivy but tends to be seasonal, corresponding to the time of pruning. Co-reaction with schefflera (*Brassaia*), a botanically related and popular houseplant, has been reported.

HYDROPHYLLACEAE (PHACELIA)

Reynolds and colleagues[198] stated that dermatitis due to *Phacelia crenulata*, or desert heliotrope, is quite common, with dermatitis frequently seen on the ankles and legs of persons walking in the desert during the spring blooms. Desert heliotrope grows during the spring months throughout the arid southwestern United States (California, Arizona, southern Utah, and southern Nevada) and is commonly found along the sand and gravel of desert highways and roadsides.

The major contact allergen of *P. crenulata* (Hydrophyllaceae) has been identified as geranylhydroquinone. A maximization test of geranylhydroquinone showed this to be a potent sensitizer comparable in degree to poison oak/ivy urushiol. Comparative patch testing on humans with urushiol established that the phacelia allergen does not crossreact with poison oak or ivy.

ASPIDIACEAE (FERN FAMILY)

Considering the wide use of ferns as houseplants, dermatitis from them is rare. Leatherleaf fern (*Arachnoides adiantiformis),* used as a background for floral arrangements, caused dermatitis on the palms and fingers of a florist. An allergen, present only during sporogenesis, has been isolated, but not identified.[199] Sporogenesis refers to the time when spore capsules are present on the under surface of the leaves.

Nursery workers are exposed to many plants, but de Cock and colleagues[200] were able to trace the source of dermatitis in a 23-year-old woman to contact with ferns. The specific plant was *Pteris ensiformis* 'Evergemiensis.' This fern is a member of the Pteridaceae family. Unlike previous fern allergy that required spores to be present, in this case the plant was allergenic without spores.

EUPHORBIACAE (CROTON, CODIAEUM VARIEGATUM)

There were several reports of allergic contact dermatitis to this plant family. Tafelkruyer and van Ketel[201] described a male flower grower with hyperkeratotic eczema localized to the tips of the thumb and index finger and onycholysis of these nails. The unknown sensitizer seems to be soluble in water but not in alcohol.

Codiaeum is often called croton by growers. The genus *Croton* and the genus *Codiaeum* are members of the large Euphorbiaceae family.

Pseudophytodermatis is a term used when an inorganic molecule such as nickel in a plant is found to be present in adequate concentration to elicit allergic contact dermatitis in a nickel-sensitive individual. Two plants have been reported to exhibit this phenomenon: *Ludwigia repens* and *Euphorbia triangularis.* In the later case, the plant was believed to contain 48.6 mg/kg of nickel, and the patient reacted to as little as 3 ppm nickel.[202]

Codiaeum variegatum is not to be confused with *Croton tiglium,* from which croton oil is derived. Croton oil, which is a brownish-yellow oil expressed from the seeds of *Croton tiglium,* is a violent purgative and irritant.

Hausen and Schulz[203] reported that one of the most decorative and popular ornamental potted plants is croton. Eczema of the hands developed in a nursery gardener who handled this plant for a period of 6 months. Patch tests with croton leaves gave positive results. Control test results remained negative. Sensitization experiments in guinea pigs with a methanolic extract of the leaves were successful.

The results of the study indicate that the latex of croton produces no primary irritant reaction and the latex is able to induce contact allergy. Further experiments are being continued in an attempt to isolate irritant and allergenic factors from the latex of various Euphorbiaceae species. Many plants of this family, particularly the genus *Euphorbea,* are irritant, having a milky sap that is injurious to the skin and the eye.

UNUSUAL PLANTS

Workers in botanical gardens may develop contact dermatitis from unusual plants. Such a worker in Italy developed allergy to *Vernonia noveboracensis* L., a member of the Compositae family. It contains germacranolides and guaianolide and the patient reacted to sesquiterpene lactone mix. Whole and chopped leaves also were used for patch testing, with positive results.[204]

GRASS

Allergy to grasses is commonly associated with repiratory allergy, but Wong and colleagues[205] found that military personnel who complained of grass allergy could have either immediate or delayed hypersensitivity. Of 23 patients, 2 were prick test positive and 3 were patch test positive to grass (*Axonopus compressus*). The authors pointed out that Bermuda grass (*Cynodon dactylon*) and crab grass (*Digitaria sanguinalis*) have also caused contact dermatitis.

Intolerance of grass was the subject of a study of patients in Singapore.[206] Of the 46 patients with this complaint, 11% were confirmed to have a positive patch test to one of five grasses: carpet grass (*Axonopus compressus*), seashore centipede grass (*Ischaemem muticum*), lalang (*Imperata cylindrica*), Guinea grass (*Panicum maximum*), or elephant grass (*Pennisetum purpureum*).

FUNGICIDE DERMATITIS

The fungicide Plondrel can cause dermatitis that appears to be caused by the plant, because positive patch tests may be obtained with leaves that still contain traces of the fungicide.[207]

Clinical and Botanical Investigation

When the dermatologist or the patient suspects that a plant is causing contact dermatitis, samples must be obtained of all the plants to which exposure may have occurred. Flowers and leaves of all the suspected plants should be brought in by the patient and stored temporarily in a refrigerator in the physician's office. The patient should be warned that he or she must be thorough and bring samples of all plants, including those considered "weeds."

The plants selected for the first set of patch tests should be those recognized as causing dermatitis. If these first tests are negative, tests with the remaining plants should be carried out. In some instances, repeated search may be required before the offending plant is detected. An absolute necessity is botanical identification of the plants used for testing. Sources of information are listed in Table 21.14. It is fruitless and misleading to look up the common or colloquial name of the plant in any book.

Table 21-14 Sources for Botanical Identification of Plants Suspected of Causing Contact Dermatitis

Botanical gardens

Botanist (plant taxonomist if possible) at national, state, or private herbarium or high school

County agricultural agents and soil conservation agents (U.S. Department of Agriculture)

Department of Botany at a university

Curator of herbarium

Table 21-16 Steps for Preserving Plants for Patch Testing

Recommended steps for patch testing with a plant:

1. Divide the plant into three parts. Air dry or freeze one part and keep for botanical identification (flowers needed).

   Label, date, source, geographic site obtained.

   Put two parts into freezer:

   a. For patch testing

   b. For making extract dilutions and for chemical studies

2. Patch test with leaf, flowerhead, stalk, and petal.

   Tests in control individuals are essential.

An expert identification of the suspected plants by a plant taxonomist is essential.

Speed is also essential in identifying a suspected plant. Wasted time leads to lack of interest by patient and physician, and important information may be lost by delay. Each case is a minor or even a major research exercise. The suspected offending plant should promptly be divided into three approximately equal portions. One portion for botanical identification should be dried or stored in the freezer. The second and third portions should be stored in a freezer, one portion for patch test purposes, and the other for possible later chemical studies.

An interested patient available for patch testing, the suspected plants reliably identified, and the samples safely frozen in three portions provide the opportunity for a significant and rewarding investigation. Armed with the names of the plants, one can turn to the literature.

AVOIDANCE OF TESTING IRRITANT PLANTS

It is useless to patch test with irritant plants; some plant families, such as the Euphorbiaceae (spurge) family, contain mostly irritant plants. A partial list of irritant plant families appears in Table 21.15.

PATCH TESTING WITH PLANTS

The steps to be carried out are summarized in Table 21.16.

There is no point in patch testing with the known irritant plants shown in Table 21.17. If irritancy seems possible, it is necessary to patch test with caution. In all cases, patch tests to plants in a patient suspected to be allergic should be accompanied by control patch tests in at least 5, preferably 20, volunteer subjects. The literature abounds with invalid reports in which alleged allergenic plants have not received the simple, but crucial, tests for irritancy in controls. No plant can be considered proven allergenic unless tests are negative in a substantial number of controls.

The actual plants to which the patient was exposed should be used for patch testing. Rarely is it possible to use dried herbarium specimens of identified species for this purpose.

To prepare a plant for patch testing, leaves and petals should be lightly crushed, and stalks and thick leaves should be cut into thin slices. Having established the allergenicity of a plant by suitable patch testing and by the use of controls, one can proceed to test more thoroughly with various parts of the plant root, stalk, leaf, flower head, and other parts of the flower. Controls are required for each part tested because the parts of a plant often vary in their chemical composition. Hausen recommends a 60-second dip in either as an all-purpose

Table 21-15 Botanical Families that Contain Many Irritant Plants[a]

Family	Genus
Araceae	Dieffenbachia
Capparidaceae (caper)	*Capparis* (Cleopatra's needle)
Cruciferae (mustard)	*Brassica* (mustard)
Euphorbiaceae (spurge)	*Euphorbia* (spurge)
Ranunculaceae (buttercup)	*Ranunculus* (buttercup)
	Clematis (pasqueflower)
	Anemone (windflower)

[a]Plants of the genera noted are often irritant.

Table 21-17 Irritant Hairy Plants

Many plants of Borage family, *Borago,* etc.

Cortusa—relative of *Primula*

Begonia rex and hybrids

Sparmannia (indoor linden) (this plant is also allergenic)

Ulmus (elm)

Cornus sanguinea (blood-twig dogwood)—T-shaped hairs

Nettles—*Urtica*

extraction procedure for plant allergens, notably sesquiterpene lactones from plant hairs.

Several methods of making plant allergens for patch testing have been suggested. The 60- to 90-second dip in diethyl ether provides for an adequate extraction. This is evaporated to dryness and resuspended in either petrolatum or acetone in a concentration of 1% to 10%. Some prefer to use acetone for the extraction. Alternatively, a 1-hour patch test can be performed.[208]

ROLE OF AGE OF PLANTS

Often, mature plants are more allergenic than immature plants. With age, secondary products of metabolism accumulate in plants because they have little or no excretory mechanisms. Therefore, mature plants should be used for patch testing. Some provisional evidence suggests that immature plants of *Asparagus* (asparagus) and *Chicorium* (chicory) may be more allergenic than flowering specimens. If this is the case, these plants are exceptions to the rule noted previously. These plants are commonly used for commercial and culinary purposes when in a state of immaturity; therefore, maximum exposure occurs to immature rather than to mature plants. Until this aspect is clarified, it is probably best to use mature plants for patch testing.

TIMING AND SITE OF PATCH TESTS

If plant dermatitis is suspected clinically but no clear lead is provided by the history, it may be useful to limit screening patch testing to plants within these commonly offending families; otherwise, patch tests with innocuous but popular plants may continue to be performed.

One should wait until acute dermatitis has subsided before patch testing, in order to avoid the risk of provoking a focal or disseminated flare. The skin site selected for patch testing should be clear of dermatitis for at least 2 weeks, preferably 1 month, before such testing is carried out—hence the usefulness of freezing plants. The irritant plant *Ranunculus* (buttercup) becomes more irritant after freezing; as the tissues are rewarmed, the cells burst and enzyme action releases an irritant compound, protoanemonin. Dried buttercups are hardly irritant at all, because protoanemonin is converted into an innocuous polymer, anemonin. There is no firm evidence that plant allergens are made innocuous by freezing. False-positive reactions can result from testing during status eczematicus—the so-called "angry back." The back is more sensitive than are the extremities. Confusion may occur from discoloration of the skin at the test site by the presence in a plant of a red

dye that simulates an erythema. An irritant patch test reaction can never be reliably distinguished from an allergic patch test reaction on morphologic grounds alone.

Patch Testing with Bulbs

The bulbs of the tulip *(Tulipa)*, hyacinth *(Hyacinthus)*, and daffodil *(Narcissus)* are important causes of contact dermatitis in the bulb-growing industry. The problem is well known to the growers, but cases are rarely seen by a dermatologist. For patch testing, the thin dried outer scale of the bulb should be removed. The moist fleshy outer layers of the bulb, which are actually leaves modified to storage, should be used for patch testing. Tests on control subjects are required to exclude irritancy.

Patch Testing with Hairy Plants

Patch testing with hairy plants can produce irritant patch test reactions. Some irritant, hairy plants are listed in Table 21.17. Indoor linden *(Sparmannia)* can produce irritant patch test reactions and is also probably allergenic. Thus, judicious patch testing with the plant and its extracts is required. The T-shaped hairs of blood-twig dogwood *(Cornus sanguinea)* produce urticarial reactions if the leaf is rubbed on the skin in the direction of its long axis. Some other commonly grown hairy plants produce irritant patch test reactions from their leaves (for example, cineraria *(Senecio)*, primrose *(Primula sinensis)*, and fig *(Ficus macrophylla)*.

PHOTOPATCH TESTING

Phytophotodermatitis is caused by a photochemical reaction mediated by psoralens and possibly by other plant chemicals. No allergic mechanism is implicated, and any individual exposed adequately to the plant juices and then to sunlight will react. Skin tests are meaningless if the suspected plant is known to contain psoralens, but they may be of interest if such information is lacking in the world literature and facilities for photochemical studies are not available. The tests can be carried out on any volunteer to avoid inconveniencing the patient, who is often a child.

PURIFICATION AND IDENTIFICATION OF PLANT ALLERGENS

Purification and identification of plant allergens have been accomplished only in a few instances. The method used has been summarized by Benezra.[209] To carry an investigation this far is a major research exercise.

Table 21-18 Patch Testing with Irritant, Suspected Allergenic Plants

1. Make 20% aqueous extract. Allergen of *Allium* (garlic), for example, is water soluble.
2. Use 10% ethanol extract. Most plant allergens are soluble in organic solvents.
3. Patch test the patient and controls.
4. If negative, try 20% or more to find a nonirritant, allergenic concentration. A variety of organic solvents can be tried.

Some plants are irritant and allergenic. When such plants are suspect, it is necessary to use plant extracts, diluted to a nonirritant level for patch testing. This complex but not unimportant problem is summarized in Table 21.18.

Control Tests

Regarding controls, synthetic primin, the allergenic quinone of *Primula obconica,* provides a useful example. Concentration 1:100 is always irritant; 1:1,000 is often irritant; 1:10,000 produces active sensitization (sensitization by patch testing); 1:50,000 elicits positive reactions only in sensitized individuals. The allergen of *Tulipa* (tulip) (alpha-methylene-g-butyrolactone) is irritant at a concentration 1:600 but produces positive patch test reactions in sensitized persons 1:20,000. An overriding consideration is that the concentrations should *not* be great enough to cause active sensitization. Twenty-five microliter pipettes may be used for applying the fluid extracts. The test response depends on the amount of allergen deposited per surface area and not on the total dose. A study of 79 patients with atopic dermatitis found 5 who were sensitive to plant allergens. Those reactions were to alpha-methylene gamma-butyrolactone (2 cases), and one case was reactive to evernic acid, one case to dandelion and tansy, and a final case to dandelion and propolis.[210]

Dermatitis Due to Spices

At least 60 spices, with their essential oils, are in use. Six of these are of particular interest to the dermatologist because they produce allergic contact dermatitis.

In the United States, the five spices that most commonly produce dermatitis are capsicum, cinnamon, cloves, nutmeg, and vanilla. In Europe, laurel is apparently the most common cause.

All these spices can produce flares at the healed sites of allergic contact dermatitis when they are ingested or inhaled. In addition, spices may produce urticaria when ingested with foods or drink or when inhaled.

Spices have been used in perfumes, cosmetics, and topical medications.

Highly seasoned foods were known to cause rosacea, particularly rhinophyma, a fact immortalized in the following poem more than three and a half centuries ago[211]:

Nose, nose, nose, nose!
And who gave thee this jolly red nose!
Nutmeg, and ginger, cinnamon and cloves,
And they gave me this jolly red nose.

All the spices contain essential oils, which can irritate the skin in concentrated form. The dust that forms when spices are ground produces an irritant dermatitis mechanically as well as chemically. Many of the essential oils also are sensitizers.[212] Spice allergy may be underdiagnosed, because 47% of patients reacting to standard substances like colophony, balsam of Peru, fragrance mix, and/or wood tars also reacted to one or more spices (paprika, cinnamon, laurel, celery seed, nutmeg, coriander, cacao, or garlic).[212] In this study, powdered spices were moistened with a little water. Of those reacting to spices, 28% were to nutmeg, 19% to paprika, and 12% to clove.[213]

Many spices, particularly mustard and capsicum, can irritate the mucous membranes of the eyes and respiratory passages. The oleoresin of capsicum is such an efficient lacrimator that it is employed in the United States as tear gas.[214,215]

CAYENNE PEPPER (*CAPSICUM FRUTESCENS*)

This pepper, from which the oleoresin of capsicum is extracted, is distributed worldwide. One patient was recently studied who had an acute eczematous dermatitis on one side of the neck after being playfully sprayed with an aerosol containing the oleoresin of capsicum at a New Year's Eve party. One year before this episode, the patient had a stiff neck and applied Capsolin Rubefacient, which contains oleoresin of capsicum, camphor, oil of turpentine, and oil of cajeput (a pungent oil from an East Indian myrtle tree). Patch tests revealed a maximal reaction to capsicum and negative reactions to the other ingredients.

On two occasions, the dermatitis of the neck flared after the ingestion of pickles that had been flavored with capsicum. Ginger ale and liqueurs flavored with capsicum can produce similar eczematous contact dermatitis in sensitized individuals.[216]

Table 21-19 Cinnamon, Cassia, and Nutmeg Terminology in Various Languages			
	Cinnamon	Cassia	Nutmeg
Spanish	Canela	Canella de la China	Nuez Moscada
French	Cannelle	Cannelle de Cochinchine	Muscade
German	Zimt	Zimtkassie	Muskatnuss
Swedish	Kanel	Kassia	Nuskot
Arabic	Qurfa	Darasini	Babbasa
Dutch	Kaneel	Kassia	Notemuskaat
Italian	Cannella	Cassia	Noce Moscata
Portuguese	Canela	(none known)	Noz-Moscada
Russian	Koritsa	(none known)	Oryekh Muskatny
Japanese	Seitron-Nikkei	Bokei	Nikuzuku
Chinese	Jou-Kuei (or Jou-Kwei)	Kuei (or Kwei)	Jou-Tou-K'ou

CINNAMON AND CASSIA

There has been a confusion between cinnamon and cassia. When we order cinnamon toast, we should, to be correct, ask for cassia toast, because cassia has almost entirely replaced cinnamon as a spice in the United States.

In Great Britain, the word "cinnamon" applies only to *Cinnamomum zeylanicum* and cassia to *C. cassia*. In the United States, the Food, Drug and Cosmetic Act of 1938 officially permitted the word "cinnamon" to be used for both *C. zeylanicum* and *C. cassia,* as well as other species of cassia. The nomenclature in various countries is listed in Table 21.19.

Cinnamon is the bark of the cinnamon or cassia tree. The flavor is derived from oil of cinnamon, which contains cinnamic aldehyde and eugenol. Oil of cinnamon is used mainly for flavoring food, toothpaste, chewing gum, tobacco, aperitifs and bitters, and cola beverages. Because of its sensitizing properties, it is used for perfumes only to a limited extent, and always in low concentrations.

Occupational dermatitis from oil of cinnamon may occur in bakers and candy makers, but cinnamon dermatitis has also been observed among cooks and homemakers.[217] Oil of cinnamon has further been reported as the cause of allergic dermatitis from ammoniated toothpaste,[218] bubble gum, and lipstick. Sensitization to balsam of Peru may result in a high degree of cross-sensitivity to oil of cinnamon.[53] Ingestion of oil of cinnamon may produce an eczematous contact type of flare-up in individuals previously sensitized by contact with the oils.[219]

NUTMEG AND MACE

The nutmeg tree, *Myristica fragrans,* produces two closely related but separate spices, nutmeg and mace. The terms for nutmeg in different countries are listed in Table 21.19.

The essential oils of nutmeg and mace contain myristicin, which is highly toxic and a powerful narcotic. The fatty oils of nutmeg are used in the manufacture of soap and perfumes and may be the cause of allergic dermatitis. Blends of mace and nutmeg are used extensively for flavoring foods. Bakers may acquire allergic dermatitis from handling these spices. Pure nutmeg oil contains eugenol, isogenol, safrole, myristicin, elemicin, and limonene.[220] Nutmeg oil has been found to inhibit prostaglandin synthesis due to its eugenol content.[220]

Connecticut is known as the "Nutmeg State." This nickname resulted from the ingenuity of Connecticut Yankee peddlers of the early nineteenth century who were charged with the sale of wooden imitation nutmegs as the genuine article to unsuspecting housewives.

When the word "mace" is mentioned in the United States, most dermatologists think of chemical Mace, referring to a tear gas. The term is an acronym derived from the chemicals involved—*M*ethylchloroform chlor-*ACE*tophenone.[221] Chemical Mace is a potent sensitizer and, of course, is unrelated to mace, the spice.

For patch test purposes, capsicum and mace are tested in a 1% alcoholic solution.

CLOVES

The word "clove" (*Syzygium aromaticum)* is derived from the French *clou,* referring to the flower bud of the tree.

Oil of clove is rich in essential oils, particularly eugenol, which are widely used in perfumes, soaps, toothpastes, and mouthwashes.

Eugenol is a pale yellow liquid with a strong smell of carnation used in zinc oxide-eugenol dental cement. It may also be combined with rosin and zinc oxide. It is the essential chemical constituent of clove oil and is also present in cinnamon oil, perfumes, soaps, and bay rum. Individuals sensitized to eugenol should avoid exposure to such products. Eugenol is both a primary irritant and a sensitizer, and for patch testing a 10% solution in olive oil or a 5% solution in petrolatum is used.

Eugenol, one of the main constituents of oil of bay, may show crossreactions with balsam of Peru. Sometimes oil of cloves and of cinnamon are added to bay rum. Both oils are sensitizers, and cinnamon oil may crossreact with eugenol and balsam of Peru. Eugenol, when used in dental preparations, such as impression pastes, surgical packings, temporary fillings, and cements, may produce stomatitis venenata and allergic eczematous eruptions in dental personnel.[222]

Oil of cloves incorporated into a liniment has been reported as a cause of allergic dermatitis.[223,224] The mucilage of postage stamps may also contain clove oil, and cause glossitis in persons who lick the stamps. Clove oil may be patch tested with a 1% alcoholic solution.

Individuals sensitized to oil of cloves or eugenol may have to avoid ingestion of foods containing the spice or the essential oil in order to avoid a flare of dermatitis. Indians use cloves to flavor the betel nut; the English use oil of cloves in apple tarts; the French love onion soup with cloves. In the United States, cloves are frequently used with pork.

VANILLA AND VANILLIN

Vanilla is a flavoring extract made from the pod of the vanilla plant. Vanillin is a crystalline compound, which is the fragrant constituent of vanilla. The vanilla bean is the dried and fermented fruit of an orchid, *Vanilla planifolia.* Vanillin, a benzaldehyde, is formed from glycosides, such as glucovanillyl alcohol and glucoconiferyl alcohol, the latter being converted into glucovanillin, glucose, and vanillin.

Contact dermatitis due to vanilla occurs in individuals used in the cultivation, trade, or industrial use of vanilla. One variety of vanilla dermatitis is a pseudophytodermatitis caused by mites, living on vanilla pods, of the same species as meal mites (*Tyroglyphus farinae),* which produce an eruption of urticarial papules, called vanilla lichen,[225] on exposed parts of the body. Vanillism, an allergic contact dermatitis acquired by workers handling the vanilla plant, produces marked edema and erythema. Rhinitis, asthma, and vertigo may accompany the eruption.

Synthetic vanillin can be produced from pine tree sap, eugenol, wood pulp, sugar, and coal tar. The U.S. Food and Drug Administration requires that the term "imitation vanilla" appear on the label if the product contains synthetic ingredients. If the label has the term "vanilla extract," the product must be derived from vanilla beans. Some individuals are sensitized to synthetic vanillin and not to the natural spice, and vice versa.[212]

An unusual source of exposure to vanillin is smoking certain types of tobacco. For patch test purposes, a 10% alcoholic extract of vanilla in acetone can be used. Vanillin may be tested 10% in petrolatum.

LAUREL

The bay tree, *Laurus nobilis,* also known as sweet bay, is native to the Mediterranean region and Asia Minor. This bay tree is not related to the West Indian bay tree *Pimenta acris,* leaves of which are distilled to produce bay rum.

Laurel oil is used in medicine and in the textile and soap industries. Laurel leaves are used in cooking because of their flavoring and antioxidant properties. They are also used in meat and fish preservation, pickled gherkins, condensed soups, and spiced sauces.

The bactericidal properties of laurel oil have been known for a long time in Germany and made use of in an ointment for abscesses. In France, laurel oil is used in only one Codex listed product (Fioravanti balsam) and in the commercial product Vegebom. Fioravanti spirit, which is also called turpentine spirit mixture, contains 0.4% of *L. nobilis* berries, 20% of larch tree turpentine, and other products. Among the Vegebom preparations, only the ointment, the suppositories, and an adhesive for prosthetic dentistry (Dental Vegebom) include appreciable quantities of laurel oil (1.2% in the ointment).

Laurel oil is often used in the textile industry to improve the luster of felt hats. In the store, the hatband becomes contaminated when the hats are stacked and produces hatband dermatitis in the wearer.

In the United States, dermatitis from laurel is apparently rare. Sensitization to laurel is not uncommon, however, in Europe. Most cases have been observed in Germany, Switzerland, and France.[226]

In Germany, sensitization occurs from the use of laurel in the felt industry. In France and Switzerland, the source of exposure is ointments containing the oil of laurel (Vegebom ointment).

Cosmetics and food may also be sources of exposure. It is surprising to learn that in Strasbourg, laurel oil is a more common sensitizer than nickel or mercury.

In the United States, bay leaves are practically never used for medicinal purposes; consequently, sensitization from topical exposure is eliminated. Bay leaves are used to season some dishes, particularly bean soup. Bay leaves are popular in French cuisine for flavoring meats, fish, poultry, vegetables, and stews. It is conceivable that such extensive use may have sensitized some individuals.

Patch tests with laurel oil may be performed with a 2% concentration in petrolatum or with a 5% solution of essential oil in alcohol.

THYME

Farmers who grow thyme (*Thymus vulgaris*) may develop airborne contact dermatitis from the dust of dried thyme. Four of 46 thyme farmers showed symptoms after exposures of 5 to 30 minutes to thyme dust.[227]

ROSEMARY

A woman who picked fresh rosemary (*Rosmarinum officinalis*) was found to be reactive to patch tests with the plant "as is" as well as to thyme (*Thymus vulgaris*). Both plants are members of the Labiatae family. Phototesting increased the degree of reactivity to both plants. No reactions were found to two other members of the Labiatae family, mint (*Menntha piperita*) and origanum (*Origanum vulgare*).[228]

Additional Foods Capable of Producing Contact Dermatitis

A dry, often fissured, fingertip dermatitis is most frequently associated with garlic. Of 155 persons tested to a slice of fresh garlic, 8 reacted.[229] Additional patch tests to garlic powder as is, 2% and 5% diallyl disulfide in petrolatum, ethanol (2%), and aqueous (10%) were conducted, and five of five women with an irritant-appearing dermatitis were positive to all of the tests confirming diallyl disulfide as an allergen and the utility of any of the materials for test purposes. Inasmuch as fresh garlic under a Finn chamber patch test unit causes irritant reactions,[230] the powder would give more reliable results.

LETTUCE

Gosta Krook of Malmo, Sweden (personal communication), reported a gardener with a dermatitis of his hands, face, arms, and legs from contact with lettuce. During the winter, when he did not work with lettuce, he did not develop dermatitis. Positive patch tests were obtained to the lettuce stalk and leaf.

Rinkel and Balyeat[231] also reported a patient with contact dermatitis due to lettuce.

Closson[232] described a patient with oral mucosal edema and swelling of the eustachian tubes due to the ingestion of lettuce.

Two patients with a gardening hobby became sensitized to sesquiterpene lactones in weeds and flowers. Ingestion of lettuce caused a flare of the patients' dermatitis and burning of the mouth. Extracts of lettuce and chicory were positive at 10% in petroleum, and these are known to be sources of sesquiterpene lactones.[233]

KIWIFRUIT

Cheilitis, pruritus, and burning tongue with accompanying swelling was seen within minutes of eating kiwifruit (*Actinidia chinensis*). The pulp gave a positive scratch test, but application to intact skin was negative.[234]

MUSHROOMS

The mushroom *Agaricus bisporus* caused an occupational hand eczema in a mushroom picker. Patch tests to the cap with spores as well as the stem were positive in the patient and negative in 25 controls.[235] The second most commonly produced mushroom in the world is the shiitake (*Lentinus edodes*).[236] The hyphae have been the source of allergic contact dermatitis among growers, and in guinea pig maximization testing, the shiitake mushroom is a moderate sensitizer.[237] A dermatitis has been described after ingestion of shiitake mushrooms. Small 1-mm papules widely disseminated occur and may be accompanied by petechia from scratching. The Koebner phenomenon may be seen. One to 2 days after eating half-baked raw shiitake, the trunk exhibits the majority of the rash, followed by the face and head. The duration ranges from 2 to 14 days and averages 8 days. The overall picture suggests a mobilliform pattern not unlike a drug eruption.[236] There are no gastrointestinal, central nervous system, or mucosal symptoms. Patch and intracutaneous tests are not helpful, and complete boiling of the mushrooms seems to eliminate the potential for dermatitis.[236]

Pleurotus ostreatus is a commercially cultivated mushroom in the order Agaricales and family Tricholomataceae. It can cause contact dermatitis in those who harvest the mushroom. Other mushrooms reported to cause contact dermatitis are *Lentinus edodes*, *Suillus*, *Agaricus*, *Boletus*, and *Ramaria flava*.[238]

Mushroom pickers are at risk for occupational contact dermatitis to shiitake mushroom (*Lentinus edodes*), white mushrooms (*Agaricus hortensis*), brown mushrooms (*Agaricus bisporus*), yellow boletus (*Boletus luteus*), finger mushrooms (*Clavaria flava*), orange agaric mushroom (*Lactarius deliciosus*), and *Suillus* and *Pleurotus ostreatus*.[239]

CHAMOMILE

Oil of chamomile is found in herbal remedies often used by lactating women for treatment of nipple eczema. A 0.1% in petrolatum concentration is adequate for patch test purposes. There are both German and Roman sources, and they come from different genera. The German source is *Matricaria recutita* and the Roman source *Chamalmelum nobile*. Both are in the Compositae (Asteraceae) family, and the Roman product appears more allergenic.[240] The ingestion of chamomile tea can exacerbate contact dermatitis from chamomile.[240]

Miscellaneous Food Dermatitis

MANGO

Contact dermatitis can be caused by the oleoresin of the mango tree sap or the skin of the fruit. Patients who are sensitized to poison ivy may acquire an allergenic cheilitis from eating mango, which contains a catechol related to that of poison ivy. Hershko and colleagues[241] observed that Americans who had prior exposure to poison ivy/oak and were working at a summer camp in Israel picking mangoes developed dermatitis on first exposure. However, Israelis doing the same task who also had a history of exposure to poison ivy/oak did not develop dermatitis. This led the authors to speculate that Israelis who grow up eating mangoes develop immune tolerance to the plants, while Americans whose diet does not typically include mangoes do not acquire tolerance.[241]

Mango and poison ivy/oak are commonly thought to crossreact. To test the chemical basis for such crossreactivity, Oka and colleagues[242] extracted 3 resorciol derivatives from Phillipine mango: heptadecandienylresorcinol, heptadecenylresorcinol and pentadecylresorcinol. Patients with mango allergy reacted to the first two at 0.05% in petrolatum. Six urushiol-sensitive patients were also tested, and 5 reacted to heptadecandienylresorcinol and 2 reacted to heptadecenylresorcinol. A chemical explanation for the crossreactivity was thus established.

Dang and Bell[243] reported an anaphylactic reaction to the ingestion of mango.

EGGPLANT

Hand dermatitis developed in a woman who had taken up the cultivation of eggplant (*Solanum melongena*). She was patch test positive to chopped leaves of the plant. Her dermatitis began 1 to 2 days after exposure to the plant and was independent of exposure to the fruit.[244]

LITCHI

Litchi or lichee or lychee (*Litchi chinensis*) is a fruit that has caused generalized urticaria, angioedema, and bronchospasm after ingestion. Positive prick tests to the mesocarp and epicarp were obtained in a 34-year-old woman who exhibited these symptoms. Additionally, a positive patch test was found to the epicarp. The patient also reacted to mango, which is in the Anacardiaceae family. Both litchi and mango are in the order Sapindales.[245]

WALNUT

Protein contact dermatitis due to immediate hypersensitivity to walnuts occurred in a baker who made walnut cakes. The presentation was chronic hand dermatitis and the prick test to walnut was positive. Oral exposure to walnuts caused dry mouth and sore throat. Reports of life-threatening food allergy to walnut have also been noted.[246]

PINEAPPLE

Pineapple juice contains bromelin, a proteolytic enzyme that can cause a primary irritant dermatitis.[247] The enzyme causes separation of the superficial layers of the skin and increases skin and capillary permeability. These effects resemble the mechanical damage produced by needle-shaped calcium oxalate crystals of tulip bulbs. Both the enzyme and the crystals produce itching and increased permeability of capillaries with the formation of wheals, which are suggestive of histamine liberation in the skin.

COFFEE

Lupton[248] described a persistent cheilitis due to coffee. In this instance, the coffee produced a positive patch test reaction on the skin. Green coffee-bean dust has been reported to cause Type I allergy in coffee manufacturing plants. It can also cause Type IV reactions and contact dermatitis. An electrician in a coffee plant was exposed to the dust, which collects on surfaces readily. He did not react to coffee grounds, roasted coffee beans, and extracted coffee beans, but only to the green bean dust.[249]

MALT FLOUR

Calnan[250] studied a 19-year-old woman who was working as a research assistant in an experimental test bakery. Once a week she used a malt flour. Patch tests were positive to malt flour on two occasions. Six control subjects were negative.

Calnan stated that cases of dermatitis from grain and flour are difficult to evaluate and quoted personal communications from Solomons, who described reactions to barley and oats, and from Malten, who described reactions to bran, maize, barley, vitamins, and beet pulp.

Hjorth[251] suggested that chefs and kitchen workers with dermatitis should be patch tested not only with the standard patch tests but also with the following foods: garlic, onions (various kinds), chives, leek, carrot, cucumber, horseradish, lemon peel, endive, lettuce, asparagus, and artichoke. Cinnamon might also be added to this list.

Botanical Nomenclature

Common names are used in this chapter, but this usage has limitations, particularly in countries where the common names vary. To assist the reader with the proper scientific names, the glossary developed by John Mitchell is provided in Table 21.20.[252]

This is a revision of a chapter written for the 3rd edition by A. A. Fisher and John C. Mitchell.

Table 21-20 Botanical Glossary

Common name	Genus, species	Family
Alstroemeria	*Alstroemeria aurantiaca*	Alstromeriaceae
Anemone	*Anemone* sp	Ranunculaceae
Angelica	*Angelica silvestris*	Umbelliferae
Angelica (garden)	*Angelica archangelica*	Umbelliferae
Arnica	*Arnica montana*	Compositae
Asparagus	*Asparagus officinalis*	Liliaceae
Burdock	*Arctium minus*	Compositae
Buttercup	*Ranunculus* sp	Ranunculaceae
Cabbage	*Brassica oleracea*	Cruciferae
Camomile, chamomile	*Matricaria chamomilla*	Compositae
Caper	*Capparis decidua*	Capparidaceae
Carrot	*Daucus carota*	Umbelliferae
Cashew nut tree	*Anacardium occidentale*	Anacardiaceae
Cauliflower	*Brassica oleracea botrytis*	Cruciferae
Celery	*Apium graveolens*	Umbelliferae
Chicory	*Cichorium intybus*	Compositae
Chrysanthemum of florists	*Chrysanthemum hortorum*	Compositae
Clematis	*Clematis* sp	Ranunculaceae
Congress weed	*Parthenium hysterophorus*	Compositae
Costus	*Saussurea lappa*	Compositae
Daffodil	See *Narcissus*	
Dock	*Rumex* sp	Polygonaceae
Endive	*Cichorium endivia*	Compositae
False ragweed	*Franseria* sp	Compositae
Feverfew	*Parthenium hysterophorus*	Compositae
Field chamomile	*Anthemis arvensis*	Compositae
Fig tree	*Ficus carica*	Moraceae
Frullania	*Frullania nisqualensis*	Jubulaceae
Garden cress	*Lepidium sativum*	Cruciferae
Gas plant, fraxinella	*Dictamnus albus*	Rutaceae
Gingko (ginkyo) tree	*Ginkgo biloba*	Ginkyoaceae
Horseradish	*Armoracia rusticana*	Cruciferae
Ivy, Algerian	*Hedera canariensis*	Araliaceae
Ivy, English	*Hedera helix*	Araliaceae
Jonquil	See *Narcissus*	
Laurel oil	*Laurus nobilis*	Lauraceae
Mango	*Mangifera indica*	Anacardiaceae
Maple	*Acer* sp	Aceraceae
Marsh elder	*Iva* sp	Compositae
Milfoil, Yarrow	*Achillea millefolium*	Compositae
Mugwort	*Artemisia* sp	Compositae
Mustard	*Brassica nigra, Sinapsis alba*	Cruciferae
Narcissus	*Narcissus* sp	Amaryllidaceae
Nettle	*Urtica* sp	Urticaceae
Norway spruce	*Picea excelsa*	Pinaceae
Ox-eye daisy	*Chrysanthemum leucanthemum*	Compositae
Parsley	*Petroselinum sativum*	Umbelliferae

From: Mitchell JC. Plant dermatitis in Vancouver. Can J Dermatol 1993;5:389. Used with permission.

References

1. Rook A. Plant dermatitis in general practice. *Practitioner* 1962;188:627.

2. Fisher AA. *Contact* Dermatitis, 3rd ed. Philadelphia: Lea & Febiger, 1986.

3. Goldstein N. The ubiquitous urushiols—contact dermatitis from mango, poison ivy, and other "poison" plants. Cutis 1968;6:679.

4. Kullavanijaya P, Ophaswongse S. A study of dermatitis in the lacquerware industry. Contact Dermatitis 1997;36:244.

5. Rademaker M, Duffill MB. *Toxicodendron succedaneum* (Rhus tree), New Zealand's poison ivy. Contact Dermatitis 1995;33:357.

6. Ale SI, Ferreira F, Gonzalez G, Epstein W. Allergic contact dermatitis caused by *Lithraea molleoides* and *Lithraea brasiliensis*: identification and characterization of the responsible allergens. Am J Contact Dermat 1997;8:144.

7. Kawai K, et al. Heat treatment of Japanese lacquerware renders it hypoallergenic. Contact Dermatitis 1992;27:244.

8. Kawai K, et al. Tetrahydrourushiol glycoside, o-monoglycosylated hydrourushiol, can be used for the investigation of contact allergy as a water-soluble urushiol. Contact Dermatitis 1994;31:59.

9. Farmer's Bulletin No. 2158, Chemical control of brush and trees. Washington, DC: US Department of Agriculture, US Government Printing Office.

10. Orchard S, Fellman JH, Storrs FJ. Poison ivy/oak dermatitis use of polyamine salts of a linolein acid dimer for topical prophylaxis. Arch Dermatol 1986;122:783.

11. Grevelink SA, Olsen EA. Efficacy of barrier creams in suppression of experimentally induced Rhus dermatitis. Am J Contact Dermat 1991;2:69.

12. Marks JG Jr, Fowler JF Jr, Sheretz EF, Rietschel RL. Prevention of poison ivy and poison oak allergic contact dermatitis by quaternium-18 bentonite. J Am Acad Dermatol 1995;33:212.

13. Gillis WT. Poison-ivy and its kin. Arnoldia 1975;35:93.

14. Guin JD. The black spot test for recognizing poison ivy and related species. J Am Acad Dermatol 1980;2:332.

15. Mallory SB, Miller OF, III, Tyler WB. Toxicodendron radicans dermatitis with black lacquer deposit on the skin. J Am Acad Dermatol 1982;6:363.

16. Kligman AM. Poison ivy (*Rhus*) dermatitis. Arch Dermatol 1974;90:535.

17. Gillis WT. Systematics and ecology of poison ivy and the poison oaks (Toxicodendron, Anacardiaceae). Rhodora 1971;73:72.

18. Shankar DSK. Contact urticaria induced by *Semecarpus anacardium*. Contact Dermatitis 1992;26:200.

19. Fisher AA. Poison ivy—the poison "Rhus" plants. Cutis 1966;2:316.

20. Epstein WL, Byers VS, Frankart W. Induction of antigen specific hyposensitization to poison oak in sensitized adults. Arch Dermatol 1982;118:630.

21. Cooley GR. The vegetation of Sanibel Island, Lee County, Florida. *Rhodora* 1955;57:268.

22. Farmer's Bulletin No. 1972, Poison ivy, poison oak and poison sumac. Washington, DC: US Department of Agriculture, US Government Printing Office, 1976.

23. Devich KB, et al. Renal lesions accompanying poison oak dermatitis. Clin Nephrol 1975;3:106.

24. Block SH. Rhus hyposensitization dermatitis. JAMA 1973;224:627.

25. Kawai K, et al. Hyposensitization to urishiol among Japanese lacquer craftsmen: results of patch test on students learning the art of lacquerware. Contact Dermatitis 1991;25:290.

26. Kawai K, et al. Hyposensitization to urishiol among Japanese lacquer craftsmen. Contact Dermatitis 1991;24:146.

27. Reginella RF, Fairfield JC, Marks JG, Jr. Hyposensitization to poison ivy after working in a cashew nut shell oil processing factory. Contact Dermatitis 1989;20:274.

28. Blumhardt R, Pappano JE, Moyer DG. Depression of poison ivy skin tests by measles vaccine. *JAMA* 1968;206:27.

29. Becker LE, Skipworth GB. Ginkgo tree dermatitis, stomatitis and proctitis. JAMA 1975;231:1162.

30. Mitchell JC, Rook AJ. Diagnosis of contact dermatitis from plants. Int J Dermatol 1977;16:257.

31. Fisher AA. The notorious poison ivy family of Anacardiaceae plants. Cutis 1977;20:570.

32. Morton JF. Brazilian pepper—its impact on people, animals and the environment. Economic Botany 1978;32:353.

33. Hurtado I, et al. Studies on the skin-sensitizing properties of the "pepeo" tree, *Mauria puberula* (Anacardiaceae). J Am Acad Dermatol 1982;7:341.

34. Mitchell JC, Dupuis G. Allergic contact dermatitis from sesquiterpenoids of the Compositae family of plants. Br J Dermatol 1971;84:139.

35. Mitchell JC, et al. Allergic contact dermatitis from ragweeds (*Ambrosia* species): the role of sesquiterpene lactones. Arch Dermatol 1971;104:73.

36. Hausen BM. A simple method of isolating parthenolide from Tanacetum and other sensitizing plants. Contact Dermatitis 1991;24:153.

37. Fitzgerald DA, English JSC. Compositae dermatitis presenting as hand eczema. Contact Dermatitis 1992;27:256.

38. Ducombs G, et al. Patch testing with the "sesquiterpene lactone mix": a marker for contact allergy to Compo-sitae and other sesquiterpene-lactone-containing plants. A multicentre study of the EECDRG. Contact Dermatitis 1990;22:249.

39. Hausen BM, et al. Peroxyachifolid and other new sensitizing sesquiterpene lactones from yarrow (*Achillae millefolium* L., Compositae). Contact Dermatitis 1991;24:274.

40. Lovell CR, Rowan M. Dandelion dermatitis. Contact Dermatitis 1991;25:185.

41. Pipker C, et al. Crossreactivity with *Tagetes* in *Arnica* contact eczema. Contact Dermatitis 1992;26:217.

42. Wrangsjo K, Ros AM, Walhlberg JE. Contact allergy to Compositae plants in patients with summer-exacerbated dermatitis. Contact Dermatitis 1990;22:148.

43. Mitchell JC. Allergy to *Frullania*. Arch Dermatol 1969;100:46.

44. Calnan CD. Dermatitis from cedar wood pencils. Trans St John Hosp Derm Soc 1972;58:43.

45. Rook A. Plant dermatitis: the significance of variety-specific sensitization. Br J Dermatol 1961;73:283.V

46. Curtis GH. Plant dermatitis. Va Med Monthly 1960;87:301.

47. Bleumink E, et al. Allergic contact dermatitis to garlic. Br J Dermatol 1972;87:6.

48. Cairns RJ. Plant dermatoses. Trans St John Hosp Derm Soc 1964;59:137.

49. Kligman AM. Poison ivy (*Rhus*) dermatitis. Arch Dermatol 1958;77:149.

50. Hjorth N, Fregert S, Schildknecht H. Cross-sensitization between synthetic primin and related quinones. Acta Derm Venereol (Stockh) 1969;49:552.

51. Puglisi V. Dermatoses caused by lemons. Gior Ital Derm e Sif 1951;92:239.

52. Pirila V., et al. Chemical nature of eczematogens in oils of turpentine: pattern of sensitivity to different terpenes. Dermatologica 1969;139;183.

53. Hjorth N. Eczematous allergy to balsams: allied perfumes and flavoring agents. Copenhagen: Munksgaard, 1961:134.

54. Fisher AA. The clinical significance of patch test reactions to balsam of Peru. Cutis 1976;13:910.

55. Hjorth N. Allergy to balsams. Spectrum 1971;8:97.

56. Pirila V. Endogenic contact eczema. Allerg Asthma 1970;16:1.

57. Veine NK. Systemically induced eczema in adults. Acta Derma Venereol [Suppl] 1989;147:9.

58. Jordan WP. Resorcinol monobenzoate, steering wheels, Peruvian balsam. Arch Dermatol 1973;108:278.

59. Jordan WP, Dahl MV. Contact dermatitis from cellulose ester plastics. Arch Dermatol 1972;105:880.

60. Karlberg A-T, et al. Maleopimaric acid—a potent sensitizer in modified rosin. Contact Dermatitis 1990;22:193.

61. Mitchell J, Rook A. Botanical dermatology. Vancouver: Greengrass, 1979.

62. Malten KE, Nater JP, van Ketel WG. Patch testing guidelines. Amsterdam: Dekker and van de Veg Nijmegen, 1976.

63. Ehrin E, Karlberg AT. Detection of rosin (colophony) components in technical products using an HPLC technique. Contact Dermatitis 1990;23:359.

64. Agrup G. Hand eczema and other hand dermatoses in South Sweden. Acta Derm Venereol (Stockh) 1969;49:1.

65. Kirk J. Colophony collar dermatitis. Contact Dermatitis 1976;2:294.

66. Fregert S. Colophony in cutting oil and in soap water used as cutting fluid. Contact Dermatitis 1979;5:52.

67. Adams RM. Occupational contact dermatitis. Philadelphia: JB Lippincott Co, 1969.

68. Wilkinson DS, Calnan CD. Rosin used for belt-drive machine. Contact Dermatitis 1975;1:64.

69. Satyawan I, Oranje AP, van Joost T. Perioral dermatitis in a child due to rosin in chewing gum. Contact Dermatitis 1990;22:182.

70. Wahlberg JE. Abietic add and colophony. Contact Dermatitis 1979;4:55.

71. Cronin E, Calnan CD. Allergy to hydroabietic alcohol in adhesive tape. Contact Dermatitis 1978;4:57.

72. Dooms-Goossens A, Degreef H, Luytens E. Dihydroabietyl alcohol (abitol): a sensitizer in mascara. Contact Dermatitis 1979;5:350.

73. Rapaport MJ. Sensitization to Abitol. Contact Dermatitis 1980;6:137.

74. Rasmussen JE, Fisher AA. Allergic contact dermatitis to a salicylic acid plaster. Contact Dermatitis 1976;2:237.

75. Fisher AA. Allergic contact termatitis in a violinist: the role of abietic acid sensitizer in rosin (colophony) as the causative agent. Cutis 1981;27:466.

76. Widstron L. Contact allergy to colophony in soldering flux. Contact Dermatitis 1983;9:205.

77. Bergmark G, Meding B. Allergic contact dermatitis from newsprint paper. Contact Dermatitis 1983;9:330.

78. Dahlquist I. Contact allergy to colophony and formaldehyde from sandcores. Contact Dermatitis 1981;7:167.

79. Fisher AA. Some plant chemicals that produce allergic reactions. Cutis 1977;20:441.

80. Fisher AA. Some immunologic phenomena in treatment of and patch testing for ragweed oil dermatitis. J Invest Dermatol 1952;19:271.

81. Hjorth N, Roed-Petersen J, Thomsen K. Airborne contact dermatitis from Compositae oleoresins simulating photodermatitis. Br J Dermatol 1976;95:613.

82. Green C, Ferguson J. Sesquiterpene lactone mix is not an adequate screen for Compositae allergy. Contact Dermatitis 1994;31:151.

83. Schumacher MJ, Silvis NG. Airborne contact dermatitis from *Ambrosia deltoidea* (triangle-leaf bursage). Contact Dermatitis 2003;48:212.

84. Paulsen E, Christensen LP, Andersen KE. Do monoterpenes released from feverfew (*Tanacetum parthenium*) plants cause airborne Compositae dermatitis? Contact Dermatitis 2002;47:14.

85. Howell JB. Contact dermatitis from weeds: facts and fallacies. Contact Dermatitis 1979;4:365.

86. Grater WC. Hypersensitivity dermatitis from American weeds, other than poison ivy. Ann Allergy 1975;35:159.

87. Burry NJ, Kuchel R, Reid KJ. Australian bush dermatitis: Compositae dermatitis in South Australia. Med J Aust 1973;1:110.

88. Crounse RG. Plant dermatitis due to the Compositae (Asteraceae) family. J Am Acad Dermatol 1980;2:417.

89. Arlette J, Mitchell JC. Compositae dermatitis: current aspects. Contact Dermatitis 1981;7:129.

90. Frain-Bell W, Johnson BE. Contact allergic sensitivity to plants and the photosensitivity dermatitis and actinic reticuloid syndrome. Br J Dermatol 1979;101:503.

91. Rietschel RL. Selected highlights of the European Contact Dermatitis Society meeting: Brussels, Belgium, October 8–10, 1992. Am J Contact Dermat 1993;4:66.

92. Mitchell JC, Calnan CD. Scourge of India: Parthenium dermatitis. Int J Dermatol 1978;17:303.

93. Lonkar A, Mitchell JC, Calnan CD. Allergic contact dermatitis from *Parthenium hysterophorus*. *Trans St John Hosp Derm Soc* 1974;60:43.

94. Shelmire B. Contact dermatitis from vegetation. South Med J 1940;33:338.

95. Rodriguez E, et al. Role of sesquiterpene lactones in contact sensitivity to some North and South American species of feverfew (Parthenium-Compositae). Contact Dermatitis 177;3:155.

96. Hausen BM. Allergy to parthenium, occupational and environmental dermatoses. Dermatosen 1978;26:115.

97. Fisher AA. Contact dermatitis due to American parthenium weed in India. Cutis 1979;23:20.

98. Mitchell JC. Parthenium pollen—parthenium dermatitis. Contact Dermatitis 1981;7:212.

99. Fisher AA. Safety of pyrethrin insecticides in ragweed sensitive patients. Contact Dermatitis 1978;22:141.

100. Feinberg SM. Pyrethrum sensitization—its importance and relation to pollen allergy. JAMA 1934;102:1557.

101. Mitchell JC, Dupuis G, Towers GHN. Allergic contact dermatitis from pyrethrum (*Chrysanthemum* spp). *Br J Dermatol* 1972;86:568.

102. Head SW. The quantitative determination of pyrethrins in gas-liquid chromatography. *Pyrethrum Post* 1966;8:3.

103. Hausen BM, Schulz KH. Experimental studies on the identification of chrysanthemum allergens. Contact Dermatitis 1975;4:244.

104. Mitchell JC, Schofield WB, Singh B, Towers GHN. Allergy to *Frullania*: allergic contact dermatitis occurring in forest workers caused by exposure to *Frullania nisquallensis*. *Arch Dermatol* 1969;100:46.

105. Storrs FJ, Mitchell JC, Rasmussen JE. Contact hypersensitivity to liverwort and the Compositae family of plants. *Cutis* 1976;18:681.

106. Tomb RR. Patch testing with *Frullania* during a 10-year period: hazards and complications. Contact Dermatitis 1992;26:220.

107. Bancons F. *L'Allergie au frullania: son role dans la "dermite du bois de chene."* Bordeaux, France: Thesis, 1967.

108. Salo H, Hannuksela M, Hausen B. Lichen picker's dermatitis [*Cladonia alpestris* (L.) Rab.]. Contact Dermatitis 1981;7:9.

109. Edwards EK Jr, Edwards EK Sr. Immediate and delayed hypersensitivity to the nettle plant. Contact Dermatitis 1992;27:264.

110. Camm EL, Gowers GHN, Mitchell JC. Ultraviolet-mediated antibiotic activity of some Compositae species. *Phytochemistry* 1975;14:2007.

111. Ashwood-Smith MJ, et al. Photosensitivity from harvesting lovage (*Levisticum officinale*). Contact Dermatitis 1992;26:356.

112. Ena P, Camarda I. Phytophotodermatitis from *Ruta corsica*. Contact Dermatitis 1990;22:63.

113. Ingber A. Primula photodermatitis in Israel. Contact Dermatitis 1991;25:265.

114. Knight TE, Boll P, Epstein WL, Prasad AK. Resorcinols and catachols: a clinical study of cross-sensitivity. Am J Contact Dermat 1996;7:138.

115. Julian CG, Bowers PW. The nature and distribution of daffodil pickers' rash. Contact Dermatitis 1997;37:259.

116. Giannattasio M, et al. Contact dermatitis from Tetrapanax papyriferum trichomes. Contact Dermatitis 1996;35:106.

117. Oka K, Saito F. Allergic contact dermatitis from *Dendropanax trifidus*. Contact Dermatitis 1999;41:350.

118. Oka K, Saito F, Yasuhara T, Sugimoto A. The major allergen of *Dendropanax trifidus* Makino. Contact Dermatitis 1997;36:252.

119. Machado S, Silva E, Massa A. Occupational allergic contact dermatitis from falcarinol. Contact Dermatitis 2002;47:113.

120. Oka K, Saito F, Yasuhara T, Sugimoto A. The allergens of *Dendropanax trifidus* Makino and *Fatsia japonica* Decne. et Planch. and evaluation of cross-reactions with other plants of the Araliaceae family. Contact Dermatitis 1999;40:209.

121. Fisher T. Bougainvillaea contact urticaria. Contact Dermatitis 1991;24:376.

122. van Hecke E, et al. Airborne contact dermatitis from coleus in a housewife. Contact Dermatitis 1991;25:128.

123. Kubo Y, Nonaka S, Yoshida H. Allergic contact dermatitis from gardenia fruit. Contact Dermatitis 1990;22:65.

124. Izu R, et al. Allergic contact dermatitis from cream containing *Centella asiatica* extract. Contact Dermatitis 1992;26:192.

125. Avenel-Audran M, Hausen BM, Le Sellin J, et al. Allergic contact dermatitis from hydrangea – is it so rare? Contact Dermatitis 2000;43:189.

126. Kuligowski ME, Chang A, Leemreize JHM. Allergic contact hand dermatitis from hydrangea: report of a 10th case. Contact Dermatitis 1992;26:269.

127. Meijer P, Coenraads PJ, Hausen BM. Allergic contact dermatitis from hydrangea [Comments]. Contact Dermatitis 1990;23:59.

128. Sharma SC, Kaur S. Contact dermatitis from Dahlia pinnata. Contact Dermatitis 1990;23:204.

129. Aberer W, Hausen BM. Active sensitization to elecampane by patch testing with a crude plant extract. Contact Dermatitis 1990;22:53.

130. Hausen BM, Helmke B. Butenylbithiophene, alphaterthienyl and hydroxytremetone as contact allergens in cultivars of marigold (*Tagetes* sp.). Contact Dermatitis 1995;33:33.

131. van Baar HMJ, van der Valk PGM. Contact allergy due to Trachelium caeruleum. Contact Dermatitis 1994;31:118.

132. Banerjee P, Rycroft RJG. A second florist with dermatitis from *Trachelium caeruleum*. Contact Dermatitis 2002;46:241.

133. Potter PC, et al. Immediate and delayed contact hypersensitivity to verbena plants. Contact Dermatitis 1995;33:343.

134. Estlander T, Kanerva L, Tupasela O, Jolanki R. Occupational contact urticaria and Type 1 sensitization caused by gerbera. Contact Dermatitis 1998;38:118.

135. Van der Waal RIF, Rustemeyer T, Kamphof WG, et al. Occupational allergic contact dermatitis and Type I sensitization caused by *Gerbera* in a greenhouse worker. Contact Dermatitis 2002;46:116.

136. Estrela F, Tapadinhas C, Pereira F. Allergic contact dermatitis from *Dittrichia viscosa* (L.) Greuter. Contact Dermatitis 1995;32:108.

137. Di Berardino L, Di Berardino F, Castelli A, et al. A case of contact dermatitis from jojoba. Contact Dermatitts 2006;55:57.

138. 138.Reider N, Issa A, Hawranek T, et al. Absence of contact sensitization to *Aloe vera* (L.) Burm. f. Contact Dermatitis 2005;53:332.

139. Majmudar V, Azam NAM, Finch T. Contact urticaria to *Cannabis sativa*. Contact Dermatitis 2006;54:127.

140. Woods B, Calnan CD. Toxic woods. *Br J Dermatol* 1976;94(Suppl 13):3.

141. Hausen BM. *Woods injurious to human health.* New York: Walter deGruyter, 1981.

142. Fisher AA, Bikowski J, Jr. Allergic contact dermatitis due to a wooden cross made of *Dalbergia Nigra*. Contact Dermatitis 1081;7:45.

143. Martin P, Bergoend H, Piette F. Erythema multiformelike eruption from Brazilian rosewood. Barcelona: 5th International Symposium on Contact Dermatitis, March 28, 1980.

144. Hausen BM, Rothenborg HW. Allergic contact dermatitis caused by olive wood jewelry. Arch Dermatol 1981;11:732.

145. Vidal C, Cabeza N. Contact urticaria due to eucalyptus pollen. Contact Dermatitis 1992;26:265.

146. de Groot AC, Weyland JW. Systemic contact dermatitis from tea-tree oil. Contact Dermatitis 1992;27:279.

147. Jolanki R, et al. Contact allergy to salicyl alcohol in aspen bark. Contact Dermatitis 1997;37:304.

148. Aalto-Korte K, Valimaa J, Henriks-Eckerman M-L, et al. Allergic contact dermatitis from salicyl alcohol and salicylaldehyde in aspen bark (*Populus tremula*). Contact Dermatitis 2005;52:93.

149. Hausen BM, Bruhn G, Koenig WA. New hydroxyisoflavans as contact sensitizers in cocus wood *Brya ebenus* DC (Fabaceae). Contact Dermatitis 1991;25:149.

150. van der Wegen-Keijser MH, Bruynzeel DP. Allergy to cane reed in a saxophonist. Contact Dermatitis 1991;25:268.

151. McFadden JP, Ingram MJ, Rycroft RJ. Contact allergy to cane reed in a clarinetist. Contact Dermatitis 1992;27:117.

152. Tanaka S, Matsumoto Y, Tamada Y. Allergic contact dermatitis due to perupok wood. Contact Dermatitis 2003;48:273.

153. Jemec GB, Hausen BM. Contact dermatitis from Brazilian box tree wood (*Aspidosperma* sp.) Contact Dermatitis 1991;25:58.

154. Pires MC, Manoel Silva dos Reis V, Mitelmann R, Moreira F. Pigmented contact dermatitis due to *Plathymenia foliosa* dust. Contact Dermatitis 1999;40:339.

155. Gamboa PM, et al. Allergic contact dermatitis from tali (missanda) wood (*Erythrophleum guianense*). Contact Dermatitis 1991;24:309.

156. Hausen BM, Bruhn G, Tilsley DA. Contact allergy to Australian blackwood (*Acacia melanoxylon* R. Br.): isolation and identification of new hydroxyflavan sensitizers. Contact Dermatitis 1990;23:33.

157. Dejobert Y, Martin P, Bergoend H. Airborne contact dermatitis from *Apuleia leiocarpa* wood. Contact Dermatitis 1995;32:242.

158. Meding B, Karlberg A-T, Ahman M. Wood dust from jelutong (*Dyera costulata*) causes contact dermatitis. Contact Dermatitis 1996;34:349.

159. Hausen BM, Knight TE, Milbrodt M. *Thespesia populnea* dermatitis. Am J Contact Dermat 1997;8:225.

160. Gonçalo S. Allergic contact dermatitis from *Bowdichia nitida* (sucupira) wood. Contact Dermatitis 1992;26:205.

161. Stingeni L, Mariotti M, Lisi P. Airborne allergic contact dermatitis from iroko (*Chlorophora excelsa*). Contact Dermatitis 1998;38:287.

162. Hinnen U, Willa-Craps C, Elsner P. Allergic contact dermatitis from iroko and pine wood dust. Contact Dermatitis 1995;33:428.

163. Kanerva L, Tuppurainen M, Keskinen H. Contact urticaria caused by obeche wood (*Triplochiton scleroxylon*). Contact Dermatitis 1998;38:170.

164. Munoz FJ, et al. Airborne contact urticaria due to mulberry (*Morus alba*) pollen. Contact Dermatitis 1995;32:61.

165. Oliwiecki S, Beck MH, Hausen BM. Occupational allergic contact dermatitis from caffeates in poplar bud resin in a tree surgeon. Contact Dermatitis 1992;27:127.

166. Gougerot H, Carteaud A. Les dermatoses professionelles. Paris: Norbert Maloine, 1952.

167. Burks JW. Classic aspects of onion and garlic dermatitis in housewives. Ann Allerg 1954;12:592.

168. Seligman EI, Key MM. Corn dermatitis. Arch Dermatol 1968;97:664.

169. Somner RG, Jillson OF. Phytophotodermatits (solar dermatitis from plants) gas plant and wild parsnip. N Engl J Med 1967;276:1484.

170. Klauder JV, Kimmich J. Sensitization to carrots. Arch Dermatol 1956;74:149.

171. Pigatto PD, et al. Ig-E-mediated contact and generalized urticaria from *Eruca sativa*. Contact Dermatitis 1991;25:191.

172. Potter TS, Hashimoto K. Butternut squash (Cucurbita moschata) dermatitis. Contact Dermatitis 1994;30:123.

173. Hausen BM, Wolf C. 1,2,3-trithiane-5-carboxylic acid, a first contact allergen from *Asparagus officinalis* (Liliaceae). Am J Contact Dermat 1996;7:41.

174. Zachariae COC. Cucumber contact dermatitis. Contact Dermatitis 2000;43:240.

175. Van Ketel WG, Mijnssen GAWV, Nerring H. Contact eczema from *Alstroemeria*. Contact Dermatitis 1975;1:323.

176. Mijnssen GAWV. Pathogenesis and causative agent of "tulip finger." Br J Dermatol 1969;81:737.

177. Merrick C, et al. A survey of skin problems in floristry. Contact Dermatitis 1991;24:306.

178. Hausen BM, Oestmann G. Untersuchungen über die Häufigkert berufsbedingter allergischer Hauter-Krangen auf einen Blumengrossmarkt. Dermatosen 1988;36:117.

179. Bajaj AK, et al. *Tabernaemontana coronaria* causing fingertip dermatitis. Contact Dermatitis 1996;35:104.

180. Mitchell JC. Contact dermatitis from plants of the caper family, Capparidaceae—effects on the skin of some plants which yield isothiocyanates. Br J Dermatol 1974;91:13.

181. Mitchell JC, Jordan WP. Allergic contact dermatitis from the radish, *Raphanus sativus*. Br J Dermatol 1974;91:183.

182. Kohl PK, Frosch PJ. Irritant contact dermatitis induced by a mustard compress. Contact Dermatitis 1990;23:189.

183. Angelini G, et al. Allergic contact dermatitis from *Capparis spinosa* L. applied as wet compresses. Contact Dermatitis 1991;24:382.

184. Ingber A, Menné T. Primin standard patch testing: 5 years' experience. Contact Dermatitis 1990;23:15.

185. Fregert S, Hjorth N, Schultz KH. Patch testing with synthetic primin in persons sensitive to *Primula obconica*. Arch Dermatol 1968;98:144.

186. Agrup G, et al. Routine patch testing with ether extract of *Primula obconica*. Br J Dermatol 1968;80:497.

187. Aplin C, Tan R, Lovell C. Allergic contact dermatitis from *Primula auricular* and *Primula denticulate*. Contact Dermatitis 2000;42:48.

188. Aplin CG, Lovell Cr. Contact dermatitis due to hardy primula species and their cultivars. Contact Dermatitis 2001;44:23.

189. Calka I, Akdeniz N, Metin A, et al. Phototoxic dermatitis due to *Chenopodium album* in a mother and son. Contact Dermatitis 2005;53:58.

190. Powell RF, Smith EB. Tumbleweed dermatitis. Arch Dermatol 1978;114:751.

191. Estrada JL, Gozalo F, Cecchini C, et al. Contact urticaria from hops (*Humulus lupulus*) in a patient with previous urticaria-angioedema from peanut, chestnut and banana. Contact Dermatitis 2002;46:127.

192. Gonçalo M, Couto J, Gonçalo S. Allergic contact dermatitis from *Nicotiana tabacum*. Contact Dermatitis 1990;22:188.

193. Brazzelli V, Romano E, Balduzzi A, Borroni G. Acute irritant contact dermatitis from *Agave americana* L. Contact Dermatitis 1995;33:60.

194. Salinas ML, Ogura T, Soffchi L. Irritant contact dermatitis caused by needle-like calcium oxalate crystals, raphides, in *Agave tequilana* among workers in tequila distilleries and agave plantations. Contact Dermatitis 2001;44:95.

195. Sanchez-Morillas L. Contact dermatitis due to Dieffenbachia. Contact Dermatitis 2005;53:172.

196. Hammershoy O, Verdich J. Allergic contact dermatitis from *Philodendron scandens* Koch et Sello subsp. oxycardium (Schott) bunting ("Philodendron scandens cordatum"). Contact Dermatitis 1980;6:95.

197. Mitchell JC, Rook A. Scindapsus dermatitis. Contact Dermatitis 1976;2:125.

198. Reynolds G, et al. A potent contact allergen of *Phacelia* (Hydrophyllaceae). Contact Dermatitis 1980;6:272.

199. Hausen BM, Schulz KH. Occupational allergic contact dermatitis due to leatherleaf fern *Arachnoides adiantiformis* (Forst) Tindale. Br J Dermatol 1978;98:325.

200. de Cock PAJJM, Vorwerk H, Bruynzeel DP. Hand dermatitis caused by ferns. Contact Dermatitis 1998;39:324.

201. Tafelkruver J, van Ketel WG. Sensitivity to *Codiaeum variegatum*. Contact Dermatitis 1976;2:288.

202. Pigatto PD, Persichini P, Kokelj F, et al. A new case of pseudophytodermatitis: allergic contact dermatitis from nickel in an ornamental plant (*Euphorbia triangularis*). Contact Dermatitis 2002;46:354.

203. Hausen BM, Schulz KH. Occupational contact dermatitis due to Croton (Codiaeum variegatum [1] A. Juss var. pictum [Lodd] Muell Arg.): sensitization by plants of the Euphorbiaceae. Contact Dermatitis 1977;3:289.

204. Fortina AB, Magno FM, Cappelletti EM, et al. Contact dermatitis from *Vernonia noveboracensis*. Contact Dermatitis 2002;46:357.

205. Wong WK, Ng SK, Goh CL. Grass allergy among national servicemen in Singapore: a preliminary report. Contact Dermatitis 1994;30:108.

206. Koh D, et al. Allergic contact dermatitis from grass. Contact Dermatitis 1997;37:32.

207. van Ketel WG. Allergic contact dermatitis from a new pesticide. Contact Dermatitis 1975;1:297.

208. Guin J. Patch testing to plants: some practical aspects of what has become an esoteric area of contact dermatitis. Am J Contact Dermat 1995;6:232.

209. Benezra C. Allergänes vegetaux. Mëthodes chimiques d'isolement et d'identification. Rev Fr Allergol 1973;13:51.

210. Nettis E, Giordano D, Soccio AL, et al. Frequency of contact allergy to Compositae extracts in patients with atopic dermatitis. Contact Dermatitis 2002;47:169.

211. Rosengarten F. The book of spices. Wynnewood, PA: Livingston Publishing Co, 1969.

212. Schwartz I, Tulipan L, Birmingham DJ. Occupational diseases of the skin, 2nd ed. Philadelphia: Lea & Febiger, 1957.

213. van den Akker TW, Roesyanto-Mahadi ID, van Toorenenbergen AW, van Joot T. Contact allergy to spices. Contact Dermatitis 1990;22:267.

214. Fisher AA. Dermatitis due to tear gases (lacrimators). Derm Int 1970;9:91.

215. Gleason MN, et al. Clinical toxicology of commercial products, 3rd ed. Baltimore: Williams & Wilkins, 1969.

216. Ormsby OS, Montgomery H. Diseases of the skin, 8th ed. Philadelphia: Lea & Febiger, 1954.

217. Kern AB. Contact dermatitis from cinnamon. Arch Dermatol 1960;87:599.

218. Leifer W. Contact dermatitis due to cinnamon. Arch Dermatol 1951;64:52.

219. Fisher AA. Systemic eczematous "contact-type" dermatitis medicamentosa. Ann Allergy 1966;24:415.

220. Rasheed A, et al. Eugenol and prostaglandin biosynthesis [Letter]. N Engl J Med 1984;310:50.

221. Fisher AA. Mace—modern acronym and an ancient nomenclature [Letter]. JAMA 1970;212:320.

222. Goransson L, et al. Some cases of eugenol hypersensitivity. Derm Venereol Tandlak T 1967;60:545.

223. Gaul LE. Dermatitis of the hands from oil of cloves. Skin 1963;2:413.

224. Gaul LE. Contact dermatitis from synthetic oil of mustard. Arch Dermatol 1964;90:158.

225. Matheson R. Medical entomology, 2nd ed. Ithaca, NY: Comstock Publishing Co, 1950.

226. Foussereau J, et al. Contact dermatitis from laurel: I. Clinical aspects. Trans St John Hosp Derm Soc 1967;53:141.

227. Spiewak R, Skorska C, Dutkiewicz J. Occupational airborne contact dermatitis caused by thyme dust. Contact Dermatitis 2001;44:235.

228. Armisen M, Rodriguez V, Vidal C. Photoaggravated allergic contact dermatitis due to *Rosmarinum officinalis* cross-reactive with *Thymus vulgaris*. Contact Dermatitis 2003;48:52.

229. Lembo G, et al. Allergic contact dermatitis due to garlic (*Allium sativum*). Contact Dermatitis 1991;25:330.

230. Lee TY, Lam TH. Contact dermatitis due to topical treatment with garlic in Hong Kong. Contact Dermatitis 1991;24:193.

231. Rinkel HJ, Balyeat RM. Occupational dermatitis due to lettuce. JAMA 1932;98:137.

232. Closson JB. Oral allergy after lettuce ingestion (questions and answers). JAMA 1974;230:113.

233. Oliwiecki S, Beck MH, Hausen BM. Compositae dermatitis aggravated by eating lettuce. Contact Dermatitis 1991;24:318.

234. Veraldi S, Schianchi-Veraldi R. Contact urticaria from kiwi fruit. Contact Dermatitis 1990;22:244.

235. Korstanje MJ, van de Staak WJM. A case of hand dermatitis due to mushrooms. Contact Dermatitis 1990;22:115.

236. Nakamura T. Shiitake (*Lentinus edodes*) dermatitis [published erratum appeared in Dermatitis 1992;27:351]. Contact Dermatitis 1992;27:65.

237. Ueda A, et al. Allergic contact dermatitis in shiitake (*Lentinus edodes* [Berk] Sing) growers. Contact Dermatitis 1992;26:228.

238. Rosina P, Cheiregato C, Schena D. Allergic contact dermatitis from *Pleurotus* mushroom. Contact Dermatitis 1995;33:277.

239. Kanerva L, Estlander T, Jolanki R. Airborne occupational allergic contact dermatitis from champignon mushroom. Am J Contact Dermat 1998;9:190.

240. McGeorge BC, Steele MC. Allergic contact dermatitis of the nipple from Roman chamomile ointment. Contact Dermatitis 1991;24:139.

241. Hershko K, Weinberg I, Ingber A. Exploring the mango-poison ivy connection: the riddle of discriminative plant dermatitis. Contact Dermatitis 2005;52:3.

242. Oka K, Saito F, Yasuhara T, et al. A study of crossreactions between mango contact allergens and urushiol. Contact Dermatitis 2004;51:292.

243. Dang RW, Bell DB. Anaphylactic reaction to the ingestion of mango. Hawaii Med J 1967;27:149.

244. Kabashima K, Miyachi Y. Contact dermatitis due to eggplant. Contact Dermatitis 2004;50:101.

245. Giannattasio M, et al. Contact urticaria from litchi fruit (*Litchi chinensis* Sonn.). Contact Dermatitis 1995;33:67.

246. Mendonca C, Madan V, Austin S, et al. Occupational contact urticaria from walnut associated with hand eczema. Contact Dermatitis 2005;53:173.

247. Polunin I. Pineapple dermatoses. Br J Dermatol 1951;63:441.

248. Lupton ES. Cheilitis due to coffee. Arch Dermatol 1961;84:798.

249. Diba VC, English JSC. Contact allergy to green coffee bean dust in a coffee processing plant worker. Contact Dermatitis 2002;47:56.

250. Calnan CD. Malt flour dermatitis. Contact Dermatitis Newsletter 1973;14390.

251. Hjorth N. Battery for testing of chefs and other kitchen workers. Contact Dermatitis 1975;2:63.

252. Mitchell JC. Plant dermatitis in Vancouver. Can J Dermatol 1993;5:389.

PHOTOCONTACT DERMATITIS

EXECUTIVE SUMMARY

The diagnosis of photocontact dermatitis is much like that of "ordinary" contact dermatitis, except for the requirement for UV light (or rarely visible light) exposure in addition to contact with an allergen or irritant. Phototoxic (photoirritant) contact dermatitis occurs when a chemical that is altered by UV wavelengths into something capable of directly damaging the skin is present on the skin surface during UV exposure. The foremost example of this is the psoralen family of substances found in various plants. The resulting skin damage is similar to a sunburn and does not require immunologic activity to occur. Anyone can suffer the reaction on first exposure. In contrast, photoallergic contact dermatitis (photo-ACD), like "ordinary" ACD, will occur only after a person has become sensitized to an allergen produced as a result of the effects of UV light on a precursor chemical.

In the past, fragrances have been the most common causes of photo-ACD, but currently sunscreen chemicals hold the spotlight. The clinical appearance is more like ACD than a sunburn, but is found predominantly in sun exposed areas. Just as the diagnosis of ICD is made based on the knowledge of exposure patterns and clinical findings, so is the diagnosis of phototoxic contact dermatitis made. For the diagnosis of photo-ACD to be made, photopatch testing is needed. The differential diagnosis of photocontact dermatitis includes systemic photoallergic or phototoxic dermatitis along with a variety of autoimmune and metabolic conditions, which will not be discussed in this text.

Dermatologic conditions resulting from exposure to light can occur in several forms and can be caused by both local and systemic processes. The differential diagnosis of a photosensitive eruption includes autoimmune diseases, such as lupus erythematosus, metabolic alterations, such as the porphyrias, photosensitivity caused by internal or external exposure to photoactive agents, and diseases of unknown mechanisms such as polymorphous light eruption and chronic actinic dermatitis. In addition, "regular" contact dermatitis can occur in a photodistribution. For example, allergy to a sunscreen chemical can give this clinical pattern. Airborne ACD can mimic photoallergy. For the purposes of this text, this chapter will concentrate on reactions to topically encountered agents, realizing that there is often overlap with systemic photosensitivity. The other cutaneous photosensitivity reactions are reviewed in several texts and articles.[1–4]

Photocontact dermatitis may be divided into two broad categories, photoallergic and phototoxic dermatitis, depending on whether the reaction is immune mediated or not. It may be difficult clinically to distinguish between the two, and sometimes a chemical can cause both types of reactions. Table 22.1 lists characteristics helpful in separating photoallergic and phototoxic reactions.

In either case, by definition, light energy, along with exposure to the chemical in question, is required to produce a reaction. It should be noted, however, that some chemicals are able to act as regular allergens as well as photoallergens. Although direct sunlight (ultraviolet light) is almost always needed to produce a photoreaction, occasionally artificial light sources may be sufficient.[5]

Photocontact dermatitis reached the proportions of a mini-epidemic in the 1960s in the United States, Europe, and Australia. Thousands of individuals developed photosensitivity after exposure to antibacterial agents in soaps and other cleaning products.[6,7] Fortunately, the causative agents were eventually recalled by the U.S. Food and Drug Administration and other regulatory agencies.

Since the 1980s, a shift has occurred to new agents causing photodermatitis. Sunscreen agents and fragrances have been responsible for the majority of photoallergic reactions in the last decades.[8–12] The plant-derived furocoumarins remain as the most frequent cause of

Table 22-1 Characteristics of Contact Photosensitivity: Phototoxic and Photoallergic Reactions

Characteristics	Reaction	
	Phototoxic	Photoallergic
Incidence low	Usually relatively high (theoretically 100%)	Usually
Clinical manifestations morphology	Usually resemble sunburn	Varied
Possibility of reaction on first exposure	Yes	No
Incubation period after first exposure	No	Yes
Development of persistent light reaction	No	Yes
Possibility of "flares" at distant previously involved sites	No	Yes
Cross-reactions to structurally related agents	No	Frequent
Broadening of cross-reactions following repeated photopatch testing	No	Possible
Concentration of drug necessary for reaction	High	Low
Chemical alteration of photosensitizer	Sometimes	Yes
Covalent binding with carrier protein	No	Yes
Cellular passive transfer abolition with anti-T-cell sera	No	Possible
Lymphocyte stimulation test	No	Possible
Macrophage migration inhibition test	No	Possible

phototoxic reactions. In some countries where topical nonsteroidal anti-inflammatory drugs (NSAIDs) are used, the NSAIDs have caused frequent phototoxicity and some photoallergy.[9]

Clinical Features of Photodermatitis

Exposed areas, such as the face, the V of the neck, the back of the hands, and the dorsal forearms, are the most frequent sites of contact photodermatitis. Any skin area receiving sufficient light and a photosensitizing chemical, however, may develop a reaction. The scalp and other densely hairy areas, the periorbital areas, and the skin immediately under the chin are rarely involved. When lesions are present on the forearms, the extensor and radial aspects are almost always the most extensively involved. The cubital fossae are frequently spared. Sharply demarcated areas of involvement may appear below the sleeves. Photodermatitis from sunlight exposure, while driving an automobile with a left-hand drive, affects the left side of the face and the uncovered left arm and forearm most severely, and therefore such a photodermatitis may present in a unilateral pattern.

Phototoxic reactions often resemble sunburn and are limited invariably to areas exposed to light. Many types of reaction patterns, however, can occur. The eruption may be eczematous, bullous, or fissured, may resemble lichen planus, or may mimic lupus erythematosus. Phototoxic dermatitis usually disappears promptly when the photocontactant is avoided. The eruption is rarely persistent. Dermatitis that is limited to, or occurs predominantly on, areas exposed to light should be investigated for the possibility of being a photosensitive reaction. Dermatitis due to airborne contactants can closely simulate photodermatitis, but usually affects shaded areas such as the anterior neck as well as exposed areas.

Phototoxic Contact Dermatitis

Phototoxic contact dermatitis can occur in virtually anyone upon first exposure to the phototoxin and under appropriate conditions, such as sufficient intensity of light (Table 22.2). Phototoxic reactions are not dependent on immunologic mechanisms, and therefore previous sensitization is not required for expression of the condition. Phototoxicity is clinically similar to a severe sunburn, with severe blistering reactions possible.

Each compound causing a photocontact dermatitis will absorb only specific wavelengths of light. Its absorption spectrum is determined by its chemical structure. This spectrum usually closely approximates the wavelengths responsible for the clinical reaction, the so-called action spectrum. Most phototoxic sensitizers have an action spectrum in the ultraviolet band between 280 and 430 nm. Certain dyes, however, such as eosin photosensitize in the visible light region. Window glass, which usually absorbs ultraviolet radiation of wavelengths shorter than 320 nm, will protect

Table 22-2 Topically Encountered Phototoxic Drugs and Chemicals

Coal-tar derivatives
    Acridine
    Anthracene
    Phenanthrene
Drugs
    Phenothiazines
    Sulfonamides
Dyes
    Anthraquinone
    Eosin
    Methylene blue
    Rose bengal
Plant derivatives—furocoumarins
    Psoralens
    Dictamnin

Table 22-3 Common Plants in the United States Known to Cause Phytophotodermatitis

Family	Botanical name	Common name
Compositae	Achillea millefolium	Milfoil, yarrow
	Anthemis cotula	Stinking mayweed
Umbelliferae	Angelica gigas	Angelica
	Ammi majus	False bishop's weed
	Anthriscus sylvestris	Cow parsley, wild chervil
	Apium graveolens dulce	Celery
	Daucus carota	Carrot
	Foeniculum vulgare	Fennel
	Heracleum lanatum	Cow parsnip
	Heracleum mantegazzianum	Giant hogweed, wild parsnip
	Pastinaca sativa	Parsnip
	Petroselinum crispum	Parsley
Papilionaceae	Psoralea corylifolia	Psoralen
Rutaceae	Citrus aurantifolia, begamia	Lime, bergamot lime
	Citrus limon	Lemon
	Citrus sinensis	Orange
	Dictamnus albus	Gas plant, burning bush, fraxinella
	Cneoridium dumosum	Coast spice bush
	Pelea anisata	Mokihana
	Ruta graveolens	Rue
Moraceae	Ficus carica	Fig

Partially adapted from Bowers[13]

patients from those phototoxic reactions that have an action spectrum below 320 nm, but fails to protect against photosensitizers with a higher action spectrum such as tar and the psoralens that produce most cases of phototoxic contact dermatitis.[5]

PHYTOPHOTODERMATITIS DUE TO FUROCOUMARINS IN PLANTS

When a phototoxic chemical is contacted by exposure to a plant, vegetable, or fruit, the resulting photodermatitis is referred to as phytophotodermatitis. Bowers[13] in a fine review of this topic, stated that as early as 1500 B.C. Egyptians used an extract from *Ammi majus* to treat vitiligo. This plant, called false bishop's weed, is a commonly seen member of the Umbelliferae family.

The most common presentation of phytophotodermatitis is linear streaks of pruritic dermatitis on sun-exposed skin surfaces. Depending on the degree of exposure to the offending plant and the level of sun exposure, painful blisters may occur. Marked hyperpigmentation develops after the acute phase heals. This usually resolves slowly after several months without sequelae. Perhaps the most commonly seen phytophotodermatitis is from limes served with beer or mixed drinks consumed in sunny areas. Wagner et al reported a case and noted that Bergapten was the most prevalent phototoxin in the lime rind.[14] Levels of furocoumarins psoralen, xanthotoxin, isopimpinellin, and limettin were also seen, and occurred in the rind at levels 20–100 times greater than in the pulp. Common phototoxic plants are listed in Table 22.3. Phytophotodermatitis is caused primarily by furocoumarin compounds, which are present in the plants. These phototoxic substances are lipid-soluble and penetrate into the epidermis with ease. Absorption of psoralens into the skin is enhanced by high humidity.[15] The most common phototoxins are activated by UVA radiation (320–400 nm).

Occupational phytophotodermatitis has been described in individuals exposed to the oil of limes and in carrot processors and celery pickers (Tables 22.3 and 22.4).[16]

Table 22-4 Occupations at Risk for Phytophotodermatitis

Occupation	Photosensitizer
Bartenders	Persian limes, lemons
Cannery packers	Celery, figs, carrots
Dairy workers	Parsnips
Vegetable harvesters, produce workers	Fennel, parsley, celery, dill, parsnips, carrots
Farmers	Many weeds
Cooks	Fruits and vegetables noted above

Therapeutically, psoralens, purified from plant materials or synthetically produced, have become common agents in the treatment of many cutaneous diseases, most notably psoriasis and vitiligo. Photochemotherapy utilizes either topical or systemic psoralens and ultraviolet radiation in the UVA (320–400 nm) range and is referred to as PUVA.[17]

Berloque Dermatitis

Certain clinical manifestations of phytophotodermatitis have been given specific names, such as Berloque dermatitis and meadow grass dermatitis. Berloque dermatitis is produced at sites exposed to a combination of certain perfumes and sunlight. The streaky erythema of the eruption is followed by pigmentation. Oil of bergamot, containing bergapten (5-methoxy-psoralen), is probably the principal cause of photodermatitis produced by perfumes and toilet waters.[18,19]

Phytophotodermatitis from Wild or Cultivated Plants

Farmworkers are probably the most likely group to be at risk for phytophotodermatitis. A major outbreak involving 11 people occurred while weeding parsnips by hand on an "organic" farm. Surreptitious use of pesticides was suspected before the true diagnosis was established.[20] Lovage and angelica have caused reactions in workers.[21,22] In Hawaii, the Mokihana bush (Pelea arisata), which grows in the mountains of Kauai, is a common cause of phytophotodermatitis.[23] The berries are used to make garlands.

Meadow grass dermatitis (dermatitis bullosa striata pratensis), another example of phytophotodermatitis, is produced by contact of the skin with meadow grass and subsequent exposure to sunlight. The eruption is a phototoxic reaction characterized by bizarre, criss-cross, linear streaks of erythema and vesicles or bullae, which heal with hyperpigmentation. The photosensitizing agent is not grass, but is either the yellow-flowered wild meadow parsnip, which belongs to the carrot family, or a common wild yellow-flowered herb of the rose family. The skin of individuals who sunbathe in meadows may become impregnated with the juices of these weeds or wild flowers containing furocoumarins. Subsequent exposure to sunlight produces the phototoxic dermatitis.

Occasionally, the bites of chiggers or other arthropods infesting grass may produce a pseudo-phytophotodermatitis that may be confused with meadow grass dermatitis. Itching is more intense and pigmentation is less marked in dermatitis produced by arthropods than in meadow grass dermatitis.

The gas plant (Dictamnus alba) has been reported to cause typical phytophotodermatitis in gardeners. In addition to psoralens, it contains an alkaloid, dictamnin, which is also a phototoxin.[24]

The coast spice bush or berry rue (Cneoridium dumosum) is a common plant in southern California and Mexico, usually growing in dry areas below 2,500 ft elevation.[25] This member of the Rutaceae family is a slender branched evergreen shrub growing 3 to 5 ft tall, with white flowers and red berries. Exposure to this plant during a field trip caused photodermatitis with severe blistering in two naturalists and multiple students. The vesicular dermatitis was experimentally reproduced later in a volunteer, with minimal exposure to the plant.[25]

Wild spinach, Chenopodium album, caused two cases of systemic (from eating the plants) phototoxic dermatitis in Turkey.[26] The plant was freshly cooked and the afflicted persons performed farming work in the sun for at least 2 hours after the meal. One of the patients required a month of hospitalization, but recovered completely.

An Italian couple applied a homemade extract of freshly ground fig leaves (Moraceae family) and sunbathed, in an effort to produce a quick tan.[27] Instead of a quick tan they received a severe burn, with an ensuing 2 weeks in hospital.

PHOTOTOXIC TAR DERMATITIS

Coal-tar derivatives are common photosensitizers. At least 400 compounds have been isolated from coal tar, many of which are used in diverse industries, including the manufacture of drugs, dyes, perfumes, synthetic resins, explosives, insecticides, and disinfectants. The known active photosensitizers of coal tar are acridine, anthracene, benzpyrene, phenanthrene, and pyridene. Wood tars generally are not photosensitizers and do not contain any of these photosensitizing chemicals. The action spectrum for coal-tar contact photosensitivity is in the 320 to 430 nm range.

Photodermatitis due to tar and pitch may appear as a severe sunburn referred to as "flashes" and "smarts" in workers exposed to tar, pitch, or creosote and sunlight. Actual contact with pitch or creosote is not necessary for the production of a photosensitive reaction, because the volatile fumes emanating from these products when heated can produce a photodermatitis. Moderate to marked pigmentation may occur at the sites of tar photodermatitis. In one series, 70% of white workers exposed to pitch fumes were affected, whereas black workers were not affected.[28] The increased pigmentation of the skin of black workers proved to be protective against pitch photosensitivity. Smarting and erythema may continue 1 to 3 days after exposure to pitch fumes. There may be a latent period of 2 weeks or more between the initial exposure to pitch fumes and the appearance of photosensitivity.

The ability of coal-tar derivatives to cause photosensitivity contributes to the treatment of psoriasis using the classic Goeckerman therapy.

Photoallergic Contact Dermatitis

Photoallergic contact dermatitis is similar to "regular" delayed hypersensitivity in that the pathogenesis is a T-cell-mediated immunologic response (Table 22.5). The concentration of the allergen needed to elicit a photoallergic reaction is often lower than that needed to produce a phototoxic reaction, and there is no clinical reaction on first exposure. Some photoallergens, especially sunscreens and fragrances, can also produce "ordinary" ACD in the absence of light.

Clinical differentiation between photoallergic and phototoxic contact dermatitis may be difficult at times. The criteria in Table 22.1 may be helpful in distinguishing between the two types.

PHOTO-ACD TO ANTISEPTICS AND DISINFECTANTS

A widespread outbreak of photoallergic reactions to topically encountered agents resulted from the use of soaps and cleansers containing halogenated salicylanilides and related compounds. Although most of these substances are no longer used in consumer products in the United States and in Western Europe, patients are

Table 22-5 Topically Encountered Photoallergenic Drugs and Chemicals
Antifungal agents
Fragrances
Methylcoumarin
Musk ambrette
Halogenated salicylanilides
Medications
Phenothiazines
Sulfonamides
NSAIDs
Sunscreens
Benzophenones
Cinnamates
Dibenzoylmethanes
Others-see text
Whiteners
Stilbenes
Others- see text

occasionally encountered with "persistent light reactions" initiated by these agents 20 or more years ago. They should, therefore, be considered as possible etiologic agents in the differential diagnosis of photosensitivity. These compounds should also be included in the group of antigens used in routine patch testing procedures.

TETRACHLOROSALICYLANILIDE (TCSA: IMPREGON)

In Great Britain, many instances of photodermatitis were reported from exposure to soap containing TCSA.[29,30] In a small U.S. market test of a product containing 0.5% tetrachlorosalicylanilide, several instances of photosensitization were reported and verified by patch tests.[31] The individuals developed intense itching and erythema in areas exposed to the sun. In some instances, papules and vesicles also appeared. This agent is still available in the United States as a surface disinfectant and mold inhibitor.

TRIBROMOSALICYLANILIDE (TBS)

This antiseptic was a favorite deodorant agent in many soaps and detergents and produced allergic photocontact dermatitis from its presence in Lifebuoy, Safeguard, and Praise soaps.[32]

DIBROMSALAN (4,5 -DIBROMOSALICYLANILIDE; DBS)

This chemical, which was present in Lifebuoy soap, also caused photoallergic contact dermatitis.

TRICHLOROCARBANILIDE (TCC)

This agent, used in the past in Dial, Zest, and Safeguard soaps, is a potent photosensitizer.[33]

There are numerous reports in the literature of these halogenated salicylanilides and related chemicals producing photodermatitis.[34–36]

JADIT (CHLOROSALICYLAMIDE)

This antifungal agent with the formula 4-chlorohydroxybenzoic acid-*n*-butilamide, used in Australia and Europe, can cause a photoallergic reaction that may be persistent. The photosensitizing action is probably related to that of the halogenated salicylanilides.[37]

BITHIONOL (BISPHENOL, ACTAMAR)

Bithionol, 2–29-thiobis (4,6-dichlorophenol), is a bacteriostatic agent related to hexachlorophene. It can produce both ordinary and photoallergic dermatitis. Bithionol often shows cross-reactions not only to the hexachlorophene but also to the halogenated salicylanilides.[38–40]

HEXACHLOROPHENE

This formerly widely used halogenated phenol antiseptic rarely produces ordinary contact allergy. Cross-contact sensitivity and photocontact sensitivity to hexachlorophene have been observed in guinea pigs with primary photosensitivity to tetrachlorosalicylanilide and tribromosalicylanilide.[6] It is not certain whether hexachlorophene is a primary photosensitizer, although such photosensitivity has been reported.[35]

CROSS-REACTION BETWEEN BITHIONOL, HEXACHLOROPHENE, AND THE HALOGENATED SALICYLANILIDES

Cross-reaction may occur with tetrachlorosalicylanilide and tribromosalicylanilide, and bithionol is apparently a primary photosensitizer engendering cross-sensitivity to both. Reactions to hexachlorophene in patients with contact photodermatitis from bithionol not requiring any light represent cross-sensitivity between a photosensitizer and a simple contact allergen.

FENTICHLOR [BIS(2-HYDROXY-5 -CHLOROPHENYL) SULFIDE] AND BROMOSALICYLCHLORANILIDE (MULTIFUNGIN, 5-BROMO-49 -CHLOROSALICYLANILIDE)

These topical antifungal agents, used in Australia, are photoallergens. Fentichlor, chemically related to bithionol, also cross-reacts with hexachlorophene.

A number of positive patch test reactions are seen to Fentichlor that defy clinical explanation. Multifungin is chemically related to tribromosalicylanilide, with which it cross-reacts.[41,42]

Photoallergic Contact Dermatitis to Medicaments

PHENOTHIAZINE AND ITS DERIVATIVES

Phenothiazine and derivatives are used as insecticides and as an anthelmintic in human and veterinary medicine, as well as antipsychotic agents. It is a parent substance for methylene blue, a dye that is a powerful photosensitizer.[43]

Orchard workers using phenothiazine as an insecticide against moths exhibited photosensitivity. Because many individuals were involved, it was presumed that the reaction was one of phototoxicity rather than of photoallergy.[43]

Chlorpromazine (Thorazine)

Allergic photocontact dermatitis occurs principally among medical and nursing personnel who contaminate their hands while injecting the drug.[44,45] Those receiving the drug systemically may acquire a phototoxic dermatitis.

Promethazine Hydrochloride (Phenergan)

This antihistamine can also produce phototoxic and photoallergic reactions. In France, where Phenergan Cream was used extensively as a topical antipruritic, many instances of photocontact dermatitis occurred. Photosensitivity seems to be induced primarily by contact with promethazine, whereas systemic administration without topical application does not appear to induce photosensitivity.[46,47] Cross-photosensitivity may occur between promethazine and chlorpromazine.[47]

Many phenothiazine compounds can also produce ordinary ACD. Cross-reactions between the phenothiazine compounds may include both the photoallergic and the ordinary allergic variety. Sometimes the cross-reactivity extends only to the photoallergic phenomenon.[48]

More recently, dioxopromethazine (in Prothanon Gel), used topically for pruritus, has been reported.[49] The acute episode was followed by development of persistent light reactivity for over 1.5 years. Cross-photoreactivity occurred to promethazine but not to chlorpromazine.

NON-STEROIDAL ANTI-INFLAMMATORY DRUGS

Topical NSAIDs may cause ACD or photo-ACD. Since first reported in 1985, ketoprofen and its derivatives have been the most common photosensitizing NSAIDs.[50] Photo-ACD is due to the benzophenone moiety in these drugs.[51] Photopatch-testing to these drugs is recommended at a concentration of 1% or 2% in petrolatum.[52] A report from Sweden gives details on 35 patients with positive photopatch tests to ketoprofen (1% ethanol).[53] Almost all reacted to the commercial topical medication as well. A large number of these patients also had positive photopatch tests to fenticlor, fenofibrate, and tetrachlorosalicylanilide. Since the chemical structures are similar, this was presumably cross-reactivity.

Diclofenac (Solareze Gel) topically has been used for treatment of actinic keratoses. Both ACD and photo-ACD have been reported to this agent.[54]

SULFANILAMIDE

This antibacterial agent can apparently produce both phototoxic and photoallergic reactions.[55] Phototoxic reactions are also produced by systemic administration of the drug. Window glass usually protects the individual from such phototoxic reactions. However, the topical application of sulfanilamide preparations may engender photoallergic contact sensitivity. Fortunately, topical sulfanilamide preparations are not commonly used at this time. Other topically applied sulfonamide compounds, such as sulfacetamide, sulfathiazole, and sulfadiazine, are apparently not common photosensitizers. Hypoglycemic sulfonamides, such as chloropropamide (Diabinese) and tolbutamide (Orinase), thiazide diuretics, such as chlorothiazide (Diuril) and hydrochlorothiazide (Esidrix, HydroDIURIL, and Oretic), and quinethazone (Hydromox), however, may produce phototoxic and photoallergic reactions when administered systemically.[56]

POTENTIAL MECHANISM OF PHOTOALLERGY OR TOXICITY TO CERTAIN MEDICAMENTS

Several photoactive agents were studied for their ability to induce apoptosis in cultured keratinocytes. TCSA, bithionol, chlorpromazine, enoxacin, and sparfloxacin were all found to induce apoptosis in irradiated as compared to non-irradiated cultures.[57]

PHOTOALLERGY TO GARLIC

There are several case reports of photo-patch test reactions to diallyl disulfide, the allergenic component in garlic. Clinical relevance has been noted, with the eruption being caused by ingestion, rather than contact usually.[58]

PHOTOALLERGY TO PSORALENS

Since psoralens are potent phototoxins, usually an adverse reactions to these agents is suspected to be phototoxic in nature. However, there are sporadic reports of true photoallergy from 8-methoxypsoralen used in phototherapy.[59]

Sunscreen Agents

Sunscreen agents have become the most common causative substances of photoallergic contact dermatitis in the United States.[10,11,60,61] These chemicals are also able to cause "regular" allergic contact dermatitis without UV light exposure. Many sunscreen lotions contain two or more active ingredients to provide a broader spectrum of photoprotection. In addition, many cosmetic products and moisturizing creams incorporate a sunscreen agent. Although in the past, PABA derivatives were the most

common sunscreen allergens, now oxybenzone is the most common.[10,11,61]

ANTHRANILATES

These are UVA absorbers, which are combined with other agents to provide broad-spectrum photoprotection. Allergy to these agents has not yet been documented.

PARA-AMINOBENZOIC ACID (PABA) AND ITS ESTERS

These chemicals are among the earliest sunscreen agents and are still used. They are primarily effective at blocking UVB light. Some persons report a transient stinging or burning reaction upon application, especially to sensitive skin areas. This is much more common than a true allergy but may lead the patient to believe that he or she is "allergic" to the chemicals. Some sunscreen lotions may be mistakenly marketed as being "hypoallergenic" because they contain no PABA and PABA esters

DeLeo and colleagues[10] found 3 of 187 patients with allergic contact dermatitis to PABA or octyldimethyl PABA (PABA-O, padimate-O), 3 with photoallergic contact dermatitis to PABA, and 2 with combined photoallergic contact dermatitis and ACD; almost 4% of the 187 patients tested and 22% of the 37 patients with any positive reaction. The researchers also reported 3 of 11 patients tested with pentyl-dimethyl PABA had a reaction of either ACD or photoallergic contact dermatitis, or both.[10] Fotiades and colleagues[62] found no cross-reactivity between PABA and the PABA esters PABA-O and amyldimethyl PABA (PABA-A, padimate-A). There were 9 positive patch tests to one of the esters (out of 138 tested) and 3 to PABA.[62] In contrast, 54 suspected photosensitive cases were tested by Lenique and colleagues[63] in France with no reaction to PABA, and only 1 to PABA-O. However, seven were positive to oxybenzone (see below). Berne and Bos[64] found only 2 positives to PABA out of 355 patients (0.6%) tested to PABA (5% alcohol). They did not test with PABA esters. However, in a report from France, photoallergic contact dermatitis to PABA was second only to oxybenzone.[61]

Some patients with positive patch tests to PABA may react due to cross-sensitivity between other para-amino substances such as paraphenylenediamine (PPDA), para-aminoazobenzene, or benzocaine.[65] Theeuwes and colleagues[66] showed that these reactions may not be clinically relevant. Fifty-four of 74 patients with positive reactions to a sunscreen agent (not photoreaction) had no history of problems from cosmetics or sunscreens. All 54 were positive to either PABA or PABA-O. Also, 46 of

328 patients reactive to PPDA and 51 of 180 benzocaine-allergic patients were positive to PABA or PABA-O.

OXYBENZONE AND OTHER BENZOPHENONES

Oxybenzone, also known as benzophenone-3 and Eusolex 4360, is the most frequently used benzophenone in sunscreens. The benzophenones may also be used for photoprotection in textiles, rubber, and plastics. Oxybenzone is also the most common sunscreen agent to cause photoallergic contact dermatitis. In an English multi-centre study, (1155 patients tested) oxybenzone accounted for 27 positive photopatch tests from a total of 128 positives (21%) in 66 patients.[67] It was the most common of all photoallergens.

Sczurko and colleagues[61] found 35 cases of photo-ACD to oxybenzone out of 283 patients tested (12.4%). In over one-third, exposure was not from a sunblock product but from a daily moisturizer. In a large Italian study of 1,050 patients, 31 showed reactions to sunscreen agents, with oxybenzone the most common at 10. Overall, oxybenzone was the fourth most common photoallergen after phenothiazines and Fentichlor.[68]

Of the 54 patients treated by Lenique and colleagues,[63] 7 (13%) reacted to oxybenzone. There were three cases of pure photoallergic contact dermatitis, two cases of allergic contact dermatitis, and two cases with both. Only two of the seven reacted to other photoallergens.[63] Photoallergy to oxybenzone has been reported in a patient with a clinical pattern similar to erythema multiforme.[69] Photocontact urticaria has been reported from benzophenone-3 and 10.[70] Use of sunscreens without oxybenzone is suggested in patients with known or presumed photoallergy.

Positive patch tests to oxybenzone (not photo-patch tests) were seen in just 0.6% of patients tested by the NACDG from 1998 to 2004.[71]

Other benzophenones, sulisobenzone and mexenone, are also used in sunscreens. There are scattered case reports of ACD and photoallergic contact dermatitis and contact urticaria from these agents.[72]

BUTYLMETHOXYDIBENZOYLMETHANE (PARSOL 1789, AVOBENZONE)

This chemical is a newer, particularly effective, UVA blocker currently used in the United States and elsewhere. In some newer studies, this agent has moved into second or third place in frequency of allergy to sunscreens. Schauder and Ippen[73] from Germany reported 15 cases of ACD and 13 cases of photoallergy from 402 patients tested in 1997. Bryden et al, from England, reported 22 of 128 (17%) positive photopatch tests were to this allergen, making it the second most common photoallergen in their

series.[67] Because it is one of the better UVA blockers, frequency of use of, and therefore photoallergy to, this agent will likely increase in the coming years.

ISOPROPYL DIBENZOYLMETHANE

This agent was withdrawn from the market in 1993 due to frequent reports of photosensitization. It was by far the most common sunscreen photoallergen in one study[73] from the 1980s to early 1990s. Cross-reactivity may result in photo-ACD to the newer dibenzoylmethane sunscreens.

CINNAMATES

These are primarily UVB absorbers and are used in many sunscreens. They are poorly soluble in water and therefore are common in "waterproof" sunscreens.72 In one study from Germany, out of 402 patients, there were 7 cases of allergy and 14 cases of photoallergy to either octylmethoxycinnamate or isoamyl *p*-methoxycinnamate.[73] In a study from France, however, only 3 of 283 reacted to a cinnamate,[61] whereas, in a study from Italy, 6 of 1,050 reacted,[68] In a recent British study, cinnamates ranked third in frequency of photoallergy, after oxybenzone and butylmethoxydibenzoylmethane.[67] Allergy to these agents is unusual. Probably the most significant feature is their cross-reactivity with fragrances and flavorings, particularly cinnamic aldehyde, alcohol, and cinnamon oil. Avoidance of perfumes and cinnamon-type spices in food may be necessary.

METHYL BENZILIDENE CAMPHOR

This UVB blocker is apparently a better allergen than a photoallergen. In Germany, there were 32 cases of allergy but only 5 of photoallergy.[73] In France, there were three positive patch tests and no positive patch tests.[61]

OCTYL TRIAZONE AND OCTOCRYLENE

These UVB blockers have caused several reported cases of photo-ACD.[74,75] Other photallergies were present in all these cases.

PHENYLBENZIMIDAZOLE-5-SULFONIC ACID (EUSOLEX 232, NOVANTISOL)

Several cases of photo-ACD to this agent have been reported from Europe.[64,73]

SALICYLATES

Although they are only weak UVB absorbers, salicylates are popular in sunscreens because of their safety, solubility, and stability. Although not used in routine patch test batteries, apparently contact allergic reactions are very rare.[76] A case of ACD and photo-ACD to octisalate with cross reactivity to cis-3-hexenyl salicylate has been reported.[77]

PHYSICAL SUNSCREENS

These "nonchemical" sun blockers act by physically blocking light rays away from the skin by virtue of their opacity. Titanium dioxide and zinc oxide are most commonly used. Allergy and photoallergy have not been reported. The opaque appearance may be either desirable or objectionable, depending on the individual.

Nonspecific Sunscreen Reactions

Many "reactions" to sunscreen products are not due to photoallergy. Additives such as fragrances and preservatives are more likely to cause ACD. Even more commonly, transient reactions such as stinging occur, especially with PABA. Other dermatologic disorders, such as acne and urticaria, may develop after sunscreen use. An Australian study of 603 adults using a single sunscreen product found that 19% complained of some sort of reaction.[78] None of these were due to photoallergy to the active agents. More than 90% were not allergic at all. Atopics were more likely to experience an adverse reaction than others.

PHOTOALLERGIC CONTACT DERMATITIS FROM PERFUMES

Contact photoallergic reactions to perfumes are due to either of two major components contained in the product: the fragrance per se or the fixative used to hold the fragrance or to enhance its scent.

Fragrances in their natural form are essential oils obtained from plants or flowers. In an attempt to reduce cost, synthetic fragrances have been produced and are widely used. These less expensive agents are organic compounds of the aldehyde, ketone, or alcohol variety.

The fixatives used in perfumes are usually secretions from the sexual scent glands of animals. They can also be synthesized, as exemplified by musk ambrette.

Musk ambrette, a synthetic fragrance fixative, is used in both the food and cosmetic industries. Its potent, floral odor has been considered quite desirable and in the past was present in concentrations as high as 15% in the final perfume product. Raugi and Storrs[79] reported localized photocontact dermatitis to men's aftershave lotions and traced the source to musk ambrette. Musk ambrette, like the halogenated salicylanilides, has also been reported to induce persistent light reaction in several patients.[80]

6-methylcoumarin, a synthetic organic lactone, is structurally related to the furocoumarins. Unlike the psoralens, however, 6-methylcoumarin was thought after initial testing to be a nonphotoactive substance. Since the early part of the last century it has been used extensively in the United States both in cosmetics and as an artificial flavoring agent in several foods. In the late 1970s, several reports of severe photosensitivity reactions occurring after patients used a suntanning preparation, in which 6-methylcoumarin had been incorporated as a fragrance, were noted in the southern United States.[81] Interestingly, in these patients, the clinical reaction had morphologic features both of phototoxicity and of photoallergy. The eruption occurred in some patients without a history of prior exposure to the suntanning product; lesions occurred within a few hours of exposure and were followed by long-lasting pigmentary changes in the skin. This finding suggested phototoxicity. Conversely, the eruption was a papulovesicular one morphologically; it occurred in a relatively small number of users of the product, and the reaction spread to areas not exposed to the product or irradiation. This pattern is associated usually with a photoallergic reaction. Reactivity could be elicited experimentally in only a small percentage of test subjects, suggestive of photoallergy.[82] Photosensitivity could be induced in guinea pigs and was immunologic.[83] Confirmation by routine phototesting in humans was unrewarding until it was discovered that to produce positive patch test reactions, the test substance must be applied shortly before irradiation rather than at the routine 24 to 48 hours. When done at the later (usual) time, false-negative results were obtained.

Since then, 6-methylcoumarin has been removed from suntanning products. It is believed that 6-methylcoumarin represents a substance of low photosensitizing potential that under most circumstances does not result in photocontact dermatitis unless used in high concentrations with adequate exposure to ultraviolet irradiation.

MISCELLANEOUS PHOTOALLERGIC SENSITIZERS

Epstein reported that ragweed pollen,[84] benzocaine,[85] and Dangard[86] are photosensitizers. Dangard, a chloromercaptodicarboximide, has been used by barbers as an antiseborrheic agent. Dangard is also a trade name for Vanicide 89 Re, which is used as an antiseptic in cosmetic and pharmaceutical preparations.

Photoallergy has been reported from Japan to three pesticides, maneb, fenitrothion, and Daconil (tetrachloroisophthalonitrile). Test concentrations were 0.01% aqueous, 0.01% aqueous, and 0.002% aqueous, respectively.

The first two were used in rice paddies and the latter in recreational gardening.[87,88]

Photosensitivity reactions from blankophores (optical brightening agents),[89] cadmium sulfide,[90,91] the yellow pigment in tattoos, fluorouracil,[92] chromate,[93] cobalt,[94] diphenhydramine,[95,96] amantadine, quindoxin, and dibucaine[97–99] have been reported.

Chronic Actinic Dermatitis

A variety of terms have been used to characterize chronic, persistent sensitivity to light, including persistent light reactivity, actinic reticuloid, and others. The diagnosis "chronic actinic dermatitis" encompasses all these conditions. Hawk has recently published an insightful overview of this condition.[100] It may appear as a sequelae of photo-ACD (persistent light reactivity) or may occur *de novo*. The term "actinic reticuloid", first used by Ive and colleagues,[101] has been used to refer to a pseudolymphomatous presentation. Actual progression to malignancy apparently occurs rarely, if at all,[102,103] although some cutaneous lymphomas may show photosensitivity.[104]

Pathophysiologically, CAD seems to share similar features with chronic ACD. It has been suggested that a photoproduct of UV irradiation, such as DNA or RNA may become "allergenic" whenever the appropriate wavelengths impact the skin.

The clinical picture is that of an eczematous photoeruption. Most patients are men over the age of 50. The clinical picture is similar to other types of photodermatitis, although generalization to non-sun-exposed areas is common. Often persistence throughout the year is seen, although worsening usually occurs in summer.[105] Most patients show extreme sensitivity to both UVB and UVA, while some react to only one wavelength. Occasionally visible light sensitivity is seen. Menage and colleagues[106] reported that 83% of 89 patients had reduced MEDs to both UVA and UVB, 9% to UVB alone, and 8% to UVA, UVB, and visible light. They also found that 36% had a positive patch or photopatch test to sesquiterpene lactone mix (0.1% pet, Hermal, Rheinbeck, Germany). Some patients reacted to other allergens, including colophony, fragrances, and sunscreens. Relevance of reactions was not always clear.

Persistent Light Reactivity

A small number of individuals who develop a photoallergic contact dermatitis to certain agents will retain a persistent reactivity to light (PLR) long after all exposure to the photosensitizing compound has ceased. This phenomenon was probably first recognized in soldiers photosensitized in North Africa after topical application of sulfanilamide in World War II. Promethazine, chlorpromazine, bithionol, and most notably the halogenated salicylanilides were reported to induce this type of reaction in the 1950s and 1960s.[107–109] The perfume component musk ambrette has caused PLR.[80] Occasionally systemic agents including quinine, NSAIDs, and thiazides may produce a PLR phenomenon.[110,111]

Regardless of the particular photosensitizers involved, patients who become affected may become incapacitated, because they cannot tolerate exposure to sunlight. In fact, they may be so exquisitely photosensitive as to react adversely even to light emitted from artificial sources, such as household fluorescent tubes.[105] An important and still puzzling feature of the phenomenon is that the action spectrum of the patient's photosensitivity extends beyond those wavelengths that initiated sensitization. Also, people who develop a PLR regularly show a markedly abnormal reaction to UVB. The persistent light reactors have no more-than-average incidence of atopy. They do include a preponderance of males in the fifth, sixth, and seventh decades of life.

The mechanism of persistent light reaction remains unclear, but a plausible theory may be that the patient has become autophotosensitized to a carrier protein that absorbs photons in the UVB range, thereby producing erythema and an eczematous response.[112] Roelandts[111] suggested that somehow a state of "conditioned hyperirritability" could develop in PLR patients due to endogenous or exogenous influences.

SUBTYPES OF PERSISTENT LIGHT REACTIVITY

Persistent photosensitivity reactions that first appear morphologically as edematous or vesicular reactions and later resemble chronic dermatitis can be differentiated according to several criteria. The following discussion outlines a working classification of these types of reactions on the bases of whether photosensitivity is localized or generalized and of the response of the patient to phototests and photopatch tests.

Localized Specific Nonimmunologic Persistence of Photosensitivity

This type of reactivity was first described in Swedish sailors tattooed with cadmium sulfide, a yellow pigment.[113] Localized swellings confined solely to the yellow portions of the tattoos occurred whenever the sailors were exposed to sunlight. Studies indicated that the action spectrum of cadmium was in the UVA and visible light ranges. All phototests and photopatch tests on nontattooed sites are normal. This type of phototoxic reactions arises from the local retention of the photosensitizer in macrophages.

Localized Specific Immunologic Persistence of Photosensitivity

This reaction was well described by Burry[114] in 1967. He studied Australian patients with photoallergic contact dermatitis. Several patients had incurred repeated topical exposure to Fentichlor and Multifungin, which were commercially available topical antibiotic preparations containing halogenated salicylanilides or closely related compounds. Burry reported that at such sites as the forearms where a severe, chronic, lichenified photodermatitis occurred, the patients remained photosensitive to UVA light for months with no continued exposure to the halogenated salicylanilides. In contrast, phototests on normal-appearing uninvolved skin exposed to UVA radiation were negative. Photopatch tests with Fentichlor and Multifungin plus UVA light on these same uninvolved sites, however, were strongly positive. A possible explanation of this phenomenon is that the damaged skin at the previously light-exposed sites retained some of the photosensitizers for more extended periods of time than did normal skin.

Polyvalent Light Sensitivity with Persistent Photosensitivity

This term describes patients who respond initially to both UV and visible light with marked erythema and who subsequently develop pruritic, lichenified plaques. No known phototoxic or photoallergic agent can be identified from the patient's history or by phototesting. Unfortunately, the disability may persist indefinitely.

PHOTOTESTING AND PHOTOPATCH TESTING

Phototesting and photopatch testing can be performed in the outpatient setting as long as a light source and photoallergens are available. The most important equipment needed to perform photopatch tests is an artificial light source with relatively good spectral irradiance in the UVA range. A combined UVB/PUVA box can be used to deliver the appropriate radiation dosages. Handheld light sources are also available. The light source should be calibrated with a UV photometer to insure that the desired dosage is accurately delivered.

The usual dose of UVA light for phototesting and photopatch testing is 5 or 10 joules (J)/cm^2. Occasionally, if extreme UVA photosensitivity is suspected, phototesting can also be performed to 1 and 5 J/cm^2. If 10 J/cm^2 or less causes erythema, the next lower dose is then used for photopatch tests. Regardless of skin color, reaction to 10 J/cm^2 of UVA indicates UVA photosensitivity.

The dosage of UVB light for phototesting is not so clear-cut. The minimal erythema dose (MED) varies normally with the skin color. An MED of 30 mJ/cm^2 may be normal in a fair-skinned person (types I or II) but would be abnormal in a dark-skinned patient. Doses between 5 and 100 mJ/cm^2 of UVB may be given in phototesting, depending on the patient's skin type.

Photopatch testing is conducted with UVA radiation because the vast majority of photo-ACD reactions are due to UVA. The chemicals currently recommended by the North American Contact Dermatitis Group (NACDG) for photopatch testing are listed in Table 22.6.

Table 22-6 Suggested Photopatch Test Allergens
Sunscreen agents
Ethylhexyl methoxycinnamate 10%
Methylbenzylidene camphor 10%
Octyl triazone 10%
Isoamyl-p-methoxycinnamate 10%
Octocrylene 10%
Drometriazole trisiloxane 10%
Para-amino benzoic acid (PABA) 10%
Octyldimethyl PABA (padimate-O) 10%
Amyldimethyl PABA (padimate A) 10%
Oxybenzone (benzophenone-3) 10%
Sulisobenzone (benzophenone-4) 10%
Butyl methoxybibenzoylmethane (parsol 1789) 10%
Octyl salicylate 5%
Homosalate 5%
Menthylanthranilate 5%
2-hydroxy-methoxy methyl benzophenone (mexenone) 10%
2-phenylbenzimidazol-5-sulfonic acid 10%
Zinc oxide 2.5%
Titanium oxide 1%
Antiseptic agents
Dichlorophene 1%
Hexachloropene 1%
Triclosan 2%
Chlorhexidine diacetate 0.5% (aq)
Bithionol 1% pet
Tribromsalicylanicide 1%
Triclocarban 1%
Fragrances
Fragrance mix-I 8%
Sandalwood oil 2%
Musk Ambrette 5%
Miscellaneous
Thiourea 0.1%
Sesquiterpene lactone mix 0.1%
Lichen acid mix 0.3%
Fentichlor 1%
Ketoprofen 5%
Promethazine 0.1%
Chlorproamzine 1%
All in petrolatum except as noted

Duplicate sets of patches are prepared and are placed on symmetrical sites of the back, as in ordinary patch-test procedures. One set of the duplicate patches will be irradiated with UVA light, whereas the nonirradiated set serves as a control.

Photopatch testing using patient-supplied or "non-standard" materials can be performed in the same fashion. Perfumes and sunscreen preparations generally can be tested full strength (as is). Pieces of plants or plant juices can be tested to prove phytophotodermatitis. Because of the likelihood of producing persistent pigmentation, however, testing on a covered area such as the buttock is recommended.

After application of the chemicals, the two sets of patches are both covered with light-opaque material, if aluminum patch-test chambers are not used. After 24 or 48 hours, both sets of patches are removed and each site is evaluated for any visible reaction. A report from England showed that more photoallergic reactions were seen with 48 hour patch occlusion than after 24 hours.[115] A positive test indicates the presence of either an "ordinary" allergic contact dermatitis or, rarely, a primary irritant reaction to the applied chemical. After the uncovered sites are evaluated, one set is irradiated with 10 J/cm^2 of UVA, as recommended by the NACDG. The British Photodermatology Group, however, recommends testing with 5 J/cm^2.[116] After completion of irradiation, the photopatch test sites are covered again with light-opaque material. Forty-eight hours later, 96 hours after initial patch application, a second reading is performed. Some authors suggest a further delayed reading of the irradiated side in another 2 to 4 days.

If the irradiated site shows a positive reaction and the nonirradiated site shows a negative one, contact photoallergy is present. If both sites show equally positive reactions, then contact allergy is present. If both are positive but the irradiated site is obviously more so, then both photo and non-photo allergy may be occurring. (Table 22.7)

Allergen Concentration in Photopatch Testing

Hasan and Jansen[117] studied a number of photo allergens in varying concentrations and with varying doses of UVA. With PABA, for example, they found allergen concentration to be very important in photocontact reactions, but less so in "regular" ACD. The dosage of UVA did not make much difference, however, so they recommend 5 joules for routine testing.. However, testing with 10 joules may result in a few more positive reactions without any increased risk.

HAZARDS OF PHOTOPATCH TESTING

It should be emphasized that photopatch testing is not always an innocuous procedure. Some hazards and complications associated with it are outlined in Table 22.8. The patient should be aware that strong reactions characterized by vesiculation may cause discomfort. Photopatch testing should be avoided, if possible, in patients with acute active dermatitis, because false-positive reactions may result from the "hyperirritability" of the skin.

Management of Photocontact Sensitivity

Individuals with an acute photosensitivity reaction with severe erythema and edema may obtain relief with ice cold compresses of Burow's solution diluted 1:10. It is often beneficial to superimpose these compresses on a thin layer of petrolatum to prevent excessive drying.

In acute phototoxic reactions (sunburn), aspirin (or possibly other NSAIDs) is very helpful if given as soon as possible after the exposure. Two or three tablets every 4 to 6 hours for about 48 hours, if tolerated, is usually sufficient. In generalized cases, systemic corticosteroid therapy may gives prompt symptomatic relief. The dosage is similar to that for any generalized acute dermatitis.

Exposure to the photosensitizing agent must be eliminated, and the patient should minimize exposure to sunlight for at least 2 weeks. It is advisable to give the patient

Table 22-7 Interpretation of Photopatch Tests		
Reading at irradiated site[a]	Reading at non-irradiated site[a]	Interpretation
0	0	Negative
1–3+	0	Contact photoallergy
1–3+ =	1–3+	Contact allergy alone
1–3+ >	1–2+	Contact photoallergy and contact allergy

[a]Evaluations are scored 0 through 3, as described by the NACDG

Table 22-8 Hazards and Complications of Photopatch Testing
1. Inadvertent sensitization to photopatch test materials
2. Mechanical or radiation injury due to improper use of light sources
3. False-positive and false-negative tests due to selection of inappropriate type or amount of light
4. Discomfort at patch test sites and "flares" at previously involved sites
5. Masked photopatch reaction
6. Persistent hyperpigmentation at test sites

a list of related drugs or chemicals that produce cross-photosensitivity and that may need to be avoided. This list is important, particularly when the salicylanilides and phenothiazines are implicated.

In chronic cases that are only responsive to systemic corticosteroids, and in which a significant morbidity is present, immunosuppressive agents may be helpful.[111] Azathioprine seems to be the most efficacious of these agents, but methotrexate or mycophenolate mofetil may be tried.

Although it may seem paradoxical, PUVA therapy has proven helpful, especially in some cases of chronic actinic dermatitis.[118] Apparently, clinical improvement is related to inhibition of T cells and Langerhans cells.

Cyclosporine, alone or with PUVA, has been noted to be beneficial in sporadic case reports, as has the anabolic steroid danazol.[119,120]

PROTECTION AGAINST LIGHT

The avoidance of sunlight must often be extended beyond the period of acute dermatitis because excretion of the photosensitive chemical from the skin may be delayed. In severe cases, confinement of the patient in a darkened room for several days may speed recovery. Window glass does not usually protect against contact phototoxic or contact photoallergic reactions.

Knowledge of the action spectrum of a photosensitizer is often of value, because ordinary window glass (3 mm thick) usually affords protection only against UV radiation less than 320 nm.[121]

Patients with a photosensitivity dermatitis may obtain protection by using adequate clothing. Closely woven dark fabrics are best. The weave pattern of the fabric is much more important than the color or fabric type.[122] White clothing becomes much more permeable to erythema-producing radiation when it is wet with water or perspiration.

Repeated, short exposures to sun have occasionally helped in desensitizing individuals. Such desensitization is probably nonimmunologic and is due to increased melanin formation and thickening of the horny layer. Dark-skinned individuals are less apt to have photosensitizing reactions than are fair-skinned people. Birmingham and colleagues[15] noted that the skin of Mexican and black harvesters affords protection against the phototoxic effects of the celery pink rot. Crow and colleagues[28] noted that dark-skinned workers are protected against photodermatitis from pitch.

USE OF SUNSCREEN AGENTS

Unfortunately, sunscreens seem to be of only modest benefit in the prevention of photodermatitis, especially the chronic varieties. For those who are allergic to the active sunscreen agents, physical sunscreens such as titanium dioxide and zinc oxide may be useful. However, some of these products produce a visible opaque coating on the skin.

The sunless tanning agents offer minimal photoprotection even though the skin darkens slightly with their use.

Birmingham and colleagues[15] reported that physical sunscreens protected celery harvesters against phototoxic reactions due to pink rot in celery, but chemical sunscreens did not.

MANAGEMENT OF CONTACT PHOTODERMATITIS DUE TO TAR THERAPY

Individuals receiving tar therapy in whom a photosensitivity reaction is to be avoided should apply the tar at night only and should remove it carefully in the morning. Patients should be warned that, even though the tars have apparently been completely removed from the skin, avoidance of exposure to strong sunlight for several days is important, because traces of the tar alone may cause phototoxic reactions. Purified or refined tars are less apt to cause photosensitivity reactions. It may be desirable occasionally to substitute wood tars (e.g., pine tar), which are not photosensitizers.

References

1. Harber LC, Bickers DR. Photosensitivity diseases: principles of diagnosis and treatment. Philadelphia: WB Saunders, 1981.

2. Gould J, Mercurio M, Elmets C. Cutaneous photosensitivity diseases induced by exogenous agents. J Am Acad Dermatol 1995;33:551.

3. Gonzalez E, Gonzalez S. Drug photosensitivity, idiopathic photodermatoses and sunscreens. J Am Acad Dermatol 1996;35:871.

4. Murphy G: Investigation of photosensitive disorders. Photodermatol Photoimmunol, Photomed 2004;20:305.

5. Baer RL, Harber LC. Photosensitivity induced by drugs. JAMA 1965;192:989.

6. Harber LC, Targouik SE, Baer RL. Studies on contact photosensitivity to hexachlorophene and trichlorocarbanilide in guinea pigs and man. J Invest Dermatol 1986;51:373.

7. Harber LC, Levine GM. Photo sensitivity dermatitis from household products. GP 1969;39:95.

8. Menz J, Muller SA, Connolly SM. Photopatch testing: a six-year experience. J Am Acad Dermatol 1988;18:1044.

9. Hölzle E, et al. Photopatch testing: the 5-year experience of the German, Austrian, and Swiss Photopatch Test Group. J Am Acad Dermatol 1991;25:59.

10. DeLeo V, Suarez S, Maso M. Photoallergic contact dermatitis: results of photopatch testing in New York, 1985–1990. Arch Dermatol 1992;128:1513.

11. Scheuer E, Warshaw E: Sunscreen allergy: a review of epidemiology, clinical characteristics, and responsible allergens. Dermatitis 2006; 17:3.

12. Bryden A, Moseley S, Ibbotson M, et al: Photopatch testing of 1155 patients: results of the U.K. multicentre photopatch study group. Br J Dermatol 2006;155:737.

13. Bowers A. Phytophotodermatitis. Am J Contact Derm 1999;10:89.

14. Wagner A, Wu J, Hansen R, et al: Bullous phytophotodermatitis associated with high natural concentration of furocoumarins in limes. Am J Contact Dermat 2002; 13:10.

15. Birmingham DJ, et al. Phototoxic bullae among celery harvesters. Arch Dermatol 1961;83:73.

16. Pathak MA, Daniels Jr F, Fitzpatrick TB. The presently known distribution of furocoumarins (psoralens) in plants. J Invest Dermatol 1962;39:225.

17. Parrish JA, Fitzpatrick TB, Tanenbaum L, Pathak MA. Photochemotherapy of psoriasis with oral methoxsalen and longwave ultraviolet light. N Engl J Med 1974;291:1207.

18. Harber LC, et al. Berloque dermatitis. Arch Dermatol 1964;90:572.

19. Sams EM. Photodynamic action of lime oil (Citrus aurantifolia). Arch Dermatol 1941;44:571.

20. Aberer W. Occupational dermatitis from organically grown parsnip (Pastinaca sativa L.) Contact Dermatitis 1992;26:62.

21. Ash-Wood-Smith MF, et al. Photosensitivity from harvesting lovage (Lesisticum officinale). Contact Dermatitis 1992;26:356.

22. Hann SK, et al. Angelica-induced phytophotodermatitis. Photodermatol Photoimmunol Photomed 1991;8:84.

23. Elpern DJ, Mitchell JC. Phytophotodermatitis from Mokihana fruits (Pelea anisata H. Mann, fa. Rutaccae) in Hawaiian lei. Contact Dermatitis 1984;10:224.

24. Schempp C, Sonntag C, Schopf E, et al. Dermatitis bullosa striata pretensis durch Dictamnus albus L. (Brennender Busch). Hautarzt 1996;47:708.

25. Tunget C, Turchen S, Manogiuerra A, et al. Sunlight and the plant: a toxic combination. Severe phytophotodermatitis from Cneoridium dumosum. Cutis 1994;54:400.

26. Calka O, Akdeniz N, Metin A, et al. Phototoxic dermatitis due to Chenopodium album in a mother and son. Contact Dermatitis 2005;53:58.

27. Bassioukas K, Stergiopoulou C, Hatzis J: Erythrodermic phytophotodermatitis after application of aqueous fig leaf extract as an artificial suntan promoter and sunbathing. Contact Dermatitis 2004;51:94.

28. Crow KD, et al. Photosensitivity due to pitch. Br J Dermatol 1961; 73:220.

29. Calnan C, Harman R, Wells G. Photodermatitis from soap. Br Med J 1961;2:1266.

30. Wilkinson DS. Photodermatitis due to tetrachlorosalicylanilide. Br J Dermatol 1961;73:213.

31. Vinson LK, Flatt RS. Photosensitization by tetrachlorosalicylanilide. J Invest Dermatol 1962;38:327.

32. Osmundsen PE. Contact photodermatitis due to tribromosalicylanilide. Br J Dermatol 1969;81:929.

33. Auerbach R, Pearlstein HH. Photosensitivity and soap. NY J Med 1971;72:747.

34. Harber LC, Harris H, Baer RL. Photoallergic contact dermatitis. Arch Dermatol 1966;94:255.

35. Freeman RG, Knox JM. The action spectrum of photocontact dermatitis caused by halogenated salicylanilides and related compounds. Arch Dermatol 1968;97:130.

36. Harber LC, Harris H, Baer RL. Structural features of photoallergy to salicylanilides and related compounds. J Invest Dermatol 1966;46:303.

37. Burry JM, Hunter GA. Photocontact dermatitis from jadit. Br J Dermatol 1970;82:224.

38. Gaul LE. Sensitivity to bithionol. Arch Dermatol 1963;87:383.

39. Epstein J, Rees W, Baughman RD. Contact photodermatitis from bithionol. Arch Dermatol 1964;90:153.

40. O'Quinn SE, Kennedy B, Isbell KH. Contact photodermatitis due to bithionol and related compounds. JAMA 1967;199:89.

41. Burry JM. Photoallergies to Fentichlor and multifungin. Arch Dermatol 1967;95:287.

42. Burry JM. Cross sensitivity between Fentichlor and bithionol. Arch Dermatol 1968;97:496.

43. DeEds F, Wilson RH, Thomas JO. Photosensitization by phenothiazine. JAMA 1940;114:2095.

44. Cahn MM, Levy EJ. Ultraviolet light factor in chlorpromazine dermatitis. Arch Dermatol 1957;75:38.

45. Epstein JH, Brunsting LA. Topical application of chlorpromazine: its effect on the erythema response to ultraviolet light. J Invest Dermatol 1958;30:91.

46. Sidi E, Hincky M, Gervais A. Allergic sensitization and photosensitization to Phenergan Cream. J Invest Dermatol 1955;24:345.

47. Newill RGD. Photosensitivity caused by promethazine. Br Med J 1960;2:359.

48. Epstein S, Rowe RJ. Photoallergy and photocross sensitivity to phenergan. J Invest Dermatol 1957;29:319.

49. Schauder S. Dioxopromethazine induced photoallergic contact dermatitis followed by persistent light reaction. Amer J Contact Derm 1998;9:182.

50. Alomar A Ketoprofen photodermatitis. Contact Dermatitis 1985;12:112.

51. Bosca F, Miranda M. Photosensitizing drugs containing the benzophenone chromophore. J Photochem Photobiol B 1998; 43:1.

52. Goday-Bujan J, Rodriguez-Lozano J, Martinez-Gonzalez M, et al. Photoallergic contact dermatitis from dexketoprofen. Contact Dermatitis 2006;55:59.

53. Hindsen M, Zimerson E, Bruze M: Photoallergic contact dermatitis from ketoprofen in southern Sweden. Contact Dermatitis 2006;54:150.

54. Kowalzick L, Ziegler H: Photoallergic contact dermatitis from topical diclofenac in Solareze Gel. Contact Dermatitis 2006;54:349.

55. Epstein S. Photoallergy and primary photosensitivity to sulfanilamide. J Invest Dermatol 1939;2:43.

56. Harber LC, Lashinsky AM, Baer RL. Photosensitivity due to chlorothiazide and hydrochlorothiazide. N Engl J Med 1959;261:1378.

57. Kurita M, Shimauchi T, Kobayashi M, et al: Induction of keratinocyte apoptosis by photosensitizing chemicals plus UVA. J Dermatol Sci 2007;45:105.

58. Alvarez M, Jacobs S, Jiang B, et al: Photocontact Allergy to Diallyl Disulfide. Am J Contact Dermat 2003;14:161.

59. Ravenscroft J, Goulden V, Wilkinson M: Systemic allergic contact dermatitis to 8-methoxypsoralen. J Am Acad Dermatol 2001;45:S218.

60. Journe F, Marguery M, Rakotondrazafy J, et al. Sunscreen sensitization: a 5-year study. Acta Derm Vener 1999;79:211.

61. Szczurko C, Dompmartin A, Michel M, et al. Photocontact allergy to oxybenzone: ten years of experience. Photodermatol Photoimmunol Photomed 1994;10:144.

62. Fotiades J, Soter NA, Lim HW. Results of evaluation of 203 patients for photosensitivity in a 7.3 year period. J Amer Acad Derm 1995;33:597.

63. Lenique P, et al. Contact and photocontact allergy to oxybenzone. Contact Dermatitis 1992;26:177.

64. Berne B, Bos A. Seven-year experience of photopatch testing with sunscreen allergen in Sweden. Contact Dermatitis 1998;38:1.

65. Uter W, Lessmann H, Geier J, et al. The spectrum of allergic cross sensitivity in clinical patch testing with para-amino compounds. Allergy 2002; 57:319.

66. Theeuwes M, Degreef H, Dooms-Goossens A. Para-aminobenzoic acid (PABA) and sunscreen allergy. Am J Contact Dermat 1992;3:206.

67. Bryden A, Moseley S, Ibbotson M, et al: Photopatch testing of 1155 patients: results of the U.K. multicentre photopatch study group. Br J Dermatol 2006;155: 737.

68. Pigatto PD, Legori A, Bigardi AS, et al. Gruppo Italiano ricerca dermatiti da contatto ed ambientali. Italian multicenter study of allergic contact photodermatitis: epidemiological aspects. Amer J Contact Derm 1996;7:158.

69. Zhang XM, Nakagawa M, Kawai K, et al. Erythema-multiforme-like eruption following photoallergic contact dermatitis from oxybenzone. Contact Dermatitis 1998;38:43.

70. Bourrain J, Amblard P, Beani J: Contact urticaria photoinduced by benzophenones. Contact Dermatitis 2003;48:54.

71. Pratt M, Belsito D, DeLeo V, et al. North American Contact Dermatitis Group patch test results, 2001–2002 study period. Dermatitis 2004; 15:176.

72. Sterling GB. Sunscreens: a review. Cutis 1992;50:221.

73. Schauder S, Ippen H. Contact and photocontact sensitivity to sunscreens: review of a 15-year experience and of the literature. Contact Dermatitis 1997;37:221.

74. Sommer S, Wilkinson SM, English J, et al: Photoallergic contact dermatitis from the sunscreen octyl triazone. Contact Dermatitis 2002;46:304.

75. Carotte-Lefebrve I, Bonnevalle A, Segard M, et al. Contact allergy to octocrylene. Contact Dermatitis 2003;48:46.

76. Fisher AA. Sunscreen dermatitis: part IV—the salicylates, the anthranilates, and physical agents. Cutis 1992;50:397.

77. Shaw D: Allergic contact dermatitis from octisalate and cis-3-hexenyl salicylate. Dermatitis 2006; 17: 152–5.

78. Foley P, et al. The frequency of reactions to sunscreens: results of a longitudinal population-based study on the regular use of sunscreens in Australia. Br J Dermatol 1993;128:512.

79. Raugi GJ, Storrs FJ. Photosensitivity from men's cologne. Arch Dermatol 1979;115:106.

80. Giovinazzo VJ, Harber LC, Bickers DR, Armstrong RB. Photoallergic contact dermatitis to musk ambrette: histopathologic features of photobiologic reactions observed in a persistent light reactor. Arch Dermatol 1981;7:344.

81. Jackson RT, Nesbitt Jr LT, De Leo VA. 6-methylcoumarin photo-contact dermatitis. J Am Acad Dermatol 1980;2:124.

82. Kaidbey KH, Kligman AM. Contact photoallergy to 6-methylcoumarin in proprietary sunscreens. Arch Dermatol 1978;114:1709.

83. Harber LC, Armstrong RB, Ichikawa H. Current status of predicting animal models for drug photoallergy and their correlation with drug photoallergy in humans. J Natl Cancer Inst 1982;69:237.

84. Epstein S. Role of dermal sensitivity in ragweed contact dermatitis. Arch Dermatol 1960;82:48.

85. Epstein S. Photocontact dermatitis from benzocaine. Arch Dermatol 1965;92:591.

86. Epstein S. Photoallergic contact dermatitis: report of a case due to Dangard. Cutis 1968;4:856.

87. Nakamura M, Arima Y, Nobuhara S, et al. Airborne photocontact dermatitis due to the pesticides maneb and fenitrothion. Contact Dermatitis 1999;40:222–223.

88. Matsushita S, Kanekura T, Sarvinatari K, et al. Photoallergic contact dermatitis due to Daconil. Contact Dermatitis 1996;35:115.

89. Burckhardt W. Photoallergic eczema due to blankophores (optic brightening agents). Hautarzt 1957;8:486.

90. Bjoernber A. Reactions of light in yellow tattoos from cadmium sulfide. Arch Dermatol 1963;88:267.

91. Goldstein N. Mercury-cadmium sensitivity in tattoos: a photoallergic reaction in red pigment. Ann Intern Med 1967;67:984.

92. Sams WM. Untoward response with topical fluorouracil. Arch Dermatol 1968;97:14.

93. Tronnier H. Photosensitivity of eczema patients (with particular reference to chromate eczema). Arch Klin Exp Derm 1970;47:494.

94. Romaguera C, Lecha M, Grimalt F, et al. Photocontact dermatitis to cobalt salts. Contact Dermatitis 1982;8:383.

95. Yamada S, Tanaka M, Kawahara Y, et al. Photoallergic contact dermatitis due to diphenhydramine hydrochloride. Contact Dermatitis 1998;38:282.

96. Horio T. Allergic and photoallergic dermatitis from diphenhydramine. Arch Dermatol 1976;112:1124.

97. Urrutia I, Jauregui I, Gamboa P, et al. Photocontact dermatitis from cinchocaine (dibucaine). Contact Dermatitis 1997;39:139.

98. Zaynoun S, Johnson BE, Frain-Bell W. The investigation of quindoxin photosensitivity. Contact Dermatitis 1976;2:343.

99. Frain-Bell W, Gardiner J. Photocontact dermatitis due to quindoxin. Contact Dermatitis 1975;1:256.

100. Hawk JLM: Chronic actinic dermatitis. Photoderm Photoimmun Photomed 2004;20:312.

101. Ive FA, Magnus LA, Warin RP, et al. Actinic reticuloid: a chronic dermatosis associated with severe photosensitivity and the histological resemblance to lymphoma. Br J Dermatol 1969;81:469.

102. Toonstra J, Henquet C, van Weelden H. Actinic reticuloid. J Am Acad Dermatol 1989;21:205.

103. Bilsland D, Crombie I, Ferguson J. The photosensitivity dermatitis and actinic reticuloid syndrome: no association with lymphoreticular malignancy. Br J Dermatol 1994;131:209.

104. Dawe R, Crombie I, Ferguson J: The natural history of chronic actinic dermatitis. Arch Dermatol 2000; 136:1215.

105. Willis I, Kligman AM. The mechanism of the persistent light reactor. J Invest Dermatol 1968b;51:385.

106. Menage H, Ross J, Norris P, et al. Contact and photocontact sensitization in chronic actinic dermatitis: sesquiterpene lactone mix is an important allergen. Br J Dermatol 1995;132:543.

107. Jillson OF, Baughman RD. Contact photodermatitis from bithionol. Arch Dermatol 1963;88:409.

108. Sidi LE, Hincky M, Gervais A. Allergic sensitization and photosensitization to phenergan cream. J Invest Dermatol 1955;24:345.

109. Wiskemann A, Wulf K. Untersuchungen uber den auslosenden spektral Bereich und die direkte licht Pigmentierung bei chronischen und akuten licht Auschlagen. Arch Klin Exp Derm 1959;209:443.

110. Guzzo C, Kaidbey K. Persistent light reactivity from systemic quinine. Photodermatol Photoimmunol Photomed 1990;7:166.

111. Roelandts R. Chronic actinic dermatitis. J Am Acad Dermatol 1993;28:240.

112. Katsamura Y, Tanaka J, Ichikawa H, et al. Persistent light reaction: induction in the guinea pig. J Invest Dermatol 1986;87:330.

113. Bjornberg A. Reactions to light yellow tattoos from cadmium sulfide. Arch Dermatol 1963;88:267.

114. Burry JN. Photoallergies to Fentichlor and Multifungin. Arch Dermatol 1967;95:287.

115. Batchelor R, Wilkinson S: Photopatch testing- a retrospective review using the 1 and 2 day irradiation protocols. Contact Dermatitis 2006;54:75.

116. British Photodermatology Group. Workshop report: photopatch testing—methods and indications. Br J Dermatol 1997;136:371.

117. Hasan T, Jansen CT. Photopatch test reactivity: effect of photoallergen concentration and UVA dosaging. Contact Dermatitis 1996;34:383.

118. Hindson C, et al. PUVA therapy of chronic actinic dermatitis: a 5-year follow-up. Br J Dermatol 1990;123:273.

119. Gareazábal J, et al. Successful treatment of musk ketone-induced chronic actinic dermatitis with cyclosporine and PUVA. J Am Acad Dermatol 1992;27:838.

120. Humbert P, et al. Chronic actinic dermatitis responding to danazol. Br J Dermatol 1991;124:195.

121. Blum HF. Sunburn. In: Hollander A, ed. Radiation biology, vol. 2. New York: McGraw-Hill, 1955.

122. Robson J, Diffey B. Textiles and sun protection. Photodermatol Photoimmunol Photomed 1990;7:32.

PARESTHESIA DUE TO CONTACTANTS

EXECUTIVE SUMMARY

In addition to irritant contact dermatitis (ICD) and allergic contact dermatitis (ACD), contactants can occasionally cause sensory symptoms that include burning, stinging, itching, and paresthesia without causing dermatitis. Examples of such contactants include pyrethroid insecticides, methacrylates, and some organic solvents. Patch testing is negative and the diagnosis is often one of exclusion. Cutaneous depigmentation can also be caused by contactants, with or without concomitant ACD. This is called chemical vitiligo or (since it often occurs in an occupational setting) occupational vitiligo. Histologically there is no difference from idiopathic vitiligo. A history of contact with known depigmenters and lack of previous vitiligo is necessary for the diagnosis, which is not always totally clear. Hydroquinones and phenolic agents are the best-known etiologic agents, but a variety of others have been reported. Sometimes pigment will return after the contact ceases, but not always. Occasionally a patch test will reproduce the depigmentation, but 2 weeks or more of contact may be needed.

Some causes of abnormal sensory symptoms without dermatitis are listed in Table 23.1.

Paresthesia from Synthetic Pyrethroid Insecticides

Knox and colleagues,[1,2] stating that occupational exposure to fenvalerate, a synthetic pyrethroid insecticide, has been reported to cause paresthesia, developed a protocol that involved the topical application of 0.05 ml of field-use diluted technical Pydrin (1:180) or a placebo (ethyl alcohol) to the ear of 36 volunteer subjects. Numbness, itching, burning, tingling, and warmth were the most commonly reported sensations. These sensations usually began after 1 hour, peaked at 3 to 6 hours, and lasted less than 24 hours. For technical Pydrin, the average score of intensity on a scale of 0 (no sensation) to 4 (markedly intense) was 1.40; the score of intensity for the placebo was 0.36. This finding demonstrates that a statistically significant sensation ($p = .001$) occurred after application of Pydrin.

As field use of fenvalerate, another pyrethroid, has increased in recent years, several reports of cutaneous paresthesias among occupationally exposed individuals have appeared.[3] These cutaneous sensations occur topically without erythema, edema, vesiculation, or any other sign of dermatitis.

LeQuesne and colleagues[3] reported that among 23 workers exposed to synthetic pyrethroids, 19 had experienced one or more episodes of abnormal facial sensation developing between 30 minutes and 3 hours after exposure and persisting for 30 minutes to 8 hours. There were no abnormal neurologic signs, and electrophysiologic studies (of the arms and legs) were normal. The sensations were variously described as "tingling," "burning," "like coming in from the cold," or like "nettle rash," but no study participants complained of loss of sensation; when directly questioned, they said it was quite different from the sensation after administration of a local anesthetic for dental treatment. The subjects were not aware of loss of sensation when they touched the affected area, and the sensation was unaffected by rubbing the skin.

The abnormal sensations were usually distributed symmetrically over the cheeks, particularly under the eyes and sometimes on the nose. In three subjects, unilateral symptoms on the face occurred after an accidental splash or direct contact with a pyrethroid solution. In other instances, subjects said they developed symptoms when working with pyrethroids in the form of a fine

Table 23-1 Contactants Producing Paresthesia
Acrylate monomers
Acrylonitrile
Pants paresthesia syndrome (from synthetic fabric?)
Physical pressure and friction
Solvents: turpentine, benzene, and acetone
Synthetic pyrethroids

powder of one- to four- particle size or dissolved in a volatile solvent, but not when working with pyrethroids in other forms.

A delay characteristically followed exposure to the pyrethroids before the onset of symptoms. The shortest delay was 30 minutes after beginning to work with pyrethroids, and the longest interval before symptoms developed was 3 hours after exposure ceased. The duration of symptoms varied from 30 minutes to 8 hours. It should be emphasized that the facial dysesthesia was not accompanied by dermatitis.

Descriptions of the facial symptoms have varied. A few subjects said the sensation that followed pyrethroid exposure resembled that after direct skin contact with some solvents, for example, dimethylsulfoxide (DMSO). However, DMSO has an immediate effect, and all sensations are rapidly relieved by washing the exposed area of skin. Similar symptoms in these patients occurred with or without exposure to a variety of solvents (the only common exposure was a pyrethroid). The delay in onset of symptoms after exposure and their duration are unlike those that follow skin contact with other irritant solutions.

It is noteworthy that one field operator found he was protected from symptoms only when wearing a full head and facial mask with breathing canister. In this group of workers, symptoms occurred only on the face. It may be that, apart from the hands, the face receives the greatest exposure and absorption occurs more easily through the facial skin than through other exposed areas. Thus, the symptoms are most likely to result from transient lowering of the threshold of sensory nerve fibers or nerve endings after exposure of the facial skin to pyrethroids. This is similar to the phenomena described after exposure of animal nerves to pyrethroids.

A field survey by Tucker and Flannigan[4] disclosed that a stinging sensation about the face and arms was reported by workers occupationally exposed to fenvalerate. Direct contact with the liquid was not necessary to induce the paresthesia. It was believed that cutaneous exposure to aerosol or vapor was responsible for several reported cases. Interestingly, a similar sensation was reported by investigators in 1941 after exposure to *Chrysanthemum*

cineariaefolium flowers.[5] The patient described tingling of his face after entering a room with an open canister of air-dried flowers. To continue his work, he was forced as a prophylactic measure to smear petrolatum over all exposed areas of his body.

Tucker and colleagues[6] performed pilot studies on various topical agents to assess their ability to prevent dysesthesia accompanying exposure to the synthetic pyrethroid, Pydrin. Six compounds were evaluated for their prophylactic efficacy on four participants on separate occasions. Nature's County Natural Vitamin E Oil (25,000 IU/2.1 fl oz) was the most effective prophylactic agent evaluated, with a prophylactic index (PI) of 97.3%. In contrast, Zinc Oxide Paste (USP 25%) appeared to be actually enhance symptoms. A cost-effective therapeutic agent would be Arrowhead Mills Brand Corn Oil, but due to the comedogenic properties of vegetable oils, it was not recommended.

Contact dermatitis in response to synthetic pyrethroids is very rare. In a survey of 230 subjects,[7] two cases of allergy to fenvalerate were reported, along with one allergic reaction to cypermethrin and two irritant reactions to resmethrin.

The Pants Paresthesia Syndrome

Fisher[8] studied four men who complained bitterly of itching, tingling, and formication of the lower extremities, particularly the inner aspects of the thighs, whenever they wore trousers not made exclusively of cotton. Examination of the skin revealed no abnormalities. Two of the patients were examined by neurologists who also found nothing objectively. Patch tests to formaldehyde and various resins and textile finishes were negative. Two of the patients believed that the "weight of the material itself" caused a burning sensation.

Dr. Frances Storrs, who interviewed two of the patients, reported to Dr. Fisher:[9]

I don't have any more ideas about those burning and itching male patients of yours than I did last year. I still think that one of the formaldehyde polymers or dyes could be causing the problem. Ask your patients to wear well-washed Levi's blue jeans for a month and only Levi's blue jeans. If they become substantially better, I think you can, in fact, look to a fabric finish or a dye as the cause of the difficulty. Perhaps they developed contact urticaria. Remember that the Levi's must be the so-called "bread and butter Levi's" that are found on whole shelves. They cannot be the so-called designer Levi's.

Dr. Calnan of London informed Fisher that several patients were "running around" in London frustrated because dermatologists were unable to come up with an answer to this problem.

Dr. Devel of Belgium sent Fisher the following information:

> Referring to your letter on "pants" problem (*Contact Dermatitis* 9:92): I have sent you the following short communication read in the Flemish newspaper *De Standaard* on Saturday 11, March 1983: "My son likes to wear velvet jean trousers, but they cause him skin irritation on the thighs, even if consisting of 85% cotton and only 15% polyester. Frequent washings, water softeners, abstinence of ironing, lining as low as the knees, ... it doesn't make any difference. Who knows what to do?[9]

One dermatologist reported that he personally suffers from this pants syndrome.

All the patients mentioned were men. Dr. L. Alston, however, writes as follows:

> Regarding contact "pants paresthesia syndrome," I have had a patient who has driven me nuts for the past year complaining bitterly of discomfort, tingling and funny sensations on her inner thighs. She is a 40-year-old slightly chubby woman who usually wears slacks. She felt the seams of her slacks were causing the problem. She would sew handkerchiefs into her slacks to cover those seams. That helped just a little. For a period of time she had a deep erythema in that region. I did patch test her to dyes, formaldehyde, etc., pieces of fabric from her slacks and could not find anything on patch testing. The rash gradually diminished with a topical steroid. She has switched to wearing dresses. She seems to fit the pattern of your male patients with the burning and itching. I cannot find anything at least in what I have patch tested her to regarding formaldehyde, resins, and textile finishes. She does not wear Levi's at all so it really is not a problem with Levi's. She usually wears brown, black, or navy polyester slacks.[9]

Paresthesia from Wool and Mohair

Wool is the natural, highly crimped fiber from sheep. Minute scales on the fiber allow interlocking to form felt cloth and mill-finished worsteds. These scales may be harsh enough to cause mechanical irritation in many persons, especially atopics.

Friction with woolen garments, particularly in association with sweating and atopic dermatitis, may produce a nonspecific pruritus and burning sensation.

Mohair is the resilient hair fiber obtained from the Angora goat. It provides a crisp, firm, and slightly scratchy feel to fabrics even when used in low percentage blends with other fibers. Its addition to clothing produces itching and discomfort in some persons, but allergic sensitivity has not been reported.

Pressure/Friction Paresthesia and Alopecia

Choy[10] reported as follows:

> A stockbroker appeared at my office with a chief complaint of hypesthesia in a palm-sized area over the left suprapatellar area of several months' duration. Another physician had ordered roentgenograms of the lumbar spine, which were normal. Physical examination showed hypesthesia and obvious hair loss over the involved area.

> Careful questioning revealed that the telephone in his office was so placed that reaching for it necessitated turning his body more than 90° to the right. This motion was always accompanied by scraping the anterior surface of his left lower thigh (the affected area) against the kneehole of the desk.

> In a follow-up visit, he reported that in discussing his now famous knee with his office colleagues, another stockbroker with the same telephone-desk configuration came forward with an almost identical complaint of hypesthesia in the left suprapatellar area.

> Perhaps an appropriate diagnosis in these two cases would be stockbroker's knee.[9]

An orthopedic surgeon reported that the pressure of a wallet in a hip pocket can produce a neuralgia-simulating sciatica.

Paresthesia from Solvents

Strong solvents, such as turpentine, acetone, and benzene, may produce dryness and fissuring of the skin accompanied by paresthesia of the fingers. Such paresthesias may persist for several weeks after the dermatitis has subsided and the patient no longer has contact with the solvents.

One consultant neurologist stated he had observed similar peripheral neuritis and paresthesia accompanying industrial dermatitis from benzene.[9]

Acrylonitrile, which is recognized as a skin irritant, was found to produce five cases of allergic contact dermatitis in an occupational setting. One of these was accompanied by paresthesia that had not previously been reported with acrylonitrile.[11]

Loss of Taste

Contact dermatitis in the form of cheilitis and perioral eczema due to anethole was associated with a loss of taste.[12] The sense of taste returned about 2 to 3 weeks after the cheilitis cleared. Anethole is found in oil of anise, star anise, and fennel. It can be found in toothpaste.

Methyl Methacrylate Monomer

Fisher[13] reported that surgeons and dentists who become sensitized to methyl methacrylate monomer in acrylic bone cement may suffer a distressing paresthesia of the fingertips in the form of a burning sensation, tingling, and slight numbness. The paresthesia may persist for several weeks to months after the dermatitis has subsided. Fisher saw this type of paresthesia in two orthopedic surgeons who became sensitized to acrylates. The paresthesia persisted for 3 months in one and 4 months in the other after the dermatitis cleared.

Five dentists who acquired an acrylic monomer dermatitis had persistent paresthesia for 3 to 6 months after the dermatitis subsided. Dermatitis and paresthesia of the fingertips of the first three fingers of both hands were found to be due to a dental acrylate containing 2-hydroxyethyl methacrylate.[14] A local effect on peripheral nerves is thought to be responsible for the paresthesia, which can last for months after exposure is discontinued.

It should be noted that the acrylic monomers can readily penetrate rubber or vinyl gloves within a few minutes. Some surgeons wear two or more pairs of gloves during surgery. Changing gloves frequently may be useful also. The brands Silvershield or 4-H chemical protective gloves should block acrylate penetration, but have little elasticity so they may impede fine manipulation skills.

Adverse Subjective Reactions to Topical Agents

Grove and colleagues[15] state that certain topical products, especially those applied to the face, can pass all the standard tests yet still be unacceptable because they induce strong, disagreeable sensations (e.g., stinging, burning, or itching). These investigators indicate that these disagreeable sensations occur frequently enough to warrant serious study. This is not an easy task, as the adverse reactions are purely subjective and generally not accompanied by any visual signs by which the degree of response can be graded. Thus, the ear, not the eye, serves as the detector regarding problems of adverse subjective reactions.

TESTING FOR "STINGING" TOPICAL AGENTS

Stinging is a problem that occurs primarily on the face, particularly on the nasolabial folds and cheeks. The enhanced sensitivity of this region is a reflection of its microanatomic features, including a more permeable stratum corneum, a high density of appendages (hair follicles and sweat glands) that serve as diffusional shunts, and an elaborate network of sensory nerves. In humans, every vellous hair is associated with specialized nerve endings that connect to an elaborate dermal nerve network.[16] Thus, it is not surprising that the face is so sensitive to touch and pain.

Stinging seems to be a variant of pain that develops rapidly and fades quickly any time the appropriate sensory nerves are stimulated. This type of response is usually quite well tolerated. Consumers have come to expect such a short burst of stinging from alcoholic formulations, for example, aftershave lotions, astringents, and toners. With the intolerable variety of stinging with which we are concerned, the response is not only more intense but somewhat delayed and sustained. Typically, it begins within 1 or 2 minutes after product application and intensifies over the next 5 to 10 minutes. This sharp stinging then fades slowly over the next 15 to 20 minutes. Despite the fact that this crescendo-type stinging may become so intense that frantic attempts are made to wash off the offending material, visual indications of the adverse response, for example, erythema, are rarely seen.

Using a 20:80 mixture of chloroform:methanol, Frosch and Kligman[16] found that the nasolabial fold is the region most sensitive to both "burning" and "stinging" sensations. Heavy users of cosmetics were most susceptible to the lactic acid "stinging" test and the chloroform:methanol "burning" test. Lactic acid was felt to provide more reliable results and is easier to use as a test material.[17] The essential features of this procedure were that the test materials were applied to the nasolabial folds and cheeks of preselected sensitive individuals who were brought to a state of profuse sweating in an environmental chamber. Once again, no strong correlation between irritancy and stinging was observed. For example, strong irritants, such as quaternary ammonium surfactants, undiluted kerosene, and 5% sodium lauryl sulfate, did not produce stinging under these conditions, whereas weak irritants or nonirritants, such as Escalol 506, provoked intense stinging.

Initially, Frosch and Kligman[16,17] thought that most persons who experienced stinging would be light-complexioned persons of Celtic ancestry who were easily sunburned. Grove and colleagues[15] reported, however, that skin type is not a reliable predictor of stinging proclivity. People with a darker complexion can also experience moderate or intense stinging in response to 10% lactic acid applied to the nasolabial folds and cheeks. Persons who experienced such positive reactions judged themselves as having unusually "sensitive" skin and usually reported a variety of past troubles with cosmetics, soaps, and related items. Thus, it is more expedient to prescreen candidates on the basis of a history of problem or sensitive skin than on the basis of a fair or dark complexion. Results of a lactic-acid sting test however, did not correlate well with self-reported skin sensitivity in one study, although capsaicin reactivity correlated better.[18]

The actual premarket testing of products for stinging capacity is performed on preselected "stingers." Test materials can be classified into one of three categories, based on results obtained with the improved facial sting test. The first class includes materials that exhibit little or no potential for stinging during normal use. The second class includes products that have a slight potential for stinging and that might pose a problem for some "sensitive-skinned" persons. The third class includes products with a strong potential for stinging; these would be intolerable to sensitive-skinned persons and perhaps other consumers as well. Manufacturers frequently employ panels of "stingers" to identify facial products that are likely to be problematic in this regard. Farage and colleagues[19] have recently reviewed sensory factors in sensitive skin.

TESTING FOR ITCHING IN RESPONSE TO COSMETICS

Frosch and Kligman[16] found that fragrances and sunscreen lotions are the major culprits of itching from cosmetics. They used a "histamine itching test" to determine which woman would itch from exposure to topical agents.

Using this test, Fisher[9] found no correlation between the size of the wheal and the sensation of itching. Frosch and Kligman[16] also found no correlation between wheal size and itching. There appears to be no correlation between itching and stinging or burning.

Status Cosmeticus (Problem Sensitive Skin)

Frosch and Kligman[17] came to the conclusion that a small but significant number of young women have "problem-sensitive skin." Fisher found that not only young women but also older women may have "problem-sensitive skin," which has long been called "status cosmeticus" or "cosmetic intolerance syndrome."[20] Any area or all of the face may be affected. Fisher[9] observed that many women with status cosmeticus are particularly

affected not only by lactic acid but also by sorbic acid, isopropyl myristate, and urea.

Contact Leukoderma (Vitiligo)

Contact leukoderma, also called contact vitiligo or contact depigmentation, may be defined as a complete depigmentation usually without preceding inflammation. This is in contrast to postinflammatory hypopigmentation, which must by definition be preceded by inflammation and in which total depigmentation does not usually occur. Because of the frequent association with workplace exposure, contact leukoderma is sometimes called occupational leukoderma or vitiligo.

Contact leukoderma may be indistinguishable from idiopathic vitiligo. Fisher[21] suggested that some cases of idiopathic vitiligo may be due to unsuspected inhalation or ingestion of chemicals that produce contact leukoderma, although such a possibility has not been studied. Table 23.2 lists the chemicals capable of producing contact vitiligo.

PARATERTIARY BUTYLPHENOL

Exposure to paratertiary butylphenol (PTBP) is widespread in industry, and consumers who use synthetic leather, plastics, glues, and germicidal phenolic detergents can also be exposed to it. Table 23.3 lists the numerous ways in which individuals can be exposed to this phenolic compound.

Table 23-2 Chemicals Capable of Producing Contact Vitiligo

Diisoptopyl fluorophosphate

Epoxy resins (phenylglycidyl ether?)

Hydroquinone

Mercaptoamines, such as N-(2-mercaptoethyl)-dimethylamine hydrochloride (MEDA) and b-mercaptoethylamine hydrochloride (MEA)

Monobenzyl ether of hydroquinone

Monoethyl ether of hydroquinone (p-ethoxyphenol)

Monomethyl ether of hydroquinone (p-methoxyphenol or p-hydroxyanisole)

N, N9, N0-triethylenethiophosphoramide (Thio-TEPA)

p-cresol

p-isoprophylcatechol

p-methylcatechol

p-nonylphenol

p-octylphenol

p-phenylphenol

p-tert-amylphenol

p-tert-butylcatechol

p-tert-butylphenol

Physostigmine (eserine)

Polyvinyl chloride plastics (plasticizers?)

Table 23-3 Exposure to Paratertiary Butylphenol
De-emulsifiers for oil field use
Deodorants
Duplicating paper
Formaldehyde resin CKR-1634
Germicidal phenolic detergent compounds
Insecticides
Latex glues
Motor oil additives
Paratertiary butylphenol formaldehyde resins
Plasticizers for cellulose acetate
Printing inks
Rubber antioxidants
Soap antioxidants
Synthetic oils
Varnish and lacquer resins
Valve plants

Malten and colleagues,[22] in a comprehensive review of "occupational vitiligo," pointed out that depigmentation may occur without preceding irritation, dermatitis, or burns. Malten,[23] distinguishing between occupational vitiligo and contact vitiligo in a "consumer," reported a case of mild contact dermatitis on a man's left wrist and later on the right wrist, after he started wearing his watch on that side. This contact dermatitis was from the glue (called Bison Kit in the Netherlands), which contains *p*-tertiary butylphenol formaldehyde resin from which "free" PTBP is released and which produced the depigmentation. This deduction was made from the fact that PTBP is a monomer that forms synthetic adhesives by polymerizing with formaldehyde.

Malten and colleagues[22] predicted that cases of occupational vitiligo can be expected in workers handling PTBP and its homologous substances in a variety of factories and occupations if measures are not taken from the beginning to avoid direct skin contact, inhalation, and ingestion of these chemicals.

Saruta and Nakamizo[24] reported occupational leukoderma on the neck, arms, hands, breast, abdomen, and hip of pharmaceutical workers exposed to PTBP. Histologic investigation revealed remarkably vacuolated cells in the basal layers. Occlusive dressings of PTBP applied to the backs of black guinea pigs resulted in experimental leukoderma. In the normal skin of two patients, occlusive dressings with PTBP produced leukoderma not only in areas in direct contact with PTBP but also beyond the occluded areas.

The *bindi*, the circular mark worn on the forehead of Indian women, has an adhesive on the back that may be coated with PTBP. Skin contact with PTBP in the adhesive led to depigmentation without dermatitis.[25,26] Some Indian synthetic wallets, commonly carried against the breast by Indian women, have also caused leukoderma. Analysis showed that monobenzyl ether of hydroquinone was the cause.[27]

ALKYLPHENOLS

Calnan[28] reported occupational leukoderma from the alkylphenols. In workers in industrial plants producing alkylphenols, patches of leukoderma developed not only on exposed skin but also on areas covered by clothing. Ingestion and inhalation of vaporized phenols may have been responsible for a systemic effect on melanocytes.

Table 23.4 lists skin color changes from occupational chemicals.

Table 23-4 Skin Color Changes Due to Occupational Chemicals	
Yellow	Dichromate
	Dinobuton
	Fluorescein dye
	Glutaraldehyde
	4,49-methylenedianiline: catalyst for epoxy and urethane resins
	Nitric acid
	Picric acid and picrates
	Sodium nitrite
Blue	Cobalt
	Indigo
	Oxalic acid in automobile radiator cleaners
	Silver nitrate in photographers
	Sulfadiazine silver (silvadene) in pharmaceutical workers and nurses in burn units
Brown	Chrysarobin and anthralin in pharmacists and nursing personnel
	Paraphenylenediamine in dye manufacture and photography developers
	Permanganates in bleach and dye makers, water purifiers, and paper pulp bleaches
	Phenothiazines (agricultural workers, veterinarians, and nurses)
Red	Soda ash
	TNT
Black	Mercury
	Osmium trioxide in histology technicians, incandescent lamp makers, organic chemical synthesizers, and platinum hardeners
	Gold from jewelry
Orange	Chlorine gas
	Phenothiazine
	Tetryl (trinitrophenylmethylnitramine)
Green	Copper dust in electrical workers, machinists, and copper smelters

Modified by personal communication with Dr. Robert Adams, Palo Alto, CA, 1998.

PARATERTIARY BUTYLCATECHOL

Gellin and colleagues[29] were among the first to recognize that some persons with "idiopathic vitiligo" may actually have an environmentally or occupationally induced leukoderma. Four workers at an assembly plant in Michigan developed leukoderma from exposure to paratertiary butylcatechol (PTBC). These workers had dermatitis on the upper limbs before the onset of leukoderma. Their depigmentation began as early as a few months to as late as 4 years after they started work in the assembly plant. In one patient, leukoderma was confined to the hands and forearms, but in the other three patients, distant areas were also affected. One of these three patients, a woman, had depigmentation over 75% of her body surface.

When patch tested with PTBC, three of the four patients had eczematous positive patch test reactions. In one man, an area of depigmentation remained for over 20 months, even though the reaction had subsided.

Experimentally, the catechol derivative was found to induce varying degrees of irritation in six volunteer subjects and to cause depigmentation in black, but not albino, guinea pigs. The related chemical, PTBP, had the same effect.

Occupational exposure to coal tar and tar products led to ACD to PTBC and subsequent progressive leukoderma in another case.[30] There was no cross-reactivity to PTBP in this case.

DEPIGMENTATION CAUSED BY PHENOLIC DETERGENT GERMICIDES

Kahn[31] reported that certain phenolic detergent germicides, used widely in hospitals and many households, may cause depigmentation of the skin. Such depigmentation occurred on the hands and forearms of five persons on the housekeeping staff of a Denver hospital, 6 months after they used the phenolic detergent-disinfectant O-Syl, containing PTBP, for cleaning. At about the same time, seven employees of an adjacent Denver hospital had a similar experience. Six months after introduction of the phenolic-disinfectant Ves-Phene, containing paratertiary amylphenol (PTAP), the skin on the patients' hands and arms also showed depigmentation.

Both PTBP and PTAP are found in germicidal disinfectants. PTAP is also used in the manufacture of oil-soluble resins, in organic synthesis, as a plasticizer, and as a fumigant. A 1% PTAP sensitized 5 of 13 patients in this report, and the 6% solution irritated the skin of every person to whom it was applied. This agent is apparently more toxic to epidermal and bacterial cells than is PTBP. A 1% ethanolic PTAP solution produces depigmentation similar to that produced by 6% PTBP solution.

Kahn found that these agents depigmented the skin of both patients and volunteers within 2 weeks without producing dermatitis. In three patients, depigmentation disappeared at the test site within 6 months. In the other two, it was still present more than 1 year after testing. The average onset of depigmentation was about 2 weeks. In a discussion of the mechanism of pigment loss, Kahn found that phenolics remain in the skin long after application.

EPOXY RESIN DILUENTS

Vitiligo on the hands of a worker, along with ACD to epoxy diluents including phenylglycidyl ether has been reported, but the positive patch test sites did not depigment.[32]

TRIGLYCIDYL-P-AMINOPHENOL

An aircraft worker developed ACD from epoxy-related allergens including this agent.[33] He developed depigmentation at the patch-test sites several months after testing. No depigmentation developed at other patch-test sites or sites of dermatitis.

PHENOLIC COMPOUNDS IN THE CERAMIC INDUSTRY

Tosti and colleagues[34] reported possible contact leukoderma in a ceramics worker heavily exposed to lacquers containing phenolic compounds, including phlobaphenes, stilbenes, flavonoids, and lignins.

POLYVINYL CHLORIDE PLASTICS

There are two reports of depigmentation from PVC medical items that had prolonged recurrent contact with skin. One was from stethoscope earpieces and the other from an oxygen nasal canula.[35,36] In both cases the PVC contained phthalates as plasticizers. The exact agent responsible for the depigmentation is uncertain.

MECHANISM OF PHENOLIC DEPIGMENTATION

Gellin and colleagues[29] state that both PTBP and PTBC are structurally related to monobenzyl ether of hydroquinone, which has long been known to induce occupational leukoderma. Thus, it appears that many phenols and catechols are capable of depigmenting mammalian skin, especially with group substitutions at the *para* position. The investigators theorized that the mechanism of pigment loss is due to competitive inhibition of tyrosine oxidase, because of the structural similarities between phenols and catechols and tyrosine, with a resultant cytotoxic effect on melanocytes.

Recent research suggests, however, that tyrosinase-related protein 1 (TYRP1), a melanogenic enzyme, is involved.[37] Intramelanocyte oxidate stress is induced by PTBP. Vitiligo melanocytes are much more susceptible to damage from this, apparently because of altered levels of TYRP1.[38]

Hydroquinone Uses and Abnormal Reactions

Hydroquinone is used widely in industry as a reducing agent, as a photographic developer, and as an antioxidant or stabilizer for certain materials that polymerize in the presence of oxidizing agents. Thus, in acrylic and polyester resin systems, its presence prevents unintended spontaneous polymerization.[39] Some occupational exposures are shown in Table 23.5. It is also used as a reagent for phosphate determination.

Hydroquinone dust is a mild primary irritant. Skin sensitization to the dry solid is rare but occurs on occasion from contact with its alkaline solutions. The skin may be depigmented by repeated applications of ointments of hydroquinone, but this virtually never occurs from contact with dust or dilute water solutions. Following prolonged exposure to elevated dust levels, brownish conjunctival stains may appear. These stains may be followed by corneal opacities, which may lead to loss of visual acuity.[40] The early skin pigmentation may be reversible, whereas the corneal changes tend to be progressive.

DEPIGMENTATION FROM HYDROQUINONE IN PHOTOGRAPHIC DEVELOPMENT

There are several reports of occupational leukoderma from exposure to hydroquinone developer in photogra-

TABLE 23-5 Occupational Exposures to Hydroquinone

Antioxidant makers
Bacteriostatic agent makers
Cosmetologists (artificial nails)
Dental personnel
Drug makers
Fur processors
Motor fuel blenders
Organic chemical synthesizers
Paint makers
Photographic developer makers
Plastic stabilizer workers
Rubber production workers
Stone coating workers
Styrene monomer workers

phy.[41,42] The concentration of hydroquinone in the various photographic processes was probably over 7%. At a dermatology meeting, Fisher[43] saw a high school student who developed contact vitiligo of the hands from exposure to hydroquinone in a school course on photographic development.

DEPIGMENTATION FROM "BLEACHING CREAMS" CONTAINING HYDROQUINONE

Numerous so-called bleaching creams containing hydroquinone are used widely in attempts to lighten hyperpigmented areas of the skin, such as melasma, freckles, senile lentigines, and other forms of melanin hyperpigmentation. These are available both by prescription and OTC.

Adverse reactions that have been reported in the past include rare instances of allergic reactions, erythema, and stinging sensations. However, a possible "toxic" reaction to hydroquinone has been noted in several patients.[44,45] Fisher[45] encountered four patients who had never used monobenzyl ether of hydroquinone but nevertheless acquired disfiguring leukoderma following the use of three popular bleaching creams containing 2% hydroquinone. The possibility of such hydroquinone preparations worsening latent idiopathic vitiligo must also be considered.

A review of the literature and personal communications from various authorities,[46–48] however, indicate that hydroquinone bleaching creams containing low concentrations of hydroquinone are safe and rarely if ever produce the depigmentation seen with the use of monobenzyl ether of hydroquinone.

ROLE OF PATCH TESTING WITH HYDROQUINONE

The few patients of Fisher[45] who developed leukoderma from hydroquinone bleaching creams had neither preceding inflammation nor a positive patch test reaction to 1% hydroquinone in petrolatum after 72 hours. In one patient, "open testing" (rubbing 1% hydroquinone in pet into one site) produced hypopigmentation on normal skin.

Hydroquinone may cross-react with resorcin and pyrocatechol.

RELATION OF MONOBENZYL ETHER OF HYDROQUINONE TO HYDROQUINONE

Van Ketel[49] stated that sensitization to monobenzyl ether of hydroquinone occurs rather frequently, whereas hydroquinone is regarded as a rather weak sensitizer. He reported that one of his patients showed sensitization to both hydroquinone and monobenzyl ether of hydroquinone. It is possible that sensitization to monobenzyl ether may be partially explained by hydrolysis to hydroquinone.

BUTYLATED HYDROXYTOLUENE (BHT) DEPIGMENTATION

Vollum[50] reported two black children, one with psoriasis and one with eczema, who developed hypopigmentation after treatment with polyethylene film (polythene) applied over a corticosteroid ointment. The area of depigmentation was limited to the skin covered by the polyethylene. Analysis of the film showed that it contained butylated hydroxytoluene (BHT) as an antioxidant to prevent decomposition, and this was deemed to be the responsible factor. In one patient, the skin gradually returned to normal 8 weeks after treatment was ceased; in the other, there was no sign of repigmentation 4 weeks after cessation of treatment. Although there have been several reports of ACD from this antioxidant in cosmetics and foods, there have been no other reports confirming depigmentation from BHT.[51] Many other factors could have caused the hypopigmentation in Vollum's report.

NONOCCUPATIONAL VITILIGO FROM CONTACTANTS

With the use of synthetic leather and shoe adhesives containing PTBP, contact vitiligo of the feet can occur.

LEUKODERMA FROM ADHESIVES

Frenk and Kocsis[52] reported depigmentation from adhesive tape. One of the adhesive tapes studied was of polyvinyl chloride, with a natural rubber base adhesive containing a derivative of dihydroxydiphenylmethane. A case of leukoderma following application of transdermal buspirone patches has been reported, but the contents of the adhesive was not documented.[53]

Neoprene adhesives and PTBP resin adhesives may produce leukoderma.[54,55]

Maibach (personal communication, January, 2006) reported a case of depigmentation on the breast induced, presumably, by monobenzyl ether of hydroquinone present in the adhesive of breast prostheses ("falsies") worn by the patient.

PARA-PHENYLENEDIAMINE

Taylor and colleagues[56] reported four cases of contact leukoderma from hair coloring agents. Another report detailed contact leukoderma with no dermatitis on the lip after use of a mustache coloring product containing para-phenylenediamine (PPDA). Patch test was negative to PPDA.[57] A report of hair dye depigmentation from India discussed a patient with allergy to PPDA with

positive patch tests. The test sites depigmented 3 months later.[58] A henna tattoo containing PPDA caused ACD with subsequent leukoderma.[59] A worker in a hair-dye plant developed ACD and leukoderma from contact with p-toluenediamine sulfate.[60]

OTHER CAUSES OF CONTACT VITILIGO

Alta, a red solution used by some Indian women to color the feet, has been reported to occasionally cause depigmentation.[61] Alta contains two azo dyes, Crocein Scarlet MOO and rhodamine B. Depigmentation occurred at patch test sites and also at the site of a patch test to PPDA.

Kanerva and Estlander[62] reported persistent (2.8 years) depigmentation at sites of patch testing with acrylates. The test substances were dental resins tested at use concentrations instead of being diluted as recommended.

Rubber "consumer" products, such as condoms, rubberized stockings, bandages, orthopedic splints,[63] and cosmetic face sponges, can produce contact vitiligo (Table 23.6).

A report of localized vitiligo following ACD from nickel in a belt buckle was recently published.[64] Cause and effect are unproven.

PERIORAL LEUKODERMA FROM CINNAMIC ALDEHYDE

Mathias and colleagues[65] described a perioral leukoderma simulating vitiligo in a 25-year-old woman. A patch test to cinnamic aldehyde was positive; depigmentation was observed at the patch test site 3 months after the initial application. No changes in pigmentation occurred from a concomitant allergic patch test reaction to neomycin sulfate. A toothpaste containing cinnamic aldehyde was implicated; perioral hypopigmentation resolved when a toothpaste without cinnamic aldehyde was substituted. A repeated patch test to cinnamic

Table 23-6 "Consumer" Products Producing "Nonoccupational" Vitiligo

Acrylates

Adhesive tapes

Bindi

Cinnamic aldehyde in a toothpaste

Dyes: Para-phenylenediamine and alta

Germicidal phenolic detergents

Latex glues

Rubber products

"Falsies," condoms, stockings, girdles, bandages, cosmetic face sponges

Shoes

Wristwatch bands

aldehyde again showed depigmentation at the patch test site 3 months after application.

DIFFERENTIATION OF IDIOPATHIC AND CONTACT VITILIGO

Fitzpatrick[66] indicated that vitiligo from contactants can readily be confused with the "idiopathic" variety. Histologic examination is of no help because melanocytes degenerate similarly in both conditions. Idiopathic vitiligo is usually permanent, whereas vitiligo from contactants may sometimes clear if the causative contactant is removed.

A careful history may reveal exposure to a depigmentary chemical listed in the tables. Fitzpatrick[66] noted that "idiopathic" vitiligo may accompany other diseases, such as thyrotoxicosis, hyperparathyroidism, and pernicious anemia.

Frenk and Kocsis,[52] in their case report of depigmentation from either a plastic strip or adhesive, stated they could distinguish contact vitiligo from the idiopathic variety by the presence in the electron microscope of "unusual clear cells." This has not been confirmed from other reports.

Fisher[67] stated that subtle ocular changes, such as pigment loss in the iris, may be found in idiopathic vitiligo. Presumably this would not occur in contact leukoderma.

EXPERIMENTAL REPRODUCTION OF CONTACT VITILIGO

Gellin and colleagues[29] found that the experimental depigmentary effect of local open application of PTBP to black guinea pigs appeared to be vehicle dependent and seemed on occasions to be related to concomitant irritancy. PTBP in concentrations of 0.005, 1.5, and 10 g/100 mL of acetone was ineffective, although the two higher concentrations were irritating. With dimethyl sulfoxide or propylene glycol, a depigmentary (and irritating) effect of PTBP was seen only in the 10 g/100 mL solutions but not in the 1 or 5 g solutions, which were not irritant.

Similarly, experimental incubation in human volunteers is dependent upon strength, vehicle, method of external application (frequency, open or closed), and site of application. Kahn[31] reported that depigmentation (after closed patch testing on alternating days with 6% PTBP in alcohol) occurred after an average of 2 weeks.

DIMINISHED CONTACT SENSITIVITY IN VITILIGINOUS SKIN

Uehara and colleagues[68] studied 30 patients with vitiligo (10 of the segmental type and 20 of the generalized type) who were sensitized with dinitrochlorobenzene (DNCB)

in a normal skin site on the upper medial aspect of the arm. Challenge tests with DNCB were performed in vitiliginous patches and in normal skin sites. In vitiliginous patches, diminished contact sensitivity reactions to DNCB were noted in both groups of patients, whereas in normal skin sites, a normal delayed hypersensitivity response to the same antigen developed in the same patients. Tuberculin reactivity was not suppressed in vitiliginous lesions. The investigators suggested that diminished contact reactivity in vitiliginous skin might be due to functional changes in Langerhans' cells or to an alteration of carrier (skin) proteins in the lesions.

Nordlund and colleagues[69] made a similar observation of diminished reactivity to monobenzone in areas of vitiligo, and a similar lack of contact dermatitis occurred with airborne exposure to parthenium in India (vitiliginous areas of the lips and fingers remained uninvolved).[70] Similarly, a lack of dermatitis has been reported within areas of nevoid depigmentation despite surrounding textile dermatitis.[71]

PROGNOSIS AND TREATMENT OF CONTACT VITILIGO

Spontaneous repigmentation of affected areas may occur occasionally. In most instances, however, the depigmentation lasts indefinitely. Ehrenfeld[72] treated a hospital orderly who acquired depigmentation from washing instruments with a solution of O-Syl detergent. Employing the technique described by Fulton and colleagues,[73] Ehrenfeld treated the patient by painting a solution of methoxsalen on the dorsum of the right hand and irradiating the area with UVA lights. The PUVA treatments were performed at weekly intervals for 2 months. Pigment about the hair follicles on the proximal phalanges of the right hand began to form after six treatments. No such repigmentation occurred on the left hand, which had not been treated. Kahn,[35] however, did not succeed in obtaining repigmenting in his cases of contact vitiligo with topical psoralens and sunlight.

POSTINFLAMMATORY PIGMENTARY CHANGES

Gellin and colleagues[29] stated that increased pigmentation may be a postinflammatory response following contact dermatitis from diverse causes. Photosensitive reactions may follow contact with tar, pitch, and psoralens, or phytodermatitis may result from contact with celery, figs, or limes. (See chapter 22.) Physical damage from chemical and thermal burns may also be responsible. Postinflammatory hyperpigmentation may occur frequently after some inflammatory skin diseases such as lichen planus or fixed drug eruption.

Decreased pigmentation may also be postinflammatory following contact dermatitis from various causes. It can result from physical damage inflicted by chemical and thermal burns, or it may occur after any inflammatory dermatosis such as psoriasis or contact dermatitis. Clinically, postinflammatory hypopigmentation manifests as a decrease in color, not total absence of melamine, as is seen in leukoderma. Recovery to normal skin color is nearly universal once the inflammation has subsided.

HYPOPIGMENTATION OR HYPERPIGMENTATION FROM RUBBER

Rubber compounds containing antioxidants, particularly hydroquinone, have long been known to produce leukoderma. Hamada and Horiguchi,[74] however, reported chronic melanodermatitis from rubber caused by contact with the rubber peephole of a ship radarscope.

Bleehen and Hall-Smith[75] reported marked depigmentation of the skin in areas in direct contact with an elasticized brassiere containing spandex yarn. They suggested that the persistent skin depigmentation that occurred in this case is an isomorphic phenomenon due to friction and pressure from the brassiere in a patient with vitiligo.

EXOGENOUS OCHRONOSIS FROM HYDROQUINONE DAMAGE TO DERMIS FROM BLEACHING CREAMS

South African dermatologists[76,77] reported an outbreak of exogenous ochronosis and colloid milium in patients who had used strong hydroquinone bleaching creams. These phenomena developed after a few years and took place when the melanocytes had overcome the bleaching influence. Sun exposure and thorough inunction of the cream were required for the more advanced changes. Analogous changes have been seen when the skin is exposed to certain crude fuels in persons who work in the sun; phenolic components in the fuels are suspected. Sarcoid-like reactions to the ochronotic material and to the lichenoid eruptions at the affected sites are also reportedly possible.

Cutaneous ochronosis from hydroquinone has been reported in the United States, even from over-the-counter products.[78,79] However, because the concentration of hydroquinone in over-the-counter products may exceed a presumed 2% concentration, as noted previously, the concentration responsible may be similar to those in the South African cases.

Exogenous ochronosis may be caused by a number of chemicals, such as phenol, hydroquinone, and resorcinol, after repeated contact with the skin. The pigmentation probably represents either a polymer of the causative chemical itself or a polymer of homogentisic acid owing to interference with tyrosine metabolism.

HYDROQUINONE BLEACHING CREAMS WRONGLY USED FOR LENTIGO MALIGNA

A report[80] warns of the danger of mistakenly using such creams in superficial malignant melanomas. In one patient, use of such a depigmenting cream delayed surgical excision of a lentigo maligna for 1 year and allowed it to grow to considerable size. Depigmentation occurred in the center of the lesion, demonstrating that hydroquinone can affect abnormal as well as normal melanocytes.

PARADOXICAL NAIL PIGMENTATION WITH HYDROQUINONE

An orange-brown to chestnut-brown color may develop on the nail plate with application of hydroquinone over the distal fingertips. Oxidation of hydroquinone has been one explanation, and this may be observed with the cream itself upon prolonged exposure to air.[81] A role for sunlight in the production of this pigmentation has also been suggested.[82] These changes can be confused with heavy metal poisoning or half-and-half nails.

PIGMENTATION OF PALMS AND SCALP FROM PHENOLIC HAIR TONICS

Forman[83] reported pigmentation of the palms and scalp that was probably from proprietary hair tonics containing various phenols and phenolic derivatives.

BENZENE HYPERPIGMENTATION

Dupre and colleagues[84] reported that a manual worker exposed to benzene derivatives developed blue to black spots confined to the hands, which represented pigmented granules in elastic and collagen fibers.

DYSPIGMENTATION FROM *PIPER BETLE* LEAVES

A report from Taiwan discusses 15 patients with areas of mottled depigmentation and hyperpigmentation in the face.[85] All had applied steamed leaves of the plant *Piper betle* (betle pepper) as a "treatment" for melasma or freckling. The patients observed stinging and erythema after leaf application. The authors stated that the leaves contain the essential oils chavical and chavibetal, which are phenolic derivatives. Patch testing was not performed.

PARADOXICAL PIGMENTARY EFFECTS OF TOPICAL MERCURY COMPOUNDS

Mercury-containing topical agents have previously been used as bleaching agents because mercury can displace copper from tyrosinase, inactivating the enzyme that plays a role in the synthesis of melanin.[86] Repeated applications of mercury-containing ointments or cosmetics, however, may give rise to gray-brown pigmentation limited to areas to which it is applied, with accentuation in the skin folds. Burge and Winkelmann,[87] using the electron microscope, demonstrated that melanin pigmentation increased secondarily to the presence of the metal.

References

1. Knox JM, Tucker SB. A new cutaneous sensation caused by synthetic pyrethroids. Clin Res 1982;30:915A.

2. Knox II JM, Tucker SB, Flannigan SA. Paresthesia from cutaneous exposure to a synthetic pyrethroid insecticide. Arch Dermatol 1984;120:744.

3. LeQuesne PM, Maxwell IC, Butterworth ST. Transient facial sensory symptoms following exposure to synthetic pyrethroids: a clinical and electrophysiological assessment. Neurotoxicology 1980;2:1.

4. Tucker SB, Flannigan SA. Cutaneous effects from occupational exposure to fenvalerate. Arch Toxicol 1983;54:195.

5. Martin TJ, Hester KHC. Dermatitis caused by insecticidal pyrethrum flowers (*Chrysanthemum cinerariaefolium*). Br J Dermatol 1941;53:127.

6. Tucker SB, Flannigan SA, Smolensky MH. Comparison of therapeutic agents for synthetic pyrethroid exposure. Contact Dermatitis 1983;9:316.

7. Lisi P. Sensitization risk of pyrethroid insecticides. Contact Dermatitis 1992;26:349.

8. Fisher AA. Contact "pants paresthesia syndrome." Contact Dermatitis 1983;9:92.

9. Fisher AA. Contact dermatitis, 3rd ed. Philadelphia: Lea & Febiger, 1986, p. 482.

10. Choy DSJ. "Stockbroker's knee." Arch Dermatol 1977;113:1300.

11. Bakker JG, Jongen SM, Van Neer FC, Neis JM. Occupational contact dermatitis due to acrylonitrile. Contact Dermatitis 1991;24:50.

12. Franks A. Contact allergy to anethole in toothpaste associated with loss of taste. Contact Dermatitis 1998;38:354.

13. Fisher AA. Paresthesia on the fingers accompanying dermatitis due to methylmethacrylate bone cement. Contact Dermatitis 1979;5:56.

14. Kanerva L, et al. Fingertip paresthesia and occupational allergic contact dermatitis caused by acrylics in a dental nurse. Contact Dermatitis 1998;38:114.

15. Grove GL, Soschin D, Kligman AM. Guidelines for performing facial sting tests. In: Proceedings of the 12th International Congress of the I.F.S.C.C., Paris.

16. Frosch P, Kligman AM. A method for appraising the stinging capacity of topically applied substances. J Soc Cosmet Chem 1977;28:197.

17. Frosch P, Kligman AM. Recognition of chemically vulnerable and delicate skin. In: Frost P, ed. Principles of cosmetics for the dermatologist. St. Louis: Mosby, 1984;287.

18. Robinson M, Perkins M: Evaluation of a quantitative clinical method for assessment of sensory skin irritation. Contact Dermatitis 2001;45:205.

19. Farage M, Katsarou A, Maibach H: Sensory, clinical, and physiologic factors in sensitive skin: a review. Contact Dermatitis 2006;55:1.

20. Fisher AA. Cosmetic actions and reactions: therapeutic, irritant, and allergic. Cutis 1980;26:22.

21. Fisher AA. Vitiligo due to contactants. Cutis 1976;17:431.

22. Malten KE, et al. Occupational vitiligo due to paratertiary butylphenol and homologues. Trans St Johns Hosp Derm Soc 1971;57:115.

23. Malten KE. Paratertiary butylphenol depigmentation in a "consumer." Contact Dermatitis 1975;1:181.

24. Saruta T, Nakamizo Y. Leukoderma due to paratertiary butylphenol. Rinsho Dermatol 1974;16:161.

25. Mathur AK, Srivastava AK, Singh A, Gupta BN. Contact depigmentation by adhesive material of bindi. Contact Dermatitis 1991;24:310.

26. Bajaj AK, Gupta SC, Chatterjee AK. Contact depigmentation from free paratertiary-butylphenol in bindi adhesive. Contact Dermatitis 1990;22:99.

27. Bajaj AK, Gupta SC, Chatterjee AK. Contact depigmentation of the breast. Contact Dermatitis 1991;24:58.

28. Calnan CD. Occupational leukoderma from alkylphenols. Proc R Soc Med 1973;66:258.

29. Gellin GA, Possick PA, Perone VB. Depigmentation from 4-tertiary butyl catechol—an experimental study. J Invest Dermatol 1970;55:190.

30. Gawkrodger DJ, Cork MJ, Bleehen SS. Occupational vitiligo and contact sensitivity to para-tertiary butyl catechol. Contact Dermatitis 1991;25:200.

31. Kahn G. Depigmentation caused by phenolic detergent germicides. Arch Dermatol 1970;102:177.

32. Silvestre J, Albares M, Escutia B, et al: Contact vitiligo appearing after allergic contact dermatitis from aromatic reactive diluents in an epoxy resin system. Contact Dermatitis 2003;49:113.

33. Jappe U, Geier J, Hausen B: Contact vitiligo following a strong patch test reaction to triglycidyl-p-aminophenol in an aircraft industry worker. Contact Dermatitis 2005;53:89.

34. Tosti A, Gaddoni G, Piraccini BM. Occupational leukoderma due to phenolic compounds in the ceramics industry? Contact Dermatitis 1991;25:67.

35. Srinivas C, Mukhi S: Stethoscope earpiece induced chemical depigmentation. Contact Dermatitis 2003;49:110.

36. Kim Y, Kim M, Park Y, et al: Nasal-canula induced chemical depigmentation. Contact Dermatitis 2006;55:113.

37. Boissy R, Manga P: On the etiology of contact/occupational vitiligo. Pigment Cell Res. 2004;17:208.

38. Manga O, Sheyn D, Yang F, et al: A role for tyrosinase-related protein 1 in 4-tert-butylphenol induced toxicity in melanocytes: implications for vitiligo. Am J Pathol 2006; 169:1652.

39. Bentley-Phillips B, Bayles MAH. Butylated hydroxytoluene as a skin lightener. Arch Dermatol 1974;109:216.

40. US Department of Health, Education and Welfare, NIOSH. Occupational diseases—a guide to their recognition. Washington, DC: US Government Printing Office, 1977;249.

41. Kersey P, Stevenson CJ. Vitiligo and occupational exposure to hydroquinone from servicing self-photographing machines. Contact Dermatitis 1981;7:285.

42. Duffield JA. Depigmentation of the skin by quinol and its monobenzyl ether. Lancet 1952;1:1164.

43. Fisher AA. Contact dermatitis, 3rd ed. Philadelphia: Lea & Febiger, 1986.

44. Smith TL. Depigmentation from 2% hydroquinone cream. Schoch Lett 1981;31:48.

45. Fisher AA. Can bleaching creams containing 2% hydroquinone produce leukoderma? J Am Acad Dermatol 1982;7:134.

46. Jimbow K, Obata H, Pathak MA, Fitzpatrick TB. Mechanism of depigmentation by hydroquinone. J Invest Dermatol 1974;62:436.

47. Spencer MC. Topical use of hydroquinone for depigmentation. J Am Acad Dermatol 1965;194:962.

48. Engasser P, Maibach HI. Cosmetics and dermatology: bleaching creams. J Am Acad Dermatol 1981;5:143.

49. Van Ketel WG. Sensitization to hydroquinone and the monobenzyl ether of hydroquinone. Contact Dermatitis 1984;10:253.

50. Vollum DI. Hypomelanosis from an antioxidant in polyethylene film. Arch Dermatol 1971;104:70.

51. Fisher AA. Contact dermatitis to antioxidants in cosmetics and foods. Cutis 1976;17:21.

52. Frenk E, Kocsis M. Depigmentation due to adhesive tape: ultrastructural comparison with vitiligo and vitiliginous depigmentation associated with a melanoma. Dermatologica 1974;148:284.

53. Chapman S, Perazyd J, Perry A, et al: Contact leukoderma caused by buspirone patches. Am J Contact Dermatitis 2002;13:46.

54. Calnan CD, Cooke MA. Leukoderma in industry. J Soc Occup Med 1974;24:59.

55. Wozniak KD, Hamm G. Allergisches Kontaktekzem und vitiligo-artige Depigmentierungen durch parateritiares Butylphenol. Berufsdermatos 1977;25:215.

56. Taylor JS, Maibach HI, Fisher AA, Bergfeld WF. Contact leukoderma associated with the use of hair colors. Cutis 1993;52:273.

57. Brancaccio R, Cohen DE. Contact leukoderma secondary to para-phenylenediamine. Contact Dermatitis 1995;32:313.

58. Bajaj A, Gupta S, Chatierjee A, et al. Hair dye depigmentation. Contact Dermatitis 1996;35:56.

59. Valsecchi R, Leghissa P, DiLandro A, et al: Persistent leukoderma after a henna tattoo. Contact Dermatitis. 2007;56:108.

60. Mahendran R, Stables G, Wilkinson S: Contact leukoderma secondary to occupational toluenediamine sulfate exposure. Contact Dermatitis. 2002;47:117.

61. Bajaj AK, Panley RK, Misra K, et al. Contact depigmentation caused by an azo dye in alta. Contact Dermatitis 1998;38:189.

62. Kanerva L, Estlander T. Contact leukoderma caused by patch testing with dental acrylics. Am J Contact Dermat 1998;9:196.

63. Nabai H, Mehregan A. Rubber induced depigmentation secondary to a wrist splint. Cutis 1994;53:295.

64. Silvestre J, Botella R, Ramon R, et al: Periumbilical contact vitiligo appearing after allergic contact dermatitis to nickel. Am J Contact Dermat 2001;12: 43.

65. Mathias CGT, Maibach HI, Conant MA. Perioral leukoderma simulating vitiligo from use of a toothpaste containing cinnamic aldehyde. Arch Dermatol 1980;116:1172.

66. Fitzpatrick T. Vitiligo. Int J Dermatol 1973;12:202.

67. Fisher A. Ask the experts: the role of ocular disturbances in the differentiation of idiopathic vitiligo from contact leukoderma. Am J Contact Dermat 1997;8:53.

68. Uehara M, Miyauchi H, Tanaka S. Diminished contact sensitivity response in vitiliginous skin. Arch Dermatol 1984;120:195.

69. Nordlund JJ, Forget Z, Kirkewood J, Lerner AB. Dermatitis produced by application of monobenzone in patients with active vitiligo. Arch Dermatol 1985;121:141.

70. Singh KK, Srinivas CR, Balachandran C, Menon S. Parthenium dermatitis sparing vitiliginous skin. Contact Dermatitis 1987;16:174.

71. Srinivas CR, Singh KK, Balachandran C. Textile dermatitis sparing nevoid depigmentation. Contact Dermatitis 1987;16:235.

72. Ehrenfeld ID. Depigmentation due to phenolic detergent germicide: treated with methoxsalen and black-lite. Arch Dermatol 1971;104:216.

73. Fulton JE, Leyden J, Papa C. Treatment of vitiligo with topical methoxsalen and black-lite. Arch Dermatol 1969;100:224.

74. Hamada T, Horiguchi S. Chronic melanodermatitis due to the rubber peephole of a ship radarscope. Contact Dermatitis 1978;4:245.

75. Bleehen SS, Hall-Smith P. Brassiere depigmentation: light and electron microscope studies. Br J Dermatol 1970;83:157.

76. Findlay GH, Morrison JGL, Simson IW. Exogenous ochronosis and pigmented colloid milium from hydroquinone bleaching creams. Br J Dermatol 1975;93:613.

77. Findlay GH, DeBeer HA. Chronic hydroquinone poisoning of the skin from skin-lightening cosmetics: a South African epidemic of ochronosis of the face in dark-skinned individuals. S Afr Med J 1980;57:187.

78. O'Donoghue MN, Lynfield YL, Derbes V. Ochronosis due to hydroquinone. J Am Acad Dermatol 1983;1:123.

79. Hoshaw RA, Zimmerman KG, Menter A. Ochronosislike pigmentation from hydroquinone bleaching creams in American blacks. Arch Dermatol 1985;121:105.

80. Savin JA, Hardie RA. Proprietary depigmenting cream used wrongly for lentigo maligna. Br Med J 1981;282:1666.

81. Garcia RL, White JW Jr, Willis WF. Hydroquinone nail pigmentation [letter]. Arch Dermatol 1978;114:1402.

82. Coulson IH. "Fade out" photochromonychia. Clin Exp Dermatol 1993;18:87.

83. Forman L. Pigmentation of the palms and scalp probably due to proprietary hair tonics, containing various phenols and phenolic derivatives. Br J Dermatol 1977;93:718.

84. Dupre A, Bonafe J-L, Virabes R, Arquie M-T. Idiopathic pigmentation of the hands: professional exogenous ochronosis? New entity? Arch Dermatol Res 1979;266:1.

85. Liao Y, Chiang Y, Tsai T, et al. Contact leukoderma melanosis induced by the leaves of Piper betle (Piperacene): a clinical and histopathologic survey. J Am Acad Dermatol 1999;40:583.

86. Levantin A, Almeyda J. Drug-induced changes in pigmentation. Br J Dermatol 1973;89:105.

87. Burge KM, Winkelmann RF. Mercury pigmentation. Arch Dermatol 1970;102:51.

OCCUPATIONAL DERMATITIS

EXECUTIVE SUMMARY

Occupational dermatitis has been reported as either predominantly irritant in nature or allergic in nature, depending on whether the population studied was drawn from a patch test clinic or a work site. The medical field is commonly over-represented in studies of occupational dermatitis.

Pre-employment patch testing is not recommended. Pre-existing skin diseases such as psoriasis can be aggravated by work friction. Persistent postoccupational dermatitis can develop in up to 10% of work-related contact dermatitis cases. Material safety data sheets can be a good source of information about occupational exposures. At times a visit to the work site by the physician may be required.

Some industries are linked to specific cutaneous eruptions, such as lichenoid eruptions and leukoderma in the photography industry. Pigmentary and purpuric eruptions are found in the textile industry. The printing industry is linked to exposure to ultraviolet cured acrylates. Contact urticaria from animal danders and secretions is common among agricultural workers.

Seemingly innocent exposure to everyday office supplies can cause contact dermatitis from sources such as carbon paper, carbonless paper, copy paper, copy machine toner, and typewriting paper. Bakers, hairdressers and dentists face many occupational exposures that can lead to contact dermatitis.

Dermatitis is by far the most frequently reported occupational disease, and patch testing with a standard screening series of allergens reveals a substantial number of relevant causes. In addition, of course, special test series may have to be performed on workers exposed to diverse contactants.

In industry, as elsewhere, patch testing is indicated only in the diagnosis of allergic eczematous contact dermatitis. Aside from investigative procedures, patch tests are of no value in the primary irritant type of contact dermatitis. The diagnosis of industrial dermatitis depends not only on the patch test results but also on the history, clinical picture, and proved exposure to the suspected contactant.[1,2]

The patch test is particularly valuable in ascertaining the cause of outbreaks of isolated cases of allergic contact dermatitis in an industry in which workers are directly or indirectly exposed to many sensitizing chemicals. Although a careful history and personal investigation of the patient's exposure to contactants often reduce the necessity for routine patch tests, such procedures are often necessary to confirm a diagnosis of allergic contact dermatitis.

Most insurance carriers and industrial boards accept a significant patch test reaction as proof of the etiologic basis of an allergic contact dermatitis. A properly performed and correctly interpreted patch test is scientific proof of the relationship of a specific contactant to a particular dermatitis.

Patch testing may also help in differentiating occupational and nonoccupational dermatitis, particularly when a person with contact dermatitis is exposed to sensitizers not only at work but also at play or in pursuit of hobbies. Properly performed patch tests may pinpoint the offending contactant quickly and efficiently, whereas reliance on history and trial and error may prolong the dermatitis while the offending allergen is being pursued.

Many workers have a superimposed allergic contact dermatitis from sensitizing topical medications. Such a complication can be proved only by patch testing.

The factory dispensary or "first aid" room is sometimes the source of a superimposed allergic contact dermatitis, because sensitizing topical medications are often dispensed or used on industrial dermatitis, burns, and other injuries. Table 24.1 lists the sensitizing medications often found in factories as well as nonsensitizing alternatives.

In an English contact dermatitis clinic, of 1,153 patients evaluated, 17% were diagnosed as having occupational dermatitis. The final diagnosis was irritant

Table 24-1 Suggested Nonsensitizing Medications for Factory First-Aid Treatment

Medication	Low sensitizers	Potent sensitizers
Anesthetics	Pramoxine HCl cream or lotion Xylocaine ointment	Topical "caine" anesthetics, especially those containing benzocaine
Antibiotics	Ilotycin ointment	Topical antibiotics containing neomycin
Antifungal agents	Micatin, Lotrimin lotion, Whitfield's ointment	Mycolog cream
Antihistamines	Oral antihistamine to relieve itching	Topical antihistamine-containing creams
Antiseptics	Hydrogen peroxide Betadine solution	Thimerosal (Merthiolate) Nitrofurazone (furacin)
Steroids	Hydrocortisone cream 0.5% to 2.5% Fluorinated corticosteroid creams 0.01% to 0.05%	Paraben-containing steroid creams
Vitamin preparations	Petrolatum	Vitamin E–containing creams

Occupational dermatitis involves both irritant and allergic contact dermatitis. When aggregated, the individuals who develop occupational contact dermatitis as compared with nonoccupational contact dermatitis are younger, less likely to be atopic, more likely to be male, to have hand and arm dermatitis, and to show positive patch test responses to metals, rubber compounds, p-phenylenediamine, epoxy, and rosin. However, when the irritant occupational contact dermatitis cases are compared with the allergic occupational contact dermatitis cases, the allergic cases are likely to be female, atopic, and to have dermatitis of the hands, arms, and eyelids.[8]

A survey of Gothenberg, Sweden, sampled 7.6% of the population by questionnaire, with an 82.9% response rate. At issue were whether the populace experienced hand eczema and what role was played by occupation. It was learned that 1,385 respondents had experienced hand eczema in the previous 12 months, and it was the result of occupational exposure in 11.8%. Cleaners had the highest period prevalence (21.3%). Most cases were irritant, and the most common allergen was nickel, followed by cobalt, fragrance mix, balsam of Peru, and colophony. Colophony, an allergen associated with paper products, increased in prevalence with administrative work.[9]

Many workers believe that their job is the source of their skin problem. In a Swedish automotive plant, 382 employees responded to a questionnaire about their skin condition during employment. There were 214 who thought they had work-related skin problems. A detailed evaluation of 163 metal workers and 19 office workers, all of whom believed their problem to be job related, found that 23 of the 163 and 1 of the 19 did have an occupational skin disease. Irritant contact dermatitis was diagnosed in 12 metal workers, and allergic contact dermatitis in 10 metal workers and 1 office worker. One metal worker had folliculitis. Neat oils, water-based cutting fluids, and various biocides were the allergens identified.[10]

Holness and Nethercott[11] surveyed 230 workers over a 5-year period and learned that 48% of their occupational cases of dermatitis were allergic and 52% irritant. Persons who did not remember their diagnosis correctly were twice as likely to have active dermatitis and dermatitis that was more severe. The majority of patients did not accurately recall their diagnosis. Wall and Gebauer[12] investigated the outcome of occupational skin disease in 771 patients, more than 60% of whom were followed more than 2 years from the initial diagnosis. Wall and Gebauer found that 50% were still suffering from the original dermatitis. Furthermore, if these patients had changed jobs, many were back in work environments that put them at the same risk as in the first job. More than 10% had persistent postoccupational dermatitis without obvious cause (11.5%).[12]

contact dermatitis in 53% and allergic contact dermatitis in 47%.[3] The most common job associated with occupational dermatitis was metal processing, followed by nursing, catering, hairdressing, cleaning, then shop work. A study of 5,839 patients referred for patch testing found that 1,097 (19%) of the referrals were deemed occupationally related. Of the occupational cases, 60% were of allergic and 32% were of irritant origin. The hands were the primary body part affected in 64% of the allergic and 80% of the irritant cases. Epoxy resin was the allergen most closely associated with an occupational exposure. The medical field was over-represented in the study compared to other occupations, and it was not clear if this was due to access to medical evaluation or reflective of a greater occupational risk.[4] A study of health care workers found that 16.5% (72/436) had allergic contact dermatitis and 44.4% (194/436) had irritant contact dermatitis (Figures 24-1 and 24-2). The most common allergens were nickel, benzalkonium chloride, glutaraldehyde, and rubber chemicals.[5] Health care workers, pharmaceutical workers, and veterinary surgeons are most likely to develop contact sensitization to drugs. The most common drugs that cause sensitization are penicillins, cephalosporins, and aminoglycosides. Also noteworthy are propacetamol hydrochloride and ranitidine hydrochloride. In a series of 33 such workers, 26 were nurses, who constitute the group at greatest risk.[6] Nurses can be occupationally exposed to airborne antibiotics. Ceftiofur, cephalexin, cefotiam and cefazolin have caused airborne contact dermatitis and contact urticaria.[7]

Persistent postoccupational dermatitis is the term for ongoing skin disease that began with a specific occupational event, but that does not improve on withdrawal from further exposures. It has been pointed out that the expectation of improvement on an occupational exposure adjustment may lead to a determination that a work-related connection is lacking, and benefits are thus terminated. Awareness of persistent postoccupational dermatitis is needed to address this problem.[13]

Patch Testing with New Industrial Compounds

Particular care must be exercised when new manufacturing processes and compounds are introduced. Under such circumstances, the dermatologic hazards of the new procedures and chemicals must be evaluated properly and as fully as possible before a large number of workers are exposed and sensitized.

Animal studies are of value when the chemical is a strong primary irritant. Preliminary human patch tests for primary irritant effects are useful, but they should be done on volunteer or paid subjects rather than on the workers to prevent undue apprehension among them, complaints from labor unions, or legal action.

The application of a new compound every day or two for 2 to 3 weeks may simulate working conditions and may prove of value in determining the irritant properties of the substance.

Whenever new chemicals are tested and the proper concentration for testing has not been established, it is much safer to perform the preliminary patch test by the open method. If the reaction is negative, it is then relatively safe to patch test by the usual covered method.

Solutions of dyes, paints, or liquid resins may be painted on the skin and left uncovered, because they evaporate and adhere to the site. Volatile solvents should be allowed to evaporate before being covered. If it is suspected that the chemical to be tested is a strong sensitizer, it is wise to observe the patient in the office for an hour or so after the patch test has been applied. Such observations may sometimes detect chemicals that are producers of nonimmunologic or immunologic contact urticaria.

Rules for Testing with Unlisted or Unknown Substances

1. Test liquid substances with litmus paper to ascertain whether they are strongly acidic or alkaline. Such substances must be tested carefully and in the proper dilutions to avoid severe irritation or burns.

2. Determine whether the substance to be tested is soluble in water, acetone, or olive oil or can be dispersed in petrolatum. Petrolatum is the preferred dispersing agent because it is suitably occlusive and nonirritating.

3. Always test unknown or unlisted substances at first by the "open" method. Start with a 0.1% concentration. If there is no reaction, test with a 1% concentration. If there is then no reaction, proceed to "closed" patch testing starting with a 0.1% concentration and then to a 1% concentration. Should a positive reaction be obtained, test three controls to rule out an irritant reaction.

4. Test substances stored in rubber-stoppered bottles or containers may be contaminated with rubber chemicals and may thus give false-positive reactions.

5. Observe the patient in the office for 1 hour after the patches are applied. Examine for evidence of contact urticaria.

Interpretation of Patch Test Results with New Compounds

The interpretation of results of patch testing with new compounds is fraught with pitfalls, because it may be difficult to distinguish an allergic from a primary irritant reaction. A neat vesicular eruption consisting of closely set, clear vesicles is probably an allergic response, particularly if the site itches and the reaction persists and spreads.

An erosion or a single bulla covering the entire patch test site and confined almost exactly to the area of application is probably a primary irritant reaction. Less marked primary irritant reactions may consist of minute papules and pustulovesicles irregularly situated at follicular or sweat gland orifices, and follicular crusts and minute superficial etched-out ulcers. Primary irritant reactions tend to disappear rapidly when the covering patch is removed, but allergic reactions often become more intense. Unfortunately, irritant reactions occasionally intensify for 1 to 2 days after a patch test is removed, so that the intensification phenomenon is not an absolute distinguishing feature.

Whenever the results of patch testing with a new compound are doubtful, the chemical should be tested on three normal controls. A primary irritant will usually cause a reaction in one or two of the controls, but an allergen should not cause a reaction in them.

Another type of irritant or false-positive reaction may occur when the skin is hyperirritable or an acute dermatitis is present. In such instances, even testing substances used in nonirritating concentrations may produce reactions that are difficult to distinguish from a true allergic response. In case of doubt, patch tests should be repeated after a week or so when the skin is less irritable or the dermatitis less acute.

Pre-Employment Patch Testing

The routine use of pre-employment patch tests should be avoided. Workers who do not have a history of allergic dermatitis or who do not present with a dermatitis that is compatible with an allergic contact dermatitis should not be subjected to pre-employment patch test procedures. Although a properly performed patch test does not usually sensitize those who would not in all likelihood have become sensitized by the occupational exposure, workers who react positively may claim that the procedure caused the sensitization.

A contrary view has been presented for people entering the hard metal industrial trades. Prescreening with patch tests showed 28 of 79 male students training for work in the metalworking industry were sensitive to nickel, cobalt, or chromate, leading the authors to conclude that screening was valuable.[14]

If the worker gives a history of allergic contact dermatitis or presents with a dermatitis compatible with such a diagnosis, pre-employment patch testing may be indicated. Such testing alerts him or her to avoid further exposure, in the new occupation, to a specific chemical to which he or she had become sensitized in the past.

A worker who shows a strongly positive patch test reaction to a chemical must avoid not only that particular chemical but also immunochemically related allergens. For example, individuals who demonstrate allergic hypersensitivity to paraphenylenediamine should also avoid azo and aniline dyes. However, a positive patch test reaction to the dichromates does not preclude exposure to other metals, such as nickel and copper, because crossreactions between these metals do not usually occur.

It is unfair to exclude a worker from employment merely because he or she has had an allergic contact dermatitis in the past. As a rule, aside from cross-sensitization reactions, allergic contact hypersensitivity is specific and is restricted to one group of chemicals. It would also be unfair to deny employment to an individual because he or she has had an allergic contact dermatitis and has an "immunologic" scar or because his or her skin had been damaged in the past.

Although strongly positive patch test reactions usually indicate that the patient will acquire severe contact dermatitis if exposed to the sensitizer, mild positive reactions, such as a 1+ rating, need not necessarily exclude a worker from handling the sensitizing compound.

In many instances in which a highly skilled worker has a minimal dermatitis with a weakly positive patch test reaction to a particular chemical, the dermatitis remains mild despite continued exposure to the allergen. Fisher[15] observed several furriers with mild test reactions to paraphenylenediamine and minimal dermatitis who continued to be exposed to the dye for years without much difficulty. Such instances are not examples of hardening, but of a low-grade sensitization, which may at any time suddenly become more marked. Fisher[15] also observed low-grade sensitizations with minimal dermatitis from dichromates and formaldehyde in patients who continued to be exposed without acquiring disabling eruptions.

Great care must be taken to dilute strong sensitizers so that a strongly positive patch test reaction may be avoided. Such reactions may produce marked itching and discomfort for several weeks and may cause a disgruntled employee to claim that he or she never had any "skin trouble" until the patch test was performed. Medicolegal complications may result from such severe reactions.

Prevention

A paradigm for occupational dermatitis prevention was developed within the medical field. Prevention of hand dermatitis among student nurses was attempted by running an educational program prior to their clinical duties. Those students who had the intervention of the educational program has significantly fewer skin problems compared to a control group who had not received the intervention. Key components of the educational program are:

- Use of protective gloves for wet work and cotton liners if the gloves are to be worn for longer than 10 minutes
- No rings worn at work
- No use of disinfectant agents unless needed for specific hygienic reasons
- Moisturizer use during the day and at the end of the work shift
- Protective gloves in wet work at home.[16]

Use of Patch Tests to Determine Hardening in Industry

The term "hardening," as originally introduced by J. Jadassohn, indicated a condition in which an allergic contact dermatitis in sensitized persons disappeared or failed to reappear on repeated exposure to the sensitizing chemical. This concept of a specific hardening has been broadened to include a nonspecific variety.

"Nonspecific hardening" refers to instances in which a patient acquires a dermatitis from a primary irritant, such as fiberglass, and subsequently can handle it without acquiring an eruption. The type of nonspecific hardening is neither proved nor disproved by patch testing.

Specific hardening may be described as a form of natural hyposensitization in which certain individuals suffering from an allergic dermatitis may become hyposensitized to the allergen in spite of continued exposure. The term "hyposensitization" is preferred to "desensitization," because in many instances the hypersensitivity returns, particularly if there is re-exposure after a period of avoidance.

Hardening is said to occur under conditions of diminished but continuous contact with the allergen, and it is more likely to occur if the allergic dermatitis appears after a short exposure than after prolonged contact. It is also claimed that hardening is less likely to occur after a severe dermatitis than after a mild attack. Hardening after allergic sensitization is more likely to occur with certain sensitizing chemicals, for example, tetryl, than with sensitizers such as the dichromates.

It was Fisher's opinion[15] that hardening, or hyposensitization, occurs only in rare instances and may be attributed to better hygiene so that contact with the allergen is avoided. In most instances in which hardening is cited in the literature, the impression is "clinical" only. Scientific proof of specific hardening would be established when the following criteria have been satisfied:

1. The patient has had an allergic contact dermatitis due to a specific chemical that caused a *strongly* positive patch test reaction.
2. The allergic contact dermatitis produced by the chemical clears and remains clear despite exposure to the chemical that caused the positive patch test reaction.
3. The previously strongly positive patch test reaction to the chemical becomes negative or only weakly positive.

Fisher's experience[15] was that hardening, or desensitization, that fulfills these criteria occurs only in rare instances and usually cannot be relied upon in the management of allergic contact dermatitis due to occupational exposures. A recent study of the persistence of allergic eczematous sensitivity to paraphenylenediamine revealed that such hypersensitivity persisted for 10 to 15 years in more than 90% of patients, and strongly positive patch test reactions were obtained in sensitized individuals even when they apparently no longer came in contact with the sensitizer.

More recent reports suggest that some form of hardening may have occurred in Japanese lacquer workers and in cashew nut shell oil dermatitis.[17,18] Rietschel and colleagues[19] tried to induce hardening with an irritant-maleic acid. After 6 weeks of daily exposure in 50 human volunteers, only about 20% demonstrated some diminution of reactivity, and nearly as many developed intense, vesicular dermatitis of sudden onset after 2 to 4 weeks of exposure, indicating the onset of true allergy. None of this latter group could be hardened, and further exposure only exacerbated the dermatitis. The investigators concluded that hardening of any type, specific or nonspecific, was the exception rather than the rule and could not be anticipated as a clinically useful outcome.

Workers who acquire an allergic contact dermatitis from a chemical that produces a strongly positive patch test reaction should not be exposed to the sensitizing compound in the hope that hardening, or desensitization, may take place. This expectation is almost never fulfilled.

Attempts at desensitization by exposing the patient's skin to gradually increasing concentrations of the contact allergen also fail. Therapeutic hardening by feeding or injecting graduated amounts of specific contact allergens has been successful only partially with poison ivy and ragweed oleoresins.

Nonspecific hardening does frequently take place with continued use of mild or moderate primary irritants because of gradual thickening and pigmentation of the skin.

Occupational Contact Psoriasis of the Hands from Trauma (Koebner Phenomenon)

Pressure and friction from occupational procedures may produce psoriasis of the hands, particularly the palms and volar surface of the fingers (the Koebner phenomenon). This was seen in a pharmacist (from the pressure of opening and closing containers with child-resistant caps), a surgeon, a dentist (from the pressure of various instruments), a bus driver (from the pressure of the steering wheel), and in an office worker (from pounding a stapler).[20]

Also, fresh lesions of psoriasis that appear after trauma from scratching, abrasions, lacerations, folliculitis, and acne have led many workers to press for compensation in the belief that the disease was caused or activated by their occupation. If a "koebnerized" lesion is followed quickly by a severe flare of the disease, the idea of occupational causation seems even more likely to the worker. Trauma may undoubtedly incite the development of new lesions of psoriasis, but only in persons who already have the disease, if only in latent form. For this reason, careful consideration should be given to the job placement of persons with active psoriasis and even to those with a history of the disease. Thus, Koebner phenomenon is medicolegally important when it follows industrial injuries. Lichen planus may occasionally also produce an industrial Koebner phenomenon.

Occupational Site Survey: Principles and Significance

The procedure of occupational site survey includes teamwork between physicians, nurses, industrial hygienists, biostatisticians, and epidemiologists. The personnel involved in data collection should be chosen so as to obtain the most information during a single visit to an industrial plant and to best interpret the data gathered. It is important to make an appointment before visiting an industrial plant and never to visit unannounced.

White and Rycroft[21] discovered, on a visit to an industrial plant in which there had been an outbreak of dermatoses among the employees of a soft lens factory, that the dermatitis was the result of low relative humidity in the ambient atmosphere.

Occupational Dermatitis that is Self-Inflicted

Meneghini and Angelini[22] state that cases of occupational dermatosis of this type fall into two pathogenetic groups: (a) dermatoses produced directly on healthy skin and (b) aggravation of pre-existing dermatoses of spontaneous origin.

The malingerer uses various noxious, usually exogenous, agents; mechanical, physical (red-hot metal objects, boiling water, or olive oil), and chemical solutions of strong acids or alkalis, (chromium salts, aqua regia, or other solvents); or substances of vegetables (capsicum and cactus) or animal (cantharides) origin.

Most of the lesions are found mainly at the sites exposed to the possible action of occupational factors. The lesions almost always show regular punched-out outlines, are monomorphic, and are surrounded by normal skin.

Fisher[15] saw patients, however, who were accused of being malingerers but who actually had porphyria cuta-

nea tarda with punched-out ulcers of the dorsum of the hands on apparently normal skin.

In many cases the morphology of the lesions alone may provide sufficient grounds for the diagnosis of dermatitis artefacta. The diagnosis is also helped by the fact that the malingerer often attempts to reproduce the clinical picture of occupational contact dermatitis on healthy skin and does not realize that this is difficult to do.

Angelini and colleagues[23] state that some patients produce persistent edema of the hand by the application of a tourniquet or by repeated self-inflicted contusion of the dorsum of the hand, the so-called Secretan's syndrome.

The diagnosis is more difficult when the malingerer seeks to aggravate or perpetuate the preexisting eczematous dermatosis. Continued observation in the hospital may be necessary to solve this diagnostic problem.

Assessment of Occupational Cutaneous Impairment and Disability

The evaluation of impairment is usually possible through the exercise of sound clinical judgment and depends on a detailed medical history, a thorough physical examination, and a judicious use of diagnostic procedures. Some articles are recommended in the reference section to help in such an assessment.[24–28] The role of a chronic allergic occupational dermatitis in a patient who develops mycosis fungoides is a difficult assessment to make. Able[29] did not find a correlation between specific industrial exposures and the occurrence of mycosis fungoids in a carefully controlled study.

A METHOD OF EVALUATION FOR PATIENTS WITH OCCUPATIONAL CONTACT ALLERGY*

"Standard" patch test series contain the most frequently encountered allergens found in the home and work environment and are especially valuable for the discovery of sensitivities to cosmetics and medications. For workplace allergens, only the rubber chemicals, epoxy resin, dichromate, rosin, nickel, and p-tert-butylphenol formaldehyde are included on the most frequently employed standard patch test series.

A search for a hidden allergen need not offer formidable difficulties or be especially time-consuming if a program of logical steps is followed.

This section is by Robert M. Adams, Clinical Professor of Dermatology, Stanford University Medical Center, and author of Occupational skin disease (Philadelphia: WB Saunders, 1990).

OCCUPATIONAL HISTORY

The cornerstone of the investigation is the occupational history, which must be obtained as soon as possible after the onset of the dermatitis. The dermatitis is often no longer present by the time of the patient's initial visit, especially if the worker is referred for evaluation by an insurance company or by a lawyer. The physician must, therefore, reconstruct the conditions surrounding the onset through detailed questioning, with sufficient time reserved for the interview, usually 30 to 45 minutes.

It is important to learn the area of skin involved at the onset of the dermatitis. This information can often provide a clue to the initial event and to the substances contacted at that time. The next regions involved and any subsequent spreading must be noted. Details of early treatment should be recorded. Improvement away from work and regular recurrence on returning to the same activity is relevant, as this is often the sole criterion required in worker's compensation law to substantiate a work relationship. Other workers may be similarly affected, which may suggest the presence of an unrecognized irritant, improper work practices, or the existence of a newly introduced allergen.

It is common for workers to have fixated on a putative cause that may or may not be correct, and they will want to direct the entire interview toward this substance. It actually saves time to ask patients to put that subject aside and go back to the beginning of their skin problem. Inquire where it occurred, what they did about it first, and what they did next. Reassure patients that you want to be comprehensive and know as much as possible about what they have been going through. This will eliminate a lot of otherwise missed information that is required for compensation forms and depositions. Keep asking "What did you do next, and what did you do after that?" until you come up to the present day.

It is important to document treatment from the plant dispensary, as well as the use of home remedies, barrier creams, special soaps, and whether gloves and other protective clothing have been worn.

Considerable questioning is usually necessary to learn the details of the work performed. Workers who do their jobs automatically, especially when the work is repetitive, often have difficulty explaining what they actually do. In these cases, it is necessary to urge the patient to recite a detailed step-by-step explanation of the exact movements required by the job. The worker should also be asked to describe the materials contacted at work, and from this the physician must estimate to what degree and in what manner they contact the skin.

Information can sometimes be gained from previous occupations and any work-related skin conditions arising from that work. A general medical history is also important, with special emphasis on a personal or family history of atopy. Previous contact dermatitis, especially reactions to cosmetics, topical medications, and jewelry, should be recorded. Also important are hobbies and other recreational activities, as well as the existence of a second job.

MATERIAL SAFETY DATA

Material safety data sheets are documents required by the U.S. Labor Code Section 6390, which provide information about particular hazardous substances or mixtures in the work environment. Every employer is required to have available, or have requested from a manufacturer, producer, or any other seller of a hazardous substance, a completed material safety data sheet (MSDS) for each hazardous substance in use at the place of employment, and to make this information available upon the request of an employee, a union representative, or an employee's physician. These documents are supposed to provide pertinent information regarding ingredients, including the chemical names, physical data, fire and explosive information, reactivity data, leak, spill, and clean-up procedures, and special protective and handling information.

Unfortunately, an MSDS frequently contains little or no information of value to dermatologists. On many of them, ingredients are not precisely listed or are not named at all. Often they are recorded only in general terms, such as "amine" or "hydrocarbon." Substances in concentrations of less than 1% are frequently not included.

This situation can create difficulties, as important skin allergens are usually found in this fraction, especially germicidal agents, antioxidants, and fragrance materials. A telephone number at the upper right-hand corner of the first sheet, however, will lead the physician to a person who can provide the required information. It is important to identify oneself as a physician, to explain that the information is required to study a patient properly, and to clarify that the knowledge gained may result in keeping the worker on the job. This approach is usually sufficient to loosen any tight reins on disclosure of any "proprietary" information.

Sometimes a company may agree to release information only after a secrecy agreement has been signed. Agreeing to this stipulation will usually open up a free-flowing dialogue of vital information.

When several ingredients are listed, a dermatologist experienced in contact dermatitis can readily identify those chemicals that are known to cause allergic reactions, as well as those usually associated solely with irritancy.

INDUSTRIAL PLANT VISITS

While material safety data sheets, when properly used, are indispensable for learning the chemical hazards of a given workplace, additional information can be obtained from an industrial plant visit, which can be profitable in many ways. Familiarity with work materials, job processes, the industrial plant environment, and the attitudes of workers and management enable physicians to more adequately diagnose and treat occupational skin diseases arising from working conditions in the plant. The physician will also be in a better position to recommend preventive measures and to assist in the placement of workers.

A visit can be arranged by the manager of a small industrial plant, or the safety or personnel departments of larger industrial plants. If the industrial plant has a part-time or full-time physician, arrangement can be made through him or her. Another method is to obtain an appointment through an industrial engineer of the local or state health department. Visits should be made early in the day, at the beginning of the day shift (at 7:00 A.M.), and can usually be completed within an hour or so.

PHYSICAL EXAMINATION

Although most cases of occupational skin disease involve only the hands and forearms, it is important to examine the entire skin to rule out other diseases or contributory conditions. It should be emphasized it is impossible to differentiate in every case between an allergic and an irritant contact dermatitis from the appearance of the eruption alone. Allergic reactions are often more explosive in onset, with marked vesiculation and itching. They are also often intermittent, appearing 1 or 2 days after contact with the allergen in a previously sensitized individual. However, mild irritant reactions develop more gradually, requiring days or weeks to evolve. In almost every case, however, it is impossible to differentiate between allergic and irritant dermatitis from appearance alone.

PATCH TESTING

The only certain way to diagnose allergic contact dermatitis in the workplace is through diagnostic patch testing. One is sometimes tempted to test with a product used by the worker without knowledge of its exact contents and potential for irritancy. Even substances that appear fairly innocuous may produce an irritant reaction when tested full strength under an occluded patch test for 48 hours, and the result can easily be interpreted incorrectly as a true allergic response.

When the history, examination, and information from the MSDS cause one to suspect one or more ingredients in a given compound as allergens, the next step is to obtain these chemicals in as pure a state as possible. If they are not present on a standard patch test series, they must be obtained from a chemical company. Catalogs are available on request. A supply company will refuse occasionally to sell a chemical to a private physician, but one can usually avoid this by appeal to higher officials of the company, or by buying the material through a hospital pharmacy or university chemical department. The costs are minor in small amounts, and after preparation any excess of the test materials can be stored for future use.

Appropriate concentrations for patch testing can be found in textbooks on contact dermatitis. A pharmacist can be found to prepare the mixtures, usually in white petrolatum, and the compensation insurance carrier can be billed for the cost, which is usually minor.

Determination of Relevance

When a positive test result is obtained with one or more known ingredients of a substance, the next step is to attempt to reproduce the dermatitis by a "use" test. The material itself, unless irritating, can be applied, in the concentration normally contacted by the patient, to a small area of skin, usually on the inner aspect of the arm just above the elbow, twice daily for 7 days, or until a reaction appears. The physician must recognize nonspecific irritant reactions due to lack of sufficient skin penetration.

Finally, relevance must be confirmed by again questioning the worker regarding the actual way the substance contacted the skin during the work process. It is reasonable that this substance could be responsible for the worker's dermatitis. If this seems to be true, one can be reasonably certain that a given substance containing an allergen to which the worker is found sensitive is indeed the cause of the dermatitis under investigation. At the same time, contributing factors such as nonoccupational activities can be placed in perspective.

A study of this magnitude is important because knowledge of the exact chemical responsible will enable the physician to help the patient avoid future contact with the allergen, either by substitution with unrelated and nonallergenic substances, or by suggesting an appropriate job change. Without this information, the worker is condemned to repeated episodes of dermatitis.

Resources for Information or Assistance in Occupational Dermatitis

The following agencies can help the physician to obtain information concerning occupational exposures and injury:

1. NATIONAL INSTITUTE FOR OCCUPATIONAL SAFETY AND HEALTH

Clearinghouse for Occupational Safety and Health Information
4676 Columbia Parkway
Cincinnati, OH 45226

2. CONSUMER PRODUCT SAFETY HOTLINE

Injury Information Clearinghouse
1111 18th Street, N.W.
Washington, DC 20207

3. OCCUPATIONAL SAFETY AND HEALTH ADMINISTRATION

Director, Office of Information and Consumer Affairs
200 Constitution Avenue, N.W.
Washington, DC 20210

4. ENVIRONMENTAL PROTECTION AGENCY

Public Information Center
401 M Street, S.W.
Washington, DC 20460

Valuable information can also be obtained from the *Dictionary of Occupational Titles*, 4th ed., US Department of Labor, 1977.

CATALOGS OF CHEMICAL COMPANIES

Eastman Organic Chemicals Catalog
Fischer Scientific Company
JT Baker Company
R & K Laboratory of Rare and Fine Chemicals
Subdivision of ICN Pharmaceuticals, Inc.
121 Express Street
Plainview, NY 11803

MANUFACTURERS OF OCCUPATIONAL PROTECTIVE MATERIALS

Protective Clothing

American Optical Corporation, 14 Mechanic Street, Southbridge, MA 01550
    Mine Safety Appliances Co., 400 Penn Center Boulevard, Pittsburgh, PA 15235
    Safety Clothing and Equipment Co., Division of Safety First Industries, Inc., 1522 East 69th Street, Cleveland, OH 44103
    Uniroyal Protective Clothing, Washington, IN 47501

Protective Sleeves and Aprons

American Optical Corp., 14 Mechanic Street, Southbridge, MA 01550
    Mine Safety Appliances Co., Penn Center Boulevard, Pittsburgh, PA 15235
    Standard Safety Equipment Co., 431 North Quentin Road, Palatine, IL 60067
    Surety Rubber Co., Box 97-G-12, Carrollton, OH 44615
    Wheeler Protective Apparel, Inc., 226 West Huron Street, Chicago, IL 60610

Industrial Rubber Gloves and Synthetic Rubber Gloves

Edmont-Wilson, 3167 Walnut Street, Coschocton, OH 43812
    Mine Safety Appliance Co., 400 Penn Center Boulevard, Pittsburgh, PA 15235
    Pioneer Rubber Co., Tiffin Road, Willard, OH 44890
    Surety Rubber Co., Box 97-G-12, Carrollton, OH 44615

Industrial Cleaners

Calgon Corp., Calgon Commercial Division, 7501 Page Street, St. Louis, MO 63133
    Dameron Enterprises, Inc., 7635 National Turnpike, Louisville, KY 40214
    Milburn Co., 3246 Woodbridge, Detroit, MI 48207
    Sugar Beet Products, P.O. Box 1387, Saginaw, MI 48605
    West Chemical Products, Inc., 4216 West Street, Long Island City, NY 11101

Waterless Hand Cleaners

Dameron Enterprises, Inc., 7635 National Turnpike, Louisville, KY 40214
    Go-Jo Industries, Inc., P.O. Box 991, Akron, OH 44309
    Sugar Beet Products, P.O. Box 1387, Saginaw, MI 48605
    West Chemical Products, Inc., 4216 West Street, Long Island City, NY 11101

Protective Ointments and Barrier Creams

Amar-Stone Laboratories, Inc., 601 East Kensington Road, Mount Prospect, IL 60056
    Ayerst Laboratories, 685 Third Avenue, New York, NY 10017
    Calgon Corp., Calgon Commercial Division, 7501 Page Avenue, St. Louis, MO 63133
    E. I. Du Pont de Nemours & Co., 1007 Market Street, Wilmington, DE 19898
    Milburn Co., 3246 E. Woodbridge, Detroit, MI 48207

Mine Safety Appliances Co., 201 North Braddock Avenue, Pittsburgh, PA 15208

West Chemical Products, Inc., 4216 West Street, Long Island City, NY 11101

Zee Medical Products, 11800 Woodruff Avenue, Downey, GA 90241

Lichenoid Eruptions and Leukoderma in the Photography Industry

Photographers may acquire lichen planus–like eruptions from CD2-type color developers. The chemicals involved are derivatives of paraphenylenediamine or aniline. Most reports incriminate Kodak CD2 and Kodak CD3.[30–34]

Roed-Petersen and Menné[35] reported that these color developers are now being used in the processing of high-speed black-and-white film. At present, there are fewer reports of lichen planus–like eruptions as a result of industrial automatization that successfully stopped the previous epidemic of dermatitis. Most film developing is performed at large-scale, fully automated plants. Sporadic skin reactions occur among amateurs, newspaper photographers, and others who develop their own films manually.

Automated photoprocessing might seem to eliminate contact with color film developer chemicals, but facial dermatitis from airborne contact from this source has occurred.[36] Color developers CD2, CD3, and CD4 were the source. Lichenoid changes were not observed in this context.

Another type of unusual reaction that may occur in the photography industry is a contact leukoderma (vitiligo). This type of depigmentation is due to hydroquinone used in the developing process.[37–39] This type of eruption also usually occurs mostly in amateurs who develop their own films. Adams[15] saw a high school student who took a course in photography and who developed a leukoderma of the hands.

Goh[40] reported allergic hand eczema due to Colorprint 101ER Developer Replenisher. The dermatitis was accompanied by onycholysis and was traced to hydroxylamine sulfite, which is tested at 2% aqueous concentration.

Photographers are exposed to many irritants and allergens, such as the following:

1. *Developers* (hydroquinone, *p*-amino-phenol, pyrocatechol, pyrogallol, metol, and paraphenylenediamine). These developers are dissolved in irritant alkaline solutions containing sodium sulfate and sodium carbonate or sodium hydroxide.

2. *"Stop bath"* (bromoresol purple). The "stop bath" consists of a weak solution of acetic acid. The concentrated acid can cause burns, and inhalation of the vapors can irritate the breathing passages and throat. Potassium chrome alum, sometimes used as a stop hardener, contains chromium and can cause ulcerations, especially in cuts and nasal membranes, and allergies.

3. *Fixers.* The fixer usually contains sodium sulfite, acetic acid, sodium thiosulfate (hypo), boric acid, and potassium alum. Hypo and the mixture of sodium sulfite and acetic acid produce sulfur dioxide, which is highly corrosive to the lungs. Potassium alum, a hardener, is a weak sensitizer and may cause some skin dermatitis.

4. *Bleaches.* Bleaches may contain potassium dichromate, hydrochloric acid, or mercuric chloride.

5. *Reducers.* Reducers may contain potassium ferricyanide.

6. *Toners.* Toners contain both irritants and allergens. Many toners contain highly toxic chemicals. These include selenium, uranium, liver of sulfur (corrosive to skin and breathing passages), gold, platinum (allergies), and oxalic acid (corrosive).

7. *Hardeners and stabilizers.* Hardeners and stabilizers often contain formaldehyde, which is poisonous and is very irritating to the eyes, throat, and breathing passages. They can cause dermatitis, severe allergies, and asthma. Some of the solutions used to clean negatives contain harmful chlorinated hydrocarbons.

8. *Print flattening solutions* (formaldehyde, hydrazine).

9. *Antifoggants* (Benzotriazole). The greatest skin hazard occurs during the preparation and handling of concentrated stock solutions of the various chemicals.

Pigmentary and Purpuric Eruptions in the Textile Industry

A survey of 72 textile workers found irritant contact dermatitis related to work exposures in 27 (38%).[41] Allergic contact dermatitis was due to occupational contactants in 21 (29%). The most frequent allergens were textile dyes in 12 workers, textile finishes in 11, and rubber-related allergens in 10. The textile finishes were formaldehyde-related permanent press finishes, and no one dye predominated.

Textile workers may acquire purpuric dermatitis presumably from formaldehyde resin and extensive hyperchromatism presumably due to naphthol compounds added to dyes in the process of preliminary dyeing.[42,43]

Dooms-Goossens and colleagues[44] describe contact dermatitis caused by dimethylthiourea, an additive in diazo-sensitized paper used for textile cutting patterns.

Table 24-2 Patch-Test Series for Dermatitis Acquired in the Textile Industry[a]

Patch test allergens	Patch test concentration
Azo dyes	
C.I. Disperse Black 2	1% pet
C.I. Disperse Yellow 35	1% pet
C.I. Disperse Red 1	1% pet
C.I. Disperse Yellow 3	1% pet
Cresol	2% pet
Dimethylolurea	10% pet
Ethylene glycol	2.5% aq
Ethylene urea	50% aq
Formaldehyde	2% aq
Hydrazine	1% pet
Melamine-formaldehyde resin	10% pet
Paraphenylenediamine	1% pet
Pentachlorophenol	3% pet
Phenylmercuric nitrate	0.05% pet
Potassium dichromate	0.5% pet
Quaternary ammonium salts	0.1% aq
Triethylene-imino-phosphine oxide	1% olive oil
Urea-formaldehyde resin	10% pet

[a]Aq, aqueous; pet, in petrolatum.

Table 24.2 shows patch test series suitable for dermatitis acquired in the textile industry.

Occupational Dermatitis in the Painting Industry

As a consequence of the decreasing use of solvent-based glues and paints and the increasing use of water-based products, manufacturers face problems with preservation.

Merthiolate, phenyl mercuric nitrate, and more recently chloracetamide have been used for this purpose. Chloracetamide has proved to be a common sensitizer in the painting industry.[45–47]

Many painters have been exposed to chloracetamide in hanging wallpaper and fiberglass fabrics. Painters are also exposed to glues that may contain chloracetamide. It should be known that chloracetamide is also used as a preservative in cosmetic creams and lotions. The pesticide chlorothalonil has been added to some paints, which has led to facial dermatitis in people inhabiting freshly painted rooms due to the vapor pressure of chlorothalonil.[48] In this case, the patch test was positive from 1% down to 0.0001% aqueous solution (0.4 ppm chlorothalonil). This potent sensitizer is used as a wood preservative and a pesticide in floriculture.[48] In addition, various acrylates found in paint are shown in Table 24.3. Table 24.4 shows the numerous compounds found in

Table 24-3 Acrylates Found in Paints[a]

Acrylate	Patch test concentration
Butyl acrylate	1% pet
Epoxy acrylate	1% pet
Ethyl acrylate	1% pet
2-ethyl-hexylacrylate	1% pet
N-methylolacrylamide	1% pet
Pentaerythritol triacrylate	0.2% pet
Trimethylolpropane triacrylate	1% pet
Tripropylene glycol triacrylate	1% pet

[a]Pet, in petrolatum.

Table 24-4 Miscellaneous Compounds Found in Paints

Pigments
  Alizarin
  Chromates
  Lithol red
  Nickel dust
  Para-red
  Phthalocyanine blue
  Rhodamine
  Thioflavin
  Toluidine toners
Vehicles (binders)
  Linseed oil (rare)
  Rosin
  Synthetic resins, catalysts, and plasticizers
  Tung oil
Miscellaneous
  Antifoam agents
  Dibutyl phthalate
  Pine oil
Antioxidants
  Hydroquinone
Driers
  Cobalt naphthenates
Paint thinners
  Diptene
  Turpentine
Plasticizers
  Acrylates
  Dibutyl phthalate
  Polyester resins
  Sulfonamides
Preservatives
  Chloracetamide
  Chlorothymol
  Mercuric oxide
  Organic mercurials
  Tetramethylthiuram disulfide
  Thimerosal
  Thymol

Table 24-5 Patch Test Tray for Painters[a]

Allergens	Patch test concentration
Acrylates	1% pet
Betanaphthol (wallpaper adhesive)	10% olive oil
D3-Carene-turpentine sensitizer	1% as peroxide in olive oil
Chloracetamide	1% pet
Chloroparanitraniline red	2% pet
Cobalt chloride (dyes and driers)	2% pet
Colophony (rosin)	20% pet
Dipentene	10% MEK (methyl ethyl ketone)
Epoxy resin	1% pet
Epoxy resin hardeners	1% pet
Ethylene glycol	2.5% aq
F4R red	2% pet
Formaldehyde	2% aq
Hansa yellow	2% pet
Hydroquinone	1% pet
Para red	2% pet
Paratoluenesulfonamide	2% pet
Phenylmercuric nitrate (germicidal)	0.5% pet
Polyester resin monomer (polyester paint)	10% pet
Potassium dichromate (green and yellow)	2% pet
Propylene glycol	5% aq
Thimerosal (germicidal)	0.1% pet
Toluidine red (helio red)	2% pet
Tricresyl phosphate	5% pet
Turpentine	20% olive oil

[a]Aq, aqueous; pet, in petrolatum.

paint,[49] and Table 24.5 lists the suggested patch test series for painters.

Painters may become sensitized to resin additives. 1,2-benzisothiazolin-3-one (BIT) is a preservative that can be found in paints and combined with ethylenediamine in a product called Proxel XL 2 or Proxel CRL. It has caused contact dermatitis in painters, and sensitization to Kathon CG is commonly seen in these cases.[50]

Another paint additive that has caused contact dermatitis is dichlofluanide, a fungicide that is also used in agriculture. Five cases of dichlofluanide allergy from glazing paints were reported by Gruvberger and colleagues.[51] One of these patients developed erythema multiforme–like dermatitis. In guinea pigs, dichlofluanide is a strong sensitizer.

Most occupational literature on diidocyanates focuses on respiratory problems, but if the workplace provides a cutaneous exposure, contact dermatitis can result. A company that produced flooring based on phenol-formaldehyde resins used a one-part polyurethane lacquer to waterproof the flooring and this material was based on diphenylmethane-diisocyanate monomers. Several workers became sensitized to 4,4'-diaminodiphenylmethane, and 1 also reacted to dicyclohexylmethane-4,4'-diisocyanate.[52]

Painters may acquire dermatitis from turpentine and dipentene, which is used as a paint thinner.

Protection for Artists and "Do-It-Yourself" Home Decorators and Painters

Dermatitis is one of the biggest dangers of working with art materials. The best way to prevent dermatitis is to prevent hazardous substance contact with the skin, particularly the hands, by wearing plastic or rubber gloves, especially when working with organic solvents, acids, and caustics. There are two basic requirements in choosing the type of glove: first, that the glove should be impervious to the materials being used; and second, that the glove should allow the degree of "feel" required for one's art.

For many purposes, polyvinyl gloves are suitable, such as cheap, disposable "surgeons' gloves" and heavier lined gloves for greater comfort. These polyvinyl gloves protect against most solvents except those containing large amounts of ketones, such as acetone.

Butyl rubber or natural rubber gloves will protect against ketones but not against aromatic solvents (toluol, xylol, and polyester resin) or most chlorinated hydrocarbons, and only provide fair protection against petroleum distillates (naphtha, mineral spirits, and kerosene) and acids. Neoprene rubber gloves have almost the exact opposite characteristics of other rubbers.

For work with acids and caustics, either polyvinyl chloride or neoprene rubber is best. For work with concentrated solutions, the gloves should be the gauntlet type with a cuff to turn back the acid or caustic. If protection from acrylates is required, the 4-H glove is better than rubber and vinyl, which provide no meaningful protection. The 4-H glove has recently been shown to provide protection for up to 1 week in electron microscopists exposed to 1-hexadecene and 2-hydroxyethyl acrylate.[53]

If one cannot wear gloves, the use of barrier creams ("invisible gloves") might help by providing an impermeable barrier between the skin and the toxic material. There are different types of barrier creams, some water soluble and others water insoluble, but silicone types are supposed to be best. These barrier creams have to be renewed regularly. After use, the barrier creams are washed off with a mild soap and water. Unfortunately, even barrier creams that test well in the laboratory do not always help in practice. A clinical study of 12 patients showed that with the use of the best laboratory-tested barrier creams, 7 experienced return of dermatitis.[54]

In cleaning hands, it is important to wash carefully and frequently with soap and water (especially before eating and smoking). Harsh or abrasive soaps must not be used, because these can cause dermatitis themselves and can just increase the problem. With some materials, including paints, ink, and oils, waterless hand cleansers are helpful. These hand cleansers are often available in hardware and art supply stores. Cleansers containing kerosene are not recommended because of their defatting action. One hand cleaner, Centrex Red, has been reported to cause allergic contact dermatitis due to a sulfosuccinate derivative tested at 5% in petrolatum. The substance was sodium ricinoleic monoethanolamido-sulfosuccinate, which was the liquid detergent present at 0.47% in the product.[55] After washing with these cleansers, one should also wash with plenty of soap and water. One should then use a hand lotion or cream containing lanolin to replace any skin oils lost.

Detailed information on the subject of art hazards is contained in the following publications: Gail Coningsby Barazani, *Safe Practices in the Arts and Crafts: A Studio Guide,* available from the College Art Association, 16 East 52nd Street, New York, NY 10022; and Michael McCann, *Artist Beware: The Hazards and Precautions in Working with Art and Craft Materials,* published by Watson-Guptil, New York. For additional information and assistance, artists may consult the *National Poison Control Network,* Pittsburgh, PA, and the *Center for Occupation Hazards and Art Hazards Information Center,* 5 Beekman Street, New York, NY 10038.

Occupational Dermatitis in the Printing Industry

The printing industry (not only newspapers, books, and magazines but also containers) has been almost revolutionized by a new drying method using polyfunctional acrylics (some also with an epoxy), a benzophenone photoactivator, and ultraviolet light. The old methods of solvent drying with all their difficulties can be dispensed with, and the time of cure is only seconds. Most cases of dermatitis have occurred in those persons who make the inks, and almost none in the users, so far.

Malten and colleagues[56] state that the manufacture of photopolymer printing plates in general is based on a light-induced curing of synthetic resin applied on a metal or plastic carrier sheet. Ultraviolet light causes a radical donor to decompose into radicals, inducing cross-linking by a hardener between (long) chains bearing reactive

sites. The irradiated parts of the plate are thus cured within a few seconds, making these parts resistant to subsequent processing (blowing or dissolving) means to remove the unirradiated parts of the plate.

The composition of the inks varies widely and consists of pigments dispersed in a vehicle that contains various resins, photoinitiators, diluents, hydrogen transfer agents, stabilizers, surfactants, flattening agents, and inhibitors. Allergic sensitization to several polyfunctional acrylic monomers, epoxy acrylate oligomers, and associated isocyanate compounds has recent been reported, as has phototoxicity from exposure to mixed isomers (ortho and para) of amyl dimethylaminobenzoate.[57–65]

In printing plants, printers, typesetters, and press operators are exposed to several irritants that include alcohols, alkalis, developers, etching solutions, grease, waxes, inks, resins, soaps, detergents, and solvents. Workers in printing operations may also be exposed to the following contact allergens: potassium dichromate, dyes, formaldehyde, hydroquinone, glues, and gums. Table 24.6 is a suggested patch test series for printers.

Table 24-6 Test Tray for Printers[a]	
Allergens	**Patch test concentration**
Brown Sudan (naphthylaminoazonaphthol)	2% pet
Chloroparanitraniline red	2% pet
Eosin	50% pet
Epoxy acrylate	1% pet
Ethylene glycol	2.5% aq
Formaldehyde	2% aq
Hexanediol diacrylate	1% pet
Impression plates (acrylics)	as is
Lake Red C	2% pet
Mercaptopropionic acid	1% pet
Methacrylics	5% pet
Other plates (polyurethane)	as is
Para red	2% pet
p-phenylene diamine	1% pet
Pentaerythritol triacrylate	0.2% pet
Polythiol (pentaerythritol + mercaptopropionic acid)	0.1% acetone
Potassium dichromate	0.5% pet
Propylene glycol	2.5% aq
Toluidine red (or helio red)	2% pet
Trimethylol propane triacrylate	1% pet
Turpentine D3-carene (peroxides)	1% pet
UV drying inks	1% pet

[a]Aq, aqueous; pet, in petrolatum.

Table 24-7 Occupational Exposures to Pesticides	
Agricultural workers	Farmers
Cattle breeders	Foresters
Dairy workers	

Occupational Dermatitis from Pesticides

Those occupations most often exposed to various pesticides that are likely to acquire pesticide dermatitis are listed in Table 24.7. A classification of the pesticides and repellents is given in Table 24.8.

Many of these pesticides are dispensed in solvents that are irritating to the skin. The pure active ingredient should be obtained if possible for patch tests. Impurities may cause more trouble than the active pesticides. Thus, Milby and Epstein[66] reported that the allergen in malathion is not the chemical itself but diethyl fumarate, which is present as a contaminant.

Both at home and abroad numerous reports indicate that pesticides produce many instances of occupational dermatitis.[67–74]

Table 24-8 A Classification of Pesticides and Repellents
Acaricides
Animal repellents, including rodenticides
Fungicides
Herbicides
Insecticides and insect repellents

Table 24-9 Patch Testing for Fungicides[a]	Patch test concentration
Chloronitrobenzenes	
DNCB	0.1% aq
Pentachloronitrobenzene	1% pet
Dicarboximides	
Captan	1% pet
Difolatan (captafol)	0.1% pet
Phaltan	0.1% pet
Dithiocarbamates (see Table 24.10)	
Mercaptobenzothiazole	1% pet
Mercury compounds	
Phenyl mercuric nitrate	0.01% pet
Nitrophenols	
4,6,-dinitro-o-cresol	0.5% aq
Dinobuton (acrex)	10% pet
Dinocap	0.5% pet
Nitrofen	0.5% pet
Organ-tin compounds (tributyltin oxide)	0.01% aq
Phenols	
Pentachlorophenol	1% aq
p-chloro-o-cresol	0.1% alcohol
Tetrachlorodihydroxydiphenyl	1% aq
Sulfide (vancide bl)	1% aq
O-benzyl-p-chlorophenol (Chlorophene, santophen 1)	1% aq
Phosphothioate	
Plondrel (ditalimfos)	0.01% pet
Quinones	
Chloranil	1% pet
Dichlone	1% pet
Dithianone	1% pet

[a]Aq, aqueous; pet, in petrolatum.

FUNGICIDES

Patch-test procedures with various fungicides are listed in Table 24.9. The dithiocarbamates listed in Table 24.10, which are widely used as fungicides, have caused numerous instances of allergic contact dermatitis.[73,75–79]

In the midwestern section of the United States, the dithiocarbamate Maneb, used widely to prevent the ginseng weed from producing potato blight, has resulted in many severe cases of allergic contact dermatitis among farmers.

If is of interest to note that the agricultural fungicides thiram and the dithiocarbamates are closely related to Antabuse, which causes "flushing" when used in the treatment of alcoholism.

Potato farmers in Ecuador have a high prevalence of dermatitis and frequent exposure to the fungicide Maneb. A comparison of farmworkers with those applying the fungicide found significant differences in dermatitis frequency.[80] Conjunctivitis was present in 7% of fungicide

applicators but in none of the workers or controls. Dermatitis was present in 68% of the workers, 55% of those applying fungicide, and 31% of controls. These findings are somewhat different from those reported from California, where dermatitis was due to vegetation in about 50% of cases and to pesticides in 20%.

Such dicarboximide fungicides as captan, phaltan, and difoltan can also produce allergic contact dermatitis.[81–83] The less widely used fungicides such as phenylmercuric nitrate and the "quinone," dithianone, have caused dermatitis[84,85] Hearn[67] analyzed 250 cases of poisoning due to pesticides that occurred between 1957 and 971. "Dermatitis" was a feature in 54 cases and chemical burns occurred in 18 cases. Many different chemicals were involved, but the most frequent causes of dermatitis were the organomercurial compounds, paraquat and thiram. The soil fumigant DD-95 is predominantly 1,3-dichloropropene, a severe irritant, but allergy can be distinguished

Table 24-10 Dithiocarbamates[a]

Chemical name	Common name	Patch test concentration
Chloro butynyl-chlorophenyl-carbamate	Barban (carbyne)	1% pet
Iron dimethyldithiocarbamate	Ferbam	1% pet
Manganese and zinc ethylene-bis-dithiocarbamate	Mancozeb	1% pet
Manganese ethylene-bis-dithiocarbamate	Maneb	0.5% pet
Methyl-butylcarbamoyl-benzimidazole carbamate	Benomyl (benlate)	0.1% pet
Mixture of polyethylene-bis-thiram sulfides	Carbatene	1% pet
Sodium methyldithiocarbamate	Metam-sodium	1% pet
Tetraethylthiurammonosulfide	Tetmosol	1% pet
Tetramethylthiuram disulfide	Thiram	1% pet
Triscopper dimethyldithiocarbamate-bis-chloride	Cuprobam	1% pet
Zinc dimethyldithiocarbamate	Ziram	1% pet
Zinc ethylene-bis-dithiocarbamate	Zineb (dithane)	1% pet
Zinc propylene-bis-dithiocarbamate	Propineb	1% pet

[a]Pet, in petrolatum

by patch testing at 0.005% in petrolatum, because 0.05% was negative in 20 volunteers.[86] Tin compounds such as tributyl tin oxide (hexa-*n*-butyl distanoxane) is corrosive at 0.1% as a patch test, and clothing contaminated by it should be discarded, as it does not wash out.[87] This compound is also found in papermaking, timber preservation, polymerization of silicon, and stabilization of plastic, and is a biocide in paint.[87]

Quinoxyfen, which is 5,7-dichloro-4-(4-fluoropenoxy)-quinoline, is a fungicide of the quinazoline class, and contact dermatitis has been reported in the facility in which it is produced.[88]

INSECTICIDES

Table 24.11 lists the insecticides. Rycroft[89] stated that the organophosphorus compounds were introduced originally as insecticides, but members of the group are now used as fungicides, herbicides, and plant growth regulators. Instances of contact dermatitis may be due to the pure chemical or to impurities in such compounds.[64,90,91]

HERBICIDES

Table 24.12 lists the herbicides in current use. Peachey[92] states that no cases of contact dermatitis due to the herbicides paraquat or diquat have been reported so far, but Sharvill[93] described skin ulceration due to contact with paraquat solution, and Samman and Johnston[94] reported softening and discoloration of fingernails due to

Table 24-11 Insecticides[a]

	Patch test concentration
Carbamates (methyl)	1% pet
Cyclodienes	
Aldrin	1% pet
Dieldrin	1% pet
Dazomet (mylone) (hydrolyzes to formalin)	0.25% aq
DDD-dichloro-bis-chlorophenyl	1% acetone
Dichloro-diphenyl-trichloro-ethane (DDT)	1% pet
Lindane	1% pet
Omite	0.05% pet
Organophosphorus compounds	
Malathion	0.5% pet
Naled (dibrominated)	1% pet
Parathion	1% alcohol
Organothiocyanates	
Rodannitrobenzine	1% pet
Inorganic insecticides	
Arsenic	1% pet
Fluorides	1% pet
Botanical insecticides	
Benzyl benzoate	5% pet
Nicotine sulfate	5% aq
Pyrethrum powder	as is
Rotenone	5% in talcum powder

[a]Aq, aqueous; pet, in petrolatum.
Note: The esters derived from pyrethrum powder are active insecticides as pyrethrens and cinerins. These do not contain sensitizers that crossreact with sesquiterpene lactones, which cause dermatitis from the chrysanthemum plant and ragweed.

Table 24-12 Herbicides in Current Use[a]

	Patch test concentration
Amides	
Propachlor	1% pet
Randox (A chloracetamine)	0.1% pet
Pentachlorophenol	1% pet
Quaternary salts	
Diquat	0.1% pet
Paraquat	0.1% pet
Triazines	
Atrazine	1% pet
Desmetryne	1% pet
Methotryne	1% pet
Prometryne	1% pet
Simazine	1% pet

[a]Pet, in petrolatum.

contact with the concentrated chemical. Spencer[95] reported contact dermatitis due to the herbicide Randox.

Pentachlorophenol, which was used in a Japanese herbicide, caused dermatitis and death.[96]

INSECT REPELLENTS

The US Department of Agriculture has tested more than 9,000 insect repellents and found that n,n9-diethyl-m-toluamide (commonly known as "DEET") is the best all-purpose repellent. Other effective agents include ethyl hexanediol, dimethyl phthalate, dimethyl carbate, and butopyronoxyl (Indalone).

More than 50 repellent preparations are available commercially: Most of them contain either DEET (Off and McKesson Mosquitone) or ethyl hexanediol (6–12 Brand and SkeetoGo). They are available in several forms, including liquid, foam, pressurized spray, stick, cream, and wipe-on tissue. Concentrations of the active ingredient vary with both type of formulation and brand. Preparations in which DEET is the only repellent contain from less than 5% (in wipe-on tissues) to more than 40% (in liquids).

Autan is an insect repellent that has rarely caused contact dermatitis. Rossi and Steffens[97] reported a case of contact allergy to this repellent that was found to be due to methyl glucose dioleate, a component of Isolan DO faction of the pump spray formula test at 3% in paraffin oil. There was no reaction to the active ingredient hydroxyethyl isobutyl piperidine carboxylate. The active ingredient is also known as picaridin, and Corazza and colleagues reported sensitization to both picaridin (a piperidine) and to methyl glucose dioleate. Picaridin was tested at 2.5% petrolatum and methyl glucose dioleate at 10% petrolatum.[98]

FACTORS AFFECTING REPELLENT ACTION

Some compounds are more effective than others against certain insects; for example, Indalone is better than DEET in preventing tick bites. The concentration of the active compound can affect both the range of susceptible effects and the duration of effect.

Cronce and Alden[99] reported a case of flea collar dermatitis. An insecticide (2,2-dichlorovinyl dimethyl phosphate and related compounds) in antiflea dog collars caused primary irritant contact dermatitis in 4 patients who handled dogs wearing these collars. The insecticide is a known poison that inhibits cholinesterase, and it is capable of producing primary irritant dermatitis and even chemical burns when it is incorporated into soft, plastic, antiflea dog collars in a 9% to 10% concentration. Fortunately, this insecticide is liberated slowly

Table 24-13 Animal Repellents[a]

	Patch test concentration
Birds	
Anthraquinone powder[b]	as is
Dogs and cats	
Citronella oil	1% pet
Diethyl phthalate	2% pet
Eucalyptus oil	1% pet
Nicotine sulfate	5% aq
Oil of lemongrass	1% pet
Pine tar	1% pet
Synthetic oil of mustard	0.1% pet
Rabbits, deer, and meadow mice	
Thiram (used up to 20%)	1% pet
Rodents	
Antu (naphthylthiourea, Antirax)	1% pet
Warfarin	0.05% pet
Squirrels	
Oil of lemongrass	1% pet
Paradichlorobenzene	1% alcohol
Synthetic oil of mustard	0.1% pet

[a]Aq, aqueous; pet, in petrolatum.
[b]Used on seeds to make them distasteful to birds.

from the collar under normal circumstances, and the dog's hair helps to prevent dermatitis on its neck.

Shell's No-Pest Strip contained the same insecticide as do flea collars. DEET may produce a bullous reaction resembling a blistering insect eruption.[100] In addition, DEET may produce contact urticaria.[101]

ANIMAL REPELLENTS

The animal repellents are shown in Table 24.13. Warfarin, which is used widely as a rodenticide, causes death by producing hemorrhage in animals.

Antu, also known as Antirax, may be patch tested 2% in petrolatum. Antu, which is a thiourea compound and is also a widely used rat poison, can cause contact dermatitis in humans.[102]

The acaricides are listed in Table 24.14. Omite, a sulfite compound, may be tested 0.05% in petrolatum, and even under this dilute concentration may produce irritant reactions.[103] Dinobuton (Acrex), a nitrophenol compound, can cause yellow staining of the hair and nails and skin irritation. This compound is closely related to picric acid, which can cause a similar type of staining. Patch testing may be performed with 10% in petrolatum.

BIRD REPELLENTS

Anthraquinone is used to make seeds distasteful to birds and thus acts as a repellent. Because some anthraquinone

Table 24-14 Acaricides[a]	
	Patch test concentration
Benzyl benzoate	5% pet
Dinobuton (Acrex)	10% pet
Omite (propargite)	1% pet
Sulfur compounds	5% pet

[a] Pet, in petrolatum.

dyes crossreact with paraphenylenediamine, contact with such seeds in a paraphenylenediamine-sensitive individual could possibly cause an eruption.

FARMERS AND AGRICULTURAL WORKERS

Not only are such workers exposed to pesticides, but also the average farmer engages in a wide variety of activities, including the rearing and feeding of animals, milking, veterinary care, treatment of soil and crops, harvesting, and maintenance of the farm building and machinery.[104] Furthermore, mechanized farming may expose the farmer to dyes in gasoline, rubber tires, various lubrications, and greases. Piglet dealers who sedate pigs going to market with Stresnil, which contains azaperone (49-fluoro-4-(4-(2-pyridyl)-1-piperazinyl) butyrophenone, may experience photocontact dermatitis. A 0.4% aqueous concentration plus 10J of UVA light can confirm this allergy.[105]

The feed additive olaquindox causes photosensitivity in white pigs that must be kept indoors when fed this substance, and it can cause photoallergic contact dermatitis in pig farmers.[106] Olaquindox forms a reactive oxyziridine on light exposure. The closely related quindoxin, which was marketed in the 1970s, was withdrawn due to persistent light reactions.

A group of 15 pig farmers were reported with photodermatitis from olaquindox airborne exposure.[107] Prolonged UVA sensitivity accompanied the photoallergic dermatitis in almost all patients and prolonged UVB sensitivity in about half of the cases.

A study of farmers in Finland found that 8.6% had hand eczema.[108] Furthermore, 70% of hand dermatitis cases were work related. Cow allergy was the main problem, and this was seen as both immediate sensitivity identified by skin prick test and delayed hypersensitivity to cow dander seen by patch tests.

Between 1990 and 1994 there were 2,759 cases of occupational allergic contact dermatitis in Finland: 30% due to contact urticaria and 70% to allergic contact dermatitis of

Table 24-15 Farmers and Agricultural Workers[a]	
Allergens	**Patch test concentration**
Antu (thiourea rat poison)	2% pet
p-dimethylaminoazobenzene (gasoline dye)	1% pet
Dithiocarbamates	
Maneb	1% pet
Thiram	1% pet
Zineb	1% pet
Ziram	1% pet
Potassium dichromate (leather gloves)	0.5% pet
Ragweed oleoresin	1% pet
Red Sudan IV (gasoline dye)	2% pet
Rubber chemicals (boots and gloves)	
Miscellaneous	
Animal feed additives (antibiotics and preservatives)	
Fertilizers	
Insecticides	
Lichens	
Mercury (organic and inorganic)	
Plants	
Wood	

[a] Pet, in petrolatum.

a delayed type.[109] Contact urticaria was found in women more commonly than men by 70% to 30%. The most common causes of contact urticaria as an occupational skin disease were cow dander (44%); natural rubber latex (24%); flour, grains, and feed (11%); foodstuffs (3%); industrial enzymes (2%); and decorative plants (2%).

Aside from the allergens listed in Table 24.15, these workers may be exposed to various plants, woods, lichens, fertilizers, insecticides, and animal feed additives.

DAIRY WORKERS

As with farmers and agricultural workers, dairy workers are exposed to many allergens besides pesticides. Rubber sensitivity is quite common in dairy workers because they are in frequent contact with water, detergents, and hypochlorite chemicals from the rubber.[110] Black[111] and Lintum and Nater[112] reported hand eczema in dairy workers due to sensitization to isopropyl-phenyl-para-phenylenediamine in the black rubber hosing of milking machines. Further cases were reported by Nurse.[110] Besides contact with hypochlorite solutions and detergents used for sterilizing the milking machinery and rubber hosing, dairy workers also have contact with iodine-containing preparations, which are used for washing the cows' teats before milking and as a teat-dip after milking. Chlorhexidine may also be used in teat care. Animals' coats (fur or wool) may also pose a source of dermatitis, as was reported[113] among ewe milkers who

Table 24-16 Dairy Workers[a]	
Allergens	**Patch test concentration**
Benzalkonium chloride (disinfectants)	0.01% aq
Chlorpromazine (medications)	1% pet
Cinnamon oil (medications)	0.5% pet
Coal tar (dust control oils)	5% pet
Cobalt chloride (animal feed additives)	1% pet
Dichlorophene (disinfectants)	1% pet
Neomycin sulfate (feed additives and medications)	20% pet
Rosin (medications)	20% pet
Rubber chemical series (milking machines and rubber gloves)	

[a]Aq, aqueous; pet, in petrolatum.

work bare-handed. A patch test to ewe's wool was positive, and there was no crossreaction with wool alcohol (30%) or lanolin (100%).

Suggested patch test allergens for dairy workers are listed in Table 24.16. It should be noted that milk samples may be preserved with dichromates that are sent for laboratory analysis for lipids and proteins. Such dichromates may cause dermatitis in laboratory workers.[114]

CATTLE BREEDERS

Cattle breeders may be exposed to insecticides, insect repellents, animal feed additives, and other allergens listed in Table 24.17.

Table 24-17 Cattle Breeders[a]	
Allergens	**Patch test concentration**
3,5-dinitro-o-toluamide	1% pet
Ethoxyquin	0.5% pet (photopatch test)
Furadantin	5% pet
Furazolidone	3% pet
Furfuraldehyde	3% pet
Isopropylparaphenylenediamine (IPPD) (rubber)	0.5% pet
Lauryl gallate	2% pet
Neomycin	20% pet
Nitrofurazone	3% pet
Penicillin	1% pet
Phenothiazine	2.5% pet
Piperazine (diethylenediamine)	5% aq
Quindoxin	0.1% pet (photopatch test)
Rubber chemicals	see standard tray
Spiramycin	10% pet
Tylan (tylosin)	1% pet

[a]Aq, aqueous; pet, in petrolatum.

Table 24-18 Forest Workers[a]	
Allergens	**Patch test concentration**
Alantolactone	0.1% pet
D3-Carene (turpentine)	1% peroxides in olive oil
Frullania, whole plant (liverwort)	as is
Parmelia (lichen)	as is
Pine bud	as is
Pine sap	10% pet
Poplar resin	10% pet
Plant extracts	Hollister-Stier in alcohol
Chrysanthemum (chrysanthemum)	
Cocklebur (xanthium)	
Feverfew (chrysanthemum parthenium)	
Marsh elder (iva)	
Sagebrush (artemisia)	
Short ragweed (ambrosia)	
Tansy (tanacetum)	
Rosin	20% pet
Usinic acid (sensitizer in lichens)	1% pet
Various sawdusts (moist with water)	as is

[a]Pet, in petrolatum.

FOREST WORKERS

Although pesticide dermatitis occurs in this group of workers, irritant dermatitis from wet work and plant dermatoses are probably more common.

Contact with the bark of trees in felling or processing the trees also often produces an allergic dermatitis due to a *d*-usnic acid found in the lichens on tree barks. In addition, sesquiterpenes in liverworts (Frullania), a primitive plant found on the surface of smooth barked trees such as the alder and hemlock, produce many instances of allergic dermatitis that may be confused with a photodermatitis.[115] These sesquiterpenes crossreact with chrysanthemum, ragweed, and other members of the Compositae family.[116–119] Table 24.18 lists the plant chemicals for patch testing forest workers who have dermatitis. A caterpillar known as the pine processionary caterpillar (*Thaumetopoea pityocampa*) poses an occupational risk to pine-cone or resin collectors, woodcutters, farmers, and stockbreeders. The most common reaction is contact urticaria but anaphylaxis has also been reported. In a study of 30 affected workers 60% also showed angioedema, 30% had papular lesions that lasted several days, and in this series 40% had anaphylactic reactions.[120]

GARDENERS

An extensive survey of Danish gardeners and greenhouse workers found 17% to have occupational allergic contact dermatitis.[121] Plants were the overwhelming source of the dermatitis compared with pesticides and rubber allergens, which were rarely the source. The Compositae plants produced most of the reactions. The 17% prevalence of dermatitis was the same as that found among tulip workers by Bruze in Sweden.[122]

Short-lived skin irritation of urticarial-type symptoms is commonly reported among gardeners and greenhouse workers. In a Danish study of such workers, 25% had short-lived symptoms.[123] When prick tested for plant sensitivity, 33% of 105 tested workers had a reaction to one or more plants. The most commonly identified reaction was to Christmas cactus (*Schlumbergera* hybrids).

Other Biologic Causes of Contact Dermatitis

A type of Italian cheese (taliggio) is wrapped in rags during its manufacture, which supports the growth of the mite *Rhizoglyphus*.[124] This mite causes rhinitis, asthma, and dermatitis on exposure. This is confirmed by prick tests and tests with other mites that proved negative.[124]

Marine organisms cause hand and forearm dermatitis among North Sea fishermen trawling the Dogger Bank. *Alcyonidium gelatinosum* or *hirsutum* causes most of the cases. Other organisms that cause what is referred to as "white seaweed" dermatitis include *Electra pilosa* and *Sertularia argentae*, which cause contact urticaria; *Flustra folicea* (a bryozoan); and *Abieturiasia abretina* and *Hydralmania falcata* (coelenteratis).[125]

A coffee worker developed dermatitis from roasted espresso coffee in powdered form and as a drink. Prior reports have been of dermatitis from green coffee beans.[126]

A worker who packaged flesh-fly larvae for use as fish bait developed hand dermatitis. He was patch test negative to the larvae of *Calliphora vomitoria*, but prick tests proved positive. This was considered a form of protein contact dermatitis.[127]

Paper Dermatitis

More than 600 products are used in the manufacture of paper from the cellulose fibers of trees (spruce, pine, and hemlock). These products include fillers, preservatives, plasticizers, whitening agents, chelators, adhesives, dispersing agents, corrosion inhibitors, and many other additives such as ammonia, hydrogen sulfide, sulfuric acid, carbon monoxide, sodium hydroxide, and chlorine.[128]

ROLE OF FORMALDEHYDE AND FORMALDEHYDE RESINS

Formaldehyde and its reactive derivatives are used in the paper industry to improve the wet-strength, water-resistance, shrink-resistance, grease-resistance, and other characteristics of paper and paper products. In addition, formaldehyde serves as a disinfectant and preservative in paper manufacture and in the preparation of finishes, sizing agents, and parchment paper.

Paper towels may contain melamine formaldehyde resin to increase resistance to water, and paper money may contain formaldehyde and its resins to prevent mildew.[129] Wrapping paper, inexpensive paper, and newspapers may produce dermatitis from the presence of free formaldehyde.[130]

Many types of paper contain formaldehyde or its resin to increase "wet strength" and to prevent mildew.

Glossy table paper contains a formaldehyde resin and free formaldehyde. The shiny, heavy, more expensive table paper is much more likely to contain formaldehyde than the thinner, less expensive, duller, more fragile type of paper. To be on the safe side, formaldehyde-sensitive patients should be protected from table paper with an all-cotton sheet.

The handling of most newspapers, magazines, both hardcover and paperback books, and glossy paper readily produces dermatitis in formaldehyde-sensitive individuals.

In connection with paper dermatitis, Black[131] reported a formaldehyde-sensitive individual who was allergic to blank newsprint. The estimation of free formaldehyde content of the newsprint showed it to be 0.02%. A similar estimation done on paper towels used in Black's hospital as an "economy" measure was 0.03%.

The formaldehyde-sensitive patient also acquires dermatitis from many types of paper tissues, paper towels, paper plates, and cups, except Marcal products. Although formaldehyde is not present in the actual ingredients of Dixie plates and cups, a minute quantity of formaldehyde is present in the lubricants used to keep the paperboard from wrinkling during its manufacture.

The formaldehyde-sensitive individual cannot tolerate any art paper used for acrylic paint or water colors, except for paper with the Grumbacher label. Incidentally, Boncour acrylic paint is tolerated by formaldehyde-sensitive individuals, but Liquitex is not.

QUATERNIUM AMMONIUM

Paper strength is increased by the addition of modified cationic starch to the pulp and sizing. The manufacture of this type of starch involves a quaternium ammonium compound known as 2,3-epoxypropyl trimethyl ammonium chloride. This potent sensitizer in guinea pigs sensitized several Finnish workers exposed to this occupationally.[132] It is also known as glycidyl trimethyl ammonium chloride. Beyond usage in paper

Table 24-19 Constituents of Carbon Papers

Oils
  Mineral and castor oils
  Stearic and oleic acids
Pigments and dyes
  Carbon black
  Methyl and crystal violet
  Miliori blue
  Nigrosine
  Victoria blue
Waxes
  Beeswax
  Cardelilla
  Carnauba
  Montan
  Oricony
  Paraffin wax

manufacture, this chemical is useful in the production of cellulose textile fibers, hair dye, dispersing and emulsifying agents, surfactants, fabric softeners, and adsorbents for the removal of dyes from wastewater. A patch test concentration of 0.5% in petrolatum was effective in identifying the cases.

COLOPHONY

Hand eczema can occur from handling paper and newsprint (without ink) due to colophony.[133] Patch tests with the paper are usually negative. A proper patch test is prepared from an acetone extract of paper at about 10% concentration.

CARBON PAPER

Calnan[134] stated that there are only two reports of proven reactions to carbon paper. Hjorth[135] described a man with a positive patch test to one type of carbon paper and to the plasticizer triphenyl phosphate, which was present at a concentration of 30% in the film emulsion. The second report by Calnan and Connor[136] described a man with dermatitis from nigrosine that was present only in a special carbon paper used for computer work.

A carbon paper ink consists basically of three elements: waxes, oils, and colors (Table 24.19). Each of these elements consists of complex mixtures. The oils are nondrying to produce softness and compactness of the ink; the waxes keep the ink hard and dry at room temperature and are a vehicle for the colors. The quality of the paper on which the ink is deposited is also important, because it must be thin and free of pinholes.[137]

CARBONLESS PAPER

Calnan[138] describes carbonless paper as pressure-sensitive paper for which either a ballpoint pen or an electric typewriter is the most suitable writing instrument. The principle consists of coating the undersurface of the top or writing sheet of paper with a thin emulsion that contains microcapsules of "ink." The "inks" are "color formers" that are colorless at one pH and colored at another. The pH inside the capsules is acid, and the pH outside the capsules is alkaline.

The top surface of the second sheet is coated with a material that absorbs the "ink" (color former) when the microcapsules are broken by the pressure of the ballpoint pen. This material is alkaline, and so the color appears.

The color formers are mostly triphenyl methane dyes such as gentian violet and malachite green, which are dissolved in organic solvents inside the microcapsules. The solvents include kerosene diarylethanes, alkyl naphthalenes, cyclohexane, and dibutyl phthalate, which may be diluted with odorless kerosene. Some of these papers contain formaldehyde, others contain ammonia.

Complaints from handling the carbonless copy papers include mild dermatitis and rather severe upper respiratory symptoms. Some individuals complain of an irritating odor emanating from handling the papers.[134,138,139]

Rycroft and Calnan[140] stated that there have been several instances of irritation of the skin, eyes, and upper respiratory tract in office workers handling carbonless copy paper. Symptoms that these carbonless copy papers produced were dismissed initially by some physicians as psychoneurotic, but their occurrence now in several different groups of employees seems to make it certain that this is a physical phenomenon. The symptoms are suggestive of an airborne irritant, and research into release of chemicals from the complex chemical system incorporated in the paper is needed. It appears at present that the most likely candidates for the cause of these irritant symptoms reside among a range of organic solvents that are an essential component of these systems. The symptoms attributed to NCR paper of skin and mucous membrane irritation, itching, headache, and fatigue have more recently been attributed to "sick building syndrome."[141] The chemicals used to manufacture NCR paper have been virtually dermatitis free even though 1.8 2106 tons are produced worldwide.[141]

Marks[142] reported an allergic reaction to a component of a carbonless paper containing a color former composed of paratoluene sulfinate of Michler's hydrol (PTSMH). Paratoluene sulfinate of Michler's hydrol is a colorless dye salt that forms a colored print on transfer to a suitable receiving paper. The reaction of Michler's hydrol and paratoluene sulfinic acid produces PTSMH.

Table 24-20 Methods of Paper Copying (Duplication)
Photocopying
Dyeline or diazo method
Thermofax (heat process)
Electrostatic or xerographic procedure

This chemical coating was developed to improve business copy papers.

COPY PAPER

Table 24.20 lists the four methods of copying or duplicating.

1. *Verifax* (Eastman Kodak) is a photocopying method. Two men were sensitized while employed making the powder for the sensitized emulsion. Both men developed severe and widespread eczema and were sensitized by 4-phenyl catechol, patch tested 0.5% in petrolatum.[143] Jensen and Roed-Petersen[144] described patients who had itchy erythema of the face and headaches from vapor evaporating from wet toners used in photocopy machines, but they were unable to identify the precise chemical. Adequate ventilation solved the problem.

2. *Diazo or dyeline process.* The dyeline or diazo process is a paper copying method. An original pattern is placed on diazo-sensitized paper and is exposed to ultraviolet light. The ultraviolet light decomposes the diazonium salts in the diazo paper, except where they are shielded by the pattern. The paper is then developed with ammonia gas, which causes a change of color in the unexposed portions of the diazo-sensitized paper. Diazonium salts interact with "coupling agents" present in the paper to give a blue, black, or brown copy by the formation of azo dyes.[143]

   The coupling agents are generally aromatic alcohols such as phenol and resorcinol derivatives. Other components such as stabilizing agents are also present. Zinc chloride and acids such as citric acid inhibit chemical interactions at room temperature, thus preventing premature coupling. Antioxidants, for example, thiourea, prevent yellowing of the white nonimage area. Ammonia is also used in the process. Nickel salts are present in some papers. The allergen in diazo paper is usually *p*-diethylaminobenzene diazonium chloride (diazodiethyl aniline hydrochloride, DDA), which is reduced to an amine that may crossreact with paraphenylenediamine. Crossreactions do not appear to occur with other azo compounds.

   The DDA is not a sensitizer when it is irradiated. Thus, patch tests with the nonirradiated paper are positive in sensitized individuals but are negative with irradiated paper. There are several reports of dermatitis from such diazo papers as Amonax, Ozalid, and Radex papers.[143, 145–147]

   An irritant dermatitis may occur from the ammonia used in the process. The DDA was tested in a 10% aqueous solution by Mijnssen and Verspyck,[145] who found that sensitized patients gave a positive reaction to the nonirradiated paper.

   Dooms-Goossens and colleagues[44] reported a textile cutter who had conjunctivitis and an erythematous itching dermatitis of the eyelids, nasal mucous membranes, and the corners of the mouth. Patch testing revealed a strong positive reaction to the textile cutting patterns that she handled, which were duplicated by diazo processing. The contact dermatitis reaction was caused specifically by thiourea (dimethyl-thiourea), an additive in diazo-sensitized paper that prevents discoloration of the paper. Sengel and colleagues[148] reported a similar case. Van der Leun and colleagues[149] described a case of photodermatitis from thiourea in copy paper. Thiourea may be tested 5% in aqueous solution.

3. *Thermofax* (heat process). This heat process used in duplication paper produced many instances of allergic sensitization to 4-tertiary butyl catechol, which may crossreact with pentadecylcatechol in poison ivy.

   Dermatitis from thermofax paper was reported by Fisher[150] and also by Harman and Sarkany.[143] Degos and colleagues[151] reported dermatitis due to methyl gallate, an antioxidant used in thermofax paper.

   Patch tests may be performed with the butyl catechol, 0.5% in petrolatum, and methyl gallate, 2% in petrolatum. The thermofax paper may be tested "as is."

   There are several reports of thermofax dermatitis that stops when the subject is no longer in contact with the duplication paper or if the subject uses a different paper. Thermofax paper allergy can be suppressed by using the two new nonsensitizing thermofax papers Jl and Jlo. Cases of allergy to the hypoallergenic thermofax paper have been reported.[152–154] Hand dermatitis that improved on job leave and vacation and relapsed on return to work was traced to colophony in telefax paper that contained 1% colophony. Patch testing with this fax paper gave only ± reactivity.[155]

4. *The electrostatic or xerographic method.* No instance of contact dermatitis has been reported from this process of duplication.

PHOTOCOPY WORK

Photocopier toner may contain quaternium-15, and this may be a source of dermatitis for those involved in photocopying.[156]

TYPEWRITING PAPER

Wikstrom[157] reported that in dermatitis due to typewriting paper the allergen appeared to occur in the "size" contained in the paper, a gum resin that consisted partly of rosin. Sensitivity to the typewriting paper can be accompanied also by sensitivity to rosin, juniper tar, and styrax. All of these substances contain mixtures of resinous acids, one of which is abietic acid. Allergic reactions to abietic acid were shown in sensitivity to typewriting paper.

TYPEWRITER CORRECTION PAPER

Jordan and Bourlas[158] found that a patient had an allergic reaction from a phenol formaldehyde resin, Arochem 455, tested 1% in alcohol. The resin is used as a binder for the powdery coating on the paper. Patch tests should be done with the powdered side of the paper.

PERFUME IN PAPER

Perfumed facial tissues, toilet paper, and sanitary napkins can produce allergic contact dermatitis, particularly if they contain cinnamic aldehyde or cinnamic alcohol.[159–161]

Parks[162] believed that perfume in toilet tissue is unlikely to cause sensitivity because of its low concentration and the manufacturing practice of applying it to the inner core of the roll. The perfume is probably there in low concentration, because it has to be carried to the paper by diffusion.

Bakers' Dermatitis

In a population-based study of occupational skin disease, bakers had a higher risk of dermatitis (191 per 10,000 employees) compared with confectioners (84 per 10,000) and cooks (34 per 10,000).[163] Irritant contact dermatitis was the most common diagnosis. Occupationally relevant type 1 allergy was found in 36% of bakers, 16% of confectioners, and 9% of cooks.

Many cases of hand dermatitis of bakers are irritant, infectious, or due to infestation: Some cases are atopic in nature or due to dyshidrosis.[164] An evaluation of 873 bakers, cooks, and butchers found that 213 (24.4%) had allergic contact dermatitis. The recommended patch test series to identify the sources of dermatitis were the standard, rubber, and Compositae series and the patients' own products.[165]

1. *Irritant dermatitis.* Most instances of hand dermatitis in bakers are due to a nonspecific dermatitis from various irritants, such as wet, sticky dough, sweetening agents, enzymes, and various flavors. Soaps and

Table 24-21 Irritants That Bakers May Encounter
Acetic acid
Ascorbinic acid (flour improver)
Bleaching agents
Calcium acetate and sulfate
Emulsifying agents
Enzymes
Fruit juices
Lactic acid
Potassium bicarbonate
Potassium iodide and bromate
Wet dough
Yeast

detergents used for cleansing the hands are also often the cause of irritant bakers' dermatitis. In such instances, the patch tests are negative. Table 24.21 lists the numerous irritants to which bakers are exposed.

2. *Paronychia.* Monilial and bacterial paronychia occurs frequently in bakers. Painting the paronychial area with a Betadine solution is often effective for both types of paronychia.

3. *Food mite dermatitis.* Food mite dermatitis may be papulofollicular rather than eczematous and most prominent on the dorsal aspect of the hands. Flour mites (Tyroglyphus) may be found in the flour and on the bakers' skin. This type of "bakers' itch" occurs particularly among workers in flour mills and bakeries in small establishments that do not use mechanical processes and have few sanitary arrangements. Pastry bakers are subject to a dermatitis due to the sugar mite.[166]

4. *Bakers' "psoriasis."* Bakers with psoriasis may develop a fissured, hyperkeratotic, psoriatic lesion on their palms due to the Koebner phenomenon from trauma to their hands. Wütrich[167] used the term "bakers' psoriasis" for palmar keratoderma of bakers due to this phenomenon.

5. *Dyshidrotic eczema.* Several bakers were observed with dyshidrotic eczema of the hands. In two bakers, however, the dyshidrosis continued after they discontinued their jobs as bakers. Young[168] reported that he observed bakers with positive intracutaneous tests to flour extracts and with skin eruptions of atopic dermatitis or dyshidrotic eczema, and that an inhalant allergy to flour may cause eczema of the hands as the only symptom.

6. *Atopic dermatitis.* Hjorth[169] stated that most bakers' dermatitis was associated with an immediate type 1 sensitivity. Herxheimer[170] found that skin sensitivity to pollen and flour often occurred together. Jarvinen

and colleagues[171] found that a disease of the atopic group was established in 25% of bakery employees investigated and that 9% had asthma, 25% had allergic rhinitis, and 5% had atopic eczema. They concluded that an individual with atopy is unsuitable for bakery work.

7. *Contact urticaria due to flour.* Flour can produce a contact urticaria of the baker's hands that the baker scratches and excoriates. When it can be seen, the hand dermatitis resembles an eczematous dermatitis. A careful history usually reveals that the baker complains of immediate burning and itching when handling flour. The hands soon become red and edematous. Patch tests are negative, but moistened flour on the scratch produces an urticarial wheal in the baker and not in controls. Fisher[172] and Odom and Maibach[173] reviewed this type of urticarial reaction to various food products.

Enzymes are added to flour because most are deficient in amylase. Enzymes such as *Aspergillus orzae* and *Bacillus subtilis* may cause contact urticaria in bakers.[174] In bakers, alpha-amylase can cause both immediate and delayed hypersensitivity[175] and has caused contact urticaria and protein contact dermatitis. Kanerva and colleagues[176] found that differences in allergenicity of alpha-amylase exist depending on whether the enzyme is of bacterial or fungal origin. Their patient was sensitive only to enzyme of fungal origin, which would allow for an allergen substitution of the bacterial alpha-amylase.

In addition to alpha-amylase, other enzymes are used industrially. Skin reactions have been reported to cellulase found in feeds, baking, brewing, detergents, pulp/paper, textile processing; glucoamylase in alcohol production and baking; papain in brewing, contact lens detergents and pharmaceuticals; and xylanase in the pulp/paper industry.[177]

8. *Sorbic acid reactions.* This preservative is sometimes added to flour, particularly in the making of rye bread. An eczematous contact dermatitis of the hands from hypersensitivity to sorbic acid with positive patch test reactions to sorbic acid and potassium sorbate can be demonstrated.

In addition, a baker developed an immediate reaction consisting of redness and slight itching of hands where he contacted flour containing sorbic acid. The 48-hour patch test was negative. The baker, however, developed an immediate wheal from the application of 5% sorbic acid in petrolatum.[178]

Potassium sorbate, which crossreacts with sorbic acid, is used as a preservative in meringue.

9. *Flour flavors.* Malten[179] reported several bakers with contact dermatitis from flavors in flours and pointed

Table 24-22 Flavoring Used by Bakers
Anise
Cardamom
Cinnamon
Cloves
Ginger
Laurel
Lemon juice
Lemon oil
Methyl salicylate
Nutmeg
Peppermint
Vanilla

out cinnamon as an occupational hazard of bakers. Table 24.22 lists the various flavors that may be used by bakers.

Five cases of occupational contact dermatitis due to spices were reported in chefs and kitchen or restaurant workers.[180] All had hand dermatitis. The incriminated spices were garlic, cinnamon, ginger, allspice, and clove. Patch tests were also positive to foods including tomato, lettuce, and carrot.

10. *Karaya gum.* Karaya gum, a vegetable gum derivative, is used as a pastry filler and as a stabilizer of meringue, which is a frothy pastry topping consisting of beaten egg whites and sugar. Patch testing reveals a positive reaction to karaya gum, which is a rare sensitizer.[181] Karaya is also widely used in hair waving lotions, denture adhesive powders, furniture polishes, and as a cement for ileostomy appliances. Karaya may occasionally produce allergic reactions.[182]

11. *Ammonium persulfate reactions.* Ammonium persulfate was used previously in certain European countries as a flour "improver" to render the flour white. In Greece, until recently, this chemical was added to flour, but it has never been permitted in flour in the United States.

Ammonium persulfate and benzoyl peroxide are still permitted in flour in the Netherlands and in Great Britain, but although benzoyl peroxide is still widely used, many millers have replaced persulfates with potassium bromate, which is equally efficient and easier to handle. Ammonium persulfate not only may produce an eczematous contact dermatitis, but in certain individuals severe urticaria and anaphylactic shock may occur.[183,184]

12. *Benzoyl peroxide.* This antioxidant flour bleaching agent may produce allergic contact dermatitis in sensitized bakers.[185]

Table 24-23 Allergens in the Baking Industry[a]

	Patch test concentration
Alpha-tocopherol (antioxidant for fats)	10% pet
Ammonium persulfate (Europe)	1% aq
Balsam of Peru (crossreacts with flavors)	25% pet
Beeswax (artificial flowers)	5% pet
Benzoyl peroxide	1% pet
Butylated hydroxyanisole [(BHA) (antioxidants for lards and greases)]	2% pet
Butylated hydroxytoluene (BHT) (antioxidants for lards and greases)	2% pet
Cinnamic aldehyde	1% pet
Cinnamon oil	0.5% pet
Eugenol	5% pet
Food dyes	1% pet
Karaya gum (sterculia gum)	as is
Lauryl gallate (antioxidant in margarines)	5% pet
Limonen, oil of	1% in alcohol
Methyl salicylate (flavorings)	2% in olive oil
p-amino-azo-benzene (indicator for azo dyes)	0.25% pet
Potassium bromate	5% aq
Potassium dichromate	0.25% pet
Sorbic acid (preservative)	5% pet
Vanilla (alcoholic extract)	10% in acetone
Vanillin	10% pet

[a]Aq, aqueous; pet, in petrolatum.
Note: Flour may be tested as is for delayed hypersensitivity. Urticarial reactions with flour should be tested with moistened flour on a scratch.

Table 24-24 A "Screening" Patch Test Series for Hairdressers

Bleaching
 Ammonium persulfate 2.0% (Caution: may cause syncope)
Fragrance[a]
 Fragrance mix no. 3 (standard tray)
Hair dyes[b]
 o-nitro-p-phenylenediamine 1%
 p-aminophenol 1%
 p-phenylenediamine 1%
 p-toluylenediamine 1%
 Pyrogallol 1%
 Resorcinol
Metals[a]
 Nickel 5% (standard tray)
Perfumes
 Balsam of Peru 25%
Permanent waving
 Ammonium thioglycolate 2.5%
 Glyceryl monothioglycolate 2.5%
Preservatives
 Formaldehyde 1% aqueous
 Proteins
 Quaternium 15 (Dowicil 200)
Rubber chemicals
 Carbamate mix
 Mercaptobenzothiazole 2%
 Thiram mix

[a]Standard tray.
[b]All these may crossreact with paraphenylenediamine except resorcinol and pyrogallol.
Note: All are tested with petrolatum except formaldehyde (1% aqueous).

13. *Antioxidants in flour.* The antioxidants, butylated hydroxyanisole (BHA), butylated hydroxytoluene (BHT), and lauryl and propyl gallate may produce contact dermatitis in bakers.[186–188]

14. *Chromates in flour.* There are no reports of dermatitis in bakers from chromium compounds in this country. Heime and Fox[189] in Germany reported, however, that they studied a baker with eczema of the hands with relapses that obviously occurred because of contact with flour. Patch testing revealed only hypersensitivity to chromate. Four sorts of flour used in Germany were analyzed, and it was found that the chromium content ranged from 0.01 to 0.09 mg/dL in these four flour samples. These authors concluded that even those comparatively low chromium levels were capable of giving rise to eczema in chromate-sensitive individuals.

Table 24.23 lists the allergens that bakers may encounter.

Dermatitis in Hairdressers

Hairdressers are exposed to several irritants and allergens.[190] In many cases, the hand dermatitis is a combination of an irritant and allergic variety. A hairdresser can acquire a dry irritant dermatitis over the metacarpophalangeal joints while shampooing a client's hair. Some hairdressers develop eczema of the fingers. In those who give up hairdressing, the dermatitis generally improves or heals; in those who continue hairdressing, the dermatitis is likely to persist especially in atopic individuals.[191–195]

Irritant hand dermatitis in hairdressers facilitates allergic hypersensitivity to hair dyes, rubber chemicals, nickel, and the allergens to which hairdressers are exposed. A "screening" patch test series for hairdressers is given in Table 24.24.

In a 4-year study of hairdressers, allergic contact dermatitis was more common than irritant contact dermatitis in this occupation.[196] The principal allergen was glyceryl thioglycolate. Avoidance of glyceryl thioglycolate proved problematic, as it contaminated the work surfaces of the shop, so that avoidance of permanent wave solution was insufficient for prevention. Other important allergens in this industry were ammonium persulfate and nickel. Also found were the shampoo ingredients cocamidopropyl betaine and sodium coco hydrolyzed animal protein, as well as the hair-dye chemicals. A comparison of patch test results in hairdressers over a 10-year period found an increase in contact allergy to multiple occupational contactants. The study analyzed data from 379 hairdressers evaluated from 1980 to 1993, compared to 300 hairdressers tested between 1994 and 2003. Positive patch tests occurred in 78.3% of the 1994–2003 group vs 58.8% of the prior group. An occupational allergen was found in 54% vs 48.8 respectively. Occupational allergens found to have increased in more recent years include p-phenylenediamine base (54 vs 45.9), 4-aminobenzene (40.7% vs 31.9%), ammonium thioglycolate (12.3% vs 2.7%), ammonium persulfate (14.3% vs 7.9%), p-toluenediamine sulfate (15.3 vs 6.8%), p-toluenediamine sulfate 15.3 % vs 6.8%), p-aminodiphenylamine (7.7% vs 2.9%), o-nitro-4-phenylenediamine (7.3% vs 2.1%), and aminophenols (9% vs 0%). The authors called for improved protective measures.[197]

When hairdressers were followed from apprenticeship to a point 8 years into their careers, dermatitis was found to be a problem in 51%, even though they had no dermatitis before entering the profession.[198] Of those who gave up practicing hairdressing, only 33% had hand eczema. In this long-term study, no relationship was found between atopy or nickel sensitivity and the development of hand dermatitis, but dry skin was a risk factor.

Dahlquist and colleagues[199] demonstrated that nickel is released from hair clips and nickel-plated metal by ammonium thioglycolate in liquids for "permanent waves." This finding might explain to some extent the high frequency of nickel allergy among hairdressers who are exposed to nickel-plated scissors, clips, pins, rollers, rods, and grips. It would, therefore, seem advisable for nickel-sensitive hairdressers to use stainless steel or plastic utensils only.

The introduction of glyceryl thioglycolate as a hair-waving chemical has produced many instances of hand dermatitis in hairdressers.[200]

Two unusual cases of contact urticaria in hairdressers to an egg shampoo have been described.[201] Both patients had had continuous contact with raw egg in the course of their work; while massaging or packing, egg emulsion was rubbed on their skin. The first patient, a 24-year-old beautician, first observed the symptoms on her palms after using quail eggs for massage, and later contact with raw hen's egg caused urticaria. After eating egg, she developed urticaria all over the body accompanied by tightness of the chest and angioedema. Epicutaneous testing showed sensitivity to both the white and the yolk of raw egg, with wheals all over the body, and also produced shock. In the case of boiled egg only, the white produced contact urticaria that was not accompanied by general symptoms. In the course of oral exposure only, the yoke of the egg produced disseminated urticaria within 30 minutes that was followed by coughing. In the other patient, a 31-year-old hairdresser, consumption of egg dishes resulted in local and generalized urticaria. Epicutaneous testing with the white of raw egg gave a positive reaction. Oral testing showed sensitivity to the white of boiled egg, causing continuous urticaria and hard breathing. Raw egg was not tested orally because of the risk of severe symptoms.

Egg is a complex albumen; thus, isolation of the material responsible for antigenicity is rather problematic and has not yet been solved. Antigenicity is influenced strongly both by pH changes and heat.[202]

Lynde and Mitchell[203] reported that over a period of 8 years, 66 hairdresser patients were patch tested to the North American Contact Dermatitis Group screening series, to a hairdressers' screening series, or to both. Paraphenylenediamine (PPD) produced positive reactions in 45% and nickel sulfate in 27% of the patients tested. Apart from the PPD substances and glyceryl thioglycolate, other chemicals tested produced allergic reactions in no more than 4 of 66 (6%) patients.

Paraphenylenediamine, nickel, and glyceryl thioglycolate were the most common causes of allergic contact dermatitis in hairdressers.

HENNA

Urticaria of the face, sinusitis, and headache can occur from airborne henna powder in hairdressers who have immediate hypersensitivity to henna. Henna is derived from Lawsonia inermis, and the allergen is thought to be 2-hydroxy-1,4-naphtoquinone (lawsone). The case reported by Majoie and Bruynzeel[204] was prick test negative to the lawsone but positive to henna 1% in ethanol and water. They cited other cases in hairdressers with similar symptoms and asthma, some of whom were positive to lawsone and others not. Therefore, another unidentified allergen is likely to also be present in henna.

HYDROGEN PEROXIDE

Two hairdressers who were allergic to multiple salon products were also found to be allergic to hydrogen peroxide used in hair bleaching and coloring operations.[205] A 3% aqueous preparation of hydrogen peroxide was used for patch test purposes. The normal use concentration in salon products is 3% to 5%.

AMMONIUM PERSULFATE

Ammonium persulfate is used in bleaching procedures in hairdressing salons, and potassium persulfate is used industrially as a bleaching, oxidizing, and antiseptic agent. It is also a polymerization promoter in the processing of textiles and in photography. Sensitization to potassium persulfate was confirmed in a laboratory assistant by 2.5% in petrolatum.[206] This patch test concentration was negative in 20 controls. Although the laboratory assistant had never dyed or bleached her hair, she had a positive reaction to ammonium persulfate.

PROTECTION OF HANDS FOR HAIRDRESSERS

Hairdressers should choose vinyl or nitrile gloves instead of the rubber variety, because many hairdressers become sensitized to the rubber gloves. In addition, the hair perming chemical glyceryl thioglycolate passes through rubber gloves more readily than through vinyl gloves. 4-H gloves are preferable for protection over rubber or vinyl but are difficult to work in. Nitrile gloves provide better protection and dexterity.

Formaldehyde and Formaldehyde-Releasing Materials

Hand eczema is a persistent occupational and nonoccupational problem. Cronin[207] pointed out the importance of formaldehyde in perpetuating this type of contact dermatitis. Her table on formaldehyde-free products can be of use to individuals with this problem (Table 24.25). Cutting

Table 24-25 Products That, to the Manufacturers' Knowledge, Do Not Contain Formaldehyde or a Formaldehyde Donor[a]

Washing-up liquids	
Fairy Liquid (both regular and lemon fresh perfumed)	Procter and Gamble
Sunlight Lemon Liquid	Unilever
Hard surface cleaners	
Impact Bathroom Cleaner	Benckiser
Impact Kitchen Cleaner	Benckiser
Mr. Muscle Kitchen Cleaner	Bristol-Myers Co. Ltd.
Mr. Muscle Bathroom Cleaner	Bristol-Myers Co. Ltd.
Shiny Sinks	Homecare Products
Flash Powder	Procter and Gamble
Flash Liquid	Procter and Gamble
Handy Andy	Unilever

Table 24-25 (Cont.)

Cooker cleaners	
Mr. Muscle Oven Cleaner	Bristol-Myers Co. Ltd.
Easy-Do Powder Cleanser	Easy-Do Products Ltd.
Hob Brite Cleanser	Homecare Products
Window cleaners	
Mr. Muscle Window Cleaner	Bristol-Myers Co. Ltd.
Windowlene Spray	Reckitt and Colman
Windowlene Plus (trigger pack)	Reckitt and Colman
Silver brass and copper polishers	
Silver Polish	Johnson Wax
Long Term Brass Polish	Johnson Wax
Long Term Copper Polish	Johnson Wax
Bleaches	
Vortex Bleach	Procter and Gamble
Domestos	Unilever
Clothes washing preparations	
Bold 3	Procter and Gamble
Bounce	Procter and Gamble
Ariel	Procter and Gamble
Fairy Snow	Procter and Gamble
Persil	Unilever
Persil Automatic nonbiological	Unilever
Persil Automatic New System	Unilever
Surf	Unilever
Surf Automatic	Unilever
Wisk	Unilever
Breeze Automatic	Unilever
Lux Flakes	Unilever
Fabric softener	
Lenor Concentrate	Procter and Gamble
Dishwasher products	
Finish Dishwasher Powder (standard and lemon)	Benckiser
Finish Concentrated Dishwasher Liquid (standard and lemon)	Benckiser
Finish Compact Dishwasher Detergent	Benckiser
Finish Rinse Agent	Benckiser
Finish Dishwasher Cleaner and Freshner	Benckiser
Sun Machine Dishwashing Liquid	Unilever
Other domestic products	
Vanish Stain Removing Bar and Stain Stick	Benckiser
Vanish Machine Carpet Shampoo with De-foamer	Benckiser
Calgon	Benckiser
Scale Away	Benckiser
Lime Away	Benckiser
Dettol Liquid	Reckitt and Colman
Harpic Dual Action	Reckitt and Colman
Shampoos	
Flex Shampoo	Revlon
Other hair preparations	
Silvikrin Styling Mousse	Beecham Products
Silvikrin Hair Spray	Beecham Products
Flex Conditioner	Revlon

[a]From Cronin E. Formaldehyde is a significant allergen in women with hand eczema. Contact Dermatitis 1991;25:276. Used with permission.

fluids remain a frequent source of formaldehyde-releasing preservatives.[207] Prevention of metalworking fluid dermatitis has been reported by applying grapeseed oil, which contains vitamin E.[208] The grapeseed oil should be removed with soft paper, then soap and water. Formaldehyde-releasing materials have been linked to hand dermatitis additionally in gum arabic in printing materials, wallpaper adhesives, tape, flame retardants, cleaners, and fabric softeners.[207]

Electronics

Six categories of skin hazards have been identified in the electronics industry.[209]

1. *Solder.* Irritant reactions are more common than allergic reactions due to acids and solvents, but rosin-based solder poses a colophony risk that can be direct contact dermatitis, airborne dermatitis, or contact urticaria. Other potential allergens are hydrazine and aminoethyl ethanolamine.
2. *Solvents* generally are irritants and include isopropanol, *n*-butyl acrylate, freon, xylene, acetone, methanol, petroleum distillates, trichloroethane, methylene chloride, tetrachloroethylene (may cause Stevens-Johnson syndrome), ethylene glycol, and methyl ethyl ketone.
3. *Hydrofluoric acid* is the most common cause of chemical burns in the semiconductor industry.
4. *Epoxy resins* are the major allergens in the electronics industry. Also of concern is triglycidyl isocyanurate.
5. *Metals* of potential concern include ammonium bichromate, adhesion of phosphor in color TV screens, cobalt (magnets), platinum (connectors), and gold.
6. *Cyanoacrylate glue* with low relative humidity can cause irritation, which is corrected by greater than 55% relative humidity.

Ceramics

A study of 139 ceramics workers making floor and wall tile found that 52 experienced dermatitis, of which 37% were allergic and 63% irritant.[210]

In pottery workers, 24 cases of hand dermatitis occurred when a change was made from Portuguese to Indonesian turpentine.[211] Oil of turpentine is still used in the pottery industry and to some extent in the perfume industry. The most common turpentine ingredient found to cause reactions was alpha-pinene rather than delta-3-carene, which has been said to be the principal allergen. These cases were in fine china workers, and heavy metals used for ceramic decoration were not a common problem. Reverting to Portuguese oil of turpentine alleviated the epidemic.

Crystal-Arsenic

In the manufacture of crystal, arsenic is added to facilitate melting of the crystal. A 29-year-old man who mixed and carried powders to make crystal became sensitized to arsenic, which was detected by 1% sodium arsenate aqueous. Avoidance was curative.[212]

Nylon Manufacture

In the manufacture of nylon, a finish is applied to the nylon to reduce friction, decrease electrostatic charge, and prevent fraying. This is referred to as a "spin finish." N,N-methylene-bis-5-methyl-oxazolidine (Grotan OX) has been reported as a source of occupational contact dermatitis in the manufacture of nylon. While this substance is a formaldehyde releaser, the patient did not react to formaldehyde or other formaldehyde-releasing preservatives. Other spin finish allergens include chloroacetamide and methylchloroisothiazolinone/methylisothiazolinone. Dimethoxane is used as a polyester spin finish, and it has been cited as both allergen and irritant. Grotan OX is present at 0.2% in spin finish and was tested at 1% in water.[213]

Nitroglycerin

In the explosives industry, contact dermatitis to nitroglycerin has occurred 4 to 24 years after initial exposure, whereas medical use of nitroglycerin topically may cause dermatitis in as little as 3 days.[214] The allergens in dynamite or nitroglycerin include dinitrotoluene and ethylene glycol dinitrate, which can be tested at 0.1% to 0.5% in petrolatum. Nitroglycerin itself can be tested at 0.5% to 2.0% in petrolatum.

Laboratory Work

Analytic chemicals produce contact dermatitis in chemists and technicians. One such example is the reagent ethyl chloro oximido acetate, which subsequent animal work has established as a strong irritant and strong allergen.[215] Cyclohexanone caused hand dermatitis in a worker whose job involved gluing tubing to polyvinyl chloride fluid-therapy bags. The exposure was to 100% cyclohexanone, and no protection of the hands was used.

Cyclohexanone facilitates the gluing process. Allergy to cyclohexanone had previously been reported from exposure in a chemistry student, from deodorant and in its use as a polyvinyl chloride adhesive.[216]

Construction

A study of Spanish construction workers found that 65% showed one or more reactions to occupationally relevant allergens.[217] Of the 268 such workers, the most common allergen was chromate (42%), followed by cobalt (20%), nickel (10%), and epoxy resin (7.5%). A total of 106 workers were allergic to rubber components, with thiuram mix being the most prevalent rubber allergen. A German study of 205 construction workers found that chromate was the most frequently encountered allergen (32%), followed by cobalt (15%), nickel (8%), thiuram (8%), and p-phenylenediamine (8%).[218]

Several studies have attempted to assess whether addition of ferrous sulfate to cement will actually lower the prevalence of contact dermatitis to chromium.[219–221] This addition reduces hexavalent chromate to trivalent chromate, which is less likely to penetrate skin and lead to adverse reactions. Studies from Denmark, Sweden, and Finland all point to favorable results with a reduction of chromium cases of occupational dermatitis to less than one-third of previous levels.[219] However, if the cement is stored for more than 6 months, the benefit tends to be lost. The lower levels of chromium dermatitis may be due to factors other than the addition of ferrous sulfate to cement. In Singapore, where no addition of ferrous sulfate to cement occurs, the chromate problems of construction workers have decreased.[220] Changes in the blast furnace process have resulted in a lower chromate content, and the amount of chromate was found to be inversely related to the amount of slag in the cement. From 1983 to 1995, the rate of contact dermatitis from chromate in cement continued to fall in Singapore.[221] However, from 1990 to 1995 the rate of chromate dermatitis increased, but not from cement; rather, the sources were leather, electroplating, welding, and metallic dyes.

The prognosis of occupational chromate dermatitis has been found to be poor.[222] Even though 40% of workers with such a condition changed jobs to avoid chromate, 69% had persistent dermatitis.[222] It has been recommended that on-site mixing of cement be done with ferrous sulfate to decrease dermatitis. This would increase cement costs 1% to 1.5% but protect those at greatest risk, in contrast to adding ferrous sulfate to premixed cement delivered to the work site.[222]

Although chromium sensitivity has a reputation for intractability, the outcome of strict avoidance of further exposure to chromates was favorable in 72% of cases followed in Switzerland.[223] Financial support of displaced workers was considered to be a factor in the more favorable outcome.

In addition to construction, chromate sensitization is an issue in the production of color television tubes.[224] Ammonium chromate is used in production as a fixer and can cause occupational contact dermatitis.

Shoemakers

A survey of 246 shoemakers found occupational contact dermatitis in 36 individuals.[225] Irritant contact dermatitis was diagnosed in 20 (8.1%) and allergic contact dermatitis in 16 (6.5%). The most common allergens were p-tert-butylphenol-formaldehyde resin and mercapto-benzothiazole. Hyperkeratosis of the fingertips was the primary morphologic presentation.

Offshore Oil Workers

Offshore oil workers are exposed to drilling mud. Ormerod and colleagues'[226] analysis of mud composition showed the mud to be made up of inorganics and hydrocarbons. The inorganics include aluminum, silicon, sulfur, potassium, calcium, barium, and iron. The hydrocarbons in the volatile phase of the mud are white spirit or low boiling point petroleum ether combined with paraffinic or naphthenic mineral oil. Fatty acid amines have been components of drilling mud, but in the last few years C16/C18 alpha olefins have become common additives, and cases of irritant contact dermatitis were seen from this component by Ormerod and colleagues.

Auto and Airplane Mechanics

A survey of automobile mechanics found that 15% reported hand eczema.[227] Patch tests performed on those mechanics with hand dermatitis found that 55% actually had irritant contact dermatitis. Only 19% had allergic contact dermatitis. The most frequent relevant reaction was to nickel, which was attributed to nickel-plated tools. One allergen not found on the standard screening series of allergens that proved helpful was d-limonene, which can be found in hand cleaners.

Automobile body repair work can involve the use of two-part unsaturated polyester cements. Contact dermatitis can result from this material, which is spread onto metal surfaces and then sanded and polished prior to painting. Diethylene glycol maleate was isolated from this material and found to be the allergen. The dust that collects from sanding also contains the allergen.[228]

Jet aviation hydraulic fluid may cause allergic contact dermatitis from a cycloaliphatic epoxy resin known as ERL 4234 [2-(3,4 epoxychlorhexyl-5,5 spiro-3,4-epoxy) cyclohexane-meta dioxane]. Patch tests should be done at 0.1% or 0.01% in petrolatum.[229]

Video Display Terminals

A variety of skin complaints have been blamed on video display terminals (VDTs). A systemic evaluation found a tendency for an increase in seborrheic dermatitis among such workers, which seems to relate to low levels of relative humidity rather than VDTs.[230] A nonspecific erythema also seen among such workers correlated with perceived high work pace and inability to take rest breaks. No association was found with electrical or magnetic fields.

Medical Equipment Production

The production of microspheres for embolization in cardiovascular or neurosurgical procedures involves the use of N-(2-(diethylamino)ethyl)acrylamide or DEAEA. This compound has proven to be highly allergenic, as it sensitized 5 workers involved in the microsphere manufacturing process. A 1% petrolatum concentration is used for patch testing.[231]

An outbreak of dermatitis in 16 workers in a medical equipment manufacturing facility was traced to aromatic diisocyanates. Dicyclohexylmethane-4,4'-diisocyanate was the main allergen identified, but some workers were also sensitive to hexamethylenediisocyanate and isophoronediisocyanate. The authors felt that aromatic isocyanates might be more reactive than aliphatic ones and the aromatic compounds might be degraded before percutaneous absorption rendering them somewhat less allergenic than aliphatic isocyanates.[232] Reported reactions to isocyanates include allergic or irritant contact dermatitis, generalized urticaria, and contact urticaria. A case of IgE-mediated contact urticaria to diphenylmethane-4/4'-diisocyanate (MDI) was reported from Finland.[233]

Performing Artists

In an investigation of opera-house artists, 50% had a history of intolerance of cosmetics, but when patch tested, contact allergy was uncommon.[234] The rate of fragrance allergy was similar in this profession to that commonly found among patch test clinic patients in general. However, fragrance sensitivity was over-represented among the cosmetic intolerant group.

Musicians

Recorders can be of boxwood, cedar, or rosewood construction. A 65-year-old man who played this instrument was found to be allergic to only his recorder made of boxwood.[235] He had a hyperkeratotic eczema of his fingertips. Boxwood is from the Buxus sempervirens of the family Buxaceae.

Allergens found among musicians include rosin (colophony) to wax string instruments, nickel in chin rests, metallic parts of bows used on string instruments, cane reeds on woodwinds, and propolis in violin varnishes.[236] Nonallergic skin changes found in musicians include soft tissue and bony changes, lip problems (hyperkeratosis and at times cheilitis), callus formation from repetitive trauma, and cutaneous hemorrhage from repetitive trauma.[237] The repetitive trauma of musical instruments has caused conditions known as fiddler's neck, fiddler's fingers, drummer's digits, piano paronychia, pizzicato paronychia, guitar nipple, cellist's chest, and broken lips (the latter known as Satchmo's syndrome, so named for Louis Armstrong).[238] Skin conditions can influence musicians' performances: Hyperhidrosis has caused musicians to change the instrument they play, xerostomia and hypersalivation can disable a wind player, and infections such as herpes labialis can impair brass and woodwind musicians.[239]

Metalworkers

Metal-working oils that operate under extreme pressure contain additives to help keep them in place between the moving metal parts. Contact dermatitis from an additive zinc, bis((O,O'-di2-ethylhexyl)dithiphosphate) was identified in 4 workers and a 6% petrolatum patch test concentration has been recommended (Figure 24-3).[240]

Dentists

A survey of dentists in Sweden found that 15% had experienced hand dermatitis in the preceding year. The survey included nearly 3,500 dentists. A subset of these dentists were evaluated and of 149 with confirmed hand dermatitis 67% proved to have irritant contact dermatitis and 28% allergic contact dermatitis. The most common allergens were nickel, fragrance, gold, thiuram, 2-hydroxyethyl methacrylate, and ethylene glycol dimetharylate.[241] In another study of Swedish dentists, 109 of 173 (63%) were found to have hand eczema, of which 67% was found to be of irritant origin and 33% of allergic origin. Of the 109, 24 had a reaction to dental acrylates, the most frequent of which were 2-hydroxyethyl methacrylate, ethylene glycol dimethacrylate, and methyl methacrylate.[242]

This chapter is the revision of a chapter written for the third edition by Robert M. Adams.

References

1. Fisher AA. Occupational, Industrial, and Plant Dermatology Symposium. San Francisco, March 26–28, 1979. Part 1: general considerations. Cutis 1979;24:143.

2. Fisher AA. Occupational, Industrial, and Plant Dermatology Symposium. Part 2: role of skin appendages, physical factors, pigment and malingering. Cutis 1979;24:249.

3. Owen CM, Gawkrodger DJ. Occupational dermatitis in Sheffield: a preliminary study. Contact Dermatitis 1999;40:223.

4. Rietschel RL, Mathias CGT, Fowler JF Jr, et al. Relationship of occupation to contact dermatitis: evaluation in patients tested from 1998–2000. Am J Contact Dermat 2002;13:170.

5. Nettis E, Colanardi MC, Soccio AL, et al. Occupational irritant and allergic contact dermatitis among healthcare workers. Contact Dermatitis 2002;46:101.

6. Gielen K, Goosens A. Occupational allergic contact dermatitis from drugs in healthcare workers. Contact Dermatitis 2001;45:273.

7. Straube MD, Freitag M, Altmeyer P, et al. Occupational airborne contact dermatitis from cefazolin. Contact Dermatitis 2000;42:44.

8. Holness DL, Nethercott JR. Comparison of occupational and nonoccupational contact dermatitis. Am J Contact Dermat 1994;5:207.

9. Meding B, Swanbeck G. Occupational hand eczema in an industrial city. Contact Dermatitis 1990;22:13.

10. Gruvberger B, Isaksson M, Frick M, et al. Occupational dermatoses in a metalworking plant. Contact Dermatitis 2003;48:80.

11. Holness DL, Nethercott JR. Is a worker's understanding of their diagnosis an important determinant of outcome in occupational contact dermatitis? Contact Dermatitis 1991;25:296.

12. Wall LM, Gebauer KA. A follow-up study of occupational skin disease in Western Australia. Contact Dermatitis 1991;24:241.

13. Sajjachareonpong P, Cahill J, Keegel T, et al. Persistent post-occupational dermatitis. Contact Dermatitis 2004;51:278.

14. Kraus SM, Muselinovic NZ. Pre-employment screening for contact dermatitis among the pupils of a metal industry school. Contact Dermatitis 1991;24:342.

15. Fisher AA. Contact Dermatitis, 3rd ed. Philadelphia: Lea & Febiger, 1986.

16. Held E, Wolff C, Gyntelberg F, et al. Prevention of work-related skin problems in student auxiliary nurses, an intervention study. Contact Dermatitis 2001;44:297.

17. Kawai K, Nakagawa M, Kawai K, et al. Hyposensitization to urushiol among Japanese lacquer craftsmen: results of patch tests on students learning the art of lacquerware [Comments]. Contact Dermatitis 1991;25:290.

18. Reginella RF, Fairfield JC, Marks JG Jr. Hyposensitization to poison ivy after working in a cashew nut shell oil processing factory [Comments]. Contact Dermatitis 1989;20:274.

19. Rietschel RL, Klemm J, Thompson M. The influence of accommodation (hardening) on the response to irritants, allergens, and mediators of inflammation in humans. Clin Res 1982;30:605A.

20. Fisher AA. Occupational palmar psoriasis due to safety prescription container caps. Contact Dermatitis 1979;5:56.

21. White IR, Rycroft RJG. Low humidity occupational dermatosis—an epidemic. Contact Dermatitis 1982;8:287.

22. Meneghini CL, Angelini G. Occupational dermatitis artefacta. Dermatosen 1979;27:163.

23. Angelini G, Meneghini CL, Vena GA. Secretan's syndrome: an artefact edema of the hand. Contact Dermatitis 1982;8:345.

24. Robblee R. The dark side of worker's compensation: burdens and benefits in occupational disease coverage. Ind Rel Law Rev 1978;2:596.

25. Whitmore CW. Cutaneous impairment, disability and rehabilitation. Cutis 1970;6:989.

26. Goldsmith J. The new ethic: the doctor's responsibility for health on the job. Environ Res 1976;11:170.

27. Whitmore CW. Workmen's compensation. Cutis 1974;13:673.

28. Robinson Jr HM. Measurement of impairment and disability in dermatology. Arch Dermatol 1973;108:207.

29. Able EA. Mycosis fungoides and occupational exposure: is there an association? Dermatol Clin 1990;8:169.

30. Buckley WR. Lichenoid eruptions following contact dermatitis. Arch Dermatol 1958;78:454.

31. Canizares O. Lichen planus–like eruption caused by color developer. Arch Dermatol 1959;80:81.

32. Fry L. Skin disease from color developers. Br J Dermatol 1965;77:456.

33. deGraciansky P, Boulle P, Quercy P, Cardol J-L. Eruptions lichenoids et lichens plans vrais chez les ouvriers du developpement des films en couleurs. Bull Soc Fr Dermatol Syphiligr 1958;65:498.

34. Knudsen E. Lichen planus-like eruption caused by color developer. Arch Dermatol 1964;89:357.

35. Roed-Petersen J, Menné T. Allergic contact dermatitis and lichen planus from black and white photographic developing. Cutis 1976;18:699.

36. Marconi PMB, Campagna G, Fabri G, Schiavino D. Allergic contact dermatitis from colour developers used in automated photographic processing. Contact Dermatitis 1999;40:109.

37. Engasser PG. Leukoderma from hydroquinone? J Am Acad Dermatol 1982;7:134.

38. Frenk E, Loi-Zedda P. Occupation depigmentation due to a hydroquinone-containing photographic developer. Contact Dermatitis 1980;6:238.

39. Kersey P, Stevenson CJ. Vitiligo and occupational exposure to hydroquinone from servicing self-photographing machines. Contact Dermatitis 1981;7:285.

40. Goh CL. Allergic contact dermatitis and onycholysis from hydroxylamine sulphate in colour developer. Contact Dermatitis 1990;22:109.

41. Soni BP, Sherertz EF. Contact dermatitis in the textile industry: a review of 72 patients. Am J Contact Dermat 1996;7:226.

42. Kiec-Swierczynski M. Occupational contact dermatitis in the workers employed in production of Texas textiles. Dermatosen 1982;30:41.

43. Romaguera C, Grimalt F, Lecha M. Occupational purpuric textile dermatitis from formaldehyde resin. Contact Dermatitis 1981;7:152.

44. Dooms-Goossens A, Boyden B, Ceuterick A, DeGreef H. Dimethylthiourea, an unexpected hazard for textile workers. Contact Dermatitis 1979;5:367.

45. Wahlberg JE, Hogberg M, Skare L. Chloracetamide allergy in house painters. Contact Dermatitis 1978;4:116.

46. Hogberg M, Wahlberg JE. Health screening for occupational dermatoses in house-painters. Contact Dermatitis 1980;6:100.

47. Pedersen NB, Fregert S. Occupational allergic contact dermatitis from chloracetamide in glue. Contact Dermatitis 1976;2:122.

48. Liden C. Facial dermatitis caused by chlorothalonil in a paint [Comments]. Contact Dermatitis 1990;22:206.

49. Calnan CD. Acrylates in industry. Contact Dermatitis 1980;6:53.

50. Ezzelarab M, Hansson C, Wallengren J. Occupational allergy caused by 1,2-benzisothiazolin-3-one in water-based paints and glues. Am J Contact Dermat 1994;5:165.

51. Gruvberger B, Bjorkner B, Bruze M. Contact allergy to dichlofluanide in humans and guinea pigs. Am J Contact Dermat 1995;6:221.

52. Frick M, Isaksson M, Bjorkner B, et al. Occupational allergic contact dermatitis in a company manufacturing boards coated with isocyanate lacquer. Contact Dermatitis 2003;48:255.

53. Tobler M, Freiburghaus AU. A glove with exceptional protective features minimizes the risks of working with hazardous chemicals. Contact Dermatitis 1992;26:299.

54. Pigatto PD, Bigardi A, Legori G, et al. Are barrier creams of any use in contact dermatitis? Contact Dermatitis 1992;26:197.

55. Reynolds NJ, Peachey RD. Allergic contact dermatitis from a sulfosuccinate derivative in a hand cleanser. Contact Dermatitis 1990;22:59.

56. Malten KE, van der Meer-Roosen CH, Seutter E. Nyloprint-sensitive patients react to NN9methylene bis acrylamide. Contact Dermatitis 1978;4:214.

57. Downham II TF, Birmingham DJ. Contact dermatitis to photographic print coating liquid. Cutis 1980;25:421.

58. Bastelain P-Y, Pirious A, Raulot-Lapointe H, et al. Sensitization to abietoformophenolic resin in printing ink. Contact Dermatitis 1980;4:145.

59. Windstrom L. Contact allergy to acrylate monomer in a printing plate. Contact Dermatitis 1982;8:68.

60. Malten KE. Cobalt and chromium in offset printing. Contact Dermatitis 1975;1:120.

61. Nethercott JR. Skin problems associated with multifunctional acrylic monomers in ultraviolet curing inks. Br J Dermatol 1978;98:541.

62. Castelain P-Y, Piriou A. New case of sensitization to Nyloprint. Contact Dermatitis 1978;4:310.

63. Pedersen NB, Chevallier M-A, Senning A. Secondary acrylamides in Nyloprint printing plate as a source of contact dermatitis. Contact Dermatitis 1982;8:256.

64. Pedersen NB. Allergy from NAPP. Contact Dermatitis 1980;6:35.

65. Bjorkner B, Dahlquist I, Fregert S. Allergic contact dermatitis from acrylates in ultraviolet curing inks. Contact Dermatitis 1980;6:405.

66. Milby TH, Epstein WL. Allergic contact sensitivity to malathion. Arch Environ Health 1967;15:89.

67. Hearn CED. A review of agricultural pesticide incidents in man in England and Wales. Br J Industr Med 1973;30:253.

68. Hjorth N, Wilkinson DS. Contact dermatitis. II. Sensitization to pesticides. Br J Dermatol 1968;80:272.

69. Kaloyanova E, Zielhuis RL. Documentation of international meetings: occupational health criteria for the evaluation of pesticides. Int Arch Arbeitsmedizin 1974;33:335.

70. Kleinman GD, West I, Augustine MS. Occupational disease in California attributed to pesticides and agricultural chemicals. Arch Environ Health 1960;1:118.

71. Rosival L, Jager KW. Documents of international meetings and activities: evaluation of various existing classifications of toxicity and hazard, as far as relevant for occupational exposure to pesticides. Report of an international workshop. Int Arch Occup Environ Health 1978;41:287.

72. Matsushita T, Nomura S, Wakatsuki T. Epidemiology of contact dermatitis from pesticides in Japan. Contact Dermatitis 1980;6:255.

73. Burry JN. Contact dermatitis from agricultural fungicide in South Australia. Contact Dermatitis 1976;2:289.

74. Fisher AA. Occupational, Industrial and Plant Symposium. Part 3: dermatitis in specific occupations. Cutis 1979;24:364.

75. Van Ketel WG. Allergic dermatitis to a new pesticide. Contact Dermatitis 1975;1:297.

76. Van Ketel WG. Sensitivity to pesticide benomyl. Contact Dermatitis 1976;2:290.

77. Schubert H. Contact dermatitis to sodium n-methyl-dithiocarbamate. Contact Dermatitis 1978;4:370.

78. Kleibl K, Rackova M. Cutaneous allergic reactions to dithiocarbamates. Contact Dermatitis 1980;6:348.

79. Matsushita T, Arimatsu Y, Nomura S. Experimental study on contact dermatitis caused by dithiocarbamates maneb, zineb and their related compounds. Int Arch Occup Environ Health 1976;37:169.

80. Cole DC, Carpio F, Math JJM, Leon N. Dermatitis in Ecuadorean farm workers. Contact Dermatitis 1997;37:1.

81. Fregert S. Allergic contact dermatitis from pesticides captan and phaltan. Contact Dermatitis Newsletter 1967;2:11.

82. Cottel WI. Difolatan. Contact Dermatitis Newsletter 1972;11:252.

83. Camarasa G. Difolatan dermatitis. Contact Dermatitis 1976;2:127.

84. Morris GE. Dermatoses from phenylmercuric salts. Arch Environ Health 1960;1:53.

85. Calnan CD. Dithianone sensitivity. Contact Dermatitis Newsletter 1969;3:119.

86. Bousema MT, Wiemer GR, Van Joost T. A classic case of sensitization to DD-95. Contact Dermatitis 1991;24:132.

87. Grace CT, Ng SK, Cheong LL. Recurrent irritant contact dermatitis due to tributyl tin oxide on work clothes. Contact Dermatitis 1991;25:250.

88. Chowdhury MMU, Chakrabarti A, Prais L, et al. Occupational allergic contact dermatitis caused by 5,7-dichloro-4-fluorophenoxy)quinoline (quinoxyfen). Contact Dermatitis 2001;45:119.

89. Rycroft RJG. Contact dermatitis from organophosphorus pesticides. Br J Dermatol 1977;97:693.

90. Edmundson WF, Davies JE. Occupational dermatitis from naled. Arch Environ Health 1967;15:89.

91. Fregert S. Allergic contact dermatitis from the pestiade Rodannitrobenzene. Contact Dermatitis Newsletter 1967;1:4.

92. Peachey RDG. Skin hazards in farming. Br J Dermatol 1981;105:45.

93. Sharvill DE. Reaction to paraquat. Contact Dermatitis Newsletter 1971;9:210.

94. Samman PD, Johnston ENM. Nail damage associated with handling paraquat and diquat. Br Med J 1969;1:818.

95. Spencer MC. Herbicide dermatitis. JAMA 1966;198:1307.

96. Watanabe S. Contact dermatitis due to the herbicides PCP and MCPB. Jpn J Clin Dermatol 1070;24:945.

97. Rossi G, Steffens W. Allergic contact dermatitis from Autan ® spray: methyl glucose dioleate as sensitizing ingredient. Contact Dermatitis 2004;50:324.

98. Corazza M, Borghi A, Zampino MR, et al. Allergic contact dermatitis due to an insect repellent: double sensitization to picaridin and methyl glucose dioleate. Acta Derm Venereol 2005;85:264.

99. Cronce PC, Alden HS. Flea collar dermatitis. JAMA 1968;206:1563.

100. Lamberg S, Mulrennan JA. Bullous eruption to diethyl toluamide (DEET) resembling a blistering insect eruption. Arch Dermatol 1969;100:582.

101. Fisher AA. Contact urticaria due to medicaments, chemicals and foods. Cutis 1982;30:168.

102. Laubstein H. Kontaktekzem durch ein Rodentizid. Berfusdermatosen 1962;10:154.

103. Nishioka K, Kozuka T, Tashiro M. Agricultural miticide (BPPS) dermatitis. Skin Res 1970;12:15.

104. Wahlberg JE. Yellow staining of hair and nails and contact sensitivity to dinobuton. Contact Dermatitis Newsletter 1974;16:481.

105. Brasch J, Hessler H-J, Cristopher E. Occupational (photo) allergic contact dermatitis from azaperone in a piglet dealer. Contact Dermatitis 1991;25:258.

106. Kumar A, Freeman S. Photoallergic contact dermatitis in a pig farmer caused by olaquindox. Contact Dermatitis 1996;35:249.

107. Schuader S, Schroeder W, Geier J. Olaquindox-induced airborne photoallergic contact dermatitis followed by transient or persistent light reactions in 15 pig breeders. Contact Dermatitis 1996;35:344.

108. Susitaival P, Husman L, Hollmen A, et al. Hand eczema in Finnish farmers: a questionnaire-based clinical study. Contact Dermatitis 1995;32:150.

109. Kanerva L, Toikkanen J, Jolanki R, Estlander T. Statistical data on occupational contact urticaria. Contact Dermatitis 1996;35:229.

110. Nurse DS. Dermatitis danger to dairy farmers. Med J Aust 1978;1:223.

111. Black H. Analysis of routine battery results in Auckland skin clinic. Contact Dermatitis Newsletter 1972;12:323.

112. Lintum JC, Nater JP. Contact dermatitis caused by rubber chemicals in dairy workers. Berufdermatosen 1973;21:16.

113. Quirce S, Olaquibel JM, Muro MD, Tabar AI. Occupational dermatitis in a ewe milker. Contact Dermatitis 1992;27:56.

114. Huriez CL, Martin P, Lefebvre M. Sensitivity to dichromate in a milk analysis laboratory. Contact Dermatitis 1975;1:247.

115. Mitchell JC, Fritig B, Singh B, Towers GH. Allergic contact dermatitis from Frullania and Compositae. J Invest Dermatol 1970;54:233.

116. Mitchell JC, Dupuis G. Allergic contact dermatitis from sesquiterpenoids of the Compositae family of plants. Br J Dermatol 1971;84:139.

117. Storrs EJ, Mitchell JC, Rasmussen JE. Contact hypersensitivity to liverwort and the Compositae family of plants. Cutis 1976;18:_681.

118. Mitchell J, Rook AI. Botanical dermatology—plants injurious to the skin. Vancouver: Greenglass, 1979.

119. Thune P. Allergy to lichens with photosensitivity. Contact Dermatitis 1977;3:213.

120. Vega J, Vega JM, Moneo I, et al. Occupational immunologic contact urticaria from pine processionary caterpillar (Thaumetopoea pityocampa): experience in 30 cases. Contact Dermatitis 2004;50:60.

121. Paulsen E. Occupational dermatitis in Danish gardeners and greenhouse workers. Part 2: etiological factors. Contact Dermatitis 1998;38:14.

122. Bruze M, Bjorkner B, Hellstrom AC. Occupational dermatoses in nursery workers. Am J Contact Dermat 1996;7:100–3.

123. Paulsen E, Skov PS, Andersen KE. Immediate skin and mucosal symptoms from pot plants and vegetables in gardeners and greenhouse workers. Contact Dermatitis 1998;39:166.

124. Pigatto PD, Bigardi A, Riboldi A, et al. Occupational atopic contact dermatitis from Rhizoglyphus. Contact Dermatitis 1991;25:193.

125. Ashworth J, Curry FM, White IR, et al. Occupational allergic contact dermatitis in east coast of England fishermen: newly described hypersensitivities to marine organisms. Contact Dermatitis 1990;22:185.

126. Piraccini BM, Bardazzi F, Vincenzi C, Tardio MP. Occupational contact dermatitis dueto coffee. Contact Dermatitis 1990;23:114.

127. Pazzaglia M, Tullo S, Tosti A. Occupational protein contact dermatitis due to Calliphora vomitoria larvae (maggots) bred as fishing bait. Contact Dermatitis 2003;48:176.

128. Fregert S. Registration of chemicals in industries slimicides in the paper-pulp industry. Contact Dermatitis 1976;2:358.

129. Fisher AA. Formaldehyde: some recent experiences. Cutis 1976;17:665.

130. Fregert S. Allergic contact dermatitis from formaldehyde in paper. Contact Dermatitis Newsletter 1974;15:459.

131. Black H. Contact dermatitis from formaldehyde in newsprint. Contact Dermatitis Newsletter 1971;10:242.

132. Estlander T, Jolanki R, Kanerva L. Occupational allergic contact dermatitis from 2,3-epoxypropyl trimethyl ammonium chloride (EPTMAC) and Kathon LX in a starch modification factory. Contact Dermatitis 1997;36:191.

133. Liden C, Karlberg A-T. Colophony in paper as a cause of hand eczema. Contact Dermatitis 1992;26:272.

134. Calnan CD. Carbon and carbonless copy paper. Acta Derm Venereol (Stockh) 1979;59:27.

135. Hjorth N. Contact dermatitis from cellulose acetate film. Berufsdermatosen 1964;12:86.

136. Calnan CD, Connor BL. Carbon paper dermatitis due to nigrosine. Berufsdermatosen 1975;20:248.

137. Carver JW. Typewriter ribbon and carbon inks. Am Ink Maker 1942;20:22.

138. Calnan CD. Unsolved problems in occupational dermatology. Br J Dermatol 1981;105:3.

139. Menné T, Asnae G, Hjorth N. Skin and mucous membrane problems from "no carbon required" paper. Contact Dermatitis 1981;7:72.

140. Rycroft RJG, Calnan CD. Occupational dermatology. Dermatol Digest 1979;18:21.

141. Murray R. Health aspects of carbonless copy paper. Contact Dermatitis 1991;24:321.

142. Marks Jr JG. Allergic contact dermatitis from carbonless copy paper. JAMA 1981;245:2331.

143. Harman RRM, Sarkany I. Studies in contact dermatitis XI. Copy paper dermatitis. Trans St John Hosp Dermatol Soc 1960;44:37.

144. Jensen M, Roed-Petersen J. Itching erythema amongst post office workers caused by a photocopying machine with wet toner. Contact Dermatitis 1979;5:389.

145. Mijnssen GAW, Verspyck X. Dermatitis from Ozalid and Radex copy paper. Contact Dermatitis Newsletter 1967;2:152.

146. Gianotti F, Meneghini GD. Observations concernant certaines dermatites eczemateuses par contact chez les travailleurs affects à la fabrication des papiers sensible. Dermatologica 1966;132:106.

147. Foussereau J, Benezra CR. Les eczémas allergiques professionnels. Paris: Masson et Cie, 1970.

148. Sengel PD, Khelladi A, Foussereau J. Allergie professionnelle au papier diazo dans l'industrie textile. Derm Veruf Umwelt 1979;27:178.

149. Van der Leun JC, de Kreek EJ, Deenstra-van Leeuwen M, van Weelden H. Photosensitivity owing to thiourea. Arch Dermatol 1977;113:1611.

150. Fisher AA. Allergic eczematous contact dermatitis due to thermofax paper. Arch Dermatol 1958;77:741.

151. Degos R, Lepine J, Akhoundzadeh H. Sensibilisation cutanée due à la manipulation de papier "reprographic." Bull Soc Française Dermatol Syphiligraph 1968;75:595.

152. Sheard CP, Spoor HJ, Abel R. Contact dermatitis from "high speed duplicator" papers. Arch Dermatol 1958;77:435.

153. Hasegawa J, Lerit F, Bluefarb SM. Contact dermatitis due to Thermo-Fax paper. JAMA 1958;166:1173.

154. Kendrick FJ. Dermatitis caused by a copying paper. Arch Dermatol 1958;77:334.

155. Kanerva L, Estlander T, Jolanki R, Henriks-Exkerman ML. Contact dermatitis from telefax paper. Contact Dermatitis 1992;27:12.

156. Zina AM, Fanan E, Bundino S. Allergic contact dermatitis from formaldehyde and quarternium-15 in photocopier toner. Contact Dermatitis 2000;43:241.

157. Wikstrom K. Allergic contact dermatitis caused by paper. Acta Derm Venereol (Stockh) 1969;49:547.

158. Jordan WP, Bourlas M. Contact dermatitis from typewriter correction paper. Cutis 1975;15:594.

159. Guin JD. Contact dermatitis to perfume in paper products. J Am Acad Dermatol 1981;4:733.

160. Keith I, Erich W, Bush IM. Toilet paper dermatitis. JAMA 1969;209:269.

161. Larsen WG. Sanitary napkin dermatitis due to the perfume. Arch Dermatol 1979;115:363.

162. Parks TD. Perfume dermatitis. JAMA 1969;210:559.

163. Tacke J, Schmidt A, Fartasch M, Diepgen TL. Occupational contact dermatitis in bakers, confectioners and cooks: a population-based study. Contact Dermatitis 1995;33:112.

164. Bauer A, Geier J, Elsner P. Type IV allergy in the food processing industry: sensitization profiles in bakers, cooks and butchers. Contact Dermatitis 2002;46:228.

165. Fisher AA. Hand dermatitis—a baker's dozen. Cutis 1982;29:214.

166. Baker EW, Wharton GW. Acarology. New York: Macmillan, 1952.

167. Wütrich B. The cause of bakers' eczema. Hautarzt 1970;21:214.

168. Young E. Dyshidrotic (endogenic eczema). Dermatologica 1964;129:306.

169. Hjorth N. Occupational dermatitis in the catering industry. Br J Dermatol 1981;105:37.

170. Herxheimer H. The skin sensitivity to flour of bakers' apprentices: a final report of a long-term investigation. Acta Allergy 1973;8:42.

171. Jarvinen KAJ, Pirila V, Njorksten F, et al. Unsuitability of bakery work for a person with atopy: a study of 234 bakery workers. Ann Allergy 1979;42:192.

172. Fisher AA. Urticarial and systemic reaction to contact varying from hair bleach to seminal fluid. Cutis 1977;19:715.

173. Odom RB, Maibach H. Contact urticaria: a different contact dermatitis. Cutis 1970;18:672.

174. Cronin E. Contact dermatitis. London: Churchill Livingstone, 1980.

175. Morren M-A, Janssens V, Dooms-Goossen AD, et al. a-Amylase, a flour additive: an important cause of protein contact dermatitis in bakers. J Am Acad Dermatol 1993;29:723.

176. Kanerva L, Vanhanen M, Tupasela O. Occupational allergic contact urticaria from fungal but not bacterial alpha-amylase. Contact Dermatitis 1997;36:306.

177. Kanerva L, Vanhanen M. Occupational protein contact dermatitis from glucoamylase. Contact Dermatitis 1999;41:171.

178. Fisher AA. Cutaneous reactions to sorbic acid and potassium sorbate. Cutis 1980;25:350.

179. Malten KE. Four bakers showing positive patch tests to a number of fragrance materials which can be used in flavors. Acta Derm Venereol (Stockh) 1979;59:117.

180. Kanerva L, Estlander T, Jolanki R. Occupational allergic contact dermatitis from spices. Contact Dermatitis 1996;35:157.

181. Figley KD. Karaya gum hypersensitivity. JAMA 1940;114:109.

182. Camarasa JMB, Alomar A. Contact dermatitis from a karava seal ring. Contact Dermatitis 1980;6:139.

183. Fisher AA, Dooms-Goossens A. Persulphate hair bleach reactions. Arch Dermatol 1976;112:1407.

184. Calnan CD, Shuster S. Reactions to ammonium persulphate. Arch Dermatol 1963;88:812.

185. Lindemavr H, Drobil M. Contact sensitization to benzoyl peroxide. Contact Dermatitis 1981;7:137.

186. Roed-Petersen J, Hjorth N. Contact dermatitis from antioxidants: hidden sensitizers in topical medications and foods. Br J Dermatol 1976;94:233.

187. Kahn G, Phanuphak P, Claman HN. Propyl gallate-contact sensitization and orally induced tolerance. Arch Dermatol 1974;109:506.

188. Brun R. Eczame de contact à un antioxidant de la margerine (gallate) et changement de métier. Dermatologica 1970;140:390.

189. Heime VA, Fox G. Baker's eczema through chromium compound in flour. Derm Beruf Umwelt 1980;28:113.

190. Crotlin E, Kullavanijaya P. Hand dermatitis in hairdressers. Acta Derm Venereol (Stockh) 1979;59:48.

191. Wahlberg JE. Nickel allergy in hairdressers. Contact Dermatitis 1981;7:358.

192. Black MM, Russel BJ. Shampoo dermatitis in apprentice hairdressers. J Soc Occup Med 1973;23:120.

193. Wahlberg JE. Nickel allergy and atopy in hairdressers. Contact Dermatitis 1975;1:161.

194. Wilkinson DS, Hambly EM. Prognosis of hand eczema in hairdressing apprentices. Contact Dermatitis 1978;4:63.

195. Marks R, Cronin E. Hand eczema in hairdressers. Aust J Dermatol 1977;18:123.

196. van der Walle HB, Brunsveld VM. Dermatitis in hairdressers. Part 1: The experience of the past 4 years. Contact Dermatitis 1994;30:_217.

197. Valks R, Conde-Salazar L, Malfeito J, et al. Contact dermatitis in hairdressers, 10 years later: patch-test results in 300 hairdressers (1994 to 2003) and comparison with previous study. Dermatitis 2005;16:28.

198. Majoie IML, von Blomberg BME, Bruynzeel DP. Development of hand eczema in junior hairdressers: an 8-year follow-up study. Contact Dermatitis 1996;34:243.

199. Dahlquist E, Fregert S, Gruvberger B. Release of nickel from plated utensils in permanent wave liquids. Contact Dermatitis 1979;5:52.

200. Warshawshki L, Mitchell JC, Storrs F. Allergic contact dermatitis from glyceryl monothioglycolate in hairdressers. Contact Dermatitis 1981;7:351.

201. Temesvari LE, Varkonyi V. Contact urticaria provoked by egg. Contact Dermatitis 1980;6:143.

202. Rudzki E, Grzywa Z. Contact urticaria from egg. Contact Dermatitis 1977;3:103.

203. Lynde CW, Mitchell JC. Patch test results in hairdressers, 1973–81. Contact Dermatitis 1982;8:302.

204. Majoie IML, Bruynzeel DP. Occupational immediate-type hypersensitivity to henna in a hairdresser. Am J Contact Dermat 1996;7:38.

205. Aguirre A, Zabala C, Sanz de Galdeano N, et al. Positive patch tests to hydrogen peroxide in 2 cases. Contact Dermatitis 1994;30:113.

206. Kanerva L, Alanko K, Jolanki R, et al. Occupational allergic contact dermatitis from potassium persulfate. Contact Dermatitis 1999;40:116.

207. Cronin E. Formaldehyde is a significant allergen in women with hand eczema. Contact Dermatitis 1991;25:276.

208. Krogsrud NE, Larsen AI. Grapeseed oil as a safe and efficient hand cleansing agent. Contact Dermatitis 1992;26:208.

209. Koh D, Foulds IS, Aw TC. Dermatological hazards in the electronics industry. Contact Dermatitis 1990;22:1.

210. Seidenari S, P Danese, A Nardo, et al. Contact sensitization among ceramics workers. Contact Dermatitis 1990;22:45.

211. Lear JT, Heagerty AH, Tan BB, et al. Transient re-emergence of oil of turpentine allergy in the pottery industry. Contact Dermatitis 1996;35:169.

212. Barbaud A, Mougeolle JM, Schmutz JL. Contact hypersensitivity to arsenic in a crystal factory worker. Contact Dermatitis 1995;33:272.

213. Batta K, McVittie S, Foulds IS. Occupational allergic contact dermatitis from N,N-methylene-bis-5-methyl-oxazolidine in a nylon spin finish. Contact Dermatitis 1999;41:165.

214. Kanerva L, Laine R, Jolanki R, et al. Occupational allergic contact dermatitis caused by nitroglycerin. Contact Dermatitis 1991;24:356.

215. Hausen BM. Occupational allergic contact dermatitis from ethyl chloro oximido acetate [published erratum appears in Contact Dermatitis 1993 May;28(5):312]. Contact Dermatitis 1992;27:277.

216. Pazzaglia M, Tullo S, Voudouris S, et al. Contact dermatitis due to cyclohexanone: a further case. Contact Dermatitis 2004;49:313.

217. Conde-Salazar L, et al. Occupational allergic contact dermatitis in construction workers. Contact Dermatitis 1995;33:226.

218. Geier J, Schnuch A. A comparison of contact allergies among construction and nonconstruction workers attending contact dermatitis clinics in Germany. Am J Contact Dermat 1995;6:86.

219. Roto P, Sainio H, Reunala T, Laippala P. Addition of ferrous sulfate to cement and risk of chromium dermatitis among construction workers. Contact Dermatitis 1996;34:43.

220. Goh CL, Gan SL. Change in cement manufacturing process, a cause for decline in chromate allergy? Contact Dermatitis 1996;34:51.

221. Wong SS, et al. Occupational chromate allergy in Singapore: a study of 87 patients and a review from 1983 to 1995. Am J Contact Dermat 1998;9:1.

222. Halbert AR, Gebauer KA, Wall LM. Prognosis of occupational chromate dermatitis. Contact Dermatitis 1992;27:214.

223. Lips R, Rast H, Elsner P. Outcome of job change in patients with occupational chromate dermatitis. Contact Dermatitis 1996;34:268.

224. Ali SA. Occupational dermatitis in the manufacture of color television tubes. Am J Contact Dermat 1997;8:222.

225. Mancuso G, Reggiani M, Berdondini RM. Occupational dermatitis in shoemakers. Contact Dermatitis 1996;34:17.

226. Ormerod AD, Dwyer CM, Goodfield MJ. Novel causes of contact dermatitis from offshore oil-based drilling muds. Contact Dermatitis 1998;39:262.

227. Meding B, Barregard L, Marcus K. Hand eczema in car mechanics. Contact Dermatitis 1994;30:129.

228. Pfaffli P, Jolank R, Estlander T, et al. Identification of sensitizing diethyleneglycol maleate in a two-component polyester cement. Contact Dermatitis 2002;46:170.

229. Maibach HI, Mathias CT. Allergic contact dermatitis from cycloaliphatic epoxide in jet aviation hydraulic fluid. Contact Dermatitis 2001;45:56.

230. Bergqvist U, Wahlberg JE. Skin symptoms and disease during work with visual display terminals. Contact Dermatitis 1994;30:197.

231. Garnier R, Levy-Amon L, Malingrey L. Occupational contact dermatitis from N-(2-(diethylamino)-ethyl)acrylamide. Contact Dermatitis 2003;48:343.

232. Frick M, Bjorkner B, Hamnerius N, et al. Allergic contact dermatitis from dicyclohexylmethane-4,4'-diisocyanate. Contact Dermatitis 2003;48:305.

233. Kanerva L, Grenquits-Norden B, Piirila P. Occupational IgE-mediated contact urticaria from diphenyl-methane-4,4'-diisocyanate (MDI). Contact Dermatitis 1999;41:50.

234. Farm G, Karlberg AT, Liden C. Are opera-house artistes afflicted with contact allergy to colophony and cosmetics? Contact Dermatitis 1995;32:273.

235. van Neer FJMA, van Ginkel CJW. Allergic contact dermatitis from a boxwood recorder. Contact Dermatitis 1997;36:305.

236. Fisher AA. Dermatitis in a musician. Part 1: allergic contact dermatitis. Cutis 1998;62:167.

237. Fisher AA. Dermatitis in a musician. Part 2: injuries to skin, soft tissue, and bone from musical instruments. Cutis 1998;62:214.

238. Fisher AA. Dermatitis in a musician. Part 3: injuries caused by specific musical instruments. Cutis 1998;62:261.

239. Fisher AA. Dermatitis in a musician. Part 4: physiologic, emotional, and infectious problems in musicians. Cutis 1999;63:13.

240. Isaksson M, Frick M, Gruvberger B, et al. Occupational allergic contact dermatitis from the extreme pressure (EP) additive zinc, bis ((O,O'-di-2-ethylheyxl)dithiophosphate) in neat oils. Contact Dermatitis 2002;46:248.

241. Wallenhammar L-M, Ortengren U, Andreasson H, et al. Contact allergy and hand eczema in Swedish dentists. Contact Dermatitis 2000;43:192.

242. Wrangsjo K, Swartling C, Meding B. Occupational dermatitis in dental personnel: contact dermatitis with special reference to (meth)acrylates in 174 patients. Contact Dermatitis 2001;45:158.

Useful Readings

Dermatology

Adams RM. *Occupational skin disease.* Philadelphia: WB Saunders, 1990.

Cronin E. *Contact dermatitis.* Edinburgh: Churchill Livingston, 1980.

Foussereau J, Ezra Benezra J, Maibach H. *Occupational contact dermatitis.* Philadelphia: WB Saunders, 1982.

Maibach HI, Gellin GA, eds. *Occupational and industrial dermatology.* Chicago: Year Book Medical Publishers, 1982.

Schwartz L, Tulipan L, Birmingham DJ. *Occupational diseases of the skin,* 3rd ed. Philadelphia: Lea & Febiger, 1957.

General Occupational

Browning E. *Toxicity of industrial metals.* London: Butterworth, 1961.

Clayton GD, Clayton FE. Patty's industrial hygiene and toxicology, vols 2 and 3. New York: John Wiley & Sons, 1991.

Encyclopedia of occupational health and safety, vols 1 and 2. Geneva: International Labor Office, 1983.

Proctor NH, Hughes JP, Fischman ML. *Chemical hazards of the workplace.* Philadelphia: JB Lippincott Co, 1988.

Ramazzini B. *Diseases of workers* (first published in 1700). New York: Hafner Publishing Co, 1974.

Rom WN. *Environmental and occupational medicine.* Boston: Little, Brown and Company, 1982.

Zenz C, ed. *Occupational medicine.* Chicago: Year Book Medical Publishers, 1975.

Technical

Hawley GG. *The condensed chemical dictionary,* 10th ed. New York: Van Nostrand Reinhold, 1983.

Kirk-Othmer encyclopedia of chemical technology, 3rd ed. New York: Wiley-Interscience, 1983.

CUTTING OILS, SOLVENTS, PETROLATUM, AND COAL-TAR PRODUCTS

EXECUTIVE SUMMARY

Metalworking fluids (MWFs) are common causes of allergic contact dermatitis (ACD). Metalworking shops (usually called machine shops or tool and dye makers in the US) are ubiquitous. Almost every community has them, from small one- or two-person operations to large factories employing hundreds. The MWFs used nowadays are mostly water-based, requiring biocides, emulsifiers, and other additives. The biocides, many of which are also used in cosmetics, are common allergens. Other MWF-specific biocides are used, many of which are formaldehyde releasers. Fragrances, anti-oxidants, and metals are usually present in the fluids. Virtually all the additives can cause ACD, at least occasionally. Fortunately for the patch tester, MWFs can usually be tested "as is." Then, if positive reactions are found, ideally the exact allergens can be identified with "aimed" testing. As usual, however, the clinician and patient must remember that Material Safety Data Sheets (MSDSs) rarely contain information on all the likely allergens in the MWF; further detective work is often necessary. The other materials covered in this chapter rarely cause ACD, but may cause irritant contact dermatitis (ICD) and other skin reactions such as acne and folliculitis. Oily materials cause follicular occlusion, with resultant pathology in the form of comedones, papules, pustules, etc. Chloracne is a special form of acne, due not to occlusion but rather to toxic effects of some halogenated hydrocarbons on the skin. It is clinically and histologically distinct from regular acne or occlusion folliculitis. Solvents, by virtue of their ability to dissolve lipids, dry the skin. Occasionally they can cause ACD, but much more frequently ICD results from the lipid-removal effect of these chemicals.

Metalworking Fluids

The various types of industrial oils and metalworking fluids (MWFs) are shown in Table 25.1. These metalworking fluids are used throughout industry to cool and lubricate metalworking operations, for example, machining and grinding.

When hard materials such as metal are cut, so much heat is generated that a metal-cutting tool can become welded to the metal being cut (workpiece). Metalworking fluids are therefore directed at the interface between cutting tool and workpiece. By reducing friction and conducting away heat, the fluid cools the cutting process.[1] Table 25.2 lists the three main types of metalworking fluids.[2]

INSOLUBLE FLUIDS

These "straight" oils are made of mineral, animal, vegetable, or synthetic oils.[1] Skin exposure to neat (insoluble) oils can cause oil acne or folliculitis and, when prolonged, hyperpigmentation, keratoses, and cancer of the scrotum and other exposed skin. Eczematous dermatitis, rather than folliculitis, occurs occasionally and is usually irritant in etiology. Allergens added to neat oils may cause allergic contact dermatitis (ACD).

SOLUBLE FLUIDS

Oil-in-water emulsions (30–85% oil) used for metalworking are commonly called "soluble oils." They

Table 25-1 Industrial Oils and Fluids
Cooling emulsions
Cutting compounds
Drilling fluids
Grinding fluids
Lubricating fluids
Metalworking fluids

Table 25-2 Make-up of Various Types of Metalworking Fluids
Insoluble fluids (neat oils)
Additives
Mineral, animal, or vegetable oils
Sulfur, chloride, and phosphorus
Soluble oils (oil in water)
Amine coupler
Emulsifiers (sulfate, rosin)
Germicides
Oils
Surfactants (carboxylic soaps)
Water
Synthetic fluids (aqueous solutions)
Amines
Anti-foaming agents (silicone)
Bactericides
Deodorizers
Dyes
Fatty acids
Soaps
Water softeners

contain not only emulsifiers, such as petroleum sulfonates and carboxylic acid soaps, but also corrosion inhibitors, phase stabilizers, extreme pressure additives, antifoams, dyes, fragrances, and microbiocides.[1,2]

Eczematous eruptions are common with exposure to soluble oils. Clinically, the early stages of soluble-oil dermatitis may be characterized by the appearance of a fine follicular erythema. This appears to be a follicular eczema rather than a pustular folliculitis as seen with neat oils. Later stages of soluble-oil dermatitis are characteristically patchy, papular, and eczematous, and sometimes resemble discoid eczema over the backs of the hands or forearms. Other typical findings of ACD such as intense pruritus and frequent recurrence are seen. Because the oils are normally splashed and aerosolized, dermatitis commonly occurs on any exposed surfaces and any areas where shoes or clothing become saturated with the fluid.

SYNTHETIC AND SEMI-SYNTHETIC (AQUEOUS) FLUIDS

Semi-synthetics may contain up to 30% oils. Otherwise they are made of water with detergent-like additives and emulsifiers to provide lubrication.[1] These fluids also commonly produce eczematous eruptions, because they tend to have the most variety of additives (Figure 15).

Allergic versus Irritant Reactions to Cutting Fluids

ACD to such oils is not uncommon, although ICD is probably more common. ACD is usually caused by biocides. corrosion inhibitors, fragrances, breakdown products, or metals (cobalt, nickel, chrome especially) from machined metals. Gellin[3] stated that primary ICD and not ACD is the major skin disorder among machinists and other workers handling cutting fluids and that prolonged immersion in watery or oil solutions produces the irritant dermatitis. Samitz and Katz[4] and Samitz[5] also found that instances of allergic contact sensitivity in association with cutting oil preparations are less common.

Hodgson,[6] however, reported that 50% of cutting oil eczemas were allergic in nature. He found that the dilution of sensitizing chemicals in the final cutting oil lubricant often obscured identification of the specific allergen. In his material, the following contact allergens produced ACD in those working with cutting oils: antimicrobials, chlorocresol, dichlorophene, formaldehyde, trisnitrol, triazine, antioxidants, azo dyes used as coloring agents, hydrazine, and deodorizers such as pine oil and balsam of Peru.

Shah and colleagues[7] sent a questionnaire to 64 patients who had contact dermatitis from metalworking fluids. Fifty-one responded to the survey. There was no difference in the outcome between those who gave up their occupation and those who continued to work with the fluids, indicating a poor prognosis. Biocides were the most common allergen found in the group.

A cutting oil used in automobile seat manufacturing produced contact dermatitis in 12 workers who were machine operators.[8] The chlorinated paraffin fraction of the oil was responsible. Half of the workers were also sensitive to epoxy resin. Because pure chlorinated paraffin was negative, an additive related to epoxy was suspected to be the actual allergen. Epoxy-related additives that have been found in cutting oils include glycidyl ester of hexahydrophthalic acid and Epoxide 7.

Nonallergic skin disorders associated with metalworking fluid are noted in Table 25.3.

Table 25-3 Nonallergic Dermatoses from Cutting Oils
Folliculitis
Hyperpigmentation
Irritant contact dermatitis
Keratosis
Leukoderma
Mechanical injury from metal fragments
Oil acne
Phototoxic dermatitis
Postinflammatory pigmentary changes
Scrotal cancer

Table 25-4 Additional Recommended Metalworking Fluid Allergens
Biocides:
Bioban CS 1135- 1%
Bioban CS 1246- 1%
Bioban P 1487- 0.5%
Grotan BK- 1% aq.
Grotan OX- 1%
Benzisothiazolinone (BIT)- 0.1%
Methylene-bis morpholine- 1%
PCMC
PCMX
Emulsifiers, Surfatants, and Others
Cocamide DEA
Diethanolamine- 2%
Diglycolamine- 1%
Monoethanolamine- 2%
Myristyl alcohol-10%
Oleyl alcohol- 10%
Polyethylene glycol- 100%
Triethanolamine

Patch Testing with Metalworking Fluids

GENERAL PRINCIPLES

Metalworking fluids may usually be tested as is, undiluted, although rarely they may show irritant reactions to such testing. Dilution, to avoid irritancy, may give false-negative reactions to allergens in the fluid. Fluids are recirculated in a continuous loop, often among several machines. To reduce rancidity and breakdown various additives are added to the circulation system. Testing with original versus "used" industrial oils diluted 1 to 25 in aqueous solution, a positive patch test reaction to the used "dirty" oil and not to the original oil would imply that additives such as corrosion inhibitors, bacteriostatic agents, or break-down products including metal salts are the sensitizers. In addition, unexpected findings in recycled MWFs include "tramp" oils, lubricants and hydraulic fluids from the machines, and cleaning products used at the work site. Because a positive patch test reaction to either the original or the used oils may be rarely be irritant in nature, the tests should be repeated on three normal controls. Table 25.4 lists potential oil and cooling fluid additive allergens, beyond those on standard series.

PATCH TESTING WITH METALWORKING FLUIDS THEMSELVES

Geier and colleagues tested 141 metal workers with their MWFs as is and in dilutions. They conclude that testing with the actual undiluted fluids is preferred. Irritation was rare and many reactions were missed if the fluids were diluted. They found no reactions from "neat" oils, but from the other MWFs they saw ACD to about 25% of the samples tested, with irritant reactions in only 5%.[9]

METALWORKING FLUID ALLERGENS ON STANDARD SERIES

Several allergens from standard patch test series are found in MWFs to cause ACD. Formaldehyde, all the FRPS, and all other preservatives can potentially be found in MWFs. German reports have emphasized the prevalence of allergy to methyldibromoglutaronitrile (MDGN) in MWFs, especially.[10,11] Fragrance mix and *Myroxylon pereirae* are common positives, as is mercaptobenzothiazole and rosin. Metals, of course, especially chromate, cobalt, and nickel may be positive. Somewhat less common are propylene glycol, lanolin, and ethylenediamine.

Some specific allergens are considered as follows.

Ethylenediamine Hydrochloride versus Amines in Cutting Oils

Angelini and Meneghini[12] reported that two engineers with dermatitis due to synthetic coolants had positive reactions to ethylenediamine and thought that this implied a cross-sensitization reaction with amines in the fluids.

Camarasa and Alomar[13] reported three cases of hand dermatitis eczema in metallurgical workers. All three workers, who improved greatly when away from work, had positive patch test results with the cutting fluids used in their work, as well as with ethylenediamine from the "standard" series.

Allergic reactions to ethylenediamine may signify cross-reactions with the other polyamines found in cutting oils—ethylenediamine (EDA), diethylenetriamine (DETA), triethylenetetramine (TETA), dipropylenetriamine (DPTA), tetraethylenepentamine (TEPA), diethylaminopropylamine (DEAPA), and trimethylhexamethylenediamine (TMDA). In a personal communication to Dr. Fisher, Fregert stated that he had seen crossreactions between ethylenediamine, diethylenetriamine, and triethylenetetramine but was not certain if these are true cross-sensitizations, because the compounds may contain traces of the other two.

Triethanolamine

Certain synthetic cutting oils contain varying amounts of mineral oil with the fatty amine triethanolamine used as an emulsifying agent. Triethanolamine is also used widely in cosmetics. Suurmond[14] showed crossreactions between triethanolamine and other tertiary amines, such as promethazine.

Monoethanolamine and Diethanolamine

Mono- or diethanolamine is present in some soluble oils and is a rare cause of ACD. A 2% in petrolatum concentration is adequate for patch testing, as it was negative in 50 controls and positive in a patient reported by Bhushan and colleagues.[15]

Alkanolamineborates

Alkanolamineborates are used as metalworking fluids and can cause both irritant and allergic contact dermatitis.[16] They are water-based fluids, and, because of their alkalinity, it is necessary to dilute them with an acidic buffer. The use concentration of these chemicals is in the range of 10% to 30%, and their primary function is corrosion inhibition.

Oleyl Alcohol

ACD to oleyl alcohol in a coolant has been reported.[17] Oleyl alcohol is added to cutting fluids to improve the solubility of other components of the final formula. This rare allergen can also be seen as a contaminant in cetyl and stearyl alcohol.

Formaldehyde

Angelini and Meneghini[12] reported two cases of dermatitis in patients who were allergic to formaldehyde due to coolants. Formaldehyde had been added to used synthetic fluid after recovery as an antibacterial agent. In addition, the same formaldehyde-releasing preservatives that are used in cosmetics may be used in metalworking fluids. (See Chapter 16).

Grotan OX

This biocide, N,N methylene-bis-5-methyl-oxazolidine, was found to cause ACD in 15 cases (4.7%) of 318 tested workers. Formaldehyde was also positive in 11 of these. Grotan OX is a formaldehyde releaser.[18]

Grotan BK

Grotan BK is a "triazine" industrial bacteriocide, added to water miscible, metalworking fluids of the oil-in-water emulsion ("soluble oil") and synthetic types. Bacterial growth in these fluids, which occurs particularly at oil-water interfaces, can cause problems of foul odor, metal corrosion, and emulsion breakdown. The active ingredient of Grotan BK is a hexahydro-1,3,5-tris(2-hydroxyethyl)-s-triazine. The recommended concentration of Grotan BK in a metalworking fluid is 0.15%. The triazine molecule liberates formaldehyde under certain conditions but, according to the manufacturers, this does not explain the antibacterial effect of Grotan BK. There is some controversy as to whether Grotan BK is a strong or weak sensitizer.[19,20]

Phenolic Compounds

These antimicrobial agents, which include cresols, phenols, hexachlorophenes and dichlorophenes, bisphenols, and chlorinated phenols, are added to cutting oils to prevent bacterial growths that may break the emulsions in producing an offensive odor. It should be noted that the bisphenols are photosensitizers, and chlorinated phenols may produce leukoderma.

Mercaptobenzothiazole (MBT)

Fregert and Skog[21] reported that ACD in seven patients had an obvious connection with exposure to cutting oil containing MBT. The patients showed positive test reactions to MBT, which is used to prevent corrosion, especially of copper and tin, by lowering the pH of cutting oil. Mercaptobenzothiazole is present in the biocide Vancide TH as an antibacterial and antifungal agent. Six of Fregert's seven patients sensitive to MBT showed negative reactions to the cutting oil itself. Without testing the ingredients separately, their dermatitis would have been considered due to the primary irritant effect.

Sodium Pyrithione (Sodium Omadine)

Sodium pyrithione may be used in semisynthetic and synthetic oils, and contact dermatitis from exposure to this product has been reported.[22] This material may also be encountered in water-based printers' ink and common antidandruff shampoos. A 0.3% aqueous solution has been recommended for patch testing.

Hydrazine

In the metal industry, there is wide exposure to hydrazine as a cleaning agent to prevent oxidation and corrosion of metallic surfaces. Hovding[23] reported that hydrazine shows cross-sensitization with Apresoline, isonicotinic acid hydrazide, phenylhydrazine, and Nardel.

Lanolin and Amerchol L 101

Lanolin and its derivatives may be present in some metalworking fluids as an antirust compound.

Deodorant Agents

Pine oil, perfumes, and *Myroxylon pereirae* may be added to industrial oils to reduce offensive odors. Hodgson[6] studied 50 patients with hand dermatitis from exposure to metalworking fluids. The most common positive reactions to pine oil, perfumes, and balsam of Peru were caused by pine oil, which produced four instances of allergic hand dermatitis.

Metals

Samitz and Katz[4] and Samitz[5] found that under ordinary working conditions in which grinding fluids were used, spot testing did not reveal the presence of nickel or chromates. Laboratory studies, however, showed that nickel can be leached from the machined metals. Either tiny particulates of metal may be carried or metal salts may be solubilized in coolants. Cobalt, chromate, and nickel have all caused ACD from exposure to coolants. Of course, the worker is usually handling and touching the hard metal objects so ACD may come from this route of contact as well.

ROLE OF BACTERIA IN CUTTING FLUIDS

Bactericides are added to protect against rancidity and preserve the cutting fluid emulsions. They may have a role in making a soluble oil more irritant, although this has not been proved. Whether they are able to cause skin infections in workers is uncertain as well.

Geretzki[24] reported that a list has been compiled showing pathogenic agents that can be isolated from oils. Under certain conditions, cutting oil may prove to be a pool of pathogenic agents.

It should be noted that the antimicrobial agents and biocides listed in Table 25.5 are used to prevent rancidity of the cutting fluids rather than to protect the worker.

Control of ACD to Metalworking Fluids

The nature of the job is usually such that the use of protective gear is usually not feasible. Gloves may easily be caught in rotating and reverberating parts, leading to serious hand injuries. Since the fluids are usually spraying around the machine and work area, anything short of a full chemical protective suit is unlikely to prevent skin contact with airborne allergens. Often, the worker will need to change jobs and even avoid the entire work area to avoid continuous allergen exposure.

Occupational Acne

Occupational acne consists of two main varieties: one caused by oils such as petroleum and its derivatives and coal-tar products and the other, chloracne, due to halo-

Table 25-5 Antibacterial Agents (Biocides) Registered for Use in Metalworking Fluids[a]

Bioban P-1487	0.1% pet
Busan 85	1% pet
Captax, dermacid, mertax, and thiotax	1% pet
Chloroxylenol	1% pet
Dowicid 1	1% pet
Dowicid A	1% pet
Dowicid 1	1% pet
Dowicil 75	2% pet
Formalin	2% aq
G-4	2% pet
G-11	0.5% pet
Givgard DXN	1% pet
Grotan BK	1% pet
Grotan HD2	1% pet
Kathon 886-MW	0.025% pet
Merthiolate	0.1% pet
Onyxide 200	1% pet
Ottafact	0.01% pet
p-tertiary butyl phenol	2% pet
Preventol D-2 and D-3	2% pet
Proxel CRL	0.1% pet
Resorcinol phthalen	1% alcohol
Rosin	20% pet
Sodium-Omadine	0.1% pet
Triadine-10	1% pet
Tris-Nitro	1% pet
Vancide 51	1% pet
Vancide TH	1% pet
XD-8254 DBNPA	1% pet
Zinc Omadine	0.1% pet

[a]Aq, aqueous; pet, in petrolatum.

genated aromatic hydrocarbons[25] (Tables 25.6 and 25.7). Table 25.8 lists certain environmental factors that may influence the severity of occupational acne.[28,29] Table 25.9 lists the differential diagnosis of chloracne.

OIL ACNE

Oil acne or oil folliculitis consists of numerous comedones, follicular papules, and pustules in areas of heavy oil exposure, such as the extensor surfaces of the arms and thighs and under oil-soaked clothing. Pustules and furuncles may also appear.

Table 25-6 Oil and Tar Acne

Coal-tar products	Petroleum and its derivatives
Coal-tar oils	Crude oil and fractions
Creosote	Cutting oils
Pitch	

Table 25-7 Halogenated Aromatic Compounds (Chloracnegens)

Contaminants of polychlorophenol compounds, especially herbicides (2,4,5-T and pentachlorophenol) and herbicide intermediates (trichlorophenol)

    2,3,7,8-tetrachlorodibenzo-*p*-dioxin (TCDD)

    Hexachlorodibenzo-*p*-dioxin

    Tetrachlorodibenzofuran

Contaminants of 3,4-dichloroaniline and related herbicides (Propanil and Methazole)

    3,4,39,49-tetrachloroazoxybenzene (TCAOB)

    3,4,39,49-tetrachloroazobenzene (TCAB)

Polyhalogenated biphenyls[a]

    Polybromobiphenyls (PBBs)

    Polychlorobiphenyls (PCBs)

Polyhalogenated dibenzofurans[a]

    Polybromodibenzofurans, especially tetrabromodibenzofuran

    Polychlorodibenzofurans, especially tri-, tetra-(TCDF), penta-, and hexachlorodibenzofuran

Polyhalogenated naphthalenes[a]

    Polybromonaphthalenes[b,c]

    Polychloronaphthalenes

Other

    1,2,3,4-tetrachlorobenzene (experimental)

    Dichlobenil (Casoron)—herbicide (clinical only)

    DDT (Crude trichlorobenzene)[c]

[a]The polychlorodibenzofurans and hexachloronaphthalenes may occur as contaminants in some PCBs.
[b]The polybromonaphthalenes may occur as contaminants in some PBBs.
[c]not confirmed as chloracnegens.

Table 25-8 Miscellaneous and Contributing Causes to Occupational Acne

Bromides and iodides

Friction

Gram-negative folliculitis (hot-tubs and swimming pools)

Greasy cosmetics

Heat with sweating and occlusion

With improved engineering and less heavy contact with oils, oil acne is not as prevalent as in the past. The people who are most often affected are machinists using insoluble cutting oils; workers in coal-tar plants who handle heavy coal-tar distillates and coal-tar pitch; auto, truck, and aircraft mechanics; roofers, oil-well drillers; coke-oven workers; petroleum refiners; rubber workers; textile mill workers; and road-maintenance workers. Melanosis and photosensitivity also may occur in these individuals. Occasionally vegetable oils may cause acne and folliculitis in cooks and kitchen workers.

Certain halogenated chemicals are potent acnegens that can produce chloracne.[26,27] Most cases result from chloronaphthalenes and diphenyl contamination (PCBs), herbicides, herbicide intermediates, flame retardants, and isomers of chlorodibenzodioxins and chlorodibenzofurans, which are the fly ashes and flue gases of industrial incinerators.

The polychloronaphthalenes, which were used primarily in insulating waxes, dielectrics, and wood preservatives, have now been replaced. The PCBs are now restricted to closed-system applications to avoid environmental contamination.

The contaminant 2,3,7,8-tetrachlorodibenzo-*p*-dioxin (TCDD) is a potent acnegen formed during the synthesis of trichlorophenol, an intermediate in the synthesis of the herbicide 2,4,5-T and also hexachlorophene.

Poisoning with TCDD may be acute, with nausea, vomiting, headache, and mucosal and skin irritation. The initial cutaneous reaction is comparable to a chemical burn, usually from a combination of trichlorophenol, TCDD, and sodium hydroxide, and is not chloracne. Chloracne is often the first and most constant finding of the *chronic* stage of TCDD poisoning. Systemic disorders may appear and include porphyria cutanea tarda, hyperpigmentation, and hypertrichosis without porphyria.

Bleiberg and colleagues[28] reported that 29 patients, who worked in a chemical factory engaged in the manufacture of 2,4-dichlorophenol (2,4-D) and 2,4,5-trichlorophenol (2,3,5-T), and who exhibited features of chloracne, were studied for the presence of porphyria cutanea tarda. In 11 cases, urinary uro porphyrins were elevated.

Taylor[26,29] reported several outbreaks of chloracne (mostly unreported in the medical literature) that

Table 25-9 Differential Diagnosis of Chloracne

	Age	Sites	Clinical appearance
Acne vulgaris	Greatest involvement between ages 13 and 26	Face, neck, chest, and back to waist	Comedones, papules, pustules, cysts, and scars
Folliculitis	Any age	Any area, especially arms, dorsa of hands, thighs, and under oil-soaked clothing	Black comedones, papules, pustules, and melanosis
Chloracne	Any age	Face, especially neck, ear lobes, shoulders, abdomen, genitalia, and legs	Straw-colored cysts, numerous comedones and milia, papules, and often pruritus

occurred among workers exposed to azo and azoxyben-zenes. In one small chemical plant, chloracne developed in more than 90% of the workers.

FEATURES OF CHLORACNE

1. Straw-colored cysts are characteristic. Comedones are often present, involving every follicular orifice in affected areas. Pruritic inflammatory pustules and abscesses also occur, but are much less common than in acne vulgaris. Although exposed body areas typically are involved, there may be lesions in covered areas. Nasal involvement is unusual whereas comedones around the ears and malar areas are typical. Edema of the eyelids and conjunctivitis may occur. A brownish discoloration of the nails may be present.

2. Chloracne lesions may continue to appear after all exposure to the inciting chemical has ceased.

3. Hyperpigmentation may follow exposure to TCDD or PCBs. Acute burns with marked facial edema and erythema with subsequent development of hyperkeratosis and chloracne may develop after explosions occurring during trichlorophenol production. "Cable rash" resembling photosensitivity preceded chloracne from exposures to cables insulated with various mixtures of chlorinated naphthalenes and biphenyls.

4. Although chloracne occurs typically from external cutaneous contact, ingestion or inhalation may be important.

5. Hirsutism, hyperpigmentation, and increased skin fragility are also common, suggesting systemic involvement with porphyria cutanea tarda, especially when the exposure is to TCDD.

6. Dibenzodioxins are potent teratogens that depress cell-moderated immunity and that have several long-range, dose-related toxicologic effects in laboratory animals, including tumor induction. PCBs, PBBs, and TCDD can also modify tumor initiation in laboratory-animal oral and skin assays.

7. The low acnegenic threshold of these chemicals is illustrated by several reports of the families of plant workers in whom chloracne developed, even though they had never been in or near the factory; exposure occurred when work clothes or tools were brought home.

8. Prevention and control of chloracne require a totally enclosed manufacturing process with no opportunities for direct skin contact, ingestion, or inhalation of the chemical. The only other alternative is alteration of the chemical synthetic process to eliminate exposure to the contaminant chloracnegens.

9. Histologic examination shows lack of inflammation and atrophy of sebaceous glands.[30]

THERAPY OF CHLORACNE

Oil folliculitis is best treated by avoiding contact with oils and grease, by wearing oil-impervious aprons, or by environmental control. The wearing of gloves is usually hazardous in machinists and should be avoided. Work clothing should be changed frequently. Local acne medications (benzoyl peroxide gels or retinoid creams or gels) and oral antibiotics (tetracyclines) are frequently helpful, along with other acne therapy.

Chloracne is refractory to therapy with the usual methods used to treat acne vulgaris. Oral tetracylines, acne surgery (manual expression of comedones and cysts with a comedone extractor), and topical retinoic acid preparations may sometimes be beneficial. Dermabrasion may be helpful later for severe scarring. Excellent results in various keratinizing disorders and in severe acne vulgaris have been achieved with the oral, synthetic retinoid, 13-*cis*retinoic acid (isotretinoin or Accutane). A trial of this drug is warranted in severe cases of chloracne.

Solvent Dermatitis

The organic solvents are indispensable in modern manufacturing processes. They are used to dissolve and thin lacquers, varnishes, and paints and to act as solvents for rubber and natural and synthetic resins. They are also used in the dry-cleaning industry and in the manufacture of organic dyes, artificial silk, glues, and cements. They act as extractives for fats, waxes, oils, and perfumes.

The physical properties of solvents influence the injurious effects they have on the skin. In general, the more poorly absorbed solvents cause more skin damage and the fewest systemic symptoms. The saturated hydrocarbon solvents and the paraffin series of solvents are stronger skin irritants than those derived from the aromatic series. The irritant effect decreases as the boiling point increases. The concentration, duration of exposure, and degree of occlusion of the area are also relevant. More irritation may be caused by washing with soaps and detergents and immersion in water.

All solvents can cause dermatitis by dissolving the natural protective barrier of oil on the skin. Some solvents are noticeably irritating on contact, but others cause no particular pain even while they are penetrating or defatting the skin.

A chronic, scaling dermatitis results when the skin comes in frequent contact with solvents, as in washing grease from the hands or when cloths moistened with solvents are used for cleansing or degreasing. Solvents dissolve and remove the surface lipids, the lipid material in the stratum corneum, and the fatty fraction of cell membranes. The percutaneous absorption of water and other substances is increased through this defatting action. Solvents may also damage the stratum corneum cells themselves.

An experiment showed that workers who contact solvents have greater absorption through the skin if they have dermatitis than if the skin is intact.[31] Twenty eight printers with exposure to the solvent butoxyethoxy ethanol (BEE) were examined and had urine tests to determine solvent absorption. BEE levels in urine of workers with hand dermatitis were almost twice as high as those without.

The most frequent cause of occupational dermatitis by solvents is the practice of washing with a solvent. Workers whose occupation predisposes them to wash with a solvent include painters, who use paint thinners and turpentine; plastic workers, who use acetone; printers, who use typewash; auto mechanics, who use gasoline and kerosene; and dry cleaners, who use trichloroethylene, perchloroethylene, and Stoddard solvent.

Employees usually clean their hands with available solvents. The workers use a variety of solvents, for example, petroleum, coal-tar derivatives, chlorinated hydrocarbons, alcohols, ketones, and turpentine, to remove materials such as ink, tar, glue, gum, cement and other mucilaginous and viscous substances, grease, oil, stain, lacquer, and varnish.

Workers who had significant exposure to gasoline had from 3 to 11 times higher incidence of hand dermatitis, nail changes, and skin dryness than non-exposed controls. In addition, stratum corneum levels of ceramides, cholesterol, and fatty acids were significantly lower in the exposed group.[32]

Solvents may also damage the peripheral nervous system. The symptoms caused by this nerve damage are numbness, tingling sensations, weakness, and paralysis in the arms and legs. Solvents may also produce a lymphangitis when they enter into a fissure or laceration and pass through the dermis and into the lymphatics.

The prevention of solvent dermatitis involves educating workers in the importance of wearing protective clothing while using solvents as cleaning agents, or, preferably, not using solvents at all. Skin contact should be avoided while moving metal parts into and out of degreasing solutions. Clothing on which solvent has been spilled should be removed as soon as possible. Solvent-proof rubber gloves under solvent-proof sleeves closed at the wrist should be worn. Glove manufacturers can supply charts with breakthrough times for different types of gloves for different solvents. Thin, disposable medical-type gloves usually degrade rapidly upon solvent exposure and therefore are not recommended for industrial use.

PATCH TESTING FOR SOLVENT ALLERGY

In patch testing with volatile organic solvents, Vail[33] showed that the highly volatile antigen-containing compounds, applied as is in an open patch test, evaporate so rapidly that they do not penetrate the stratum corneum in sufficient concentration to evoke a reaction. It is, therefore, advisable to use a modified open patch test, that is, covering the test area several minutes after application of the solvent in order to allow the solvent to penetrate the stratum corneum. Such evaporation, however, does not take place when the organic solvents are tested in olive oil; the usual patch test procedure may be used.

Aliphatic hydrocarbons may be tested 50% in olive oil.

ALCOHOL SOLVENTS

The following alcohol solvents may be tested ''as is'' undiluted:

1. Ethanol (ethyl or grain alcohol)
2. Methanol (wood or methyl alcohol, carbinol, wood spirit)
3. N-propyl alcohol
4. Isopropyl alcohol (rubbing alcohol, 2-methylpropanol)
5. Isobutyl alcohol
6. Isoamyl alcohol (fusel oil)

Kurwa[34] pointed out that contact sensitization to primary alcohols such as ethanol and methanol usually occurs from occupational exposure, as in nurses, doctors, and laboratory technicians, and occasionally from cosmetic use. Some cases have been recorded in which ingestion of alcohol has produced a reaction in the mouth; in others, asthma, angioedema, and urticaria were aggravated by drinking alcoholic beverages.

Isopropyl alcohol is used extensively in general and hospital practice in the form of prepacked swabs for cleansing the skin before injections are given. Alcohol swab use caused ACD in a girl which was initially thought to be a vaccine allergy.[35] Positive ROAT to the swab was diagnostic.

Fregert and colleagues[36] demonstrated that patients with hypersensitivity to primary alcohols (in which the carbon atom attached to the hydroxyl group is also attached to two hydrogen atoms) are also hypersensitive to secondary alcohols (the hydroxyl group that is attached to a carbon atom linked to two other carbon atoms).

ACD to alcohols can be of the delayed, eczematous variety and the urticarial type.[37–39] (See also the section on alcohol dermatitis in Chapter 26.)

Berlin and colleagues[40] reported a woman who experienced eye and respiratory irritation with erythema of the face and swollen eyelids when in buildings that had been recently painted with water-based paints. She was patch test positive to Euxyl K 400 0.1% in petrolatum and to the solvent 2–butoxyethoxyethanol (BEE). The BEE, also known as diethyleneglycol mono-*n*-butyl ether, was blamed for the symptoms. The authors noted one other case of allergy to the similar compound butoxyethoxyethyl acetate.

French workers tested ethanol at 10% and 70% in water and identified 4 cases of ethanol allergy. Only 3 reacted to the 10% solution. 140 controls were negative. Exposure was from transdermal therapeutic systems in 2 and disinfectants in 2.[41]

Alcohol-based hand disinfectants

Instead of frequent hand washing, many health-care facilities suggest use of waterless hand disinfectants. A repeat irritant patch test study with one gel in 53 subjects showed no irritant or allergic responses.[42] Another study examined skin tolerance of 5 ethanol based gels in atopics and non-atopics. All were tolerated well and no difference was seen between the 2 groups.[43]

ALIPHATIC HYDROCARBONS

Aliphatic hydrocarbons may be tested 50% in olive oil. These compounds refer to any organic compound that has an open chain of carbon atoms, whether normal or forked, saturated or unsaturated. Besides their use as solvents, these chemicals are also used as follows:

Pentane—Use: in thermometers, as an anesthetic

N-hexane—Use: determining refractive index of materials: filling for thermometers instead of mercury, usually with a blue or red dye

Benzine (petroleum naphtha, ligroin, petroleum ether, and petroleum benzine)

Gasoline (petrol)—Use: fuel, in paint mixing and rubber cements

Diesel—May contain enough water to support the growth of microorganisms; therefore, biocides may be added to diesel. Kathon FP is one such biocide, which has caused contact dermatitis. Positive patch tests were found to methylchloroisothiazolinone and 2-methyl-4-isothiazolin-3-one.[44] This is the same combination found in Kathon CG.

Dyes added to diesel have been thought by the public to possibly be responsible for rashes, but patch tests have not confirmed this. Rather, the more environmentally friendly diesel fuels that contain low concentrations of aromatic compounds and a lower sulfur content than traditional high viscosity, high aromatic and sulfur content oils are more irritating than the older product.[45] Cocamide DEA may be added to diesel fuel.

VMP naphtha—Use: varnishes and paint thinner

Mineral spirits (petroleum spirits and ligroin)

Stoddard solvent (white spirits)

Kerosene (kerosine, coal oil, jet fuel, and range oil) (paraffin—British term)—Use: kerosene lamps, flares, and stoves; as a degreaser and cleaner; and in insecticides

Kerosene is a strong skin irritant. A Japanese report describes extraction of kerosene from the roof of an epidermal blister in an affected woman, proving the diagnosis.[46] Barnes and Wilkinson[47] described an eruption similar to that of toxic epidermal necrolysis without systemic symptoms in a boy whose clothing became contaminated with kerosene.

AROMATIC HYDROCARBONS

The chemicals included under the heading of aromatic hydrocarbons are a small segment in the broad category of organic solvents. They are classified as aromatics because of the presence of the benzene ring in their chemical structure.

Benzene (benzol, cyclohextriene, phenyl hydride, coal naphtha, phene, and benzole)—Test 5% olive oil. Use: manufacture of medicinal chemicals, dyes and many other organic compounds, artificial leather, linoleum, oil cloth, airplane dopes, varnishes, and lacquers; as solvent for waxes, resins, and oils

Skin contact with liquid benzene may cause erythema and blistering, with prolonged or repeated contacts responsible for the development of a dry, scaly dermatitis. Any evaluation of exposure must also consider the absorption through the skin following contact with liquid benzene.[48]

Coal-tar naphtha (naphthalene)—Test "as is." Use: dyes and moth repellent

Nitrobenzene (nitrobenzol, oil of mirbane, and oil of bitter almonds)—Test 25% olive oil

Tetrahydronaphthalene (tetralin) should be tested at 2.5% in olive oil, as higher concentrations were reported to cause irritant reactions.[49]

Aniline is obtained from the reduction of nitrobenzene, and the two chemicals are often used in the same industrial process. This compound is used in shoe dyes and as an artificial flavor in foods, soaps, and perfumes because its odor is like that of oil of bitter almonds. It is a volatile, yellowish fluid also used for refining lubricating oils and the manufacture of pyroxylin compounds.

Toluene (toluol, methylbenzene, phenylmethane, and methylbenzol)—Test 50% olive oil. Use: manufacture benzoic acid, benzaldehyde, perfumes, explosives, dyes, and many other organic compounds; also as a solvent in the extraction of various principles from plants

Styrene (cinnamene, cinnemenol, cinnamal, phenethylene, phenylethylene, styrol, styrene monomer, styrolene, and vinyl benzene)—Test 1% olive oil. Use: manufacture of synthetic rubber, modifier of alkyd acrylic and polyester resins, extractive of storax balsam, preparation of compound tincture of benzoin, and fixative for soap in the cosmetic industry.

Styrene liquid is sometimes used in acrylic resin powder to form a denture. Polystyrenes may be used for denture material. Styrene not only is a synthetic industrial compound but can also occur in nature, for example, in raspberries.

Sjoborg and colleagues[50] described contact allergy to styrene with crossreaction to vinyltoluene.

Xylene (xylol and dimethylbenzene)—Test 50% olive oil. Use: raw material for production of benzoic acid, phthalic anhydride, isophthalic and terephthalic acids, as well as their dimethyl esters used in the manufacture of polyester fibers; manufacturing dyes and other organics: sterilizing catgut; with Canada balsam as oil immersion in microscopy; cleaning agent in microscope technique

Altman[51] described allergic contact urticaria due to xylene. Testing with 1% and 100% xylene revealed an immediate, acute, urticarial patch (25 mm) to the 100% xylene and, in 15 minutes, a similar but smaller, urticarial patch (15 mm) to the 1% xylene. All other patches were negative. Three controls were negative to the 1% and 100% xylene.

CHLORINATED HYDROCARBONS

Carbon tetrachloride (tetrachloromethane and perchloromethane)—Test 10% olive oil. Use: as fire extinguisher; for cleaning clothing; for rendering benzine nonflammable; as azeotropic drying agent for wet spark plugs in automobiles; as solvent for oils, fats, lacquers, varnishes, rubber waxes, and resins; for extracting oils from flowers and seeds; for exterminating destructive insects; as solvent; for starting material in manufacture of many organic compounds

Chloroform Test 40% olive oil. Use: as solvent for fats, oils, rubber, alkaloids, waxes, gutta-percha, resins; as cleansing agent; in fire extinguishers to lower the freezing temperature of carbon tetrachloride; in the rubber industry

Ethylene dichloride (1,2-dichloroethane, symdichloroethane, ethylene chloride, glycol dichloride, and b-dichloroethane)—Test 50% olive oil. Use: solvent for fats, oils, waxes, gums, resins, and particularly for rubber: irritation of respiratory tract and conjunctiva, corneal clouding, equilibrium disturbances, narcosis, and abdominal cramps

Methylene chloride (dichloromethane, methylene dichloride, and methylene bichloride)—Test 1% acetone. Use: solvent for cellulose acetate: degreasing and cleaning fluids, and as a paint stripper

Methyl chloroform (1,1,1-trichloroethane)—Test 1% olive oil. Use: in cold-type cleaning; also in cleaning

plastic molds. Caution: irritating to eyes, mucous membranes, and, in high concentrations, narcotic

Occupational allergic contact dermatitis to methyl chloroform was detected with concentrations down to 0.01% in olive oil.[52] Fowler reported contact urticaria in an eyeglass maker from this substance.[53]

Trichloroethylene (trichloroethene, trilene, trethylene, and tri-clene)—Test 50% olive oil. Use: widely used as a dry-cleaning agent.

Trichloroethylene is also used to degrease metal, as a solvent for oils, resins, sulfur, and phosphorus, and medicinally as a wound cleanser and for relief of angina pectoris. It may sensitize the patient to alcohol. A combination of alcohol ingestion and trichloroethylene exposure may produce an "aldehyde syndrome," with flushing of the skin, nausea, and vomiting. Alcohol-induced flushing has also been reported by skin absorption of dimethylformamide.[54] This organic solvent caused such flushing in 19 of 102 workers up to 4 days after exposure and also caused contact dermatitis.[54]

An irritant reaction may occur from contaminated clothing, also an exfoliative dermatitis or scarlatiniform eruption may result from contact with trichloroethylene.[55]

Epstein[56] reported that epichlorhydrin used as a stabilizer in trichloroethylene can cause an allergic contact dermatitis in metalplate workers. Patients were tested 0.01% in alcohol.[56]

Perchloroethylene (perc, tetrachloroethylene, carbon dichloride, and ethylene tetrachloride)—Test 25% olive oil. Use: dry cleaning and degreasing metals

Exposure to perchloroethylene causes flushing of the skin with ingestion of alcohol. This reaction is similar to an Antabuse reaction.

Sparrow[57] reported a 19-year-old male who had a connective-tissue type of disease similar clinically to vinylchloride disease. It is suggested that this may have been caused by abnormal sensitivity to perchloroethylene, to which he was exposed in his occupation.

Tetrachloroethane (1,1,2,2-tetrachloroethane, sym-tetrachloroethane, acetylene tetrachloride, and ethanetetrachloride)—Test 1% olive oil. Use: nonflammable solvents for fats, oils, waxes, resins, cellulose acetate, rubber, copal, phosphorus, sulfur, as solvent in certain types of Friedel-Crafts reactions or phthalic anhydride condensations; in the manufacture of paint, varnish, and rust removers; in soil sterilization, weed killer, and insecticide formulations; in the determination of theobromine in cacao; as immersion fluid in crystallography; in the biologic laboratory to produce pathologic changes in the gastrointestinal tract, liver, and kidneys; intermediate in the manufacture of trichloroethylene and other chlorinated hydrocarbons that have two carbon atoms

ESTERS

Esters are formed by a reaction of an alcohol and an acid. These esters are rare sensitizers.

Methyl acetate Test 10% olive oil. Use: solvent for nitrocellulose, acetylcellulose, and many resins and oils; manufacture of artificial leather

Ethyl acetate (acetic ether and vinegar naphtha)—Test 5% methyl ethyl ketone. Use: artificial fruit essences; solvent for nitrocellulose, varnishes, lacquers, and airplane dopes; manufacture of smokeless powder, artificial leather, photographic films and plates, artificial silk, perfumes; cleaning textiles

Isopropyl acetate—Test 10% olive oil. Use: solvent for cellulose derivatives, plastics, oils, and fats; in perfumery

Amyl acetate (isoamyl acetate, pear oil, banana oil, amyl acetate ester, and pentyl acetate)—Test 10% olive oil. Use: in alcohol solution as a pear flavor in mineral waters and syrups; as solvent for old oil colors, for tannins, nitrocellulose, lacquers, celluloid, and camphor; swelling bath sponges; covering unpleasant odors, perfuming shoe polish; manufacture of artificial silk, leather or pearls, photographic films, celluloid cements, waterproof varnishes, bronzing liquids, and metallic paints; dyeing and finishing textiles. A special grade of the amyl acetate has been used for burning in the Hefner lamp serving as a photometric standard.

GLYCOLS

The glycols may be tested 5% in alcohol.

Ethylene glycol (1,2-ethanediol, glycol alcohol, glycol, and EG)—Use: antifreeze in cooling and heating systems; in hydraulic brake fluids; industrial humectant; ingredient of electrolytic condensers (where it serves as solvent for boric acid and borates); solvent in the paint and plastics industries; in the formulation of printers' inks, stamp pad inks, and inks for ballpoint pens; softening agent for cellophane; stabilizer for soybean form used to extinguish oil and gasoline fires; in the synthesis of safety explosives, glyoxal, unsaturated ester–type alkyd resins, plasticizers, elastomers, synthetic fibers (terylene and dacron), and synthetic waxes, and lens-cutting industry.

There are two reports of ethylene-glycol sensitivity.[58,59] In both instances, the dermatitis occurred from exposure to ethylene glycol used to bathe glass lenses while they were being cut. In one instance, there was primary sensitization to ethylene glycol with cross-sensitivity to propylene glycol.[59]

Most glycol ethers were found to be either nonirritating or only mildly irritating when studied by Draize testing and nonsensitizers by guinea pig maximization.[60] Two glycol ethers were irritants: 2-butoxyethanol and isopropoxyethanol.

Cellulosolve (2-ethoxy ethanol, ethyl cellosolve, ethylene glycol, and monoethyl ether)—Use: solvent for nitrocellulose, lacquers, and dopes; in varnish removers, cleansing solutions, dye baths; finishing leather with water pigments and dye solutions; increasing stability of emulsions

Methyl cellosolve (ethylene glycol monomethyl ether and 2-methoxy ethanol)—Use: solvent for low-viscosity cellulose acetate, natural resins, some synthetic resins, and some alcohol-soluble dyes; in dyeing leather, sealing moisture-proof cellophane; in nail polishes, quick-drying varnishes and enamels, and wood stains. Readily absorbed through the skin

Butyl cellosolve (ethylene glycol monobutyl ether and 2-butoxyethanol)—Use: solvent for nitrocellulose, resins, grease, oil, and albumin; dry cleaning

KETONES

Ketones are substances with the characterizing atom group —CO—, linking two carbon atoms. The ketones apparently are sensitizers very rarely, if at all.

Acetone (2-propanone, dimethyl ketone, beta-ketopropane, and pyroacetic ether)—Test 10% olive oil. Use: solvent for fats, oils, waxes, resins, rubber, plastics, lacquers, varnishes, rubber cements, manufacture of methyl isobutyl ketone, mesityl oxide, acetic acid (ketene process), diacetone alcohol, chloroform, iodoform, bromoform, explosives, aeroplane dopes, rayon, photographic films, isoprene; extraction of various principles from animal and plant substances; in paint and varnish removers; purifying paraffin; hardening and dehydrating tissues

Methyl ethyl ketone (buranone, 2-buranone, MEK, ethyl methyl ketone)

Methyl butyl ketone (2-hexanone, N-buryl methyl ketone, propyl acetone, MBK)

Methyl isobutyl ketone (hexone, isopropylacetone, 4-methyl-2-pentanone, MIBK)—Test as is. Use: solvent for gums, resins, nitrocellulose; in the surface coating industry; manufacture of smokeless powder; colorless synthetic resins

MISCELLANEOUS SOLVENTS

N-methyl-2-pyrrolidone. This solvent was reported to cause acute irritant contact dermatitis in 10 of 12 workers after 2 days of exposure.[61]

d-limonene. The oil of several citrus, caraway, dill, and celery is now being used as an environmentally friendly alternative to halogenated hydrocarbons in up to 95% concentration. Uses include degreasing metals before painting, as a hand cleaner, as a substitute for xylene, and as a solvent for asphalt, heavy oil, and rosin.[62] Allergic potential increases with air oxidation.[62]

In guinea pigs *d*-limonene of high purity is not a sensitizer, but when exposed to air, oxidized *d*-limonene contains limonene oxide, carvone, and hydroperoxides, which can lead to sensitization.[63]

Phenyl-alpha-naphthylamine (PAN). This substance has been incorporated into fire-resistant grease used on conveyor belts at a 1% concentration.[64] PAN produced contact dermatitis confirmed by testing at 1% in petrolatum. PAN did not crossreact with phenyl-beta-naphthylamine or di-beta-naphthyl-*p*-phenylenediamine.[63]

Carbon disulfide (carbon bisulfide and dithiocarbonic anhydride)—Test 10% olive oil—Use: in the manufacture of rayon, carbon tetrachloride, xanthogenates, soil disinfectants, electronic vacuum tubes; solvent for phosphorus, sulfur, selenium, bromine, iodine, fats, resins, and rubbers

Tetrahydrofuran (diethylene oxide and tetramethylene oxide)—Test 10% olive oil. Use: solvent for high polymers, especially polyvinyl chloride; as reaction medium for Grignard and metal hydride reactions; in the synthesis of butyrolactone, succinic acid, 1,4-butanediol diacetate; solvent in histologic techniques; may be used under US Federal Food, Drug and Cosmetic Act for fabrication of articles for packaging, transporting, or storing of foods if residual amount does not exceed 1.5% of the film

Dioxane (1,4-diethylene dioxide, diethylene ether, 1,4-dioxane, and para-dioxane)—Test 0.5% aqueous. Use: solvent for cellulose acetate, ethyl cellulose, benzyl cellulose, resins, oils, waxes, oil and spirit-soldyes, and many other organic as well as some inorganic compounds

Fregert[65] reported an allergic contact dermatitis from dioxane in a solvent for cleaning metal parts.

Turpentine (gum turpentine, oil of turpentine, spirit of turpentine, gum spirit, pine resin gum, wood turpentine, and sulfate wood pulp waste)—Oil of turpentine, a variable mixture of numerous terpenoid compounds, is derived from various sources, such as balsam of pine trees, and is a by-product in the manufacture of sulfate cellulose. The main components are alpha-pinene, beta-pinene, delta-3-carene, and dipentene (limonene). These are monoterpenes with a common chemical formula of $CH_{10}H_{16}$.

According to Pirila and colleagues,[66] practically all oils of turpentine contain large amounts of 2-pinene. However, the 3-carene content varies in different types, being high (30% to 40%) in most sulfate oils and low or negligible in many balsam oils, for example, French oil of turpentine. The eczematogenic effect of 3-carene depends on its hydroperoxide content.

Hjorth and Wilkinson[67] confirmed that with turpentine the patch test reactions provoked by the same dilution are related to the source, the method of manufacture (sulfate process or gum distillation), the amount of delta-3-carene present, and the concentration of peroxides formed during storage. These factors vary, as do the relative quantities of alpha-pinene and beta-pinene present. Because some patients may be sensitized by alpha-pinene and others by delta-3-carene, turpentine for testing should contain both of these ingredients and a suitable concentration of their peroxides.

Pirila and colleagues[66] used a mixture of 3-carene, 2-pinene, and limonenes containing 1% peroxides in olive oil for testing turpentine sensitivity.

Turpentine is both a primary irritant and a sensitizer. As an irritant, it usually acts by defatting the skin and causing dryness and fissuring. It is universally used as a cleanser for removing paints and waxes and is one of the most common causes of hand eczema.

Opportunity for contact with turpentine is widespread, both in industry and elsewhere. It may be applied externally in the form of liniments, ointments, and "rubbing" compounds, and in some countries it is prescribed internally as an anthelmintic and laxative. Other compounds containing turpentine include varnishes, lacquers, floor waxes, cleansers, shoe and floor polishes, paint thinners, printers' ink, dry-cleaning preparations, and various adhesives, including adhesive tape. The skin of citrus fruits contains oleoresins related to turpentine.

Old, oxidized turpentine is more irritating and sensitizing than is the freshly made product. When turpentine is allowed to stand, especially with exposure to light, oxidation results in the formation of formic acid and aldehydes. Pinenes and limonene, which are also formed in the oxidation process, may cause allergic sensitization and crossreact with the oils in orange peels and other essential oils.

The terpenes in turpentine have also been incriminated as active sensitization agents. Similar terpenes are present in citrus fruits and celery, and the possibility of crossreaction must be kept in mind. Cross-sensitivity reactions may also occur between turpentine and ragweed oleoresin, chrysanthemum, pyrethrum, and various balsams, such as those of pine, spruce, and Peru. Wood tars in general have been found to co-react with fragrance mix 43% of the time and balsam of Peru 31% of the time.[68] This suggests a shared fragrance material may be present. Co-reactions between wood tar and coal tar occurred only 18.5% of the time.[68]

The residue remaining after distillation of crude oil of turpentine is rosin, or colophony, which consists mainly of abietic acid and 1-pinearic acid. Rosin obtained from turpentine is present in many adhesives and may cause dermatitis in sensitized individuals (see Chapter 30).

Olive oil—This oil is generally safe for patch test purposes and is widely used as a diluent for other solvents in this chapter. However, when used on stasis dermatitis, allergic contact dermatitis may occur; 13 cases were reported within a 4-year period.[69] While tests of multiple brands of olive oil were positive, individual tests to the nine components of olive oil listed in the Merck Index were negative.

References

1. <www.ccohs.ca/oshanswers/chemicals/metalworking_fluids.html> (accessed June 4, 2007).

2. Fisher AA. Allergic contact dermatitis of the hands due to industrial oils and fluids. Cutis 1979;23:131;134,138, passim.

3. Gellin GA. Cutting fluids and skin disorders. Industr Med Surg 1970;39:65.

4. Samitz MH, Katz SA. Skin hazards from nickel and chromium salts in association with cutting oil operations. Contact Dermatitis 1975;1: 158.

5. Samitz MH. Effects of metalworking fluids on the skin. Prog Dermatol 1974;8:11.

6. Hodgson G. Eczemas associated with lubricants and metalworking fluids. Dermatol Digest 1976;10:11.

7. Shah M, Lewis FM, Gawkrodger DJ. Prognosis of occupational hand dermatitis in metalworkers. Contact Dermatitis 1996;34:27.

8. Scerri L, Dalziel KL. Occupational contact sensitization to the stabilized chlorinated paraffin fraction in neat cutting oil. Am J Contact Dermat 1996;7:35.

9. Geier J, Uter W, Lessmann H, et al: Patch testing with metalworking fluids from the patients workplace. Contact Dermatitis 2004;51:172.

10. Geier J, Lessmann H, Dickel H, et al: Patch test results with the metalworking fluids series of the German contact dermatitis research group. Contact Dermatitis 2004;51:118.

11. Geier J, Lessmann H, Becker D, et al: Patch testing with components of water-based metalworking fluids. Contact Dermatitis 2006;55:322.

12. Angelini G, Meneghini CL. Dermatitis in engineers due to synthetic coolants. Contact Dermatitis 1977;3:219.

13. Camarasa JM, Alomar A. Ethylenediamine sensitivity in metallurgic industries. Contact Dermatitis 1978;4:178.

14. Suurmond D. Patch test reactions to phenergan cream, promethazine and triethanolamine. Dermatologica 1966;133:503.

15. Bhushan M, Craven NM, Beck MH. Contact allergy to 2-aminoethanol (monoethanolamine) in a soluble oil. Contact Dermatitis 1998;39:321.

16. Bruze M, et al. Occupational allergic contact dermatitis from alkanolamineborates in metalworking fluids. Contact Dermatitis 1995;32:24.

17. Koch P. Occupational allergic contact dermatitis from oleyl alcohol and monoethanolamine in a metalworking fluid. Contact Dermatitis 1995;33:273.

18. Madan V, Beck MH. Occupational allergic contact dermatitis from N,N methylene-bis-5-methyl-oxazolidine in coolant oils. Contact Dermatitis 2006;55:39.

19. Keczke K, Brown PM. Hexahydro, 1,3,5, tris (2-hydroxyethyl) triazine, a new bacteriocidal agent as a cause of allergic contact dermatitis. Contact Dermatitis 1976;2:92.

20. Poitou P, Marignac B. Sensitizing effect of Grotan BK in the guinea pig. Contact Dermatitis 1978;4:166.

21. Fregert S, Skog E. Allergic contact dermatitis from mercaptobenzothiazole in cutting oil. Acta Dermatovener (Stockh) 1962;42:235.

22. Tosti A, Piraccini B, Brasile GP. Occupational contact dermatitis due to sodium pyrithione. Contact Dermatitis 1990;22:118.

23. Hovding G. Occupational dermatitis from hydrazine hydrate used in boiler protection: cross sensitization to a presoline, isoniazid and phenelzine. Acta Derm Venereol (Stockh) 1967;47:293.

24. Geretzki P. Pyodermia in metalworking industry [German]. Dermatosen 1982;30:116.

25. Taylor JS. The pilosebaceous unit. In: Maibach HI, Gellin GA, eds. Occupational and industrial dermatology. Chicago: Year Book Medical Publishers, 1982, p. 131.

26. Taylor JS. Environmental chloracne: update and overview. Ann NY Acad Sci 1979;320:295.

27. Fowler J: Occupational Dermatology. Curr Prob Dermatol 1998;10:214.

28. Bleiberg J, et al. Industrially acquired porphyria. Arch Dermatol 1964;89:793.

29. Taylor JS. Occupational dermatoses: method of James S. Taylor, M.D. In: Conn HF, ed. Current therapy. Philadelphia: WB Saunders, 1979, p. 635.

30. Moses M, Prioleu P. Cutaneous histologic findings in chemical workers with and without past exposure to TCDD. J Am Acad Dermatol 1985;12:497.

31. Korinth G, Goen T, Lakemeyer M, et al. Skin strain and its influence on systemic exposure to a glycol in offset printing workers. Contact Dermatitis 2003;49:248.

32. Jia X, Xiao P, Jin X, et al. Adverse effects of gasoline on the skin of exposed workers. Contact Dermatitis 2002;46:44.

33. Vail JT Jr. False-negative reaction to patch testing with volatile compounds. Arch Dermatol 1974;110:130.

34. Kurwa AR. Contact dermatitis from isopropyl alcohol. Contact Dermatitis Newsletter 1970;8:168.

35. Storer E, Marshman G, Kupa A. Contact dermatitis to alcohol swabs masquerading as vaccine allergy. Australas J Dermatol 2004;45:149.

36. Fregert S, et al. Hypersensitivity to secondary alcohols. Acta Derm Venereol (Stockh) 1971;51:271.

37. Stotts J, Ely WJ. Induction of human skin sensitization to ethanol. J Invest Dermatol 1977;69:219.

38. Rilliet A, Hunziker N, Brun R. Alcohol contact urticari syndrome (immediate-type hypersensitivity): case report. Dermatologica 1980;161:361.

39. Karvonen J, Hannuksela M. Urticaria from alcoholic beverages. Acta Allerg 1976;31:167.

40. Berlin K, Johanson G, Lindberg M. Hypersensitivity to 2-(2-butoxyethoxy)ethanol. Contact Dermatitis 1995;32:54.

41. Barbaud A, Trechot P, Reichert-Penetrat S, et al. Ann Dermatol Venereol 2000;127:484.

42. Kampf G, Muscatiello M, Hantschel D et al. Dermal tolerance and effect on skin hydration of a new ethanol based gel. J Hosp Infect 2002;52:297.

43. Kampf G, Wigger-Alberti W, Wilhelm K. Do atopics tolerate alcohol-based hand rubs? Acta Derm Venereol 2006;86:140.

44. Bruynzeel DP, Verburgh CA. Occupational dermatitis from isothiazolinones in diesel oil. Contact Dermatitis 1996;34:64.

45. Fischer T, Bjarnason B. Sensitizing and irritant properties of 3 environmental classes of diesel oil and their indicator dyes. Contact Dermatitis 1996;34:309.

46. Tsujino Y, Hieda Y, Morita E. A rapid and definitive diagnosis of kerosene dermatitis. Arch Dermatol Res 2005;297:91.

47. Barnes RL, Wilkinson DS. Epidermal necrolysis from clothing impregnated with paraffin. Br Med J 1973;4:466.

48. Gasper AL. Aromatic hydrocarbons. Occupational Medicine, Current Concepts (NYS Dept Health) 1980;3:1.

49. Heine A. Is tetrahydronaphthalene an allergen? Contact Dermatitis 1991;24:303.

50. Sjoborg S, et al. Contact allergy to styrene with cross reaction to vinyltoluene. Contact Dermatitis 1982;8:207.

51. Altman AT. Facial dermatitis. Arch Dermatol 1977;113:1460.

52. Ingber A. Occupational allergic contact dermatitis from methyl chloroform (1,1,1-trichloroethane). Contact Dermatitis 1991;25:193.

53. Fowler J: Contact urticaria to I,I,I trichloroethane. AM J Contact Dermatitis 1991;2:239.

54. Cox NH, Mustchin CP. Prolonged spontaneous and alcohol-induced flushing due to the solvent dimethylformamide. Contact Dermatitis 1991;245:69.

55. Bauer M, Rabens SF. Trichloroethylene toxicity. Int J Dermatol 1977;16:113.

56. Epstein E. Allergy to epichlorohydrin masquerading as trichloroethylene allergy. Contact Dermatitis Newsletter 1974;16:475.

57. Sparrow GP. A connective tissue disorder similar to vinyl chloride disease in a patient exposed to perchloroethylene. Clin Exp Dermatol 1977;2:17.

58. Dawson TA. Ethylene glycol sensitivity. Contact Dermatitis 1976;2:233.

59. Hindson C, Ratcliffe G. Ethylene glycol in glass lens cutting. Contact Dermatitis 1975;1:386.

60. Zissu D. Experimental study of cutaneous tolerance to glycol ethers. Contact Dermatitis 1995;32:74.

61. Leira HL, et al. Irritant cutaneous reactions to N-methyl-2-pyrrolidone (NMP). Contact Dermatitis 1992;27:148.

62. Karlberg AT, Magnusson K, Nilsson U. Air oxidation of d-limonene (the citrus solvent) creates potent allergens. Contact Dermatitis 1992;26:332.

63. Chang Y-C, Karlberg A-T, Maibach HI. Allergic contact dermatitis from oxidized d-limonene. Contact Dermatitis 1997;37:308.

64. Carmichael AJ, Foulds IS. Isolated naphthylamine allergy to phenyl-alpha-naphthylamine. Contact Dermatitis 1990;22:298.

65. Fregert S. Allergic contact dermatitis from dioxane in a solvent for cleaning metal parts. Contact Dermatitis Newsletter 1974;15:438.

66. Pirila V, et al. On the chemical nature of the eczematogens in oil of turpentine (V). Pattern of sensitivity to different terpenes. Dermatologica 1969;139:183.

67. Hjorth N, Wilkinson DS. Turpentine sensitivity. Br J Dermatol 1968;80:22.

68. Roesyanto ID, van den Akker TW, van Joost TW. Wood tars allergy, cross-sensitization and coal tar. Contact Dermatitis 1990;22:95.

69. Malmkvist Padoan S, Pettersson A, Svensson A. Olive oil as a cause of contact allergy in patients with venous eczema, and occupationally. Contact Dermatitis 1990;23:73.

CHAPTER 26

GASES AND PROPELLANTS

EXECUTIVE SUMMARY

Gases and propellants are rare causes of dermatitis. Irritant contact dermatitis (ICD) is more common than allergic contact dermatitis (ACD) in this regard. Chemical lacrimators (tear gases) have as their method of action direct irritant effects on the skin and mucous membranes. Rare ACD to these agents can occur. Ethylene oxide, a potent sterilizing agent, has caused frequent outbreaks of ICD from exposure to inadequately ventilated hospital garments and equipment.

Tear gas, ethylene oxide, and propellants may produce irritant and allergic contact dermatitis.

Dermatitis Due to Tear Gases (Lacrimators)

The term "tear gas" includes not only gases but also liquids and solids that at ordinary temperatures give off vapors that produce so much irritation of the conjunctivae with lacrimation and photophobia that the affected individual is temporarily blinded and can more readily be subdued.[1]

Most of the tear gases used by military and law enforcement officers are synthetic organic compounds. Citizens in the United States, and elsewhere, may carry tear gas, or "pepper spray," containing oleoresin of capsicum.[2]

THE CHEMICAL NATURE OF TEAR GASES

Chloracetophenone

This lacrimator, known in the United States as CN, was first used in World War I and has become a tear gas weapon used worldwide by the military and the police. Chloracetophenone ($C_6H_5COCH_2Cl$) is made by chlorinating acetic acid to form monochloracetic acid, which is further chlorinated with sulfur monochloride and chlorine gas to form chloroacetyl chloride. This compound is treated with benzene in the presence of

aluminum chloride. It consists of colorless crystals that melt at 59°C and smells like apple blossoms.[3,4]

Mace

Chloracetophenone is available in a compound called Mace, which is an acronym derived from the chemicals methylchloroform and chloracetophenone. Methylchloroform, a solvent, is 1,1,1-trichlorethane.[5] Mace also contains kerosene. The chemical mixture is dissolved in an ether-alcohol combination and emitted under pressure from a grenade cartridge by one of the freon propellants.

CS

This term refers to the lacrimator *ortho*-chlorobenzylidene malononitrile,[6] a white powder that is often combined with ethyl bromacetate, a dispersing agent. The letters are rumored to represent Carson and Stoughton, the chemists who invented the chemical. It has been used in thermal grenades by the United States military in Vietnam, by American police in domestic disturbances, and by British forces in the north of Ireland. CS is available in the United States in aerosol form.

CR

This chemical, dibenz 1,4 oxazepine, is the most potent lacrimator and has the least systemic toxicity.[7]

Miscellaneous Synthetic Tear Gases

Much less widely used lacrimators include the following: Brombenzyl cyanide ($C_6H_5CHBrCN$) is known as CA in the United States and as Chamite in France

534

Ethyliodoacetate ($CH_3ICOOC_2H_5$) is the British SK
Bromacetone (CH_3COCH_2Br) is the American BA, the
French Martinite, and the German B-Stoff
Xylyl bromide ($C_6H_4CH_3CH_2Br$) is the German T-Stoff
Benzyl iodide ($C_6H_5CH_2I$) is the French Fraissite
Ethyl bromoethanoate ($CH_2BrCOOC_2H_5$)
Phenyl carbylamine chloride ($C_6H_5CNCl_2$)
Benzyl bromide ($C_6H_5CH_2Br$) is the French Cyclite
Acrolein (CH_2CHCHO) is the French Papite
Bromo-methyl ethyl ketone ($BrCH_2COC_2H_5$)
Chloracetone (CH_3COCH_2Cl) is the French Tonite
Iodoacetone (CH_3COCH_3I) is the French Bretonite.

Oleoresin of Capsicum

For some time, the US government has issued aerosol
sprays containing this oleoresin to postal carriers for
repelling animals, particularly dogs. Similarly, individuals may arm themselves with capsicum aerosols in
containers varying in size from that of a lipstick to a
fountain pen.

The oleoresin is a dark red, extremely acrid and pungent liquid that is extracted from cayenne pepper pods
with alcohol or ethyl ether. It irritates the conjunctivae
and the nasal and oral mucosa and can be classified as a
tear gas or lacrimator. Although organic synthetic lacrimators do not affect dogs and other animals as much as
they do humans, the oleoresin of capsicum is an efficient
repellent for both man and beast.

Cayenne pepper *(Capsicum frutescens)*, from which the
oleoresin of capsicum is extracted, is distributed worldwide and has the following names in different countries:
pimenton (Spain); *poivre rouge* (France); *cayennepfeffer*
(Germany); *kajennepeppar* (Sweden); *cayennepeper*
(Holland); *pepe di caienna* (Italy); *pimentao-de-caiena*
(Portugal); *kayenski pyerets* (Russia); *la-chiao* (China);
and *filfil ahmar* (Arabic). In Japan, cayenne pepper is
not known, but the closely related chili pepper *(togara-
shi)* is available. Cayenne pepper may colloquially be
called Guinea pepper, Spanish pepper, African pepper,
chilies, or bird pepper.[8]

PRIMARY IRRITANT REACTIONS TO TEAR GASES

All lacrimators in high concentrations are powerful skin
irritants and can produce first- and second-degree chemical burns. Third-degree burns with ulceration may
result, particularly with CS, in the presence of moisture
and occlusion. Stinging and erythema are produced
when CS is wetted.

Technicians and others handling lacrimators, particularly CS, may acquire an irritant dermatitis, especially
where there is constriction from wearing apparel, such

as at the neck and waist, or in intertriginous areas, such
as the axillae and vulva.[9]

Irritant and possible allergic contact dermatitis may be
severe in those on the wrong end of riot control sprays
containing CS. One report from France found that an
average of 6 days was needed in the hospital following
exposure.[10]

INDUSTRIAL CONTACT DERMATITIS DUE TO TEAR GAS

Shmunes and Taylor[11] reported that 25 of 28 workers in
a chemical plant manufacturing *ortho*-chlorobenzylidene
malonitrile (CS) gave a history of dermatitis involving
the arms and neck. Two of 25 workers showed positive
patch test reactions when tested with a 1:1,000 dilution
of CS in olive oil. The study reveals that in the industrial
setting, a significant sensitizing potential exists, but irritancy was the major factor in the production and perpetuation of the dermatitis.

Kanerva and colleagues[12] reported two cases of sensitization to CN and CS in workers following only one
accidental exposure.

LOCALIZED OCCUPATIONAL DERMATITIS IN POLICE OFFICERS FROM TEAR GAS

Tear gas is supplied to police in canisters and holsters.
Occasionally, such canisters may leak or become self-
activated, and discharge the tear gas. Such localized dermatitis occurs usually on the hip near the belt line of the
police officer who is wearing a can of Mace. Watson and
Rycroft[13] reported 7 cases of reactions to CS in police-
men. Three had ACD, documented by patch tests diluted
to 0.0001% in acetone. The others had ICD along with
worsening of seborrheic dermatitis (1 case), rosacea (2),
or leukoderma (1).

The manufacturers of chemical Mace aerosol tear gas
projectors state that the projectors should be carried with
the firing actuator downward in the pocket to make
them less conspicuous and to reduce the chances of
acciden7tal discharge. It is important to have the firing
actuator in the lock or safe position when carrying the
projector to reduce the chance of an accidental discharge.

ALLERGIC CONTACT DERMATITIS FROM TEAR GASES

ACD from chloracetophenone has been reported occasionally since as early as 1942.[14–17] It has been emphasized that the CN in Mace is a potent sensitizer, which
cross-reacts with dichloracetophenone but not with

para-chloracetophenone or bromoacetophenone. Although CS is also a sensitizer, it is not as potent as CN.

ACD from synthetic tear gas is typical eczematous dermatitis, often accompanied by marked edema. Contact sensitization to the oleoresin of capsicum is not common, but it suggests the possibility that ingestion of foods containing capsicum (spicy and ethnic foods, such as Mexican and Chinese) may produce an eczematous contact–type dermatitis. Diffuse erythema has been reported from the ingestion of capsicum.

PATCH TESTING WITH TEAR GASES

Great care must be taken in performing patch tests with tear gases, because the minimum irritating concentration is as low as 1 part in 100,000.

In Mace, CN is present in a 0.9% concentration. Patch tests may be performed with chemical Mace diluted 1 part with 100 parts acetone, which gives a 0.009% concentration of chloracetophenone. This concentration is not an irritant under a closed patch test and is sufficient to produce a positive allergic eczematous patch test reaction in sensitized individuals.

Patch tests with CS should be commenced with a 1:100,000 dilution in acetone. (It should be noted that CS dissolves with difficulty.) The other tear gases should be tested in a 1:100,000 dilution in ethanol to determine a concentration that is not irritating under a closed patch.

Capsicum may be tested in a 1% solution in ethanol.

MANAGEMENT OF TEAR GAS DERMATITIS

In sensitized individuals, the skin should be irrigated with copious amounts of water within a few minutes or dermatitis is inevitable. The lacrimator CS should also be removed with water as soon as possible. Although dry skin is unharmed initially by it, prolonged exposure may produce first- and second-degree burns and even ulceration. As soon as the individual begins to wash the powder off, a burning sensation and erythema occur but usually subside in an hour or so.

Barrier creams and petrolatum do not offer much protection from tear gas. Plastic clothing, including plastic helmets and visors, are the best protective devices available. Aluminum and or magnesium hydroxide (as found in antacid) apparently bind these agents and reduce bioavailability.

The treatment of primary irritation, burns, or allergic dermatitis from the tear gases is similar to the treatment of these conditions from other causes.

Ethylene Oxide Dermatitis

The most common types of cutaneous reactions to ethylene oxide gas are irritant reactions or burns, which may at times be severe. There are also a few reports of allergic reactions to this gas.

NATURE OF ETHYLENE OXIDE STERILIZATION

Ethylene oxide is a colorless, gaseous, simple epoxy compound whose sterilizing ability depends on its inherent toxic effect on all living cells. This is most likely because of ethylene oxide's ability to replace a hydrogen atom in protein molecules with hydroethyl (alkyl group), a process known as alkylation. Because this process is irreversible, the cell is killed. It is important, therefore, to remove all traces of ethylene oxide from the item sterilized before it comes into contact with human tissues. In addition, it is genotoxic.[18]

Gaseous ethylene oxide has become one of the major sterilizing agents of medical equipment and materials. Sterilization can be accomplished at low temperatures and humidity, thus avoiding damage to heat- or moisture-sensitive materials, as might occur with autoclave sterilization. Its highly diffusive nature and its permeability make it possible to sterilize through hermetically sealed plastic wrapping films, shipping cartons, and containers.

The ethylene oxide gas sterilization process consists of two essential parts: (a) sterilization by ensuring penetration of a sufficient concentration of the gas into all parts of load and (b) aeration until one is certain that all gas residues are eliminated from the sterilized items.

The Ethylene Oxide Subcommittee of the American National Standards Institute recommends the following precautions be taken to avoid the hazards of ethylene oxide sterilization:

1. Polyvinyl chloride or rubber materials sterilized with ethylene oxide should not be used within 7 days following sterilization, if stored at room temperatures.
2. Polyethylene (3 to 5 mL) and paper wrap are the best packaging materials. Nylon and polyvinylidine chloride are less permeable to ethylene oxide.
3. Polyvinyl chloride objects that have been gamma-irradiated should not be resterilized with ethylene oxide because large amounts of ethylene chlorohydrin will be formed.
4. "Disposable" items should be discarded after use because the by-products of later ethylene oxide sterilization may include ethylene chlorohydrin, which is a severe skin irritant.
5. Water droplets should be removed from material to be sterilized, to prevent the formation of ethylene glycol, a powerful irritant.

6. Ethylene oxide gas sterilization is indicated for equipment (e.g., ventilators) that is too bulky for steam sterilization and for certain plastics, whereas syringes, instruments, drapes, gowns, rubber, and some heat-resistant plastics can all be steam sterilized. It should be emphasized that the key to safety with ethylene oxide is proper aeration following sterilization.

IRRITANT DERMATITIS AND BURNS FROM ETHYLENE OXIDE

La Dage[19] reported a severe facial irritation from excess ethylene oxide in anesthesia masks. Hanifin[20] described six cases of contact dermatitis that were traced to residual ethylene oxide in prepacked nitrofurazone dressings. Ippen and Mathies[21] observed three workers who suffered from third-degree burns of the hands, forehead, axillae, periumbilical region, and the genitalia after cleaning a storage container that had traces of ethylene oxide. These authors suggest that, if an industrial case is seen, immediate treatment should be to rinse the affected area with water under pressure, such as may be obtained from using a hose. Contaminated garments should also be cleaned thoroughly.

Biro and colleagues[22] and Fisher[23] reported that 19 hospitalized women suffered postoperatively from severe burns of the buttocks and back from contact with reusable surgical gowns and drapes that had been sterilized with ethylene oxide and had not been properly aerated. Initially, an "epidemic" of bullous impetigo was suspected. Severe irritant reactions to detergents and antiseptics were also considered. The burned skin resembled a localized form of toxic epidermal necrolysis.

Testing samples of reusable gowns that had been worn by the patients showed that the amount of ethylene oxide residue varied from 3,600 ppm ethylene oxide to 10,800 ppm ethylene oxide. The safe level for ethylene oxide gas recommended by both the Health Industries Association (HIA) and the Z-79 Committee of New York Mount Sinai Hospitals is 200 ppm (maximum). The levels of residual ethylene oxide in the implicated gowns were thus determined to be 16 to 50 times the safe level for skin contact. Percutaneous absorption of ethylene oxide can be significant, especially under occlusion.[18]

OCCUPATIONAL EXPOSURE TO ETHYLENE OXIDE

Sporadic reports of irritant contact dermatitis (ICD) to ethylene oxide (ETO) have been published. A group of pharmaceutical workers in Israel, totalling 9 of 34 exposed persons, developed ETO ICD from overalls that were improperly aerated after ETO sterilization.[24] A level of 500 ppm ETO

was found in the garment bags. All patients developed severe pruritus, vesicles, and erythema around the wrists, which resolved after about 3 weeks. Hospital workers are not uncommonly affected, as discussed in a report by Romaguera and Vilaplana.[25] The four workers were exposed to ETO from a leaking sterilizing unit. Patch tests were not performed in either case.

Taylor[26] reviewed the effects of industrial exposure to ethylene oxide. He stated that cutaneous exposure to ETO usually occurs during production of the liquid chemical or as a result of its use as a gas sterilizing agent. Because of its importance as an industrial compound, ETO is among the top chemicals produced in the United States. It is used widely as a raw material in the synthesis of many organic chemicals, as a solvent and plasticizer in the production of high-energy fuels, and in large quantities for the manufacture of ethylene glycol, the main ingredient of permanent antifreeze.

Taylor[26] pointed out that ETO (C_2H_4O) is a clear, colorless liquid below its boiling point of 10.7°C; above this temperature it is a clear, colorless gas with a sweetish odor. Ethylene oxide is miscible with water in all proportions. The explosive decomposition of ETO vapors is a major industrial hazard. As little as 3% ETO vapor in the air will support combustion and will be violently explosive if confined. When ETO is used as a sterilizing agent, this hazard is prevented by dilution of the vapor with various inert gases.

If liquid ETO is spilled directly on the skin, it should be allowed to vaporize before being washed with water. All clothing contaminated with liquid ETO should be removed at once, especially shoes and gloves, and washed immediately with large quantities of water. First aid for acute inhalation exposure and protective measures to prevent exposure are available from local poison control centers and usually from hospital safety offices.

The hazards associated with production of ETO—well known to industrial toxicologists—include cutaneous burns, allergic contact dermatitis, mucosal irritation, acute inhalation toxicity, explosions, and fire. Pure anhydrous liquid ETO does not produce primary injury to the dry skin of workers, but solutions of ETO have a vesicant action and may cause conjunctivitis if splashed in the eye. Burns are more likely to occur when the solution is held in contact with the skin by clothing, gloves, and shoes. In common with other cutaneous irritants, repeated exposure may result in delayed allergic contact hypersensitivity.

Acute inhalation toxicity to high concentrations may manifest as mucosal irritation and pulmonary edema. Lower concentrations of vapor result in delayed nausea and vomiting. A threshold limit value of 50 ppm ETO by volume in air is said to offer an adequate margin of safety

Table 26-1 Hazards from Industrial Exposure to Ethylene Oxide
Allergic contact dermatitis
Acute inhalation toxicity
Cutaneous burns (irritant contact dermatitis)
Explosions
Fire
Mucosal irritation

from ostensible systemic effects.

Table 26.1 lists the hazards to industrial exposure, according to Taylor.[26] Table 26.2 lists medical supplies sterilizable by ethylene oxide.

ALLERGIC REACTIONS TO ETHYLENE OXIDE

Sexton and Henson[27] first experimentally produced ACD to ETO. Dolovich and Bell reported allergy to a product of ethylene oxide gas with demonstration of IgE and IgG antibodies and hapten specificity.[28] Their patient, on chronic hemodialysis, developed severe allergic reactions after exposure to articles such as plastic tubing and hemodialysis supplies that had undergone cold sterilization with ETO gas. It was shown that human serum albumin, exposed to ethylene oxide in the usual sterilization procedure, selectively elicited positive skin tests and *in vitro* histamine release.

Poothullil and colleagues[29] studied a patient who developed an anaphylactic reaction to ETO, and Bronk and van Ketel[30] described a patient with a postoperative delayed allergic contact reaction from a reusable operating room lift mat that had been sterilized with excessive ETO. Positive patch tests to ethylene oxide-sterilized patches and polyethylene glycol 300 were obtained. It

Table 26-2 Medical Supplies Sterilizable by Ethylene Oxide
Hospital central supply sterilizers
1. Telescopic instruments: bronchoscopes and endoscopes
2. Plastic goods: catheters, syringes, gloves, petri dishes, parts for heart-lung machines, and renal dialysis units
3. Rubber goods: tubing, surgical gloves, catheters, sheeting, and anesthesia face masks
4. Instruments: knives, needles, and speculae
Commercial sterilizers
1. Supplies listed above
2. Drugs and medication: anesthetic, otic, and ophthalmic solutions; surgical jellies; and nitrofurazone dressings
3. Implantable devices: sutures, prostheses, valves, and pacemakers

was suggested that the ACD could also be due to polyethylene glycol, a polymer of ethylene oxide and water. The breakdown products of ETO are ethylene glycol and ethylene chlorohydrin. Some allergic reactions to ETO may possibly be due to these breakdown products.

The Spanish investigators Romaguera and Grimalt[31] and Alomar and colleagues[32] reported allergic reactions from face masks sterilized with ETO. Allergic contact dermatitis to ETO has been reported in a nurse from a surgical gown and from suture material.[33,34]

PATCH TESTING FOR ALLERGIC REACTIONS TO ETHYLENE OXIDE

Romaguera and Grimalt[31] showed that their patient was allergic to ethylene oxide by exposing gauze to ethylene oxide. The gauze was ventilated for 8 hours and produced a strong reaction (+++) in the patient. Gauze that was ventilated for 24 hours had the same reaction, but the gauze that was properly ventilated for 48 hours produced no reaction.

Similarly, Alomar and colleagues[32] showed that in their patient, gauze and all materials sterilized with ethylene oxide at 24, 48, and 72 hours of ventilation showed positive reactions of ++ and +++ at 92 hours. Twelve controls tested simultaneously gave negative results.

One gauze sterilized 48 hours beforehand was introduced into a sterile glass tube with 15 mL of double distilled water, and 48 hours later a patch test with the water showed a ++ positive reaction at 96 hours.

Shupack and colleagues[35] reported patch materials that rapidly lose ethylene oxide, such as fabric or rubber, produced few reactions even at ethylene oxide levels as high as 5,000 ppm. A patch material that loses ethylene oxide more slowly in polyvinyl chloride (PVC) film produced reactions at ethylene oxide levels above 1,700 ppm. The patch materials that retained ethylene oxide the longest, thick PVC blocks and petrolatum applied to Webril pad, produced the most reactions. When the ethylene oxide level in those materials approximated 1,000 ppm or higher, irritant skin reactions usually appeared after 4 to 8 hours' contact. The level of reactivity among the volunteers was quite consistent. One subject, however, who developed allergy to ethylene oxide, showed a mild delayed reaction to approximately 1,000 ppm of ethylene oxide in PVC. Because little or no reaction developed to the patches containing ethylene oxide by-products, ethylene oxide itself was assumed to be the etiologic agent. The experiments support the conclusion that the lowest level of ethylene oxide that produces skin irritation in nonsensitized subjects approximates 1,000 ppm, when retained in slow-airing material against the skin for 4 hours or more.

Birnie and English noted that ethylene oxide and epoxypropane differ only by the addition of one methyl group in the latter. They propose that testing with this substance (1% pet) might be useful to detect ACD to ETO.[36] However, currently there are no reports of this having been done.

COMPOUNDS RELATED TO ETHYLENE OXIDE

Ethyl Chloride

This substance is used as a propellant and skin cooling agent. Allergy has been reported from its use in deodorants and in a local anesthetic spray.[37]

A single case report from Switzerland discussed a 30-year-old woman with patch test proven ACD to both ethyl chloride and Freon 12 (CFC 12), which was caused by use of these agents in a medical aerosol.[38]

Ethylene Glycol

This glycol is used in antifreeze solutions as a solvent and in lacquer, adhesives, resins, inks, and stains. Allergic reactions have been reported in its use in eyeglass lens manufacture. Patch testing is best performed with 3% in alcohol.[39]

Ethylene Chlorohydrin (Chloroethanol)

Ethylene chlorohydrin is a toxic solvent in polymers, lacquers, and insecticides. Wahlberg and Boman[40] stated that it can be absorbed through the skin.

Cellosolves (Methyl, Ethyl, Butyl, and Diethyl)

These cellosolves are monoalkyl ether of ethylene glycol, which are readily absorbed through the skin and can therefore produce poisoning by absorption as well as by inhalation. They are also strong solvents for paints, varnishes, plastics, and dyes and can cause defatting and drying of the skin.

Methylene Chloride (Dichlormethane, Carene)

This chemical may be added to freon sprays or may be used as an aerosol propellant by itself. It is a solvent and a degreasing agent and is a mild skin irritant because it can release hydrochloric acid in small amounts.

Trichloroethane (Methyl Chloroform)

This chemical may also be added to some freon sprays. It is a chlorinated hydrocarbon solvent and is used in the synthesis of many organic compounds.

Fowler[41] reported a case of contact urticaria in an eyeglass factory worker caused by trichloroethane. Immediate patch tests were positive, with negative delayed hypersensitivity tests. Ingber[42] reported a case of a metalworker exposed to trichloroethane used for cleaning metal plates.

Positive patch tests were seen at 1%, 0.1%, and 0.01% in olive oil with five negative controls.

Trichloroethylene

There have been reports worldwide of idiosyncratic reactions to trichloroethylene that resemble systemic drug hypersensitivity. This has been reviewed in the occupational medical literature.[43] The syndrome includes exfoliative dermatitis which may be as severe as toxic epidermal necrolysis.

Propellant Dermatitis

Halogenated hydrocarbons (freons), which were widely used in the past, have now been largely replaced either voluntarily or because of government restriction, because they have been shown to cause damaging effects on the earth's ozone layer. The following propellants are commonly used: propane, butane, isobutane liquified petroleum gases (LPGs), compressed gases (e.g., nitrogen or carbon dioxide), and gelled propellants.

DEODORANT SPRAY ALLERGY DUE TO FREONS

Occasional case reports of allergy to freons have been published.

Three patients with an acute eczema in the axillae after the use of a deodorant spray were investigated by van Ketel.[44] All three patients reacted positively to (open) patch tests with the propellant Freon 11 (trichloromonofluoromethane). One patient also reacted to Freon 12 (dichlorodifluoromethane). Of the other two patients, one developed an eczematous eruption after ethyl chloride had been sprayed onto the skin before biopsy was taken. Patch tests with ethyl chloride were performed on the other two patients and were found to be positive.

FEMININE "HYGIENE" (DEODORANT) SPRAYS

Feminine hygiene sprays, a euphemism for female genital deodorants, are more delicately called abroad "intimate" or "intime" sprays. These sprays are packaged mainly in an aerosol form consisting essentially of a fragrance, an emollient, and a propellant. Some sprays, in addition, contain an antibacterial agent.

Vulvitis and dermatitis produced by the sprays have been reported, principally by gynecologists, without distinguishing between irritant and allergic reactions.[45–47] Gowdy[47] stated that 26 instances of dermatitis were reported to the US Food and Drug Administration (FDA), principally the irritant variety, but surmised that some of the reactions may have been due to "allergic" reactions to hexachlorophene or perfumes. There is no mention of patch testing procedure in these 26 cases. Gowdy also cited three instances of the reaction in the genital area of the "consorts" of women who had used the sprays.

Fisher[48] reported that 30 women were patch tested to the individual ingredients in 12 different feminine hygiene sprays that had produced a vulvar and inguinal or thigh dermatitis. In addition, two men were tested who had acquired penile and scrotal dermatitis after having sexual intercourse with women who used the sprays just prior to sexual intercourse.

The propellants used were the fluorinated hydrocarbons. These include trichloromonofluoromethane (Freon 11), dichlorodifluoromethane (Freon 12), and tetrafluoromethane (Freon 14). The propellants are rare sensitizers but were probably the most common cause of an irritant dermatitis when the spray is applied too closely to the vulvar area.

Four positive patch test reactions were obtained. The specific ingredients that produced the positive patch test reactions and caused an allergic contact dermatitis and vulvitis from their presence in the sprays were benzethonium chloride, chlorhexidine, isopropyl myristate, and perfume.

References

1. Fisher AA. Dermatitis due to tear gases (lacrimators). Int J Dermatol 1970;9:91.

2. Hu H, Fine J, Epstein P, et al. Tear gas: harassing agent or toxic chemical weapon. JAMA 1989;262:660.

3. Stein AA, Kerwin WE. Chloracetophenone (tear gas) poisoning: a clinicopathological report. J Forensic Sci 1964;9:379.

4. Schwartz I, Tulipan L, Birmingham DJ. Occupational diseases of the skin, 2nd ed. Philadelphia: Lea & Febiger, 1957:466.

5. Fisher AA. Mace, a modern acronym and an ancient nomenclature. JAMA 1970;212:320.

6. Gleason MN, et al. Clinical toxicology of commercial products, 3rd ed. Baltimore: Williams & Wilkins, 1969, p. 301.

7. Blain P: Tear gases and irritant incapacitants. 1-chloroacetophenone, 2-chlorobenzylidene malononitrile, and dibenzyl(b,f)-1,4-oxazepine. Toxicol Rev 2003;22:103.

8. Rosengarten F. The book of spices. Wynnewood, PA: Livingston Publishing, 1969:129.

9. Penneys NS, Israel RM, Indgin SM. Contact dermatitis due to 1-chloracetophenone and chemical mace. N Engl J Med 1969;281:413.

10. Parneix-Spake A, et al. Severe cutaneous reactions to self-defense sprays. Arch Dermatol 1993;129:913.

11. Shmunes E, Taylor JS. Industrial contact dermatitis. Arch Dermatol 1973;107:212.

12. Kanerva L, Tarvainen K, Pinola A, et al. A single accidental exposure may result in a chemical burn, primary sensitization, and allergic contact dermatitis. Contact Dermatitis 1994;31:229.

13. Watson K, Rycroft R: Unintended cutaneous reactions to CS spray. Contact Dermatitis 2005;53: 9.

14. Frazier CA. Contact allergy to mace. JAMA 1976;236:2526.

15. Natrop KHE, Pinzer B, Hornk K. Skin lesions due to tear gas. Hautschaden Tranengas Dermatol Monatsschr 1975;161:678.

16. Holland P, White RG. The cutaneous reactions produced by o-chlorobenzyl-idenmalononitrile and w-chloroacetophenone when applied directly to the skin of human subjects. Br J Dermatol 1972;86:150.

17. Ingram JT. Dermatitis from exposure to tear gas. Br J Dermatol 1942;54:319.

18. Wester R, Hartway T, Serranzana, et al. Human skin in-vitro percutaneous absorption of gaseous ethylene oxide from fabric. Food-Chem-Toxicol 1997;35:513.

19. La Dage LH. Facial "irritation" from ethylene oxide sterilization of anesthesia face mask. Plast Reconstr Surg 1970;45:179.

20. Hanifin JM. Ethylene oxide dermatitis. JAMA 1971;271:213.

21. Ippen H, Mathies V. Protracted chemical burns (ethylene oxide). Berufsdermatosen 1970;18:6.

22. Biro L, Fisher AA, Price E. Ethylene oxide burns: a hospital outbreak involving 19 women. Arch Dermatol 1974;110:924.

23. Fisher AA. Post-operative ethylene oxide dermatitis. Cutis 1973;12:177.

24. Lerman Y, Ribak J, Skulsky M, et al. An outbreak of irritant contact dermatitis from ethylene oxide among pharmaceutical workers. Contact Dermatitis 1995;38:280.

25. Romaguera C, Vilaplana J. Airborne occupational contact dermatitis from ethylene oxide. Contact Dermatitis 1998;39:85.

26. Taylor JS. Dermatologic hazards from ethylene oxide. Cutis 1977;19:189.

27. Sexton RJ, Henson EV. Experimental ethylene oxide human skin injuries. Arch Ind Hygiene Occup Med 1950;2:549.

28. Dolovich J, Bell B. Allergy to product(s) of ethylene oxide gas: demonstration of IgE and IgG antibodies and hapten specificity. J Allergy 1978;62:30.

29. Poothullil J, Shimizu A, Day RP, Dolovich J. Anaphylaxis from the products of ethylene oxide gas. Ann Intern Med 1975;82:58.

30. Bronk WJ, van Ketel WG. A possible case of delayed hypersensitivity to ethylene oxide. Clin Exp Dermatol (Oxford) 1981;6:4.

31. Romaguera C, Grimalt F. Irritant dermatitis from ethylene oxide. Contact Dermatitis 1980;6:351.

32. Alomar A, Camarasa JMB, Noguera J, Aspinolea F. Ethylene oxide dermatitis. Contact Dermatitis 1981;7:205.

33. Ulrich M, Berner D, Volz T, et al. Delayed-type hypersensitivity dermatitis to ethylene oxide. Contact Dermatitis 2005;53:303.

34. Dagregorio G, Guillet G: Allergic suture material contact dermatitis induced by ethylene oxide. Contact Dermatitis 2004;49:123.

35. Shupack JL, Andersen SR, Romano SJ. Human skin reactions to ethylene oxide. J Lab Clin Med 1981;98:723.

36. Birnie A, English J: Ethylene oxide allergy may have been confirmed by patch testing to a similar compound. Contact Dermatitis 2006;55:126.

37. Kriechbaumer N, Hemmer W, Focke M, et al. Sensitization to ethyl chloride in a handball player. Contact Dermatitis 1998;38:227.

38. Bircher A, Hampl K, Hirsbrunner P, et al. Allergic contact dermatitis from ethyl chloride and sensitization to dichlorodifluoromethane (CFC 12). Contact Dermatitis 1994;31:41.

39. Dawson TAJ. Ethylene glycol sensitivity. Contact Dermatitis 1976;2:233.

40. Wahlberg JE, Boman A. 2-chloroethanol—percutaneous toxicity of a solvent. Dermatology 1978;156:299.

41. Fowler JF. Contact urticaria to 1,1,1-trichloroethane. Am J Contact Dermat 1991;2:239.

42. Ingber A. Occupational allergic contact dermatitis from methyl chloroform (1,1,1-trichloroethane). Contact Dermatitis 1991;25:193.

43. Kamijima M, Hisanaga N, Wang H, et al. Occupational Trichloroethylene exposure as a cause of idiosyncratic generalized skin disorders and accompanying hepatitis similar to drug hypersensitivity. Int Arch Occup Environ Health. 2007;80:357.

44. Van Ketel WG. Allergic contact dermatitis from propellants in deodorant sprays in combination with allergy to ethyl chloride. Contact Dermatitis 1976;2:115.

45. Kaye BM. Hazards of feminine hygiene sprays for women. JAMA 1970;212:2121.

46. Davis BA. Irritancy from feminine hygiene sprays. Obstet Gynecol 1970;36:812.

47. Gowdy JM. Feminine deodorant sprays. N Engl J Med 1972;287:203.

48. Fisher AA. Allergic reaction to feminine hygiene sprays. Arch Dermatol 1973;108:801.

CHAPTER 27

PLASTICS, ADHESIVES, AND SYNTHETIC RESINS

EXECUTIVE SUMMARY

Plastics consist of large numbers of long chainlike molecules made from small molecules (called monomers) linked together. These chainlike molecules are called polymers, and the process of linking the monomers together is called polymerization. Adhesives and surface coatings are often composed of the same types of polymers. Depending on their nature, these materials can set or cure (polymerize) on their own or with application of heat or mixing with curing agents. In the vast majority of cases, once a material is completely polymerized it is no longer allergenic. While in theory chemical reactions generally follow to a conclusion, in practice some non-polymerized material may remain in certain plastics. Allergic contact dermatitis (ACD) occurs primarily to the uncured monomers, diluting agents, or setting agents. Accordingly, most cases of ACD to these chemicals are occupational in origin. Workers involved with manufacturing plastic vehicle components and sporting goods, and manufacturing or applying adhesives and paints are at risk for ACD to these agents. One notable non-occupational exposure is allergy to acrylates in dental and medical devices. The constant contact with a hearing aid, prosthesis, or denture allows for occasional ACD to these types of finished products to occur.

The main allergens in this category are epoxy resins, epoxy hardeners, acrylates, and formaldehyde resins. Many other plastic components have been occasionally reported to cause allergy, however. Effective patch testing usually requires supplemental allergen series tailored to the known exposures of the patient. Testing with patient-supplied materials may be necessary, but must be done cautiously to avoid false positive irritant reactions.

Plastics chemicals that commonly cause dermatitis are epoxy resins and phenol-formaldehyde plastics, which can cause allergic and irritant dermatitis. Carbamidformaldehyde and acrylic plastics can cause allergic reactions. Polyester plastics may produce irritant and rarely allergic dermatitis. Rare causes of dermatitis among the plastics are polypropylene, polyurethane, Teflon, furene, polycarbonates, silicones, carbonyls, coumarone, cellulose derivatives, polystyrene, polyvinyl chloride (PVC), polypropylene chloride (PPC), polyvinyl acetate (PVA), polybutadiene nitrile alkyds, and polyethylene.

The various types of plastics are presented here on the basis of their chemical composition. Other ways of considering plastics include the way they set and the way they are polymerized (addition or condensation).

Cellulose-based plastics were discovered by Alex Parkes (Birmingham, UK) in the 1860s and the first synthetic, Bakelite, was invented in 1907 by Leo Baekeland.[1] Bakelite's first use was as an electrical insulator. Modern plastics have improved on the flexibility and workability of Bakelite. Polystyrene and polyvinyl plastics came along, followed by polyamide (nylon). More recently, epoxies, acrylics, and other plastics have been invented.

Cellulose Ester Plastics

These plastics are used in eyeglass frames, hearing aids, steering wheels, toothbrush and hairbrush handles, tool handles, pens, and toys. In addition, the following are cellulose products: cellophane, rayon, cellulose nitrate (celluloid), collodion, pyroxylin, gun cotton, and cellulose film. These products, particularly eyeglass frames, may produce both irritant and allergic reactions.[2]

Industrial sensitization readily develops in workers exposed to the additives used in the manufacture of the cellulose ester plastics. More rarely, the finished products can produce allergic contact dermatitis.

Jordan and Dahl[2] found the principal sensitizers in these plastics to include the following:

1. *Resorcinol monobenzoate.* An ultraviolet absorber, which may crossreact with balsam of Peru but not with resorcinol. This chemical is not widely used at present.
2. *Azobenzene dyes*
3. p-*tert-butylphenol.* A sensitizer and depigmenting agent used for heat stabilizing.
4. *Ethylene glycol monoethyl ether acetate.* A solvent used to weld nosepads to eyeglass frames and laminate plastic sheets.
5. *Plasticizers.* The phthalates are the most common plasticizers in cellulose ester plastics and are rare sensitizers. The plasticizer triphenyl phosphate, which is used for cellulose acetate and nitrocellulose, has been found to cause allergic contact dermatitis in a plastic glue. A 5% in petrolatum concentration is recommended for testing.[3]

Table 27.1 lists the materials that should be used for patch testing individuals suspected of having allergic dermatitis from cellulose ester plastic.

Epoxy Resins

The epoxy resins are one of the most important causes of occupational dermatitis in plastics and coatings industries, both in the United States and in other countries.

The versatile epoxy (epoxide or ethoxylene) resins are used widely in manufacturing electrical equipment for enclosing transformers, condensers, and other components; in vehicle manufacturing plants to make many automobile, boat, and aircraft components; in construction of many sporting goods such as tennis rackets, skis, etc.; in production of many other plastic materials; in paints for surface coating; and in many industries for adhesive purposes (Figure 27-1).

INGREDIENTS OF EPOXY RESIN SYSTEMS

In the manufacture and use of epoxy resins, individuals may acquire dermatitis from one or more of the follow-

Table 27-1 Patch Tests for Cellulose Ester Plastic Sensitivity	
Substance	Percentage in vehicle
Cellulose acetate flakes	As is
Cellulose acetate flakes ethyl ketone (MEK)	10% in methyl
Cellulose acetate plastic	As is
Cellulose acetate propionate plastic	As is
Cellulose acetate butyrate plastic	As is
Carbon black	1% pet
Black dye mixture	1% pet
Solvent yellow 3 (Color Index No. 11160)	1% pet
Solvent red 26 (Color Index No. 26102)	1% pet
Other colorants of black dye mixture	1% pet
Ethylene glycol monoethyl ether acetate	5% in MEK
Potassium acid oxalate	0.5% aq
p-tert-butylphenol	2% pet
Dimethyl phthalate	As is
Diethyl phthalate	As is
Tricresyl phosphate	5% pet
Triphenyl phosphate	5% pet
Phenyl salicylate	2% pet
Resorcinol monobenzoate	1% pet
2,29-dihydroxy-4,49-dimethoxybenzophenone	1% in MEK

ing chemicals, which may be incorporated in the epoxy resin system:

Blends of other resins

Catalytic agents consisting of amines and anhydrides, which are called converters, hardeners, or curing agents

Fillers

Pigments

Plasticizers

Reactive diluents

Solvents

Uncured epoxy resin (liquid or solid)

The most frequently encountered sources of occupational dermatoses from epoxy resins have been diglycidyl ether of bisphenol A (DGEBA), which is the standard patch test screening substance, 4,49-diaminodiphenylmethane, phenyl glycidyl ether, or o-cresyl glycidyl ether.[4] Epoxy systems based on Bisphenol F (DGEBF) have also been reported to cause ACD, less commonly. A series of compounds and patch test concentrations have been recommended (Table 27.2).

Uncured Epoxy Resins

At least 90% of epoxy resins used worldwide are based on diglycidyl ether of bisphenol A (DGEBA). A typical uncured epoxy resin is obtained by the condensation

Table 27-2 Patch Testing of Patients Exposed to Epoxy Resin Compounds

Test substance	Concentration % (w/w) in pet
Epoxy resins (ER)	
Standard epoxy resin (DGEBA-ER)	1
DGEBF	1
Amine hardeners (AHs)	
Ethylenediamine (EDA)	1
Diethylenetriamine (DETA)	1
Hexamethylenetetramine	1–2
Triethylenetetramine (TETA)	0.5
4,49-diaminodiphenylmethane (MDA)	0.5
Isophoronediamine (IPDA)	0.5
Reactive diluents (RDs)	
n-butyl glycidyl ether (BGE)	0.25
phenyl glycidyl ether (PGE)	0.25
o-cresyl glycidyl ether (o-CGE)	0.25
Allyl glycidyl ether (AGE)	0.25
Butanediol diglycidyl ether (BDDGE)	0.25
Hexanediol diglycidyl ether (HDGE)	0.25
Neopentyl glycol diglycidyl ether (NPGDE)	0.25
Glycidyl ester of synthetic fatty acids (Cardura E 10)	0.25
Glycidyl ether of aliphatic alcohols (Epoxide 8)	0.25
Others	
Bisphenol A	1
Epichlorohydrin	0.1–0.3
BIS-GMA	2
BIS-MA	2

w/w = by weight; pet = petrolatum.

of epichlorohydrin and p,p9-isopropylidenediphenol (bisphenol A). Other epoxy resins such as DGEBF, are condensates consisting of a mixture of polyglycidyl ethers. Epoxy resins are of little use in the form in which they are supplied to the market. They must be further polymerized or cured by the addition of curing agents, such as amines, amides, anhydrides, or inorganic fluoride compounds. Cured epoxy resins are hard, relatively insoluble materials that are nonirritating and nonsensitizing. Epoxy resin (DGEBA) is a well-known allergen. ACD has also been reported with other resins including heterocyclic dimethylhydantoin epoxy resin, phenol novolate epoxy resin (DGEBF), and brominated epoxy resin.[5] These latter substances are found in electrical insulation, coil winding and cleaning of work sites, respectively. DGEBF has superior heat resistance properties. The Dow Chemical Company's website states the global epoxy market is: building and construction 21%, power coatings 16%, industrial coatings 15%, structural composites 15%, electrical 12%, can coatings 12%, auto coatings 9%.

One of the largest surveys of allergy to epoxy resins in a single industry reported that 66 (20%) of 325 patch-tested workers had positive patch tests to occupational allergens.[6] Allergy to the epoxy resin in the standard series (DGEBA) was found in 34 workers, while 26 reacted to both DGEBA and DGEBF. Only two had reactions to DGEBF without reacting to DGEBA. There were several reactions to other epoxy resins while 9 workers had 14 positive patch tests to various reactive diluents (diglycidyl ethers). Hand dermatitis was the primary complaint.

Pratt and colleagues reported on 100 patients with dermatitis from a company in Ottawa involved in assembly of fiberoptic devices.[7] While 56 had hand dermatitis, 84 had facial and/or neck dermatitis, suggesting airborne ACD. Thirty-six reacted to DGEBA and 45 reacted to one or more DGEBF resins, 10 of whom were negative to DGEBA. There were assorted reactions to other epoxy resins and diluents and to acrylic resins.

A report from Finland detailed occupational epoxy allergy seen over 22 years.[8] Of 182 workers, 146 reacted to DGEBA. Reactions to other resins were seen in 17, and there were 85 positive patch tests to diluents, hardeners, etc. Single reactions were seen in 130 patients. It is unclear how many were tested to DGEBF, however.

In a study of industrial painters in Norway working in the petroleum industry, 23 workers had ACD to epoxy systems, an incidence rate of 4.5/1000 person-years.[9] Seventeen were allergic to DGEBA, with the others reacting to various hardeners.

A report from several North American centers discussed cross reactivity among various epoxy resins.[10] Forty-one patients (24 females) known to be allergic to DGEBA were tested to 23 epoxy-related allergens. The great majority (92–95%) reacted to DGEBF and/or epoxy phenol novolac resin. Eight patients (20%) reacted to one or more epoxy acrylates while 13 (32%) reacted to tosylamide epoxy resin. Twelve reacted to phenylglycidyl ether.

Wind turbine rotor blade production is a significant industry in Sweden. A report of 325 workers who were patch tested found ACD in 20%. DGEBA (1% pet) accounted for half of this number. Twenty-six were allergic to DGEBF (all but 2 also to DGEBA). A number also reacted to various hardeners.[11]

A contact dermatitis puzzle was solved when it was found that a patient was allergic to his public transit pass—a plastic card. He carried the card in his shirt pocket, which corresponded to the site of dermatitis. He was allergic to cycloaliphatic epoxy resin in the coating of the card.[12]

For patch testing purposes, bisphenol A may be used in a 1% concentration in petrolatum. This is a standard patch testing substance on most series. It must be emphasized that a negative reaction to bisphenol A does not rule out epoxy dermatitis, because the epoxy dermatitis may be due to curing agents.

Catalysts and Curing Agents

These chemicals speed the polymerization of epoxy resin. Liquid epoxy compounds can be cured to form hard, insoluble products by polymerization in the presence of catalysts or by polyaddition with cross-linking agents containing active hydrogen atoms. These curing agents or hardeners may act at either room or elevated temperatures and have been divided into the following four categories:

1. Amine hardeners (e.g., aliphatic polyamines and aminopolyamides)
2. Acid hardeners (e.g., polycarboxylic acids and dicarboxylic acid anhydrides)
3. Aldehyde condensation products (e.g., phenol, melamine, and urea-formaldehyde resins)
4. Inorganic or organic metallic compounds (e.g., boron trifluoride, titanium acid ester, and aluminum alcoholate)

Of this host of chemicals, amine hardeners appear to be the most frequent sensitizers.

Epoxy Amine Hardeners

The amines are used particularly when the epoxy resin is cured, catalyzed, or self-hardened at room temperature. These agents are usually aliphatic amines, such as diethylenetriamine, triethylenetetramine, and metaphenylenediamine, an aromatic amine hardener. In the uncombined state, they are caustic and can produce severe burns on contact with the skin. In addition, they can cause severe ACD characterized by severe redness, edema, and itching of the exposed skin. The aliphatic hardeners, diethylenetriamine and triethylenetetramine, are powerful water-soluble skin irritants. Airborne ACD has been reported from the widely used hardener isophoronediamine (3-aminomethyl-3,5,5-trimethylcyclohexylamine). A 0.5% petrolatum patch test concentration was used.[13]

There are several reports of ACD due to epoxy resin curing agents. (see Table 27.2 for patch test recommendations).[14–17]

Reactive diluents used in epoxy resin systems include the glycidyl ethers. De Groot[17] identified three chemical plant employees who were sensitized to alpha-naphthyl glycidyl ether and *p*-fluorphenyl glycidyl ether. A patch test concentration of 1% in petrolatum was positive in all sensitized workers. A guinea pig maximization assay of alpha-naphthyl glycidyl ether sensitized all 20 animals.

Other reactive diluents that have been reported to cause contact dermatitis are listed in Table 27.2.

Marble workers who were exposed to both epoxy resin and reactive diluents developed contact dermatitis more commonly to the diluent than the resin.[18] The most frequent diluent was ortho-cresyl glycidyl ether in 10 of 22 workers. In this same group, only four patients reacted to epoxy resin.

A group of subway construction workers were allergic to m-xylene diamine or hexanediol glicidyl ether. Only a few reacted to the epoxy resins themselves.[19]

A study from Germany looked at allergy to epoxy resins and especially to the hardeners and diluents. Among the reactive diluents, 1,6 hexanediol diglycidyl ether 1,4 butanediol glycidyl ether were most commonly positives (after the resins) at almost 20%. Other glycidyl ethers were occasionally positive. M-xylene diamine was the most common hardener allergen at 14%.[20]

Other Hardeners

Another class of epoxy hardeners is the phthalic anhydrides. Kanerva and colleagues[21] reported a patient who was allergic to methylhexahydrophthalic anhydride. This compound and methyltetrahydrophthalic anhydride have been associated with contact urticaria and immunologically mediated respiratory disease. Their patient had coexistent immediate and delayed hypersensitivity.

Unusual Epoxy Allergies

At times a product will produce contact dermatitis, but upon product analysis it has been found that the ingredients are not the stated ingredients and the contaminant present in the material is the actual allergen. This is somewhat common in the plastic/acrylate type of resin systems. A case of this type was reported by Dooms-Goossens and colleagues.[22] A 43-year-old man who worked in the plastics industry was allergic to epoxy silane, but the actual allergen was a contaminant allyl glycidyl ether, which is a reactive epoxy diluent.

An aircraft factory worker developed urticaria and angioedema when working around epoxy resins.[23] Delayed-type patch tests were negative, but patch tests applied for 30 minutes, removed, and read showed immediate whealing from epoxy resin 1% in petrolatum, phenyl glycidyl ether 0.25% in petrolatum, and cresyl glycidyl ether 0.25% in petrolatum. In discussing his case, Sasseville[23] pointed out that aliphatic polyamine hardeners, phthalic anhydrides, and epoxy resins have caused immediate reactions. The reactive diluents, which are highly volatile, was an unexpected additional finding.

The fact that patients sensitized to ethylenediamine hydrochloride from exposure to original formula

Table 27-3 Uses of Epoxy Resins

Adhesives
  All-purpose, aircraft, electrical, constructional, domestic, ceramic, metallic, waterproof, furniture, furnace gaskets, fiberglass, and metal cements
Product finishing
  Aircraft, road and bridge coating, appliance finishes, appliance primers, automotive primers, can and drum linings, chemical resistant finishes, pipe and tank linings, flame retardants, industrial floorings, equipment (marine, masonry finished), and wall panel coatings
Laminates
  Structural, electrical, and fibrous reinforcements, and filament windings
Electrical
  Encapsulations for transformers, coils, and motors
Polyvinyl chloride films in which epoxy resins have been used as stabilizers and plasticizers
  For example, in plastic gloves, adhesive tapes, plastic panties, handbags, chamber pots, and beads in necklaces
Miscellaneous industrial
  Applications: toolings and die casting, model making, jigs and fixtures, molding and patterns, marine varnishes, artistic and sculptural use

Mycolog cream may show crossreactions with certain "amine" hardening agents may be important.[15,24]

Lachapelle and Lachapelle-Ketelaer[25] reported cross-sensitivity between an isophorone amine and isophorone disocyanate.

Table 27.3 shows the numerous exposures from the use of epoxy resins. Epoxy resin dermatitis has been described from a pacemaker and from a hemodialysis set.[26,27] There are several reports of epoxy resin adhesives and glues that have produced unusual forms of contact dermatitis.[28]

Fregert and colleagues[29] traced a hand dermatitis in a patient who had a contact dermatitis of the hands due to an unhardened epoxy resin that he had applied to certain sign boards. These authors emphasized that epoxy resin hardened at room temperature is seldom if ever completely cured.

At times a product will produce contact dermatitis, but upon product analysis it has been found that the ingredients are not the stated ingredients and the contaminant present in the material is the actual allergen. This is somewhat common in the plastic/acrylate type of resin systems. A case of this type was reported by Dooms-Goossens and colleagues.[22] A 43-year-old man who worked in the plastics industry was allergic to epoxy silane, but the actual allergen was a contaminant allyl glycidyl ether, which is a reactive epoxy diluent.

Microscope immersion oil containing epoxies and hardeners caused a mini-epidemic of ACD in Canadian laboratory technicians.[30]

Epoxy-Induced Contact Vitiligo

This has been reported to the resin and/or the diluents, in only 2 cases.[31]

Epoxy-Induced Scleroderma?

Two cases of scleroderma allegedly due to inhalation of an epoxy plasticizer, bis (amino methyl cyclohexyl) methane have been reported.[32]

Occupational Contact Urticaria

Hardeners for epoxy resins include dicarboxylic anhydrides. Inhalation of such compounds has led to urticaria, and skin contact with methylhexahydrophthalic anhydride and methyltetrahydrophthalic anhydride caused contact urticaria in patients with only airborne exposure.[33]

Polyfunctional aziridine hardener (PFA), which is used in paints, primers, lacquers, and other protective coatings, has caused both contact urticaria and contact dermatitis.[34] PFA hardener is synthesized from ethyleneimine or propyleneimine and a multifunctional acrylate such as pentaerythritol triacrylate or trimethylolpropane triacrylate (TMPTA). PFA hardener has been found as a contaminant in some TMPTA. In cases of dermatitis, no reactions were found to the materials from which PFA hardener is synthesized. A 1% aqueous concentration of PFA hardener is recommended for patch testing. Aziridine hardeners are associated with polyurethane plastics.

The epoxy hardener 2,4,6-tris(dimethylaminomethyl) phenol is a sensitizer but is not commonly found on commercially available resin series. Brooke and Beck[35] found a 0.5% concentration free of irritant reactions in 50 controls and suitable for identification of allergy.

Amine hardeners were a source of contact dermatitis in a Finnish painter.[36] Over the years he was followed, he reacted to multiple hardeners, one of which had not previously been reported to cause contact dermatitis: tetraethylenepentamine.

Dermatitis rather than urticaria occurred after airborne exposure to the epoxy resin hardener 3-amino-methyl-3,5,5-trimethylcyclohexylamine.[37] A patch test concentration of 1% in petrolatum is recommended.

Dahlquist and Fregert[38] proposed that when the face and eyelids are involved in an epoxy dermatitis, it is probable that there has also been sensitization to the curing agent or hardeners. The volatility of epoxy resin is so low that it is unlikely that sufficient fumes are in the air to involve the face. This indicates the importance of patch testing patients with suspected epoxy resin dermatitis with the hardeners. A greater emphasis on patch testing with the hardeners that the patient has actually used should enable further preventive recommendations to be made.

Blends of Other Resins

Epoxy resins may be blended with urea-formaldehyde, phenol-formaldehyde, and melamine-formaldehyde resins, all of which are potential sensitizers and irritants.

Non-occupational Exposure to Epoxy Resins

Epoxy glues are available for household use. They come in two parts, the hardener and the resin. The labels on the containers state that ingredients contacting the skin should immediately be removed with soap and water. Artists and sculptors find many uses for these glues, and some have acquired epoxy resin dermatitis.

Allergic contact stomatitis may occur from acrylic dental filling materials, and some contain epoxy portions.[39] A patient was allergic to an acrylic material and was also allergic to epoxy resin from the standard tray. In the product, the main acrylic compounds were triethylene glycol dimethacrylate and 2,2-bis-[4-(2-methacryloxypropoxy)-phenyl]propane (bis-GMA). Because both epoxy resin and bis-GMA are derivatives of bisphenol A, it is likely that the positive patch test to epoxy resin was due to cross-sensitivity to the bisphenol A derivatives in the dental resin.

Taylor[40] identified the source of epoxy resin positive patch tests in three children who had been wearing certain sizes of Sears, Roebuck and Co. Toughskin or Roughouser jeans with knee patches. Each child had eczema about the knees and also had positive patch tests to pieces of knee patches. Epon 828 (4,4-isopropyledene diphenylepichlorhydrin) was added to the knee patch adhesive as an adhesion promoter. One child had a positive patch test to Epon 828 at a dilution of 1:20,000. Sears substituted a nonepoxy adhesive for the knee patch of its jeans.[40]

In years past, approximately 5% to 10% of the underwear produced in Japan was said to be treated with an epoxy-lanolin softener.[41] Epidemics of genital dermatitis were not reported, at least in the English language literature.

LOW AND HIGH MOLECULAR EPOXY RESINS

The low molecular resins are more potent sensitizers than the high molecular variety. The low molecular epoxy resins have a lower viscosity and have a much greater ability to wet and penetrate the skin than do the higher variety. It is mainly the epoxy resin oligomer of molecular weight 340 that is responsible for epoxy resin allergy.[42] Occasionally, however, an epoxy resin of high molecular weight may produce sensitization, and some products regarded as safe because of high average molecular weight may contain significant quantities of the molecular weight 340 oligomer.[43] When this oligomer and the oligomer of molecular weight 624 are absent, the product can usually be regarded as relatively safe for practical purposes.

It should be emphasized that patch testing with the various epoxy resins in a "routine" series may fail to detect epoxy resin sensitivity unless one tests with the patient's own sample of epoxy resin and with one of many epoxy hardeners or diluents.

PREVENTION OF EPOXY RESIN DERMATITIS

Sigfrid Fregert, who made outstanding contributions to the study of various types of contact dermatitis, suggested that the following criteria should be met to help prevent epoxy resin dermatitis (International Symposium in Lund, Sweden, 1977):

1. Epoxy oligomer of molecular weight 340 should not be included, or at least only in a low concentration.
2. Epoxy oligomer of molecular weight 624 should probably be present only in a low concentration.
3. Reactive diluents should be of the high molecular weight type, probably over 1,000.
4. Hardeners should be of the adduct type and should not contain remains of aliphatic amines. It is probable that even polyaminoamides are free from risk when they do not contain remains of aliphatic amines.

Estlander and colleagues[44] found that the epoxy chemical bisphenol A can be found in some PVC gloves (see below).

Formaldehyde Resins

Formaldehyde may be combined with the chemicals listed in Table 27.4 to produce various types of resins. Individuals allergic to a formaldehyde-based resin, except for textile resins, usually do not react to formaldehyde itself.

Table 27-4 Types of Formaldehyde Resins

Cashew nut shell oil
Melamine
Phenols (including *p*-tert-butylphenol)
Resorcin
Urea (dimethylene urea)

PHENOL-FORMALDEHYDE RESINS

The phenols listed in Table 27.5 are used in phenol-formaldehyde resins.

Products such as paper laminates and Bakelite are examples of phenol-formaldehyde resins. Fregert[45] reported that Bakelite may produce both allergic and irritant dermatitis. Two patients gave a positive patch test to Bakelite powder 10% in petrolatum.

Table 27-5 Phenols Used in Phenol-Formaldehyde Resins	
Alkyl phenols	Phenol
Bisphenol A	Resorcinol
Cresol	Xylenol
p-tert-phenylphenol	

P-TERT-BUTYLPHENOL-FORMALDEHYDE RESINS

These resins are used in many adhesive and glue formulations, particularly in shoes, and are common sensitizers.[45–50] As a rule, the sensitizing agent in these phenol-formaldehyde resins is the p-tert-butylphenol or the entire resin, and not the phenol or formaldehyde.

Occupational groups at greatest risk are adhesive workers, plywood and box makers, foundry workers, dental personnel, brake-lining workers, textile manufacturers and handlers, insulation makers, leather finishers, automobile industry workers, and shoemakers.

Table 27.6 lists some of the wide variety of exposure to p-tert-butylphenol. An unusual case of occupational aphonia and dyspnea with type 1 and type 1 hypersensitivity to p-tert-butylphenol-formaldehyde in glass-wool was described by Kalimo and colleagues.[51]

p-tert-butylphenol has proved to be a depigmenting agent in several patients.[49,52] (See Chapter 22.)

p-tert-butylcatechol (PTBC) has been incorporated into both acrylic and polyester prosthetic devices. It was found in PVC manufacturing, where occupational leukoderma can occur.[53] Styrene frequently contains PTBC at a final concentration of 0.005%

Table 27-6 p-tert-Butylphenol: Uses and Where Found
Antioxidant and heat stabilizer in neoprene cements
Color film developers
Demulsifier for oil field drilling use
Deodorants and commercial disinfectants
Duplicating paper
Germicide detergents
Insecticides
Intermediate for rubber antioxidants
Intermediate in manufacture of varnish and lacquer resins
Leather articles laminated with neoprene contact cement
Motor and synthetic oils
Plasticizer for cellulose acetate
Printing inks
Resins to give latex glues initial adhesive force
Rubber cements, especially in shoes
Stabilizer in some cellulose ester plastics

in cured resin, which has been reported to cause dermatitis.[53]

The resin systems in marking pens can cause contact dermatitis.[54] Ingredients identified include ninhydrin, arochean (phenolic formaldehyde maleic anhydride resin), 2-hydroxy-5-tert-butyl benzylalcohol, and 2,6-bis (hydroxymethyl)-4-tert-butylphenol. The latter compound is thought to crossreact with the common screening allergen 4-tert-butylphenol formaldehyde resin.

Edwards and Edwards[55] reported that a Styrofoam flotation device known as "spoodles" due to a physical resemblance to noodles caused eight cases of axillary dermatitis, three of which were patch tested to the device with positive results. They incriminated polystyrene as the allergen, but no chemical analysis for contaminate or uncured resins was done. One of their patients exhibited contact urticaria to the patch test as well as delayed vesicular reaction.

Use of a standard group of allergens to screen for plastic and glue sensitization was evaluated in 839 patients over a period of 7 years.[56] Only 52 had any reaction to this collection of 31 allergens, and the most prevalent was p-tertiary-butylphenol-formaldehyde resin (9 cases). There were 7 cases of diaminodiphenyl methane sensitivity and 5 colophony sensitive cases.

The standard patch test material p-tert-butylphenol formaldehyde resin can be a clue to sensitization to p-tert-butyl catechol. Zimerson and Bruze[57] were able to identify p-tert-butyl catechol as present in some brands of p-tert-butylphenol formaldehyde resin. Phenyl formaldehyde resin–sensitive patients were found to be commonly allergic to 2-methylol phenol and at times to other closely related methylol phenols.[58]

Patch testing with PTBC has been usually performed at 1% in petrolatum. German investigators are concerned that this may actively sensitize, so a lower concentration may be recommended.[59]

UREA-FORMALDEHYDE RESINS

These thermosetting resins may be used in textile resins, wood glues, pressed-wood products, foam insulation, and surface coatings. Formaldehyde may be released from some of these materials, especially when new.[60] Hjorth and Fregert[61] reported that of 67 patients sensitized by urea-formaldehyde, 51 (76%) also reacted to formaldehyde.

MELAMINE-FORMALDEHYDE RESIN

Melamine-formaldehyde is a rare sensitizer. It is used extensively in tableware because the polymerized resin

Table 27-7 Patch Testing with Formaldehyde Resins
1. Phenol-formaldehyde resins 10% in pet
2. *p*-tert-butylphenol-formaldehyde resin 10% in pet
3. *p*-tert-butylphenol 10% in pet
4. Formaldehyde 2% in water
5. Hexamethylenetetramine 1% in pet
6. Furfuraldehyde 5% in water

has good heat and water resistance and does not stain readily.

There is one report of an orthopedic cast reinforced with melamine-formaldehyde resin that produced a formaldehyde dermatitis in several patients.[62] Fregert[63] described formaldehyde dermatitis from gypsum molds containing melamine-formaldehyde. Romaguera and colleagues[64] reported purpura from formaldehyde-urea-melamine resin. Patch testing allergens for formaldehyde resins are listed in Table 27.7.

CASHEW NUT SHELL OIL–FORMALDEHYDE RESIN

Cashew nut shell oil has been combined with formaldehyde to form brake linings and clutch facings. ACD may occur due to the presence of urushiol in the cashew nut shell in patients sensitive to poison ivy, oak, or sumac.

Acrylic Plastics

The widely used acrylic resins, like the epoxy resins, may produce many instances of allergic and irritant dermatitis (Figure 27-2). Specific exposures, such as in dental materials or artificial fingernails, are discussed more thoroughly in other chapters.

GENERAL USES OF ACRYLIC RESINS

There are a multitude of uses for acrylates. Many plastic household and industrial components are acrylic-based. Many adhesives and inks are made from acrylates. Dentures and other dental materials, artificial joints, hearing aids, artificial eye lens implants, and prostheses may be made of acrylics or use acrylic cements. Artificial fingernails and many nail hardeners are made of acrylic. Acrylate polymers are used in hair sprays and other cosmetics. Some possible exposures to acrylic compounds are listed in Table 27.8. Acrylates and methacrylate compounds are used in leather finishing, as a textile size, in adhesives, paints, oil additives, and windows, and to produce artificial rubber and synthetic fibers. Moreover, diacrylates can be used as cross-links between polycondensates of unsaturated polyesters, for example, electron beam copolymerization in spray paints to multiple large surfaces such as doors,

Table 27-8 Possible Exposures to Acrylic Compounds
Construction
Paint, adhesive, sealer and stopper, additive to concrete
Cosmetics
Hair spray, fragrance, dentifrice, nail polish, and insecticide
Medical
Eye, dental, vascular, prostheses, heart valve, artificial joint, contact lens, eyeglasses, adhesive plaster, wound spray, infusion system, and splint
Printing
Ultraviolet curable ink, photopolymer and flexographic printing plate
Textile
Fiber, finish (and on leather)
Utensils
Plexiglas, veneer, and synthetic rubber
Miscellaneous
Plastic foam, molecular, sieve, gel electrophoresis, additive to lubricant, mineral sedimentation, soil improver, and water purification

or in the production of photopolymer printing plates. Ethyl acrylate has been used for decades as a basic material in compounding perfumes, but the Research Institute for Fragrance Materials discourages its use for this purpose.

CYANOACRYLATE GLUES (CRAZY GLUE, SUPER GLUE)

These glues contain no solvents. Although they are irritating to the eyes and respiratory tract when vaporized, allergic reactions are considered unlikely because of the immediate bonding of the acrylate to surface keratin. The liquid glues are hygroscopic but do not mix with water; the rapid polymerization reaction with water is exothermic. Nylon, vinyl, or rubber gloves should not be used, but polyethylene or polypropylene gloves are satisfactory.

Cyanoacrylates polymerize readily in air at room temperature and are used as adhesives for metal, rubber, glass, and plastics, and also in surgery to bind tissues and to seal wounds. Cyanoacrylates bond strongly to keratin, and isobutyl cyanoacrylate, which polymerizes when moist, has been used to fix vertebral discs and to prevent leakage from ileostomy appliances.

Calnan[65] reported patients with a slight irritant facial contact dermatitis and eye irritation, which was attributed to a vapor generated from a cyanoacrylate glue when spoiled parts of the glue were heated during soldering. The complaints were dropped after the humidity of the environmental air was raised. What would have been present in the vapor as alkyl cyanoacrylate monomer became polymerized by the water content of the air to an inert material.

Ethyl cyanoacrylate is used as a contact adhesive for metal, glass, rubber, plastics, and textiles. It is used to seal human tissues and is commonly referred to as "super glue". When contact dermatitis is suspected, the monomer may polymerize on Finn chambers and give false-negative reactions. Suspension in petrolatum retards the polymerization. A concentration of 0.032% to 10% has been found adequate.[66]

Only a few cases of contact dermatitis due to cyanoacrylates have been reported. Belsito[67] found three patients who were allergic to ethyl cyanoacrylate in artificial nail "wraps," and Tombs and colleagues[68] reported finger and eyelid dermatitis from occupational use of ethyl cyanoacrylate used to glue on artificial hairs. A 10% concentration in petrolatum is used for patch testing. Artificial nails made of cyanoacrylate glue have caused dermatitis in clients of nail salons as well as in nail technicians. Cases are relatively infrequent. One worker achieved adequate protection by wearing polypropylene gloves.[69] Contact dermatitis to ethyl cyanoacrylate has also been reported to mimic small plaque parapsoriasis.[70]

First-Aid Treatment for Skin Bonded with Cyanoacrylate Adhesive

Human skin can become accidentally bonded to itself by a cyanoacrylate adhesive. One manufacturer states, "In the event of such an accident, surgery should never be necessary to separate the bonded skin—simple first aid procedures are the best treatment." Do not try to pull the bonded surfaces apart with a direct opposing action. Immerse the surfaces in warm, soapy water. Peel or roll the surfaces apart by using a blunt edge such as a spoon handle. Wash adhesive off the skin with soap and water. Another manufacturer advises the use of acetone to dissolve the adhesive bond.

Margo and Trobe[71] noted that cyanoacrylate adhesives have been used for a wide range of industrial and domestic purposes since they were first commercially introduced. Their widespread availability in plastic containers resembling ophthalmic medicinal dispensers in size and shape has created a new consumer safety problem. Three patients mistakenly instilled cyanoacrylate adhesives into the eyes, resulting in firm upper-to-lower lid adhesion and transient keratoconjunctivitis. In one patient, the "tarsorrhaphy" had to be undone with scissors.

ACRYLIC NAILS

The original concerns about acrylic nails focused on methyl methacrylate. Freeman and colleagues[72] reported four cases of acrylic nail–related changes consisting of nail fold, fingertip, and hand dermatitis, as well as face and neck reactions and dystrophic nails and fingertip paresthesias. Three of their cases were due to ethylene glycol dimethacrylate, and these cases did not react to methyl methacrylate. Although current artificial nail products may be free of methyl methacrylate, the other acrylates are excellent sensitizers as well. (See Chapter 16.)

A study of 11 patients with acrylate allergy associated with artificial nails found the most frequent sensitizers to be ethyl acrylate, 2-hydroxyethyl acrylate, ethylene glycol dimethacrylate, ethyl alpha cyanoacrylate, and triethylene glycol diacrylate.[73]

PRESSURE-SENSITIVE ADHESIVES

The term "pressure-sensitive adhesive" (PSA) refers to a type of adhesive that, when in a dry state, adheres to a variety of surfaces merely by application of light bond pressure.[74–79] PSAs were first developed in the mid-1980s for use on surgical tapes. Many products now utilize PSAs. The major markets are the tape and label industries. All of these products are combinations of two components: backing and the adhesive. Several backing materials are used, such as fabric, paper, and plastic films. PSAs are usually classified by the chemical nature of the elastomer. Natural rubber was the first elastomer used in PSAs and is still commonly used today, along with acrylates. Major applications for natural rubber adhesives include packaging, masking, electrical, and double-sided tapes.

There are several methods of applying PSAs[80]: (a) organic solvent solutions, (b) water-based emulsions, (c) hot melts, and (d) radiation (UV or electron beam). Solvent-based PSAs predominate. Solvent-based adhesives consist typically of various elastomers in conjunction with tackifiers, plasticizers, ultraviolet inhibitors, fillers, antiozonants, and antioxidants. In acrylic PSAs, the most commonly used monomers are 2-ethylhexyl acrylate, butyl acrylate, ethyl acrylate, and acrylic acid. Some nonacrylic monomers, such as vinyl acetate, are also used to modify the polymer properties. Many other compounds have been used in the synthesis of acrylic PSAs.

Allergy to Pressure-Sensitive Adhesives

Following a positive patch test from a PSA (e.g., a piece of a tape or label tested closed for 48 hours), testing with the standard screening tray may point to an allergen such as rubber, acrylate, colophony, or epoxy resin. It may be necessary, however, to identify the specific PSA components. It is possible some industrial PSAs, not normally intended for skin contact, might irritate the skin following a 48-hour patch test occlusion.

Acrylic Medical Pressure-Sensitive Adhesives

Single component adhesives were developed to avoid the allergic reactions and irritability associated with rubber-based adhesives. These adhesives are usually formed by combinations of an acrylic ester monomer with a polar monomer. The acrylic ester monomer is replaced occasionally with an acrylic monomer combined with another type of monomer, such as vinyl acetate. These acrylic-based adhesive tape glues are less allergenic than the rubber-based glues, because the amounts of uncured monomers are negligible in the acrylic tapes.[81]

Heskel and colleagues[76] reported two patients with eczematous reactions to Curad brand medical adhesive plastic bandages who were found to be allergic to the N-dodecyl maleamic acid monomer (5% in pet). Vehicle-specific patch test reactions also occurred from N-octodecyl maleamic acid (1% aqueous and alcohol but not 1% in pet), undecyl polyethylene oxymaleic acid ester (1% aqueous and alcohol but not 1% in pet), and octylmaleic acid ester (1% in pet but not 1% aqueous and alcohol). Two patients of Heskel and colleagues[76] were patch test negative to 3 ethylhexyl acrylate (3-EHA).

In 1975, Jordan[82] reported seven volunteers who developed contact sensitivity to Curad adhesives that were used to hold testing materials in place during the course of predictive patch testing. All seven volunteers were allergic to 2-EHA (5% in olive oil); three also reacted to N-tert-butyl maleamic acid (1% in pet), whereas none reacted to the remaining two acrylate components (acrylonitrite 5% in olive oil and ethyl acrylate 5% in olive oil). N-tert-butyl maleamic acid is not used in Curad adhesives, and Jordan's subjects may have demonstrated a crossreaction to a chemical in the same generic class as dodecyl maleamic acid. Jordan's patients tolerated another adhesive tape (Dermicel Hypoallergenic Cloth Tape; Johnson & Johnson, New Brunswick, NJ).

Scanpore tape also contains 2-EHA.[83] In one guinea pig study, sensitized animals failed to show reactions to Scanpore tape because the concentration of free penetrable 2-EHA was very low.[83]

Other acrylic glues used in adhesive tape include cyanoacrylates and tetraethylene glycol dimethacrylate. When methyl 2-cyanoacrylate polymer, used as a medical adhesive, degrades, one of the products is formaldehyde.[74]

Backing (Facing) of Medical Pressure-Sensitive Adhesives

Fregert and colleagues[81] reported 28 patients, reacting to an adhesive tape (Leukoflex-Beiersdorf AG, Hamburg) used in routine patch testing, who had positive patch test reactions to diphenylthiourea (DPTU) and phenylisothiocyanate (PITC) present in the PVC backing (not the adhesive) of the tape. These 28 positive reactors represented 1.1% of 2,491 patients who were routinely tested with DPTU 1% (w/w) in petrolatum. Fifteen of the 28 had positive patch tests to higher dilutions, one at 0.000001% (w/v) of DPTU. PITC was positive at 0.1% (v/v) in acetone and in four patients at 0.0001% (v/v).

Some of the subjects also had positive reactions to diethyl- or dibutylthiourea, thiram mix, colophony, or abitol. DPTU is a heat stabilizer in the PVC and is partly decomposed to PITC. The two substances were also found in a PVC blister package for salt and pepper shakers. As a result of Fregert's report, DPTU was removed from the tape backing. It has not been established, however, if other sensitizers are present in the PVC used as backing.[81]

Foussereau and colleagues[84] described a patient who reacted to polythene in the patch unit and was sensitive to colophony and abietic acids. Similar reactions have occurred with the Al-test.

ULTRAVIOLET-CURED ACRYLATE GLUES

Television manufacturing workers may be exposed to acrylate glues. In a report from Poland, 21 of 81 workers had dermatitis related to the use of acrylate glues cured by UV radiation. ICD was found in 12 and ACD in 9. None reacted to methacrylates, but all were allergic to various acrylates and diacrylates.[85]

ANAEROBIC ADHESIVES

Anaerobic sealants are liquid, thermosetting industrial adhesives that polymerize rapidly in the absence of air.[86] Chemically, they are based primarily on esters of acrylates and methacrylates. Anaerobic adhesives are packaged in small volumes in low molecular weight polyethylene containers. The free passage of oxygen through the container walls inhibits cure during shipping and storage. These single component adhesives also contain initiators, accelerators, and other additives.

Anaerobic adhesives are used for locking screws firmly in position, as gaskets, as paper sealants, and for retaining and mounting cylindrical parts, particularly in the automotive industry. Industrial exposure is most common, but occasional exposure occurs from home or hobby use. The Loctite brand is one of the most popular in the USA.

Most early cases of contact allergy from anaerobic sealants emanated from Europe. Allardice,[87] Magnusson and Mobacken,[88] and Jansen[89] each reported hand dermatitis among European automotive assembly workers handling acrylic or methacrylic acid ester adhesives. Cronin[90] reported three men and one woman who were allergic to dimethacrylate screw sealants. Cronin described the dermatitis as affecting principally the pulps of the fingers, causing a dry, scaly eczema, which was chronic and uncomfortable rather than incapacitating. Positive patch tests included dimethacrylate ester (5%) and tri- (5%), tetra- (1%), and polyethylene glycol dimethacrylate (5%).

In 1982, Dempsey[91] in the United States described two cases of allergic hand eczema from Loctite compounds and one case from Sta-Loc 1250 Green anaerobic sealant and Sta-Loc 600 Redi-Form Gasket. The allergen in one product was polyurethane dimethacrylate and in another was glyceryl methacrylate. Each allergen was positive at 1%. One patient was tested with ethyl and methacrylate, each at 1%, and was positive to both.

Mathias and Maibach[92] saw three electronic assembly workers with eczema of the fingers who were allergic to polyethylene glycol dimethacrylate found in an anaerobic sealant. Onycholysis developed in one worker, and no crossreactions to methyl methacrylate developed. This again emphasizes the necessity for patch testing with the specific resin to which an individual has been exposed. In some instances, disposable plastic gloves and careful handling techniques (e.g., application of sealant to the screw socket rather than the screw) may permit affected individuals to continue work duties with the sealant. Automatic dispensing devices are used in some operations.

New materials continue to be used as acrylic sealants. An anaerobic sealant contact dermatitis is most commonly traced to dimethacrylates, but 1-acetyl-2-phenylhydrazine has also been reported.[93] This latter substance should be tested at 1% in petrolatum.

CIRCUIT BOARDS

The manufacture of circuit boards involves the use of silk-screen application of inks. Allergens identified in this process include diaminodiphenylmethane, 2-hydroxyethyl methacrylate, and triglycidyl isocyanurate.[94] The latter is a trifunctional epoxy compound made from epichlorohydrin and isocyanuric acid. It is a hardener in thermosetting one-component polyester powder coatings, and it has been patch tested at a concentration of 0.1% to 10% w/w in petrolatum.

ACRYLATE IN PRINTING PLATES

Various acrylates are used to make printing plates. Positive patch tests were obtained to 2-hydroxyethyl methacrylate (0.1% in alcohol), diethylene glycol dimethacrylate (1% in methyl ethyl ketone), and tetraethylene glycol dimethacrylate (1% in methyl ethyl ketone).[95]

Tetraethylene glycol dimethacrylate, acting as an irritant and a sensitizer, caused an outbreak of dermatitis in a newspaper plant.[96] Beurey and colleagues[97] recommended 0.5% to 0.1% of the resin for patch testing with these compounds.

IV INFUSION SETS

Needles are secured to plastic supports for IV infusion sets, with glues that may cause ACD. Allergens include epoxy resins and acrylates. The UV-cured acrylates that have caused contact dermatitis in IV infusion sets include isobornyl acrylate, betacarboxyethyl acrylate, and 1-benzoylcyclohexanol.[98]

ACRYLIC BONE CEMENT USED IN ORTHOPEDIC PROSTHESES

Orthopedic surgeons, surgical personnel, and dental workers have developed ACD of the hands from exposure to the methyl methacrylate monomer, which passes through rubber gloves.[99–101] Better protection may be obtained by wearing two pairs of gloves and discarding them immediately.

Fisher[102] reported that paresthesias in the involved fingers of the medical personnel sometimes lasted months after discontinuation of contact with the cement. Monomethyl methacrylate, after it penetrates the skin, may have an untoward effect on naked myelinized nerve fibers and on the Ranvier nodes.[103] Acrylamide neurologic effects have also been described.[104] Such effect on the peripheral nervous system in individuals with acrylic monomer dermatitis of the hands may explain the prolonged burning and tingling sensations that accompany the dermatitis.

ALLERGIC REACTIONS TO ACRYLIC BONE CEMENT IN ARTIFICIAL JOINT REJECTION

Metals in joint replacement have been implicated rarely in failure of an orthopedic implant. It seems possible that a rare case of allergy to acrylates could also cause dermatitis, poor wound healing, or joint failure. Delayed-type allergy to methyl methacrylate monomer has been found rarely in patients undergoing hip surgery,[105] perhaps because the sensitizers in these cements come in contact initially with the bloodstream.[106] This situation may promote the production of T suppressor cells.

ULTRAVIOLET-CURED ACRYLATES IN THE PRINTING INDUSTRY

The usefulness of the acrylates to the printing industry comes about because certain acrylic compounds can be made to polymerize almost instantaneously by exposure to ultraviolet light. They can therefore be used both in quick-drying inks and in the rapid production of printing plates from photographic negatives. Polymerization by ultraviolet light in one instance dries the ink and, in the other, hardens the plate where the photographic negative allows light through. The popularity of the UV-cured inks has grown because they are efficient and simple to use. Exposure to ultraviolet light rapidly cured

Table 27-9 Acrylate Inks: Light-Sensitive or UV Cured Acrylates: Components of UV Cured Inks

Multifunctional acrylic monomers (MFAs) (these bind together acrylate resins)

Photoinitiator

Benzophenone, benzoin, or chlorinated aromatic compound

Reactive base prepolymer with terminal acrylate group: acrylated polyesters, polyethers, urethanes, or epoxy resins

the liquid solution into a plastic coating, eliminating the need for heating or the use of a solvent evaporator.

Reports of ACD have come from both applications. In almost all cases the acrylate involved did not crossreact with methyl methacrylate. Also, irritant reactions are common, necessitating patch test concentrations sometimes as low as 0.1% to avoid false-positive reactions. Individuals with negative patch tests to acrylates have been reported as having a phototoxic dermatitis from mixed isomers of amyl dimethylaminobenzoate, which are used as absorbers of ultraviolet light to initiate the reaction.

Ultraviolet (UV)-cured inks are based on three components (Table 27.9). The first component is a reactive base prepolymer with terminal acrylate groups that may make up 80% of the formulation. They are usually acrylated polyesters, acrylated polyethers, acrylated urethanes, or acrylated epoxy resins. The second component is a photoinitiator, often benzophenone, benzoin, or a chlorinated aromatic compound. The third component is the multifunctional acrylic monomers (MFAs) that are used as diluents with cross-linking properties to bind together the acrylated resins.[107]

The polyfunctional acrylic monomers should be regarded as relatively potent allergic sensitizers, and care should be taken accordingly to minimize their contact with the skin in their industrial use. Good industrial hygiene practices to minimize direct skin contact with the inks are critical to reducing the incidence of ACD in workers.

There are several reports of allergic reactions to the various acrylic compounds used in ultraviolet-cured inks.[107–110] Although not often reported these days, cases are still seen to the UV inks, either with or without UV exposure.

Goossens and colleagues[111] reported on a man exposed to a UV ink in the printing of athletic shirts. He washed off UV-irradiated screens and was found allergic to ethylene glycol dimethacrylate and bis-GMA (an epoxy acrylate). He also reacted to tripopylene glycol diacrylate. Airborne contact dermatitis occurred from urethane diacrylate used as part of an ultraviolet-cured ink process in printing of lottery tickets.[112]

PHOTOTOXIC REACTION ASSOCIATED WITH ULTRAVIOLET-CURED ACRYLIC INKS

Emmett and colleagues[113] described four workers employed in the manufacture of ultraviolet-cured inks who complained of photosensitivity characterized by an intense burning sensation during sun exposure. Dermatitis developed on exposed areas in three of these workers following sun exposure. Six compounds used as photoinitiators in the ink formulations were found to absorb solar ultraviolet radiation. Two preparations of mixed isomers (ortho and para) of amyl dimethylaminobenzoate were found to be phototoxic.

These responses could be prevented in two subjects by the application of a 10% sulisobenzone sunscreen prior to sun exposure. Two other photoinitiators, Michler's ketone and thioxanthone, were phototoxic *in vitro* but not after topical application *in vivo*.

The phototoxic reactions, observed with the two industrial preparations of undiluted mixed isomers of amyl dimethylaminobenzoate, were considered surprising as purified amyl *p*-dimethylaminobenzoate is demonstrably effective as a sunscreen at a 5% concentration. No phototoxicity was observed in these employees when a 5% concentration of amyl *p*-dimethylaminobenzoic acid was applied.

MISCELLANEOUS CASES OF ALLERGIC CONTACT DERMATITIS TO ACRYLATES

Windshields are repaired with acrylates, and contact dermatitis to common acrylate allergens has been seen in workers exposed to this material. Hydroxyethyl methacrylate is one of the allergens likely to be found in this setting.[114] Chemists are exposed to novel compounds and concentrations of compounds that may not occur widely in the environment. A 31-year-old chemist developed contact dermatitis to glycidyl methacrylate and ethoxyethyl acrylate used to make textiles and paper water resistant.[115] A concentration of 0.05% in acetone was positive to both compounds, and nitrile gloves were protective if used for no more than 1 day.

Since the late 1980s, Australian money has been printed with UV acrylate inks. Two cases of ACD from the banknotes were reported. Both patients reacted to multiple acylates, diacrylates, and methacrylates. The Australian government unsurprisingly did not divulge the exact composition of the inks.[116]

Both hydroxyethyl acrylate (HEA) and hydroxyethyl methacrylate (HEMA) have been the source of acrylate problems among medical and dental-related fields. 2-hydroxyethyl acrylate was found to be the primary sensitizer in Lowicryl embedding medium.[117] Protection was afforded by 4-H gloves but not vinyl or latex gloves. The hydropad of a transcutaneous electrical nerve stimulation (TENS) unit caused contact dermatitis due to its HEMA content.[118]

Irritant Acrylate Reactions

Bullous irritant reactions in workers in the platemaking industry may be due to the irritant effect of tetraethylene glycol diacrylates. These diacrylates can also produce allergic reactions in sensitized persons who were unable to continue their work even when protected by gloves. The 4-H glove has been recommended for protection against acrylates.[119] This same glove has been found to be effective in epoxy resin exposure for up to 8 hours.[120]

PATCH TESTING WITH ACRYLIC COMPOUNDS

The most recent NACDG patch test series includes 2-HEMA, methyl methacrylate (MMA), and ethyl acrylate(EA). The most recent data finds a rate of positive reactions of 1.6% of 5143 patients to MMA and 1.1% to EA.[121]

Use of a screening series of 30 acrylates in 275 patients over a 10-year period of time in Finland revealed that the most commonly encountered allergenic substances were 2-hydroxyethyl acrylate (12%), 2-hydroxypropyl methacrylate (12%), and 2-hydroxyethyl methacrylate (11%).[122] This should not be taken to imply that these substances are the most allergenic, as frequency of use and likelihood of contact with skin or mucous membranes have a controlling influence in the type of patient seen in patch test clinics. Further investigation from Sweden showed that both 2-HEMA and ethylene glycol dimethacrylate should be tested at 2% petrolatum; that about half the patch test reactions persisted for at least 1 month; and that a rare reaction did not appear until day 10.[123]

Cavelier and colleagues[124] reported that the irritancy of the whole group of acrylates makes them difficult compounds with which to patch test. Concentrations that are too high irritate and even actively sensitize.[125] In order to avoid too low a dilution, the patch test concentrations recommended may be on the borderline of irritancy, and reactions are difficult to interpret.

Thus, methyl methacrylate monomer may be tested 1% in olive oil or petrolatum, whereas pentaerythritol triacrylate should be tested 0.2% in petrolatum. The hazards of patch testing with too high a concentration include an increased likelihood of sensitization. Kanerva and colleagues[99] reported that 14% (3 of 21) patients screened for acrylate allergy were actively sensitized by the patch test procedure. A 0.5% concentration of ethyl acrylate, 2-hydroxyethyl acrylate, and 2-hydroxypropyl acrylate was incriminated, and the concentration was lowered to 0.1%. When a patient became sensitized by the 0.1% concentration, these three acrylates were dropped from the screening series of (meth)acrylates.[99]

Glycidyl methacrylate may give reactions to methacrylate-sensitive patients as well as to those sensitized to epoxy resins. The same holds true for a diacrylate ester of an epoxy resin (e.g., diglycidyl ether of bisphenol A), a member of a class of products called epoxy acrylate resins. These may be used for applications involving ultraviolet light or electron beam–initiated cross-linking.

With guinea pig test methods, monoacrylates are more potent sensitizers than corresponding monomethacrylates, and this is reflected in human experience.[83] The allergic tendency of acrylic ester monomers decreases as the size of the acrylic ester group increases. The di- and tri-acrylate esters are potent allergens whose frequency of sensitization increases as the number of unsaturated groups in the monomer increases.[74–76,126,127]

The ingredients declared on material product safety data sheets can be unreliable in terms of a full disclosure of the true components of acrylic resins. Henriks-Eckerman and Kanerva[128] used gas chromatography and mass spectrometric methods to analyze 10 acrylic products.

ACRYLIC RESIN SYSTEM COMPONENTS

The resin accelerator N,N-dimethyl-paratoluidine has been widely used and is reported as a cause of burning, sore mouth in patients with acrylic dental plates.[129] A 1% to 5% petrolatum patch test concentration has been used. Benzoyl peroxide is a common curing agent and has also been a source of prosthesis dermatitis.[130]

Plastics frequently contain ultraviolet light-absorbing materials to protect them from photodegradation. One such material, Tinuvin (P-(2-(2-hydroxy-5-methylphenyl) benzotriazole)) has been added to spandex, ostomy bags, and plastic watch straps and is also in cosmetics. In spandex, its concentration drops >80% with washing. No crossreactions have been noted to other benzotriazoles, and patch tests at 0.01%, 0.1%, 1.0%, and 5.0% in petrolatum have all been positive.[131] Phenyl salicylate is another photoprotectant used in plastics. It is a UV blocker at 230 to 330 nm, and is used as an antiseptic and intestinal disinfectant as well as an occasional ingredient in some skin creams.[132] Plastic safety glasses have been found to cause contact dermatitis due to the presence of this allergen.[132]

INITIATORS

Acrylates often include initiators to propagate the production of free radicals needed for chain production. One such compound is 2.29-azobis(2-amidinopropane) dihydrochloride [AAPH], which caused an outbreak of dermatitis in workers manufacturing this substance. Eight cases of dermatitis were reported by Takiwaki and colleagues.[133] Both 1% and 5% aqueous solutions of AAPH were positive in all eight cases and negative in six controls. AAPH is also being used in biomedical research concerning lipid peroxidation and antioxidants.

Another free radical donor is methyl ethyl ketone peroxide. This crossreacts with benzoyl peroxide, and both irritant and allergic contact dermatitis can result from exposure. Keratitis is another potential exposure hazard of methyl ethyl ketone peroxide. This chemical is used in plastic resin systems such as fiberglass-reinforced plastics.[134]

SOLVENTS

Nitromethane is a solvent used for acrylics and other adhesives, and also in fuels. Webb and Fowler saw four cases of ACD to this in automotive workers from one company. Avoidance was curative.[135]

Polyester Resins

There are many uses for polyester resins, ranging from casting and laminating to the manufacture of bathtubs to automobile bodies. Most of the workers at risk for contact dermatitis are employed in the manufacturing industries. The incidence of allergic sensitization is small compared with the extensive skin contact that occurs among these workers. Dermatitis results usually from irritation by solvents and fiberglass. The irritating components or inclusions of the polyester plastics are polybasic acids (phthalic anhydride), polybasic alcohols (propylene glycol), styrene (vinyl benzene), fiberglass, and acetone. The chief sensitizers have been reported as peroxide catalysts and cobalt.[136–138]

Table 27.10 lists the ingredients of a polyester resin system and the concentration for patch testing. The unsaturated polyester is a condensation product of an unsaturated dibasic acid and glycol that may be tested 10% in acetate.

Diethyleneglycol maleate, a hardener in a polyester resin system caused ACD in a car body repairman.[139]

Burrows and Campbell[140] reported on spin finishes, liquid dressings applied to synthetic fibers in the course of manufacture to facilitate their processing. Fourteen cases of dermatitis possibly due to spin finishes were found in a factory that manufactured polyester yarns. Patch testing with all of the constituents of the spin finishes being used during the period excluded any allergic cause. A direct irritant effect from the oils and surfactants was probably responsible.

Table 27-10 Patch Testing Polyester Resin Systems

Unsaturated polyester resin 10% in acetone
Cross-linking agents
  a-methylstyrene 1% pet
  Methyl methacrylate 5% pet
  Styrene (vinyl benzene) 1% in olive oil
  Vinyl toluene 1% in olive oil
Inhibitors
  Hydroquinone 5% pet
  Quinone 5% pet
  p-tert-butylcatechol 1% in acetone
Organic peroxide catalysts
  Benzoyl peroxide 5% pet
  Cumene hydroperoxide 0.5% pet
  Cyclohexanone peroxide 0.5% pet
  Methyl ethyl ketone peroxide 0.5% pet
Activators (accelerators)
  Cobalt naphthenate 5% pet
  Cobalt octate 5% pet
  Diethylaniline 10% in alcohol
Ultraviolet energy absorbers
  Benzophenone 5% pet
  Benzotriazoles 1% pet
Reinforcers
  Fiberglass—do not patch

Triglycidyl isocyanurate is used primarily in polyester coatings as a hardener, but it is also found in electrical insulation, inks, adhesives, and circuit boards. To identify this allergen in a paint factory worker, 5% in methyl ethyl ketone was used.[141]

POLYETHYLENE

Contact urticaria has been reported from polyethylene gloves. Multiple positive scratch tests were reported to plasticizers and stabilizers, but only 3 controls were reported.[142]

POLYSTYRENES

Polystyrene is available as sheets that can be cut and shaped, as molding pellets that can be fused, as foam sheets (Styrofoam) that can be cut with hot wire cutters, and as expandable polystyrene beads for foam molding. Cutting or sewing of factory-fresh or large slabs of Styrofoam releases the colorless, odorless gas methyl chloride and can release any trapped styrene monomer. In small amounts, methyl chloride can cause symptoms of drunkenness; in large amounts, it can cause dizziness, staggering, and even death. Open flames should be avoided when using expandable polystyrene beads because they contain flammable pentane gas. Some styrene cements used in cement Styrofoam contain styrene monomer.

STYRENE (VINYL BENZENE, STYROL)

This chemical, sometimes used to modify polyester monomer, is an unsaturated hydrocarbon obtained from storax (styrax) balsam. Styrene may have an irritating, drying, and defatting effect on the skin, but it rarely produces allergic dermatitis. Because storax is used in the preparation of compound tincture of benzoin, and in some perfumes and soaps, allergic sensitization to styrene carries with it the possibility of crossreaction with benzoin compounds and some soaps. Styrene can be removed from the skin with acetone. For patch testing purposes, either 1% styrene in olive oil or 2% styrene in petrolatum can be used.

Styrene liquid is also sometimes used in acrylic resin powder to form dentures. The polystyrenes may also be used for denture material. Styrene not only is a synthetic industrial compound, used in polyester and other resins, but can also occur in nature, for example, in raspberries, in which it is formed by enzymatic decarboxylation of cis-cinnamic acid.

It has caused ACD from vinyl toluene,[143] and may produce occupational dermatitis.[144]

Polyurethanes (Isocyanate Resins)

Table 27.11 lists the occupational exposures to isocyanates that are chemicals with the general formula R-(N=C-O)n. They react with hydroxyl groups of polyols and form polyurethane. The isocyanates used in industry include several compounds. The most common is toluene diisocyanate (TDI).[145] TDI is a strong irritant but is not a common sensitizer.

Table 27-11 Occupational Exposure to Isocyanates

Adhesive workers
Casts for splints
Foundry core binders
Insulation workers
Lacquers
Organic chemical synthesizers
Paints
Polyurethane flexible and rigid foams
Polyurethane sprayers
Ship welders
Spray painters
Surface coatings
Synthetic rubber
Toluene diisocyanate (TDI)
Wire coating workers

PATCH-TESTING PROBLEMS WITH ISOCYANATES

TDI and 4,4-diphenylmethane diisocyanate (MDI) can both be patch tested at 1.5% in petrolatum Swedish investigators, however, have shown that MDI degrades within several months down to almost nothing, if kept at room temperature. Storage in a freezer prevented the degradation.[146]

ALLERGIC CONTACT DERMATITIS TO ISOCYANATES

A medical equipment factory saw an outbreak of eczema in 16 workers. An isocyanate adhesive, dicyclohexylmathane-4,4-diisocyanate (DMDI) was positive in 13, with several more positives to other isocyanates.[147] All the positives were to aliphatic isocyanates and none to the more common aromatic isocyanates.

In a series of six patients sensitive to polyurethane, binding agents TDI and MDI were the most commonly identified as causative.[148] Also of note is 1,6-hexamethylene diisocyanate (HDI). Sensitivity to diaminodiphenyl methane may also be found.[148]

Goossens and colleagues identified 22 occupational polyurethane-allergic patients. Nine reacted only to diaminodiphenylmethane (MDA) and the others to this and/or isocyanates. Occupations included laboratory technicians, and auto workers primarily.[149]

When airborne patterns of contact dermatitis are commonly seen with epoxy resins, isocyanates are a rare cause of this pattern of dermatitis. One such case was due to a polyurethane resin in a glue used to make sandpaper for belt sanders.[150] The patient was sensitive to MDI and TDI.

Emmett[151] reported that at least eight persons, employed as molders in the manufacture of polyurethane plastics in a small factory, developed dermatitis within 6 months. Three employees who were examined had eczematous eruptions on exposed areas. Patch testing on two employees revealed positive reactions to methylene bis(4-cyclohexylisocyanate), 1% in petrolatum, and to methylenedianiline, 1% in olive oil. These concentrations were not irritating when tested on four normal volunteers. The distribution of the eruption suggested that airborne materials may have elicited the allergic contact dermatitis. After the institution of rigid hygienic measures to avoid further skin contact, no further instances of dermatitis occurred over the ensuing year.

Dicyclohexylmethane-4,49-diisocyanate, also known as Desmodur W, PICM, reduced MDI (RMDI), saturated MDI, or methylene bis(4-cyclohexylisocyanate), is used in wool processing. In this use, contact dermatitis occurred when wool saturated with this chemical was handled by a 47-year-old textile worker. Fully cured resin was nonallergenic.[152]

Polyurethane sculpting materials have caused ACD in artists.[153]

Whereas the diisocyanates are strong pulmonary sensitizers and relatively weak cutaneous sensitizers, the reverse may be true of the aliphatic diisocyanates.[25]

Isocyanates are associated with occupational asthma, and in less than half of the cases with positive bronchial challenge test will a positive IgE-mediated reaction be found. Contact urticaria is not commonly reported with these agents, but Kanerva and colleagues[154] reported contact urticaria from diphenylmethane-4,49-disocyanate (MDI) in a carpenter exposed to MDI in a polyurethane glue. They speculated that contact urticaria is more common than reported and their case was IgE-mediated.

PREVENTION OF IRRITATION FROM LIQUID ISOCYANATES

The liquid monomer can produce a marked inflammatory reaction characterized by edema and redness if it is not removed immediately from the skin. Contaminated skin, therefore, should be washed copiously and thoroughly with water, and the affected area should be treated with 30% isopropyl alcohol and should then be washed with soap and water.

All contaminated clothing should be removed, preferably in a safety shower.

Vinyl Plastics

The vinyl polymers (polyvinyl chloride, polyvinyl acetate, and polyvinyl alcohol) are rarely, if ever, sensitizers, but certain additives may cause dermatitis. These polymers are thermoplastics. Table 27.12 lists the various additives that may sensitize and also the concentration for patch testing. There are very few contemporary reports of vinyl ACD, most reports are from decades ago.

SARAN AND OTHER VINYL PLASTICS

Saran, the generic name for certain polyvinylidene resins, may be used in flexible plastics such as belts, suspenders, and raincoats. Saran Wrap is used for occlusive dressings and may produce miliaria and maceration, particularly in patients who have atopic dermatitis. Dermatitis due to Saran Wrap has been reported.[155] Plastics closely related to saran include the polyvinyl resins.

There have been reports of contact dermatitis caused by watchbands, garters, and suspenders made of Elastiglass, which is a vinyl acetate and a chloride polymerization product. The dermatitis in these cases was ascribed

Table 27-12 Patch Testing with Vinyl Resins and Additives
Vinyl resins 10% aq[a]
Additives
Plasticizers
Dibutyl phthalate 5% pet[a]
Diethyl phthalate 5% pet
Dioctyl phthalate 5% pet
Stabilizers
Dibutyl tin dilaurate 0.5% pet
Dibutyl tin maleate 0.5% pet
Epoxy resin 2% pet
Ultraviolet light absorbers
Benzophenones 1% pet
Resorcinol monobenzoate 1% pet
Aldehydes
Glyoxal (dialdehyde) 1% aq

to traces of the plasticizer or stabilizer (dibutyl tin maleate or dibutyl sebacate) that was not removed properly during the production of Elastiglass.[156]

Plastic mittens and tablecloths made of vinyl plastic may produce ACD.[157] Allergic skin reactions to epoxy resins used as plasticizers and stabilizers in polyvinyl chloride films have also been reported.[158] PVC is used in leather cloth for clothes, shoes, upholstery packaging tags, and electrical insulation. The PVC chair fabric caused ACD in a Japanese patient, with a pyridine derivative implicated as the allergen.[159]

Hindson and Lawlor[160] reported an allergic reaction to glyoxal, a dialdehyde used in vinyl acetate to form an aqueous emulsion of an adhesive. This resin emulsion system is used in the manufacture of paints, adhesives, carpet backing, paper backing, wallpaper finishing, and as a plastic additive. A 10% aqueous solution of the resin emulsion gave a positive reaction, as did a 10% aqueous solution of the glyoxal.

PVC glove allergy has been traced to bisphenol A in several reports. Bis-A is used as an antioxidant and polymerization inhibitor.[161,162]

PHTHALATES

Schulsinger and Mollgaard[163] reported seven cases of contact dermatitis in children due to identification bracelets made of polyvinyl chloride plastic. Patch tests with the bracelets were negative in the five cases tested. It is concluded that the reactions were irritant due to some unknown chemical in the bracelets. Only one positive patch test was found in 1,532 patch tests with phthalate mK, performed as a joint study by the International Contact Dermatitis Research Group.

Two cases of contact dermatitis to the mouse attached to computers were found to be due to phthalates present in the plastic.[164] One patient was sensitive to diethyl phthalate and the other to dimethyl phthalate, both tested at 5% in petrolatum. The manufacturers confirmed the presence of phthalates in the mice, and a cloth over the mice was preventive. Diethyl phthalate is used in most cellulose ester plastic commonly used to manufacture eyeglasses and hearing aids, although many are made of acrylics now. Contact dermatitis to diethyl phthalate has been reported from these sources.[165] The allergens in eyeglasses were reviewed by Nakada and Maibach.[166] The allergens break down into metals, plastics, plasticizers, solvents, UV stabilizers, antioxidants, dyes, and waxes. The plastics include butyl acrylate, cellulose acetate, epoxy resin, and phenol-formaldehyde. The plasticizers include abietic acid, diethyl phthalate, tricresyl phosphate, triphenyl phosphate, and tritolyl phosphate. UV stabilizers include resorcinol monobenzoate and phenyl salicylate. Another source of allergy to plastic eyeglass frames is colophony, which is used to polish the plastic.[167]

Fisher in previous editions of this text, reported plastic identification bracelets as a cause of PVC dermatitis in infants.

TOXIC VINYL CHLORIDE DISEASE

Walker[168] reported that angiosarcoma of the liver and acro-osteolysis (Raynaud's phenomena, lytic lesions of bone, and sclerodermatous skin changes) are recognized as occupational hazards in men engaged in the process of polymerization of vinyl chloride to PVC.

Over a 1-year period, 30 men from a local PVC plant were treated for symptomatic complaints of coldness and paresthesia of the hands or feet. Additional symptoms included undue fatigue, muscle and joint pains, dyspnea, and impotence. A severe but variable acrocyanosis of the hands and feet was observed in at least 10 patients. Skin histology revealed fragmentation of the elastic tissue in the dermis and abnormal staining of the collagen. Sclerodermatous skin changes were not present.

Arteriograms in the more severely affected patients demonstrated narrowing of the digital vessels. Finger blood flow and skin temperature fell dramatically when the patients were subjected to cool environments. Immunologic investigations in 20 patients revealed cryoglobulins or cryofibrinogen in 14 patients. Respiratory investigations suggested a perfusion impairment that is unexplained as yet.

Ward and colleagues[169] stated that a metabolite of vinyl chloride binds to plasma or tissue protein to form an antigen that is the possible toxin in toxic vinyl disease.

Fiberglass

NATURE OF FIBERGLASS AND FIBERGLASS DERMATITIS

Glass fibers are prepared usually in one of two forms: wool fibers or textile fibers. Wool fibers are of varying lengths, whereas textile fibers are continuous filaments of yarns. The elements of fiberglass are shown in Table 27.13. Nearly all glass fibers are coated with binders, lubricants, or coupling agents that serve to bind individual fibers together, to protect the fiber surface, or to serve as a bonding agent if the fibers are to be eventually incorporated into a matrix of resins. Among the chemicals used for this purpose are phenyl-formaldehyde resins, urea-formaldehyde resins, melamine-formaldehyde resins, polyvinyl acetate, silicones, dyes, starch, epoxy resins, ammonium hydroxide, and mineral oils. Despite the addition of these materials, allergic sensitization is rare because these resin systems are in the fully cured state prior to human exposure.[170]

Workers in composite plastic production develop predominantly irritant contact dermatitis based on data collected over 20 years by Tarvainen and colleagues.[171] They found that 49% of their cases were ICD, predominantly to synthetic mineral fibers (e.g., fiberglass). ACD was seen in 42% of workers and was mainly epoxy resin dermatitis. Contact urticaria was present in 9%, mostly due to natural rubber latex.

The handling of glass fibers may cause an intense pruritic reaction, because fine particles and glass dust may readily penetrate the skin and cause a characteristic miliarial eruption consisting of small, erythematous follicular papules. Other skin lesions, including purpura, telangiectasis, folliculitis, urticaria, and linear erosions in the skin creases, may also be produced, particularly in fair-complexioned individuals with dry skin. In addition, paronychia may result from the penetration of glass spicules beneath the nail fold.[172]

Workers involved in the manufacture of glass fibers may also develop a pustular, follicular acneiform eruption from hydrogenated vegetable oils and coating emulsions. In addition, glass fibers and resins may coat and interfere with the porosity of leather footwear, often producing maceration and dermatitis of the feet.

Glass fiber particles may penetrate clothing and underwear and may produce dermatitis on covered portions of the body. Glass particles may be brought home and transferred from the worker's clothing and skin to other members of the family. This type of "contagious" glass fiber dermatitis may be mistaken for scabies.

The washing of clothing contaminated with fiberglass in a washing machine with the family underwear may produce a family "epidemic" of itching. Lucas[173] stated that fiberglass dermatitis could spread among family groups through the cross-contamination of clothing with glass spicules from curtains or other fibrous glass items during washing. This cause of pruritus should always be suspected when several family members begin almost simultaneous complaints of intense itching. In several instances, Lucas traced the apparent source to commercially operated self-service coin laundries. Sufficient carryover was present to contaminate the clothing of the next customer using the machine. Such items should be washed separately from other clothing items and in a basin or tub that can be rinsed thoroughly after use. Rubber gloves should be worn in the procedure.

Elby and Jetton[174] reported a case of school desk dermatitis due to a primary irritant contact reaction to fiberglass present in reinforced plastic chairs and school desks.

Fiberglass made from a mixture of polyvinyl alcohol, polyethylene glycol, acetic acid, and organosilane solution (Dow Corning Z-6032 silane) was produced in a facility where eight workers developed dermatitis on part areas exposed to the material.[175] Four of the eight were found patch test positive to the organosilane, which was positive in all four at 0.3% aqueous. A contaminant in the organosilane was suspected to be the actual allergen, but this was not definitively ascertained.

VARIATIONS IN FIBERGLASS DERMATITIS

A few workers handling fiberglass suffer from dermatitis as long as they are exposed to it. They generally seek other work fairly promptly. Those who stay in the job usually become "hardened" with continual exposure to fiberglass and eventually no longer develop dermatitis from contact with it.

Bjornberg and colleagues[176] studied 98 workers who were patch tested with glass fibers and six chemical irritants in a glass-wool factory. A rubbing test was done with the fibers and with Trafuril.

Trafuril is an ester of nicotinic acid that is a histamine-releasing agent when rubbed into the skin. The subjects with strong patch test reactions to one quality of fiber also reacted strongly to the other types of fibers, but they did not show any increased sensitivity to other tests. The subjects with intense skin reactions to rubbing with the fibers showed an increased skin reactivity to the patch tests with fibers. These subjects had fair skin and blue eyes. In another study, these authors reported that 33 workers at a glass-wool factory were tested (patch test with glass fibers and chemical irritants, epicutaneous tests with Trafuril, and intracutaneous tests with hista-

mine) before starting work at the factory. They were then retested after at least 4 weeks of exposure to glass fibers.[177] No statistically significant differences in the intensity of the skin reactions before and after exposure were found. Thus, no general increased irritancy of the normal skin was induced by the continuous exposure to glass fibers.

Bjornberg and colleagues[178] also studied workers in a glass-wool factory who were divided into three comparable groups: those with persistent troublesome itching from the fibers, those without itching, and those who had become "hardened" to the itching. The three groups were compared with respect to the results of patch testing with glass fibers and six chemical irritants, a rubbing test with fibers and six chemical irritants, and the Trafuril test. Anamnestic data with respect to atopy, itching from wool and synthetic fibers, sweating, and reactions to the sun were evaluated, as was also the general skin pigmentation. No statistically significant differences between the three groups were found in respect to any of these tests or factors except for a subjectively increased sensitivity in the rubbing test with fibers for the itching group.

ECZEMATOUS NATURE OF CERTAIN FIBERGLASS DERMATOSES

In some individuals, fiberglass dermatitis has a distinctly nummular eczema-like appearance, and at times even a more widespread eczematous reaction may occur that closely resembles a diffuse allergic contact dermatitis. Cuypers and colleagues[179] studied a control group of 36 normal persons who were patch tested with glass fibers. The tested filaments had a length of about 3 to 5 mm and a diameter of 9 to 13 mm. The glass fibers were obtained from the normal production process and had been coated with cured epoxy resin. A control group of 29 normal persons was tested with the same type of fibers from which the epoxy finish had been burned off. Another group of 36 persons was patch tested with coated and uncoated ultra-small glass globules with a diameter of 10 to 50 mm. On every person, five patch tests with the same material were done. They were removed after 1, 5, 24, 48, and 72 hours. On the coated fibers, 12 of 36 tested people reacted with either a 1+ or 2+ reaction. On the uncoated fibers, a reaction could be noted in 10 of 29 persons.

The patch tests with coated as well as uncoated glass globules all gave negative results. A total of 60 biopsies were performed in those cases in which a 1+ or 2+ reaction was noted. The histologic examination of the biopsies showed no difference between the reactions on coated and uncoated fibers. The skin reactions to glass fiber showed, besides microtraumatic changes, several histologic characteristics of an eczematous reaction like spongiosis and perivascular lymphocytic infiltration. It was concluded that the microtraumatic influence of fiberglass spicules may produce histologic reactions of an eczematous nature closely mimicking an allergic contact dermatitis.

DERMATITIS DUE TO FIBERGLASS RESIN FINISHES

As a rule, the formaldehyde and epoxy resins applied to certain glass fibers are completely cured and do not produce allergic contact dermatitis. Occasionally, however, dermatitis caused by these resin finishes have been reported.[180]

Kalimo and colleagues[51] described a patient who had both immediate type 1 and delayed type 4 hypersensitivity reactions to p-tert-butylphenol-formaldehyde resin in glass fiber finishes, and who developed aphonia without skin symptoms in connection with exposure to glass wool.

The patient, a 46-year-old truck driver, had been employed by a glass-wool delivery firm since 1972. The driver's work was to load and deliver glass-wool rolls (masses of glass fibers resembling wool), used for thermal insulation and air filters.

An urticarial reaction was seen in 60 minutes at the site of the patch test application, and in 3 days a delayed type 4 reaction also developed. The patient's own glass-wool material was tested repeatedly with identical immediate and delayed type skin reactions. Tests with the same wool in 10 control persons were not due to irritation of the wool. Formaldehyde caused no reaction.

Rockwool

NATURE OF ROCKWOOL AND ROCKWOOL DERMATITIS

Rockwool is a type of mineral wool made by blowing a jet of steam through molten rock (such as limestone or siliceous rock) or through slag and is used for heat and sound insulation in the building industry. Such "wool" is usually transparent in appearance and has thin, sharp fibers of different diameters. Mineral oil, a silicone compound, and phenyl-formaldehyde resin may be added. The resin is then cured by heat. Mineral cotton, silicate cotton, and slag wool are other names for rockwool.

Rockwool may cause severe itching and skin reactions on direct contact with the skin. The two varieties of

dermatitis that develop from rockwool are mostly irritant in nature. Rockwool, which is produced from slag, often contains free lime and can produce a severe diffuse irritant reaction due to its alkalinity, particularly on wet or perspiring skin. The other is a more or less punctate or follicular eruption that can become eczematous due to penetration of the sharp spicules.

Bjornberg and Lowhagen[181] patch tested 225 eczematous patients with rockwool. A total of 25 (11%) had positive 2+ or 3+ reactions. Rockwool powder without spicules did not produce any patch test reactions. The authors concluded that the typical sharp properties of the fibers produce these skin reactions mechanically. The reactions often have the macroscopic appearance of a true allergic response. Even microscopically, some showed subcorneal bullae with spongiosis and dermal mononuclear infiltrate. In some reactions, spongiosis dominated the picture, and in others a dermal infiltrate was present without epidermal changes.

In a later study, Bjomberg and Lowhagen[182] reported that 25% of 315 subjects exhibited skin reactions when patch tested with mineral wool. Coating of the mineral fibers with phenyl-formaldehyde did not influence the skin reactions. The reactions seem to be induced mechanically, as the mineral without the fibers did not give any reactions. No allergic reactions to the chemical additives were demonstrated.

Parts of this chapter were originally contributed by James S. Taylor, MD, Cleveland, Ohio, in the third edition of this book as Chapter 37, Adhesives, Gums, and Resins.

References

1. <http://en.wikipedia.org/wiki/plastics> Accessed October 20:2007.

2. Jordan WP, Dahl MV. Contact dermatitis from cellulose ester plastics. Arch Dermatol 1972;105:880.

3. Camarasa JG, Serra-Baldrich E. Allergic contact dermatitis from triphenyl phosphate. Contact Dermatitis 1992;26:264.

4. Jolanki R, Kanerva L, Estlander T, et al. Occupational dermatoses from epoxy resin compounds. Contact Dermatitis 1990;23:172.

5. Kanerva L, Jolanki R, Estlander T. Allergic contact dermatitis from non-diglycidyl-ether-of-bisphenol-A epoxy resins. Contact Dermatitis 1991;24:293.

6. Ponten A, Carstenen O, Rasmessen K, et al. Epoxy-based production of wind turbine rotor blades: Occupational contact allergies. Dermatitis 2004;15:33.

7. Pratt M, et al—presented at American Contact Dermatitis Society, Hershey, PA. July, 2005.

8. Jolanki R, Estlander T, Kanerva L:182 patients with occupational allergic epoxy contact dermatitis over 22 years. Contact Dermatitis 2001;44:121.

9. Romhyr O, Nyfors A, Leira H, et al. Allergic Contact Dermatitis caused by epoxy resin systems in industrial painters. Contact Dermatitis 2006;55:167.

10. Lee H, Pokorny C, Law S, et al. Cross-reactivity among epoxy acrylates and bisphenol F epoxy resins in patients with bisphenol A epoxy resin sensitivity. Am J Contact Dermat 2002;13:108.

11. Ponten A, Carstensen O, Rasmussen K, et al. Epoxy-based production of wind turbine rotor blades. Dermatitis 2004; 15:33–40.

12. Sasseville D, Hakim M, Muhn C. Bus pass dermatitis. Am J Contact Dermat 2003;13:146.

13. Guerra L, Vincenzi C, Bardazzi F, et al. Contact sensitization due to isophoronediamine. Contact Dermatitis 1992;27:52.

14. Dahlquist I, Fregert S. Contact allergy to Cardura E, and epoxy reactive diluent of the ester type. Contact Dermatitis 1979;5:121.

15. Rudzki E. Dermatitis from epoxy resin, triethylenetetramine and ethylenediamine. Contact Dermatitis 1978;4:53.

16. Dahlquist I, Fregert S. Contact allergy to the epoxy hardener Isophoronediamine (IPD). Contact Dermatitis 1979;5:120.

17. de Groot AC. Occupational contact allergy to alpha-naphthyl glycidyl ether. Contact Dermatitis 1994;30:253.

18. Angelini G, et al. Occupational sensitization to epoxy resin and reactive diluents in marble workers. Contact Dermatitis 1996;35:11.

19. Chu C, Ponten A, Sun C, Jee S: Concomitant contact allergy to the resins, reactive diluents, and hardener of a bisphenol A/F based epoxy resin. Contact Dermatitis 2006;54:131.

20. Geier J, Lessmann H, Hillen U, et al. An attempt to improve the diagnostics of contact allergy to epoxy resin systems. Contact Dermatitis 2004;51:262.

21. Kanerva L, et al. Delayed and immediate allergy caused by methylhexahydrophthalic anhydride. Contact Dermatitis 1997;36:34.

22. Dooms-Goossens A, et al. Contact allergy to allyl glycidyl ether present as an impurity in 3-glycidyloxypropyltrimethoxysilane, a fixing additive in silicone and polyurethane resins. Contact Dermatitis 1995;33:17.

23. Sasseville D. Contact urticaria from epoxy resin and reactive diluents. Contact Dermatitis 1998;38:57.

24. Fisher AA. Cross-reactions between epoxy resin ''amine'' hardeners and ethylenediamine. Cutis 1976;17:839.

25. Lachapelle JM, Lachapelle-Ketelaer MJ. Cross-sensitivity between isophorone diamine (IPD) and isophorone diiocyanate (IPDI). Contact Dermatitis 1979;5:55.

26. Anderson KE. Cutaneous reaction to an epoxy coated pacemaker. Arch Dermatol 1979;115:97.

27. Mork NJ. Contact sensitivity from epoxy resin in a hemodialysis set. Contact Dermatitis 1979;5:331.

28. Bjorkner B. Allergic contact dermatitis from (foxy) epoxy. Contact Dermatitis 1980;6:499.

29. Fregert S, Persson K, Trulsson L. Allergic contact dermatitis from unhardened epoxy resin in a finished product. Contact Dermatitis 1979;5:277.

30. Sasseville D, Moreau L, Brassard J, et al. Allergic contact dermatitis to epoxy resin in microscopy immersion oil. Am J Contact Dermat 2000;11:99.

31. Silvestre J, et al. Contact vitiligo appearing after contact dermatitis from aromatic diluents in an epoxy resin system. Contact Dermatitis 2003;49:113.

32. Ishikawa O, Warita S, Tamura A, et al. Br J Dermatol 1995;133:786–9.

33. Tarvainen K, et al. Immunologic contact urticaria due to airborne methylhexahydrophthalic and methyltetrahydrophthalic anhydrides. Contact Dermatitis 1995;32:204.

34. Kanerva L, et al. Occupational allergic contact dermatitis and contact urticaria caused by polyfunctional aziridine hardener. Contact Dermatitis 1995;33:304.

35. Brooke R, Beck MH. Contact allergy to 2,4,6-tris(dimethylaminomethyl)phenol. Contact Dermatitis 1998;38:284.

36. Kanerva L, Jolanki R, Estlander T. Occupational epoxy dermatitis with patch test reactions to multiple hardeners including tetraethylenepentamine. Contact Dermatitis 1998;38:299.

37. Patussi V, Kokelj F, Buttazzi P. Occupational airborne contact dermatitis due to 3-amino-methyl-3,5,5-trimethylcyclohexylamine. Contact Dermatitis 1995;32:239.

38. Dahlquist I, Fregert S. Allergic contact dermatitis from volatile epoxy hardeners and reactive diluents. Contact Dermatitis 1979;5:406.

39. Nijnemaki A, et al. Allergic stomatitis from acrylic compounds. Contact Dermatitis 1983;9:148.

40. Taylor JS, et al. Contact dermatitis to knee patch adhesive in boys' jeans: a nonoccupational cause of epoxy resin sensitivity. Cleve Clin Q 1983;50:123.

41. Nakayama H, et al. As referenced by Malten KE, Nater JP, van Ketel WG. Patch testing guidelines. Nijmegen, Netherlands: Dekker and Van de Vegt, 1976:91.

42. Fregert S, Thorgeirsson A. Patch testing with low molecular oligomers of epoxy resins in humans. Contact Dermatitis 1977;3:301.

43. Bokelund F, Fregert S, Trulsson L. Sensitization from epoxy resin powder of high molecular weight. Contact Dermatitis 1980;6:144.

44. Estlander T, Jolanki R, Henriks-Eckerman M-L, Kanerva L. Occupational contact dermatitis to bisphenol A. Contact Dermatitis 1999;40:52.

45. Fregert S. Irritant dermatitis from phenolformaldehyde resin powder. Contact Dermatitis 1980;6:493.

46. Adams RM. "Spontaneous flare" to p-tert-butyl-phenol formaldehyde resin. Contact Dermatitis 1975;1:321.

47. Mobacken H, Hersle K. Allergic contact dermatitis caused by para-tertiary-butyl-phenol-formaldehyde resin in watch straps. Contact Dermatitis 1976;2:59.

48. Burrows D, Rycroft RJ. Contact dermatitis from PTBP resin and tricresyl ethyl phthalate in a plastic nail adhesive. Contact Dermatitis 1981;7:336.

49. Romaguera C, Grimalt F. Occupational leukoderma and contact dermatitis from paratertiary-butylphenol. Contact Dermatitis 1981;7:159.

50. Fregert S. Contact allergy to phenoplastics. Contact Dermatitis 1981;7:170.

51. Kalimo K, Saarni H, Kytta J. Immediate and delayed type reactions to formaldehyde resin in glass wool. Contact Dermatitis 1980;6:496.

52. Malten KE. Paratertiary butylphenol depigmentation in a "consumer." Contact Dermatitis 1975;1:181.

53. MacFarlane AW, Yu RC, King CM. Contact sensitivity to paratertiarybutyl-catechol in an artificial limb. Contact Dermatitis 1990;22:56.

54. Hagdrup H, Egsgaard H, Carlsen L, Andersen KE. Contact allergy to 2-hydroxy-5-tert-butyl benzylalcohol and 2,6-bis(hydroxymethyl)-4-tert-butylphenol, components of a phenolic resin used in marking pens. Contact Dermatitis 1994;31:154.

55. Edwards EK Jr, Edwards EK Sr. Unusual cutaneous reaction to polystyrene in an otherwise healthy population. Contact Dermatitis 1998;38:50.

56. Tarvainen K. Analysis of patients with allergic patch test reactions to a plastics and glue series. Contact Dermatitis 1995;32:346.

57. Zimerson E, Bruze M. Demonstration of the contact sensitizer p-tert-butylcatechol in p-tert-butylphenol formaldehyde resin. Am J Contact Dermat 1999;10:2.

58. Bruze M, Zimerson E. Cross-reaction patterns in patients with contact allergy to simple methylol phenols. Contact Dermatitis 1997;37:82.

59. Hillen U, Frosch P, John S, et al. Patch test sensitization caused by para-tertiary butylcatechol. Contact Dermatitis 2002;45:193.

60. Malten KE. Old and new, mainly occupational dermatologic problems in the production and processing of plastics. In: Maibach HI, Gellin GA, eds. Occupational and industrial dermatology. Chicago: Year Book Medical Publishers, 1982:255.

61. Hjorth N, Fregert S. Sensitivity to formaldehyde and formaldehyde resins. Contact Dermatitis Newsletter 1967;2:18.

62. Logan WP, Perry H. Cast dermatitis due to formaldehyde sensitivity. Arch Dermatol 1972;106:717.

63. Fregert S. Formaldehyde dermatitis from a gypsum-melamine resin mixture. Contact Dermatitis 1981;7:56.

64. Romaguera C, Grimalt F, Lecha M. Occupational purpuric textile dermatitis from formaldehyde resins. Contact Dermatitis 1981;7:152.

65. Calnan CD. Cyanoacrylate dermatitis. Contact Dermatitis 1979;5:165.

66. Bruze M, Bjorkner B, Lepoittevin J-P. Occupational allergic contact dermatitis from ethyl cyanoacrylate. Contact Dermatitis 1995;32:156.

67. Belsito DV. Contact dermatitis to ethylcyanoacrylate-containing glue. Contact Dermatitis 1987;17:234.

68. Tombs RR, Lepoittevin J-P, Duprepaire F, et al. Ectopic contact dermatitis from ethyl cyanoacrylate instant adhesives. Contact Dermatitis 1993;28:206.

69. Fitzgerald DA, Bhaggoe R, English JSC. Contact sensitivity to cyanoacrylate nail-adhesive with dermatitis at remote sites. Contact Dermatitis 1995;32:175.

70. Shelley ED, Shelley WB. Chronic dermatitis simulating small plaque parapsoriasis due to cyanoacrylate adhesive used in fingernails. JAMA 1984;252:2455.

71. Margo CE, Trobe JD. Tarsorrhaphy from accidental instillation of cyanoacrylate adhesive in the eye. JAMA 1982;247:660.

72. Freeman S, Lee M-S, Gudmundsen K. Adverse contact reactions to sculptured acrylic nails: 4 case reports and a literature review. Contact Dermatitis 1995;33:381.

73. Koppula SV, Fellman JH, Storrs FJ. Screening allergens for acrylate dermatitis associated with artificial nails. Am J Contact Dermat 1995;6:78.

74. Malten KE. Recently reported causes of contact dermatitis due to synthetic resins and hardeners. Contact Dermatitis 1979;5:11.

75. Emmett EA. Contact dermatitis from poly-functional acrylic monomers. Contact Dermatitis 1977;3:245.

76. Heskel NS, Samour CM, Storr FT. Allergic contact dermatitis from dodecyl maleamic acid in Curad adhesive plastic bandages. J Am Acad Dermatol 1982;7:747.

77. Calnan CD. Diethyldithiocarbamate in adhesive tape. Contact Dermatitis 1978;4:61.

78. Murphy JC, Reit AE, January HL. Cutaneous hypersensitivity to adhesive and Scotch tapes. J Invest Dermatol 1958;31:45.

79. Cronin E, Calnan CD. Allergy to hydroabietic alcohol in adhesive tape. Contact Dermatitis 1978;4:57.

80. Hagan J, Steuben K: Pressure sensitive adhesives. In: Schneberger EL, ed. Adhesives in Manufacturing. New York. Marcel Dekker, 1982:189.

81. Fregert S, Trulson L, Zimerson E. Contact allergic reactions to diphenylthiourea and phenylisothiocyanate in PVC adhesive tape. Contact Dermatitis 1982;8:38.

82. Jordan WP. Cross-sensitization patterns in acrylic allergens. Contact Dermatitis 1975;1:13.

83. Waegemaekers TLH, Van Der Walle HB. The sensitizing potential of 2-ethylhexyl acrylate in the guinea pig. Contact Dermatitis 1983;9:372.

84. Foussereau J, et al. L'allergie à la colophane des rondelles en polyethylene des patch tests. Bull Soc Fr Dermatol Syphiligr 1971;78:604.

85. Kiec-Swierczynska M, Krecisz B, Swierczynska-Machura D, et al. An epidemic of occupational contact dermatitis from an acrylate glue. Contact Dermatitis 2005;52:121–5.

86. Malten KE. Dermatological problems with synthetic resins and plastics in glues. Berufs-Dermatosen 1984;32:81.

87. Allardice JT. Dermatitis due to an acrylic sealer. Trans St John's Hosp Dermatol Soc 1967;53:86.

88. Magnusson B, Mobacken H. Contact allergy to a self-hardening acrylic sealer for assembling metal parts. Berufs-Dermatosen 1972;20:199.

89. Jansen K. Zur Haufigkeit unt Prophylaxe Allergischer Kontaktekzeme durch Acrylat-Klebstoffe. Berufs-Dermatosen 1975;23:183.

90. Cronin E. Contact dermatitis. Edinburgh: Churchill Livingstone, 1980:3.

91. Dempsey KJ. Hypersensitivity to Sta-Lok and Loctite anaerobic sealants. J Am Acad Dermatol 1982;7:779.

92. Mathias CGT, Maibach HI. Allergic contact dermatitis from anaerobic acrylic sealants. Arch Dermatol 1984;120:1202.

93. Foulds IS, Koh D. Contact allergy to 1-acetyl-2-phenyl-hydrazine in a dimethacrylate adhesive. Contact Dermatitis 1991;25:251.

94. Jolanki R, Kanerva L, Estlander T, Tarvainen K. Concomitant sensitization to triglycidyl isocyanurate, diaminodiphenylmethane and 2-hydroxyethyl methacrylate from silk-screen printing coatings in the manufacture of circuit boards. Contact Dermatitis 1994;330:12.

95. Malten KE, van der Meer-Roosen CH, Seutter E. Nyloprint-sensitive patients react to N,N9-methylene bis acrylamide. Contact Dermatitis 1978;4:214.

96. Malten KE, Bende WJM. 2-hydroxy-ethyl-methacrylate and di- and tetraethylene glycol dimethacrylate: contact sensitizers in a photoprepolymer printing plate procedure. Contact Dermatitis 1979;5:214.

97. Beurey J, Mougeolle JM, Weber M. Accidents cutanes des résines acryliques dans l'imprimerie (Cutaneous manifestations due to acrylic resins used in printing [French]). Ann Dermatol Venereol 1976;103:423.

98. Busschots AM, Meuleman V, Poesen N, Dooms-Goossens A. Contact allergy to components of glue in insulin pump infusion sets. Contact Dermatitis 1995;33:205.

99. Kanerva L, Estlander T, Jolanki R. Double active sensitization caused by acrylics. Am J Contact Derma 1992;3:23.

100. Pegum JS, Medhurst FA. Contact dermatitis from penetration of rubber gloves by acrylic monomer. Br Med J 1971;2:141.

101. Fries JB, Fisher AA, Salvati EA. Contact dermatitis in surgeons from methyl methacrylate bone cement. J Bone Joint Surg 1975;57A:547.

102. Fisher AA. Acrylic bone cement sensitization and dermatitis. Cutis 1973;12:333.

103. Bohling HG, Borchard U, Drouin H. Monomeric methyl-methacrylate (MMA) acts on desheathed myelinated nerve and on the node of Ranvier. Arch Toxicol 1977;38:307.

104. Edwards PM. Filling in the acrylamide picture. Br J Ind Med 1975;32:31.

105. Monteney E, Oleffe J, Donkerwolke M. Methylmethacrylate hypersensitivity in a patient with cemented endoprosthesis: a case report. Acta Orthop Scand 1978;49:554.

106. Pahuja K, Lowe H, Chand K. Blood methyl methacrylate levels in patients having prosthetic joint replacement. Acta Orthop Scand 1974;45:737.

107. Bjorkner B. Sensitization capacity of acrylated prepolymers in ultraviolet curing inks tested in the guinea pig. Acta Dermato-Venereol 1981;61:7.

108. Nethercott JR. Skin problems associated with multifunctional acrylic monomers in ultraviolet curing inks. Br J Dermatol 1979;98:541.

109. Bjorkner B, Dahlquist I, Fregert S. Allergic contact dermatitis from acrylates in ultraviolet curing inks. Contact Dermatitis 1980;6:405.

110. Emmett EA, Kominsky JR. Allergic contact dermatitis from ultraviolet cured inks: allergic contact sensitization to acrylates. J Occup Med 1977;19:113.

111. Goossens A, Coninx D, Rommens K, Verhamme B. Occupational dermatitis in a silk-screen maker. Contact Dermatitis 1998;39:40.

112. Guimaraens D, Gonzalez MA, Del Rio E, Conde-Salazar L. Occupational airborne allergic contact dermatitis in the national mint and fiscal-stamp factory. Contact Dermatitis 1994;30:172.

113. Emmett EA, Taphorn BR, Kominsky JR. Phototoxicity occurring during the manufacture of ultraviolet-cured ink. Arch Dermatol 1977;113:770.

114. Bang Pedersen N. Allergic contact dermatitis from acrylic resin repair of windscreens. Contact Dermatitis 1998;39:99.

115. Matura M, et al. Glycidyl methacrylate and ethoxyethyl acrylate: new allergens in emulsions used to impregnate paper and textile materials. Contact Dermatitis 1995;33:123.

116. Mohamed M, Delaney T, Horton J: Allergic contact dermatitis to plastic banknotes. Austral J Dermatol 1999;40:164.

117. Tobler M, Wüthrich B, Freiburghaus AU. Contact dermatitis from acrylate and methacrylate compounds in Lowicryl® embedding media for electron microscopy. Contact Dermatitis 1990;23:96.

118. Marren P, DeBerker D, Powell S. Methacrylate sensitivity and transcutaneous electrical nerve stimulation (TENS). Contact Dermatitis 1991;25:190.

119. Fisher AA. A glove for protection against acrylates. Am J Contact Dermat 1990;1:149.

120. McClain DC, Storrs FJ. Protective effect of both a barrier cream and a polyethylene laminate glove against epoxy resin, glyceryl monothioglycolate, frullania, and tansy. Am J Contact Dermat 1992;3:201.

121. Pratt M, Belsito D, DeLeo V, et al. North American Contact Dermatitis Group patch-test results. 2001–2002 period. Dermatitis 2005;15:176.

122. Kanerva L, Jolanki R, Estlander T. 10 years of patch testing with the (meth)acrylate series. Contact Dermatitis 1997;37:255.

123. Isakkson M, Lindberg M, Sundberg K, et al. The development and course of patch-test reactions to 2-HEMA and EGDMA. Contact Dermatitis 2005;53:292–7.

124. Cavelier C, Jelen G, Herve-Bazin B, Foussereau J. Irritation et allergie aux acrylates et methacrylate. Premiere partie: monoacrylates et monomethyacrylates simples (Irritation and allergy to acrylates and methacrylates. Part 1: polyfunctional acrylic monomers [French]). Ann Dermatol Venereol 1981;108:549.

125. Cavelier C, Jelen G, Herve-Bazin B, Foussereau J. Irritation et allergie aux acrylates. Deuxieme partie: monomeres acryliques polyfonctionels (Irritation and allergy to acrylates and methacrylates. Part 2: polyfunctional acrylic monomers [French]). Ann Dermatol Venereol 1981;108:559.

126. Rycroft RJG. Contact dermatitis from acrylic compounds. Br J Dermatol 1977;96:685.

127. Marks JG, Bishop ME, Willis WF. Allergic contact dermatitis to sculptured nails. Arch Dermatol 1979;115:100.

128. Henriks-Eckerman M-J, Kanerva L. Product analysis of acrylic resins compared to information given in material safety data sheets. Contact Dermatitis 1997;36:164.

129. Nerschueren GLA, Bruynzeel DP. Allergy to N,N-dimethyl-p-toluidine in dental materials. Contact Dermatitis 1991;24:149.

130. Vincenzi D, Camelli N, Vassilopoulou A, et al. Allergic contact dermatitis due to benzoyl peroxide in an arm prosthesis. Contact Dermatitis 1991;24:66.

131. Arisu K, Hayakawa R, Ogino Y, et al. Tinuvin® P in a spandex tape as a cause of clothing dermatitis. Contact Dermatitis 1992;26:311.

132. Fimiani M, Casini L, Bocci S. Contact dermatitis from phenyl salicylate in galenic cream. Contact Dermatitis 1990;22:239.

133. Takiwaki H, Arase S, Nakayama H. Contact dermatitis due to 2,29-azobis(2-amidinopropane) dihydrochloride: an outbreak in production workers. Contact Dermatitis 1998;39:4.

134. Bhushan M, Craven NM, Beck MH. Contact allergy to methyl ethyl ketone peroxide and cobalt in the manufacture of fiberglass-reinforced plastics. Contact Dermatitis 1998;39:203.

135. Webb K, Fowler J: Occupational contact dermatitis to nitromethane. Am J Contact Dermat 20;13:201.

136. Adams RM. Polyester resins. In: Maibach HI, Gellin GA, eds. Occupational and industrial dermatology. Chicago: Year Book Medical Publishers, 1982:291.

137. Key MM, Discher DP. Polyester resins: their dermatologic aspects in industry. Cutis 1966;2:1.

138. 139. Pfaffli P, Jolanki R, Estlander T, et al. Identification of sensitizing diethyleneglycol maleate in a two-component polyester cement. Contact Dermatitis 2002;46:170.

139. Bourne LB, Milner FJ. Polyester resin hazards. Br J Ind Med 1963:20:100.

140. Burrows D, Campbell HS. Contact dermatitis to polyester spin finishes. Contact Dermatitis 1980;6:362.

141. Wigger-Alberti W, Hofmann M, Elsner P. Contact dermatitis caused by triglycidyl isocyanurate. Am J Contact Dermat 1997;8:106.

142. Suguira K, Suguira M, Shiraki R, et al. Contact urticaria due to polyethylene gloves Contact Dermatitis 2002;46:262.

143. Sjoborg S, Dahlquist I, Fregert S, Trulson L. Contact allergy to styrene with cross reaction to vinyltoluene. Contact Dermatitis 1982;8:207.

144. Fregert S. Outbreak of irritant dermatitis from dial-lyl-phthalate (and styrene) in polyester resin. Contact Dermatitis Newsletter 1971;10:234.

145. Mowe G. Health risks from isocyanates. Contact Dermatitis 1980;6:44.

146. Frick-Engfeldt M, Zimerson E, Karlsson D, et al. Is it possible to improve the patch test diagnostics for isocyanates? Contact Dermatitis 2007;56:27.

147. Frick M, Bjorkner B, Hamnerius N, et al. Allergic contact dermatitis from dicyclohexylmethane-4,4-diisocyanate. Contact Dermatitis 2003;48:305–98.

148. Estlander T, Keskinen H, Jolanki R, et al. Occupational dermatitis from exposure to polyurethane chemicals. Contact Dermatitis 1992; 27:161.

149. Goossens A, Detienne T, Bruze M: Occupational allergic contact dermatitis caused by isocyanates. Contact Dermatitis 2002;47:304.

150. Schroder C, Uter W, Schwanitz HJ. Occupational allergic contact dermatitis, partly airborne, due to isocyanates and epoxy resin. Contact Dermatitis 1999;41:117.

151. Emmett EA. Allergic contact dermatitis in polyurethane plastic moulders. J Occup Med 1976;18:802.

152. Thompson T, Belsito DV. Allergic contact dermatitis from a diisocyanate in wool processing. Contact Dermatitis 1997;37:239.

153. Mitello G, Sasseville D, Ditre, et al. Allergic contact dermatitis from isocyanates among sculptors. Dermatitis 2004;15:150

154. Kanerva L, Grenquist-Norden B, Piirila P. Occupational IgE-mediated contact urticaria from diphanylmethane-4,49-diisocyanate (MDI). Contact Dermatitis 1999;41:50.

155. Osbourn RA. Contact dermatitis caused by Saran Wrap. JAMA 1964; 188:1159.

156. Morris GE. Vinyl plastics; their dermatological and chemical aspects. AMA Arch Ind Hyg 1953;8:535.

157. Templeton HJ. Contact dermatitis from plastic mittens. Arch Dermatol Syphilol 1950;61:854.

158. Fregert S, Rorsman H. Hypersensitivity to epoxy resins used as plasticizers and stabilizers in polyvinyl chloride (PVC) resins. Acta Dermato-Venereol 1963;43:10.

159. Hu W, Masuji Y, Tada J, et al. Allergic contact dermatitis from a pyridine derivative in polyvinyl chloride leather. Am J Contact Dermat 2001;12:35.

160. Hindson C, Lawlor F. Allergy to glyoxal in a polyvinyl resin emulsion. Contact Dermatitis 1982;8:213.

161. Aalto-Korte A, Alanko K, Henriks-Eckerman M, et al. Allergic contact dermatitis from bisphenol-A in PVC gloves. Contact Dermatitis 2003;49:202.

162. Matthieu L, Godoi A, Lambert J et al. Occupational allergic contact dermatitis from bisphenol-A in vinyl gloves. Contact Dermatitis 2004;49:281

163. Schulsinger C, Mollgaard K. Polyvinyl chloride dermatitis not caused by phthalates. Contact Dermatitis 1980;6:477.

164. Capon F, et al. Occupational contact dermatitis caused by computer mice. Contact Dermatitis 1996;35:57.

165. Oliwiecki S, Beck MH, Chalmers RJG. Contact dermatitis from spectacle frames and hearing aid containing diethyl phthalate. Contact Dermatitis 1991;25:264.

166. Nakada T, Maibach HI. Eyeglass allergic contact dermatitis. Contact Dermatitis 1998;39:1.

167. Thorneby-Andersson K, Hansson C. Allergic contact dermatitis from colophony in waxes for polishing spectacle frames. Contact Dermatitis 1994;31:126.

168. Walker AE. Preliminary report of vascular abnormality occurring in men engaged in manufacture of polyvinyl chloride. Br J Dermatol 1975;93:22.

169. Ward AM, Udnoon S, Watkins J, et al. Immunological mechanisms in the pathogenesis of vinyl chloride disease. Br Med J 1976;1:936.

170. Fisher AA. Fiberglass vs mineral wool (rock-wool) dermatitis. Cutis 1982;29:412, 415–416, 422 passim.

171. Tarvainen K, et al. Occupational dermatoses from the manufacture of plastic composite products. Am J Contact Dermat 1995;6:95.

172. Heisel EB, Hunt FE. Further studies in cutaneous reactions to glass fibers. Arch Environ Health 1968;17:705.

173. Lucas JB. Common industrial dermatoses. *Cutis* 1974;13:33.

174. Eby CS, Jetton RL. School desk dermatitis. Primary irritant contact dermatitis to fiberglass. Arch Dermatol 1972;105:890.

175. Heino T, Haapa K, Manelius F. Contact sensitization to organosilane in glass filament production. Contact Dermatitis 1996;34:294.

176. Bjornberg A, Lowhagen GB, Tengberg JE. Relationship between intensities of skin test reactions to glass-fibres and chemical irritants. Contact Dermatitis 1979;5:171.

177. Bjornberg A, Lowhagen GB, Tengberg JE. Does occupational exposure to glass-fibres increase the general skin reactivity to irritants? Contact Dermatitis 1979;5:175.

178. Bjornberg A, Lowhagen GB, Tengberg JE. Skin reactivity in workers with and without itching from occupational exposure to glass fibres. Acta Dermato-Venereol 1979;59:49.

179. Cuypers JMC, Hoedemaeker PJ, Nater PJ, de Jong MC. The histopathology of fiberglass dermatitis in relation to von Hebra's concept of eczema. Contact Dermatitis 1975;1:88.

180. Dahlquist S, Fregert S, Trulsson L. Allergic contact dermatitis from epoxy resin finished glass fiber. Contact Dermatitis 1979;5:190.

181. Bjornberg A, Lowhagen GB. Patch test reactions to rock-wool. Contact Dermatitis 1975;1:242.

182. Bjornberg A, Lowhagen GB. Patch testing with mineral wool (rockwool). Acta Dermato-Venereol 1977;57:257.

FOOD ADDITIVES AND DYES

EXECUTIVE SUMMARY

Sorbic acid added to foods as a preservative has caused eczematous contact dermatitis of the hands of bakers from flour exposure, contact urticaria of a non-allergic type on the faces and perioral skin of children exposed to it in mayonnaise, and vesicular hand and foot eczema from ingestion of yogurt with prunes, strawberries, and margarine.

Other food additives include antioxidants such as butylated hydroxanisole, butylated hydroxytoluene, sodium bisulfite, tocopherols, and gallates. Flavor ingredients that most commonly cause oral symptoms include peppermint oil, cinnamon, anise, coriander, garlic, sesame, and cashew. Emulsifying agents can include propylene glycol, and stabilizers include gum Arabic and other gums. Systemic contact dermatitis can occur via ingestion of foods with such additives.

Other food additives of interest include ammonium persulfate, benzoyl peroxide, natural and synthetic dyes, curcumin, and halogens. A variety of dyes is added to pharmaceuticals and this type of exposure has been associated with urticaria, purpura, asthma, and fixed drug eruptions. D & C Yellow No. 11 has been particularly problematic.

Food Additives

About 400 additives are included in the US Food and Drug Administration's list of additives "generally recognized as safe," except for large groups of natural flavors and oils. To be on this list, an additive must have been in use before 1958 and must have met certain safety specifications. Additives brought into use since 1958 must be approved individually. Substances are removed occasionally from the list by the FDA in light of new evidence.

Many additives to foods, cosmetics, and topical medications can produce contact dermatitis, including preservatives, antioxidants, dyes, flavoring agents, "spoilage retarders," "dough conditioners," "flavor protectors," and "cloudiness preventatives"[1] (Table 28.1).

The dermatitis that these chemical additives produce can be of several varieties, including irritant dermatitis, allergic eczematous contact dermatitis, and contact urticaria, both allergic and nonspecific in nature. The most common food additive dermatitis is a hand dermatitis in certain sensitized individuals, particularly homemakers, food handlers, bakers, and cooks. Often the same agents have also proved to be sensitizers in topical medications and cosmetics.[2–4]

PRESERVATIVES AND FLAVORS ADDED TO FOODS

Table 28.2 lists the preservative antibacterial and antimold agents that are added to many foods. Of these preservatives, the parabens and sorbic acid are the most common causes of contact dermatitis.

The Parabens

These agents are used not only in many topical medications and cosmetics but also in many foods. Thus, methylparaben and propylparaben may be added in the amount of 1,000 parts per million to tomato pulp, puree, catsup, pickles, relishes, fruit juices, syrups, jams, marmalades, fruit jellies, mincemeat, milk preparations, soft drinks, and candy, and packaged fish, meat, and poultry. The ingestion of paraben-containing foods does not seem to produce flares in paraben-sensitive individuals.

Sorbic Acid

This preservative food additive is unique in that it can rarely produce both allergic eczematous contact dermatitis in sensitized individuals and a nonspecific contact urticaria in 5% of the population.[5] The presence of

Table 28-1 Food Additives

Additive	Comment
Benzoyl peroxide	Flour "improver"
Butylated hydroxyanisole	Oxidizer—prevents rancidity
Butylated hydroxytoluene	Oxidizer—prevents rancidity
Calcium disodium EDTA	Stabilizer, chelating agent
Calcium propionate	Antimold for bread
Chlorophyll	Color for pastry
Citric acid	Preservative
Dodecyl gallate	Antioxidant
Dyes, certified	Cause urticaria
Flavoring agents and spices	Cause contact dermatitis
Gum arabic (acacia)	Cream and cheese additive
Gum benzoin	Antioxidant
Karaya	Pastry filler
Lauryl and propyl gallate	Antioxidant
Lanolin	Chewing gum
Monoglycerol citrate	Preservative
Nordihydroguaiaretic	Antioxidant
Paraben	Preservative
Polysorbate	Preservative
Potassium persulfate	Sprayed on some fruits
Propylene glycol alginate	Filler
Sodium benzoate	Preservative
Sodium bisulfite	Antioxidant
Sodium silicon aluminate	Lump preventer in cake mix
Sorbic acid	Preservative
Tetramethylthiuram	Sprayed on bananas
Tocopherols	Antioxidant
Tragacanth	Vegetable gum filler

sorbic acid in red fruits and in foods such as yogurt with prunes and strawberries and margarine has been said to provoke vesicular hand and foot eczema in sorbic acid–sensitive patients. Avoidance was curative and oral challenge was provocative.[6]

Sorbic acid may be added to flour, particularly in the making of rye bread. Fisher[7] reported one baker who had an eczematous contact dermatitis of the hand from hypersensitivity to sorbic acid and positive patch test reactions to sorbic acid and potassium sorbate and to flour.

Another baker developed an immediate reaction consisting of redness and slight itching of hands when he came in contact with flour containing sorbic acid. His

Table 28-2 Preservatives Added to Foods

Benzoic acid	Monoglycerol citrate
Calcium propionate	Parabens
Citric acid	Sodium benzoate
Guaiac gum	Sorbic acid

48-hour patch test gave negative results. However, he developed an immediate wheal from the application of 5% sorbic acid in petrolatum. This is a "nonspecific" contact urticaria from sorbic acid (Figure 28–1).

Clemmensen and Hjorth[8] also observed contact urticaria in 18 of 20 kindergarten children following the intake and accidental perioral application of mayonnaise salad dressing. In healthy adult controls, stinging tests and closed 20-minute patch tests with the salad dressing were positive in 9 out of 12 and 4 out of 10 cases, respectively. Twenty-minute "open" tests with the different components of the salad dressing were positive only to sorbic acid and benzoic acid. Urticaria was provoked by inunction of the salad dressing periorally in two healthy boys. Serial 20-minute closed patch testing with varying concentrations of sorbic acid in 91 patients and benzoic acid in 41 patients gave almost identical results. The response was only partially blocked by antihistamine applied locally before testing. The authors pointed out that nonimmunologic mechanisms are probably responsible for the transient reaction, and no restriction in the extensive use of sorbic acid or benzoic acid as preservatives in food should be considered. Lahti and colleagues[9] showed these types of reactions to be inhibited by prostaglandin-inhibiting agents, such as aspirin and indomethacin.

Fisher[5] observed the same type of nonspecific erythema and urticarial response in many individuals using a hydrocortisone cream containing sorbic acid as a preservative. In such individuals, it is preferable to use hydrocortisone ointment to avoid this uncomfortable stinging effect from the sorbic acid in the hydrocortisone cream, or to use a hydrocortisone cream free of sorbic acid.

ANTIOXIDANTS IN FOODS

Table 28.3 lists the antioxidants that may be used in various foods to prevent a common type of food spoilage—an undesirable change in color or flavor caused by oxygen in the air. For example, sliced fresh apples and peaches turn brown when exposed to air, and

Table 28-3 Antioxidant Food Additives

Ammonium persulfate (flour color improver used in some European countries)

Benzoyl peroxide (flour color improver)

Butylated hydroxyanisole (BHA)

Butylated hydroxytoluene (BHT)

Dodecyl gallate

Gum benzoin

Lauryl and propyl gallate

Nordihydroguaiaretic acid (NDGA)

Sodium bisulfite

Vitamin E (tocopherols)

fatty foods, such as mayonnaise and lard, become rancid if kept unprotected too long. Both of these conditions are caused by oxidation and can be retarded by using antioxidants.

The darkening of some fruits and vegetables is known as "enzymatic browning." If foods containing certain enzymes are cut, bruised, or overripe and are exposed to air, the tissues turn brown. Apples, apricots, bananas, cherries, peaches, pears, and potatoes contain such enzymes. Antioxidants prevent or delay this enzymatic browning.

Oxidation also causes the rancid taste and odor that sometimes develop in fats, oil, mayonnaise, and lard. Processed foods that contain these materials are thus protected with antioxidants from possible oxidation in order to maintain their best flavor during storage.

At present, antioxidants, such as butylated hydroxyanisole and butylated hydroxytoluene, are replacing gum benzoin. These antioxidants, which may also be present in cosmetics, can be tested 2% in petrolatum for patch test purposes.

With a few exceptions, the lipid-soluble antioxidants are phenols. Those favored by industry are butylated hydroxytoluene (BHT), butylated hydroxyanisole (BHA), nordihydroguaiaretic acid (NDGA), esters of gallic acid (propyl-, octyl-, and dodecyl-gallate), and tocopherols. NDGA is not used extensively in the United States.

Butylated Hydroxyanisole (BHA)

Other names for this antioxidant include Tenox GHA (Eastman), 2-t-butyl-4-methoxyphenol, 4-methoxy-2-t-butylphenol, Embanox (May & Baker), and Nipantiox 1-F (Nipa).

BHA is used as an antioxidant for oils and fats either alone or with a gallate and a synergist, such as citric or phosphoric acid. It may be dissolved in many oils at room temperature or warmed slightly. BHA dissolves readily in molten fats.

Up to 200 ppm of BHA or BHT, or a mixture of these, may be used for the preservation of fixed oils, fats, or vitamin oil concentrates in pharmaceutical practice and food. Up to 100 ppm of BHA or BHT may be added to essential oils used in food; its use is not allowed in essential oils of the British Pharmacopeia.

BHA is used in a wide variety of products, including beverages, ice cream, candy, baked foods, gelatin, soup bases, potatoes, glazed fruits, potato flakes, dry breakfast cereals, dry yeast, dry mixes for desserts and beverages, shortening, smoked dry sausage, and emulsions as stabilizers for shortenings.

Roed-Petersen and Hjorth,[10] in a search for contact sensitivity to antioxidants, patch tested consecutive patients referred with eczematous dermatitis. Six cases

of allergic contact sensitivity to NDGA were observed. Three had been sensitized by one brand of cream containing 0.1% NDGA; in three other patients, the source of sensitization could not be traced.

Four patients had positive patch tests to BHA or BHT. In two cases, the positive patch tests were relevant because both patients remained asymptomatic when antioxidants were avoided in foods. They both had acute flares of vesicular eczema on the fingers after oral administration of small amounts.

Butylated Hydroxytoluene (BHT)

This antioxidant, which is substituted for toluene, has several names: Catalin CAO-3 (Ashland), DBPC, 2,6-di-t-butyl-p-cresol, Ionol (Shell), Ionol CP (Shell), Tenox BHT (Eastman), 4-methyl-2,6-di-t-butyl-phenol, Annulex BHT, Embanox BHT (May & Baker), Topanol OC, and O (ICI).

BHT, like BHA, is used as an antioxidant for oil and fats. In foods, BHT may be used to a 0.02% concentration, whereas in cosmetics it is used in a 0.01% to 0.1% concentration.

Reactions from Ingestion of Antioxidants BHA and BHT

Fisherman and Cohen[11] reported that a group of patients developed a "positive sequential vascular response" to BHA and BHT. These patients, upon ingestion of BHA and BHT, had an intensification of rhinitis and asthma. Other symptoms noted on challenge were marked diaphoresis, somnolence, headaches, occasionally high retrosternal pain radiating to the back, flushing, and suffusion of the conjunctivae. In addition, all of the BHA-BHT patients, when tested with aspirin in doses of 100 mg, not only did not exacerbate clinically, but they often improved.

One investigation of BHT found none of 1,336 patients patch tested to be positive to 2% BHT in petrolatum.[12] Other uses for BHT are given in Table 28.4. The table lists the product category only.

Sodium Bisulfite in Salads

Epstein[13] described hand eczema in a salad maker caused by Veg-White, an antioxidant used to prevent discoloration of fruits and vegetables in salads. The specific sensitizer in this preparation was sodium bisulfite. Patch tests can be performed with a 1% aqueous solution of sodium bisulfite.

Patch tests with sodium bisulfite must be interpreted with care because many test results are irritant in nature. Several controls should always be tested. Toxic effects from the ingestion of sodium bisulfite in foods have been reported recently.[14-16]

Product category	No. of products*	Typical concentration
Paints and lacquers (1- and 2-component)	141	< 25 ppm
Hardeners for 2-component paints, glues, fillers, etc.	100	< 10 ppm
Binders for paints, glues, fillers, etc.	34	0–2000 ppm
Adhesives/glues	33	200–1000 ppm
Toiletries	31	200–1000 ppm
Industrial oil and grease (including cutting fluids)	23	300–10,000 ppm
Fillings and mouldings	23	< 25 ppm
Cleaning agents	11	< 200 ppm
Printing/offset products (inks, stabilizers, etc.)	9	—
Thinners and solvents	8	—
Flooring materials	5	—

*Some products are registered in two or more product categories. Categories with fewer than four products were omitted. Used with permission from Flyvolm, M-A., and Menné, T. Sensitizing risk of butylated hydroxytoluene based on exposure and effect data. Contact Dermatitis 23:341, 1990.

Gallates (Gallic Acid Esters)

The esters most commonly used as antioxidants are the propyl, octyl, and dodecyl esters. The latter two are easily soluble in fats. Propyl ester is more soluble in water than in fats. These antioxidants are often used in the cosmetic and food industry, particularly in bakery goods and frying oils. In guinea pigs all three gallates are moderate to strong sensitizers, with dodecyl being the strongest.[17] A 0.3% concentration in petrolatum is recommended for patch testing. Octyl gallate, when mixed with heated chicken fat, has caused an airborne contact dermatitis.[18]

Lauryl Gallate

Brun[19] reported contact dermatitis in a baker due to lauryl gallate present as an antioxidant in margarine.

Postendorf[20] speculated that the topical application of cosmetics and pharmaceuticals containing gallates may produce dermatitis in certain individuals, "perhaps because they are sensitized by gallates in foodstuffs."

ORAL SYMPTOMS AND ADDITIVES

Lip swelling and oral ulceration are symptoms that at times can be caused by food additives. Menthol, peppermint oil, dodecyl and octyl gallate, and butylated hydroxyanisole were identified as causative factors in five patients reported by Lewis and colleagues.[21] For menthol and peppermint oil, restrictions were placed on toothpaste, mouthwashes, inhalers, and confections. For the gallates, margarine, oils, cosmetics, and lip balms were restricted. Butylated hydroxyanisole sensitivity was treated with avoidance of margarine, fats, soups, sauces, cakes, and pastries.

Peppermint Oil

The ingredients in peppermint oil include menthol, menthone, menthyl esters (acetate and isovalerate), l-limonene, pinene, phellandrene, and cineole. Wilkinson and Beck[22] emphasized the role of menthol as an allergen in peppermint oil and noted that menthol joins l-limonene, alpha-pinene, and phellandrene as causes of contact dermatitis.

Detection of menthol and peppermint oil allergy may be missed if patch test readings are not taken beyond day 4. Fleming and Forsyth[23] found day 5 to be the correct time to read for these allergens.

Morton and colleagues[24] reported 12 cases of allergy to peppermint oil and/or menthol sensitivity in patients with burning mouth syndrome, recurrent oral ulceration, or lichenoid oral reactions. Avoidance of the identified substance was clearly beneficial in at least half of these individuals.

Cinnamon

Malten[25] reported several bakers with contact dermatitis and identified cinnamon as the causative agent. It should be noted that cinnamon and balsam of Peru often cross-react. Fisher[26] observed a baker with allergic hypersensitivity in whom hand dermatitis flared whenever he drank vermouth containing cinnamon. This patient also developed a cheilitis from the use of a cinnamon-containing toothpaste.

Spices used in cooking may produce systemic contact dermatitis.[27]

Tocopherols or Vitamin E

These natural substances are themselves rather prone to oxidation and are therefore not quite as suitable as the synthetic antioxidants already mentioned. Yet they are widely used as a result of the urge to produce pure natural foodstuffs. The smell of oxidized tocopherols is slightly reminiscent of fish, which can be a disadvantage in some foods. Most vegetable oils in their natural state contain considerable amounts of tocopherols, for example, 0.1% to 0.01%. Animal fats also contain tocopherols, but to a far lesser degree.

It is worthwhile to note that there are no reports of allergic reactions from the ingestion of vitamin E. Topical application of vitamin E, however, can readily produce allergic contact dermatitis. Thus, so many cases of dermatitis were produced by Mennen's "E" deodorant that it was withdrawn from the market. In addition, patients who pierce vitamin E capsules and rub the contents into their skin or apply various vitamin E creams or topical agents not infrequently acquire allergic contact dermatitis (see Chapter 9).

Topical vitamin E may also cause contact urticaria (see Chapter 16).

Nordihydroguaiaretic Acid (NDGA)

This antioxidant, no longer used in food in the United States, is used in pharmaceutical and cosmetic preparations. It may be made synthetically or extracted from guaiac and desert plants. Roed-Petersen and Hjorth[10] reported allergic reactions to this antioxidant.

Anise

Cakes baked with anise caused contact dermatitis in two women reported from Seville who were proven to be sensitive to the allergen in anise, anethole.[28] The chemical name for anethole is 1-methoxy-4-(1-propenyl) benzene, and it is closely related to eugenol, but cross-reactivity does not occur.

Coriander

Coriander in curry powder has caused a variety of skin problems, including stomatitis, hand dermatitis, and contact urticaria. It is derived from the dried fruit of *Coriander sativum*. A chef presented with hand dermatitis and was found to have a negative patch test to coriander, but a positive prick test. This is considered protein contact dermatitis. He was also found to have a positive prick test to celery, carrot, and mugwort; the addition of a spice made his case fit a syndrome that is called "celery-carrot-mugwort-spice syndrome." This is an oral allergy syndrome.[29] A similar case of mugwort-spice syndrome was reported in a butcher who had chronic hand dermatitis but rather than delayed hypersensitivity, he manifested immediate reactions to cumin, curry, paprika, and mugwort. He was prick test negative to celery and carrot. This is another example of protein contact dermatitis.[30]

Compositae

Wintzen and colleagues[31] pointed out the difficulty of differentiating atopic dermatitis from dermatitis due to an endogenous food source. Their patient was a 35-year-old woman who was patch test positive to Compositae mix. When their patient avoided food products from the Compositae family, she improved dramatically. She avoided chamomile tea, lettuce, chicory, and endive. Initially the patch test seemed related to past rather than present events, but allergen avoidance led to her no longer requiring topical corticosteroids.

Propolis

While honey does not normally contain propolis, a known contact allergen, some home-made honeys may have propolis added for "therapeutic" purposes. This proved to be the cause of cheilitis and perioral dermatitis in a woman who ingested home-made honey containing propolis. She did not demonstrate any stomatitis.[32]

Garlic

Contact dermatitis to garlic has been associated with fingertip dermatitis but caused a pompholyx pattern of dermatitis when ingested orally as a commercially available garlic extract to treat hyperlipidemia.[33] A 5% aqueous patch test to garlic extract was positive. Cooked garlic did not cause a reaction, as this denatures the allergens diallyldisulfide, allylpropyldisulfide, and allicin. In a review of 7 years of patch test experience, 69 cases of positive reactions to plants could be identified. Of these, 47 were diallyl disulfide and most commonly the patient was a middle-aged housewife with chronic hand eczema.[34]

A garlic herb coating mix applied to potato wedges caused a worker to develop dermatitis of the forearms. She was patch test positive to diallyl disulfide and *Myroxylon pereirae* (balsam of Peru), and also to a 25% dilution of the garlic herb mix. It was not clear if the herbs in the mix were linked to the balsam of Peru reaction.[35] Cheilitis, accompanied by dermatitis of the antecubital fossae, lower back, and periorbital skin, was found to be due to diallyl disulfide in a woman who ate raw garlic but did not prepare foods with garlic and thus the fingers were spared.[36] Exposure to pure garlic powder in a food-industry worker led to both type I and type IV allergy symptoms. The patient had a high IgE level to garlic, but patch tests to diallyl disulfide, the usual garlic allergen, were negative. Instead, the patient reacted to garlic powder in arachis oil 10%, which was negative in 13 controls.[37] Eczema of the lip brought on by sunlight exposure was traced to diallyl disulfide in garlic proven by photopatch testing to diallyl disulfide 1% in petrolatum and exposure to 15J of UVA light.[38]

MISCELLANEOUS ADDITIVES

Sesame

Sesame oil in food and cosmetics caused urticaria from ingestion and skin contact in two French patients.[39] Prick tests were positive to crushed sesame seeds, sesame oil, or their own products.

Cashew

Allergen may be added to foodstuffs and provoke systemic reactions that clinically display flexural, groin, and/orbuttock erythema. Hamilton and Zug[40] reported

Table 28-5 Emulsifying Agents in Foods
Cholic acid
Desoxycholic acid
Discetyl tartaric acid esters of mono- and diglycerides
Glycocholic acid
Mono- and diglycerides
Monosodium phosphate derivatives of above
Ox bile extract
Propylene glycol
Taurocholic acid

Table 28-6 Foods Containing Propylene Glycol
Bakers Coconut
Dream-Whip Whipped Topping Mix
Duncan Hines cake mixes
Durkee Coconut
Durkee Real French Fried Onions and Potato Sticks
Hellman's Big H (sandwich mix)
Jello Cheesecake Mix
Kraft Thousand Island, Creamy Cucumber, Russian Dressing
Mountain Dew Beverage
Pepperidge Farms—pineapple n'cream, strawberry n'cream, and most of its frosted cakes
Pfeiffer Russian, cole slaw, French dressing
Pillsbury Plus cake mixes
Sara Lee chocolate n'cream layer, strawberry n'cream layer cake, French cheesecake, chocolate Bavarian, and strawberry cheesecake
Wise Butter Flavored Popcorn

this type of reaction in a Toxicodendron-sensitive patient who ingested a pesto sauce that contained raw cashew nuts. When cashew nuts are roasted, the allergen is inactivated, but the pesto had the raw nuts.

EMULSIFYING AGENTS IN FOODS

Propylene Glycol

Propylene glycol is the only emulsifying agent (Table 28.5) that has been shown to be a sensitizer. Individuals sensitized to propylene glycol from topical agents may exhibit a "systemic" contact dermatitis when they eat foods containing this emulsifier.[41] Many prepared food salads contain propylene glycol. Table 28.6 lists some of the foods that contain significant amounts of propylene glycol.

Propylene Glycol Dermatitis Due to Ingestion of Certain Foods

Fisher[41] reported three women, with exquisite allergic hypersensitivity to propylene glycol, who were certain that otherwise unexplained flares of their dermatitis were caused by the ingestion of foods containing propylene glycol. These women implicated the propylene glycol–containing foods shown in Table 28.6 as the cause of their flare-ups.

Flares of dermatitis were produced in two patients who deliberately ate propylene glycol–containing foods. Patch tests with the implicated foods gave negative results, however.

Hannuksela and Forstrom[42] performed double-blind tests with ingestion of capsules containing propylene glycol. Eight of 10 patients sensitive to a 2% propylene glycol patch test and seven of 28 sensitive to 10% to 100% patch tests exhibited an exanthem 3 to 16 hours after ingestion of 2 to 15 mL of propylene glycol.

Sodium Stearoyl Lactylate

Sodium stearoyl lactylate is an emulsifier that can be added to dough to improve texture, or as an emulsifier in whipped foods such as whipped cream, salad dres-

sings, soups, and coffee creamers. It has stabilizer and emulsifier properties in egg-white products. It can also be used as an emulsifier in cosmetics and was reported as a contact allergen in ostrich oil cream. When tested at 2% in petrolatum there may be irritant reactions.[43]

STABILIZERS IN FOODS

Table 28.7 is a list of food stabilizers. Some of the stabilizers also include waxes and gums, guaiac, guar, karaya, acacia (gum arabic), tragacanth, benzoin, spermaceti, carnauba, and beeswax; the last four are used to glaze confectionery. Acacia (gum arabic) is used in chocolate drinks, creams, French dressing, malt liquors, milk, mustard, pickles, cheese, ice cream, and sherbet. Guaiac gum is used as a preservative for fats and oils, guar gum for a preservative in milk products. Guar gum is also used as a stabilizer and as a thickening and film-forming agent for cheese, salad dressings, ice cream, and soups, and as a binding and disintegrating agent in tablet formulations in suspensions, emulsions, lotions, creams, and toothpastes.

Because some of these waxes and gums crossreact with balsam of Peru, routine patch testing with balsam of

Table 28-7 Stabilizers in Foods	
Acacia (gum arabic)	Ghatti gum
Agar-agar	Guar gum
Ammonium alginate	Potassium alginate
Calcium alginate	Sodium alginate
Carbo bean gum	Sterculia (or karaya) gum
Chondrus extract	Tragacanth

Peru may be valuable in discovering the cause of hand dermatitis in food handlers.

Karaya Gum Dermatitis

A baker complained that whenever he prepared meringue pies he developed a dermatitis on his hands. It was learned that karaya gum is used as a pastry filler and stabilizer of the meringue. Potassium sorbate is sometimes also used as a preservative in meringue. Patch testing revealed a positive reaction to karaya gum, which is a rare sensitizer. Karaya, a vegetable gum derivative, is also used widely in hair-waving lotions, denture adhesive powders, and furniture polishes, and as a cement for ileostomy appliances. It may occasionally produce allergic reactions from such exposure.[44] (See also Chapter 10.)

BLEACHING AGENTS TO "IMPROVE" FLOUR

The "persulfates" in Europe and occasionally benzoyl peroxide, in the United States, added to flour have produced contact dermatitis in bakers.[45,46]

Ammonium Persulfate Reactions

Ammonium persulfate was previously used in certain European countries as a flour "improver" to render the flour white. This flour "improver" was especially used in Greece. In the United States, this chemical has never been used in flour but is used widely in hair bleaches to enhance the bleaching action of hydrogen peroxide. Interestingly, a woman who formerly baked bread in Greece and who had acquired a severe hand dermatitis from the presence of ammonium persulfate in flour developed a severe reaction and a flare-up of her hand dermatitis when she had her hair bleached in the United States.[45]

Ammonium persulfate may not only produce an eczematous contact dermatitis, but in certain persons severe urticaria and anaphylactic shock may occur.

Cronin[47] stated that in the 1920s ammonium and potassium persulfates and benzoyl peroxide were added to flour to inhibit proteolytic enzymes from attacking the gluten films that surround the carbon dioxide bubbles that form during fermentation and make bread light. Both chemicals are sensitizers, and their introduction increased the incidence of baker's eczema. Persulfates, thought to be the greater hazard, were banned first in Switzerland, Belgium, and Denmark, and in 1957, in Germany, where persulfate sensitivity had become a considerable problem. After their use was prohibited in Germany, the incidence of baker's eczema fell.

Ammonium persulfate and benzoyl peroxide are still used to make flour in the Netherlands and Britain, but, although benzoyl peroxide is still widely used, many millers have replaced the persulfates with potassium bromate, which is equally efficient and easier to handle.

Benzoyl Peroxide Dermatitis

A young baker had acquired a contact dermatitis of the hands from the presence of benzoyl peroxide used as a flour bleach. When he applied a benzoyl peroxide acne preparation to his face, a severe facial dermatitis developed in addition to a flare-up of his hand dermatitis.[4]

IRRITANT AND ALLERGIC HAND DERMATITIS IN BAKERS DUE TO FOOD ADDITIVES

Table 28.8 lists the food additives to flour, bread, or pastry that can produce a nonspecific irritant dermatitis. Thus, most instances of hand dermatitis in bakers that Fisher[48] observed were due to nonspecific dermatitis from various irritants, such as wet, sticky dough, sweetening agents, and various flavors. Soaps and detergents used for cleansing the hands are also often the cause of irritant bakers' dermatitis. In such instances, patch tests give negative results.

Bakers may also react to enzymes added to flour to facilitate the rising of dough. These additives also make bread lighter and extend shelf life. The enzymes used include alpha- and beta-amylase, cellulase, proteases, and lipoxygenases. Alpha-amylase has been identified as a cause of hand eczema and respiratory allergy (rhinitis and asthma) in bakers.[49] Of 32 bakers tested, 7 were found to have immediate hypersensitivity and 2 had delayed hypersensitivity.

Table 28.9 lists the allergen food additives encountered by bakers and the concentration for patch test purposes.

Table 28-8 Food Additive Irritants That Bakers May Encounter

Acetic acid

Ascorbinic acid (flour improver)

Bleaching agents

Calcium acetate and sulfate

Emulsifying agents

Lactic acid

Potassium bicarbonate

Potassium iodide and bromate

Yeast

Table 28-9 Food Additive Allergens in the Baking Industry

Allergen	Patch test concentration
Benzoyl peroxide	1% pet
Potassium bromate	5% in water
Cinnamon oil	0.5% pet
Limonene, oil of	1% alcohol
p-amino-azo-benzene (indicator for azo dyes)	0.25% pet
Eugenol	5% pet
Vanilla (alcoholic extract)	10% in acetone
Sorbic acid	5% pet
Karaya gum (sterculia gum)	As is
Ammonium persulfate (Europe)	1% in water

Pet = in petrolatum.

INSECTICIDE SPRAYS ON FRUITS

Table 28.10 lists insecticides that may adhere to foods. Such insecticides may produce contact dermatitis in those handling such fruits.

MISCELLANEOUS FOOD ADDITIVES

Quillaja is used as a foaming agent for soft drinks, and sodium alginate is listed for a wide variety of foods. Aluminum sulfate, admittedly a rare skin sensitizer, is permitted in canned fish, pickles, relishes, and starch.

COLORS ADDED TO FOODS

Several "natural" and 10 synthetic organic dyes are permitted in the United States. Citrus Red No. 2 and Sunset Yellow have formulas that indicate possible crossreactions with paraphenylenediamine and sulfanilamide. The synthetic colors are permitted for the dyeing of oranges, apples, jam, butter, cheese, and fish.

Chlorophyll may be added to certain pastries.

Citrus Red No. 2, used to color Florida oranges, may crossreact with clothing dyes.[50]

Curcumin

A pasta worker whose job it was to add food color to pasta and collect the fresh pasta from the machine was found allergic to curcumin food color.[51] Curcumin is used to color butter, margarine, cheese, spaghetti, macaroni, and liqueurs. *Curcuma longa* is the source for turmeric, which is derived from the rootstock of the plant. The *Curcuma*

Table 28-10 Insecticides Sprayed on Fruits

Potassium persulfate (many fruits)
Tetramethylthiuram disulfide (bananas)
Thiabendazol (citrus fruits)

Table 28-11 Metals in Foods*

Aluminum sulfate
Chromium (from water)
Cobalt
Nickel (may also be added to hydrogenated fats)

*Ethylenediamine tetra-acetate (EDTA) is often added to foods to chelate these metals.

rootstock is also the source for curcumin, the yellow food dye that produced positive patch test responses down to 0.001%. This is also a component of curry powder, and the patient reacted to curry powder at 1% concentration. She also reacted to ginger which is from *Zingiber officinale*, a member of the same family as *Curcuma longa*.

POTATO CHIP DERMATITIS

Inman[52] traced three cases of contact dermatitis of the hands occurring in a potato chip factory that were due, respectively, to cheese powder, wheat filler, and onion powder.

METALS IN FOODS

Most foods contain traces of metals, including nickel and chromium (Table 28.11). Ethylenediamine tetra-acetate (EDTA) is added to many foods to chelate such metals. It must be emphasized that EDTA is not a sensitizer and does not crossreact with ethylenediamine hydrochloride, which is a notorious sensitizer.

Nickel may be added to act as a catalyst in hydrogenating fats. In addition, it has been reported that the ingestion of nickel in foods could produce pompholyx and flares of nickel dermatitis in sensitized individuals.[53]

SULFATES IN FOODS

Sodium lauryl sulfate is used in egg white, sodium sulfate is added to biscuits and tuna fish, and sodium thiosulfate is added to table salt. The hands of food handlers with atopic or eczematous skin may be irritated by these sulfates. Aluminum sulfate is a permitted additive in canned fish, pickles, relishes, and starch.

HALOGENS IN FOODS

It should be noted that vegetable oil for citrus-flavored beverages is "brominated," and calcium iodate is used for some bakery products. Such iodine or bromine additives may produce "fixed" drug eruptions or eruptions of a pustular nature.

Several patients developed a pustular eruption from eating kelp in a salad or in vitamin preparations.

Norwegian Kelp Tablets are described as a dietary supplement. Each tablet is said to contain "0.225 mg of iodine, which supplies 22.5% of the Adult Minimum

Daily Requirement in a base of organically grown alfalfa, for which no nutritional claims are made."

Kelp, a giant brown seaweed, is one of the largest algae and may grow as long as 300 feet. The ashes of this seaweed are used as a source of iodine and sometimes potash.[54]

SILICATES AS ANTICAKING AGENTS

The silicates listed in Table 28.12 have not been implicated as contact allergens.

Table 28-12 Anticaking Agents
Aluminum calcium silicate
Calcium silicate
Magnesium silicate
Sodium aluminosilicate
Sodium calcium aluminosilicate
Tricalcium silicate

SYNTHETIC FLAVORING AGENTS

Table 28.13 lists these agents, many of which are sensitizers.

Table 28-13 Synthetic Flavoring Substances
Acetaldehyde
Acetoin
Aconitic acid
Anethole
Benzaldehyde
N-butyric acid
d- or l-carvone
Cinnamaldehyde
Citral
Decana
Diacetyl
Ethyl acetate
Ethyl butyrate
Ethyl vanillin
Eugenol
Geraniol
Geranyl acetate
Glycerol tributyrate
Limonene
Linalool
Linalyl acetate
1-malic acid
Methyl anthranilate
3-methyl-3-phenyl glycidic acid ethyl ester
Piperanol
Vanillin

Table 28-14 "Natural" Food Colors	
Anthocyanins	Flavonoids
Carotenoids	Metals
Chlorophyll	Turmeric spice

Food Dyes and Colors

Dyes added to foods, drugs, cosmetics, and textiles may produce contact dermatitis.

Dyes and various colors are added to foods for the following reasons: (a) to ensure uniform color; (b) to replace colors changed by preservatives, various processes, heat, light, and cold; and (c) to augment color of pale foods.

Table 28.14 lists the various natural colors that may be added to foods; Table 28.15 lists synthetic dyes that may be added to food. Allergic contact dermatitis from such food dyes and colors is rare; however, three of the food dyes listed in Table 28.16—amaranth, Sunset Yellow, and tartrazine—have been implicated as causing contact urticaria and purpura. Another dye, neococcine (a carrine red dye), has been similarly implicated.[55-60]

The food dyes that produce urticaria often occur in aspirin-sensitive individuals.[58,61]

Table 28-15 Food Synthetic Dyes	
Anthraquinone	Quinolene
Azo	Triarylmethane
Artificial caramel	Xanthene
Indigoid	

NATURE OF FD&C AZO FOOD DYES

Food, Drug and Cosmetic (FD&C) azo dyes, derived from coal tar, are "certified." "Certification" refers to lack of toxicity and not to allergenicity (Figure 28-2). These dyes rarely crossreact with paraphenylenediamine and are widely used to color many foods, including gelatin desserts, oleomargarine, other edible fats and oils, maraschino cherries, sausage casings, frozen desserts, carbonated beverages (FD&C Blue No. 2 is used for

Table 28-16 Food Dye Patch-Test Series	
Test 2% petrolatum	Fast green
Amaranth	Indigotine
Benzyl violet	Ponceau SX
Brilliant blue	Sunset Yellow
Citrus Red No. 2	Tartrazine
Erythrosine	

special grape shades), candy and confectionery products, bakery products, spaghetti, and puddings.

The incidence of hypersensitivity to FD&C dyes in the general population is not known. An association, however, between hypersensitivity to aspirin and tartrazine has been described.[59-69] Juhlin and colleagues[58] reported that seven of eight aspirin-sensitive patients were also allergic to tartrazine. Smith[62] found two of five aspirin-sensitive patients to be allergic to tartrazine. On the other hand, Samter and Beers,[63] in 1967, reported 3 of 40 aspirin-sensitive patients to also be allergic to tartrazine. The following year, these authors[64] reported 14 of 182 aspirin-sensitive patients to also be allergic to tartrazine. The reported incidence of aspirin hypersensitivity varies among different authors but seems to be in the range of 1% to 5% of the population, the higher percentage found in patients with asthma.[66,67] It would appear that tartrazine hypersensitivity is relatively uncommon, although it probably occurs with greater frequency in individuals with a documented history of allergy.

FOOD DYES

Mitchell[50] tested with a food-dye series shown in Table 28.16[50] (see also Chapter 16.) He found that a chef with a foot dermatitis, who was mistakenly tested with a food patch test series, was found to react to Citrus Red No. 2 that apparently crossreacted with the dye in his socks, which remained unidentified. Citrus Red dermatitis is rare. Bandmann and Nasemann[68] observed sensitization to a Ponceau (Red 6R) in a pastry cook. Citrus Red is now used to color Florida oranges, but not the California variety.

Dyes Used in Drugs

Pharmaceutical manufacturers add dyes to the liquid or solid formulation, the tablet coating, or the hard gelatin capsule of most of their products for purposes of drug identification and dosage form differentiation. These are valid reasons for the addition of coloring agents in drugs, and their continued inclusion is a necessity. Some manufacturers have employed vegetable dyes to color their products, but these agents have fallen into relative disuse because of a lack of stability resulting in a loss of uniformity of color.

For this reason, most companies now use one or more of the FD&C azo dyes (-N=N-group) that are derived from coal tar. These include FD&C Red No. 2, Red No. 3, Red No. 4, Blue No. 1, Blue No. 2, Violet No. 1, Green No. 3, Yellow No. 3, Yellow No. 5, Yellow No. 6, Yellow No. 10, and Yellow No. 11.

In addition to the pure FD&C dyes, various combinations of two or more may be employed to produce

another color (e.g., Velo Dark Green dye contains FD&C Yellow No. 5). FD&C Lake dyes are also used, prepared by extending, on a substratum of alumina, a salt prepared from one of the water-soluble, pure FD&C dyes by combining the color with aluminum or calcium. Drug and Cosmetic dyes, such as D&C Red No. 40, are added occasionally to pharmaceutical products as coloring agents. This group, unlike the pure FD&C dyes, is not used to color food products. FD&C Red No. 2, Red No. 4, Blue No. 1, Yellow No. 5, and Yellow No. 6 are the dyes that have been used most frequently in drugs.

Several dyes used in pharmaceutical products have demonstrated the potential for inducing allergic reactions in hypersensitive patients. It should be noted that the population at large is exposed to potentially allergenic FD&C dyes in foods to a greater extent than in drugs. This reflects the obviously greater ingestion of food compared with drugs, as well as the greater amounts of dye included in food products compared with drugs. In addition, foods contain potentially allergenic vegetable dyes rarely present in pharmaceutical preparations. Nevertheless, a problem resulting from coloring agents in drugs has been identified and cannot be disregarded.

Chafee and Settipane[65] in 1974 reported a case of recurrent asthma due to tartrazine. Tartrazine was finally implicated when the patient noted an exacerbation of symptoms upon taking 1.25-mg tablets of Premarin (conjugated estrogen), which also contain this dye. After elimination of tartrazine-containing products, the patient did well.

Criep[56] in 1971 reported a case of nonthrombocytopenic vascular purpura resulting from hypersensitivity to tartrazine in an adult. The patient gave a history of repeated episodes of bleeding into the skin and from various mucous membranes following ingestion of the dye.

TESTING FOR REACTIONS TO DYES IN DRUGS

Lockey[59] described sublingual testing with diluted samples of pure FD&C dyes to challenge the patient and reported the technique in detail. The patient was observed for 20 minutes following sublingual administration for signs of hypersensitivity. Feingold[55] employed a method of clinical screening to diagnose and treat suspected allergy to FD&C dyes. Patients were divided into four groups based on their pattern of allergy and skin testing, and various elimination diets were prescribed for each group, in an attempt to identify and isolate offending allergens.

Juhlin and colleagues[58] administered tartrazine in an oral solution and observed patients for signs of hypersensitivity. Allergic patients responded significantly to quantities as little as 0.75 mg. (The amount of tartrazine present in various pharmaceutical preparations is variable, but may range from 0.002 mg to greater than 2.5 mg per dosage unit in those preparations that contain the dye.)

Michaâlsson and colleagues[60] were able to provoke purpuric reactions in their hypersensitive patients by administering allergenic dyes orally in colorless gelatin capsules. A topical vasodilator was applied to a skin test site, causing a localized nonpurpuric erythema before dye administration. In some trials, purpura developed only in this test area upon ingestion of the allergenic dye. In others, purpura was more widespread. Dyes to which the patient was not hypersensitive produced no purpura.

Fiedelman and Martens[61] suggested full disclosure in labeling of all additives present in drugs. This would help prevent exposure in those patients with known hypersensitivity to coloring agents, but would do little to prevent the occurrence of new cases. Another solution is the removal of coloring agents from certain drugs, particularly those used frequently in the treatment of atopic patients (e.g., antihistamines, antiasthmatics, and corticosteroids). As an alternative, pharmaceutical companies could selectively produce dye-free preparations for those patients with known or suspected hypersensitivity to coloring agents. Indeed, for this reason, tartrazine has been removed from one antiasthmatic preparation that is available both with and without dye (Marax syrup and Marax DF syrup).

In addition to their inclusion in medication meant for oral administration, coloring agents may be present in topical preparations. Often, hospital pharmacies will add coloring agents to solutions that were originally dye-free for purposes of identification. These preparations may cause contact dermatitis in hypersensitive individuals, a reaction not uncommonly seen after application of cosmetics that contain allergenic dyes.

D&C YELLOW NO. 11

D&C Yellow No. 11 (CAS No. 8003-22-3) is the FDA designation for a color additive certified for use in drugs and cosmetics. The dye component is principally 2-(2 quinolyl)-1,3-in-dandione, synthesized by the condensation of quinoline with phthalic anhydride at 200°C in the presence of zinc. The dye substance is also known as CI Solvent No. Yellow 33, CI No. 47,000, Quinoline Yellow SS, Quinoline Yellow Base, Quinoline Yellow Spirit Soluble, Waxoline Yellow T, and Arlosol Yellow SS.

Rapaport stated that quinazaline yellow SS (D&C Yellow No. 11), a quinoline chemical, elicited interest because of a potential for sensitization.[69-72] This is an FDA-approved dye that is used widely in cosmetics. However, D&C Yellow No. 10, a closely related quinoline chemical, is more widely used in cosmetics and topical

preparations, and there has been some concern about possible cross-sensitization between these two drugs.

Noster and Hausen[73] reported one case of occupational allergic contact dermatitis due to D&C Yellow No. 11 that was present in colored smoke used in a detonator. The authors attempted sensitization experiments on guinea pigs but were unsuccessful. Börkner and Magnusson,[74] studying D&C Yellow 11 in 1981, commented on its use in spirit, lacquers, polystyrenes, polycarbonates, polyamides, acrylic resins, cosmetics, colored smokes, and hydrocarbon solvents. They patch tested 88 subjects with a 1% preparation in polyethylene glycol and found four positive patch test responses at 72 hours. One subject had a crossreaction to D&C Yellow No. 10 when patch tests to that dye were carried out.

These dyes are used extensively to impart a green-yellow shade to cosmetics and topical preparations. More than 300 cosmetic preparations incorporate D&C Yellow into their formulas; usage of D&C Yellow No. 10 is even more widespread. In 1977, in the United States alone, 8.16 tons of D&C Yellow No. 10 and 2.23 tons of D&C Yellow No. 11 were used. Although in Europe D&C Yellow No. 10 is used as a food-coloring agent, especially in soft drinks, in the United States its use is not allowed in foods but is, however, allowed in drugs.

Many other quinolines are used in medical products. Oral drugs, for example, iodochlorohydroxyquin, chloroquin, oxolinic acid (an antimicrobial used for urinary tract infections), and oxamniquine (an antischistosomal drug), are typical. In addition, coccidiostat, an animal feed, and ethoxyquin, an antioxidant in animal feed, have widespread usage and similar formulas. The contents of all of these preparations allow for the possibility of crossreaction between the yellow dyes and chemically related topical and oral drugs.

Jordan[75] reported that a patient with D&C Yellow No. 11 sensitivity developed an allergic dermatitis from a yellow Irish Spring Soap containing this dye. She did not react, however, to green Irish Spring Soap.

Pink Dove and Caress also contain Yellow D&C No. 11. Rapaport[69] stated that Yellow D&C No. 11 does *not* crossreact with Yellow D&C No. 10. This investigator was able to sensitize 15 subjects of a panel of 56 (27%) to Yellow D&C No. 11. Some of these patients, however, did not show any reactions on retesting. They could also use cosmetics containing the dye without difficulty. There were no crossreactions with D&C No. 10. Rapaport commented that much stress is given to prophetic patch testing in terms of predicting difficulties with topically applied chemicals. Some of the chemicals in cosmetics are weak sensitizers, and detailed prophetic patch testing is necessary to seek out sensitization. Some subjects who showed positive sensitization patch test patterns 2 years earlier did not show positive reactions again to repeated insult patch tests after this rest period. Only 50% of the subjects showed positive reactions on repeated insult patch testing 2 years later. Long-term usage of the dyes in great amounts on large areas of the body does not induce dermatitis, even though a positive patch test reaction was noted in several of the subjects. Positive prophetic patch test reactions to new or existing chemicals usually imply allergenicity for positive patch test subjects on environmental contact. Possibly contact was not maintained for a long enough period in this study.

Jordan[75] stated that the eliciting of a dye allergy from showering with a soap and his predictive tests show that D&C Yellow No. 11 is a significant allergen.

Palazzolo and DiPasquale[76] found a high sensitization frequency in guinea pigs with predictive testing with D&C Yellow No. 11.

Phototoxic Dyes

Table 28.17 lists phototoxic dyes (see also Chapter 22.) The phototoxic reaction may be dependent on oxygen or visible light .[77]

NEUTRAL RED

This dye is no longer used for the treatment of herpes simplex because not only it has proved ineffective, but it is also a contact sensitizer.

Mitchell and Stewart[78] reported that a woman developed allergic contact dermatitis from neutral red chloride that had been applied to the skin for herpes simplex of the nose in three episodes over 3 months. She also had contact dermatitis of the skin of the foot from contamination with the dye. The patient's patch test to the dye, which she had used in a 3% aqueous solution, was strongly positive. A patch test given to five control subjects was negative.

Dahlquist and Fregert[79] reported neutral red added as a pH indicator to a quaternary ammonium salt solution produced an allergic contact dermatitis.

Conant and Maibach[80] also reported allergic contact dermatitis from neutral red, as did Goldenberg and Nelson,[81] from its use in the treatment of herpes genitalis.

Table 28-17 Phototoxic Dyes	
Acridine orange	Methylene blue
Acriflavine	Neutral red
Dibromofluorescein	Rose Bengal
Disperse blue 35	Toluidine blue
Eosin	

"Natural" Dyes

People first turned to plants for dyes. Among the best known and most widely used were woad (*Isatis tinctoria*) and indigo (*Indigofera tinctoria*), which gave a blue color. Yellows were provided by safflower (*Carthamus tinctorius*) and curcuma (*Curcuma ssp.*); madder (*Rubia tinctorium*), henna (*Larosonia*), and annatto (*Bixa orellana*) gave reddish hues.

Dyestuffs of animal origin were apparently developed later. It is interesting that all of these dyes were in the red color range, such as the Tyrian purple of the purpura shellfish (*Murex* spp., *Purpura* spp.) and carmine or crimson from the insects kermes (*Kermococcus vermilius*) and cochineal (*Dactylopius coccus*).[82]

The increasing mechanization of the textile industry in Europe from about the middle of the eighteenth century resulted in enormous growth in production and demanded large amounts of chemical aids, such as bleaches, detergents, and dyestuffs. This demand created the basis of the chemical industry. Originally, the chemical industry was very much textile-oriented but was only able to supply bleaches and detergents. Consequently, the cultivation of plants or insects yielding natural dyestuffs grew into a big business. Madder was produced in great quantities in southern Europe, but indigo, logwood, cattu, annatto, and cochineal had to be imported in large amounts.[83]

The birth of synthetic organic chemistry replaced nearly all the traditional dyes of botanic and animal origin, but cochineal has managed to survive up to the present, even if only on a moderate scale. It is no longer used in the textile industry, even though no synthetic dye has yet surpassed it in brilliance or fastness, but it costs more. The use of cochineal today is restricted to food, drinks, cosmetics, and pharmaceutical products.

CARMINE

Carminic acid, the red dye made by the cochineal insect, is the essential constituent of carmine. If we squash the body of a live cochineal insect, a dark red liquid (containing the blood and the internal organs) squirts out; the dye in the liquid is the cochineal carmine. The dried insects of the commercial cochineal have to be immersed in hot water, or other solvent, to extract the dye.[84] Nowadays only Peru and the Canary Islands are producing cochineal in an organized industrial manner.

Following the invention and manufacture of synthetic red dyes, mainly aniline derivatives, the cochineal dyes were gradually ousted from the textile industry, not because the synthetic colors were superior in color or fastness, but because they were cheaper and could be delivered in any quantity. The only places remaining for these magnificent natural products were the food, drink, cosmetic, and pharmaceutical industries. Even there, the synthetic red dye called Red No. 2, also known as amaranth (a coaltar dye), proved to be a serious competitor to the more costly natural products.[85] In the United States alone, about 1 million pounds of this synthetic dye, valued at up to $55 million, is used annually in about $10 billion worth of food, drugs, and cosmetics.

Most of us would be surprised to learn how wide the use of red coloring matter is in the food, drink, cosmetic, and drug industry. Cochineal carmine is used widely in the most diverse products, but the bulk goes into pork sausage, dried fish, shrimps, ice cream, jams, jellies, yogurt, fruit in syrup, alcoholic and soft drinks, chocolate fillings, sweets, cider, and vinegar. In addition, it is found in millions of pink and red medicinal pills, syrups, and cosmetic products.[74] In all of these products, cochineal serves no directly beneficial purpose except to make the products more attractive; this it does very effectively.[86]

Carmine appears to be a rare contact sensitizer. Sarkany and colleagues[87] reported that its use in lipstick produced allergic contact cheilitis in three patients.

References

1. Fisher AA. Contact dermatitis from food additives. Immunol Allergy Pract 1983;10:316.

2. Fisher AA. Contact dermatitis due to food additives. Cutis 1975;16: 961.

3. Mitchell JC. The skin and chemical additives to foods. Arch Dermatol 1971;104:329.

4. Fisher AA. Dermatitis of the hands from food additives. Cutis 1982;30:304.

5. Fisher AA. Cutaneous reactions to sorbic acid and potassium sorbate. Cutis 1980;25:350.

6. Dejobert Y, Delaporte E, Piette F, et al. Vesicular eczema and systemic contact dermatitis from sorbic acid. Contact Dermatitis 2001;45:291.

7. Fisher AA. Hand dermatitis—a "baker's dozen." Cutis 1982;29:214.

8. Clemmensen O, Hjorth N. Perioral contact urticaria from sorbic acid and benzoic acid in a salad dressing. Contact Dermatitis 1982;8:1.

9. Lahti A, et al. Acetylsalicyclic acid inhibits non-immunologic contact urticaria. Contact Dermatitis 1987;16:133.

10. Roed-Petersen J, Hjorth N. Contact dermatitis from antioxidants. Br J Dermatol 1976;94:233.

11. Fisherman EW, Cohen G. Chemical intolerance to butylated-hydroxyanisole (BHA) and butylated-hydroxytoluene (BHT) and vascular response as an indicator and monitor of drug intolerance. Ann Allergy 1973;31:126.

12. Flyvholm M-A, Menné T. Sensitizing risk of butylated hydroxytoluene based on exposure and effect data. Contact Dermatitis 1990;23:341.

13. Epstein E. Sodium bisulfite. Contact Dermatitis Newsletter 1970;7:115.

14. Riggs BS, Harchelroad FP Jr, Poole C. Allergic reaction to sulfiting agents. Ann Emerg Med 1986;15:77.

15. Prenner BM, Steven JJ. Anaphylaxis after ingestion of sodium bisulfite. Ann Allergy 1976;37:180.

16. Wolf SI, Nicklas RA. Sulfite sensitivity in a seven-year-old child. Ann Allergy 1985;54:420.

17. Hausen BM, Beyer W. The sensitizing capacity of the antioxidants propyl, octyl, and dodecyl gallate and some related gallic acid esters. Contact Dermatitis 1992;26:253.

18. deGroot AC, Gerkens F. Occupational airborne contact dermatitis from octyl gallate. Contact Dermatitis 1990;23:184.

19. Brun R. Eczema de contact à un antioxydant de la margarine (gallate) et changement de métier. Dermatologica 1970;140:390.

20. Postendorf J. Oxidative deterioration in cosmetics and pharmaceuticals. J Soc Cosmet Chem 1965;16:203.

21. Lewis FM, Shah M, Gawkrodger DJ. Contact sensitivity to food additives can cause oral and perioral symptoms. Contact Dermatitis 1995; 33:429.

22. Wilkinson SM, Beck MH. Allergic contact dermatitis from menthol in peppermint. Contact Dermatitis 1994;30:42.

23. Fleming CJ, Forsyth A. D5 patch test reactions to menthol and peppermint. Contact Dermatitis 1998;38:337.

24. Morton CA, et al. Contact sensitivity to menthol and peppermint in patients with intra-oral symptoms. Contact Dermatitis 1995;32:281.

25. Malten KE. Four bakers showing positive patch-tests to a number of fragrance materials, which can also be used as flavors. Acta Derm Venereol (Stockh) 1979;59:117.

26. Fisher AA. Contact dermatitis due to cinnamon and cinnamic aldehyde. Cutis 1975;16:383.

27. Neering H, van Ketel WG. Allergy from spices used in Indonesian cooking. International Symposium on Contact Dermatitis. Gentofte, Denmark, 1974.

28. Garcia-Bravo B, Perex Bernal A, Garcia-Hernandez MJ, Camacho F. Occupational contact dermatitis from anethole in food handlers. Contact Dermatitis 1997;37:38.

29. Kanerva L, Soini M. Occupational protein contact dermatitis from coriander. Contact Dermatitis 2001;45:354.

30. Anliker MD, Borelli S, Wuethrick B. Occupational protein contact dermatitis from spices in a butcher: a new

presentation of the mugwort-spice syndrome. Contact Dermatitis 2002;46:73.

31. Wintzen M, Donker AS, van Zuuren EJ. Recalcitrant atopic dermatitis due to allergy to Compositae. Contact Dermatitis 2003;48:87.

32. Pasolini G, Semenza D, Capezzera R, et al. Allergic contact cheilitis induced by repeated contact with propolis-enriched honey. Contact Dermatitis 2004;50:322.

33. Burden AD, Wilkinson SM, Beck MH, Chalmers RJ. Garlic-induced systemic contact dermatitis. Contact Dermatitis 1994;30:299.

34. Cabanillas M, Fernandez-Redondo V, Toribio J. Allergic contact dermatitis to plants in a Spanish dermatology department: a 7-year review. Contact Dermatitis 2006;55:84.

35. Hughes TM, Varma S, Stone NM. Occupational contact dermatitis from a garlic and herb mixture. Contact Dermatitis 2002;47:48.

36. Pereira F, Hatia M, Cardoso J. systemic contact dermatitis from diallyl disulfide. Contact Dermatitis 2002;46:124.

37. Bassioukas K, Orton D, Cerio R. Occupational airborne allergic contact dermatitis from garlic with concurrent Type I allergy. Contact Dermatitis 2004;50:39.

38. Scheman AJ, Gupta S. Photoallergic contact dermatitis from diallyl disulfide. Contact Dermatitis 2001;45:179.

39. Pecquet C, Leynadier F, Saiag P. Immediate hypersensitivity to sesame in foods and cosmetics. Contact Dermatitis 1998;39:313.

40. Hamilton TK, Zug KA. Systemic contact dermatitis to raw cashew nuts in a pesto sauce. Am J Contact Dermat 1998;9:51.

41. Fisher AA. The management of propylene glycol-sensitive patients. Cutis 1980;25:24.

42. Hannuksela M, Forstrom L. Reactions to peroral propylene glycol. Contact Dermatitis 1978;4:41.

43. Jensen CD, Andersen KE. Allergic contact dermatitis from sodium stearoyl lactylate, an emulsifier commonly used in food products. Contact Dermatitis 2005;53:116.

44. Camarasa JM, Alomar A. Contact dermatitis from a karaya seal ring. Contact Dermatitis 1980;6:139.

45. Fisher AA, Dooms-Gossens A. Persulphate hair bleach reactions: cutaneous and respiratory manifestations. Arch Dermatol 1976;112:1407.

46. Calnan CD, Shuster S. Reactions to ammonium persulphate. Arch Derm 1963;88:812.

47. Cronin E. Contact dermatitis. London: Churchill Livingstone, 1980:181.

48. Fisher AA. Contact dermatitis, 3rd ed. Philadelphia: Lea & Febiger, 1988:591.

49. Morren M-A, et al. a-amylase, a flour additive: an important cause of protein tact dermatitis in bakers. J Am Acad Dermatol 1993; 29:723.

50. Mitchell JC. Allergic contact dermatitis from a certified food dye presenting as "sock dermatitis." Contact Dermatitis Newsletter 1972;11: 247.

51. Kiec-Swierczyunska M, Krecisz B. Occupational allergic contact dermatitis due to curcumin food colour in a pasta factory worker. Contact Dermatitis 1998;39:30.

52. Inman PM. Dermatitis in a crisp factory. Acta Dermatovener (Stockh) 1965;45:295.

53. Fisher AA. Possible role of diet in pompholyx and nickel dermatitis: a critical survey. Cutis 1978;22:412.

54. Fisher AA. Water-related dermatoses: I. Cutis 1980;25:132.

55. Feingold BF. Recognition of food additives as a cause of symptoms of allergy. Ann Allergy 1968;26:309.

56. Criep LH. Allergic vascular purpura. J Allergy 1971;48:7.

57. Lockey S. Reactions to hidden agents in foods, beverages and drugs. Ann Allergy 1971;29:461.

58. Juhlin L, Michaålsson G, Zetterstrom O. Urticaria and asthma induced by food-and-drug additives in patients with aspirin hypersensitivity. J Allergy Clin Immunol 1972;50:92.

59. Lockey S. Drug reactions and sublingual testing with certified food colors. Ann Allergy 1973;31:423.

60. Michaålsson G, Pettersson L, Juhlin L. Purpura caused by food and drug additives. Arch Dermatol 1974;109:49.

61. Fiedelman W, Martens J. Hypersensitivity to tartrazine (FD&C Yellow No. 5) and other dyes present in pharmaceutical products. Cutis 1975;15:576.

62. Smith AP. Response of aspirin-allergic patients to challenge by some analgesics in common use. Br Med J 1971;2:494.

63. Samter M, Beers RF Jr. Concerning the nature of intolerance to aspirin. J Allergy 1967;40:281.

64. Samter M, Beers RF Jr. Intolerance to aspirin: clinical studies and consideration of its pathogenesis. Ann Intern Med 1968;68:975.

65. Chafee FH, Settipane GA. Aspirin intolerance. I: frequency in an allergic population. J Allergy Clin Immunol 1974;53:193.

66. Settipane GA, Chafee FH, Klein DE. Aspirin intolerance. II: a prospective study in an atopic and normal population. J Allergy Clin Immunol 1974;53:200.

67. Yuninger JW, O'Connell EJ, Logan GB. Aspirin-induced asthma in children. J Pediatr 1974;82:218.

68. Bandmann HJ, Nasemann T. Dermatitis to Ponceau Red 6R dye. Berufsdermatosen 1961;9:79.

69. Rapaport MJ. Allergy to yellow dyes. Arch Dermatol 1984;120:535.

70. Calnan C. FD and C Yellow 11 in lipstick. Contact Dermatitis 1975;1:121.

71. Larson W. Cosmetic dermatitis due to a dye (D and C Yellow 11). Contact Dermatitis 1974;1:61.

72. Rapaport MJ. Allergy to D and C yellow dye 11. Contact Dermatitis 1980;6:364.

73. Noster U, Hausen BM. Berufsdebingtes Kontaktekzem durch gelben Chinophthalonfarbstoff (solven Yellow 33: CI 47000) (Occupational dermatitis due to a yellow quinophthalone dye (solvent yellow 33: C.I. 47000)). Hautarzt 1977;29:153.

74. Börkner B, Magnusson B. Patch test sensitization to D & C Yellow No. 11 and simultaneous reaction to quinoline yellow. Contact Dermatitis 1981;7:1.

75. Jordan W. Contact dermatitis from D & C yellow 11 Dye in a toilet bar soap [letter]. J Am Acad Dermatol 1981;4:613.

76. Palazzolo MJ, DiPasquale LC. The sensitization potential of D & C Yellow No. 11 in guinea pigs. Contact Dermatitis 1983;9:367.

77. Morikawa F, Fukuda M, Naganuma M, Nakayana Y. Phototoxic reaction to xanthine dyes induced by visible light. J Dermatol 1976;3:59.

78. Mitchell JC, Stewart WD. Allergic contact dermatitis from neutral red applied for herpes simplex. Arch Dermatol 1973;108:689.

79. Dahlquist I, Fregert S. Allergic contact dermatitis from neutral red in quaternary ammonium salt solution. Contact Dermatitis Newsletter 1967;2:16.

80. Conant M, Maibach HI. Allergic contact dermatitis due to neutral red [letter]. Arch Dermatol 1968;109:735.

81. Goldenberg RL, Nelson K. Dermatitis from neutral red therapy of herpes genitalis. Obstet Gynecol 1975;46:359.

82. Baker JT. Dyes of animal origin. Endeavour 1974;33:11.

83. Brunello F. The art of dyeing in the history of mankind. Vincenza: Neri Pozza, 1973.

84. Baranovits FLC. Cochineal carmine: ancient dye with a modern role. Reading, PA: Department of Zoology, University of Reading.

85. Fisher AA. Contact Dermatitis, 3rd edition. Lea & Febiger, Philadelphia, 1986, p. 600.

86. Pelham Wright N. A thousand years of cochineal. Am Dyestuff Reporter, 19 Aug 1963, p. 635.

87. Sarkany I, Meara RH, Everall J. Cheilitis due to carmine in lip salve. Trans St John's Hosp Dermatol Soc 1961;46:39.

RUBBER

EXECUTIVE SUMMARY

Humans are exposed to a variety of allergens in rubber materials, including natural rubber latex (NRL) and a host of chemical additives. Most NRL comes from southeast Asia, whereas synthetic rubber is made worldwide. NRL protein is well known as a leading cause of immunologic contact urticaria. This IgE-mediated reaction can cause not only skin-related findings but also acute respiratory symptoms and even anaphylaxis. At least one recent report suggests that delayed allergy to latex may exist more commonly than previously expected, especially in atopic individuals. Latex immediate allergy should not be confused with the more common, but usually less severe T-cell mediated delayed hypersensitivity reaction seen clinically as allergic contact dermatitis (ACD). Both types of allergy may co-exist in a single patient, however. Not all types of rubber contain NRL. It is most often found in dipped and blown rubber articles such as gloves, balloons, and medical devices and also in some heavy-duty rubber items like tires and conveyor belts.

A variety of additives is found in rubber. Accelerators, including thiurams, carbamates, thioureas, and mercaptobenzothiazoles, enhance the polymerization of raw rubber into a functional product. Antioxidants and antiozonants, such as paraphenylenediamine derivatives, retard environmental degradation. Other chemicals increase the softness and pliability of rubber, reduce ultraviolet light degradation, and so on. Many of these additives can cause ACD. Synthetic rubber that does not contain NRL often contains these chemical additives. Some gloves (eg, nitrile) are fully synthetic and many "heavy-duty" and industrial rubber materials are made of non-latex rubber types. Nonetheless, they still cause ACD from the various additives, both in manufacturing workers and in others who have reason to come into contact with them.

It is impossible to state in absolute terms or with complete assurance which types of rubber goods will contain which allergens. Some generalizations are possible, however. Allergic contact dermatitis to rubber gloves is most often due to carbamates and hiurams. Mercaptos and paraphenylenediamine derivatives are usually found in shoes, industrial materials, and tires. Thioureas are a common ingredient in neoprene rubber, used in medical and sporting goods. Since rubber allergy is so common, screening allergens are necessary on patch-test series. If there is a high index of suspicion of rubber allergy, a number of other allergens, and even rubber pieces themselves, are useful for testing.

A note on the tables in this chapter: Previous editions of this text contained extensive tables listing various types of rubber and many rubber additives. This information is of limited value to the practising dermatologist and is impossible to keep totally current. Those readers with a special interest in detailed descriptions of these items may wish to consult internet sites of manufacturers of these materials, including those listed in the reference section.

Rubber is an organic substance, obtained from natural sources or synthesized artificially, that has the properties of extensibility, stretchability, and durability. Rubber acquired its name from its ability to erase ("rub out") pencil marks.[1] Before the last decade of the last millennium, when one talked of rubber allergy, the usual causes were the chemical additives such as vulcanizers and antioxidants. Although these are still major causes of rubber allergy, the focus among health care workers and public alike has been type 1 allergy to natural rubber latex. While it is an interesting intellectual exercise to attempt to link specific allergens with specific types of rubber, in practice this is generally not helpful. An exception may be made in occupational cases.

Types of Rubber

NATURAL RUBBER

Natural rubber occurs in over 200 species of plants, including dandelions and goldenrod. Only two species are commercially significant: the *Hevea braziliensis* tree and the guayule bush, *Parthenium argentatum*. Today, the Hevea tree accounts for virtually all of the world's natural rubber (cis-1,4-polyisoprene) supply. *H. braziliensis* is cultivated primarily in Southeast Asia (Malaysia, Indonesia, and Thailand), with less than 20% of the world supply coming from South America and West Africa. A productive tree can supply 30 to 35 grams of rubber per day. Each acre of about 150 trees will produce in 1 week enough latex for 1,500 pairs of surgical gloves. Harvesting the liquid natural rubber latex (NRL) is accomplished by cutting a groove in the tree and collecting the "sap" in a cup. Coagulation rapidly occurs; to prevent this ammonia, thiurams or other preservatives are added to the collection vessels.[2,3] The major hydrocarbon in rubber is cis-1,4-polyisoprene, which makes up 30% to 40% of natural latex.

NRL is processed in the liquid form or allowed to dry into sheets. The term "natural rubber latex" is used to describe products such as gloves and condoms formed from concentrated liquid natural latex. Dry rubber latex refers to natural latex that is processed into a solid "dry" form of sheets that are able to be stored or shipped for processing into other products, such as tires, springs, hoses, and belts.

NRL is used in a variety of applications including dipped articles such as gloves, condoms, and balloons. The NRL sap is usually centrifuged to reduce water content. This process also reduces extractable latex protein.[3]

Ammonia is the primary latex preservative added to prevent coagulation. Low ammonia latex utilizes three secondary preservative systems: (a) sodium pentachlorophenate, (b) tetramethylthiuram disulfide (TMTD) and zinc oxide, and (c) sodium dimethyldithiocarbamate and zinc oxide.[2]

BALATA AND GUTTA-PERCHA

The rubber from the Hevea tree occurs only in the cis form, whereas both balata and gutta-percha occur in the trans forms (trans-1,4-polyisoprene). Balata is harvested from wild bushes and trees in Surinam and Guiana. Raw balata is high in dirt and resin and must be purified by a solvent extraction process. Gutta-percha is obtained from trees of the family *Sapotaceae* native to Malaysia, Borneo, and Sumatra.

GUAYULE

Guayule (*Parthenium argentatum*) is a member of the sunflower family, which grows in northern Mexico and the Big Bend area of Texas. There are no significant structural differences between guayule and Hevea rubber, but guayule contains a contaminate resin that must be removed. The resin contains volatile essential oils such as alpha-pinene and dipentene, and nonvolatiles like carotenoids, palmitic acid, linolenic acid, and transcinnamic acid.[3]

A project to commercialize rubber production from the guayule plant is under development in the Southwestern USA. One major advantage to guayule rubber is that the latex protein content (responsible for causing contact urticaria) is only 0.2 to 2.0% of the level in Hevea latex.[4] A drawback is the presence of a potent contact allergen. Rodriguez et al.[5] using the guinea pig maximization test, identified the allergen in an acetone extract of the dried leaves of the plant; the sensitizer was a sesquiterpene cinnamic acid ester (guayulin A).

Synthetic Rubbers

The first synthetic rubbers were developed in the late 1920s. During World War II, the need for synthetic rubber spurred further research, leading to the synthesis of government rubber-styrene (GR-S), a butadiene-styrene polymer. Now called SBR (for styrene-butadiene rubber), it has better heat resistance but less tensile strength and flexibility than NR.

Polyisoprene rubber (IR) is a synthetic that is very similar in structure to NRL, but does not contain the allergenic proteins. Butadiene rubber (BR) is the most elastic of the rubbers, with superior wear resistance. Butyl rubber (IIR) consists of isoprene and isobutene and offers very low gas permeability. It is useful in tire inner tubes. Chloroprene rubber (CR) is the most resistant to oil and weathering. Ethylene-propylene rubber (EPDM) is highly ozone resistant and is used in the construction and automotive industries. Nitrile rubber (NBR) is a polymer of butadiene and acrylonitrile. It is often used for oil and fuel handling and in nitrile medical gloves.

Other synthetic rubbers include neoprene, silicone, urethane, thiokol, and Hypalon rubbers. In addition, compounds often thought of as plastics, such as polyethylene and polyvinyl chloride, have certain properties of rubber and may contain chemical additives used in rubber. These different rubbers all have varying qualities, such as chemical resistance, temperature tolerance, elasticity, and tear resistance, that make each more or less suitable for certain applications.

In addition to the rubber polymer itself, a rubber article may also contain many additives. The most important for the dermatologist include the vulcanizing agents and the anti-aging compounds (antioxidants, antiozonants, UV protectors). Others include fillers, such as carbon black or clays, to reinforce the compound; softeners, such as mineral oil or plasticizers to improve processing and regulate hardness; pigments; blowing agents; and flame retardants.[6]

Guin and colleagues have written an excellent review of the history, production, and uses of rubber.[3] The Olmec ("rubber people") of Central America are credited with the use of rubber as early as 1600 BC. By the early 19th century, it was mostly a novelty item, other than for its use in waterproofing.

Compounding and Vulcanization

Raw rubber in the dry state has few commercial applications, because of its lack of strength, durability, and elasticity. For most uses, the rubber must be modified, usually by the addition of vulcanizing (curing) agents and other materials, followed by vulcanization (Table 29.1). The exceptions include such uses as crepe rubber shoe soles, rubber adhesives, and masking tape.[7]

The main uses of rubber require that the polymer chains be cross-linked after being formed into the shape of the final product. After cross-linking of the polymer chains, which is called curing or vulcanization, the article is elastic.

In 1844, Charles Goodyear described the process of vulcanization using lead and sulfur, which he claimed to have invented in 1839. The process was patented by Thomas Hancock in England in November, 1843.[8] A second major breakthrough occurred in 1905 when George Oenslager discovered that sulfur-containing organic molecules were able to dramatically reduce vulcanization time, as compared to sulfur alone.

The process helped to overcome the weaknesses of untreated natural rubber that occur with aging. Vulcanization is an irreversible process and was employed originally to denote heating rubber with sulfur, but it has been extended to include any process, with any combination of materials, that produces this effect. About 4 to 5 pounds of additives go into each 100 pounds of finished rubber. The accelerators and antidegradants account for about 90% of these additives.

Rubber Accelerators: Accelerators speed up the slow process of vulcanization by acting as catalysts and undergoing chemical changes. The major accelerators include thiurams and carbamates, which act quickly, diphenylguanidine and mercaptobenzothiazoles, which act at moderate speed, and thioureas, which work more slowly. Carbamates are often complexed with heavy metals such as zinc, cadmium, lead, and others. The metal content of rubber is not enough to cause ACD in the metal-allergic patient.

The benzothiazolesulfenamides prevent premature curing and are called delayed-action accelerators. They

Table 29-1 Selected Rubber Additives

Accelerators
 Aldehyde-amine reaction products, e.g. hexamethylenetetramine
 Benzothiazoles, e.g., 2-mercaptobenzothiazole (MBT)
 Dithiocarbamates, e.g., zinc diethyldithiocarbamate (ZDEC)
 Dithiomorpholines
 Dithiophosphates
 Guanidines, e.g., 1,3-diphenylguanidine
 Isophthalate
 Sulfeneamides
 Thioureas, e.g., -dibutylthiourea
 Thiurams, e.g., tetramethylthiuram disulfide (TMTD)
 Xanthates
Antidegradants
 Amines. e.g., diphenyl-*p*-phenylenediamine
 Benzotriazoles (UV)
 Cinnamates (UV)
 Hindered Amines (UV), e.g., pentamethyl piperidinyl sebacate
 Hydroquinolines, e.g.,dihydrotrimethylquinolone
 Phenols, e.g., butylated hydroxy toluene (BHT)
 Sulfides
Peroxide Curing Agents
 Benzoyl peroxide
 Perbenzoates
Plasticizers
 Thiophenols
 Natural resins, e.g., rosin
Retarders
 N-(cyclohexylthio)phthalimide (CTP)
 Benzoic acid

also donate sulfur for curing. Ethylenethiourea is used widely for special-purpose elastomers such as polychloroprene (neoprene) and polyepichlorhydrin.[9] Others include propylpyridines, isophthalates, cyanurates, hexamethylenediamine, dithiomorpholines, benzoyl peroxides, other peroxides, and xanthates.[10]

Anti-degradation agents: Antioxidants and antiozonants prevent rubber from drying or cracking by preventing oxidation by atmospheric oxygen or by decreasing the effect of ozone.[11] These substances are used widely in polymers such as rubber, adhesives, and plastics, and also in gasoline and lubricants. The paraphenylenediamine-type antioxidants are usually the most effective in rubber and are used in the largest volume. Most are discoloring and staining and are used in applications in which this property can be ignored. Phenolic antioxidants are less discoloring than amines and include many of the newer antioxidants. Butylated hydroxytoluene (BHT) and polybutylated bisphenol A are examples of these. Others include hydroquinolones and the carbamates.

Ultraviolet light stabilizers protect from the degradation of rubber by sunlight. These include amines such as piperadines and triazines and benzotriazoles.

OTHER ADDITIVES

There is a seemingly endless list of other chemicals used in rubber production. Some examples are given here. They are almost never implicated in rubber ACD.

Retarders prevent premature vulcanization of rubber compounds during mixing, calendering, and other processing steps. N-(cyclohexylthio)-phthalimide is the predominant agent used.

Dispersing agents including sulfonates are used for the production of dipped goods.

Blowing agents are foam-producing agents used for cellular rubber, such as sponges and latex. Blowing can be compared to baking a cake with yeast; the blowing agent decomposes and causes the compound to expand, followed by curing. Inorganic substances, such as sodium or ammonium bicarbonate and ammonium nitrite, may be used; they generally release carbon dioxide gas.[9]

Peptizers, also called chemical plasticizers or softeners, soften rubber and lower the viscosity of uncured rubber. Examples include naphthols, phenols, anilides, and resins. Some peptizers have been reported to produce ACD from contact with the finished product.[11]

Processing agents do not affect physical or performance properties of rubber. Some are low molecular weight polyethylenes. N,N9-ethylenebis(stearamide) functions as a mold-releasing agent and detackifier.[7]

Reinforcing agents and fillers for rubber include carbon black, zinc oxide, calcium carbonate, calcium silicate, silicon dioxide, clay, and magnesium carbonate.[12] Some of these also act as heat stabilizers.

Bonding agents are used for adhering rubber to reinforcing agents, such as glass, textile, or steel, as used in tires, hoses, and belts. Resorcinol, resorcinol-formaldehyde, 2-naphthol, isocyanates, and tetrachlorobenzoquinone are examples.[7]

WORLD RUBBER PRODUCTION

In 2005, over 8.8 million tons of NR and 12 million tons of synthetic rubbers were produced. Both amounts have been increasing fairly steadily since 1996, when production was about 6.4 and 9.8 million tons respectively.[13]

Immediate Hypersensitivity to Latex

Nutter,[14] in 1979, and Förström.[15] a year later, were the first to definitively report type 1 latex allergy. Since then, frequent reports of NRL allergy have dramatically increased the awareness of this problem among health care workers as well as the general public. The US Food and Drug Administration issued a medical bulletin in 1991 identifying the risk of life-threatening anaphylaxis associated with latex contact.[16] The American Academy of Dermatology has issued a position paper on latex allergy and has published a review of the topic by Warshaw.[17,18] (Figure 29-1)

IDENTIFICATION OF THE ALLERGEN

At least 13 different latex protein antigens have been identified, and several appear to be important in human allergy[19] (Table 29.2). These are characterized as Hev b 1 through 13. It is possible that different patients will react to different antigens. Hevein, also known as Hev b 6.02, a 4.7kd protein, may be a major allergen in health care workers.[20] Alenius and colleagues[21] stated that "rubber elongation factor" (Hev b 1, 14.6kd) is allergenic in 18% of their NRL immediate hypersensitivity patients. Yeang, in a recent review, states that the major allergens are now thought to be Hev b 2, Hev b 5, Hev b 6, Hev b 13, and maybe Hev b 4.[19] Hamann,[2] in an excellent reference paper on latex IH, suggests that factors such as latex harvesting and preservation methods, seasonal variation, and other factors may affect antigenicity. Further substantiating the concept that natural latex processing plays an active role in antigen development is the observation that workers handling raw natural latex are not known to suffer from latex IH (C Hamann, personal communication, 1993).

FACTORS INFLUENCING LATEX IH

Many individuals that must frequently wear latex exam gloves report that the powder irritates the skin. To date, actual allergy to the powders, principally cornstarch, has been documented very rarely.[22] However, it has been shown that cornstarch glove powder absorbs latex protein. This may increase the aerosolization of the latex allergen and enhance the development of both skin and respiratory symptoms.[23]

Atopic individuals, especially those with hand eczema, are at higher risk for developing latex IH. Also spina-bifida patients with meningomyelocele, possibly because of frequent operative and genitourinary latex exposure, are at high risk. In addition, anyone with frequent occupational exposure to latex gloves, such as health-care workers and food-service workers are at risk.

Why large numbers of cases have been reported only since the mid- to late 1980s has been debated. There are most likely multiple factors, but the main reason may be the entry into the marketplace of quickly and poorly made latex products coincident with the increased need

Table 29-2 NRL Allergens[19]

Name	Trivial Name	Predicted Physiological Roles
Hev b 1	Rubber elongation factor	Rubber biosynthesis
Hev b 2	Beta-1,3-glucanases	Defense-related protein
Hev b 3	Small rubber- particle protein	Rubber biosynthesis
Hev b 4	Microhelix component	Defense-related protein
Hev b 5	Acidic latex protein	–
Hev b 6.01	Prohevein, hevein Preprotein	Defense-related protein (latex coagulation)
Hev b 6.02	Hevein	–
Hev b 6.03	Prohevein C-terminal fragment	–
Hev b 7.01 = Hev b 13 (renamed)	Patatin homologue from B-serum	Defense-related protein inhibitor of rubber biosynthesis
Hev b 7.02	Patatin homologue from C-serum	–
Hev b 8	Latex profilin	Structural protein
Hev b 9	Latex enolase	Glycolytic enzyme
Hev b 10	Mn-superoxide dismutase	Destruction of radicals
Hev b 11	Class I endochitinase	Defense-related protein
Hev b 12	Lipid transfer protein	Defense-related protein
Hev b 13 = Hev b 7.01	Latex esterase Early Nodule Specific Protein (ENSP)	Defense-related protein

for protection from HIV and other infectious diseases. Inexperienced manufacturers produced great quantities of latex products that may not have been well compounded or leached of allergens. Once individuals are sensitized by high allergen concentrations, even low levels of latex protein can cause a reaction.

LATEX ALLERGY IN HEALTH CARE WORKERS

Health care workers have the greatest likelihood of developing latex IH, other than the meningomyelocele patients noted above. Those with atopy and prior hand eczema are at highest risk. Several studies summarized by Hamman[2] have shown the prevalence overall in hospital-based physicians and nurses to be in the range of 5% to 10%. DeGroot and colleagues[25] studied laboratory workers in the Netherlands and found that 5.0% were NRL RAST positive and 8.3% were prick test positive.

Hamann and colleagues[26] tested 2,166 dental workers at national meetings with prick testing to glove extracts. Positive tests were found in 6.2%.

More recent reports suggest that the rate of latex allergy in health care workers is declining. A report from Germany reviewed records of reported cases of NRL allergy among 1.8 million health-care workers and also records of the purchase of powdered and powder-free latex exam gloves over the period 1996 to 2002.[27] They found that since 1998, the use of powder-free gloves has been increasing and suspected cases of NRL allergy decreased by 80% during that period. Unfortunately, diagnosis of NRL allergy was only suspected, not confirmed in this report.

NRL allergy also may wane if patients avoid allergen contact. Nettis and colleagues reported on 17 NRL-allergic workers who were reevaluated at a later time.[28] Only 11 (65%) remained positive on prick testing and 4 of 9 who previously had elevated latex IgE levels became negative. For obvious reasons, the workers were not rechallenged with latex contact.

LATEX ALLERGY IN OTHERS

Ylitilo and colleagues[29] screened 3,269 children for latex allergy as part of a routine prick test panel. Positives were found in 55 (1.7%). Thirty (1.0%) were further positive with both RAST and glove use tests. A number of these children had not undergone surgery, and one-third were asymptomatic. In Spain, 29 of 100 children with myelomeningocele were latex allergic.[30]

A Spanish report compared ICU to latex in health-care and other workers.[31] They found evidence of latex allergy in 17% of healthcare workers and also in 17% of food workers, as compared to 2.3% in workers overall.

CLINICAL FINDINGS

The initial presentation of latex IH may be confused with ICD or ACD by both the patient and physicians. Indeed, eczematous changes are almost always seen in the case of repeated latex exposure as occurs when wearing latex gloves. A critical point is to question the patient concerning whether itching, burning, swelling, or other symptoms occur within 1 hour or less of donning gloves or whether changes are noted only after chronic use. Also, other history of reactions to balloons, condoms, and so on, should be obtained. Even in the absence of positive history, patients with hand eczema who wear latex gloves frequently should be considered candidates for further investigation.

Respiratory and mucosal symptoms are the next most common complaint in latex IH. Symptoms may be mild to severe and even fatal. Repeated exposure may lead to worsening of the allergy.

The most severe findings occur when the route of exposure is mucosal or parenteral. Deaths have been reported due to latex anaphylaxis from exposure to barium enema tube cuffs. Exposure of a latex-sensitive patient to gloves during surgery, dental work, or vaginal or rectal examination may cause anaphylaxis.

DIAGNOSIS

The diagnosis must first be suspected on clinical grounds. No test is both totally specific and sensitive, so several procedures may be required. Anti-latex IgE RAST tests are very specific and relatively sensitive, so these tests are the first step in making a diagnosis. Use of a blood test avoids the possibility of an adverse reaction to a skin test and may be obtained by practitioners unable to do skin testing. Patch, prick, or use tests may still be necessary, however, if the RAST is negative and clinical suspicion is high. Inasmuch as standard allergens are not now available in the USA, a test solution can be easily made, as noted in Table 29.3. Also, testing to pieces of latex gloves can be done. Because testing may rarely provoke a severe reaction, resuscitation equipment should be near at hand. Testing should involve a stepwise increase in exposure, discontinuing if a positive reaction occurs. First, a finger cot can be worn on normal skin for up to 30 minutes. The next step would be contact with latex on eczematous skin. Then a piece of latex can be applied over a prick or scratch site.

It is important to note that latex allergy, despite its current popularity, still accounts for only a portion of reactions to rubber products. Additives such as accelerators and antioxidants are the causes of many, if not most, cases of rubber allergy. Therefore, even patients who are suspected of having latex IH should have "regular" patch testing to determine delayed hypersensitivity to these allergens.

Table 29-3 Preparation of "Latex Allergen" for Skin Testing

1. Place about 20 1-cm² pieces of latex glove in 5 mL of sterile saline.
2. Shake occasionally over a 2-hour period.
3. Transfer to a sterile, clean container without a rubber top.
4. Make a fresh supply weekly.

In addition, to further complicate the matter, Belsito[24] reported type 1 immediate reactions to carbamates.

SPECIAL CONSIDERATIONS FOR LATEX-ALLERGIC PATIENTS

As is always the case, avoidance of an allergen is the most reliable form of treatment. For those who must wear exam or surgical gloves, vinyl or totally synthetic rubber gloves can be used safely. Other rubber gloves, such as nitrile gloves, may still contain the additives discussed below that cause ACD, even if they are "latex free".

Crossreactivity in latex-allergic patients has been demonstrated to banana, kiwi, avocado, passion fruit, and chestnut, and occasionally to other fruits and nuts, but is apparently an uncommon occurrence.[32]

Latex-allergic patients should inform their dentists and physicians of their problem, especially if undergoing obstetrical or surgical procedures, endoscopy, or barium enema exams. Contact with any latex-containing medical device, even an insulin syringe, can cause a reaction.[33] Wearing a "medical alert" bracelet or necklace may be advisable in case the person is incapacitated.

IMMUNOTHERAPY FOR LATEX ALLERGY

In the past, desensitization therapy has not been found to be very successful. A recent report of a blinded, placebo-controlled study, however, claimed that 12 months of sublingual immunotherapy improved symptoms in all treated patients, although latex IgE levels did not go down.[34]

Delayed Hypersensitivity to Latex

Wakelin and colleagues[35] tested 608 patients with various preparations of NRL. Only 24 reactions were seen, all ranked at ± or 1+. Of the nine 1+ reactions, six were felt to be due to concomitant thiuram allergy, and the other three faded at the second reading. The author's conclusions were that patch testing with NRL gave a very low yield and was not recommended for routine use.

A French report found that 32 of 55 children who were very strongly expected to have rubber allergy were patch test positive with an NRL extract.[36] It was made by a French company from Malaysian latex sap and was said to contain 0.1 mg/mL of latex proteins. Five of the children had immediate reactions, the rest delayed only. All were negative to rubber additives and 30 were atopic. Ten developed positive latex RAST tests over the next 2 years.

Wilkinson and Burd[37] reported that 7 of 117 patients (6.0%) with hand dermatitis and glove use were positive on patch testing with NRL. The tests were done with

NRL containing no additives using 0.7% ammonia as an anticoagulant. Three of these seven had a negative prick test for latex IH. None reacted to rubber additives.

A German study found 4 of 167 patients with hand eczema and rubber exposure allergic to NRL on a delayed basis.[38] Patch and prick tests were positive only at 24 to 48 hours in 3, but positive at both immediate and delayed readings in one. Only that patient had elevated serum IgE to latex.

The reasons for these discrepancies are uncertain but may be due to patient selection and allergen factors. At this time, the value of testing for DH with NRL is uncertain.

Rubber Additive Sensitivity

Although immediate reactions to NRL are now common, delayed hypersensitivity to rubber additives, leading to ACD, has been recognized for many years. Most of the rubber additives, which are firmly entrenched in the rubber industry, have been used satisfactorily for years and are unlikely to be replaced in the near future. These include carbamates, thiurams, mercaptobenzothiazoles, para-phenylenediamine derivatives, and others. Studies of the rubber industry and commercial products have shown the current rubber patch test chemicals to be the major sensitizers. Rubber is a common cause of ACD, and in 1976 Malten and colleagues[39] stated the incidence of sensitization to rubber was increasing. The best data on the frequency of rubber sensitivity come from various patch test clinics throughout the world. The North American Contact Dermatitis Group (NACDG) reported on rates of patch test reactions over several time periods (Table 29.4).[40–42] The current data suggest that allergy to the rubber allergens is declining across the board, at least in North America.[42] The thiurams and carbamates are the most common rubber allergens in each year analyzed.

Most persons who react to carbamates also react to thiurams, most likely representing a true crossreaction, because these two agents are chemically similar. The most recent NACDG data shows a rate of positive patch tests as follows: thiuram mix- 4.6%, carba mix-4.0%, MBT-1.6%, PPDA-mix- 1.0%, thiourea mix- 1.0%, and MBT mix-0.9%.[42]

A report from Israel indicates thiuram mix was positive in 1.2% and MBT mix in 0.4% of 2,156 patients.[43]

One can speculate that the increase in the 1970s to the 1990s was due to increasing rubber glove use in many occupations, while the current decline mirrors a reduction in rubber glove use in favor of synthetics. Also, better modern manufacturing processes may reduce the amount of allergen in finished rubber products. A new concern, of unknown significance, is the increasing use of iodopropynyl butylcarbamate, a preservative for topical agents and industrial fluids. Whether this agent crossreacts with the carbamates used in rubber is currently unclear.

A comprehensive review of rubber allergy was undertaken by Conde-Salazar and colleagues in Spain.[44] Seven thousand patients were evaluated and 4,680 were tested over a 10-year period to five rubber mixes: thiuram mix, carba mix, black rubber mix, mercapto mix, and naphthyl mix. Of the 4,680 tested, 686 (14.7%) had one or more positives to rubber chemicals, 119 of these were allergic only to rubber additives. Almost half of the positives (336) were construction workers. A breakdown of the individual allergens is given in Table 29.5.

A German study showed a lower rate of rubber allergy than either Spain or North America.[45] Only 3.8% of 3,851 reacted to one or more rubber allergens (thiourea and naphthyl mix were not used as screens on all patients). Although the total number of reactors was lower, relative proportions were similar, with thiuram positive in 72% and carba positive in 25.

AGE AND GENDER IN RUBBER ALLERGY

Allergy to rubber chemicals is usually more frequent in men than women. Presumably, much of this is due to the

Table 29-4 Positive Patch Test Reactions to Rubber Chemicals from the NACDG

Chemical	Year					
	1972	1982	1985	1996	1998	2004
Black rubber mix 0.6%	NT	1.4%	1.4%	2.3%	1.5%**	1.0%
Carba mix 3%	NT	3.8%	3.3%	5.7%	7.3%	4.0%
MBT 1%	4.8%	4.8%	2.7%	2.1%	1.8%	1.3%
Mercapto mix 1%	NT	2.5%	2.9%	2.2%	1.8%	0.9%
Mixed thioureas 1%	NT	NT	NT	0.7%	1.3%	1.0%
Thiuram mix 1%	4.2%	4.3%	3.9%	6.8%	6.9%	4.6%

*Concentrations are in petrolatum.
** N-I-NP-PPDA tested instead of black rubber mix
NT = not tested.

Table 29-5 Distribution Positive Patch Test to Rubber Mixes in 686 Patients with Rubber Allergy*

Allergy	Number +	Association
Thiuram mix	569 (82.9%)	20% carba +
Carba mix	153 (22.3%)	76% thiuram +
Black rubber mix	122 (17.8%)	14% thiuram +
Mercapto mix	111 (16.0%)	14% thiuram +
Naphthyl mix	17 (2.5%)	18% black rubber +

*Adapted from Conde-Salazar, et al., ref. 44.

Table 29-6 Reactions to Rubber Allergens in Males and Females (NACDG)

	Percent positive	
Allergen	Men (*N* = 2000)	Women (*N* = 2900)
Thiuram mix	4.2	5.9
Carba mix	3.8	2.8
Mercapto mix	2.8	1.5
MBT	3.2	1.3
Black rubber mix	2.1	1.6

MBT, mercaptobenziothiazole

correlation between rubber allergy and work exposure. Conde-Salazar and colleagues[44] found that 18% of men and only 7% of women reacted to rubber allergen mixes. The NACDG has found statistically significant differences in rubber allergy between men and women as well (Table 29.6).[46] In this group, dermatitis of the hands and feet were more common in men than women, although face and neck dermatitis was more frequent in women.

A report from Sweden indicated a significant reduction in allergy to thiuram mix from 2.0% in 1992 to 1.2% in 2000.[47] The reduction was most obvious in men over 40 years old and women under 40. Positive patch-test rates to MBT and black-rubber mix also declined, although not as dramatically.

Rubber sensitivity is also well documented in children.[48,49] Leyden and Kligman[48] found that rubber chemicals were the most common contact allergens in children. Of 653 children tested with a standard battery, 98 had positive reactions, of which 41 were from thiuram or mercaptobenziothiazole (MBT). Veien and colleagues[49] reported five boys and four girls (11.7% of 77 children with one or more positive patch tests to all standard series chemicals) who reacted to rubber chemicals. Six of the nine reactions were considered currently relevant.

Mechanism of Contact Allergy from Rubber Additives

In many products that undergo polymerization or curing, such as epoxies, acrylates, other plastics, adhesives, etc., the final product is rarely allergenic. Those at risk for ACD to these items are almost always workers involved in their production, not consumers of finished goods. Why then does ACD often occur to finished rubber products?

ACD to rubber is (except as noted above) not caused by the natural rubber latex itself. Rather, the chemicals added in the manufacturing process are the sensitizers.[12]

Allergens are usually present in some chemical form in the final product, and both consumer and manufacturer are at risk of being sensitized. Even fully cured rubber products often cause ACD.[12] There are several possible explanations. According to Fregert,[50] many of the rubber additives are decomposed partially or totally during vulcanization, but others, such as antioxidants, are intended to be present in the cured product. Small quantities of accelerators and antioxidants may not be consumed in curing and may "bloom" or migrate to the surface. Contact allergy may be enhanced by local heat and sweating. Other reasons may include incomplete curing at lower temperatures, presence as an exposed chemical side group rather than in the linear structure of the rubber polymer, and the degradation of rubber by heat, friction, ozone, and other factors. Stankevich and colleagues[51] demonstrated the migration of thiuram and a mercapto compound (*n*-cyclohexyl-2-benzothiazolsulfenamide) from rubber in food containers.

Occupational Rubber Dermatitis

Contact dermatitis is fairly common among rubber workers.[3,50,52] Prevalence rates from industrial studies are 3.1, 3.7, and 5.6 cases per 1,000 workers in Great Britain, Australia, and Finland, respectively. California's rate of 7 per 1,000 workers included plastics workers.[53–54]

In a Finnish study, 56% of the cases represented irritant dermatitis, especially from solvents and bulk rubber. More than half of the ACD cases were caused by PPDA compounds. Many workers acquired dermatitis through work that did not permit use of protective gloves. It was possible to transfer workers with PPDA who were handling black rubber to a job with colored rubber. Workers could often handle cured rubber if the dermatitis was caused by uncured rubber.[52]

In a highly selected male construction worker population from Brazil, of 83 patients tested, 35% and 28% reacted to carba-mix (3% pet) and thiuram mix (1% pet) respectively.[55] The authors speculate that much of this was due to rubber glove use.

It is interesting to note that Conde Salazar and colleagues[44] found that almost half of 686 rubber allergic patients were construction workers. Presumably, this is due to use of rubber boots, gloves, and other protective gear. Rubber industry workers were not included in the study, and construction work was the only occupational rubber association.

In an NACDG report, MBT, mercapto mix, and thiuram mix reactors were more often to be occupationally exposed than otherwise.[46] Individual occupations

Table 29-7 Rubber Allergens on the NACDG Series*

Allergen	Components
Mercaptobenzothiazole (MBT) 1%	N/A
Carba mix 3%	DPG, ZDEC, ZDBC 1% each
Thiuram mix 1%	TMTM, TMTD,TETD, PTD 0.25% each
Mercapto mix 1%	MBT, DBTD, MMBT, CHBTS 0.25% each
Black Rubber mix 0.6%	IPPDA, CPPPDA, DPPDA 0.2% each
Mixed dialkyl thioureas 1%	Diethyl, dibutyl each 0.5%
Dithiomorpholine 1%	N/A

*As of 2007, all in petrolatum

were not recorded in this study. Although carba mix and black rubber mix were also more often work-related, the difference was not statistically significant. More recently, the NACDG reported that about 30% of 101 patients positive to either MBT or the MBT mix were occupationally related.[56] In contrast, 17% of patients allergic to mixed thioureas had occupational exposure.[57]

SELECTED REPORTS OF OCCUPATIONAL ACD TO RUBBER

4,4-dithiodimorpholine[58] was one of several chemicals that caused dermatitis in a Danish rubber factory. Subsequently, it was tested at 1% concentration in an investigation of 110 patients with contact dermatitis, and 6 had positive results.

Table 29.7 lists the current rubber chemicals tested by the NACDG. Other rubber allergens are listed in Tables 29.8 and 29.9.

A worker in a foam rubber plant developed a pustular reaction to hexafluorosilicate, a gelifier used to maintain the foam structure.[59] Patch tests were negative. Testing on rabbits confirmed that the chemical is able to induce pustules, presumably a type of irritant response.

Sensitivity to components of synthetic elastomers should also be suspected. A student technologist was sensitized to Hylene W (4,49-diisocyanate dicyclohexyl methane), an aliphatic monomer used in the manufacture of polyurethanes.[60] Hypalon (chlorosulfonated polyethylene) "20" and "30" rubbers, which contained epoxy resin as a stabilizer, sensitized a rubber worker who applied the

Table 29-8 T.R.U.E. Test Rubber Allergens

Allergen
Carbamate mix 0.2 mg/patch
Thiuram mix 0.61 mg/patch
Mercaptobenzothiazole mix 0.61 mg/patch
MBT 0.61 mg/patch
Black rubber mix 0.61 mg/patch

Table 29-9 Other Commercially Available Rubber Allergens

Allergen	Available from Supplier*		
	Brial	Chemotechnique	Hermal
p-tert-Butylcatechol 0.25%			X
Cyclohexylthiophtalimide 1%	X	X	X (0.5%)
Dipentamethylenethiuram tetrasulphide 0.25%	X		
Diphenyl-p-phenylenediamine 0.25%	X	X (1%)	X
Dephenylthiourea 1%	X	X	X
Diaminodiphenylmethane 0.5%		X	
Dibenzothiazyl disulphide 1%	X	X	X
Dibutylthalate 5%	X		
Dibutylthiourea 1%	X	X	X
Diethylthiourea 1%		X	
Dihydroxybiphenyl 0.1%	X		X
Dipentamethylenethiuram disulfide 0.25%	X	X (1%)	X
Diphenylguanidine 1%	X	X	X
Dodecyl mercaptan 0.1%	X	X	
Ethylenediamine dihydrochloride 1%	X		
Hexamethylenetetramine 1%	X	X (2%)	X
Hydroquinone monobenzylether 1%	X		
Latex 4%	X		
Mercaptobenzimidazole 1%	X		
Mercaptobenzothiazole 2%		X	
Morpholinyl mercaptobenzothiazole 0.5%		X (1%)	X
N,n,-di-beta-naphtyl-4-phenylenediamine 1%		X	
n-cyclohexyl-2-benzothiayl sulphenamide 1%	X	X	X
n-cyclohexyl-n-phenyl-4-phenylenediamine 1%		X	
n-isopropyl-n-phenyl-4-phenylenediamine 0.1%		X	
n-phenyl-b-napthylamine 1%	X	X	
Tetraethylthiuram disulphide 0.25%	X	X (1%)	X
Tetramethylthiuram disulphide 0.25%	X	X (1%)	X
Tetramethylthiuram monosulphide 0.25%	X	X (1%)	X
Thiourea 0.1%	X		
Trimethyl-1,2-dihydroquinoline 1%		X	
Zinc dibenyldithiocarbamate 1%			X
Zinc dibutyldithiocarbamate 1%	X		X
Zinc dimethyldithiocarbamte		X	
Zinc diethyldithiocarbamate 1%		X	X

polymer as a lacquer for rubber boots. Patch tests were positive to the two Hypalon rubbers and to epoxy resin.[61]

Adams[62] suggested that mercaptobenzimidazole (MBI) be substituted for MBT because it is probably less allergic. He observed that in subjects allergic to MBT, the MBI patch test was negative in 44 of 46 (95%) cases. This was substantiated by Foussereau and colleagues.[62]

TIRES

It is often difficult to learn the identity of the additives in various rubber products. Tires represent such an example, with compounding formulas considered proprietary information by manufacturers. Although formulations vary among different manufacturers, the same additives are used in both natural and synthetic tire components.

Study of Tire Workers in the United States

The list of chemicals patch tested by Suskind, in his unpublished 1979 study of workers in a large US tire factory, gives a clue to some of the rubber additives used in the United States tire industry (RR Suskind, Cincinnati, OH, personal communication, 1984). Suskind tested 502 employees with 36 rubber and 12 nonrubber materials. The rubber-related materials that elicited the most reactions and the number of employees reacting were 4,4-dithiodimorpholine 1% in 45 employees, 4,4-dithiodimorpholine 0.5% in 4 employees, oil-extended polybutadiene rubber in 11 employees, paraphenylenediamine 1% in 8 employees, diphenylguanidine 2% in 7 employees, nickel sulfate 2.5% in 7 employees, and n-cyclohexylthiophthalimide 1% in 8 employees.

Most of the reactions to nonrubber-related chemicals occurred from balsam of Peru 25% (in 17 people), potassium dichromate 0.5% (in 15 people), ethylenediamine 1% (in 10 people), and neomycin 20%, which probably mirror the level in the general population.

The lists of allergens that Suskind tested provide epidemiologic information on chemical exposure in a tire production plant. The sources of occupational exposure to the nonrubber chemicals were not specified.

Other Cases of Contact Dermatitis from Tires

Most reports of contact allergy from tires are from paraphenylenediamine-related antioxidants. Bieber and Foussereau,[64] in 1967, reported nine cases of n-isopropyl-n-phenylparaphenylenediamine contact dermatitis, including four men who handled finished tires at work. Subsequently, Hervö-Bazin and colleagues[65] studied 42 men who were sensitized to isopropylparaphenylenediamine (IPPD) by handling tires: 17 men in the tire manufacturing industry, 5 among tire dealers, and 20 men in the automobile transport and servicing sectors. All of the men were patch test positive to n-phenyl-n-cyclohexyl-paraphenylenediamine (CPPD) and 37% to paraphenylenediamine. Fifteen men were tested with n-dimethyl-1,3-butyl-n-phenylparaphenylene-diamine (DMPPD), and all reacted to it.

Cronin[66] reported 20 men and 1 woman with rubber sensitivity acquired by handling finished tires between 1966 and 1976. The dermatitis affected the palms and flexor surfaces of the wrists and was easily mistaken for constitutional hand eczema. Patch test results were IPPD (19/19 positive), CPPD (14/18 positive), and PPDA (7/21 positive).

The incidence of sensitization from IPPD has been reduced in a British tire plant by automation in tire building and by limiting the amount of IPPD used to 2% or less of the total rubber mix.[67]

RUBBER ALLERGY IN SHOEMAKERS

Mancuso and colleagues[68] reported on rubber allergy in 240 workers at five factories in Italy. Only 16 (6.5%) had ACD. MBT and the adhesive paratertiary butylphenol formaldehyde resin were the main allergens. Workers assembling the shoes were at greatest risk for ACD.

Patch Testing for Rubber Allergy

With the exception of mercaptobenzothiazole (MBT), the NACDG recommends that patch test screening for rubber allergy be performed with "mixes" of rubber chemicals rather than a single substance.[39–41] This testing strategy is accepted worldwide. In addition, several individual rubber allergens may be useful for patch testing in selected cases (Tables 29.7, 29.8, 29.9).

There is considerable literature describing the use of mixtures in patch testing.[69] Their usefulness lies in one patch covering several test substances. Bonnevie,[69] in 1939, pioneered the use of patch test mixes employing four wood tars and also chrysarobin with anthrarobin. Epstein,[70] in 1967, reviewed the literature and reported his findings with mixes of caines, antihistamines, rubber chemicals, and antibacterial agents, respectively. He found concordance between patch test–positive results in seven rubber-sensitive patients from a mix consisting of rubber chemicals (mercaptobenzothiazole [MBT]), tetramethylthiuram disulfide, and monobenzyl ether of hydroquinone each 1% in petrolatum) and from the individual chemicals. Less than half of his patch test–proven rubber-sensitive patients reacted to the mix, however, and he added thio-beta-naphthol and phenyl-beta-naphthylamine, each 1%, to broaden the scope of the rubber-additive screening. This new mix with five components gave frequent false-positive reactions and was discarded. These irritant reactions were caused by thio-beta-naphthol, which was found to be less irritant in the mix than when it was tested separately.

Subsequent refinement of rubber patch test mixtures has occurred. To minimize irritant reactions, the concentration of the individual mix constituents was reduced to less than 1%; carba mix is an exception.

Carba mix is the only rubber allergen mix that still gives a fairly high rate of irritant reactions. Almost always these dissipate by 48 hours after patch removal.

CARBAMATES AND DIPHENYLGUANIDINE (CARBA MIX)

Simultaneous reactions to thiuram mix and carba mix are not infrequent and occur probably because thiurams are derivatives of dithiocarbamates. Doubtful (irritant?) reactions are more likely to occur with carba mix than with most other patch test allergens. Subsequent testing with the separate components of the mix may clarify whether the weak response is an irritant or an allergic reaction. Malten and colleagues[39] list probable crossreactions for carbamates as substances derived from thiocarbamate, which are used as pesticides.

DIAMINODIPHENYLMETHANE (DDM)

Used in rubber as an anti-oxidant and anti-ozonant, DDM is also used as an epoxy hardener and in the manufacture of some dyes, plastic, fibers, and adhesives. A report from Italy found 132 positive patch tests in 6809 patients.(1.9%) There was a 2 to 1 female predominance and most patients had hand eczema. Relevance was found in 31. Other allergens often positive in these patients were the "para" compounds including PPDA, benzocaine, parabens, and Disperse Yellow dye #3. Sources of contact were not delineated.[71]

MERCAPTOBENZOTHIAZOLE (MBT)

Mercaptobenzothiazole and related chemicals, as noted previously, have long been known to cause ACD. Currently, however, positive patch tests to MBT are less common than to the other usual rubber allergens. MBT and its relatives all possess at least 2 sulfur atoms linked to nitrogen as part of 2 or more 5 or 6 carbon rings. The contribution of sulfur is essential to the vulcanization process. Adams and Warshaw have recently reviewed the uses and sources of MBT exposure.[72] ACD from MBT may occur from contact with virtually any rubber product, including rubber gloves, shoe rubber, industrial rubber products, medical devices, and even common rubber bands (Figure 2-8).

Mitchell and colleagues,[73] in 1976, reported the results of patch testing with MBT 1% in petrolatum and with MBT mix containing MBT and three derivatives, each at 0.25%. The results, showing 48 patients MBT positive and mix negative, suggested that the concentration of MBT in the mix was too low compared with MBT itself in the standard screen. Accordingly, MBT 1% in petrolatum was retained separately in subsequent screening trays.

Fregert[74] studied the pattern of crossreactions among the mercapto group of chemicals. He found that a combination of a benzene and a thiazole ring and a thiol group in the 2-position were necessary for cross-sensitivity. Cronin[66] tabulated the results of testing with separate constituents of mercapto mix. In both men and women the greatest number of reactions was to MBT, and in both sexes there was a decreasing incidence of reactions to morpholinyl MBT (MMBT), CBS, and dibenzothiazyl disulfide (MBTS). Hansson and Agrup[75] have shown, however, that what is put into a mix may not be what is still there when we do a patch test. They showed that, in reality, MBTS is the major chemical left in the MBT mix after only a few weeks storage time. This is due to the other mix ingredients reacting together to form the MBTS. Only about 25% to 30% of the other agents was present at the 3-week analysis.

The German contact dermatitis group (IVDK) showed that the mercapto mix (1% pet) missed about 30% of patients who reacted to individual components at higher concentrations of 0.5 to 1% each.[76] When considering the mix plus MBT, 23% were missed. In cases of strongly suspected allergy, therefore, testing with the individual chemicals should b considered.

A more recent report from the EECDRG of 32,475 patients gave a positive rate to MBT (2% pet) and/or the MBT mix (2% pet) of 1.0%.[77] Each allergen missed about 20% of the positives to the other allergen, so the authors concluded that both should be kept on standard series.

THIURAM MIX

Van Ketel, in the Netherlands, found thiuram mix to be a good indicator of thiuram sensitivity,[78] and there was good correlation between testing with thiuram mix and its components. Tetramethylthiuram disulfide (TMTD) alone was not an adequate indicator of thiuram allergy. Other European investigators[79] have found that reactions to tetramethylthiuram monosulfide TMTM and TMTD were highest when components of the mix were tested. These variations between countries may reflect differences in usages by manufacturers for rubber goods.

Cronin[66] found the four thiuram mix chemicals do not always crossreact one with another. Malten and colleagues[38] list crossreactions for thiuram mix components, indicating that thiurams and carbamates often cross react.

Geier and colleagues[80] found that TETD was positive in about 80% of thiuram-sensitive patients, TMTM in 60%, TMTD in 55%, and DPTD in about 40%.

Thiuram mix crossreacted with the preservative iodopropynyl butylcarbamate (IPBC) in 2 of 7 cases in one report.[81]

PPDA MIX (BLACK RUBBER MIX)

The term "black rubber mix" is somewhat unfortunate. Although these chemicals may indeed be found in dark-colored rubber materials, they also may crossreact with textile and hair dyes. The term "PPDA mix" or "PPDA-derivatives" may be more chemically correct.

The St. John's results of testing the separate constituents in most of the 53 patients positive to PPDA mix were isopropyl-paraphenylenediamine (IPPD) positive in 45 of 48, phenylcyclohexyparaphenylenediamine (CPPD) positive in 38 of 45, and diphenylparaphenylenediamine (DPPD) positive in 17 of 43 (65). Paraphenylenediamine itself was usually negative and so a poor detector of sensitization to this group of chemicals. Crossreactions may also occasionally occur with the hair dye chemical paraminodiphenylamine.[82] About 20% of those who react to PPDA mix may be allergic to certain textile dyes, especially the disperse dyes. (See Chapter 18.)

MIXED THIOUREAS

In response to the appearance of case reports of allergy to the thioureas in rubber materials, especially sporting goods and shoes, the NACDG began testing with a mix of di-alkyl thioureas in 1991. The recent review of NACDG thiourea data showed that of about 22,000 patients tested between 1994 and 2004, 225 (1.0%) reacted to mixed dialkyl thioureas (1% petrolatum).[57] The NACDG data are shown in Table 29.4.

NAPHTHYL MIX

Naphthyl mix was removed from the NACDG standard screening tray in 1979 because of a low rate of reactivity (JS Taylor and colleagues: Unpublished data on epidemiology of contact dermatitis in North America, 1976–1982, Task Force on Contact Dermatitis, American Academy of Dermatology, Evanston, IL). Van Ketel,[83] in 1983, also reported a low sensitization rate for naphthyl mix from the Netherlands. Naphthyls apparently are commonly used in tire production, however, so testing in patients with tire exposure may be worthwhile.

N-(CYCLOHEXYLTHIO) PHTHALIMIDE

This chemical, a pre-vulcanization inhibitor, has caused rare cases of ACD, especially from "heavy-duty" items like tires, hoses, rubber tiles, and belts. Patch test concentration of (0.5% petrolatum) is recommended, as 1% has caused frequent irritant reactions.[84,85]

FALSE NEGATIVE PATCH TESTS WITH RUBBER MIXES

A weak positive reaction to one of the mixes may be due either to a mild irritant effect of the total mixture or to a weak allergy to one of the components. When in doubt about the significance of such a weak reaction, the components of the mix should be tested separately. Separate testing of the components, along with other commercially available rubber allergens, should also be done if the patch test mix is negative (possibly because the components are not present in sufficient concentration to elicit a positive reaction) but rubber allergy is strongly suspected. In that case, it may be important to test with a thin shaving from the suspected rubber article or with other individual rubber chemicals suspected of causing the allergy.

Bleached rubber syndrome should also be suspected when rubber dermatitis is suspected but patch tests to rubber chemicals are negative.[86]

PATCH TESTING WITH PIECES OF RUBBER

Veien[87] reported results of patch testing with substances not in the standard series. These additional items were tested along with the standard tray chemicals. Specific rubber items eliciting relevant reactions among 24 patients included 17 gloves, 3 finger stalls, 2 rubber tubing, 1 rubber sponge, and 1 bra strap. The rubber allergies demonstrated by testing with items supplied by the patients themselves could, in many instances, have been identified by the standard series. Only 9 of the 17 patients reacting to gloves, however, had concomitant reactions to rubber chemicals.

Thioureas

Contact dermatitis from the thiourea rubber accelerators has been reported more frequently in the last two decades. Thioureas are used especially in neoprene rubber materials. This includes many orthopedic supports such as knee sleeves, and many rubber recreational and sporting goods such as wetsuits and swim goggles. Fowler's experience is that allergy to neoprene is usually due to thioureas. It is unclear whether thiourea may be in the neoprene itself, the adhesive used in a product, or both. Clinically it probably makes little difference.

A unique feature of thiourea allergy is that patients with this allergy seem to have a propensity to develop papular and vesicular dermatitis at sites distant from direct skin contact with the offending article. Fowler has seen a patient with hand eczema and scattered generalized dermatitis from thiourea contact in a weatherstripping material used in windows (unpublished observation. A report from Finland described vesicular hand eczema after wearing a neoprene ankle brace with patch test reactivity to diethylthiourea.[88]

The NACDG reviewed thiourea allergy seen from testing almost 22,000 patients.[57] Of these, 225 were positive to mixed thioureas (MDTU) (diethylthiourea and dibutylthiourea, each at 0.5% petrolatum). Significantly more men were positive than women. Footwear was the most common single source of exposure, in 20%. Current relevance (definite, probable, or possible) was positive in 173. Of these, 25% were allergic to other rubber allergens. Those allergic to MDTU were about twice as likely as others to react to thiuram, carbamate, or MBT, but not to black rubber mix.

There has been a variety of prior case reports and small series of thiourea allergy. Diethylthiourea (DTU), present as an accelerator in neoprene foam weather strips used in a new car factory for hood and door seals, also caused an outbreak of dermatitis in 15 car assembly workers and mechanics. The rashes occurred primarily on the hands, forearms, and sometimes the face, corresponding to the sites of contact with the rubber. Workers who fitted the strips in another factory were not affected. This difference was explained by White and Vickers[89] according to the way the two groups of men came into contact with the seals. The fitters who applied them handled the strips only with their palms, whereas the assembly workers and mechanics touched the rubber with all parts of their hands and arms.

Diphenylthiourea (DPTU), which was found to be present in PVC adhesive tape backing, caused dermatitis in 28 people using the tape. Fregert[90] routinely patch tested 2,491 subjects with DTU 1% in petrolatum and found that all were negative. Fregert[91] identified DPTU in other PVC objects and in certain brands of rubber gloves.

Meding and colleagues[92] reported 11 cases of allergy to DPTU in rubber orthopedic knee or elbow sleeves. A range of symptoms, including dermatitis, purpura and urticaria, were seen. All seven that were tested reacted to DPTU 1% petrolatum, six reacted to ETU 1% petrolatum, and two reacted to carbamates. The DPTU was present in an adhesive used in the sleeves. ETU was apparently not present in the products, so it was probably a crossreactor.

Ethylbutylthiourea (EBTU) contact allergy produced severe plantar foot dermatitis in 10 patients who wore Nike athletic shoes with insole material prepared by Spenco Medical Corp. The identification of EBTU as the allergen by Roberts and Hanifin in 1979 must be considered a classic example of the sleuthing sometimes required to identify a contact allergen.[93] Spenco Corp. obtained the innersole material from Rubatex Corp., which assembled the nylon-foam rubber innersole with a neoprene-based adhesive obtained from General Adhesive and Chemical Co. EBTU was used as an accelerator in the adhesive and was supplied to General Adhesive by Pennwalt Corp. A new innersole without EBTU has been marketed since then in Spenco and Nike innersoles. None of these patients reacted to a large series of known

rubber or adhesive allergens. Cross-sensitivity was later demonstrated between EBTU and other substituted thioureas: DTU, DBTU, DMTU, trimethylthiourea, and thiourea. No crossreaction occurred with ethylene thiourea. This cross-sensitivity may be important because several of Robert's and Hanifin's original patients continued to have dermatitis after discontinuing the Nike shoes and alkylthioureas may be present in other shoes.[94]

Gloves—Household, Industrial, and Surgical

The rubber product that most often causes dermatitis is gloves. Any patient with hand dermatitis and who wears rubber gloves may be sensitive to rubber, either NRL or chemical additives or both. Although this typical pattern may have an abrupt cutoff above the wrist, the classical distribution of rubber glove dermatitis was seen in few of Cronin's patients.[66] Many had a nonspecific pattern of hand eczema, and, in most patients, diagnosis could not have been made with certainty without patch testing.

Even when the patient is not allergic to rubber, gloves may make an existing hand dermatitis worse from occlusion and maceration. To avoid this, thin, white cotton lining gloves worn inside unlined rubber or vinyl gloves are suggested. The cotton liners should be changed during long tasks. Wearing two pairs of gloves, however, is not always feasible in workers requiring fine touch or dexterity. Also, rubber gloves may allow penetration of some allergens and then trap the allergen against the skin, resulting in a worsening of ACD. Especially in occupational settings, it is critical to recommend gloves that are actually protective against the chemicals that a worker encounters. Industrial glove suppliers have charts which indicate breakthrough times of various chemicals for each glove material. In individuals with hand eczema from any cause, it may be wise to recommend vinyl or other synthetic gloves to prevent the future development of rubber allergy.

Rubber glove allergy can cause a large amount of occupational dermatitis. A report from the IVDK showed that over 20% of occupational ACD cases were tested due to suspected rubber glove allergy.[80] In this group, thiurams were by far the most common rubber allergen at 16 % positive. In contrast, carbamates and MBTs reacted at a rate of about 3%, diphenyguanidine 2%, an thioureas 0.4%. The values were essentially unchanged for all the rubber allergens from 1995 to 2001.

Most of Cronin's patients also were allergic to dipentamethylenethiuram disulfide (PTD) present in thiuram mix.[66] Of 257 women and 91 men with rubber glove dermatitis, more than 80% of each group reacted to a thiuram. Ninety-six percent of the men reacted to thiuram mix, indicating it is essential to use several chemicals of a group, or a mixture of them, for testing.

Knudsen and colleagues[95] studied several types of rubber household and surgical gloves for release of thiurams and carbamates. They found wide ranges of release of these chemicals, with household gloves generally releasing less than the surgical gloves. There was a definite correlation of being patch test positive to a glove and the amount of allergen released.

According to Fisher,[96] any hand dermatitis in a surgeon should be considered as stemming from sensitization to ingredients in rubber gloves until proved otherwise. In a study by Fisher[96] of 11 surgeons who acquired allergic contact dermatitis of the hands from surgical gloves, patch testing revealed that 7 had positive patch tests to mercaptobenzothiazole. The other four were allergic to various other rubber chemicals.

A report from Oregon identified two antioxidants in latex exam gloves that caused isolated cases of ACD.[97] Two patients reacted to 4,49-thiobis (6-tert-butylmetacresol) (Lowinox 44536). One also reacted to BHA and BHT. Both were negative to rubber allergens but positive to gloves.

A good substitute for household use for those allergic to rubber is the Allerderm vinyl glove and similar products. Vinyl exam gloves are safe but lack elasticity and are therefore poorly suited to tasks requiring fine touch sensitivity. Synthetic gloves, such as the nitrile glove contain rubber additives just like latex gloves. Therefore they should only be recommended for individuals allergic to NRL but not the additives.

OTHER GLOVE REACTIONS

Endotoxins

Shmunes and Darby[98] reported dyshidrosis of the hands in a hospital phlebotomist. The source of the irritation, which occurred clinically and on usage tests 12 to 24 hours after wearing gloves for 10 to 20 minutes, was linked to bacterial endotoxin in latex gloves. Sterilization of the gloves by gamma irradiation increased endotoxin levels. When the bacterial count is elevated, the endotoxin is water soluble and is absorbed onto powder inside the gloves. Sweating under the gloves may enhance entry into the skin with subsequent dyshidrosis. No systemic symptoms were reported as may occur in cases of endotoxin reactions from contaminated biologicals intended for intravenous or intramuscular use.

Eyelid Dermatitis/Edema: ''On Call'' Dermatitis

Jordan[99] in an astute observation, described eyelid dermatitis in the absence of hand eczema in obstetric physicians and nurses who are allergic to rubber gloves. These personnel frequently use and then remove gloves after a few minutes. Brief contact with the eyelids allows the rubber accelerator (e.g., thiuram), which is leached into the donning powder, to remain on the eyelids; the rubber accelerator can be removed from the hands by washing.

Eyelid edema without hand eczema was reported by Calnan[100] to occur in a patient every time he was in contact with rubber. The reported attack occurred after laying a rubber-backed carpet. Penile edema was also present. Patch tests were positive to thiuram and carba mixes; scratch tests with the mixes were both negative.

Dermatitis from Consumer Rubber Articles

Malten and colleagues[39] pointed out that contact with most rubber articles is casual, except for the wearing of rubber gloves. Rubber is therefore often not suspected as a cause of dermatitis by the patient. Rubber sensitivity may be the entire cause of a dermatitis, or it may be superimposed upon a preexisting eczema. Rubber allergy often has no distinctive clinical pattern and cases will be missed unless patients are patch tested with standard tray rubber chemicals.[65] A positive reaction to a rubber chemical is significant and is usually relevant.[12]

CONDOMS

Contact dermatitis from rubber condoms is usually easy to diagnose, because there is a clear relationship with intercourse and it is often accompanied by marked penile or vulvar edema. In 1966, Hindson[101] reported 33 men and 2 women with dermatitis due to rubber condoms. The women presented with pruritus vulvae. In 1980, Cronin[66] identified English condoms as containing the accelerators zinc MBT, PTD, and ZDC and the antioxidant polytrimethylhydroquinolone. Condoms, like latex gloves, can cause immediate hypersensitivity in addition to ACD.

Fisher[12] identified two instances in which a preservative powder that had been dusted on the condom was the cause of dermatitis. Removal of the powder by washing allowed the patients to use the condom without acquiring dermatitis. In one instance, the powder contained 10% monobenzyl ether of hydroquinone. Fisher reported that several of his rubber-sensitive patients found by trial and error that only certain brands of condoms produced dermatitis.

Severe penile dermatitis developed in a patient after 25 years of wearing a condom catheter.[102] Allergy to thiuram and MBT was documented. Switching to a silicone device was curative.

Nonrubber condoms are made of processed sheep intestine (caecum). It should be noted that nonrubber condoms may not be completely protective against the spread of HIV.[103]

The differential diagnosis of condom allergy includes dermatitis and vulvitis from other contraceptive agents, such as spermicidal jellies, creams, foams, diaphragms, and lubricants.[104,105] Fisher[104] described connubial contact dermatitis from propylene glycol in K-Y Jelly and from feminine hygiene sprays. Vulvitis may also occur from irritants and sensitizers in douches, nail polish, nickel-plated zippers, sanitary napkin clasps, soaps, perfumes, clothing, and bubble baths.[105]

DIAPHRAGMS AND PESSARIES

Fisher[12,104,105] mentioned the occurrence of vaginitis and vulvitis from rubber diaphragms and pessaries in rubber-sensitive individuals.

MEDICAL DEVICES AND EQUIPMENT

Thiobetanaphthol, a peptizing agent added to rubber to facilitate its flow during molding, was identified as the sensitizer in a tourniquet applied to an arm before an intravenous injection.[106]

Cronin[66] reported three patients who had ACD from hot water bottles. All three were patch test positive to MBT as well as the bottle. In an 81-year-old man with dorsal hand eczema, however, the cause of the dermatitis was initially covert. The positive MBT patch test was the clue to diagnosis, and it was eventually determined, with some difficulty, that he lay in bed with his hands under a hot water bottle.

Cronin[66] also reported severe contact dermatitis in an incontinent man who always slept on a rubber sheet. He required hospitalization to clear the eczema, and on patch testing he reacted to the sheet and to dioxydiphenyl 1% in petrolatum.

Individuals with sleep apnea may be treated with a continuous positive airway pressure device (CPAP). This involves wearing a breathing mask, held in place by rubber straps. Both Reynaerts and colleagues[107] and Scalf and Fowler[108] have reported thiourea allergy and dermatitis from the straps.

Rubber Dental Plates

Rubber dentures are rarely, if ever, used today, but such dentures have caused stomatitis.[12]

Dialysis Unit

In an investigation of pruritic skin rashes in a hemodialysis unit, eight patients, four of whom had dermatitis, were patch test positive to various thiurams.[109] It was postulated that thiurams were eluted from the hemodialysis apparatus and sensitized the patients, some of whom developed dermatitis.

ATHLETIC GEAR

Swim Goggles

Goette[110] reported a "raccoon-like" periorbital leukoderma from contact with swim goggles. The patient, a 12-year-old female, had worn the same goggles the preceding year without ill effects and then had reused them after the leukoderma had cleared without any ill effects. A toxic reaction is postulated to have occurred from chemicals that leaked from the goggles and were eventually exhausted. Three of the substances present in the goggles were identified: ZDEC, phenol 2,29-methylene bis(6-(1-dimethylethyl)-4-methyl), and diethylthiourea. Goette stated that a representative of the Canadian manufacturer of the goggles was aware of 12 similar cases.

Other goggles made of silicone rubber are now available, which do not contain common allergens.

Scuba Face Masks

Maibach[111] described a mini-epidemic of facial dermatitis among scuba divers using face masks containing IPPD. Patch testing was positive to thinly shaven 2-cm^2 patches of the rubber from the mask, as well as to IPPD 0.5% in petrolatum. Tuyp and Mitchell[112] reported a dermatologist who had a recurrent facial dermatitis after scuba diving and who had a positive patch test from IPPD.

Other Swim Gear

Adams[113] reported dermatitis in a diver from DTU incorporated into a rubber wet suit. There were positive patch tests to a piece of the wet suit and DTU 0.1% in petrolatum. Other rubber allergens were negative. The diver wore a substitute suit without DTU for 8 years without recurrence, except on one occasion when he borrowed a friend's wet suit, resulting in a severe recurrence requiring hospitalization.

Squash Balls

Cronin[66] reported palmar dermatitis in a carpenter who played squash. He was patch test positive to PPD mix, and IPPD was confirmed by the manufacturers to be present in the ball.

Rubber Wishbone

Palmar eczema in two windsurfers was reported after contact with the rubber wishbone, which is held by the surfer to remain afloat. The wishbone is sometimes held continually over many hours. Both surfers were patch test positive to PPD mix. A substitution of aluminum for the black rubber was curative.[114]

CLOTHING AND RELATED ARTICLES

Garters

Garter belt dermatitis has become a clinical rarity since the introduction of pantyhose. In England, Cronin[66] identified the sensitizing chemicals as either a thiuram or MBT.

Surgical Support Stockings

Allergic contact dermatitis commonly complicates stasis dermatitis. Rubber chemical allergy may be caused by support stockings. Spandex usually is safe for those allergic to rubber.

Hairnet Elastic

Dermatitis due to elastic in hairnets may mimic seborrheic dermatitis. In such instances, wrap-around hairnets without elastic may be substituted; hair ribbons are another alternative.[12]

Dress Shields

In 1960, Schulz and Hermann[115] reported 12 cases of dress shield eczema affecting the axillae. All 12 patients were patch test positive to 4,49-dioxydiphenyl (DOD), and 6 of the 12 also reacted to other rubber chemicals. Cronin[66] also reported a case in a man. One wonders why he did not wear dresses without the shields. Differential diagnosis of dress shield eczema includes contact allergy from clothing and antiperspirants.

Rubber Panties

In addition to irritation and maceration from occlusion in the diaper area, rubber panties have caused contact allergy.[12]

Brassieres

One case of allergy to the spandex rubber used in a brassiere was reported from Japan.[116] The patient reacted to 2-hydroxy-methyl-phenyl benzotriazole (Tinuvin-P) contained in the spandex; she did not react to other benzotriazoles.

COSMETIC ITEMS

Rubber Headrest

Women with rubber sensitivity are reported to have developed an eruption resembling nuchal neurodermatitis from contact with the rubber kidney-shaped headrest attached to the shampoo tray in beauty parlors. Dermatitis was prevented by placing a plastic sheet or towel over the headrest.[12] Many such headrests today are plastic.

Rubber Cosmetic Sponges

In 1950, Furman and colleagues[117] reported 26 women with cosmetic sponge contact dermatitis involving the face and especially the eyelids. Such cases are still routinely seen. Usually the patient suspects allergy to the cosmetics, but patch testing gives the correct answer. Alternatives for cosmetic application are tissues and brushes. An adhesive is used to hold the brush bristles in the holder, but this is an unlikely cause of dermatitis. Fisher,[118] in 1993, reported three new cases of dermatitis from cosmetic sponges, all of which were caused by tetramethylthiuram.

Eyelash Curler

In 1945, Curtis[119] reported eyelid dermatitis from phenyl beta naphthylamine after use of eyelash curlers with rubber edges. A more recent report of eyelash curler allergy was due to PPDA mix components.[120]

Earplugs

Dermatitis limited to the ears occurred in a Japanese woman who wore rubber earplugs in the bath.[121] She was allergic to both MBT and thiurams.

OTHER RUBBER ITEMS

Rubber Pillows and Cushions

Cronin[66] reported two cases of facial dermatitis traced to rubber pillows and one case of a man with a dermatitis, beginning on his buttocks and spreading to his groin, abdomen, and legs, that was caused by a sponge rubber cushion he used at work.

BALLOONS AND RUBBER TOYS

NRL allergy causing immediate reactions is the classic finding in balloon allergy. However, ACD may occur as well. Balloons may cause intermittent episodes of eczema involving the lips and the lower half of the face, and the cause may not be obvious to the patient or physician.[66] Gaul[122] reported two cases that were traced to monobenzyl ether of hydroquinone. Cronin[66] described three patients each of whom was thiuram sensitive.

In the 1960s, dermatitis occurred on the face of 40% of the children playing with toys made of semisolid rubber called Flubber. Referred to as flubberitis, the condition was thought to be an irritant dermatitis and folliculitis phenomenon caused by an oil used in the production of Flubber. These products, also sold as Roobly Rubber and Plubber, were easily molded into any shape, and their resiliency enabled them to be used as bouncing toys. Flubber was composed of partially polymerized butadiene and mineral oil (70:30 ratio) with minor amounts of polymerization catalysts, antioxidants, and stoppers. Patch testing was inconclusive.[123,124]

Bleached Rubber Syndrome

Jordan and Bourlas[86] reported six patients who reacted to the elastic of their bleached underwear but not to new unbleached elastic supplied by the manufacturer. The components of the elastic and standard tray rubber chemical were also patch test negative. Washing the elastic with full-strength commercial bleach (5% sodium hypochlorite in water), however, gave the patients allergic responses due to the effect of bleach on the rubber accelerator, zinc dibenzyldithiocarbamate (ZDC). Using superb detective work to identify the allergen, ZDC was made to react with bleach, and the resultant gum was extracted with diethyl ether. Eight compounds were identified in the reaction mixture by gas chromatography/mass spectrometry. The individual components were tested on volunteers after sensitization to the reaction mixture was produced in 14 of 25 volunteers. One component, *n,n*-dibenzylcarbamyl chloride, produced an allergic response in each sensitized volunteer.

In practice, a presumptive diagnosis of bleached rubber dermatitis can be made if the patient is patch test positive to rubber from his or her underwear and negative to the screening rubber allergens. Treatment is simple; the patients must buy new underwear, and no bleach should be added to the wash. All of Jordan's original patients remained free of this dermatitis without changing to other brands of underwear. Similar reactions may take place with other bleached rubber apparel such as sneakers.

Rubber Purpura and Lichenoid Dermatitis

Both Fisher[125] and Shmunes[126] reviewed purpuric contact dermatitis, including rubber purpura. Fisher[125] referred to the PPPP syndrome as an allergic dermatitis characterized by pruritus, petechiae, and purpura produced by IPPD. Cases have been reported associated with wearing elasticized underwear, rubber boots, a rubber diving suit, and a rubberized support bandage for the leg.[125,127,128] The petechial, purpuric, eczematous dermatitis has been located typically at the exact sites of rubber contact with skin, but has also been generalized, similar to the eruption caused by sensitivity to carbromal and meprobamate.[125,128,129] Positive patch tests have been recorded from IPPD and DPPD, and in one report concomitant reactions occurred from MBT, MBTS, and phenyl-beta-naphthylamine (PBN).[128] In some cases, the patch test sites have been purpuric.[129,130] Fisher[131] saw a case of ACD that progressed to a pigmented purpura appearance from nylon stockings.

Shmunes[126] described a 59-year-old hat saleswoman with a severe purpuric eruption of the exposed areas of the face, neck, and arms. Patch testing to paraphenylenediamine produced a purpuric, eczematous response. Shmunes determined that IPPD was added to elastic material used in some elastic trim on undergarments in the United States.

Lichenoid pigmented contact dermatitis from IPPD has also been reported. Calnan[132] observed a case in a truck driver who contacted rubber tires, and Ancona and colleagues[129] described a case in a tire assembler.

Meding and colleagues[91] reported purpura in association with diphenylthiourea allergy.

Depigmentation from Rubber Chemicals

The first report of chemically induced leukoderma was by Oliver and colleagues[133] in 1939 from monobenzyl ether of hydroquinone (MBH), as an antioxidant used in rubber gloves. Half the workers wearing them were affected. After use of the gloves was discontinued, repigmentation began in some workers several months later, and within 3 years almost all the workers had regained their normal skin color. One of the commercial designations for MBH was Age Rite Alba. MBH is a potent depigmenting chemical. Its only therapeutic application is the rare need to depigment normal skin in persons with extensive vitiligo. MBH may produce pigment loss at distant, untreated sites. It is also an allergen.[122,134,135] Gaul[122] reported several severe cases of vesicular contact dermatitis from MBH. In 1984, van Ketel[135] observed sensitization from a depigmenting cream containing MBH, which was accompanied by sensitivity to hydroquinone.

Hydroquinone produces only local skin lightening and is used pharmacologically for melasma, postinflammatory hyperpigmentation, and similar disorders. Hydroquinone rarely produces complete depigmentation. It is a weaker allergen than MBH.[136] Concomitant sensitivity to hydroquinone and *p*-methoxyphenol has been observed in the guinea pig.[137]

Related chemicals producing depigmentation include monomethyl ether of hydroquinone (*p*-methoxyphenol or *p*-hydroxyanisole) and monoethyl ether of hydroquinone (*p*-ethoxyphenol).[64] Other depigmentors are listed by Gellin.[138] *p*-tert-butylphenol, *p*-tert-butylcatechol, *p*-isopropylcatechol, *p*-octylphenol, *p*-nonylphenol, *p*-phenylphenol, *p*-tert-amylphenol, *p*-cresol, dimethylamine hydrochloride (MEDA), b-mercaptoethylamine hydrochloride (MEA)], physostigmine (Eserine), diisopropylfluorophosphate, and *n,n,n*0-triethylenethiophosphoramide (Thio-TEPA). Paratertiary butylphenol caused 100 cases of local depigmentation from the use of bindi in India. Fifteen patients were patch tested, and all were negative.[139]

A more extensive discussion of chemical vitiligo is found in Chapter 23.

Nonrubber Sources of Rubber Chemicals

CARBAMATES AND THIURAMS

Thiurams are used extensively in fungicides[140] and have also been found in some oils and paints,[141] animal repellents,[141] seed disinfectants, soaps,[12,142] and Antabuse.[12,52]

Other rubber chemicals with nonrubber uses include dithiocarbamates as lawn and garden fungicides,[12,143] carbamates as heat stabilizers for polyethylene,[141] paraphenylenediamine compounds as retarders for acrylates and as inhibitors or sweeteners in gasoline,[141] diaminodiphenylmethane as a cross-linker in epoxy resins and polyurethanes,[11] and antioxidants and other rubber additives in plastics.[12] Boman and colleagues[144] reported a case of sensitivity from phenyl-alpha-naphthylamine present at 1% concentration in a grease used by an aircraft worker. Morpholine may be present as an antioxidant in coolants, and trimethyldihydroquinoline may be used as an antioxidant in high pressure lubricants (FJ Storrs, Portland, OR, personal communication, 1983).

Schulz and Hermann[145] reported dermatitis in dock workers unloading produce treated with thiuram. Shelly[146] reported a golfer who developed dermatitis after contact with TMTD used as a fungicide on a golf course. The fungicide was applied to his skin for 15 minutes and produced a large eczematous reaction 30 hours later, coupled with a generalized flare despite the continuance of systemic steroids. Cronin[147] mentioned a man who developed dermatitis after applying a thiuram insecticide in his garden. When patch tested, he reacted to TMTD and to three related thiurams.

Copeman,[148] in 1966, recorded a case of toxic epidermal necrolysis (TEN) caused by cutaneous hypersensitivity to monosulfiram (tetraethylthiuram monosulfide), which was applied as a scabicide. The patient, who had been treated for rubber sensitivity 28 years previously, began developing the TEN within 3 hours of application of monosulfiram and later had a positive patch test to TMTD.

The carbamate fungicides Zineb and Maneb have also caused contact allergy.[142,149] In the cases of Maneb allergy reported by Nater and colleagues,[149] patch tests to standard tray carbamates and thiurams and Zineb were negative. Two of the three patients were positive to ammonium dithiocarbamate and one to sodium-ethylene-bis (dithiocarbamate).

Cronin[147] reported the results of testing of both Zineb and Maneb by the International Contact Dermatitis Research Group. There were three nonrelevant positives of 655 eczematous patients tested with Zineb 1% in petrolatum. Maneb was an irritant at 1% in petrolatum concentration with a reaction from 35 of 655 patients; one of these reactions in a florist with hand eczema was thought to be clinically relevant.

Methiocarb, also called 3,5-dimethyl-4-(methylthio)-phenol carbamate, is an insecticide and molluscicide. It was found to be the cause of hand dermatitis in a flower farmer. Tests to the carbamate mix were negative. Methiocarb, trade name Mesurol, was tested at 0.5% petrolatum.[150]

Thioureas

DBTU was the cause of airborne ACD in two patients with dermatitis on exposed surfaces. Both were exposed to BTU in a paint-removing solvent. The product is a strong irritant that may have predisposed to the development of the allergy.[151]

Thiourea and derivatives are used in almost all kinds of photocopy paper as antioxidants to prevent discoloration (Table 29.10). Dimethylthiourea (DMTU) sensitivity was reported in a textile cutter with conjunctivitis and dermatitis of the eyelids, corners of the mouth, and nasal mucous membranes. There was a strong positive patch test to the textile cutting patterns she handled; these had been duplicated by diazo processing that contained DMTU. In another case, a

Table 29-10 Thiourea and Derivatives: Nonrubber Exposures
Diazo copy paper, especially blueprints, clothing patterns
Commercial detergents
Adhesive tapes
Paint and glue removers
Fruits and vegetables (metabolized from carbamate fungicides)

Table 29-11 Main Uses of Paraphenylenediamine and Related Chemicals in Industry
Antioxidants in rubber industry (used to prevent deterioration; retards surface cracking and flaking)
Antiozonants
Retarder in manufacture of acrylates
May be in gasoline as inhibitor or sweetener

construction designer had dermatitis of the hands, face, and neck from diazo copy paper. He reacted to DMTU, thiourea, and ammonium paper developers.[152] Thiourea contact sensitivity was reported by Nurse[153] in a man exposed to paper used for printing architectural and printing plans. He was patch test positive to both undeveloped and developed paper, as well as Diazo 580 1% aqueous and thiourea 1% aqueous. Sensitivity to thiourea was described by Van Der Leun and colleagues,[154] in 1977, in two patients working with photocopy paper and presenting with photodermatitis. Patch testing with thiourea was positive, in one case with exposure of the test site to light and in the other without light exposure.

Maneb and other ethylenebisdithiocarbamate fungicides and slimicides may be metabolized to thioureas. Accordingly, carbamates and ETU may be found on or in fruits, berries, potatoes, and vegetables; whether sensitivity could be maintained by exposure to these low concentrations is uncertain.[155]

Mercaptobenzothiazoles

Many rubber chemicals may be present not only in rubber or adhesives, but also in other products, such as plastics, pesticides, oils, and organic dyes.[12] Contact dermatitis has occurred from some of these sources.

MBT may be found in antifreeze,[12] cutting oils,[141] heavy duty greases,[141] black tire paints,[141] special detergents,[141] pottery mold releasing fluid,[156] photographic film emulsion,[157] fungicides,[12] and veterinary medications.[158] Salts of MBT, when used to prevent mildew in fabrics or as an algicide or slimicide, may not be as prone to cause ACD as MBT in rubber.[140]

Paraphenylenediamines

In addition to textile and hair dyes, these chemicals may be used as antioxidants and corrosion inhibitors in antifreezes and other fluids, in fuels, and in the manufacture of some plastics (Table 29.11).

Rubber, Antabuse, and Alcohol

THIURAM-ALCOHOL REACTIONS

Erythema, urticaria, and pruritus (along with severe nausea and vomiting) may develop shortly after alcohol is consumed by persons who have ingested disulfiram (Antabuse, tetraethylthiuram disulfide). According to Webb[159] and van Ketel,[160] this reaction, first observed in the rubber industry, was applied to the treatment of alcoholism. Administered by mouth or by subcutaneous implantation, disulfiram interaction with ethanol is based on the inhibition by disulfiram of the enzyme aldehyde dehydrogenase. This block in the metabolism of imbibed ethanol results in the accumulation of toxic levels of the substrate for this enzyme, acetaldehyde.

The alcohol-disulfiram reaction is nonallergic and occurs in all individuals so exposed. Topical exposure to thiuram can also produce an Antabuse-like reaction when drinking alcohol.[161] Shelly[146] reviewed two cases, one of which was in a woman who experienced facial flushing every Sunday night after her bath. Bathing on weekdays had no such effect. Investigation revealed that she had cocktails only on Sunday and regularly used a thiuram-containing soap.

Erythematous skin reactions have also been reported in patients taking disulfiram and contacting alcohol-containing substances, specifically an aftershave lotion,[162] an alcohol-containing tar gel used to treat psoriasis,[163] and a beer-containing shampoo.[164]

It is claimed that ingested ethanol can exacerbate lesions of ACD from thiurams. The basis for this observation is Van Ketel's description[160] of three homemakers with tetramethylthiuram disulfide allergy who developed severe aggravation of eczema a few hours after consuming alcohol. Webb and colleagues[159] reported a patient who noted that the rash on the dorsa of his feet worsened with alcohol ingestion. The basis for these observations deserves further study.

ANTABUSE REACTIONS IN THIURAM-SENSITIVE PATIENTS

Webb and colleagues[159] stressed that patients should be questioned carefully regarding possible rubber contact allergy prior to administration of Antabuse. They reported a severe, widespread dermatitis developing in a 32-year-old man 5 hours after beginning treatment with Antabuse. Similar systemic eczematous reactions have been reported by Pirila,[165] and Goitre and colleagues.[166]

Lachapelle[167] reported ACD in two persons with disulfiram implants that extended out onto the skin. Although one patient could tolerate disulfiram by mouth, oral administration to the other patient caused a widespread eczematous dermatitis. Van Hecke and Vermander[168] reported on a 35-year-old alcoholic man who developed an eczematous dermatitis of the extremities as well as at a 2-year-old disulfiram implantation site on his abdomen following treatment with 400 mg of oral disulfiram (Antabuse). Patch tests were positive to thiuram mix, TMTD, TMTM, TETD, and a crushed Antabuse tablet. Alcohol intolerance after an implant usually lasts no longer than 6 months.

Other reported Antabuse reactions are fixed drug eruptions and acne.[12]

ANTABUSE "REACTION" IN NICKEL-ALLERGIC PATIENTS

Ingestion of disulfiram may provoke a flare-up of nickel dermatitis at sites previously contacted by nickel. Klein and Fowler[169] reported an alcoholic who developed dermatitis on the wrist (watch) and abdomen (belt buckle) shortly after Antabuse was started. No nickel had recently contacted the areas, but prior dermatitis to nickel had occurred. Patch test was positive only to nickel.

Exposure to other chemicals can produce a flushing reaction when associated with alcohol ingestion. These chemicals include calcium cyanamide, trichloroethylene, and butyral doximine.[170]

TREATMENT OF NICKEL DERMATITIS WITH DISULFIRAM

Several reports from Europe and one from Fowler in the United States have indicated that disulfiram is effective in treating some nickel-allergic patients.[171] (See Chapter 32.)

James S. Taylor, MD, Cleveland, Ohio, wrote the chapter on rubber allergy for the 3rd edition of Fisher's Contact Dermatitis. Much of his work was retained for the 4th and 5th editions and a portion of it remains in this text.

References

1. Rubber. In: The New Encyclopedia Britannica, vol. 15, 15th ed. London: Macropaedia, 1982.

2. Hamann CP. Natural rubber latex protein sensitivity in review. Am J Contact Dermat 1993;4:4.

3. Adams RM, Goin J, Hamann C, Sullivan K. Natural and synthetic rubber. In: Occupational skin disease, 3rd ed. Philadelphia: WB Saunders, 1999, pp. 501.

4. <www.yulex.com> (accessed May 10, 2007).

5. Rodriguez E, Reynolds GW, Thompson JA. Potent content allergen in the rubber plant guayule (Parthenium argentatum). Science 1981; 211:1444.

6. <www.trelleborg.com> (accessed May 10, 2007).

7. Barnhart, RR. Rubber compounding. In: Kirk-Othmer encyclopedia of chemical technology, vol. 20, 3rd ed. New York: John Wiley and Sons, 1982.

8. <www.wikipedia.org/wiki/vulcanization> (accessed May 10, 2007).

9. Taylor R, Son PN. Rubber chemicals. In: Kirk-Othmer encyclopedia of chemical technology, vol. 20, 3rd ed. New York: Wiley Interscience, 1982.

10. <www.rtvanderbilt.com> (accessed May 10, 2007.

11. Nicholas PP, Luxeder AM, Brooks LA, Hammes PA. Antioxidants and antiozonants. In: Kirk-Othmer encyclopedia of chemical technology, vol. 3, 3rd ed. New York: Wiley Interscience, 1978.

12. Fisher AA. Dermatitis from rubber, adhesives and gums. In: Fisher AA, ed. Contact dermatitis, 2nd ed. Philadelphia: Lea & Febiger, 1973.

13. www.lgm.gov.my/nrstat/Tl.htm, accessed May 15, 2007.

14. Nutter AF. Contact urticaria to rubber. Br J Dermatol 1979;101:597.

15. Förström L. Contact urticaria from latex surgical gloves. Contact Dermatitis 1980;6:33.

16. Food and Drug Administration. Allergic reactions to latex-containing medical devices. FDA Med Bull 1991.

17. Warshaw EM. Latex allergy. JAAD 1998;39:1.

18. Cohen D, Scheman A, Stewart L, et al. American Academy of Dermatology's position paper on latex allergy. JAAD 1998;39:98.

19. Yeang H: Natural rubber latex allergens: new developments. Curr Opin allergy Clin Immunol 2004;4:99.

20. Gidrol X, Chrestin H, Tan HL, Kush A. Hevein, a lectin-like protein from *Hevea brasiliensis* (rubber tree) is involved in the coagulation of latex. J Biol Chem 1994;269:9278.

21. Alenius H, Kalkkinen N, Yip E, et al. Significance of rubber elongation factor as a latex allergen. Int Arch Allergy Immunol 1996;109:262.

22. Guin J, et al. Occupational protein contact dermatitis to cornstarch in a paper adhesive. Am J Contact Dermat 1999;10:83.

23. Seaton A. Latex as aeroallergen. Lancet 1990;336:808.

24. Belsito DV. Contact urticaria caused by rubber: analysis of seven cases. In: Dermatology clinics, Adams R,

Nethercott J (eds.), vol. 8. Philadelphia: WB Saunders, 1990, p. 61.

25. DeGroot H, DeJong NW, Duijster E, et al. Prevalence of natural rubber latex allergy (type I and type IV) in laboratory workers in the Netherlands. Contact Dermatitis 1998;38:159.

26. Hamann CP, Turjanmaa K, Rietschel R, et al. Natural rubber latex hypersensitivity: incidence and prevalence of type I allergy in the dental professional. J Am Dent Assoc 1998;129:43.

27. Allmers H, Schmengler J, John S: Decreasing incidence of occupational contact urticaria caused by natural rubber latex allergy in German health care workers. J Allergy Clin Immunol 2004;114:347.

28. Nettis E, Colanardi M, Ferrannini A: Type I latex allergy in health care workers with latex induced contact urticaria. Allergy 2004;59:718.

29. Ylitilo L, Turjanmaa K, Palosuo T, Reunala T. Natural rubber latex allergy in children who had not undergone surgery and children who had undergone multiple operations. J Allergy Clin Immunol 1997;100:606.

30. Estornell-Moragues F, Nieto-Garcia A, Mazon-Ramos A, et al. Latex allergy in children with myelomeningocele: incidence and associated factors. Actas Urol Esp 1997;21:227.

31. Valks R, Conde-Salazar L, Cuevas M: Allergic contact urticaria from natural rubber latex in healthcare and non-healthcare workers. Contact Dermatitis 2004;50:222.

32. DeCorres LF, et al. Contact urticaria: sensitization to chestnuts and bananas in patients with contact urticaria from latex. Contact Dermatitis 1990;23:277.

33. Towse A, O'Brien M, Twarog FJ, et al. Local reaction secondary to insulin injection: a potential role for latex antigens in insulin vials and syringes. Diabetes Care 1995;18:1195.

34. Nettis E, Colanardi M, Soccio A, et al: Double-blind, placebo-controlled study of sublingual immunotherapy in patients with latex-induced urticaria. Br J Dermatol 2007;156:674.

35. Wakelin S, Jenkins R, Rycroft J, et al. Patch testing with natural rubber latex. Contact Dermatitis 1999;40:89.

36. Guillet G, Guillet M, Dagregorio G: Allergic contact dermatitis from natural rubber latex in atopic dermatitis and the risk of later type I allergy. Contact Dermatitis 2005;53:46.

37. Wilkinson S, Burd R. Latex: a cause of allergic contact eczema in users of natural rubber gloves. JAAD 1998;38:36.

38. Gottlober P, Gall H, Peter R: Allergic contact dermatitis from natural latex. Am J Contact Dermat 2000;12:135.

39. Malten KE, Nater JP, van Ketel WG. Patch testing guidelines. Nijmegen, Netherlands: Dekker & van de Vegt, 1976.

40. Marks JG, Belsito DV, DeLeo VA, et al. North American Contact Dermatitis Group patch test results for the detection of delayed-type hypersensitivity to topical allergens. JAAD 1998;38:911.

41. Marks JG, Belsito DV, DeLeo VA, et al. North American Contact Dermatitis Group patch test results, 1996–1998. Arch Dermatol 2000;136:534.

42. Warshaw E, Rietschel R, Saseville D, et al: NACDG patch test results 2003–2004 study period. Dermatitis 2007.

43. Lazarov A: European standard series patch test results from a contact dermatitis clinic in Israel during the 7-year period from 1998 to 2004. Contact Dermatitis 2006;55:73.

44. Conde-Salazar L, et al. Type IV allergy to rubber additives: a 10-year study of 686 cases. J Am Acad Dermatol 1993;29:176.

45. Von Hintzenstern J, et al. Frequency, spectrum and occupational relevance of type IV allergies to rubber chemicals. Contact Dermatitis 1991;24:244.

46. Nethercott JR, et al. Patch testing with a routine screening tray in North America, 1985–1989: gender and response. Am J Contact Dermat 1991;2:130.

47. Lindberg M, Edman B, Fischer T, et al: Time trends in Swedish patch test data from1992 to 2000. Contact Dermatitis 2007;56:205.

48. Leyden JJ, Kligman AM. Contact dermatitis to Neomycin sulfate. JAMA 1979;242:1276.

49. Veien NK, et al. Contact dermatitis in children. Contact Dermatitis 1982;8:373.

50. Fregert, S. Manual of contact dermatitis, 2nd ed. Chicago: Year Book Medical Publishers, 1981.

51. Stankevich VV, et al. Hygienic assessment of organosulfur accelerators for vulcanization of rubbers for the food industry. Gig Sanit 1980;10:88.

52. Fregert, S. Chemicals used in both rubber and plastic. Contact Dermatitis Newsletter 1971;9:204.

53. Kilpikari I. Occupational contact dermatitis among rubber workers. Contact Dermatitis 1982;8:359.

54. Varigos GA, Dunt DR. Occupational dermatitis: an epidemiological study in the rubber and cement industries. Contact Dermatitis 1981;7:105.

55. Macedo M, Alchorne A, Costa E, et al: Contact allergy in male construction workers in Sao Paolo Brazil, 200–2005. Contact Dermatitis 2007;56:232.

56. Rietschel R, Mathias C, Fowler J, et al: Relationship of occupation to contact dermatitis. Am J Contact Dermat 2002;13:170–6.

57. Warshaw E, Cook J, Belsito D, et al. Positive patch test reactions to mixed dialkyl thioureas. Dermatitis 2007.

58. Calnan CD. Rubber sensitivity presenting as eyelid oedema. Contact Dermatitis 1975;1:1

59. Dooms-Goossens A, et al. Pustular reactions to hexafluorosilicate in foam rubber. Contact Dermatitis 1985;12:42.

60. King CM. Contact sensitivity to Hylene W. Contact Dermatitis 1980;6:353.

61. Kilpikari I, Home H. Contact allergy to Hypalon rubber. Contact Dermatitis 1983;9:529.

62. Adams RM. Possible substitution for mercaptobenzothiazole in rubber. Contact Dermatitis 1975;1:246.

63. Foussereau J. Allergy to MBT and its derivatives. Contact Dermatitis 1983;9:514.

64. Bieber PL, Foussereau J. Role de deux amines aromatiques dans l'allergie au caoutchouc; PBN et 4010 NA, amines antioxidantes dans l'industrie due pneu. Bull Soc Dermatol Syphil 1968;75:63.

65. Herve-Bazin B, et al. Occupational eczema from n-isopropyl-n-phenyl-paraphenylenediamine (IPPD) and n-dimethyl-1,3 butyl-n-phenylpara-phenylenediamine (DMPPD) in tyres. Contact Dermatitis 1977;3:1.

66. Cronin E: Rubber. In Cronin E, Contact Dermatitis, Churchill Livingstone, 1980. ("66a") Munn A. In: Cronin E, ed. Contact dermatitis. New York: Churchill Livingstone, 1980.

67. Livesley B, Lambelle J. Perichondritis helicis: an industrial hazard—two case reports. J Laryngol Otol 1967;81:1063.

68. Mancuso G, Reggiani M, Berdondini RM. Occupational dermatitis in shoemakers. Contact Dermatitis 1996;34:17.

69. Bonnevie P. Aetiologie und Pathogenese der Ekzemkrankheiten. Leipzig: Barth, 1981.

70. Epstein E. Simplified patch test screening with mixtures. Arch Dermatol 1967;95:269.

71. Belloni Fortina A, Piaserico S, Larese F, et al: DDM: frequency of sensitization, clinical relevance, and concomitant positive reactions. Contact Dermatitis 2001;44: 283–8.

72. Adams A, Warshaw E: Allergic contact dermatitis from mercapto compounds. Dermatitis 2006;17:56.

73. Mitchell JC, et al. Patch testing with mercaptobenzothiazole and mercapto-mix. Contact Dermatitis 1976;2:123.

74. Fregert S. Cross-sensitivity pattern of 2-mercaptobenzothiazole (MBT). Acta Derm Venereol (Stockh) 1969;49:45.

75. Hansson C, Agrup G. Stability of the mercaptobenzothiazole compounds. Contact Dermatitis 1993;28:29.

76. Geier J, Uter W, Schnuch A, et al. Diagnostic screening for contact allergy to mercaptobenzothiazole derivatives. Am J Contact Dermat 202;13:66.

77. Diepgen T, Bruynzeel D, Andersen K. Mercaptobenzothiazole or the mercapto-mix: which should be included in the standard series? Contact Dermatitis 2006;55:36.

78. van Ketel WG. Thiuram mix. Contact Dermatitis 1976;2:232.

79. Themido, R, Brandaõ FM. Contact allergy to thiurams. Contact Dermatitis 1984;10:251.

80. Geier J, Lessmann H, Uter W, et al. Occupational rubber glove allergy: results from the IVDK, 1995–2001. Contact Dermatitis 2003;48:39.

81. Bryld L, Agner T, Menné T. Allergic contact dermatitis from IPBC-an update. Contact Dermatitis 2001;44:276.

82. Schonning L, Hjorth N. Cross sensitization between hair dyes and rubber chemicals. Berufsdermatosen 1969;17:100.

83. van Ketel WG. Low sensitization rate of naphthyl mix. Contact Dermatitis 1983;9:77.

84. Geier J, Lessmann H, Frosch P, et al. Contact sensitization ton-(cyclohexyl) phthalimide. Contact Dermatitis 2003;48:1.

85. Loffeld A, Foulds I. Allergic contact dermatitis from n-(cyclohexylthio) phthalimide in a playground fitter. Contact Dermatitis 2004;51:212.

86. Jordan Jr WP, Bourlas MC. Allergic contact dermatitis to underwear elastic. Arch Dermatol 1975;111:593.

87. Veien NK. Patch testing with substances not included in the standard series. Contact Dermatitis 1983;9:304.

88. Haapasaari K, Niinimaki A. Vesicular palmar eczema from the neoprene tongue of an ankle support. Contact Dermatitis 2000;42:248.

89. White WG, Vickers HR. Diethylthiourea as a cause of dermatitis in a car factory. Br J Ind Med 1970;27:167.

90. Fregert S, Trulson L, Zimerson E. Contact allergic reactions to diphenylthiourea and phenyl isothiocyanate in PVC adhesive tape. Contact Dermatitis 1982;8:38.

91. Fregert S, Dahlquist I, Trulson L. Sensitization capacity of diphenylthiourea and phenylisothiocyanate. Contact Dermatitis 1983;9:87.

92. Meding B, et al. Allergic contact dermatitis from diphenylthiourea in Vulkan heat retainers. Contact Dermatitis 1990;22:8.

93. Roberts JL, Hanifin JM. Athletic shoe dermatitis, contact allergy to ethyl butyl thiourea. JAMA 1979;241:275.

94. Roberts JL, Hanifin JM. Contact allergy and cross reactivity to substituted thiourea compounds. Contact Dermatitis 1980;6:138.

95. Knudsen BB, et al. Release of thiurams and carbamates from rubber gloves. Contact Dermatitis 1993;28:63.

96. Fisher AA. Contact dermatitis in surgeons. J Derm Surg Oncol 1975;1:63.

97. Rich P, et al. Allergic contact dermatitis to two antioxidants in latex gloves: 4,49-thio bis(6-tert-butyl-meta-cresol) (Lowinox 44536) and butylhydroxyanisole. J Am Acad Dermatol 1991;24:37.

98. Shmunes E, Darby T. Contact dermatitis due to endotoxin in irradiated latex gloves. Contact Dermatitis 1984;10:240.

99. Jordan WP. 24-, 48-hour patch tests. Contact Dermatitis 1980;6:151.

100. Calnan CD. Rubber sensitivity presenting as eyelid oedema. Contact Dermatitis 1975;1:124.

101. Hindson TC. Studies in contact dermatitis: (16): Contraceptives. Trans St Johns Hosp Derm Soc 1966;52:1.

102. Harmon CB, Connolly SM, Larson TR. Condom-related allergic contact dermatitis. J Urol 1995;153:1227.

103. Fisher AA. Condom conundrums: part 1. Cutis 1991;48:359.

104. Fisher AA. Vulvitis due to contactants. Cutis 1974;13:725.

105. Fisher AA. Consort contact dermatitis. Cutis 1979;24:595.

106. Schamberg IL, Flesch P. Contact dermatitis from rubber caused by allergic sensitivity to thio-beta-naphthol. J Invest Dermatol 1953;21:59.

107. Reynaerts A, Bruze M, Erikstam U, Goossens A. Allergic contact dermatitis from a medical device, followed by depigmentation. Contact Dermatitis 1998;39:204.

108. Scalf LA, Fowler JF. Allergic contact dermatitis caused by dialkyl thioureas in a patient with sleep apnea. Am J Contact Dermat 1999;10:169.

109. Pennys NS, Edwards LS, Katsikos JL. Allergic contact sensitivity to thiuram compounds in a hemodialysis unit. Arch Dermatol 1976; 112:811.

110. Goette DK. Raccoon-like periorbital leukoderma from contact with swim goggles. Contact Dermatitis 1984;10:129.

111. Maibach HI. Scuba diver facial dermatitis: allergic contact dermatitis to n-isopropyl-n-phenylparaphenylenediamine. Contact Dermatitis 1975;1:330.

112. Tuyp E, Mitchell JC. Scuba diver facial dermatitis. Contact Dermatitis 1983;9:334.

113. Adams RM. Contact allergic dermatitis in a wetsuit. Contact Dermatitis 1982;8:277.

114. Tennstedt D, Lachapelle JM. Windsurfer dermatitis from black rubber compounds. Contact Dermatitis 1981;7:160.

115. Schulz KH, Hermann WP. 4,49-dioxydiphenyl als ursache von schweib blattekzemen. Derm Woschenchr 1960;141:124.

116. Arisu K, et al. Tinuvin® P in a spandex tape as a cause of clothing dermatitis. Contact Dermatitis 1992;26:311.

117. Furman D, Fisher AA, Leider M. Allergic eczematous contact–type dermatitis caused by rubber sponges used for the application of cosmetics. J Invest Dermatol 1950;15:223.

118. Fisher AA. Allergic contact dermatitis (caused by rubber cosmetic sponges) simulating cosmetic dermatitis. Cutis 1993;51:320.

119. Curtis GH. Contact dermatitis of eyelids caused by an antioxidant in rubber fillers of eyelash curlers. Arch Dermatol 1945;52:262.

120. McKenna KE, McMillan C. Facial contact dermatitis due to black rubber. Contact Dermatitis 1992;26:270.

121. Deguchi M, Tagami H. Contact dermatitis of the ear due to a rubber earplug. Dermatology 1996;193:251.

122. Gaul LE. Results of patch testing with rubber antioxidants and accelerators. J Invest Dermatol 1957;29:105.

123. Jacobziner H, Raybin HW. The rise and decline of flubberitis. NY State J Med 1963;1:2562.

124. Sauer GC. Flubber dermatitis. Arch Dermatol 1965;91:465.

125. Fisher AA. Purpuric contact dermatitis. Cutis 1984;33:346.

126. Shmunes E. Purpuric allergic contact dermatitis to paraphenylenediamine. Contact Dermatitis 1978;4:225.

127. Batschvarov B, and Minkov DM. Dermatitis and purpura from rubber in clothing. Trans St Johns Hosp Dermatol Soc 1968;54:178.

128. Calnan CD, Peachy RDG. Allergic contact purpura. Clin Allergy 1971;1:287.

129. Ancona A, Monroy F, Fernandez-Diez J. Occupational dermatitis from IPPD in tires. Contact Dermatitis 1982;8:91.

130. Fregert S, Skog E. Allergic contact dermatitis from mercaptobenzothiazole in cutting oil. Acta Derm Venereol (Stockh) 1962;42:_235.

131. Fisher AA. Nonoccupational dermatitis to "black" rubber mix: part 2. Cutis 1992;49:229.

132. Calnan CD. Lichenoid dermatitis from isopropylaminodiphenylamine. Contact Dermatitis Newsletter 1971;10:237.

133. Oliver EA, Schwartz L, Warren LH. Occupational leukoderma: preliminary report. JAMA 1939;113:927.

134. Dorsey CS. Dermatitic and pigmentary reactions to monobenzylether of hydroquinone. Arch Dermatol 1960;81:245.

135. van Ketel WG. Sensitization to hydroquinone and the monobenzylether of hydroquinone. Contact Dermatitis 1984;10:253.

136. Adams RM. Depigmentation from occupational chemicals. In: Occupational skin disease. 3rd ed., Philadelphia: WB_Saunders Co., 1999, pp. 15–20.

137. van der Walle HB, et al. Contact sensitization to hydroquinone and p-methoxyphenol in the guinea pig, inhibitors in acrylic monomers. Contact Dermatitis 1982;8:147.

138. Gellin GA. Pigment responses: occupational disorders of pigmentation. In: Maibach HI, Gellin GA, eds. Occupational and industrial dermatology. Chicago: Year book Medical Publishers, 1982.

139. Bajaj AK, Gupta SC, Chatterjee AK. Contact depigmentation from free paratertiary-butylphenol in bindi adhesive. Contact Dermatitis 1990;22:99.

140. Cronin E. Pesticides. In: Contact dermatitis. New York: Churchill Livingstone, 1980.

141. Task Force on Contact Dermatitis (North American Contact Dermatitis Group). Exposure lists—contact dermatitis antigens. Evanston, IL: American Academy of Dermatology, 1982.

142. Dick DC, Adams RH. Allergic contact dermatitis from monosulfiram (Tetmosol) soap. Contact Dermatitis 1979;5:199.

143. Adams RM, Manchester RD. Allergic contact dermatitis to Maneb in a housewife. Contact Dermatitis 1982;8:271.

144. Boman A, et al. Phenyl-alpha-naphthyl-amine—case report and guinea pig studies. Contact Dermatitis 1980;6:299.

145. Schulz KH, Hermann WP. Tetramethylthiuramdisulfide, ein thioharnstoffderivat als Ekzemnoxe bei Hafenarbeitern. Berufsdermatosen 1958;6:130.

146. Shelly WB. Golf-course dermatitis due to thiram fungicide. JAMA 1964;188:415.

147. Cronin E. Pesticides. In: Contact dermatitis. New York: Churchill Livingstone, 1980.

148. Copeman PWM. Toxic epidermal necrolysis caused by skin hypersensitivity to monosulfiram. Br Med J 1968;1:623.

149. Nater JP, Terpstra H, Bleumink E. Allergic contact sensitization to the fungicide Maneb. Contact Dermatitis 1979;5:24.

150. Willems PW, Geursen-Reitsma AM, van-Joost T. Allergic contact dermatitis due to methiocarb (Mesurol). Contact Dermatitis 1997; 36:270.

151. Kanerva L, Estlander T, Alanko K, Jolanki R. Occupational airborne allergic contact dermatitis from dibutylthiourea. Contact Dermatitis 1998;38:347.

152. Torres V, et al. Occupational contact dermatitis to thiourea and dimethylthiourea from diazo copy paper. Am J Contact Dermat 1992;3:37.

153. Nurse DS. Sensitivity to thiourea in plan printing paper. Contact Dermatitis 1980;6:153.

154. Van der Leun JC, et al. Photosensitivity owing to thiourea. Arch Dermatol 1977;113:1611.

155. Bruze M, Fregert S. Allergic contact dermatitis from ethylene thiourea. Contact Dermatitis 1983;9:208.

156. Wilkinson SM, Cartwright PH, English JSC. Allergic contact dermatitis from mercaptobenzothiazole in a releasing fluid. Contact Dermatitis 1990;23:70.

157. Rudzki, E, et al. Dermatitis from 2-mercaptobenzothiazole in photographic films. Contact Dermatitis 1981;7:43.

158. Adams RM. Mercaptobenzothiazole in veterinary medications. Contact Dermatitis Newsletter 1974;16:514.

159. Webb PK, et al. Disulfiram hypersensitivity and rubber contact dermatitis. JAMA 1979;241:2061.

160. Van Ketel WG. Rubber, alcohol and eczema. Dermatologica 1968; 136:442.

161. Gold S. A skinful of alcohol. Lancet 1966;2:1417.

162. Mercurio F. Antabuse-alcohol reaction. JAMA 1952;149:82.

163. Ellis CN, Mitchell AJ, Beardsley GR. Tar gel interaction with disulfiram. Arch Dermatol 1979;115:1367.

164. Stole D, King LE. Disulfiram-alcohol skin reaction to beer-containing shampoo. JAMA 1980;244:2045.

165. Pirila V. Dermatitis due to rubber. Proceedings of the 11th National Congress of Dermatology. Acta Derm Venereol (Stockh) 1957;11:252.

166. Goitre M, Bedello PG, Cane D. Allergic dermatitis and oral challenge to tetramethyl-thiuram disulphide. Contact Dermatitis 1981;7:272.

167. Lachapelle JM. Allergic "contact" dermatitis from disulfiram implants. Contact Dermatitis 1975;1:218.

168. van Hecke E, Vermander F. Allergic contact dermatitis by oral disulfiram. Contact Dermatitis 1984;10:254.

169. Klein LR, Fowler JF. Nickel dermatitis recall during disulfiram therapy for alcohol abuse. JAAD 1992;26:645.

170. Birmingham DJ. Occupational dermatoses. In: Clayton GD, Clayton FE, eds. Patty's industrial hygiene and toxicology, vol. 1, 3rd rev. ed. New York: John Wiley and Sons, 1978.

171. Fowler, JF: Disulfiram is effective for nickel allergic hand eczema. Am J Contact Dermat 1992;3:175.

GUMS, ROSIN, AND NATURAL RESINS

EXECUTIVE SUMMARY

Natural gums and resins have been used for centuries in gels, emulsifiers, adhesives, lubricants, foods, and medications. Gums often are hygroscopic and act as thickening agents. Allergies to these agents are rare. However, in addition to occasional allergic contact dermatitis (ACD), urticaria and anaphylaxis have been reported from systemic administration or ingestion. Resins are more likely allergens, the hallmarks of which are *Myroxylon pereirae* (balsam of Peru) and other balsams. Fragrance allergy is often detected with this allergen family. Tincture of benzoin, used in surgical preparations and dressings, frequently crossreacts with fragrances and balsams. Other natural resins include cashew-nut shell resin and resin from the Japanese lacquer tree, both of which contain urushiols.

Rosin, extracted from pine and other soft-wood trees, is also a common allergen. It is produced in solid, liquid, and powdered forms. It occurs naturally in paper, cardboard, and related materials. It is commonly used as a "tackifier" and viscosity enhancer in making glues, adhesive tapes, inks, varnishes, waxes, soldering flux, and many other products. It is a necessity to the violinist and is helpful for gripping sports equipment like baseballs, bowling balls, tennis rackets, and baseball bats.

Natural gums are produced principally in Africa and Asia and include seaweed extracts, plant exudates, gums from seed or root, and gums obtained by microbial fermentation. These resinous polysaccharides or their derivatives are water soluble and swell substantially in water.[1] Gums are used in industry because their aqueous solutions or dispersions possess suspending and stabilizing properties. Gums may produce gels or act as emulsifiers, adhesives, flocculants, binders, film formers, lubricants, or friction reducers. The principal natural gums are listed in Table 30.1. Reports of contact allergy to these gums are quite rare.[2] These gums may be used "as is" for patch testing.

Carrageenan

Carrageenans are a family of polysaccharides extracted from seaweed, especially from Irish moss. They have many uses in foods, dental products, skin and hair-care products, and some industrial uses. Much of the world's supply comes from the Philippines.

Guar Gum

This mannose- and galactose-based gum is extracted from the guar bean, *Cyamopsis tetragonoloba*. It is used in textiles and printing as a finishing agent, as a thickener in foods, and in personal-care products like toothpastes. A case of contact anaphylaxis to guar gum in a topical anesthetic gel applied to oral mucous membranes has been reported.[3]

Gum Arabic

Gum arabic (also called gum acacia) is a dried exudate containing polysaccharides and glycoproteins, from several species of acacia tree, produced under the adverse conditions of lack of moisture, poor nutrition, and hot temperatures. Most commercial gum comes from *Acacia senegal or sayal*, found in the Sudan and West Africa. It has wide and varied industrial uses but is normally a stabilizer and thickener in foods. It is used specifically as an adhesive in bakery icings and toppings, as a foam stabilizer in beer, in "gummy" candies and marshmallows,

Table 30-1 Principal Natural Gums	
Gum	Source
Algine	*Phaeophyceae* seaweed extract
Carrageenan (Agara)	*Rhodophyceae* seaweed extract
Guar gum	*Cyanaposis tetragonolibus* seed
Gum arabic (acacia)	*Acacia senegal* plant exudate
Gum ghatti	*Anogeissus latifolia* tree exudate
Gum karaya (sterculia)	*Sterculia urens* plant exudate
Gum mastic	*Pistacia lentiscus*
Gum tragacanth	*Astralagus* plant exudate
Large gum	*Larix occidentalis* tree extract
Locust bean gum	*Ceratonia siliqua* plant exudate
Pectin	Extracts from cell walls of plants
Psyllium gum	*Plantago ovata* seed extract
Quince seed gum	*Cydonia vulgaris* or *oblonga* seed
Tamarind gum	*Tamarindus indica* seed extract
Xanthan gum	Microbial fermentation of *Xanthomas capestris*

and as a crystallization inhibitor in sugar syrups. Gum arabic has limited application in the cosmetic and pharmaceutical industries as a binder and emulsion stabilizer, but the main nonfood uses are in the formulation of inks and adhesives, in shoe polish, in postage-stamp adhesive and in the textile industries, where it is used as a sizing agent.[4,5] Acacia syrup is listed in the *US National Formulary.*[6] Gum arabic has been reported to cause respiratory allergy, especially in the printing trades. Dermatitis has also been reported. A gum from cashew (*Anacardium*) may be used to adulterate gum arabic.[7]

Three renal transplant recipients found to be hypersensitive to prednisone tablets had reacted to the tragacanth and acacia used in their manufacture. Their symptoms subsided when a formulation using methylcellulose was substituted.[8]

Gum arabic adhesive may be preserved with formaldehyde, which was the cause of contact allergy in a lithoplater. Patch tests with gum arabic (as is) were positive (but negative at 1% and 10%), and formaldehyde (2%) was also positive.[9] A similar case was reported due to 1,2-benzisothiazolin-3–1 used as a preservative in gum arabic.[10]

Gum Mastic

Mastic is an evergreen shrub (*Pistacia lentiscus*) found in the Mediterranean region. It is used in various food and dental products. A Chinese orthopedic medicine, meant to be used either topically or orally, has been reported to cause ACD. The product contains both myrrh and mastic gum, each at a 12.5% concentration. One patient reacted to mastic, one to myrrh, and one to both on patch testing.

None reacted to balsam of Peru or colophony.[11] It has caused ACD when used as a postoperative dressing.[12]

Gum Tragacanth

Gum tragacanth is an exudate from the root of several species of tree, of the genus *Astragalus,* found in the dry, mountainous regions of Iran, Syria, and Turkey, known also as "locoweed." Tragacanth is used in pharmaceuticals and cosmetics, as an emulsifier, thickener and stabilizer. It has been used as a bulk laxative, an excipient for pills , and as the basis of lubricants for catheters and surgical instruments.[8] In the food industry, it is used as a thickening or stabilizing agent; in the textile industry as a sizing agent and print paste thickener; and as an emulsifier in furniture, floor, and auto polishes.[4]

An immediate life-threatening allergic reaction in a 35-year-old woman was attributed to the tragacanth present in the beef burger that she was eating.[8] Contact dermatitis in a 4-year-old boy at the sites of electrocardiogram electrodes was due to tragacanth in the electrode jelly.[8]

Karaya Gum

Karaya, or sterculia gum, is the dried extract of the *Sterculia urens* tree, which is primarily cultivated in India. Gum karaya is the least soluble gum exudate; it is used in foods as a thickening and suspending agent and as a stabilizer in salad dressings, ice cream, sherbets, and frozen desserts, in which it prevents the formation of large ice crystals. Gum karaya is also used in cheese spread, sausages, and bakery goods, sometimes in combination with carageenan.[13]

A large proportion of karaya is used by the pharmaceutical industry as a bulk laxative. It is also used as a dental adhesive and adhesive for ostomy appliances. Ulcerations, fibrous lesions, and accelerated bone resorption have been reported with inappropriate use of denture adhesives and ill-fitting dentures. In the paper industry, gum karaya is used as a binder for pulp in the preparation of long-fibered, lightweight papers. Gum solutions are used as thickening agents for printing dyes as well as textile sizes.[4] Karaya is rarely found in cosmetics, particularly hair-waving lotions and in toothpastes. Contact dermatitis from a karaya ostomy seal ring has been reported. (See Chapter 19.) The patient was not tested to the individual components of the ring.[14]

Respiratory allergy has been reported, with cross-sensitivity to gum arabic and karaya gum.[7]

Psyllium

Psyllium, primarily used as a stool-softener, comes from the seed of the genus Plantago. It is produced mostly in Europe, Russia, Pakistan, and India. Although not reported as a cause of ACD, respiratory allergy and anaphylaxis have been described.[15] Atopic individuals may be at greater risk for this. Anaphylaxis from psyllium in a laxative and airborne dermatitis and asthma in a psyllium factory worker have been reported.[16,17] IgE antibodies to psyllium were found in both patients.

Xanthan Gum

This polysaccharide gum is produced by fermentation of sugars by the bacterium *Xanthomonas campestris*. Like other gums mentioned above, it has uses in the food and pharmaceutical industry as a thickener. It is also used extensively in oil drilling.

Carboxymethylcellulose

Although not a "natural" resin, this substance has commercial uses similar to those of emulsion stabilizers and viscosity enhancers. It is synthesized from cellulose and sodium chloroacetate. Moreau and colleagues provide a good review of its uses.[18] They report a case of contact urticaria from the substance in a student handling chalk. Other cases of contact urticaria, anaphylaxis from injection or ingestion, and ACD have been reported.[19]

Natural Resins

Natural resins are derived from many sources and have diverse properties. They are mainly oleoresins from tree saps and related fluids, and they occur secondarily from other sources such as insect exudations (shellac) and minerals (Utah coal resin). Table 30.2 lists the major resins, their class (of industrial use), country of origin, source, and uses.[20,21] Natural resins used in medicines, perfumes, and flavors are listed in Table 30.3. Another term applied to these resins is "copal" (a Mexican word meaning "incense"), which describes hard oleoresins, particularly of fossil origin. Such resins are useful in varnish making. Copal resin is dug from the remains of trees long dead. Several plants yield copals, for example, *Agathis, Bursera, Canarium, Copaifera,* and *Hymenaea.* Contact sensitivity to copal occurs, and dermatitis has

Table 30-2 Natural Resins				
Resin	Class	Country of origin	Source	Uses
Accroides (yacca)	—	Australia	*Xanthorrhoea* tree leaves	Paper and wallboard lacquer, wood mahogany stains, picric acid
Amber	—	Baltic shores	Fossils of *Pinus succinifera*	Ornamental beads and jewelry, rubefacient
Canada balsam	—	United States and Canada	*Abies balsamera*	Microscope slide mounting, cement for optical glass, varnish
Cashew nutshell oil	—	—	*Anacardium occidentale*	Varnish, cutting oils, brake pads
Chinese, Thai, and Japanese lacquer	—	—	*Rhus verniciflua, Melanorrhea usitata*	Artwork, furniture lacquer
Congo	Amber, dark, white, and pale	Zaire	Fossil trees	Varnishes, flavors, perfumes, pharmaceuticals
Copals	—	South America	*Caesalpinacea*	Varnishes
Damar	Bativia, Singapore	Indonesia, India, Malaysia	*Dipterocarpaceae*	Resin modifier or nitrocellulose
East India	Batu, black, pale macassar, and pale Singapore	Indonesia	Fossil trees	Coatings
Elemi, gum	—	Philippines, India, Utah	*Burseraceae*	Solvent and plasticizer in lacquers, coatings
Gilsonite	—		Mineral	Coatings
Kauri	Brown, pale	New Zealand	Fossil trees	Coatings
Manila	Boea, Loba, and Macassar, Philippines	Indonesia, Philippines	*Caraucariacean Agathis alba* tree	Coatings, polishes
Rosin	Gum, tall oil, and wood	United States	Poinus tree	See section on colophony
Sandarac	—	Morocco	*Tetraclinis articulata* tree	Artistic coatings
Shellac	—	India	Insect *Kerria laca*	Coatings, cosmetics
Utah coal resin		Utah	Mineral	Paint, medicine

Table 30-3 Natural Resins in Perfumes and Flavors

Resins	Point(s) of origin	Source
Balm of Gilead (Mecca balsam)	Saudi Arabia and Abyssinia	*Commiphora opobalasmum* tree
Balsam of Peru*	Central America	*Myroxylon pereirae* tree bark
Balsam of Tolu*	Equatorial America	*Myroxylon punctatum* tree
Benzoin*	Thailand, Sumatra, and Java	*Styrax* tree
Copaiba**	West Indies and Brazil	*Copaifera landsdorfi* tree
Frankincense* (olibanum)	Saudi Arabia and environs	*Boswellia* tree
Guaiac*	West Indies and South America (north coast)	*Guaiacum officinale* tree
Labdanum	—	*Cistus ladaniferus* and related shrubs
Myrrh*	Saudi Arabia and East Africa	Commiphora tree
Opopanax* (sweet myrrh)	—	Commiphora tree, Burseraceae family
Storax**	Asia Minor	*Liquidambar orientalis* tree

*Allergic contact dermatitis or positive patch tests (some crossreactions).
**Crossreaction with benzoin derived from Styrax (Styracaceae).

been seen in workers during its production.[7] Copal became a designation for quality in an attempt to distinguish between botanic and commercial points of origin. It applies mainly to Congo, kauri, pontianak, and Manila resins. Amber and Utah coal resins may be the oldest of the copals.[20]

Jost and colleagues[21] published a treatise on the nomenclature and chemistry of various resins that may be of interest to readers wishing to have a detailed understanding of these substances. They also discussed 16 cases of allergic contact dermatitis from a Manila resin used in a surgical adhesive called Alpharopal. Interestingly, 13 of the 16 reacted to colophony (20% pet). Six reacted to abietic acid, and several crossreactions with other resins were noted.[21]

Allergic contact dermatitis or positive patch tests have been documented from many of these natural resins. Copal in a dental root canal has been reported to cause stomatitis.[22]

Cashew Nut Shell Resin

Cashew nutshell resin is used in the manufacture of vehicle brake components and waterproof coatings. It was introduced commercially into the USA in 1926.[23] It contains approximately 90% anacardic acid and 10% cardol, but the composition varies.[7,14] These are resorcinol derivatives that share a common molecular skeleton with the 3-pentadecyl phenols of poison ivy. In

South America, timber from the cashew nut tree (*Anacardium occidentale*) is used for house and boat building. The tree, a native of Brazil, is grown principally for its nuts, oil, and gum. Cashew nutshell oil has been used in medicine as a rubefacient and vesicant and in the past has been found in many sources in industry: on fishing lines, as an insect repellent, in book bindings, cloth markers, varnishes, and cutting oils. It has also been used as a gum arabic substitute, and in combination with formaldehyde as a resin. Dermatitis in workers in brake manufacturing plants is not unusual (Fowler J, personal communication).

Marks and colleagues reported on an epidemic of poison-ivy like dermatitis in 54 patients that they traced to ingestion of cashew nut shell fragments along with the nuts themselves.[24] More recently, systemic ACD in a "baboon-syndrome" pattern from cashews in a pesto sauce has occurred.[25]

Japanese Lacquer Tree

The history, chemistry, and allergic contact dermatitis from urushiol-containing Japanese lacquer has been reviewed by Mitchell and Rook.[7] Dermatitis has been reported from a Chinese jar buried for 1,000 years. The Thai lacquer tree (*Melanorrhoea usitata*) contains thitsiol ($C_{23}H_{36}O_2$). Three cases were reported, two nonoccupational, from Bangkok. All reacted to 10% lacquer in petrolatum. The Japanese lacquer contains urushiol ($C_{21}H_{32}O_2$) and the Vietnamese tree laccol ($C_{18}H_{26}O_2$).[26] Kawai and colleagues[27] reported that heating Japanese lacquer reduces its allergenicity.

Shellac

Shellac is a resinous excretion of the insect *Coccus lacca* exuded as a protective cover onto certain host trees, primarily in India and Thailand.[28] Shellac has irritant and sensitizing properties. Its main use is as a coating lacquer in fine wood products. Other uses are in cosmetics (especially eye and lip products), dental impression material, waxes, and cementing book covers. Pharmaceutical Glaze (*US National Formulary*) is a denatured solution containing 20% to 51% anhydrous shellac, prepared with alcohol (95%) or dehydrated alcohol.[6]

Shellac and colophony both caused allergic cheilitis from a lipstick sealant.[29] Shellac was tested at 100%, and 50 controls were negative. Mascara and eyeliner have been the sources of shellac ACD in a number of reported cases.[30,31] Le Coz and colleagues reported 5 cases of eyelid ACD from shellac from several sites over a 2-year period.[32] They used shellac (20% eth) for testing. A report from England implicated shellac allergy as a cause of allergic cheilitis in 4 patients.[33]

Benzoin

Benzoin is present in tincture of benzoin (10% alcohol). Compound tincture of benzoin contains 10% benzoin, 2% aloe, 8% storax, and 4% balsam of Tolu in ethyl alcohol. Compound tincture of benzoin is known by at least 27 other names (e.g., Balsamum Equitus Sancti Victorius, Guttate Nader, and Jerusalem Balsam).[6] Arning's tincture contains tincture of benzoin, ammonium tumenol, anthrarobin, and ether.

Sources of exposure to benzoin have been listed as adhesives, cosmetics (nail polish, perfumes, and cuticle removers), inks, benzoinated lard (BPC 1954), antioxidants in creams, expectorants, throat lozenges, raw beeswax, bee glue (propolis), and water-repellent barrier creams. Many of these uses were discovered by Hjorth in 1961.[34] Benzoin is still used in medicine as an adhesive (either alone, as a tincture, or as an adhesive for another medicament, such as podophyllum), as a photoinitiator for acrylates, rarely in cosmetics, and as a skin-toughening agent in grease-paint makeup.[35]

Benzoin may be a more frequent sensitizer than previously thought, especially when used as a medical adhesive, and should be used with caution for this purpose. Fowler has seen positive patch tests in both patients and medical personnel. Fairly severe local reactions and a generalized eruption have been reported with benzoin allergy.[36,37] Hollister medical adhesive or Mastisol may be substituted with less chance of allergic reactions.

BENZOIN PATCH TESTING

Benzoin often crossreacts with balsam of Peru and related resins, including balsam of Tolu, styrax (storax),[34] myrrh, locust, galbanum, gamboge and olibanum, and other group-specific substances listed by Malten and Fisher (J Mitchell, personal communication, December 1983). An Australian report noted positive patch test reactions to compound tincture of benzoin in 10% of 477 consecutive patients, an unusually high number.[38] Only 2, however, were clinically relevant. Crossreactivity with balsam, fragrance mix, and others probably accounted for many of the positives.

Hjorth[34] found 2.3% positive reactions among 1,421 consecutive patients patch tested with compound benzoin tincture USP. He also found that benzoin (10% alc) would react almost without exception in patients sensitive to balsam of Peru. It may be useful to do an open patch test first; if the test is negative, proceed to a closed patch test to minimize severe reactions. Benzoin in petrolatum may give false-negative results.

Podophyllin and Cantharidin

Podophyllum (extracted from the plant, *Podophyllum peltatum*) and cantharidin (extracted from the blister beetle, *Lytta vesicatria*) are two other resins used frequently in dermatology. Both are strong vesicants used for the treatment of warts and molluscum and may produce severe irritant reactions. Severe systemic toxicity may occur upon ingestion or application over large surfaces or open areas.[7]

Rosin

Rosin (colophony) is a product of pine tree oleoresin. Depending on the method of extraction, three kinds of colophony may be identified: (a) gum rosin, obtained by topping living trees and distilling the resin to yield turpentine oil and the gum rosin residue; (b) wood rosin, a distillate from dead pine tree stumps; and (c) tall oil rosin (liquid rosin), a by-product of pulping pine wood (*tall* is the Swedish word for pine).[7,18,19] An interesting review of the uses and chemical analysis of rosin is available.[41] According to Mitchell and Rook,[7] rosin produced in the United States is obtained from the longleaf pine *(Pinus palustris)* and the loblolly pine *(P. taeda)* of the south Atlantic and eastern Gulf states. In 1988, the estimated total production of rosin was over 1.2 million metric tons, whilst in 1995 production was about 1.5 million tons. Gum rosin accounted for about 60% of this total, tall oil rosin 35%, and wood rosin the remainder. In the United States, tall oil accounts for three-fourths of the total rosin produced. Rosin used in paper products, rubber, adhesives, and inks accounts for the majority of the total rosin produced. China, Latin America, and Portugal produce much gum rosin, and Scandinavia, France, Russia, and the United States produce mostly tall oil rosin.

Hausen reviewed more than 60 articles reporting contact dermatitis to colophony; epidemiologic studies demonstrate an increasing number of cases since 1980.[42] A more recent review from England is also available.[43] A person has many opportunities to become exposed to colophony and modified products and thus sensitized to them. One of the largest single uses is in the sizing of paper and paperboard. Rosin is added to paper to increase its water resistance. It serves as a protective coating for glossy paper, price labels, plastics, and stickers and prevents feathering and spreading of ink. Small quantities of rosin acids can be transferred from paper to articles packed in it, for example, food substances. Examples of other uses include the manufacture of soaps, varnishes, sealing wax, printing inks, driers (for paints), adhesives, binders, soldering fluxes, gloss oils for paints, pitch for lager beer casks, and rosining bows of violins and other string instruments. Rosin is used on the shoes of dancers and on floors of studios and stages to prevent slipping. In sports, powdered rosin is applied to the hands to improve grip on tennis rackets, bowling balls, baseballs, etc. A detailed list of potential sources of rosin exposure is provided in Table 30.4.

In the most recent data from the North American Contact Dermatitis Group (NACDG), rosin (20% pet) gave positive patch tests in 2.8% of patients (M Pratt, personal communication, Ottawa, Ontario, 2007). In Zurich in 1994, 3.6% of 1,062 patients were positive.[44]

Rosin consists of about 90% resin acids and 10% neutral matter; of the resin acids, about 90% are isomeric with abietic acid. Gas chromatographic analysis of resin acids in colophony from different sources included varying amounts and distributions of dehydroabietic, neoabietic, pimaric, isopimaric, sandaracopimaric, palustric, tetrahydroabietic, and dehydroabietic acids.[7,45] Rosin is used in a crude form, which is a soft, sticky, amber-colored material, or in chemically modified forms: hydrogenated, disproportionated, esterified, polymerized, as a salt, or reacted with maleic anhydride or formaldehyde.[21]

Esterification of rosin reduces its allergenicity, as does hydrogenation.[46] Cronin[47] reported patch test results of patients with colophony allergy at St. John's Hospital (London, England). Twenty-nine patients who were negative to a maleic ester of colophony reacted to colophony (each 20%

Table 30.4 Source of Exposure to Rosin and Rosin Derivatives

Rosin is not necessarily present in any given product noted below, but MAY be present in these types of products

Adhesives

Adhesive tapes, surgical incision drapes, bandages

Rubber cements
Shoe cements
Glues, mastics, and sealants

Building, Construction, and Industrial Products

Asphaltic products, emulsions, and foundry supplies

Caulking compounds

Cements for linoleum and tile
Concrete additive
Fillers (putty and wood dough)
Grease and lubricant thickener
Inks- printing and marking

Insulations- electrical and thermal insulating tapes
Jointing tapes
Oils: tall oil, cutting oil, core oil

Resins- adulterant or modifier of some alkyd, synthetic, ester, and phenolicresins
Rubber- tire-compounding aid, reclaiming agent, and emulsifier for synthetic rubber
Sawdust and resin of pine and spruce
Sealants, wood swellers

Soldering fluxes, soldering agents
Solvents
Waterproofing agents for cardboard, walls, oil cloth
Waxes- sealing, shoemakers, tree, grafting, car, floor, and furniture

Human Use Products (Medical, dental, food, cosmetic, etc.)
Chewing gum

Cosmetic products- brilliantine, wax depilatories, eyeshadow, mascara, rouge, hair pomade, nail polish, hair spray

Dentistry- dressings (dental and periodontal); dental cements (zinc-eugenol cement); cavity varnishes; impression pastes; sealing pulp canals

Flexible colloidion BP (not USP)- topical medications
Medicaments (human and veterinary)- disinfectants, component of plasters and ointments for its stiffening and adhesive qualities; wart removers
Ostomy appliances
Shoes (adhesive)

Paper Products
Banknotes
Cardboard
Coating and waterproofing agent, especially "slick or glossy" papers labels, stickers, etc.
Newspaper
Photographic papers
Sizing for many papers- reduces spreading of ink, improves wear

Surface Coatings
Brewery pitch
Polishes- floor, furniture, metal, shoe, car, etc
Rust-resistant paints and surface coatings
Varnishes- maleic resin adducts used extensively in oil and spirit varnishes and lacquers

Miscellaneous Uses
Athletic grip aids- wrestlers, gymnasts, ball players, bowlers (rosin bag); handles for sports equipment—golf and tennis racquets
Clay- modeling clay
Cleaners and lubricants for leather and office machines, grease remover for clothes
Dancers' shoes- floor of studios and stages
Fireworks
Inks- ceramic, marking, mimeographic, printing, some pens
Insecticides
Match tips
Non-fretted stringed instrument bows (violinist's rosin)
Postage stamp glue

Sticky fly papers

in pet); 4 patients reacted to both, and 2 gave equivocal reactions to the ester and were negative to colophony.

Karlberg[48,49] has extensively studied rosin and has succeeded in identifying at least two allergenic chemicals present in both tall oil and gum rosin. She states that purified abietic acid is nonallergenic. However, abietic acid is easily oxidized by air unless special handling precautions are taken. A major oxidation product of abietic acid, 15-hydroperoxyabietic acid, is a strong allergen.[50] Oxidation products of dehydroabietic acid are also allergenic.[51] It is possible that previous reports of allergy to abietic acid were actually identifying allergy to the oxidation products present in patch test material. Wahlberg,[52] for example, found that 9 of 15 patients who reacted to colophony also reacted to abietic acid (5% pet). Karlberg's data suggest that the allergens in tall oil and gum rosin are very similar, so that it is unlikely to matter which type is used for patch testing and to which type a patient is exposed.

Commercially modified rosins are more allergenic than natural rosins. Maleopimaric acid in modified rosin has been shown to be a strong sensitizer.[53] It may be necessary to patch test with various modified rosin products because crossreactivity with natural rosin may not always occur.[54]

Hausen and colleagues,[42] in guinea pig testing, further documented the allergenicity of several rosin oxidation products.

Clinical Presentations of Rosin Allergy

It may be difficult to find the product responsible in an individual patient with a positive routine patch test reaction to rosin. Accordingly, Table 30.4 may be useful in educating the patient about potential exposure sources.

Farm[55] has extensively reviewed clinical aspects of rosin allergy. She studied 180 workers in a tall oil rosin factory and 132 members of an opera company who had extensive exposure to rosin. Only 7 (3.9%) and 3 (2.3%), respectively, reacted to rosin on patch testing. In another portion of her report, 10 of 13 patch test positive patients had a positive repeated open application test (ROAT) to 20% rosin applied for several days.

Evaporated colophony from soldering tin threads may cause facial dermatitis.[56] Eight of 149 workers (5.4%) in the electronics industry in Singapore reacted to rosin in solder.[57] However, soldering flux can also cause ICD that can be mistaken for rosin allergy if patch-tests are not performed.[58] Rosin has been documented as a cause of perioral dermatitis from chewing gum and hand eczema from newspaper.[59,60]

Kanerva and colleagues[61] reported a female secretary with hand dermatitis that repeatedly worsened at work and cleared when away from the office. Allergy to rosin

was documented. The rosin content of the fax paper was 1%. The patient also reacted to balsam of Peru.

Although crossreactions between rosin and balsam of Peru are said to occur, Mitchell believes the evidence is scanty (J Mitchell, personal communication, December 1983). Malten lists other crossreactions for rosin as oil of turpentine, wood tar, pine resin, and spruce resin. Crossreaction with tea-tree oil (*Melaleuca*) has been reported.[62] In a review of NACDG data, 35 of 144 patients (24%) allergic to rosin also reacted to *Myroxylon Pereirae*, but only 6 (4%) reacted to tea-tree oil (personal communication, M Pratt, Ottawa, Ontario, January 2007).

Three patients reacted to rosin in the adhesive of a hydrocolloid dressing (DuoDerm or DuoDerm-E, Bristol-Myers-Squibb Co., Princeton, NJ).[63] A girl reacted to rosin in a sanitary pad and also to the patch-test marking ink that contained rosin.[64] Rosin allergy was over-represented in a population of elderly patients with lower leg dermatitis, possibly from exposure to dressings and Unna boots.[65] The adhesive of a transdermal medication caused ACD; patch test to rosin was negative, but to glyceryl hydrogenated rosinate was strongly positive.[66] Modified rosin (hydrogenated or glyceryl rosinate) accounted for ACD in most of 33 patients using a depilatory wax in Belgium and France.[67] Only 4 reacted to standard rosin.

Rosin has been reported to cause allergy in lipsticks,[68,69] lottery tickets,[70] sawdust,[71,72] floor polish,[73] cardboard dust,[73] depilatory wax,[74] paper money,[75] Portuguese shoes,[76] and bindi.[77] It may occur in musicians.[78] Rosin may be present in the ink of "permanent" markers, causing ACD with skin contact.[79]

Photocontact allergy to rosin has been noted.[80]

One of the main sources of rosin exposure is paper. Karlberg and colleagues[81] found that "environmentally friendly" paper made from mechanical pulp contains more rosin and is more allergenic than paper made from other pulps. A decrease in the manufacturing of paper from chemically treated pulps may be better for the ecology but may be worse for contact dermatitis sufferers.

Modified rosins are often used as paper sizing and in printing inks. Nilsson and colleagues[82] showed that rosin modified with malic anhydride or fumaric acid produces maleopimaric acid, a potentially important allergen.

Asthma may be caused by airborne occupational exposure to colophony.[2] Colophony-specific IgE has been demonstrated in soldering workers with occupational asthma.[83]

Zinc oxide apparently exerted an inhibitor, or "quenching," effect on allergic contact dermatitis reactions to rosin from adhesive tape in one study.[84] Farm,[55] however, found no such inhibition of rosin allergy by zinc oxide in seven subjects tested specifically for this.

Baltic Amber

Karlberg and colleagues[85] studied allergenicity of Baltic amber and determined that abietic acid and dehydroabietic acid are present in amber. Five of seven rosin-allergic patients reacted to amber (10% pet) on patch testing, but wearing an amber necklace produced no reaction.[85]

References

1. Teot AS. Resins, water soluble. In: Kirk-Othmer encyclopedia of chemical technology, 3rd ed. New York: Wiley Interscience, 1982;20:207.

2. Nilsson DC. Sources of allergenic gums. Ann Allergy 1960;18:518.

3. Roesch A, Haegele T, Vogt T, et al: Severe contact urticaria to guar gum included as a gelling agent in a local anesthetic. Contact dermatitis 2005;52:307.

4. Cottrell IW, Baird JK. Gums. In: Kirk-Othmer encyclopedia of chemical technology, 3rd ed. New York: Wiley Interscience, 1980;12:45.

5. <http://en.wikipedia.org/wiki/Gum_arabic> (accessed December 2006).

6. Martindale J. The extra pharmacopoeia. London: The Pharmaceutical Press, 1982:314.

7. Mitchell J, Rook A. Botanical dermatology. Vancouver: Greenglass, 1979:66, 84,145, 381, 385, 435, 521.

8. Rubinger D, Friedlander M, Superstine E. Hypersensitivity to tablet additives in transplant recipients on prednisone. Lancet 1978;2:689.

9. Cooke MA, Wilkinson JF. Formalin sensitivity in gum arabic. Contact Dermatitis Newsletter 1973;13:379.

10. Freeman S. Allergic contact dermatitis due to 1,2-benzisothiazolin-3-one in gum arabic. Contact Dermatitis 1984;11:146.

11. Lee TY, Lam TH. Allergic contact dermatitis due to a Chinese orthopaedic solution tieh ta yao gin. Contact Dermatitis 1993;28:890.

12. Wakelin S: Allergic contact dermatitis from mastic in compound mastic paint. Contact Dermatitis 2001; 45:118.

13. <www.willy-benecke.com/karaya> (accessed December 2006).

14. Camarasa JMG, Alomar A. Contact dermatitis from a karaya seal ring. Contact Dermatitis 1980;6:139.

15. Khalili B, Bardana E, Yunginger J: Psyllium-associated anaphylaxis and death: a case report and review. Ann Allergy Asthma Immunol. 2003;91:579.

16. Gauss WF, Alarie JP, Karol MH. Workplace allergenicity of a psyllium-containing bulk laxative. Allergy 1985;40:73.

17. Zaloga GP, Hierlwimmer UR, Engler RJ. Anaphylaxis following psyllium ingestion. J Allergy Clinical Immunol 1984;74:79.

18. Moreau L, Alomer G, Dube N, Sasseville D: Contact urticaria from carboxymethylcellulose in white chalk. Dermatitis 2006;17: 29.

19. Bigliardi P, Izakovic J, Weber J, et al: Anaphylaxis to the carbohydrate carboxymethylcellulose in parenteral corticosteroid preparations. Dermatology 2003;207: 100.

20. Weaver JC. Resins, natural. In: Kirk-Othmer encyclopedia of chemical technology, 3rd ed. New York: Wiley Interscience, 1982;20:197.

21. Jost T, Sell Y, Foussereau J. Contact allergy to Manila resin. Contact Dermatitis 1989;21:228.

22. Kimura M, Miura S, Ozawa S, et al. Allergic contact stomatitis from paraformaldehyde and copal in a dental root canal filling. Contact Dermatitis 2003;49:164.

23. < www.cardolite.com> (accessed December 2006).

24. Marks JG, DeMelfi T, McCarthy M, et al. Dermatitis from cashew nuts. J Am Acad Dermatol 1984;10:627.

25. Hamilton T, Zug K: Systemic contact dermatitis to raw cashew nuts in a pesto sauce. Am J Contact Dermat 1988;9:51.

26. Kullavanijaya P, Ophaswongse S. A study of dermatitis in the lacquerware industry. Contact Dermatitis 1997;36:244.

27. Kawai K, Nakagawa M, Kawai K, Miyakoshi T, et al. Heat treatment of Japanese lacquerware renders it hypoallergenic. Contact Dermatitis 1992;27:244.

28. <http://en.wikipedia.org/wiki/shellac> (accessed December 2006).

29. Rademaker M, Kirby JD, White IR. Contact cheilitis to shellac, Lanpol 5 and colophony. Contact Dermatitis 1986;15:307.

30. Magerl A, Pirker C, Frosch P. Allergic contact dermatitis from shellac and 1,3 butylene glycol in an eyeliner. J Dtsch Dermatol Ges 2003;1:300.

31. Scheman AJ. Contact allergy to quaternium-22 and shellac in mascara. Contact Dermatitis 1998;38:342.

32. Le Coz C, Leclere J, Arnoult E, et al. Allergic contact dermatitis from shellac in mascara. Contact Dermatitis 2002; 46: 149.

33. Strauss R, Orton D: Allergic contact cheilitis in the United Kingdom. Am J Contact Dermat 2003;14:75.

34. Hjorth N. Balsam of Tolu, styrax and benzoin. Acta Derm Venereol (Stockh) 1961;41[Suppl 46]:61.

35. Hoffman TE, Adams RM. Contact dermatitis to benzoin in grease paint makeup. Contact Dermatitis 1978;4:379.

36. Coskey RJ. Contact dermatitis owing to tincture of benzoin. Arch Dermatol 1978;114:128.

37. Spott DA, Shelley WB. Exanthem due to contact allergen (benzoin) absorbed through skin. JAMA 1970;214:1181.

38. Scardamaglia L, Nixon R, Fewings J. Compound tincture of benzoin: a common contact allergen? Australas J Dermatol 2003;44:180.

39. Widstrom L. Contact allergy to colophony in soldering flux. Contact Dermatitis 1983;9:205.

40. Arlt HG Jr. Tall oil. In: Kirk-Othmer encyclopedia of chemical technology, 3rd ed. New York: Wiley Interscience, 1983;22:531.

41. Sadhra S, Foulds I, Gray C, et al. Colophony - uses, health effects, airborne measurement and analysis. Ann Occup Hyg 1994;38:385.

42. Hausen BM, Krohn K, Budianto E. Contact allergy due to colophony (VH). Contact Dermatitis 1990;23:352.

43. Downs A, Sansom J: Colophony allergy: a review Contact Dermatitis 1999;41:305.

44. Bangha E, Elsner P. Sensitization to allergens of the standard series at the Department of Dermatology in Zurich 1990–1994. Dermatology 1996;193:17.

45. Karlberg AT, Boman A, Wahlberg JE. Allergenic potential of abietic acid colophony and pine resin-HA. Contact Dermatitis 1980;6:481.

46. Karlberg AT, Boman A, Nilsson JLG. Hydrogenation reduces the allergenicity of colophony (rosin). Contact Dermatitis 1988;9:22.

47. Cronin E. Contact dermatitis. Edinburgh: Churchill Livingstone, 1980:3.

48. Karlberg AT. Air oxidation increases the allergenic potential of tall-oil rosin: colophony contact allergens also identified in tall-oil rosin. Am J Contact Dermat 1991;2:43.

49. Karlberg AT. Contact allergy to colophony: chemical identifications of allergens, sensitization experiments and clinical experiences. Acta Derm Venereol (Stockh) 1988;139[Suppl 1].

50. Karlberg AT, et al. Identification of 15-hydroperoxyabietic acid as a contact allergen in Portuguese colophony. J Pharm Pharmacol 1988;40:42.

51. Karlberg AT, et al. Contact allergy to dehydroabietic acid derivatives isolated from Portuguese colophony. Contact Dermatitis 1988;19:166.

52. Wahlberg J. Abietic acid and colophony. Contact Dermatitis 1978;4:55.

53. Karlberg AT, et al. Maleopimaric acid—a potent sensitizer in modified rosin. Contact Dermatitis 1990;22:193.

54. Hausen BM, Mohnert J. Contact allergy due to colophony (V). Patch test results with different types of colophony and modified-colophony products. Contact Dermatitis 1989;20:295.

55. Farm G. Contact allergy to Colophony. Acta Dermato-Venereologica 1997[Suppl 201].

56. Handbook of nonprescription drugs, 7th ed. Washington, DC: American Pharmaceutical Corp., 1982:73.

57. Hiok-Hee T, Madellynn Tsu-Li C, Chee-Leok G. Occupational skin disease in workers from the electronics industry in Singapore. Am J Contact Dermat 1997;8:210.

58. Yakota K, Minami T, Michitsuji H, et al: Occupational dermatitis from soldering flux. Ind Health 2004;42:383.

59. Satyawan I, Oranje AP, Van Joost TH. Perioral dermatitis in a child due to rosin in chewing gum. Contact Dermatitis 1990;22:182.

60. Lidén C, Larberg AT. Colophony in paper as a cause of hand eczema. Contact Dermatitis 1992;26:272.

61. Kanerva L, et al. Contact dermatitis from telefax paper. Contact Dermatitis 1992;27:12.

62. Selvaag E, Eriksen B, Thune P. Contact allergy due to tea tree oil and cross-sensitization to colophony. Contact Dermatitis 1994;31:124.

63. Sasseville D, Tennstedt D, Lachapelle JM. Allergic contact dermatitis from hydrocolloid dressings. Am J Contact Dermat 1997;8:236.

64. Rademaker M: Allergic contact dermatitis to a sanitary pad. Australas J Dermatol 2004;45:234.

65. Uter W, Geier J, Pfahlberg A, et al. The spectrum of contact allergy in elderly patients with and without lower leg dermatitis. Dermatology (Switz) 2002;204:266.

66. Foti C, Bonamonte D, Conserva A, et al: Allergic contact dermatitis to glyceryl-hydrogenated rosinate in a topical plaster. Contact Dermatitis 2006;55:120.

67. Goossens A, Armingaud P, Avenel-Audran M, et al: An epidemic of allergic contact dermatitis due to epilating products. Contact Dermatitis 2002;46:67.

68. Inoue A, Shoji A, Aso S. Allergic lipstick cheilitis due to ester gum and ricinoleic acid. Contact Dermatitis 1998;39:39.

69. Batta K, Bourke JF, Foulds IS. Allergic contact dermatitis from colophony in lipsticks. Contact Dermatitis 1997;36:171.

70. Pereira F, Manuel R, Gafvert E, et al. Relapse of colophony dermatitis from lottery tickets. Contact Dermatitis 1997;37:43.

71. Watsky KL. Airborne allergic contact dermatitis from pine dust. Am J Contact Dermat 1997;8:118.

72. Meding B, Ahman M, Karlberg AT. Skin symptoms and contact allergy in woodwork teachers. Contact Dermatitis 1996;34:185.

73. Karlberg AT, Gafvert E, Meding B, et al. Airborne contact dermatitis from unexpected exposure to rosin (colophony): rosin sources revealed with chemical analyses. Contact Dermatitis 1996;35:272.

74. de-Argila D, Ortiz-Frutos J, Iglesias L. Occupational allergic contact dermatitis from colophony in depilatory wax. Contact Dermatitis 1996;34:369.

75. Koch P. Occupational contact dermatitis from colophony and formaldehyde in banknote paper. Contact Dermatitis 1995;32:371.

76. Strauss R, Wilkinson S: Shoe dermatitis due to colophonium used as a leather finishing agent in Portuguese shoes. Contact Dermatitis 2002;47:59.

77. Koh D, Lee BL, Ong HY, et al. Colophony in bindi adhesive. Contact Dermatitis 1995;32:186.

78. Fisher A. Allergic contact dermatitis in a violinist. Cutis 1981;27:466.

79. Fesquet E, Guillot B, Raison-Peyron N. Allergic contact dermatitis to rosin after a single accidental permanent marker skin contact. Contact Dermatitis 2006;55:58.

80. Kuno Y, Kato M. Photosensitivity frsom colophony in a case of chronic actinic dermatitis. Acta Derm Venereol 2001;81:442.

81. Karlberg AT, Gafvert E, Liden C. Environmentally friendly paper may increase risk of hand eczema in rosin sensitive persons. J Am Acad Dermatol 1995;33:427.

82. Nilsson AM, Gafvert E, Nilsson L, et al. Different physical forms of maleopimaric acid give different allergic responses. Contact Dermatitis 2002;46:38.

83. Elms J, Fishwick D, Robinson E, et al. Specific IgE to colophony? Occup Med (Lond) 2005;55:234.

84. Sóderberg TA, et al. Inhibitory effect of zinc oxide on contact allergy due to colophony. Contact Dermatitis 1990;23:346.

85. Karlberg AT, Boman A, Liden C. Studies on the allergenicity of Baltic amber. Contact Dermatitis 1992;27:224.

CONTACT URTICARIA

EXECUTIVE SUMMARY

Urticaria and even (in very rare cases) anaphylaxis can occur upon contact of various substances with the skin. Some substances, such as cinnamic aldehyde and benzoic acid, produce non-immunologic contact urticaria by their direct effect on such skin components as blood vessels or mast cells. This reaction is very common and results in a tingling, stinging, or possibly itching sensation. No pre-sensitization is required. Immunologic contact urticaria (ICU), requiring an IgE mediated inflammatory response, is far less common. However, many substances can produce ICU. Proteins are most commonly implicated. Latex is the most common cause of ICU in the United States (see Chapter 29). Many foodstuffs have been noted to cause ICU. Since the cause is usually obvious, the patient rarely seeks dermatologic treatment. Cooked foods are less likely to cause a reaction than the raw material. Atopic individuals appear to be at higher risk of developing ICU than non-atopics. Components of many topical medicaments can cause ICU. Examples include antibiotics, preservatives, excipients and fragrances. Animal and insect components (dander, blood, saliva, etc) and even human seminal fluid can cause ICU. Testing for CU is done by applying the suspected material to the skin for 15 to 30 minutes, with immediate observation. Nonimmunologic contact urticaria (NICU) agents usually react on intact skin. Agent that cause ICU, however, react more readily on dermatitic skin or with a prick or scratch through the material. Some chemicals can cause both ICU and allergic contact dermatitis, so patch testing is usually indicated even in suspected cases of contact urticaria.

Contact urticaria (CU) is a wheal-and-flare reaction that appears where certain agents contact the skin and may be allergic (immunologic) (ICU) or nonallergic (nonimmunologic) contact urticaria (NICU). Some contactants affect normal, intact skin, whereas others require damaged (eczematized or fissured) skin to produce urticaria.[1–3] In the nonallergic variety, the reaction is produced without any previous sensitization and can be provoked in almost all exposed individuals. The allergic variety appears only in previously sensitized individuals. CU is probably much more common than might be expected. Most cases may never present to the dermatologist, since the cause is usually fairly obvious to the affected individual (Figure 31-1).

A third variety of contact urticaria is due to an uncertain mechanism, in which both allergic and nonallergic mechanisms can be found. For example, the stings and bites of arthropods that pierce the skin may initially produce NICU. Some individuals, however, become sensitized. Subsequent exposure to these arthropods produces an allergic urticaria. Some contactants are "ambidextrous," in the sense that they seem capable of being primarily urticariogenic in most individuals, but in certain sensitized patients they can also produce delayed eczematous reactions (contact dermatitis).

Nonimmunologic Contact Urticaria (NICU)

This nonimmunologic type of urticaria, occurring without previous sensitization in nearly all individuals exposed, is the most common and potentially least serious form of contact urticaria because severe systemic reactions are not evoked (Table 31.1). A direct influence on dermal vessel walls or a nonantibody-mediated release of vasoactive substances such as histamine, slow-reacting substance A, and bradykinin is the probable cause.[2] The fact that nonsteroidal anti-inflammatory drugs (NSAIDs), including aspirin, have an inhibitory effect on NICU suggests that prostaglandins may also play some role in the reaction.

Certain agents commonly used as preservatives, fragrances, or flavoring agents in foods, soft drinks, ice cream, chewing gum, soaps, shampoos, perfumes, mouthwashes,

Table 31-1 Agents That Can Produce Nonimmunologic Contact Urticaria

Acetic acid	Dimethylsulfoxide
Alcohol	Insect stings†
Myroxylon Pereirae	Methyl nicotinate
Benzoic acid	Moths†
Caterpillar hair†	Sodium benzoate
Cinnamic acid	Sorbic acid
Cinnamic aldehyde	Nicotinic acid ester

†Can also produce allergic contact urticaria.

or pharmaceutical products, such as creams or ointments, are primary urticants in many non-sensitized people. These agents include the widely used benzoic acid, sodium benzoate, sorbic acid, cinnamic acid, cinnamic aldehyde, Myroxylon *pereirae*, acetic acid, butyric acid, and ethyl-, butyl-, isopropyl-, or cetyl alcohol.

The strongest urticariogenic agents are benzoic acid, sorbic acid, cinnamic acid, and cinnamic aldehyde. Most individuals will react with a localized urticarial response less than 45 minutes after application of relatively high concentrations to intact skin, such as 5% in petrolatum. Lower concentrations considerably lessen the urticarial reactions, although many will still react with some degree of erythema.

Kligman[4] showed clearly that a given agent may cause NICU at one concentration and may produce only erythema or itching at lower concentrations. Ten volunteers developed NICU to benzoic acid 2%, sorbic acid 2%, and cinnamic aldehyde 0.5% after a 10-minute exposure to normal skin of the face. After a one to 5 dilution, all 10 reacted with only erythema without a wheal. Finally, with another fivefold dilution to 0.08% or 0.02%, respectively, several, but not all, reacted with pruritus only without objective skin findings. This may help to explain the frequent occurrence of facial irritation in some people from cosmetics and topical products with negative patch tests.

Lahti[2] found that most of the skin reactions in an open test to benzoic acid 5.0%, sorbic 2.5%, and cinnamic acid 5.0% in petrolatum appeared within 45 minutes and disappeared within 2 hours. Atopic persons were no more liable to get NICU from these substances than nonatopic individuals, and scratching or stripping the skin did not seem to alter the urticarial response.

The feeding of capsules with benzoic acid, sorbic acid, cinnamic acid, and sodium benzoate to patients resulted in objective symptoms in 15% and subjective symptoms in 33% of the 106 patients tested. Most of the reactions were nonspecific and comparable to placebo reactions.

No correlation was seen between the reactivity in the skin test and that in the peroral test.

Rosenhall and Zetterstron[5] challenged 100 asthma patients with benzoic acid and elicited asthma, rhinitis, or urticaria in 47 of them.

Psoralen + UVA treatment (PUVA) has been shown to suppress NICU to benzoic acid and methyl nicotinate.[6]

Shriner and Maibach[7] reported on regional and age-based variations in reactivity to benzoic acid. Elderly subjects reacted less vigorously than younger ones. Eight sites on the neck, face, and forearm were tested with benzoic acid 2.5% petrolatum with greater to lesser reactivity in that order.

TESTING FOR NICU

The most common test for nonimmunologic contact urticaria is the open test, in which a small amount of test substance is applied to the volar aspect of the intact skin of the forearm. The result is recorded after 30 to 45 minutes. The patient should be off all NSAIDs and antihistamines for at least 48 hours. Lahti and colleagues[8] have shown that the best vehicle for testing substances for NICU is an alcohol-water or alcohol- propylene glycol mixture.

BENZYL ALCOHOL

Emmons and Marks found CU on open patch testing with benzyl alcohol (5% pet) in15 of 19 normal subjects and 7 of 15 patients with dermatitis.[9]

DIMETHYLSULFOXIDE (DMSO)

Dimethylsulfoxide is also known as Sulfinylbis(methane) and methyl sulfoxide. DMSO is used therapeutically as a local analgesic, an anti-inflammatory agent, and a promoter for percutaneous penetration of certain chemicals. Although not approved in the United States for use in humans, it is often used on horses, especially for treatment of inflamed joints and tendons. DMSO may cause erythema or whealing on contact.

Stoughton and Fritsch[10] reported that DMSO 20% caused transient erythema at the site of application in most subjects. True CU is frequently caused by DMSO at higher concentrations.[11]

Industrial and veterinary grades of DMSO may not be safe for humans. Furthermore, according to Drug Therapy (1980;11:60), the US Food and Drug Administration has warned that, because it is such a powerful solvent, DMSO may act as a "carrier" for many internally poisonous substances that do not ordinarily get through the skin. Camphor and menthol, for example, which are present in many arthritis "rubs," are quite safe when applied topically but may cause unpleasant and dangerous effects when transported through the skin and into the bloodstream by the supersolvent DMSO.

Kellum[12] reviewed the literature on DMSO and reported that no allergic contact sensitization to DMSO was noted in a study of several hundred people. When patch tests were occluded with plastic tape, however, the primary irritant effects of DMSO were greatly enhanced. Epidermal vesiculation, histologic evidence of epidermal cell death, and a perivascular dermal infiltrate were observed. With repeated and continuous applications of DMSO to the skin (90% concentration, daily continuous application with occlusion), "hardening" (acquired tolerance to irritating compounds) was achieved by the skin of most individuals within approximately 1 month.

TRAFURIL

In Europe, the tetrahydrofurfuryl ester of nicotinic acid (Trafuril, Ciba-Geigy, Basel, Switzerland) has been used as a rubefacient in inflammatory joint diseases and in the management of mild disorders of the blood circulation of the hands and feet.[13] Trafuril probably exerts symptomatic relief due to a direct microcirculatory effect from the erythema or a wheal and flare that follows topical application in most individuals. The erythema lasts usually from 2 to 4 hours, and varies greatly in different individuals.

Vaillancourt[14] tested 72 apparently healthy subjects with Trafuril and found a local hyperemic reaction with or without edema on the application site within 5 to 10 minutes in 69 subjects. Patients suffering from atopic dermatitis, acute rheumatic fever, and rheumatoid arthritis had a blanching reaction instead of urticaria and erythema.

SORBIC ACID

Sorbic acid, like benzoic acid, is a widely used antimicrobial agent and is a natural preservative occurring, for example, in berries of the mountain ash (Sorbus).[15] It is active against molds and yeasts and to a lesser degree against bacteria. Below pH 6.5 (optimal pH 4.5) it is used as a preservative for many pharmaceutical products and foods at a concentration of up to 0.2%.

Fryklof[16] noticed that creams and ointments containing sorbic acid caused erythema and slight itching and sometimes slight edema on the face in about half of the 20 persons tested. Hjorth and Trolle-Lassen[17] confirmed the results of Fryklof and reported erythema reactions in 18 of 26 persons tested. Rietschel[18] saw a female patient who had contact urticaria from shampoo containing sorbic acid. Rietschel's patient had both skin and respiratory symptoms and was sensitive to both sorbic acid and synthetic oil of cassia. The contact urticaria could only be elicited on intact skin of the face by open testing. The source of the patient's contactants was both her shampoo and toothpaste.

BENZOIC ACID

Benzoic acid occurs in *Myroxylon pereirae* (MP) and balsam of Tolu, in many essential oils from flowers and spices, and in berries (cranberries and other berries).[19–21] It has antibacterial and antifungal properties and is commonly used as a preservative in acidic food products. Whitfield's ointment, containing benzoic acid 6% as an antifungal agent and salicylic acid 3%, can be used in the treatment of fungal infections of the skin.[22]

Repeated applications of benzoic acid in petrolatum to the same skin site diminished the whealing gradually and finally abolished it in most cases. After the disappearance of reactivity to benzoic acid, the skin was fully capable of reacting to histamine (in a scratch test). This indicates that the decreasing reactivity to benzoic acid in repeated applications was due to the emptying of the storage of mediator(s) in the skin rather than to fatigue of the dermal vessels and thus caused a failure to react. NICU from benzoic acid is probably mediated by vasoactive substances other than histamine, because the reaction was not inhibited by oral antihistamine (hydroxyzine) before the test or by emptying the histamine storage in the skin with compound 48/80.[23]

According to Lahti,[23] scratching the skin did not strengthen the reactions to benzoic acid. The absorption of benzoic acid from intact skin of the back is apparently sufficient for maximal contact urticarial reactivity, and therefore the damage done to the barrier of the corneal layer did not have any enhancing influence.

Severe systemic immediate allergic reactions have been reported after occupational handling of materials containing benzoic acid, showing that some of the compounds, which are capable of evoking nonallergic urticaria, may exceptionally also be true sensitizers under proper conditions.[19]

NICU in the perioral area from sodium benzoate has been reported.[24]

CINNAMIC ACID

Cinnamic acid has been found among the constituents of the essential oils of basil, Chinese cinnamon, Styrax, oil of cinnamon, coca leaves, and MP.[25] It is used as a flavoring and fragrance ingredient in pharmaceutical preparations, food products, and perfumery.[26] Cinnamic acid has antibacterial and antifungal properties similar to those of benzoic acid. Contact urticaria from cinnamic acid 5% in petrolatum occurs in most normal individuals.

Cinnamic acid may be present in sunscreens that contain cinnamates. The stinging, burning sensation that occurs from the application of such sunscreens may be due to the primary urticariogenic properties of the esters of the cinnamic acid, such as menthyl and benzyl cinnamates. In addition, the coniferyl alcohol esters of cinnamic acid may be present in benzoin.

CINNAMIC ALDEHYDE

Cinnamic aldehyde is a constituent of cinnamon and is one of the substances responsible for the typical odor and flavor of this spice. Its oxidation occurs readily on exposure to air, yielding cinnamic acid. Cinnamic aldehyde is used as a flavoring agent in soft drinks, chewing gum, ice cream, baked goods, dentifrices, mouthwashes, and as a fragrance component in many products.

Nater and colleagues[27] found CU in three patients and erythema alone in three other patients from cinnamic aldehyde 10% in alcohol. Rudzki and Grzywa[28] noted immediate reactions to both MP and cinnamic aldehyde in two patients. Cinnamic aldehyde is also a potent sensitizer, and delayed-type allergic contact dermatitis (ACD) caused by this substance has been described by many authors.[29–31]

Cinnamic aldehyde at concentrations as low as 0.01% may evoke an erythematous response associated with a burning, tingling feeling of the skin.[32] Such weak, transient reactions from cinnamic aldehyde–containing products are hardly clinically significant and probably go unrecognized by the consumer in most instances; however, mild adverse effects may be an intended positive selling point, adding a "lively sensation" produced in the mouth for some oral hygiene products or chewing gums.

On patch testing, cinnamic aldehyde often causes an immediate stinging reaction with or without a visible wheal and flare. Patients may mistakenly believe this is an allergic reaction. The symptoms usually dissipate within a few hours of application of the patch.

MYROXYLON PEREIRAE (MP)

This balsam, which contains many aromatic substances, can produce both NICU and ACD.[20,33,34]

Forsbeck and Skog[35] state that closed patch tests with MP gave rise to nine immediate reactions among 121 patients with different dermatoses and to 10 reactions among 57 patients with chronic urticaria. Among components of MP, cinnamic aldehyde, cinnamic acid, benzoic acid, and benzaldehyde also gave the same reactions. The reactions, which could not be transferred passively with serum from patients, were abolished by antihistamine given before testing and by pretreatment with

compound 48/80. MP and cinnamic aldehyde did not provoke new symptoms when given orally to patients.

QUENCHING EFFECT OF EUGENOL

Eugenol, when applied before cinnamic aldehyde, sorbic acid, or benzoic acid to intact skin, was capable of diminishing or "quenching" the subject's NICU response to these agents.[36] The mechanism is unknown, but apparently is unrelated to histamine release. The same phenomenon does not occur with delayed hypersensitivity. The clinical ramifications of this phenomenon deserve exploration.

"STINGERS" AND NONIMMUNOLOGIC CONTACT URTICARIA

The cosmetic industry is concerned with the sensory irritation interpreted as "stinging" by some individuals. Those with sensitive skin "stingers" may be unable to tolerate most topicals and cosmetics, wrongly believing that they are allergic to the products.[37]

The application of 10% lactic acid to the nasolabial fold is one way to separate stingers from non-stingers. Coverly and colleagues[38] reported that the frequency of NICU to various agents such as DMSO and benzoic acid was no different in stingers and nonstingers, nor in males and females.

Allergic (Immunologic) Contact Urticaria

The usual criteria for regarding a reaction as allergic are (a) a history of previous exposure, (b) the degree of specific sensitization, which tends to increase with further exposure, and as a rule, (c) a low proportion of exposed subjects that are affected. An increasing number of chemicals are being reported as being responsible for immunologic CU.

The most common immediate immunologic mechanism is probably the one mediated by IgE. Nonspecific elevation of IgE has been reported frequently in association with immunologic CU, and IgE specific for the offending antigen has been found in some cases. Although the prevalence of NICU is the same in atopic and nonatopic individuals, it is likely that immunologic contact urticaria is more common among atopic patients.[1] Urticaria, however, may also be caused by allergic mechanisms not requiring IgE; specific IgG and perhaps also IgM might be responsible by activation of the complement flow through the classical pathway.[2]

PASSIVE TRANSFER

This procedure in some instances may prove that a contact urticarial reaction is immunologic. Passive transfer is accomplished by injecting 0.1 mL of freshly obtained serum from the patient into the forearm of a human volunteer or into a test animal, such as a monkey. After 24 hours, 0.1 ml of the eliciting agent is applied topically to the injection site and to a contralateral saline control site. A positive result, indicated by a wheal-and-flare response only at the donor serum injection site, is considered proof of a reaction being mediated by humoral immunologic mechanisms.

At present, the "proof" of allergic CU is done mostly by patch testing, with a reading within 15 to 30 minutes, with the suspected contactant. Perhaps in the future in vitro testing will help identify specific agents in food and other contactants that are common causes of allergic CU.

Allergic Contact Urticaria to Latex Rubber

Immediate IgE-mediated contact hypersensitivity to natural latex, derived from the *Hevea brasiliensis* tree, has over the last two decades become one of the most important "new" dermatologic afflictions, particularly among health care workers and certain predisposed patients. Respiratory symptoms are not uncommon. Rarely, contact urticaria to additives in rubber has also been reported (see Chapter 29 for a full discussion).

Allergic Contact Urticaria Due to Foods and Plants

A number of foods have been shown to cause ICU. Often, cases present as an occupational hand eczema, so careful questioning may be necessary to uncover the possibility of food ICU.

It should be stressed that in these cases of "immediate" food ICU the classic delayed 48-hour patch tests are negative, and therefore scratch or immediate patch tests with the raw foods may be necessary to prove the cause of this "immediate" contact food dermatitis.

At least three control subjects should also be tested when performing scratch tests with "whole" foods. A positive reaction in the patient that is not duplicated in three controls makes it likely that the reaction is allergic in nature. Usually patients with ICU due to food handling can eat such foods without a problem, if the food I thoroughly cooked. It is most likely that either cooking of the foods or the action of digestive juices denatures the protein components and renders the food "hypoallergenic" for these patients. At present, however, it is not clear whether the food antigens that allergists use in testing for allergic rhinitis, asthma, and gastrointestinal allergy are also the antigens that are responsible for the ICU of hands from handling those foods.

MILK AND DAIRY PRODUCTS

Edwards[39] described ICU that developed in a child as a reaction to cow's milk. After heating the milk to 80°C for 30 seconds, the child did not have a similar reaction. This 8-month-old girl presented with urticaria on the neck, perioral, and chest areas that had developed immediately after her diet was changed from an infant formula without iron to commercial, pasteurized cow's milk. A few minutes after first drinking warm cow's milk, the baby developed a red eruption on the face that disappeared after 30 minutes. There were no systemic manifestations of allergy.

Lecks[40] reported that a child developed a severe urticarial reaction of the diaper area with an anaphylactoid reaction from the use of Diaparene Neonatal Ointment, which contained a milk protein (casein).

Parmesan cheese caused CU in an Australian sandwich maker.[41]

A veterinarian developed CU to canine milk, but not to cow's milk.[42]

EGG

Rudzki and Gryzwa[43] described a patient with contact urticaria from egg. Temesvari and Varkonyi[44] had two patients who acquired contact dermatitis from egg. One patient was a beautician who used eggs in shampoo: She was allergic to both the white and yolk of raw eggs. The ingestion of the yolk of the egg produced generalized urticaria. The second patient, who was also a hairdresser, was allergic to the white of a raw egg on epicutaneous testing.

Ushijima and colleagues[45] reported that a 1-year-old boy had previously experienced transient red swelling of the lips after ingestion of raw egg white. He became hoarse and vomited immediately after he took some powder from medicines containing Leftose for the treatment of a common cold. About 20 minutes later, an urticarial rash developed on the peroral and mandibular regions where the vomited materials had accumulated. The rash disappeared spontaneously within 20 minutes. (Leftose is a commercial name of lysozyme chloride, which is used as a medicine in Japan for the common cold, because of its mucolytic activity. Leftose is extracted from egg white, which contains a large amount of lysozyme.) The serum IgE level was within normal limits.

The RAST score to egg white was 3. An open patch test with Leftose was positive, but the test with commercially obtained antigen of egg white was negative. The Prausnitz-Küstner reaction was performed and the patient's mother, and two healthy volunteers were used and was negative. Challenges with Leftose by topical and oral application were negative. Challenge with raw egg white by oral administration, however, induced a wheal-and-flare reaction.

POTATOES

Sensitivity to potatoes may be so severe that merely rubbing the intact skin with a raw potato may cause a wheal to form.[46,47] Scratch tests with cooked potatoes usually give negative results. Potato sensitivity can cause "housewife's hand eczema" and can be classified as an "occupational allergy" in cooks. These patients who have allergic contact sensitivity can usually eat cooked potatoes without any reaction. Pearson,[47] who reported potatoes to be a cause of ICU and asthma, demonstrated positive passive transfer and decreased respiratory function after potatoes were scraped by the patient and the fine liquid from the ruptured potato cells was inhaled.

An atopic individual with coexistent allergy to potato and latex has been reported. IgE to both was present. Both skin and respiratory symptoms occurred.[48]

SEAFOOD

Hjorth and Roed-Petersen[49] reported that some homemakers with atopic dermatitis remarked on an aggravation of their eczematic lesions after contact with fish, particularly white haddock and herring, that caused an itching erythema within 30 minutes after contact with the allergen. An open epicutaneous test with fish on the site of a preceding eczema produced a blister in the sensitized patient. On normal skin (on which there was no preceding eczema) an open epicutaneous test with fish (mostly haddock) resulted in an urticarial reaction. These patients noted that their eczema got worse in contact with fish and showed a high IgE serum level with fish (Figure 31-2).

Mitchell[50] reported that a woman with chronic hand eczema attributed the dermatitis to handling fresh shrimp. Scratch tests were carried out on the forearm flexure to the flesh (edible portion) of the shrimp (Pandalus). The raw and the boiled shrimp flesh was applied to the scratch site without covering; a drop of sea water (millipore filtered) was applied to a scratch test site as a control. Five physicians served as concomitant controls. Evidently some agent in uncooked shrimp flesh was capable of evoking localized ICU, but only when the epidermal barrier was broken by dermatitis or by an experimental scratch. The agent is heat-labile.

Lombardi and colleagues[51] cited the case of a 12-year-old boy with atopic dermatitis who acquired ICU from cod. The patch test with pieces of raw cod and an intradermal test with antigenic extract of cod both provoked an immediate specific wheal reaction. Immersion of the boy's hands and forearms in a basin of water in which a cod had been washed was followed by the appearance of urticaria, first on the contact areas and almost immediately thereafter on the face. Results of the RAST were negative, as were those of a placebo-controlled, blinded oral challenge.

Beck and Nissen[52] stated that atopic individuals have a higher frequency of contact urticaria to fish than do nonatopic individuals.

Fowler has seen ICU from handling a live crab. On an educational boating trip, a 43-year-old non-atopic woman was shown by a guide how to hold the crab. Within 3 minutes, urticarial wheals developed in a linear pattern where the seawater from the crab had flowed down her arm. She has not eaten crab since.

Squid (*Loligo japonica*) may also cause contact urticaria.[53]

Dominguez and colleagues,[54] in Spain, evaluated 29 children who all had IgE-mediated fish sensitivity. Although the children were avoiding fish in the diet, incidental contact with fish produced urticaria in all and respiratory symptoms in one.

Maibach[55] reported a female atopic food-service worker who had facial irritation that she thought was related to handling seafood. Testing on the arm and hand gave no reaction, but a wheal and flare developed when shrimp was applied to the forehead. This demonstrates the need to use extraordinary testing methods at times.

MEAT

The following meats have been reported as causing ICU, particularly in individuals with chronic hand dermatitis: chicken, lamb, turkey, calves' liver, beef, venison, and sausage.[55–61]

Fisher and Stengel[57] reported a 50-year-old butcher who had chronic dermatitis of the hands for 6 years. History revealed that the dermatitis became worse when he handled raw calves' liver. When the calves' liver was placed at the site of a scratch on the forearm, a large wheal and flare was produced in 15 minutes. Six control subjects showed no such reaction. Chicken liver did not produce a reaction.

Fisher[58] reported a 60-year-old woman who stated that her chronic hand dermatitis was made worse by wearing rubber gloves. Routine patch testing revealed positive patch tests to nickel and mercaptobenzothiazole. The patient stated emphatically that whenever she prepared beef hamburgers the hand dermatitis flared severely. In addition, when she ate a medium rare beef hamburger her lips swelled and she developed fissuring of the angles of the mouth resembling perlèche. She did not have any symptoms, however, when she ate a well-done hamburger. The patient was patch tested on normal skin, and she had no reaction to beef, pork, or chicken. Scratch tests were then performed on normal skin of the back. Each meat was gently rubbed in with a Q-Tip. Within 15 minutes an urticarial wheal without any flare appeared only at the site at which the beef had been applied. The patient did not react to cooked beef.

Moseng[59] reported that a male butcher's assistant, who was feeding a machine daily with pig's gut (Taiwanese import) as part of sausage production, developed urticarial, crusted, erosive lesions mainly on the extremities. Eating hot dogs produced urticaria in the patient. A New Zealand meat inspector had positive scratch tests and ICU to venison parts.[60]

Usually individuals with CU to meat react to only one animal product. One case, however, has been reported where allergy (CU) to beef, lamb, horse, and pork meat coexisted. All were positive on scratch testing, but cooked meats could be eaten with no ill effect.[62]

FRUIT

Lombardi and colleagues[51] reported that a 14-year-old boy had an immediate positive reaction to both the patch (with evolution to delayed eczematous reaction) and intradermal tests with peach skin; the same results with the pulp of the fruit provoked no reaction. The RAST results were negative, and the patient tolerated repeated ingestion of peeled peach and capsules containing pulp and peel (20 g), whereas handling the fruit provoked ICU on the hands and glottal edema.

Andersen and Lowenstein[63] reported the possibility of ICU from handling apples. They stated that most of the patients with reactions to raw potatoes and apples are atopics. The authors found that cross-reactivity between various vegetables and fruits may occur.

One case of CU to strawberry was seen in a fruit picker.[64] RAST testing was negative. Kiwi fruit was implicated as causing CU in an Italian woman.[65] Rather than hand eczema, her complaints were cheilitis and stomatitis. CU to litchi fruit has been reported.[66]

Latex-allergic patients occasionally experience cross-reactions from handling or eating certain fruits including banana, peach, and kiwi.[67]

GREEN VEGETABLES

Krook[68] reported four patients, with occupational contact dermatitis to lettuce (*Lactuca sativa*), who had cross-sensitivity to endive (*Cichorium endivia*). One of the patients also had ICU to lettuce and endive, and another reacted positively to scratch tests with these vegetables. In two cases such immediate allergy was considered the cause of a vesicular, intense itching eruption within a few minutes of contact with fresh leaves of Lactuca on previously eczematous skin. The severe chronic dermatitis of the hands of these patients is ascribed to combined delayed and immediate allergy. Another salad green, *Eruca sativa*, has also been reported to cause CU.[69] Artichoke[70] and asparagus have been reported to cause CU,[71]

In what is undoubtedly the largest single series of ICU to a green vegetable, Tabar and colleagues[71] reported 27 patients allergic to asparagus. Ten had ICU, and 5 of those had respiratory symptoms. ACD also occurred. Many of the cases were occupational.

CARROTS

Munoz and colleagues[72] reported a case of urticaria and upper respiratory tract symptoms caused by contact with carrots. Scratch tests were positive.

BEANS

The winged bean (*Psophocarpus tetragonolobus*) produced facial edema in a food chemist who worked extracting the bean oil.[73] In addition to a strong reaction to this bean, he reacted weakly to soybean, which is related. No other positive patch or scratch tests were found, and the patient cleared after avoiding both beans. CU, dermatitis, and rhinitis were caused in one patient by dust from castor beans.[74]

RICE

A young woman developed widespread urticaria and dyspnea after a wedding ceremony at which she had thrown rice.[75] She had no problem eating cooked rice. Prick tests were positive to rice, with weak reactions to corn, peanut, and beans. Apparently, these other foods did not provoke symptoms.

CORN

A patient had ICU to corn, proved by a strongly positive prick test. Protein contact dermatitis to corn was also present.[76] IgE was found to bind to a salt-soluble corn protein fraction.

BEER

Van Ketel[77] reported ICU from beer, but not from other alcoholic beverages. A 30-year-old woman, after entering a bar, noted that her face became red, swollen, and itchy after staying for 1 or 2 minutes. She showed the same symptoms in a room where visitors were drinking beer.

After her husband had drunk a glass of beer, kissing him on the mouth provoked redness and itching of the lips and surrounding skin within a few minutes. When her husband drank any other alcoholic drink she tolerated kissing without any trouble. The patient herself tolerated drinking other alcoholic beverages very well. She refused to drink any kind of beer because on one occasion she developed shock after drinking a mouthful of beer. A scratch test with beer was performed on the forearm. The reaction was positive in a few minutes and was strong after 20 minutes. The edema around the test site spread to the upper arm, which became swollen within 30 minutes after the test. These symptoms disappeared after 2 hours.

WHEAT

Nine women with CU to cosmetics containing hydrolyzed wheat protein (HWP) were studied.[78] Six also reacted to ingested wheat products. All had positive immediate skin tests to HWP and to cosmetics containing HWP. Three of 7 had elevated IgE levels to wheat and gluten.

PLANTS AND SEEDS

Heygi and Dolezalova[79] described a female patient who was so allergic to caraway seeds that patch tests with this spice and the use of toothpastes and a soap containing caraway seed oil produced urticaria and syncope. Sunflower seeds, poppy flowers, mulberry pollen, lupin (pea), and gerbera have been reported to cause CU.[80–84]

In a study of Danish gardeners, 35 of 105 (33%) tested had an immediate reaction to one or more plants. Most were atopic. Symptoms tended to be rather minor and short-lived.[85]

A forensics worker developed CU to marijuana (Cannabis sativa).[86] One wonders how much of this goes unreported?

OTHER FOOD-RELATED ALLERGENS

Cellulase enzyme used in the production of starch and amylase can cause occupational CU.[87,88]

Occupational CU has been reported from paprika.[89]

Sesame seed oil has been reported to cause CU in two nonatopic subjects. In both cases, both CU from cosmetic products and generalized urticaria from foods with sesame seed or oil occurred.[90]

An atopic woman had symptoms of CU from handling dill plants, with positive prick tests to dill, anise, carrot, and cumin.[91]

Curcumin, a component of the spice turmeric (Curcuma longa) was reported to cause CU in two patients, with generalized pruritus in one and both skin and

respiratory reactions in the other. From the report, it is uncertain if the mechanism was immunologic or NICU or both.[92] A pizzamaker had a weak positive prick test to olives and a relevant history of lip swelling when eating olives.[93]

Immunologic Contact Urticaria from Topical Medications

ICU may occur from the active ingredient in topical medications or from preservatives, solvents, and emulsifying agents in the topical medication.

ANTIBIOTICS

Most of the antibiotics shown in Table 31.2 that have produced ICU have also produced anaphylactic reactions when tested in various ways.

Penicillin

Penicillin is no longer used topically in the United States because it is such a common and potent sensitizer. Maucher[94] and Haustein[95] produced urticaria followed by systemic allergic reactions in three patients with severe hypersensitivity to systemic penicillin by patch testing with penicillin. Boonk[96] has shown that "hidden contacts" with penicillin may produce contact urticaria.

Sulbactam gave a positive scratch test in a nurse, who also had positive patch test to ampicillin and amoxicillin (but negative to sulbactam).[97]

Neomycin

This antibiotic, which is a common cause of delayed eczematous contact dermatitis, can also cause ICU and even anaphylactic shock when used topically, and even by a patch test procedure.[94,98] Pippen reported a patient with delayed hypersensitivity to neomycin in whom anaphylaxis developed after this chemical was applied inadvertently to a stasis ulcer.[99]

Bacitracin

Roupe and Strannegard[100] cited a case of anaphylactic shock after topical administration of an ointment

Table 31-2 Antibiotics Capable of Producing Immunologic Contact Urticaria and/or Anaphylaxis	
Bacitracin	Neomycin
Cephalosporins	Penicillin
Chloramphenicol	Rifamycin
Gentamycin	Streptomycin
Sulbactam	

containing bacitracin and neomycin. Antibacitracin reagins were demonstrated in sera from this patient with atopic dermatitis, and there is strong evidence that the anaphylactic reaction was due to hypersensitivity to bacitracin.

Comaish and Cunliffe[101] reported that bacitracin applied to a varicose ulcer may also produce an anaphylactic reaction; circulating antibacitracin reagins could be demonstrated, and intracutaneous testing may produce anaphylaxis.

Bjorkner and Moller,[102] however, studied three patients allergic to bacitracin, all of whom also had positive tests to neomycin. After intracutaneous injection of bacitracin, the three patients showed a delayed eczematous reaction. A strong immediate wheal-and-flare reaction was also induced. This was inhibited by a simultaneous local injection of the antihistamine mepyramine, which also abolished the vascular response to histamine and to the histamine liberator polymyxin B. Depletion of cutaneous histamine by pretreatment with polymyxin B diminished the wheal and flare induced by bacitracin. The authors concluded that the vascular effects of intracutaneous bacitracin in human skin are due to a release of histamine. The immediate wheal and flare was the same in healthy controls as in the three patients with delayed hypersensitivity to bacitracin. Thus, the intracutaneous test with bacitracin did not disclose any signs of circulating reagins.

Haustein's case[95] of anaphylactic shock elicited by topical administration of bacitracin would implicate circulating reagins against bacitracin.

Anaphylaxis in the operating room from bacitracin irrigation has been reported in relation to several different surgical procedures.[102]

Streptomycin

Levene and Withers[103] demonstrated anaphylaxis to topical streptomycin. The patient had an anaphylactic reaction from intradermal testing. Rudzki and colleagues[104] described a nurse who worked in a tuberculosis sanatorium who developed a contact urticaria from streptomycin. Two minutes after several drops of streptomycin prepared for injection were placed on her forearm, a large wheal appeared; a few minutes later, rhinitis and lacrimation developed, which required hydrocortisone administration.

Chloramphenicol

Kosakava[105] cited a patient sensitized to chloramphenicol who had an anaphylactoid reaction from a closed patch test.

Cephalosporins

Tuft[106] studied an instance of ICU that resulted from an acquired sensitization to cephalosporin compounds in a chemist. Patch tests elicited an immediate urticarial response. Similar control tests with other antibiotics gave negative results. Although the patient's primary complaint was urticaria, prolonged or excessive contact with the cephalosporin also caused coryza and syncope.

A number of cases of occupational CU to cefotiam dihydrochloride have been observed in Japan.[107]

Rifamycin

Rifamycin is an antibiotic derived from *Streptomyces mediterranei*. It has twice been reported to cause CU after use on a cutaneous ulcer. In one instance anaphylaxis and shock occurred.[108] In this case, an open test produced urticaria and a Prausnitz-Küstner test was positive, indicating a serum factor, probably IgE, was causative.

Gentamicin

Maucher[94] reported that patch testing with this antibiotic can produce an urticarial reaction in sensitized individuals.

MISCELLANEOUS TOPICAL OR INJECTED MEDICATIONS

Aescin

Aescin, an extract of the horse chestnut (*Aesculus hippocastanum*), caused CU in a patient who was using a product containing this substance as a topical balm for knee pain. A prick test was positive but was negative in 10 controls.[109]

Aminopyrine (Pyramidon)

Camarasa and colleagues[110] described an unusual case of ICU. A boy had had a Cibalgine suppository inserted, which is composed of aminophenazone and allobarbital. The mother developed a strong, itching sensation on one hand immediately after touching her son upon his return from the operating room after a tonsillectomy. Within a few minutes, a pronounced edema of the face and eyelids commenced and became generalized to an alarming degree. She was admitted to an intensive care unit (ICU). Patch tests with a Cibalgine suppository resulted in a 3+ urticarial reaction (wheal) after 5 minutes, which evolved into an acute generalized urticaria after a further 5 minutes, requiring treatment with epinephrine. Patch testing with the aminopyrine gave an immediate strong urticarial reaction. Testing with allobarbital was negative. The lymphocyte transformation test was positive for aminopyrine. The mechanism of transfer from the son's skin to the patient's hand remains unknown in this case.

Benzocaine

This topical anesthetic, which is not an uncommon cause of ACD, can also on rare occasions produce ICU.

Ryan and colleagues[111] reported that a 39-year-old man developed edema and vesiculation of the oral mucosa after the application of benzocaine (Hurricaine) gel. Open testing demonstrated an immediate urticarial reaction. Closed patch tests were also positive.

Rudner[112] described a 77-year-old woman who developed swelling of lips 2 days after applying Anbesol (alcohol, benzocaine, phenol, and iodine) pomade. There was no prior dermatitis or prior "caine" exposure. Anbesol was applied to the patient's forearm after her original lip lesion had cleared up. Several hours later, there was localized redness and swelling at the site of application of the Anbesol. The possibility exists that the reaction was due to benzocaine.

Benzophenone

Ramsay and colleagues[113] found a man with a broad-spectrum light sensitivity who demonstrated simultaneously an urticarial and contact sensitivity to a preparation containing 5-benzoyl-4-hydroxy-2-methoxybenzene sulfonic acid (sulisobenzone). Both the benzophenone and the sulfonic acid parts of the molecule were required for elicitation of the contact dermatitis reaction, although benzophenone alone elicited only the urticarial reaction. Storrs and colleagues reported a patient with simultaneous ACD, photo ACD, and ICU from oxybenzone (BZP-3).[114]

Chloramine-T

CU and rhinitis have been reported from use of this agent, which is a topical disinfectant. A hospital bath attendant in Finland with hand dermatitis from using a cleaner containing this agent had greatly elevated IgE antibodies to the agent. Allergic asthma also can be caused by this agent.[115]

Chlorpromazine and Promethazine

Horio[116] described a 54-year-old woman who had a recurrent pruritic eruption in light-exposed areas. She had a combination of three types of hypersensitivity to chlorpromazine: ACD, photocontact dermatitis, and immediate allergic photosensitivity. Immediate wheal reactions were found after long-wave ultraviolet light irradiation of photopatch test and intradermal injection sites with chlorpromazine. These responses were differentiated from phototoxic reactions. A positive passive transfer reaction was also observed.

Haustein[95] stated that promethazine produced shock and urticaria after patch testing with promethazine.

Chlorhexidine

Numerous reports of ICU to chlorhexidine have been published.[117–120] One person had both ACD and ICU. The other developed respiratory symptoms as well as urticaria. Contact anaphylaxis has been reported from exposure to chlorhexidine during a skin graft procedure and from a wound care cleanser. In both cases, prick tests were positive.[118,119]

By far the most comprehensive report comes from Finland, where 33 patients with positive prick tests to chlorhexidine (either 0.5 % or 1% in aqua) were reviewed.[120] Ten had severe systemic symptoms, 11 had a local reaction only and the rest were asymptomatic. Six of 14 tested for specific IgE were positive.

Chlorocresol

This disinfectant, in an aviary incubator cleaning solution, caused CU in a 28-year-old worker.[121]

Cisplatin

A nurse developed CU thought to be due to this anti-cancer drug. Open tests were positive to two platinum salts.[122]

Diphenylcyclopropenone (DPC), Dinitrochlorobenzene (DNCB), and Squaric Acid Dibutyl Ester (SADBE)

DPC is used as a topical immunotherapeutic agent in the treatment of viral warts and alopecia areata. Tosti and colleagues[123] reported generalized urticaria in four patients using DPC for alopecia. Concentrations as low as 0.05% were enough to produce symptoms. A total of 127 patients were treated with DPC during this period. DNCB caused CU and dyspnea in one unrelated case also used for alopecia.[124] Fowler has observed occasional instances of CU in patients treated with squaric acid immunotherapy for warts.

Vitamin E Oil Used Topically

Many individuals pierce vitamin E capsules and rub the contents into their skin to "remove" wrinkles and to improve the "tone" of the skin. Such efforts are, of course, in vain, because there is no therapeutic effect from such inunctions. Several patients have developed ACD and also ICU from the application of vitamin E oil.[125]

Mitchell[126] described two boys who developed localized then partially generalized urticaria from application of a vitamin E preparation for thermal burns. The mother had pricked a capsule of vitamin E and applied the oil from the capsule twice daily for 3 days. One week after the last application, confluent papular erythema appeared around the burn site. This erythema became urticarial and disseminated widely on the trunk in a diffuse pattern, extending to a patchy pattern, but was maximal around the burn site. In addition, erythematous urticarial wheals appeared on the face. The eruption faded during 1 week with peeling of the skin. Patch tests to the vitamin E and the vehicle were not carried out.

Vitamin K Injection

A case of both ICU and ACD to IM vitamin K (phytomenadione) has been reported.[127]

Lidocaine

Lidocaine is a rare contact allergen and even more rare cause of CU. A case of ACD, CU, and anaphylaxis to topical lidocaine in a hemorrhoid treatment has been reported.[128]

Menthol

Papa and Shelley[129] described a case of menthol hypersensitivity that produced a chronic urticaria and a diagnostic basophil response.

Nitrogen Mustard

Grunnet[130] studied a 36-year-old woman and a 16-year-old boy, both suffering from mycosis fungoides, who developed urticaria and an anaphylactoid reaction after topical whole-body application of nitrogen mustard. Prick tests with nitrogen mustard solution produced a wheal-and-flare response. Both patients had previously been treated intermittently with total body applications of nitrogen mustard for 2 years and 1 year, respectively, without complications.

Daughters and colleagues[131] reported a 68-year-old woman with mycosis fungoides en plaque who had severe dyspnea, urticaria, pruritus, and swelling of her hands 5 minutes after topical total body application of nitrogen mustard. In the preceding 5 years, she had been treated at least 100 times with this chemical topically without having allergic manifestations. Six weeks after her reaction, open epicutaneous application of nitrogen mustard produced a wheal-and-flare response at the test site, followed by signs of anaphylaxis.

Povidone (polyvinylpyrrolidone-PVP)

Immunologic contact urticaria was seen after application of hair-care products and later severe anaphylaxis occurred in a woman following a gynecologic procedure. Prick tests were positive to both povidone and polyvinylpyrrolidone, but negative to iodine. The povidone had been used as a disinfectant before the gynecologic procedure and PVP was present in both a shampoo and permanent-wave solution.[132]

Table 31-3 Contact Urticaria—Vehicle Ingredients of Topical Medicaments

Benzyl alcohol	Petrolatum (extremely rare)
Cetostearyl alcohol (Emulgade F)	Phenoxyethanol
Polyethylene glycol	
Guar Gum	
Monoamylamine	Polysorbate 60
Organic mercurials	Sorbitan sesquioleate
Parabens	

CONTACT URTICARIA DUE TO VEHICLE INGREDIENTS OF TOPICAL MEDICATION

Various solvents and preservatives in topical medications listed in Table 31.3 may produce allergic contact urticaria.

Benzyl Alcohol

Edwards[133] presented a patient with immediate urticaria and delayed hypersensitivity to benzyl alcohol present in a sunscreen. There have been other case reports of ICU and/or ACD from benzyl alcohol used as a preservative in topical and injectable medications.[134]

Emulgade F

This emulsifier, containing cetyl stearyl alcohol, was suspected of causing ICU and anaphylaxis.[135] Later patch testing reproduced the anaphylactoid symptoms.

Guar gum

Anaphylaxis and ICU was documented to be caused by guar gum in a dental topical anesthetic gel. Prick tests were positive to various guar gum extracts, especially to the component of the gel (tradename: Meyprogat-60).[136]

Monoamylamine

Tharp[137] reported that monoamylamine, an ingredient of tolnaftate (Tinactin) cream, produced both ICU and a delayed eczematous response. The monoamylamine in the Tinactin is an organic neutralizing agent that is being used specifically to adjust the pH of the cream so that it will thicken.

Organic Mercurials

Mercurochrome (thimerosal) has been reported to cause CU and anaphylaxis after use on superficial abrasions.[138]

Mathews[139] studied a physician who had asthma and urticaria, which was traced to hospital-laundered bed linens and uniforms. Scratch tests with phenylmercuric propionate, present as an antibacterial fabric softener used in the hospital laundry, produced a wheal-and-flare response. Provocative inhalation tests produced asthma within 5 minutes.

Parabens

Henry and colleagues[140] stated that this preservative, which can cause delayed eczematous hypersensitivity, can also produce ICU, such as developed in a patient after topical application of paraben-containing compounds. Positive open patch test results and a positive passive transfer (Prausnitz-Küstner reaction) test demonstrated an immunologic mechanism for the patient's skin reaction.

Petrolatum

CU with a positive open application test and positive delayed patch tests to all allergens in petrolatum has been reported.[141]

Phenoxyethanol

There are several reports of CU from phenoxyethanol.[142]

Polyethylene Glycol (PEG)

Fisher[143] reported that two patients had an immediate contact reaction from polyethylene glycol 400 used as a solvent in Tinactin and Lotrimin antifungal lotions. A third patient had a similar reaction to PEG 300 in Americaine Otic Solution. In all three instances, a wheal and flare occurred by rubbing in the PEG into the intact skin of the forearm of the sensitized patients. It was reported again recently from France.[144]

Polysorbate 60

Maibach and Conant[145] studied an adult male patient who noted redness on his forehead when applying 1% hydrocortisone cream. Testing revealed that application of the hydrocortisone cream produced urticaria only on the forehead but not on the back or forearm. The chemical responsible in the cream was determined to be polysorbate 60, an emulsifying agent that is a mixture of stearate esters of sorbitol and sorbitol anhydrides, consisting predominately of the mono ester. It is also known as Tween 60 (ICI America), Polyoxyethylene 20 sorbitan monostearate, Emsorb 6905 (Emery), and Armotan-20 (Armak). It should be noted that polysorbate 60 is not related to sorbic acid, which is a primary urticariogenic agent.

Sorbitan Sesquioleate

This emulsifier in a corticosteroid ointment has caused ICU.[146]

Allergic Contact Urticaria from Various Metals

ALUMINUM

An atopic woman with simultaneous CU and ACD to nickel and aluminum has been reported. Symptoms were controlled by chronic antihistamine use (cetirizine 10 to 20 mg/day).[147]

IRIDIUM

A worker in an electrochemical factory developed CU to iridium. A prick test with iridium chloride was weakly positive, but a scratch test produced anaphylaxis. Testing with platinum, a potential contaminant of the iridium solution, was negative, as was testing in controls.[148]

NICKEL

Osmundsen[149] reported two patients in whom urticaria was elicited by contact with nickel-containing objects. A 48-hour delayed patch test reaction was positive in these patients. A 20-minute patch test with nickel sulfate 2.5% in petrolatum on normal appearing skin on the forearm was negative. A chamber-prick test elicited in 20 minutes a strong urticarial reaction with pseudopods and a large flare, measuring 8 by 15 cm. The patient experienced an intense itching starting about 1 minute after the application of the test material.

Chamber-prick tests with nickel sulfate 2.5% in petrolatum, performed in five patients with ordinary nickel dermatitis (and with positive patch tests) and in three patients with chronic urticaria, revealed no immediate reaction. These responses to nickel were apparently clinically relevant, but it is uncertain whether they are due to immunologic or nonimmunologic mechanisms. If an immunologic mechanism is accepted, immediate hypersensitivity is coexistent with delayed hypersensitivity to nickel.[149]

RHODIUM

Nakayama and Imai[150] reported that 17 of 50 workers at a major precious metal factory had suffered from contact urticaria, contact dermatitis, and asthma for the preceding 9 years. Scratch patch test for 1 hour using a Finn chamber revealed that 9 of 12 patients were sensitized with platinum and 7 of 12 patients with rhodium as far as the immediate-type hypersensitivity was concerned. A closed patch test for 48 hours revealed that the patients were sensitized to rhodium, platinum, and mercury.

PLATINUM

Several reports document ICU from industrial platinum exposure. Respiratory reactions may occur and may be more significant.[149,151]

Nonallergic Contact Urticaria from Metals

The only metal that has been implicated in such a reaction is cobalt chloride. Cobalt chloride is often used as a color indicator in experimental sweat tests. It produces ACD, tuberculin-like reactions, and urticaria when injected intradermally. Smith and colleagues[152] reported contact urticaria from cobalt chloride and suggested that histamine or other vasoactive substances are at least partially responsible for the reaction.

Contact urticaria from cobalt chloride is evidently not a rare event. The precise mechanism causing urtication is unknown, but it is suggested that cobalt chloride in an alcoholic solution induces the release of vasoactive amines from mast cells through a nonimmunologic means.[153]

Immunologic Contact Urticaria from Chemicals

Several types of chemicals have been implicated as causing ICU. Occasionally, chemicals can cause generalized urticaria by cutaneous contact and percutaneous absorption. Exposures that have been productive of occupational urticaria are shown in Table 31.4.

ACRYLIC ACID

Although acrylates are common causes of ACD, acrylic acid is not thought of as a sensitizer. Acrylic acid, also known as 2-propenoic acid, is a basic monomer used in

manufacturing more complex molecules. Fowler[154] reported a chemical laboratory worker who developed CU on exposed surfaces while at work. Respiratory symptoms did not occur. Immediate testing revealed severe pruritus and a 3-cm wheal within 60 seconds after application of acrylic acid in 2% olive oil. Six controls were negative. A typical 2+ patch test reaction was present at the site after 48 hours, although the material had been wiped off the arm after 2 minutes (Figure 31-3).

ALCOHOL

Ophaswongse and Maibach[155] have reviewed cutaneous reactions to alcohols. Both NICU and immunologic CU have been reported, primarily from ethanol. Exposure may occur in medical and restaurant personnel and from recreational use.

Fowler has seen a case of anaphylaxis induced by drinking champagne, with a positive prick test to grape (personal communication, Dr. Hobert Pence, Louisville, KY, 1998).

CARBOXYMETHYLCELLULOSE

This agent is a cellulose polymer used as a binder, viscosity enhancer and stabilizer in a multitude of applications. It has been reported to cause ICU from contact with chalk in a 17-year-old student with positive open immediate test and prick test.[156] Systemic ingestion or injection can cause urticaria and anaphylaxis also.[157]

CHLOROTHALONIL

This agent is an agricultural fungicide and wood preservative. A tree nursery worker suffered CU and respiratory symptoms from handling seedlings that were treated with it.[158] Anaphylaxis was reproduced by patch testing.

DIETHYLTOLUAMIDE (DEET)

Maibach and Johnson[159] showed that DEET, a popular insect repellent, can cause an allergic contact urticaria syndrome.

DENATONIUM BENZOATE (DENATURING AGENT FOR ALCOHOL)

Bjorkner[160] reported that a 30-year-old housekeeper developed asthma and pruritus after using an insecticidal spray (Pyrex). The same symptoms appeared with an alcoholic skin disinfectant (M-sprit) and other preparations denatured with denatonium benzoate (Bitrex). An open epicutaneous test (20 minutes) showed a wheal and erythema to Pyrex, M-sprit, and Bitrex.

Denatonium benzoate was first used as a denaturant for alcohol in toilet preparations in 1960. M-sprit consists of 70% ethanol in water; denatonium benzoate was a commonly used skin disinfectant in many Swedish hospitals.

Table 31-4 Materials Causing Contact Urticaria in Industry

Materials	Industrial exposures
Acrylic acid	Plastics workers
Aliphatic polyamines	Epoxy resin workers
Aminothiazole	Pharmaceutical workers
Ammonia	Ammonia workers
Castor bean pomade	Castor oil extractors, fertilizer workers, and farmers
Chlorothalonil	Nursery or forestry workers
Complex platinum salts	Platinum refiners
Epoxy resins and related hardeners	Plastics, aircraft, and electronics workers
Formaldehyde	Phenolic and amino resin workers, fumigators, and laboratory workers
Glyceryl thioglycolate	Hairdressers
Lindane insecticide	Workers and cotton dusters
Penicillin	Pharmaceutical workers and nurses
Sodium sulfide	Photographers, workers with dyes, tanning, and hides
Spices	Spice workers, bakers, and sausage makers
Sulfur dioxide	Paper mill workers
Trichloroethane	Glass and metal cleaners
Vinyl pyrilidine	Chemistry research workers
Xylene	Chemistry research workers

FORMALDEHYDE

Formaldehyde and related compounds are extremely common causes of ACD. CU from formaldehyde has been reported in a dialysis patient. Prick and patch tests were positive. Specific IgE was present.[161] Immediate reactions have also rarely been reported from dental procedures and from topical exposure.[162,163]

Formaldehyde vapors may also cause allergic asthma.

GASES

Ammonia and sulfur dioxide gas have been shown to produce contact urticaria.[164,165]

GLYCERYL THIOGLYCOLATE

Although a common cause of ACD in hairdressers, CU is unusual. A case with positive prick test and negative patch tests has been reported.[166]

NAPHTHYLACETIC ACID

This agent, used as a plant growth regulator, produced one case of CU.[167]

PARAPHENYLENEDIAMINE (PPDA) AND OTHER DYES

Temesvari[168] reported that PPDA caused CU in three patients; two reacted to hair dye and one to colored cotton thread. Contact anaphylaxis has also been reported.[169]

Basic Blue Dye No. 99 caused CU in an elderly woman from a semipermanent hair coloring product. The dye (CI 56059; CAS 68123–13–7) is an aminoketone.[170]

PERSULFATES

Ammonium persulfate was first reported to cause ICU in 1963.[171] Persulfates are frequently used as hair bleaches and also may be found in photographic, pharmaceutical, and textile processes. In a more recent investigation, 6 of 7 prick-test positive patients had symptoms from contact with hair bleaches. Two of five had specific IgE antibodies. All patients were hairdressers. Four of them had respiratory symptoms.[172]

PLASTICS

In one case plastic folders and PVC provoked strong urticarial reactions on unbroken skin after 20 minutes.[149] These reactions correlated with the clinical history. The plastic materials that provoked the CU contained BHT or oleylamide. A 20-minute patch test with several articles of plastic (polyethylene and PVC) and with butylhydroxytoluene (BHT) 1% in ethanol elicited urticarial reactions. BHT is used as an antioxidant in plastic. Furthermore, open patch test with oleylamide (amide of oleic acid) 0.1% in ethanol elicited a strong urticarial reaction in 20 minutes. This chemical is used as a slipping agent in plastic.

A patient working with electronic components was proven to have CU to polypropylene used in capacitors.[173]

Epoxy resin and the diluents phenylglycidyl ether and cresylglycidyl ether caused CU and respiratory symptoms in an aircraft factory worker.[174] Phthalic anhydrides, epoxy resin hardeners, can also produce CU and respiratory symptoms.[175] Polyfunctional aziridine, used as a cross-linker in epoxy systems, caused ACD in two and CU in one patient.[176]

Diphenylmethane-4,4-diisocyanate (MDI) caused CU in an atopic carpenter. RAST tests were positive to MDI and to related isocyanates.[177]

Multiple allergenic antioxidants were identified from polyethylene gloves that caused ICU in a cook. These included BHT among others.[178]

Protein Hydrolysates

These substances, which are derived from natural proteins such as collagen, keratin, and silk, are used to "repair" broken hairs or split ends. Niinimaki and colleagues[179] studied 11 hairdressers with hand dermatitis by prick testing them to 22 protein hydrolysates. All were atopic, and all reacted to Crotein Q, hydroxypropyl trimonium hydrolyzed collagen.

A nonoccupational case with anaphylactoid symptoms has also been reported in a nonatopic woman.[180]

Sodium Silicate

Tanaka and colleagues[181] described an unusual combination of a primary irritant effect from sodium silicate with an ICU reaction and the production of ulcerative contact dermatitis. The patient had had recurrent ulcerative lesions on his left hand for 2 years. The ulcers were associated with chronic eczematous changes resulting from primary irritant contact dermatitis. The patient also had CU from sodium silicate. An immediate wheal-and-flare reaction was found 15 minutes after application of sodium silicate to a scratch test site. This response was not seen in healthy control subjects.

SOLVENTS

Xylene

Altman[182] described an acute urticarial reaction to xylene in a patient who was allergic to this solvent in her work. More recently, cases have been reported in medical laboratory technicians and in several factory workers.[183,184]

CU and a serum sickness–like reaction have been reported from exposure to a cleaning solvent used in a clothing factory (N355) containing xylene, cumene, and trimethylbenzene.[185]

Methyl Ethyl Ketone (MEK)

An Australian painter showed a positive open patch test to MEK and had severe irritation from occupational contact.[186]

Trichloroethane (TCE)

Fowler[187] reported a woman employed at an eyeglass manufacturer who developed urticaria on exposed surfaces when working with TCE cleaning glass lenses. Routine patch testing was negative. A positive 1-cm wheal developed after a 20-minute closed patch test on the forearm. Six controls were negative. The patient eventually had to change jobs because she could not find an area of the factory where she was free of symptoms.

WOOD

Hausen[188] stated that some species of wood or wood shavings may produce nonimmunologic types of reactions, although immediate reactions based on immunologic mechanisms are more characteristic. Species that have induced such immunologic reactions include obeche, larch, limba, and occasionally teak. A state of allergic sensitivity is proved by rubbing the patient's skin, moistened slightly before by water, with a piece of the suspected wood species 20 to 30 times on the forearm. By this process, urticarial reactions are produced within several minutes, yielding a large wheal and flare, while the nonoffending species remain negative.

Mukali wood (*Aningeria robusta*), a member of the Sapotaceae family, produced occupational asthma and CU in a woodworker.[189]

Immunologic Contact Urticaria from Animals, Insects, and Their Secretions

ICU may occur from animal hair, dander, saliva, serum, placenta, and even human seminal fluid (Table 31.5).

RAT TAILS

Rudzki and colleagues[104] showed that a psychologist who experimented with rats developed urticaria, rhinitis, and conjunctivitis. He developed contact urticaria 5 minutes after his forearm touched a rat's tail.

Table 31-5 Allergic Contact Urticaria from Animals and Animal Products

Saliva (dog, rat)
Hair
Seminal fluid (human)
Dander (human, cow)
Serum
Placenta
Jellyfish, Portuguese man-of-war
Bovine blood and amniotic fluid (cow)
Cockroach, mites, midges
Rat's tail
Guinea pig

GUINEA PIGS

Rudzki and colleagues[104] described a nurse who developed contact urticaria from handling guinea pigs.

SALIVA (DOG AND RAT)

Calnan[190] reported a patient who acquired allergic CU from dog saliva. Fowler has seen a case in a veterinarian who reacted to dog saliva but not to dog hair.

Burrows[191] stated that in companies in which large numbers of rats are used experimentally, asthma, hay fever, and urticaria are common among research workers. The problem seems to occur particularly with rats. The people carrying out experiments rather than the animal-house attendants are affected. This finding would suggest that the allergen is contained in internal secretions such as saliva rather than in hair or skin. This problem is so great in some laboratories that a labor problem is created.

HAIR AND DANDER

ICU was reported by Rudzki and Gryzwa[192] from animal hair, and Uehara and Ofuji[193] obtained positive patch test reactions to human dander in 120 of 181 (66%) patients with atopic dermatitis, in 2 of 28 (7%) patients with ACD, and in 1 of 31 (3%) normal controls. The frequency of positive reactions was significantly higher in patients with atopic dermatitis. The reactions consisted of erythema and papules, which showed histologically an eczematous change at the upper parts of hair follicles. It is suggested that certain patients with atopic dermatitis exhibit contact hypersensitivity to human dander. Whether or not the hypersensitivity has any relationship to the pathogenesis of the dermatitis was not determined by this study.

HUMAN SEMINAL FLUID

The first report of a case of an allergic reaction in a woman to male semen was published by Halpern and colleagues[194] in 1967. They showed that the condition was mediated by a skin-sensitizing antibody now known as IgE. Additional patients with allergy to seminal fluid have been reported in the literature.[195–197] Mikkelsen and colleagues[196] reported a woman who acquired an urticarial and anaphylactic reaction to male semen. Skin tests with her husband's semen produced a wheal and flare. An IgE reaginic antiseminal plasma antibody was found. No agglutinating antibody for suspensions of washed spermatozoa was found when the husband's dead spermatozoa or living or dead spermatozoa of a group O donor were used.

Mathias and colleagues[197] studied a woman with atopic dermatitis who experienced anaphylactic episodes after intercourse with her husband, with subsequent exacerbations of her atopic dermatitis. Skin testing and an in vitro leukocyte histamine release assay established the diagnosis of immediate hypersensitivity to her husband's seminal fluid; delayed hypersensitivity to seminal fluid could not be demonstrated. Antigen was found in the seminal fluid of nonrelated men. Radioallergosorbent testing detected the presence of circulating IgE antibodies specific for seminal plasma protein. Immunotherapy with seminal plasma may have limited the severity of a subsequent reaction. Serum from the husband and nonrelated men also contained antigen that provoked histamine release from the patient's leukocytes in vitro. The antigen in serum was associated with the globulin fraction and had a temporal relationship to ejaculation, appearing within 12 hours of ejaculation and disappearing within 4 days.

BOVINE DANDER

ICU to cow dander in Finland is common.[198] Presumably this is due to the fact that the cows are kept indoors for about 9 months of the year and are groomed frequently by the farmers.

BOVINE BLOOD AND AMNIOTIC FLUID

Degreef[199] reported a case of protein contact dermatitis with positive RAST to fresh bovine blood and amniotic fluid in a veterinary surgeon who suffered for 2 years from itching skin lesions on his arms and face, which were aggravated when he performed a cesarean section on a cow.

The following RASTs clinched the diagnosis:

1. Bovine amniotic fluid: 1,889 counts +++ (control: 380 counts)
2. Bovine blood: 1,623 counts +++ (control: 662 counts)
3. Bovine blood and amniotic fluid: 1,153 counts +++ (control: 372 counts)

PLACENTA OF COW

Schmidt[200] observed a "verified" case of ICU in a veterinary surgeon. After 2 years in his job, the patient started to feel itching localized to his arms and only occurring when he loosened the placenta from cows. The placenta is normally removed between 12 and 24 hours after delivery. He did not observe any trouble when working with horses, pigs, or other domestic animals. His total IgE in serum was 91 mg/mL, and he showed a positive RAST to a cow but a negative RAST to a cat and a horse. With a prick test, a +++ reaction to cow was produced. The patient showed a 3-mm reaction to amniotic fluid and a large 25-mm reaction to chorion-allantoic fluid and to the placenta from a cow. His reaction worsened to the point that he had to leave his job as a veterinary surgeon.

Fowler observed a similar case in a veterinarian who developed CU when delivering calves and the placenta. Prick test to bovine vaginal secretions was positive.

JELLYFISH AND PORTUGUESE MAN-OF-WAR

The stings of these coelenterates will produce a nonimmunologic linear papular urticaria in almost all individuals. Hartmann and colleagues[201] stated that the results of a preliminary screening of serum from patients varying in their reaction to envenomations indicate the potential of these toxin proteins to induce an allergic state in humans and illustrate the use of the RAST as a screening device to detect persons sensitive to coelenterate stings.

The coelenterate venom produces nonspecific damage to human skin and also lyses human basophils in vitro. This experiment demonstrates the immunogenicity of the toxins and their potential for inducing an allergic state, a previously unrealized aspect of coelenterate envenomation.

INSECTS

Cockroach

Zschunke[202] states that cockroaches are used to investigate insect hormones and analogous compounds. The aim of such research is to develop new insecticides. This investigator observed dermatitis, urticaria, rhinitis, bronchitis, and asthma in four research assistants whose job was breeding cockroaches. These patients had patch tests with a cockroach extract on the volar aspect of the forearms. Dilutions of 1:1,000 produced wheals (diameter 5 to 10 mm) within approximately 15 minutes, which disappeared in about 30 minutes. Zschunke concluded that dermatitis due to cockroaches should be classified as ICU.

Chironomid

These are small midges used by aquarists as fish food. A case of CU with positive prick test and IgE was reported.[203]

Mites

Tetranychus urticae, a large mite, may be a frequent cause of CU and contact dermatitis in farm workers.[204]

Caterpillars

Thirty cases of ICU to the pine processionary caterpillar (*Thaumatopoea pityocampa*), have been reviewed.[205] Apparently the insect is widely distributed throughout forests in Mediterranean and Central European countries. Most of the affected individuals were forest workers or farmers. In addition to ICU, 18 patients experienced angioedema and 12 had anaphylactic symptoms.

Contact of the intact skin with certain caterpillar hairs, moths, and plant nettles may produce a nonimmunologic contact urticaria.

Immunologic Contact Urticaria Due to Textiles

Silk, wool, rubber, and nylon may produce ICU.

Rudzki[206] reported that, in 1928, a 7-year-old girl developed wheals similar to those from contact with nettles after putting on a silk coat. It was observed soon afterward that any contact with silk elicited similar symptoms, so she endeavored to avoid any contact with this material. Over the years, each contact with silk produced increasingly severe urticaria. At the age of 56 she was still allergic to silk. When silk was applied to the flexor aspect of her right forearm, typical contact urticaria appeared.

Three divergent views are held as to the nature of the silk allergen: the silk fiber itself, the gum or glue (sericin) contained in raw silk, and the silkworm. The silkworm pupa contains 10 times more allergen than does the cocoon. Because there is undoubted sensitization to silk cloth that contains no pupa and relatively little sericin, some of the allergen must persist in finished silk.[207] Silk allergy may manifest itself as inhalant symptoms, urticaria, or dermatitis.[208]

WOOL

Many atopic individuals do not "tolerate" wool (i.e., woolen clothing exacerbates their itching). Some atopic individuals will occasionally acquire "itchy bumps," which somewhat resemble small urticarial wheals where woolen clothing is worn.[209]

SPRAY STARCH FOR CLOTHING

McDaniel and Marks[210] discovered that contact urticaria in a commercial spray starch for clothing was due to a dual sensitivity to formaldehyde and terpinyl acetate. A 20-year-old nonatopic woman had a 1-year history of pruritus and hives that occurred within minutes of wearing spray-starched clothes. New "wash-and-wear" clothes produced similar symptoms, but washed, unstarched clothes were worn without difficulty. Open tests were applied at different times to her forearm and back with the commercial spray starch and its ingredients. Within 15 minutes, urticaria was observed resulting from the spray starch, formaldehyde, and perfume. Further testing with 34 undiluted ingredients of the perfume produced hives that were due to one substance, terpinyl acetate, which was present in the perfume in a 0.25% concentration. The perfume and terpinyl acetate were formaldehyde-free, according to the manufacturer. A dozen control subjects had negative open test results to formaldehyde and terpinyl acetate.

FORMALDEHYDE IN LEATHER

Helander[211] described a patient who developed contact urticaria after she handled leather used to make leather dresses that was found qualitatively to contain minimal amounts of formaldehyde. The patient worked as a carver and model setter in a factory that made leather dresses. She had had urticaria almost daily, most severely on the hands, and occasionally, edema of the lip. During the weekends and vacations when the patient had no contact with leather, there was no evidence of skin eruption. The patient was transferred to another department in which she handles only domestic leather that does not contain formaldehyde.

The patient initially developed urticaria around a formaldehyde test site in less than 1 hour after the tests were applied; the urticaria became generalized in a few hours.

NYLON

Nylon was the apparent cause of CU in a nursing student.[212] She reacted to nylon underpants and stockings. Extensive testing found an urticarial reaction to nylon above. No reaction was seen to dyes, finishes, or other materials. She was not atopic.

TINOFIX S

Urticaria and anaphylaxis occurred in a 55-year-old man due to a textile finish used on his pants.[213] Tinofix S is described by deGroot and Gerkens[213] as a condensation product of dicyandramide, formaldehyde, ammonium chloride, and ethylenediamine. The patient did not react to the individual ingredients, only to the Tinofix S.

Contact Urticaria Due to Cold, Heat, Sun, Water, and air

The various physical urticarias due to cold, heat, sun, and water may be immunologic and nonimmunologic in nature.[214] It is not within the scope of this text to review the topic, but some mention will be made because these types of urticaria may be in the differential diagnosis of CU.

COLD URTICARIA

Essential acquired cold urticarial lesions appear usually within minutes after cold exposure, especially upon re-warming. Swimming in cold water or exposure to a cold wind may produce a shocklike syndrome, presumably due to histamine release.

HEAT URTICARIA

This rare type of urticaria may be related to exercise-induced urticaria.

SOLAR URTICARIA

Solar urticaria is a rare physical urticaria. Solar urticaria may occur after exposure to both ultraviolet and visible light; a range of reactions including syncope is possible.[215]

Monfrecola and colleagues[215] from Italy reported on 57 Caucasian patients with solar urticaria. There was a slight female preponderance (56%) and about half the patients presented between the ages of 20 and 30. Two-thirds reacted to visible light, the others mostly to UVA. Atopic dermatitis was present in 21%. Treatment with antihistamines helped 63%, while PUVA treatment abolished or reduced the sensitivity in almost all.

AQUAGENIC URTICARIA

In aquagenic urticaria, perifollicular hives appear on skin exposed to tap water or distilled water, saline, and the patient's own sweat or sebum. It is very rare and the pathophysiology is unknown. Greaves[216] stated that aquagenic urticarial eruptions appear to depend on acetylcholine release from sympathetic cholinergic nerve endings and involve histamine release, at least in part from skin mast cells. A solution of scopolamine, a potent anticholinergic agent, was applied to areas of skin, and the test sites were challenged with water. In four of five experiments, there was a complete blockade of water-provoked whealing, indicating that acetylcholine is involved in the genesis of aquagenic urticarial lesions. The acetylcholine is derived presumably from sympathetic cholinergic nerve endings in the affected skin.

A "skin-protective" foam, called Pro-Q in the United States and ProDerm elsewhere, has been anecdotally reported to provide dramatic relief from aquagenic urticaria in a child (personal communication, Thomas Skold, Ponsus Pharma, Stockholm, Sweden, 1999).

ATMOKNESIS

Bernhard[217] commented on the phenomenon, reported by some patients, that they itch upon removal of clothing and "exposure" to air. He termed this "atmoknesis," after the Greek roots atmos (air) and knesis (itching). Fowler hypothesizes that the reaction is triggered by a sudden change in skin temperature, rather than any atmospheric constituents.

Combined Eczematous and Urticarial Reactions

Many compounds can produce an acute allergic contact urticarial reaction, which may be followed by a typical delayed type of eczematous reaction (see Table 31.6). Such compounds will produce initially an immediate wheal-and-flare reaction within 30 to 45 minutes, followed by a delayed eczematous response at 48- to 72-hour readings.[1,113,154]

Testing for immediate reactions on previously eczematous skin can result in prompt itching followed within a few minutes by either urticarial responses alone or combined with eruptions of vesicles and all macroscopic features of delayed eczematous dermatitis.[50,218]

Some primarily urticariogenic compounds, such as sorbic acid, cinnamic aldehyde, and balsam of Peru, can produce NICU in many individuals and delayed eczematous reactions in some patients.

CU to natural latex may present as hand eczema that may be indistinguishable from allergic or irritant contact dermatitis. This may occur with chronic exposure to other contact urticants. Whether the eczematous appearance is due to primary immunologic factors or result from acute rubbing and scratching of the wheals is uncertain.

Table 31-6 Contactants That May Cause Combined Delayed Eczematous and Urticarial Reactions	
Acrylic acid	Lettuce
Ammonium persulfate	Metals
Benzocaine	Nickel
Castor bean	Rhodium
Cinnamic aldehyde	Platinum
Endive	Rubber
Epoxy resin	Sorbic acid
Latex	Teak
Lemon perfume	Vinyl pyridine

CONTACT ANAPHYLAXIS

Skinner and Fowler[219] have reviewed the reported causes of anaphylaxis precipitated by skin contact with an allergen. Natural rubber latex has been identified as an extremely important allergen able to cause contact anaphylaxis. (See Chapter 29).

Ammonium Persulfate—A Cause of Contact Urticaria of Uncertain Mechanism

This type of CU refers to reactions elicited by chemicals for which neither an allergic nor a direct influence on vessels or release of vasoactive substances can be proven currently. Ammonium persulfate, an oxidizing agent used in hair bleaches, is the classic example. The fact that some individuals react on the first exposure and the finding of negative passive transfer attempts favor a nonimmunologic mechanism, whereas negative tests in most controls dispute the concept of direct release of vasoactive substances.[220] The variety of reaction patterns, including toxic dermatitis, localized or generalized urticaria, rhinitis, asthma, and even vascular collapse, is puzzling.

Ammonium persulfate is used widely to "boost" peroxide hair bleaches to obtain a platinum blond effect. The persulfates can produce a variety of cutaneous and respiratory responses, including allergic eczematous contact dermatitis, irritant dermatitis, localized edema, generalized urticaria, rhinitis, asthma, and syncope.[221] Some of these reactions appear to be truly allergic, whereas others appear to be due to the release of histamine on a nonallergic basis.

Patch tests may be performed with 2% to 5% aqueous solution of ammonium persulfate. Scratch tests may result in asthma and syncope. In some patients, merely rubbing a saturated solution of ammonium persulfate into the skin will evoke a large urticarial wheal. Hairdressers should be made aware that these ammonium persulfate hair bleach preparations may provoke severe reactions and should seek medical attention if the client complains of severe itching, tingling, a burning sensation, hives, dizziness, or weakness.

TESTING WITH AMMONIUM PERSULFATE

The method of testing with ammonium persulfate is the one suggested by Brun and colleagues[222] as follows: Put 0.4 g of dry persulfate in 20 mL vials, then close the vials with gum stoppers (like antibiotic vials). Inject 20 mL of water in each vial and keep them no longer than 1 day. Always use fresh 2% solution of ammonium persulfate.

Principles of Skin Testing for Contact Urticaria

The following procedures may be followed when it is suspected that a contactant may be producing contact urticaria.

1. Test the substance on normal skin that has apparently never before been the site of dermatitis.
2. If negative, test on previously affected skin even though the skin at present appears to be normal. Previously affected skin may remain for a long time in a state of increased responsiveness as compared with skin that has never been the site of dermatitis.
3. Testing on eczematous skin may be worthwhile, providing the tested area shows only light erythema, so that an urticarial reaction may be readily perceived on the eczematous skin.
4. If all these test procedures are negative, the suspected contactant should be rubbed gently into a small scratch.
5. It should be noted that, as a rule, those substances that produce NICU will show reactions on normal skin that has never been the site of dermatitis.
6. The use of controls is much more significant in ICU than in the nonimmunologic variety. Tests for ICU should be negative in at least three to five controls.
7. The upper back, the antecubital space, and the volar aspect of the forearm are suitable sites for testing. Some agents causing NICU, however, such as benzoic acid, may react only on the face and not elsewhere.
8. Precautions: Because anaphylactoid reactions may occur in highly allergic patients from skin testing, epinephrine and resuscitation equipment should be available.
9. Local and systemic NSAIDs may inhibit NICU, and antihistamines may inhibit both forms of CU.

Pretreatment Adjuncts to Testing for Contact Urticaria

BLOCKING AGENTS

Pretreatment of the test site with 0.1 ml of atropine in 1:1,000 solution or lidocaine in 1:100 dilution indicates that a cholinergic mechanism is involved if blockade of the test site is achieved. The use of antihistamine agents via oral administration or via local pretreatment can provide evidence of a histamine-mediated reaction if successful inhibition of the skin test is achieved. Local anesthesia induced by lidocaine decreased the reactivity to benzoic acid significantly with concentrations of both 1.0% and 0.25%.[223]

COMPOUND 48/80

When compound 48/80 (Sigma Chemical Co., St. Louis, MO) is injected intradermally, mast cells at the site will release histamine and a hive will form. If 0.1 mL of a 0.05-mg/mL solution is injected into the same site on a patient's ventral forearm at 8-hour intervals, usually no response can be elicited by the third injection, as mast cells have been depleted of their histamine. Twenty-four hours after the initial injection, 0.1 mL of the incriminated substance is applied to the pretreated site and to a control site. If a typical wheal occurs at the control site but not at the prepared site, the response may, in part, be mediated by histamine. The refractory period of reactions mediated by histamine produced by compound 48/80 has been reported to last 2 to 6 days.

Contact Urticaria Statistics

Kanerva and colleagues[198] presented comprehensive occupational statistics regarding CU in Finland from 1990 to 1994. Other than this report, and except for latex allergy, comprehensive data on prevalence of CU are woefully inadequate. Kanerva et al. found that 2,759 cases of occupational contact dermatoses were reported to the Finnish Register of Occupational Disease, of which 815 (29.5%) were CU. Women accounted for 70% of the cases. The top allergens were cow dander (362 cases); latex (193 cases); flour, grains, and feed (92 cases); foodstuffs (25 cases); and industrial enzymes (14 cases). Farmers and animal attendants were the most common occupational group with CU, followed by bakers, nurses, chefs, and dental assistants.

Katsarou and colleagues[224] studied the incidence of immediate reactions to patch test allergens of the European standard series. No attempt was made to differentiate NICU from ICU, but presumably the majority of reactions were of the NICU variety. Of 664 patients, balsam of Peru reacted in 113, fragrance mix in 112, paraben mix in 30, and clioquinol in 13. A total of 328 reactions were seen to the 24 test substances. Presence of atopy was not increased in the reactive group.

References

1. Von Krogh G, Maibach HI. The contact urticaria syndrome. Semin Dermatol 1982;1:59.

2. Lahti A. Non-immunologic contact urticaria. Acta Derm Venereol 1980;60[Suppl 91].

3. Odom RB, Maibach HI. Contact urticaria: a different contact dermatitis in dermatotoxicology and pharmacology. In: Marzulli FN, Maibach HI, eds. Advances in modern toxicology, vol 4. Washington, DC: Hemisphere Publishing, 1977.

4. Kligman AM. The spectrum of contact urticaria-wheals, erythema, and pruritus. Derm Clin 1990;8:57.

5. Rosenhall L, Zetterstron O. Asthmatic patients with hypersensitivity to aspirin, benzoic acid and tartrazine. Tubercle 1975;56:168.

6. Larmi E. PUVA treatment inhibits nonimmunologic immediate contact reactions to benzoic acid and methyl nicotinate. Int J Dermatol 1989;28:9.

7. Shriner D, Maibach H. Regional variation of nonimmunologic contact urticaria: functional map of the human face. Skin-Phamacol 1996;9:312.

8. Lahti A, Poutiainen AM, Hannuksela M. Alcohol vehicles in tests for non-immunological immediate contact reactions. Contact Dermatitis 1993;29:22.

9. Emmons W, Marks J: Immediate and delayed reactions to cosmetic ingredients. Contact Dermatitis 1985;13:258.

10. Stoughton RB, Fritsch W. Influence of dimethylsulfoxide (DMSO) on human percutaneous absorption. Arch Dermatol 1964;90:512.

11. Kligman AM. Topical pharmacology and toxicology of dimethyl sulfoxide—part 1. JAMA 1965;193:796.

12. Kellum RE, ed. Selected reviews of the literature. Arch Dermatol 1966;93:135.

13. McCabe RJ. Studies with the local use of the furfuryl ester of nicotinic acid. Arch Dermatol 1956;74:522.

14. Vaillancourt de G. The cutaneous application of a nicotinic acid cream as a diagnostic aid in various rheumatic diseases. Can Med Assoc J 1954;71:283.

15. Windholz M, ed. The Merck index: an encyclopedia of chemicals and drugs, 9th ed. Rahway, NJ: Merck & Co, 1976.

16. Fryklof L-E. A note on the irritant properties of sorbic acid in ointments and creams. J Pharm Pharmacol 1958;10:719.

17. Hjorth N, Trolle-Lassen C. Skin reactions to preservatives in creams. Am Perfum 1962;77:43.

18. Rietschel RL. Contact urticaria from synthetic cassia oil and sorbic acid limited to the face. Contact Dermatitis 1978;4:347.

19. Pevny I von, Rauscher E, Lechner W, Metz D. Excessive allergie gegen Benzoesaure mit anaphylaktischem Schock nach Expositionstest. Dermatosen 1981;29:123.

20. Hjorth N. Eczematous allergy to balsams, allied perfumes and flavouring agents. Acta Derm Venereol (Stockh) 1981;41[Suppl 46]:216.

21. Juhlin L, Michaelsson G. Forbjudet och tillatet vid overkanslighet for konserveringsmedel och fargamnen. Lakartidningen 1973;70:1414.

22. Martindale W. The extra pharmacopoeia, 27th ed. Wade A, ed. London: The Pharmaceutical Press, 1977.

23. Lahti A. Skin reactions to antimicrobial agents. Contact Dermatitis 1978;4:302.

24. Munoz F, Bellido J, Moyano J, et al. Perioral contact urticaria from sodium benzoate in a toothpaste. Contact Dermatitis 1996;35:51.

25. Opdyke DLJ. Cinnamic acid. In: Monographs on fragrance raw materials. Food Cosmet Toxicol 1978;16[Suppl 1]:687.

26. Collins FW, Mitchell JC. Aroma chemicals. Reference sources for perfume and flavour ingredients with special reference to cinnamic aldehyde. Contact Dermatitis 1975;1:43.

27. Nater JP, De Jong MCJM, Baar AJM, Bleumink E. Contact Dermatitis 1977;3:151.

28. Rudzki E, Grzywa Z. Two types of contact urticaria and immediate reactions to patch-test allergens. Dermatologica 1978;157:110.

29. Calnan CD. Cinnamon dermatitis from an ointment. Contact Dermatitis 1976;2:167.

30. Magnusson B, Wilkinson DS. Cinnamic aldehyde in toothpaste: (1) clinical aspects and patch tests. Contact Dermatitis 1975;1:70.

31. Schorr WF. Cinnamic aldehyde allergy. Contact Dermatitis 1975;1:108.

32. Mathias CGT, Chappler RR, Maibach HI. Contact urticaria from cinnamic aldehyde. Arch Dermatol 1980;116:74.

33. Temesvari E von, Soos G, Podanyi B, et al. Contact urticaria provoked by balsam of Peru. Contact Dermatitis 1978;4:65.

34. Rudzki E, Grzywa Z. Immediate reactions to balsam of Peru, cassia oil and ethyl vanillin. Contact Dermatitis 1976;2:360.

35. Forsbeck M, Skog E. Immediate reactions to patch tests with balsam of Peru. Contact Dermatitis 1977;3:201.

36. Safford RJ, et al. Immediate contact reactions to chemicals in the fragrance mix and a study of the quenching action of eugenol. Br J Dermatol 1990;123:595.

37. Maes D, Marenus K, Smith W. Invisible irritation: a new look at product safety. Cosmet Toilet 1990;105:43.

38. Coverly J, Peters L, Whittle E, Basketter D. Susceptibility to skin stinging, non-immunologic contact urticaria and acute skin irritation: is there a relationship? Contact Dermatitis 1998;38:90.

39. Edwards EK. Contact urticaria to cow's milk. Cutis 1981;28:450.

40. Lecks HE. Anaphylaxis from milk protein in diaper ointment. JAMA 1980;244:1560.

41. Williams J, Moyle M, Nixon R: Occupational contact urticaria from Parmesan cheese. Contact Dermatitis 2007;56:113.

42. Foti C, Antelmi A, Mistrello G, et al: Occupational contact urticaria and rhinoconjunctivitis from dog's milk. Contact Dermatitis 2007;56:169.

43. Rudzki E, Gryzwa Z. Contact urticaria from egg. Contact Dermatitis 1977;3:103.

44. Temesvari E, Varkonyi V. Contact urticaria provoked by egg. Contact Dermatitis 1980;6:43.

45. Ushijima N, Miyanaga K, Yoshimura S, et al. Allergic contact urticaria to lysozyme. Report 6th International Symposium on Contact Dermatitis and Joint Meeting between ICRD and JCDRG, Tokyo, 1982.

46. Jemmel-Peter N, Piletta-Zanin P, Hausr C: Facial dermatitis, contact urticaria, rhinoconjunctivitis, and asthma induced by potato. Am J Contact Dermat 1999;10:40.

47. Pearson RSB. Potato sensitivity. An occupational allergen in housewives. Acta Allergol 1966;21:507.

48. Jeannet-peter N, Piletta-Zanin P, Hauser C. Facial dermatitis, contact urticaria, rhinoconjunctivitis, and asthma induced by potato. Am J Contact Dermat 1999;10:40.

49. Hjorth N, Roed-Petersen J. Berufsekzeme durch proteine. Z Hautkr 1975;50:851.

50. Mitchell JC. Contact urticaria from a shrimp, Pandalus. Contact Dermatitis Newsletter 1974;16:486.

51. Lombardi P, Campolmi P, Giorgini S, Spallanzani P. Food contact urticaria. Report 6th international symposium on contact dermatitis and joint meeting between ICRG and JCDRG, Tokyo, 1982.

52. Beck HI, Nissen K. Contact urticaria to commercial fish in atopic persons. Acta Dermatol 1982;63:257.

53. Coverly J, Peters L, Whittle E, Basketter D. Susceptibility to skin stinging, non-immunologic contact urticaria and acute skin irritation: is there a relationship? Contact Dermatitis 1998;38:90.

54. Dominguez C, Ojeda I, Crespo J, et al. Allergic reactions following skin contact with fish. Allergy-Asthma-Proc 1996;17:83.

55. Maibach HI. Regional variation in elicitation of contact urticaria syndrome (immediate hypersensitivity syndrome): shrimp. Contact Dermatitis 1986;15:100.

56. Maibach HI. Immediate hypersensitivity in hand dermatitis. Role of food-contact dermatitis. Arch Dermatol 1976;112:1289.

57. Fisher AA, Stengel F. Allergic occupational hand dermatitis due to calves' liver. An urticarial "immediate" type hypersensitivity. Cutis 1977;19:561.

58. Fisher AA. Allergic contact urticaria to raw beef—histopathology of the specific wheal reaction at the scratch test site. Contact Dermatitis (in press).

59. Moseng D. Urticaria from pig's gut. Contact Dermatitis 1982;8:135.

60. Reiche L: Venison contact dermatitis. Australas J Dermatol 2002;43:72.

61. Geyer E, Kranke B, Derhaschnig J, et al. Contact urticaria from roe deer meat and hair. Contact Dermatitis 1998;39:34.

62. Iliev D, Wuthrich B. Occupational protein contact dermatitis with type I allergy to different kinds of meat and vegetables. Int Arch Occup Environ Health 1998;71:289.

63. Andersen KE, Lowenstein H. An investigation of the possible immunological relationship between allergen extracts from birch, pollen, hazelnut, potato, and apple. Contact Dermatitis 1978;4:73.

64. Grattan CEH, Harman RRM. Contact urticaria to strawberry. Contact Dermatitis 1985;13:191.

65. Veraldi S, Schianchi-Veraldi R. Contact urticaria from Kiwi fruit. Contact Dermatitis 1990;22:244.

66. Giannattasio M, Serafina M, Guarrara P, et al. Contact urticaria from Litchi fruit. Contact Dermatitis 1995;33:67.

67. DeCorres L, et al. Contact urticaria. Sensitization to chestnuts and bananas in patients with contact urticaria from latex. Contact Dermatitis 1990;23:277.

68. Krook G. Occupational dermatitis from Lactuca sativa (lettuce) and Cichorium (endive). Contact Dermatitis 1977;3:27.

69. Pigatto PD. Ig-E-mediated contact and generalized urticaria from Eruca sativa. Contact Dermatitis 1991;25:191.

70. Quirce S, Tabar A, Olaguibel J, Cuevas M. Occupational contact urticaria syndrome caused by globe artichoke. J Allergy Clin Immunol 1996;97:710.

71. Tabar A, Alvarez-Puebla M, Gomez B, et al. Diversity of asparagus allergy: clinical and immunologic features. Clin Exp Allergy 2004;34:131.

72. Munoz D, et al. Anaphylaxis from contact with carrot. Contact Dermatitis 1985;13:345.

73. Lovell CR, Rycroft RJG. Contact urticaria from winged bean (Psophocarpus tetragonolobus). Contact Dermatitis 1984;10:314.

74. Kanerva L, Estlander T, Jolanki R. Long-lasting contact urticaria from castor bean. J Am Acad Dermatol 1990;23:351.

75. DiLernia V, Albertini G, Bisighini G. Immunologic contact urticaria syndrome from raw rice. Contact Dermatitis 1992;27:196.

76. Cristaudo A, Simonato R, Pasini G, et al. Contact urticaria and protein contact dermatitis from corn. Contact Dermatitis 2004;51:84.

77. Van Ketel WG. Immediate type allergy to malt in beer. Contact Dermatitis 1980;6:279.

78. Lauriere M, Pecquet C, Bouchez-Mahiout I, et al. Hydrolysed wheat proteins present in cosmetics can induce immediate hypersensitivities. Contact Dermatitis 2006;54:283.

79. Heygi E, Dolezalova A. Urticarial reaction after patch tests of toothpaste with a subshock condition: hypersensitivity to caraway seed. Cesk Dermatol 1976;51:19.

80. Duran S, Delgado J, Gamez R, et al. Contact Urticaria from sunflower seeds. Contact Dermatitis 1997;37:184.

81. Gamboa P, Jaurequi I, Urrutia, et al. Allergic contact urticaria from poppy flowers. Contact Dermatitis 1997;37:140.

82. Munoz F, Delgado J, Palma J, et al. Airborne contact urticaria due to Mulberry (Morus alba) pollen. Contact Dermatitis 1995;32:61.

83. Gutierrez D, Conde A, Duran S, et al. Contact urticaria from Lupin. Contact Dermatitis 1997;36:311.

84. Estlander T, Kanerva L, Tupasela O, Jolanki R. Occupational contact urticaria and type I sensitization caused by gerbera. Contact Dermatitis 1998;38:118.

85. Paulsen E, Stahl-Skov P, Andersen K. Immediate skin and mucosal symptoms from pot plants and vegetables in gardeners and greenhouse workers. Contact Dermatitis 1998;39:166.

86. Majmudar V, Azam N, Finch T: Contact urticaria to Cannabis sativa. Contact Dermatitis 2006;54:127.

87. Kannerva L, Vahanen M, Tupasela O. Occupational contact urticaria from cellulase enzyme. Contact Dermatitis 1998;38:176.

88. Kanerva L, Tarvainen K. Allergic contact dermatitis and contact urticaria from cellulolytic enzymes. Am J Contact Dermat 1990;1:244.

89. Foti C, Carino M, Cassano N, et al. Occupational contact urticaria from paprika. Contact Dermatitis 1997;37:135.

90. Pecquet C, Leynadier F, Saiag P. Immediate hypersensitivity to sesame in foods and cosmetics. Contact Dermatitis 1998;39:313.

91. Monteseirin J, Perez-Formoso J, Hernandez M, et al. Contact urticaria from dill. Contact Dermatitis 2003;48:275.

92. Liddle M, Hull C, Liu C, Powell D: Contact urticaria from curcumin. Dermatitis 2006;17:1967.

93. Williams J, Roberts H, Tate B. Contact urticaria to olives. Contact Dermatitis 2007;56:52.

94. Maucher OM. Anaphylaktische reaktionen beim epicutantest. Hautarzt 1972;23:139.

95. Haustein UF. Anaphylactic shock and contact urticaria after the patch test with professional allergens. Allerg Immunol 1976;22:349.

96. Boonk WJ. Dermatologic hazards from hidden contact with penicillin. Dermatosen 1981;29:131.

97. Kwon H, Kim M, Kim H, Park Y: The simultaneous occurrence of contact urticaria from sulbactam and allergic contact dermatitis from ampicillin in a nurse. Contact Dermatitis 2006; 54: 176.

98. Eriksen HC. Anaphylactic shock caused by neomycin treated with external cardiac massage. Ugeskr Laeg 1963;125:1077.

99. Pippen R. Anaphylactoid reaction after chymacort ointment. Br Med J 1966;5496:1172.

100. Roupe G, Strannegard O. Anaphylactic shock elicited by topical administration of bacitracin. Arch Dermatol 1969;100:450.

101. Comaish JS, Cunliffe WJ. Absorption of drugs from varicose ulcers: a cause of anaphylaxis. Br J Clin Pract 1967;21:97.

102. Sood A, Taylor J: Bacitracin: Allergen of the year. Am J Contact Dermat 2003;14:3.

103. Levene G, Withers A. Anaphylaxis to streptomycin and hyposensitization. Trans St Johns Hosp Dermatol Soc 1969;55:184.

104. Rudzki E, Rebandel P, Rogozinski T. Contact urticaria from rat tail, guinea pig, streptomycin and vinyl pyridine. Contact Dermatitis 1981;7:186.

105. Kosakava M. Sub-Schock bei der Epikutan-probe mit Chloramphenicol. Berufsdermatosen 1977;25:134.

106. Tuft L. Contact urticaria from cephalosporins. Arch Dermatol 1975;111:1609.

107. Shimizu S, Chen K, Miyakawa S. Cefotiam-induced contact urticaria syndrome. Dermatology 1996;192:174.

108. Mancuso G, Masara N. Contact urticaria and severe anaphylaxis from rifamycin SV. Contact Dermatitis 1992;27:124.

109. Escribano M, Munoz-Bellido F, Velazquez E, et al. Contact urticaria due to aescin. Contact Dermatitis 1997;37:233.

110. Camarasa JMG, Alomar A, Perez M. Contact urticaria and anaphylaxis from aminophenazone. Contact Dermatitis 1978;4:243.

111. Ryan ME, Davis BM, Marks Jr JG. Contact urticaria and allergic contact dermatitis to benzocaine gel. J Am Acad Dermatol 1980;2:221.

112. Rudner EJ. Contact urticaria. Int J Dermatol 1979;18:418.

113. Ramsay DL, Cohen HJ, Baer RL. Allergic reaction to benzophenone. Arch Dermatol 1972;105:906.

114. Landers M, Law S, Storrs F: Contact urticaria, allergic contact dermatitis, and photoallergic contact dermatitis from oxybenzone. Am J Contact Dermat 2003;14:33.

115. Kanerva L, Alanko K, Estlander T, et al. Occupational allergic contact urticaria from chloramine-T solution. Contact Dermatitis 1997;37:180.

116. Horio T. Chloropromazine photoallergy: coexistence of immediate and delayed type. Arch Dermatol 1975;111:1469.

117. Heinemann C, Sinaiko R, Maibach H: immunologic contact urticaria and anaphylaxis to chlorhexidine: overview. Exog Dermatol 2002;1:186.

118. Okano M, Nomura M, Hata S, et al. Anaphylactic symptoms due to chlorhexidine gluconate. Arch Dermatol 1989;125:50.

119. Cheung J, O'Leary J. Allergic reaction to chlorhexidine in an anesthetized patient. Anaesth Intern Care 1985;13:429.

120. Aalto-korte K, Makinen-Kiljunen S: Symptoms of immediate chlorhexidine sensitivity in patients with a positive prick test. Contact Dermatitis 2006;55:173.

121. Freitas JP, Brandao FM. Contact urticaria to chlorocresol. Contact Dermatitis 1986;15:252.

122. Schena D, Barba A, Costa G. Occupational contact urticaria to cisplatin. Contact Dermatitis 1996;34:220.

123. Tosti A, Guerra L, Bardazzi F. Contact urticaria during topical immunotherapy. Contact Dermatitis 1989;21:196.

124. VanHecke E, Santosa S. Contact urticaria to DNCB. Contact Dermatitis 1985;12:282.

125. Fisher AA. Urticarial and systemic reactions to contactants varying from hair bleach to seminal fluid. Cutis 1977;19:715.

126. Mitchell JC. Contact urticaria from a vitamin E preparation (vitamin E-vegetable oil) in two siblings. Int J Dermatol 1975;14:246.

127. Gimenez-Arnau A, Toll A, Pujol R: Immediate cutaneous hypersensitivity response to phytomenadione induced by Vitamin K1. Contact Dermatitis 2005:52:284.

128. Jovanovic M, Karadaglic D, Brkic S: Contact urticaria and allergic contact dermatitis to lidocaine. Contact Dermatitis 2006;54:124.

129. Papa CM, Shelley WB. Menthol hypersensitivity: diagnostic basophil response in a patient with chronic urticaria, flushing and headaches. JAMA 1964;189:549.

130. Grunnet E. Contact urticaria and anaphylactoid reaction induced by topical application of nitrogen mustard. Br J Dermatol 1976;94:101.

131. Daughters D, Zackheim H, Maibach H. Urticaria and anaphylactoid reactions after topical application of mechlorethamine. Arch Dermatol 1973;107:429.

132. Adachi A, Fukunaga A, Hayashi K, et al. Anaphylaxis to polyvinylpyrrolidine after vaginal application of povidone-iodine. Contact Dermatitis 2003;48:133.

133. Edwards Jr EK. Allergic reactions to benzyl alcohol in a sunscreen. Cutis 1981;28:332.

134. Curry E, Warshaw E: Benzyl alcohol allergy: importance of patch testing with personal products. Dermatitis 2005;16:203.

135. Ring J, Galosi A, Przybilla B. Contact anaphylaxis from Emulgade F. Contact Dermatitis 1986;15:48.

136. Roesch A, Haegele T, Vogt T, et al. Severe contact urticaria to guar gum included as gelling agent in a local anesthetic. Contact Dermatitis 2005;52:307.

137. Tharp CK. Contact urticaria. Arch Dermatol 1973;108:135.

138. Torres J, DeCorres F. Anaphylactic hypersensitivity to mercurochrome (Merbromium). Ann Allergy 1985;54:230.

139. Mathews KP. Immediate-type hypersensitivity to phenylmercuric compounds. Am J Med 1968;44:310.

140. Henry JC, Tschen EH, Becker LE. Contact urticaria to parabens. Arch Dermatol 1979;115:1231.

141. Grin R, Maibach H. Long-lasting contact urticaria from petrolatum mimicking dermatitis. Contact Dermatitis 1999;40:110.

142. Birnie A, English J: 2-phenoxyethanol-induced contact urticaria. Contact Dermatitis 2006;54:349.

143. Fisher AA. Immediate and delayed allergic contact reactions to polyethylene glycol. Contact Dermatitis 1978;4:135.

144. Co-Minh H, Demolly P, Guillot B: Anaphylactic shock after oral intake and contact urticaria to polyethylene glycols. Allergy 2007;62:92.

145. Maibach HI, Conant M. Contact urticaria to a corticosteroid cream: polysorbate 60. Contact Dermatitis 1977;3:350.

146. Hardy H, Maibach H. Contact urticaria syndrome from sorbitan sesquioleate in a corticosteroid ointment. Contact Dermatitis 1995; 32:114.

147. Helgesen A, Austad J. Contact urticaria from aluminum and nickel in the same patient. Contact Dermatitis 1997;37:303.

148. Bergman A, Svedberg U, Nilsson E. Contact urticaria with anaphylactic reactions caused by occupational exposure to iridium salt. Contact Dermatitis 1995;32:14.

149. Osmundsen PE. Contact urticaria from nickel and plastic additives (butylhydroxytoluene, oleylamide). Contact Dermatitis 1980;6:452.

150. Nakayama H, Imai T. Occupational contact urticaria, contact dermatitis and asthma caused by rhodium hypersensitivity. 6th International Symposium on Contact Dermatitis and Joint Meeting between ICRG and JCDRG. Tokyo, 21 May 1982.

151. Levene GM. Platinum sensitivity. Br J Dermatol 1971;85:590.

152. Smith JD, Odom RB, Maibach HI. Contact urticaria from cobalt chloride. Arch Dermatol 1975;111:1610.

153. Maibach HI, Johnson H. Contact urticaria syndrome. Arch Dermatol 1975;111:726.

154. Fowler JF. Immediate contact hypersensitivity to acrylic acid. Derm Clin 1990;8:193.

155. Ophaswongse S, Maibach H. Alcohol dermatitis: allergic contact dermatitis and contact urticaria syndrome. Contact Dermatitis 1994;30:1.

156. Moreau L, Alomer G, Dube N, et al. Contact urticaria from carboxymethylcellulose in white chalk. Dermatitis 2006:17;29.

157. Muroi N, Nishibori M, Fujii T, et al. Anaphylaxis from the carboxymethylcellulose component of barium sulfate suspension. N Engl J Med 1997;337:1275.

158. Adams RM. Occupational skin disease, 2nd ed. Philadelphia: WB Saunders, 1990.

159. Maibach HI, Johnson HL. Contact urticaria syndrome: contact urticaria to diethyltoluamide immediate-type hypersensitivity. Arch Dermatol 1975;111:726.

160. Bjorkner B. Contact urticaria and asthma from detonium benzoate (Bitrex). Contact Dermatitis 1980;6:466.

161. Maurice F, Rivory J, Larsson P, et al. Anaphylactic shock caused by long term hemodialysis. J Allergy Clin Immunol 1986;77:594.

162. Tas E, Pletscher M, Bircher A. IgE mediated urticaria from formaldehyde in a dental root compound. J Investig Allergol Clin Immunol 2002;12:130.

163. Wei Lim S, Smith W, Gillis G: IgE mediated allergy to formaldehyde from topical application. Contact Dermatitis 2006;54:230.

164. Morris GE. Urticaria following exposure to ammonia fumes. AMA Arch Health 1956;13:480.

165. Zschunke E. Occupational urticaria due to sulfur dioxide. Berufsdermatosen 1967;15:23.

166. Shelley W, Shelley E, Talanin N. Urticaria due to occupational exposure to glyceryl monothioglycolate permanent wave solution. Acta Derm Venereol 1998;78:471.

167. Camarasa J. Contact urticaria to naphthylacetic acid. Contact Dermatitis 1986;14:113.

168. Temesvari E. Contact urticaria from paraphenylenediamine. Contact Dermatitis 1984;11:134.

169. Pasche-Koo F, French L, Piletta-Zanin P. Contact urticaria and shock to hair dye. Allergy 1998;53:904.

170. Jagtman B. Urticaria and contact urticaria due to Basic Blue 99 in a hair dye. Contact Dermatitis 1996;35:52.

171. Calnan C, Shuster S. Reactions to ammonium persulfate. Arch Dermatol 1963;88:812.

172. Aalto-Korte K, Makinen-Kiljunen S. Specific immunoglobulin E in patients with immediate persulfate hypersensitivity. Contact Dermatitis 2003;49:22.

173. Tosti A, et al. Contact urticaria from polypropylene. Contact Dermatitis 1986;15:51.

174. Sasseville D. Contact urticaria from epoxy resin and reactive diluents. Contact Dermatitis 1998;38:57.

175. Kanerva L, Hyry H, Jolanki R, et al. Delayed and immediate allergy caused by methylhexahydrophylactic anhydride. Contact Dermatitis 1997;36:34.

176. Kanerva L, Estlander T, Jolanki R, Tarvainen K. Occupational allergic contact dermatitis and contact urticaria caused by polyfunctional aziridine. Contact Dermatitis 1995;33:304.

177. Kanerva L, Grenquist-Norden B, Piirila P. Occupational IgE mediated contact urticaria from diphenylmethane-4,4-diisopcyanate (MDI). Contact Dermatitis 1999;41:50.

178. Suguira K, Sugiura M, Shiraki R, et al. Contact urticaria due to polyethylene gloves. Contact Dermatitis 2002;46:262.

179. Niinimaki A, Niinimaki M, Makinen-Kiljanen S, Hannuksela M. Contact urticaria from protein hydrolysates in hair conditioners. Allergy 1998;53:1078.

180. Pasche-Koo F, Claeys M, Hauser C. Contact urticaria with systemic symptoms caused by bovine collagen in a hair conditioner. Am J Contact Dermat 1996;7:56.

181. Tanaka T, Miyachi Y, Horio T. Ulcerative contact dermatitis caused by sodium silicate: co-existence of primary irritant contact dermatitis and contact urticaria. Arch Dermatol 1982;118:518.

182. Altman AT. Facial dermatitis (xylene). Arch Dermatol 1977;113:1443.

183. Palmer KT, Rycroft RJG. Occupational airborne contact urticaria due to xylene. Contact Dermatitis 1993;28:44.

184. Weiss R, Mowad C. Contact urticaria from xylene. Am J Contact Dermat 1998;9:125.

185. Mader R, Fowler J. Contact allergy to an organic solvent: immediate sensitivity and a serum sickness-like reaction. Am J Contact Dermat 1995;6:32.

186. Varigos GA, Nurse DS. Contact urticaria from methyl ethyl ketone. Contact Dermatitis 1986;15:259.

187. Fowler JF. Contact urticaria to 1,1,1-tricholoroethane. Am J Contact Dermat 1991;2:239.

188. Hausen B. Woods injurious to human health—a manual. New York: Walter de Gruyter, 1981.

189. Garces-Sotillos M, Blanco-Carmona J, Juste-Picon S, et al. Occupational asthma and contact urticaria caused by mukali wood dust. J Investig Allergol Clin Immunol 1995;5:113.

190. Calnan CD. Allergy to dog saliva. Contact Dermatitis Newsletter 1968;3:41.

191. Burrows D. Urticaria from rats. Contact Dermatitis 1979;5:122.

192. Rudzki E, Grzywa A. Two types of contact urticaria and immediate reactions to patch test allergens. Dermatologica 1978;157:110.

193. Uehara M, Ofuji S. Patch test reactions to human dander in atopic dermatitis. Arch Dermatol 1976;112:951.

194. Halpern BN, Ky T, Robert B. Clinical and immunological study of an exceptional case of reaginic type sensitization to human seminal fluid. Immunology 1967;12:247.

195. Schultz KH, Schirren C, Kuepper I. Allergy to seminal fluid. N Engl J Med 1974;260:916.

196. Mikkelsen EJ, Henderson LL, Leiferman KM, et al. Allergy to human seminal fluid. Ann Allergy 1975;34:239.

197. Mathias CGT, Frick OL, Caldwell TM, et al. Immediate hypersensitivity to seminal fluid and atopic dermatitis. Arch Dermatol 1980;116:209.

198. Kanerva L, Toikkanen J, Jolanki R, Estlander T. Statistical data on occupational contact urticaria. Contact Dermatitis 1996;35:229.

199. Degreef H. Protein contact dermatitis with positive RAST tests to fresh bovine blood and amniotic fluid in a veterinary surgeon. 6th International Symposium on Contact Dermatitis and Joint Meeting between ICRG and JCDRG. Tokyo, 21–22 May 1982.

200. Schmidt H. Contact urticaria. Contact Dermatitis 1978;4:230.

201. Hartmann KR, Calton GJ, Burnett JW. Use of the radioallergosorbent test for the study of coelenterate toxin-specific immunoglobulin E. Int Arch Allergy Appl Immunol 1980;61:389.

202. Zschunke E. Contact urticaria, dermatitis and asthma from cockroaches. Contact Dermatitis 1978;4:313.

203. Galindo P, Melero R, Garcia R, et al. Contact urticaria from chironomids. Contact Dermatitis 1996;34:297.

204. Astarita C, Di-Martino P, Scala G, et al. Contact allergy: another occupational risk to Tetranychus urticae. J Allergy Clin Immunol 1996;98:732.

205. Vega J, Vega JM, Moneo I, et al. Occupational immunologic contact urticaria from pine processionary caterpillar (Thaumatopoea pityocampa). Contact Dermatitis 2004;50:60.

206. Rudzki E. Contact urticaria from silk. Contact Dermatitis 1977;3:53.

207. Urbach E, Gottlieb PM. Allergy. New York: Grune & Stratton, 1946.

208. Sheldon JM, Lovell RG, Mathews KP. A manual of clinical allergy. Philadelphia: WB Saunders, 1953.

209. Hambly EM, Levia L, Wilkinson DS. Wool intolerance in atopic subjects. Contact Dermatitis 1978;4:240.

210. McDaniel WR, Marks JG. Contact urticaria due to sensitivity to spray starch. Arch Dermatol 1979;115:628.

211. Helander I. Contact urticaria from leather containing formaldehyde. Arch Dermatol 1977;113:1443.

212. Dooms-Goossens A, et al. Contact urticaria due to nylon. Contact Dermatitis 1986;14:63.

213. DeGroot AC, Gerkens F. Contact urticaria from a chemical textile finish. Contact Dermatitis 1989;20:63.

214. Dice J: Physical urticaria: Immunol Allergy Clin North Am 2004;24:225.

215. Monfrecola G, Masturzo E, Riccardo A, et al. Solar urticaria: A report on 57 cases. Am J Contact Dermat 2000;11:89.

216. Greaves MM. Pharmacologic basis of aquagenic urticaria. Report of Annual Meeting of the European Society for Dermatologic Research. Amsterdam Skin Allergy News 1980;11:3.

217. Bernhard J. Nonrashes: Atmoknesis: pruritus provoked by contact with air. Cutis 1989;44:143.

218. Rothenborg HW, Menne T, Sjølin KE. Temperature dependent primary irritant dermatitis from lemon perfume. Contact Dermatitis 1977;3:37.

219. Skinner S, Fowler JF. Contact anaphylaxis. Am J Contact Dermat 1995;6:133.

220. Calnan CD, Shuster S. Reactions to ammonium persulfate. Arch Dermatol 1968;88:812.

221. Fisher AA, Dooms-Goossens A. Persulfate hair bleach reactions. Arch Dermatol 1976;112:1407.

222. Brun R, Jadassohn W, Paillard R. Epicutaneous test with immediate type reaction to ammonium persulfate. Dermatologica 1966;133:89.

223. Johansson J, Lahti A. Topical non-steroidal anti-inflammatory drugs inhibit nonimmunologic immediate contact reaction. Contact Dermatitis 1988;19:161.

224. Katsarou A, Armenaka M, Ale I, et al. Frequency of immediate reactions to the European standard series. Contact Dermatitis 1999;41:276.†Can also produce allergic contact urticaria.

METALS

EXECUTIVE SUMMARY

As a group, metals are the most common contact allergens. Nickel is the most common cause of metal allergy, and in most series ranks as the most common of all screening allergens.[1] Reactions to gold, chrome, cobalt, and organic forms of mercury are also frequently seen. Most other metals can cause some form of skin reaction, such as allergic or irritant dermatitis.[1] Allergic sensitivity to a metal is usually highly specific, but cross-sensitivity with other metals is common in certain instances. Nickel and palladium are good examples of apparent crossreactivity. Many reports of crossreactions between metals are actually co-reactions, which occur because of simultaneous exposure to two or more metals. This is particularly the case with cobalt, nickel, and chromium. For example, cement, which is a common cause of chromate allergy, also contains cobalt, which may contribute to allergic contact dermatitis (ACD) from cement.

ACD to metal generally occurs only if the metal salts are in solution, as occurs with perspiration or exposure with bodily fluids. It is, not unusual for individuals who show marked allergic contact sensitivity to gold on patch testing to be able to enjoy wearing gold jewelry without difficulty, for example. Similarly, contact with stainless steel containing nickel usually does not produce nickel dermatitis in a nickel-sensitive individual, because the alloy binds the nickel so firmly that sweat cannot liberate nickel salts. In most cases, however, if exposure is intense enough and long enough, eventually allergen will penetrate the stratum corneum and ACD will occur.

In addition to direct skin contact with metals, dermatitis from metal allergy may manifest itself due to ingestion or implantation of metals. Systemic contact dermatitis from dietary nickel intake is well recognized. The classic manifestation is a dyshidrosiform hand eczema, but dermatitis in any location can occur. Dental metal allergy may cause oral lichenoid lesions, indistinguishable from idiopathic lichen planus. Metals in orthopedic implants may cause dermatitis and/or joint complications. Metals in endovascular stents may lead to skin changes and possibly to stent restenosis. These topics are more fully considered in chapters 8, 19, and 31.

In addition to ACD, metals may cause many other dermatologic reactions. Irritant contact dermatitis (ICD) is common in workers exposed to metal salts, dusts, and fumes. Contact urticaria has been reported. Cutaneous granuloma formation seems to be fairly common if heavy metals like gold or palladium penetrate the skin.

Patch testing with metals is usually straightforward, at least with common metal allergens. With less common metals, salts are used and irritant reactions are not unusual. All metal allergens may give false positive pustular reactions, especially when tested in atopics or on dermatitic skin. Two common metal allergens produce patch test reactions of note. Cobalt usually produces a non-allergic "poral" reaction due to toxicity to the acrosyringium. Gold may produce long-lasting reactions that may take several months to recede. Lymphocyte testing for metal allergy has been studied. Unfortunately, non-specific reactions seem to be very common and correlation of "positive" tests with clinical findings is sorely lacking. Currently, patch testing remains the "gold standard" for diagnosis of metal allergy.

Overview of Metal Allergy

The latest data from the North American Contact Dermatitis Group (NACDG) show that nickel was positive in 18.7% of patients tested over a 2-year period, ranking first overall, gold (8.7%), cobalt (8.4%), and chromate (4.3%) ranked seventh, eighth, and thirteenth in overall prevalence.[2] Thimerosal was positive at a rate of about 11% previously, but is no longer tested routinely by the NACDG because of lack of relevance. Children, as well as adults, are commonly sensitized by metals. Analysis of recent NACDG data showed that of 391 patients under the age of 18, 28% reacted to nickel, 18% to cobalt, and 15% to thimerosal.[3]

Body piercing has been directly correlated with development of nickel allergy, and likely to other jewelry metals. Larsson-Stymne and Windstrom[4] found that 13% of 960 schoolgirls age 8 to 15 with pierced ears were nickel allergic, whereas only 1% of those without pierced ears were allergic. Ehrlich and colleagues tested 118 males to nickel, gold, cobalt, and palladium and assessed number of piercings.[5] Reactions to one or more metals were seen in 4% of unpierced, 3 of 27 (11%) with one piercing, and 6 of 41 (15%) with multiple piercings. A large study by the NACDG is underway to look at this in more detail.

Kanerva and colleagues have discussed occupational ACD from metals. Among over 2,500 cases of occupational ACD seen throughout 6 years, chromate caused 143 (5.6%) cases, nickel 176 (6.9%) and cobalt 41 (1.6%). Other metals were not considered. In their population, nickel occupational ACD was more common in women, while the others were more common in males.[6]

The paper by Ruff and Belsito points out a number of patient factors relating to metal allergy.[7] They reviewed 208 patients who were allergic to at least one metal, with 69 allergic to more than one. Of 156 allergic to nickel, 78% were female. With cobalt, 72% were female and with chromate 60% were male. Of those allergic to cobalt, 63% were also allergic to nickel while 38% of the chromate-allergic were allergic to nickel. They found a relatively high number of chromate allergic to be occupationally related. Overall there was a tendency for more metal-allergic patients to be atopic than those in their overall population. This has not necessarily been seen in other studies.

Table 32.1 summarizes the various reactions to metals.

Plated Metals

So-called plated metals consist of electrodeposited metallic coatings embracing various metals and alloys with widely varying physical and chemical properties.[8] The metals range in hardness from soft materials, such as lead and tin, to those as hard as nickel and chromium. Chemically, these substances range in reactivity from electronegative (anodic) metals, such as zinc and cadmium, to the relatively inert nodal metals, exemplified by gold and platinum. In color, electrodeposited coatings vary from the white of zinc, cadmium, and silver, through the yellows of brass, and the greens and reds of the gold alloys, to the black of platinum black and black nickel. Liden and colleagues[9] tested a number of nickel-containing alloys.

Table 32-1 Reactions to Metals
Miscellaneous reactions
Metal fume fever—cadmium and zinc
Metallic dust and moisture folliculitis—antimony spots
Smelters itch—arsenic trioxide
Coin rubbing dermatitis (çao-gio)
Zinc "pox"
Baboon syndrome
Primary irritant dermatitis and chemical "burns"
Allergic contact dermatitis
Systemic contact dermatitis
Granulomas
Erythema multiforme
Platinosis (respiratory allergy)
Pompholyx
Tattoo granulomas
Urticaria
Photosensitization dermatitis
Cadmium sulfide in tattoos
Chromates
Cobalt
Pigmentation and discoloration
Accidental tattoos
Argyria (silver)
Black dermographism
Chrysiasis
Hair: copper (green), cobalt (white), and silver (black)
Iron siderosis, endogenous or exogenous
Nails: mercury, lead, silver, and chromate
Rusting
Lichen planus

Many alloys and nickel liners under gold, silver, or chrome plating gave positive reactions in test subjects. This confirms that plating will not prevent nickel allergy in most cases.

Small, inexpensive metallic items, such as buttons, zippers, and other cheap fasteners, generally are simply nickel-plated. Metallic watch bands most costume jewelry may be flashed with bright chromium (or some other electrodeposit, e.g., gold, silver, or rhodium) after nickel-plating. In general, the thin deposits of chromium and other metals over the nickel are not continuous but contain many microscopic discontinuities, sometimes referred to as pinholes or pores. The nickel in a chrome-plated object, for example, may come through the pinholes of the plated object after being dissolved out by sweat and produce dermatitis in individuals with allergic hypersensitivity to nickel. The extent to which the underlying nickel may be attacked by sweat will, of course, depend on the degree of porosity of the overlying metal coating. Accordingly, one cannot assume that the underlying nickel will not come through a chrome-plated object, even though it appears not to have been worn off.

Except for industrial plating, in which the chrome coating is used because of its own unique mechanical and chemical properties, chrome-plated objects generally carry a much thicker deposit of nickel than of chromium, the ratio generally being at least 100:1. Nickel-plated objects are pinkish white, whereas chrome plating imparts a bluish white color (Figure 32-1).

Stainless Steel

The dermatologist, the allergist, and often the orthopedic surgeon are concerned with stainless steel because it may contain sensitizing metals, such as chromium, nickel, cobalt, molybdenum, and other trace metals.

Stainless steel is an iron-based alloy usually containing at least 12% chromium. Basically, the chromium content imparts the stainless property. The addition of nickel is said to create a hard, smooth surface, which increases resistance to corrosion, wear, and abrasion. Some stainless steels contain as much as 26% chromium; others contain as much as 37% nickel. (see chapter 19.)

Various other ingredients may be added, such as molybdenum, magnesium, silicon, carbon, phosphorus, cobalt, and sulfur. The molybdenum helps prevent pitting by body chlorides.

The term "solid solution" as applied to stainless steel means that an element is dispersed homogeneously and is not a separate phase, such as a precipitant. When stainless steel is manufactured, all the metals are contained in a solution at a temperature of 2,400°C. As it cools, a crystalline lattice is formed, which locks in the various metals. Stainless steel manufacturers may claim that nickel, chrome, and other metals are bound so tightly in the alloy that they can't leach out in sufficient quantity to cause allergy. In instances of casual, brief contact this may be true. However, under continuous contact with the skin along with perspiration or in an implant or in a piercing, enough of the metal can escape to cause ACD in sensitized persons.

Liden and colleagues[10] showed that 27% of 565 metal hand tools available in Sweden released significant nickel as measured by the dimethylglyoxine test.

Corroded steel may show pit marks, which may be produced by acids and sodium chloride. Rust may be formed when there is high humidity in the presence of salt.

Metals in Soap and Detergents

Ingber and colleagues[11] have shown that detergents and bleaches may be significant sources of chromium exposure. Of 38 detergents and surface cleaners and 12 bleaches, 90% of patients had over 1 ppm of chromium and 56% had over 7 ppm of chromium. Irritant effects from the cleaners may potentiate ACD from the low level of chromium. Palmolive dish washing liquid (Colgate-Palmolive, United States) was the highest, at 546 ppm.[11]

Several European studies have stressed that nickel and chromium present in detergents are factors in the production of dermatitis, particularly hand eczemas, in individuals sensitized to these metals. Nickel was found in amounts as great as 9 mg/kg in Dutch phosphate-containing detergents.[12] In order to eliminate nickel-sensitization from detergents, ethylenediamine tetra-acetate (EDTA) was added during manufacture, because the nickel-EDTA complex has no sensitizing properties.[13] The Dutch investigators concluded that nickel in detergents plays a minor role in nickel dermatitis. A Spanish report, however, concluded that the amount of nickel and chromium in detergents is sufficient to account for the persistence of contact dermatitis due to these metals after the more obvious contacts have been eliminated.[14] In a later report, also from Spain, 30 domestic detergents and cleaners were analyzed for cobalt and nickel. Of these, 78.6% showed "considerable" amounts of cobalt, and most also contained nickel. Whether the levels were high enough to cause ACD is uncertain.[15]

More recently Basketter and colleagues reported that European cleaning products they tested had levels of metals at or below 1 ppm.[16] The source of nickel in detergent compounds is the raw materials used in the manufacturing process, and the most likely source of chromates in trace quantities is phosphate.

Considering the fact that detergents and other cleaners are diluted in use, it seems unlikely to this author that these materials will be a major factor in the production of metal ACD. A study by the NACDG with a laundry detergent seems to confirm this (see Chapter 18.)

Metal Salts in Cosmetics

The following metallic salts are permitted color additives, according to the US Food, Drug, and Cosmetic Act regulations:

- Iron oxide—brownish yellow and ochre
- Chlorophyllin copper complex—green
- Chromium oxides—olive and bluish green
- Cobalt blue—blue
- Lapis lazuli—reddish blue
- Ultramarine blue—reddish blue
- Manganese violet—violet
- Potassium ferrocyanide—yellow solution

Nickel may also be present in cosmetics as a contaminant. Because the facial, and especially the eyelid, skin is very sensitive, it would seem possible that metals in cosmetics could cause ACD there in very sensitive individuals. Fowler has seen patients with strong nickel sensitivity who seem to have reactions from some cosmetics, especially eye make-ups, even though nickel is never listed on ingredient labeling. Chromium allergy is usually due to hexavalent chromate, but trivalent chromium may cause allergy occasionally. Skin that is already dermatitic is at greater risk for further sensitization.

Zugerman[17] reported a case of eyelid dermatitis due to yellow iron oxide. Considering the vast usage of color cosmetics, reactions to the coloring agents seem to be rare.

Metal Salts in Hair Dyes

Hair dyeing with metallic dyes is incompatible with permanent waving and coloring with the oxidation type of dyes. The great popularity of such hair treatment has noticeably curtailed the use of the metallic dyes by women. Large quantities of all types of metallic dyes, however, are still used by men. In the United States, the most popular metallic dyes are lead, silver, and copper. Allergic reaction or argyria rarely occurs from the use of metallic silver hair dyes. In other countries, cobalt and manganese may be used as hair dyes.

The US Food, Drug, and Cosmetic Act imposes no restriction on the use of metallic hair dyes, because such products are generally considered harmless to the intact skin. Metallic dyes may be absorbed through abrasions, however, and produce toxic effects. Men who use metallic color restorers on mustaches should be warned about the danger of accidental ingestion.

Allergic reactions to metallic hair dyes are rare. In this sense, they are much safer than the oxidation-type dyes.

Metal Salts in Tattoos

Allergic reactions to metal salts used for tattooing are not infrequent. Mercury, chromium, cobalt, and cadmium have been reported as producing various types of reactions in tattooed areas in sensitized individuals.[18]

The salts of tattoo metals that may have an allergic effect and the corresponding colors are as follows: (a) red—mercury sulfide (cinnabar and vermilion), (b) green—chromium and chromic oxide, (c) blue—cobalt aluminate, iron and (d) yellow—cadmium (e) black—iron, zinc, cobalt, nickel.

MERCURY

In the form of red cinnabar in a tattoo, mercury may produce itching, swelling, and eczematous and granulomatous reactions in sensitized individuals. Often the red tattooed areas are quiescent for many years, then suddenly an acute allergic reaction occurs. In one instance, the red portions of a tattoo began to itch and swell following intradermal injections of a vaccine containing thimerosal, a complex organic mercurial compound used as a preservative.[19] In another instance, Fisher observed an itchy swelling of the red areas in an individual who ingested calomel (mercurous chloride) and who showed a positive patch test reaction to ammoniated mercury and Mercurochrome. A generalized eczematous eruption may result from laceration of a tattoo in a mercury-sensitive patient.[20] Aside from mercury sulfide, nonmetallic red colors in tattoos include an organic pigment (scarlet lake), carmine (dried insect bodies), cochinilla, and cadmium red (selenide).

CHROMIUM

Chromium oxide powder is one of the principal green dyes used in tattooing. This powder is known as chrome green or Casalic green, and it is very stable, resistant to acids, and insoluble in water, alcohol, and acetone. Guignet's green is a closely related green pigment that contains a mixture of hydrous chromium oxides. Lowenthal[21] cited a case of persistent eczema of the extremities that did not clear until five green areas were excised from a tattoo on the arm. Apparently, these chrome particles may lie latent in tattoos for 20 years or more, then suddenly produce an allergic eczematous dermatitis.

Chromium sesquioxide (viridian), emerald green, may also be used in tattoos. In addition, chlorinated copper (phthalocyanine) may be employed in green tattoos.

COBALT

In the form of cobalt blue (azure blue and cobaltous aluminate), cobalt has been reported as causing a sarcoidal allergic reaction in areas in which it was used as a light blue tattoo pigment.[22] A patch test with cobalt evoked a positive reaction, and cobalt was also demonstrated in the pathologically altered parts of the tattoo. A tattoo test with cobalt blue elicited an inflammatory tissue reaction. In some blue tattoos copper phthalocyanine may be used. Indigo is occasionally added.

CADMIUM

This substance, in the form of cadmium sulfide, is sometimes used as a yellow pigment in tattoos, and these areas may itch and swell on exposure to sunlight. Experimental areas tattooed with cadmium sulfide showed an edematous reaction only when exposed to light of 3,800, 4,000, and 4,500 Å wavelengths.[23] The swelling reaction to cadmium sulfide in yellow tattoos seems to be phototoxic. Occasionally, commercial red tattoo pigment shows traces of cadmium sulfide, which may induce a photosensitive reaction after exposure to sun.[24] Aside from cadmium sulfide in yellow tattoos, chrome zinc and lemon yellow (chrome salts) may be present. Yellow ochre (hydrate of ferric oxide) may be added.

In one patient a reaction to a red tattoo was not caused by mercury or cadmium but to an azo dye in the tattoo.[25]

Scutt and Gotch[26] list other tattoo colors that may or may not contain metals.

Black:

1. Logwood (containing chrome)
2. Black waterproof ink (containing charcoal suspended in ammoniacal solution containing phenol)

Brown:

1. Venetian red (hydrate of ferric oxide)
2. Cadmium salts

White:

1. Titanium or zinc oxide
2. Lead carbonate (flake white)

Purple:

1. Manganese

Nguyen and Allen[27] attributed itching in a purple tattoo to manganese, but they did not patch test the patient. Scutt and Gotch[26] warn that tattoos occasionally become inflamed and pruritic, only to clear without any therapy.

SARCOIDAL TATTOO REACTIONS

Rubianes and Sánchez[28] reported one case of a woman who developed a granulomatous response to iron oxide used for cosmetic permanent eyebrow tattooing. The reaction developed 4 weeks after the implantation. Systemic corticosteroids were required to clear the reaction. Another report described a patient with a sarcoidal reaction to the black, but not blue, portion of a tattoo.[29] Patch tests were positive to nickel, cobalt, and cadmium. The black pigment, analyzed by spectrophotometry, contained iron, zinc, cobalt, and nickel.

Action of Sodium Chloride and Sweat on Metals

A ring dermatitis due to primary irritation from the action of salt on jewelry alloys may be produced. The sodium chloride acting on the metal may come from sweat or from table salt that has become trapped between the ring and the finger. The salt discolors and corrodes the metal, which may produce a primary irritant dermatitis.

It is likely that, in most cases, dissolution of metal in sweat or other liquids is important before clinical allergic manifestations will develop. A discussion of metals, alloys, and relationship to sweating has been published.[30]

In addition, a greenish black smudge due to sulfur in the sweat of some people may be produced with all types of metallic jewelry. These persons should remove rings frequently and powder their fingers with an absorbent powder that is free of zinc oxide to prevent both black dermographism and sulfide discoloration. Many individuals sensitized to nickel or gold acquire contact dermatitis from such metallic objects only when they perspire freely, thus showing the importance of the leaching action of sweat.

RELATIONSHIP OF SWEAT TO "RUSTING"

A "ruster" is an individual who produces a corrosive effect by fingering a freshly polished metallic surface. Abnormally high concentrations of chloride ion in sweat are responsible for these adverse effects.[31] Although patients with cystic fibrosis may sweat profusely, there is no direct evidence that "rusters" have the disease.

The main problem occurs in workers in the precision engineering industry. Burton and colleagues[32] pointed out that experienced workers in the precision engineering industry recognize that some people secrete sweat that readily corrodes metal. Polished metal surfaces touched by these persons will show rusty fingerprints within a few days, causing unsightly blemishes on the metal. The rust can cause the malfunction of complex small components, such as the tumblers of locks and equipment used in the electronic industry. The following measures may enable the "ruster" to continue his or her work: (a) keeping as cool as possible by wearing light clothing; (b) remaining on a low-salt diet; (c) washing the hands frequently to remove sodium chloride from the surface of the skin; (d) removing sweat from the metal immediately after it is handled, because rusting begins quickly; and (e) using Drysol, aluminum chloride in alcohol, to help reduce palmar and finger sweating.[33]

Metals in Coins

Coins contain other metals beside the metal from which they take their names.

The US Coinage Act, passed 23 July 1965, changed the composition of the dime, quarter, and half dollar. These denominations formerly contained 90% silver and 10% copper. The nickel, dime and quarter are manufactured from strips composed of three layers of metal bonded together and rolled to the required thickness. This is called cladding. The face is 75% copper and 25% nickel, and the core of the dime and quarter is pure copper, which is visible on the edges of the coins. Pennies are made of copper-plated zinc.

For students of numismatics and handlers of old coins who may be nickel-sensitive, it is of interest that nickel is present in the following US coins: (a) Flying Indian Head cent series, 1856 to 1864; (b) three-cent pieces, 1865 to 1888; (c) five-cent nickels, 1866 to date, except for those issued from 1942 to 1945.

Liden reported that nickel is easily released from Euro coins in artificial sweat within 2 minutes.[34] All denominations of Euro coinage contains high amounts of copper. The 1 and 2 Euro coins also contain about 25% nickel, while the smaller coins contain iron, aluminum, zinc, and/or tin.

METAL DERMATITIS FROM COINS

Nickel dermatitis of the hands from normal handling of nickel coins rarely occurs because of inadequate exposure and the protection of the thick, horny layer of the palm. Fisher has observed two patients, however, with nickel dermatitis of the fingers due to unusual circumstances. One patient habitually carried coins in the finger portion of her glove; the other rubbed her nose with coins, producing dermatitis not only of the fingers but also of the side of the nose that resembled seborrheic eczema. Both sites cleared promptly when contact with nickel coins was avoided.

Experimentally, when nickel coins were kept on the palms under occlusion for 24 hours, allergic dermatitis did occur in two nickel-sensitive individuals that Fisher tested.

Bang Pedersen and colleagues[35] found that much more nickel was released from coins in water and synthetic sweat than from nickel-plated metal. This indicates that silver-colored coins may be a more relevant source of allergen in everyday life than plated objects, apart from those objects that are in more or less permanent contact with the skin, such as zippers and earrings. It is thus possible that the contamination of the hands, as found in this study, is sufficient to maintain an already established eczema from nickel.

Historically, some practitioners have used coins for patch testing patients for nickel allergy. Patch testing with nickel coins is not a substitute for testing with a standard allergen preparation and should not be used for routine diagnosis. It may be of some educational value to the patient.

"THERAPEUTIC" COIN-RUBBING DERMATITIS (ÇAO GIO)

Yeatman and van Dang[36] report that coin rubbing (çao gio) is the Vietnamese practice of rubbing the skin with a coin to alleviate various common symptoms of illness. The back, neck, head, shoulders, and chest are common sites of application. Although mimicking the lesions of trauma, it is not a harmful procedure. The back and chest are massaged with a medicated substance, such as mentholated ointment or oil. Firm downward strokes with a coin, comb, or spoon over the spine and ribs produce petechiae and ecchymoses. For headache, the head is massaged in a temporofrontal direction, and the skin between the eyebrows is pinched until reddened. For cough, nausea, and vomiting, the neck and chest are preferred sites, and the sternomastoid muscle is compressed at the point of its insertion into the sternum. At first appearance, the patient may appear to be a "battered" or abused child.[37–39] Yeatman and van Dang[36] believe that when treating Vietnamese patients, the physician should discuss the practice of çao gio in neutral, if not favorable, terms. The patient or parent may initially deny the practice. Better understanding and acceptance by the physician, however, should improve rapport, compliance, and subsequent appointment keeping.

Tan[40] stated that coin rubbing is also popular in Indonesia as part of traditional medicine and is known under several names, including kerok and kerik. Coin rubbing has a definite connection with China and is practiced frequently by the Chinese and those of Chinese ancestry, especially among the older generations.

Coconut oil or cajuput oil is usually used as a skin lubricant and is applied most often to the back and the neck and less frequently to the chest. The oil is used as a home remedy for children as well as adults. The darker the color of the oil and the more ecchymoses that develop as a result of this rubbing, supposedly the greater the extent of the patient's cold.

RELATIONSHIP BETWEEN COBALT, NICKEL, AND OTHER METAL ALLERGIES

Kranke and Aberer[41] analyzed positive patch test reactions to metal in 11,516 patients. Their results are shown in Table 32.2. The most striking findings were that 95% of those allergic to palladium also reacted to nickel and that 79% of cobalt-allergic patients reacted to nickel.

Table 32-2 Metal Co-Reactivity

(Percentage of patients allergic to other metals of those positive to the metal listed in the top line)

	Nickel	Cobalt	Palladium	Chromate
Nickel	—	78.9%	94.6%	39.6%
Cobalt	23.4%	—	36.2%	31.3%
Palladium	33.0%	42.5%	—	NS
Chromate	5.5%	14.7%	NS	—

NS, Not stated Adapted from Kranke and Aberer, Ref. 41.

In England, studies of chromate-sensitive patients in two different time periods showed that 41% and 34% of patients in the two groups also reacted to cobalt.[42] The authors postulated that cosensitization to these two metals often results from cement exposure.

Rystedt[42] concluded that nickel sensitivity, in combination with irritant eczema, induces a high risk of developing cobalt allergy. From her investigation, it is not possible to conclude which are the primary and secondary events, but most facts indicate that nickel sensitivity followed by irritant dermatitis of the hands appears first, and that cobalt sensitivity is a secondary phenomenon. It is possible that a pre-existent nickel allergy increases the risk of developing cobalt allergy, because of the high frequency of hand eczema among nickel-sensitive individuals. The cobalt allergy then seems to aggravate the hand eczema. All the hard-metal workers in Rystedt's study with simultaneous nickel and cobalt sensitivity had severe dermatitis of the hands. Eight hundred fifty-three hard-metal workers were examined and patch tested. Nickel sensitivity was found in 2 men and 38 women. Eighty-eight percent of the nickel-sensitive individuals had developed a jewelry dermatitis before use in the hard-metal industry or before the appearance of hand eczema. Twenty-nine percent of the hard-metal workers gave a history of irritant dermatitis. In the nickel-sensitized group, 40% had had severe hand eczema that generally appeared 6 to 12 months after starting employment. In 25% of the cases, nickel-sensitive individuals developed cobalt allergy, compared with 5% in the total population investigated.

The relationship of cobalt and nickel allergy was also studied by Lammintausta and colleagues.[43] An increase in positive patch tests to either metal was found in guinea pigs sensitized to both metals as compared to those sensitized with only one. For example, 4 of 13 sensitized only to nickel later had positive patch tests to nickel, whereas 7 of 13 that were first sensitized to cobalt and then to nickel later reacted to nickel.

Most individuals that react to palladium on patch tests also react to nickel. This is discussed in the section on palladium below.

Patch Tests with Metals and Their Salts

Table 32.3 lists the concentrations of metal salts recommended for patch test purposes.

Table 32-3 Suggested Patch Test Concentrations for Metals

Aluminum (Al)	Aluminum chl	2%
Arsenic (As)	Sodium arsenate	10% aq
Beryllium (Be)	Beryllium chl	1%
Cadmium (Ca)	Cadmium chl	0.5%
Chrome (Cr)	Pot. dichromate	0.25% USA
		0.5% other
Cobalt (Co)	Cobalt chl	1%
Copper (Cu)	Copper sulfate	2%
Gallium (Ga)	Gallium oxide	1%
Gold (Au)	Gold sodium thiosulfate	0.5%
Indium (In)	Indium chl	1%
	Indium sulfate	10%
Iridium (Ir)	Iridium chl	1%
Iron (Fe)	Ferric chl	2%
	Ferrous sulfate	5%
	Red iron oxide	2%
	Yellow iron oxide	2% aq
Lead (Pb)	Lead acetate	0.5% aq
	Lead chl	0.2% aq
Manganese (Mn)	Manganese chl	5%
Mercury (Hg)	Mercury (metal)	0.5%
	Thimerosal	0.1%
	Amm mercury	1%
	Mercuric chl	0.01% aq
Molybdenum (Mo)	Amm heptamolybdate	1% aq
Nickel (Ni)	Nickel sulfate	2.5% USA
		5% other
Palladium (Pd)	Palladium chl	1%
Platinum (Pt)	Amm tetrachlorplatinate	0.25% aq
	Amm hexachloroplatinate	0.1% aq
Rhodium (Rh)	Rhodium sulfate	2%
Rubidium (Rb)	Rubidium iodide	1%
Ruthenium (Ru)	Ruthenium metal	0.1%
Selenium (Se)	Sodium selenium oxide	0.1% aq
Silver (Ag)	Silver, colloidal	0.1%
	Silver nitrate	1% aq
Tantallum (Ta)	Tantallum metal	1%
Tin (Sn)	Tin chl	0.5%
Titanium (Ti)	Titanium oxalate	1% aq
	Titanium oxide	0.1%
	Titanium dioxide	10%
	Amm titanium lactate	10%
Uranium (U)	Sodium uranate	2%
Vanadium (Va)	Vanadium pentoxide	10%
Zinc (Zn)	Zinc sulfate	2%
	Zinc chl	1%
	Zinc metal	1%
	Zinc pyrithione	1%
Zirconium (Zr)	Zirconium oxide	0.1%

All allergens in petrolatum unless otherwise noted.

In performing patch tests with metal salts, one must be careful not to interpret the pustular or follicular patch test reactions as allergic responses. Such reactions are not uncommon and should be considered as a nonspecific, irritant response.

A number of metal salts are now available commercially for patch testing (Table 32.3). If testing with non-standardized materials, it may be more convenient to test in water rather than petrolatum. False-positive reactions may be more likely than with standardized allergens.

NEGATIVE PATCH TEST REACTION IN SUSPECTED METAL DERMATITIS

Occasionally a person may have a true allergy but show a negative response on patch testing. This occurs with any allergen, not just metals. In such a case, repeat testing may often give the correct answer. However, with metal allergy, there may be other reasons for true negative findings. Nickel is such a common allergen that many dermatologists and patients alike suspect it whenever metal allergy seems likely from a clinical standpoint. For example, many women in Dr. Fisher's time were suspected of having nickel dermatitis because of an eruption in the garter area presumably due to a nickel-plated garter buckle or clasp. In several instances, a negative nickel test result was obtained, and further investigation revealed that the dermatitis was actually due to sensitivity to the rubber of the garter.

Whenever nickel sensitivity is suspected but not confirmed by a positive patch test reaction, one must make certain that some other substance is not the cause of the dermatitis. Cobalt, palladium, and gold especially may cause jewelry dermatitis, even in the absence of nickel allergy.

Some discordance in patch test reactivity is well known and is referred to by Rietschel as the "twinkling back" syndrome. Simonetti and colleagues[44] found a fairly high discordance with nickel sulfate (5% pet) in 612 consecutive patients. They tested allergens from two different suppliers and found that only 78% of patients reacted to both allergens, with almost equal numbers reacting to only one or the other test material. This illustrates the variability among patch test materials.

Seidenari and colleagues[45] studied 58 women with a history of nickel allergy but negative screening tests. On repeat testing, 6 (10%) exhibited a positive reaction, but 19 (21%) developed a positive reaction when the test site was occluded for one day before testing with an empty Finn chamber. Also, pretreatment of the test site with the surfactant sodium lauryl sulfate increased the number of positive reactions.[46]

In contrast, the addition of a commercial detergent to nickel patch test materials in petrolatum did not significantly increase the test sensitivity.[47]

FALSE-POSITIVE METAL PATCH TEST RESULTS

On several occasions Fisher has observed that if metal salts are tested close to each other, a strong positive patch test reaction to nickel will be accompanied by false-positive patch test reactions to the adjacent metal salts, particularly cobalt and copper. These same cobalt and copper salts may show a negative reaction when tested at least 6 inches from the nickel patch test site. Apparently, a strong positive nickel reaction creates a nonspecific hypersensitivity of the surrounding skin and induces false-positive reactions to the other metals.

INTRADERMAL TESTING WITH METAL SALTS

Meneghini and Angelini[48] studied a group of patients with clinically evident contact dermatitis and with a history suggestive of contact with metals (patch test reactions to metals were negative). The positive reactions obtained in several cases suggested that intradermal tests may reveal specific sensitivities, which patch tests using standard concentrations are not always capable of demonstrating. The authors claimed that the results of this study confirm that, in certain special situations and with easily soluble chemicals not irritant to the tissues, intradermal tests may demonstrate specific sensitivities that cannot be revealed by patch tests employing technically suitable concentrations. A more likely explanation for their findings may have been the aforementioned "twinkling back" syndrome or may have been due to inadequate patch test allergens.

Marcussen[49] compared the diagnostic value of the patch and intradermal tests with particular reference to nickel hypersensitivity and concluded that the intradermal test with nickel sulfate, 1:10,000, appeared to be more sensitive and more specific than a patch test using 5% nickel sulfate. Marcussen also found that intradermal testing improves the diagnostic results in nickel allergy by approximately 14%. Marcussen, however, admitted that there was a closer conformity than expected with nickel sulfate, 1:10,000, and with patch tests with 5% nickel sulfate. He further stated that five nickel-sensitive patients showed negative patch test reactions and positive intradermal reactions with nickel sulfate, but four of these patients showed positive patch test reactions when they were retested.

Möller[50] also believes intradermal testing may be of occasional value, especially in cases of uncertain patch test reactions. He reviewed 49 patients with 78 equivocal reactions to chromate, cobalt, and/or nickel. Positive tests at 72 hours were seen in 24 of the 78 injections. Among 10 other patients suspected of metal allergy by history but with negative patch tests, only 3 reacted to ID testing.[50]

In the opinion of Fisher and Fowler, intradermal testing with metal salts should be considered an investigative procedure, because there is no general agreement about its significance, advantages, or disadvantages. In addition there is no allergen standardization. Fisher has not observed individuals with allergic hypersensitivity to a metal or its salts in whom he was not able to obtain a positive patch test reaction.

Testing for sarcoidal reactions to zirconium salts or other metals may be performed by rubbing the zirconium preparation into a test site prepared by multiple scratches or denuded by a dermal curet. In addition, an intracutaneous test may be performed with a 1:10,000 solution of sodium zirconium lactate.

Local Lymph Node Assay (LLNA) for Metal Allergenicity

Basketter and colleagues used the murine LLNA to assess sensitization potential of 13 metal allergens.[51] Nickel showed a surprisingly very low level of reactivity, which clearly differs from clinical experience, while platinum and tin showed positive reactivity. Otherwise, the data was pretty much in line with clinical experience. High sensitizers included beryllium, chromate, cobalt, copper, gold, and mercury, while aluminum, manganese, lead, and zinc were minimally reactive.

Granulomatous Reactions to Metals

Many metals are capable of inducing a granulomatous reaction when introduced into the skin of sensitized individuals. Mercury, chromates, and cobalt in tattoos may produce sarcoidal granulomas. Mercury granulomas of the skin can be caused by a broken thermometer. Beryllium may produce not only a localized but also a systemic sarcoidal reaction. Zirconium compounds, used in poison ivy medications, readily induce a granulomatous response. Silicon in powders can form granulomas in injured skin. Aluminum, an adsorbent in injectables, may produce granulomas at injection sites. Cerium, palladium, and gold in jewelry have produced allergic granulomas.

An intralesional injection of corticosteroids in the concentration of 5 to 10 mg/mL often causes involution of such metal granulomas.

Role of Metals in Black Dermographism

Urbach and Pillsbury[52] clearly defined black dermographism 60 years ago. Black dermographism, the most common cause of skin discoloration from metal jewelry, literally means "black writing on the skin." The discoloration is a thin deposit of metallic powder produced by the friction of a metallic object on skin contaminated by powders or abrasives.[53]

Black dermographism is really a misnomer because the phenomenon is not confined to the skin and is not physiologic. It is purely a physical phenomenon, which can readily be produced on paper or fabrics.[54]

Black dermographism is explained on the basis of the relative hardness of powders dusted on the skin and of metals rubbing on it. (Hardness is defined as the capacity of a substance to abrade another.) By plotting the hardness of common powders used in cosmetics and medications with metals used in jewelry, it is noted that zinc oxide and pumice are harder than nickel, iron, platinum, silver, gold, copper, and tin. Carbon is the hardest of all and is abundant in urban and industrial dust. Carbon is dirtying in itself and adds to the discoloration of metals by abrading them. In general, any powder listed in Table 32.4 will abrade any metal on the scale below it, and the effect will be streaks of color in the pattern of the friction.[55]

Only stainless steel and chromium are harder than cosmetic powders and other makeup, and black dermographism cannot be produced with jewelry made of these metals. Often the more expensive the jewelry and the more precious the metal, the more discoloration produced by makeup. Twenty-four-karat (pure) gold and platinum readily produce black dermographism.

Calamine lotion, face powders containing zinc oxide, titanium dioxide and ferric oxide, and certain dentifrices (both toothpastes and powders) readily remove a fine metallic powder from jewelry and other metallic objects, staining the skin black. The powder is always black,

Table 32-4 Comparison of Hardness of Metals and Powders

Scale of Powders	Hardness	Metals
Carbon	10	
	9.5	Chromium
	7	Steel
Zinc oxide and pumice	5.5	
	5	Nickel
	4.5	Iron
	4	Platinum
Boric acid	3	Antimony
Magnesium and bismuth	2.5	Silver, gold, and copper
Kaolin, aluminum, and sulfur	2	Tin
Calcium salts	1.5	Lead
Talcum and zinc stearate	1	

because the particles are so fine that they do not reflect light.

Putting zinc oxide powder or pancake makeup containing it or titanium dioxide on the skin and rubbing with a gold or silver ring immediately produces black lines on the skin. No such effect is obtained with zinc stearate, which is a soft powder.

When an individual applies makeup to the face or body or uses a dentifrice (containing pumice), some of the substances may lodge under rings or other jewelry worn on the neck or wrist.

In order to avoid black dermographism, metallic ornaments should be removed and the skin that will be in contact with the jewelry should be cleansed with soap and water to make certain that no makeup or dentifrice remains at these sites.

Rapson[56] thoroughly reviewed black dermographism related to gold.

Black dermographism from cosmetics or dentifrices is the most common discoloration under a ring. Another source of discoloration may be skin secretions and perspiration that contain sulfides and chlorides. These chemicals combine with the molecules of silver and copper that are usually present in a gold alloy to form black salts, such as silver chloride and copper sulfate. This reaction sometimes occurs only when a woman is pregnant, apparently because of changes in body chemistry.

In some maritime, semitropical climates the chlorides from the sea may combine with normal skin secretions to form corrosive chemicals.

Workers in rubber factories may be exposed to sulfides, which may tarnish rings. Heavy industrial smog is often thick with sulfides from the burning of low-grade, sulfur-laden coal and fuel oil or with other corrosive chemicals, such as phosphates. These air pollutants can attack gold alloys directly, even when jewelry is not being worn. When the tarnishing ring is slipped back on the finger, or a bracelet onto the arm, the thin film or tarnish rubs off in a black smudge.

Contact Allergy to Individual Metals: Aluminum

Aluminum is a fairly inert metal with a multitude of uses based on its strength and light weight. It is produced from bauxite ore and is second only to iron in usefulness in the modern world economy. Irritant folliculitis from aluminum salts in antiperspirants is not unusual. Steinegeer[57] attributed unusual, transient grayish brown and blue skin lesions to air pollution from an aluminum factory. Hemmer and colleagues[58] routinely tested 1,922 patients with aluminum chloride hexahydrate (2% aq). Only four reacted (0.21%), and none of these reactions were reproducible with a dilution series.

Allergic granulomas and nodules have been reported in children following vaccinations containing aluminum and in adults after hepatitis B vaccination. Essentially, these reactions occur at the site of vaccination, although ACD to aluminum may occur elsewhere as well. Slater and colleagues[59] found aluminum hydroxide in granulomas by X-ray microanalysis. In a report from Denmark, 21 children developed granulomas, and all were positive on patch tests.[60]

ACD to aluminum salts may occur from prior sensitization by vaccinations or hyposensitization injections or may arise rarely from exposure to deodorants or topical aluminum containing medications. Aluminum acetate in eardrops has caused ACD.[61] Considering the wide use of aluminum salts in antiperspirants, aluminum allergy is rare.

Aluminum allergy is usually detected on patch testing when virtually all the Finn chamber test sites exhibit a reaction, usually with a prominent annular component corresponding to the chamber edge. Aluminum chloride (2% aq) or other salts such as aluminum oxide (10% pet) can be tested for confirmation. Aluminum hydroxide apparently gives less accurate results and probably should not be used.

PATCH TEST PROBLEMS WITH ALUMINUM FINN CHAMBERS

Although generally inert, the aluminum in Finn chambers may interact with metal salts in patch test preparations. Mercury salts were first reported to show this interaction.[62] Nickel and cobalt in water may interact as well.[63] However, because these metals are routinely tested in petrolatum rather than water, there is probably no practical consequence to the clinician.

POSSIBLE SYSTEMIC CONTACT DERMATITIS FROM ALUMINUM IN TOOTHPASTE

Veien and colleagues[64] described 3 children with generalized itching, all positive to aluminum chloride 2% aqueous. They were all using the same toothpaste that contained 30% to 40% aluminum oxide.

Antimony Irritation and Allergy

Antimony and its compounds are used in alloys, type metal, batteries, foil, ceramics, safety matches, ant paste, textiles, and medicinals (such as tartar emetic, Fuadin, and antimony sulfide).

Antimony is strongly irritating to tissues, including mucous membranes. Chronic antimony poisoning is similar to chronic arsenic poisoning, with symptoms of itchy skin, pustules, stomatitis, and conjunctivitis.

Antimony may produce "antimony spots," an irritant folliculitis in freely perspiring workers exposed to antimony trioxide dust that is due to penetration of the dust into the sweat follicles.[65] Three employees making antimony brazing rods developed pustules and papules from antimony dust and fumes.[66] In addition, lichenoid and eczematous eruptions resembling atopic dermatitis may occur.[67] Antimony trioxide (as is) gave positive reactions in 2 of 190 ceramics workers.[68]

Antimony trioxide may be present in fireproof packaging, and antimony pentasulfides are used in fireworks and matches.

Arsenic

Contact dermatitis due to arsenic is rare in the general population, but not in industry. The roasting of lead, copper, gold, and cobalt ores that contain arsenic exposes the worker to arsenic trioxide (white arsenic). Arsenic exposure may also take place in the manufacture of insecticides, fungicides, weed killers, poisons used for baits, glasses, enamels, and alloys.

Irritant and ACD may be produced. Folliculitis with secondary pyoderma and furunculosis is not uncommon. So-called smelter's itch, due to arsenic trioxide, occurs in smelt workers who may develop eczematous eruptions, folliculitis, furunculosis, and ulcerative lesions on the extremities and nasal septum. Birmingham and Key[69] described similar lesions in children exposed to arsenic trioxide in a mining community. The presence of sweat, excoriations, or wounds facilitates the formation of arsenical ulcers.

A 10% aqueous solution of sodium arsenate may be used for patch testing. Arsenic not infrequently produces nonspecific, pustular patch test reactions.

True allergic reactions to contact with arsenical compounds are rare. Holinquist[70] reported dermatitis from exposure to arsenic in a refinery. He obtained positive patch tests with nonirritant concentrations of arsenic compounds. Patients with arsenical keratoses and cancers from the use of Fowler's solution did not give positive patch tests with arsenical preparations.

Allergy to sodium arsenate (1% aq) caused dermatitis on exposed surfaces of a glass factory worker in France.[71]

Beryllium Dermatitis and Granulomas

Beryllium is a light metal that forms an oxide and several soluble and insoluble solutions. It is used in the manufacture of alloys for electrical equipment and ceramics, and it is present in some phosphorus used in cathode ray tubes and a few fluorescent lights. It may be used in orthodontic devices. Soluble beryllium salts are easily hydrolyzed, with the formation of the free acids, causing severe irritations of the skin with papulovesicular eczematoid, weeping, and itchy lesions. When particles penetrate the skin, ulcers and necrosis may occur.

The primary target tissue for beryllium injury is the lung. Allergy is common among beryllium production workers and may progress to a chronic inflammatory and granulomatous disease.[72] Progression to chronic disease, but not initial allergic sensitization, have been shown to be related to genetic variations in glutathione metabolism.[73] The skin may be an important route of beryllium exposure and sensitization.[74] Reportedly, up to 16% of workers exposed to beryllium metal or dust may develop this condition that mimics sardoidosis.[75] However, only 1 of 100 workers in a beryllium distribution center, with little airborne exposure developed chronic beryllium disease.[76]

Curtis,[77] after an exhaustive evaluation, reported 13 cases of beryllium dermatitis among workers in two beryllium extraction plants near Cleveland, Ohio. The criteria for establishing the dermatitis as an allergic eczematous type were fulfilled. Pure beryllium metal is insoluble with respect to the skin and sweat and therefore cannot be used for patch testing. Beryllium fluoride sensitizes the skin to a high degree, which accounts for the high incidence of dermatitis among these workers in the fluoride process of beryllium extraction. Beryllium sulfate and beryllium chloride have less capacity to sensitize the skin, and beryllium nitrate has little or none, according to these experiments.

For patch tests, a 1% aqueous unbuffered solution of beryllium sulfate or beryllium chloride is recommended.

When beryllium phosphors were widely used in fluorescent tubes, many instances of beryllium granulomas occurred after people had received cuts from the broken tubes.[78]

Surgical excision was the only cure for beryllium granuloma before adrenocorticotrophic hormone (ACTH) or corticosteroid treatment was found to bring about improvement.[79]

Jones Williams[80] presented a case report of a 48-year-old man who, following a relatively trivial finger injury, developed systemic chronic beryllium disease. Initially, he cut his finger on a grinding wheel contaminated with beryllium oxide. This injury developed into a chronic skin ulcer that failed to respond to corticosteroids and later necessitated amputation of the affected finger. Noncaseating granulomas were present in the ulcer, and spectroscopic analysis revealed the presence of beryllium.

The diagnosis was further confirmed by a positive patch test. Six months later, two granulomas together with beryllium containing nodules were removed from the lymphatics of the same forearm. The wounds healed, chest symptoms were absent, and there was no radiologic evidence of disease. The patient remained apparently well but in June 1970, nearly 7 years after the original injury, he presented with multiple firm nodules along the course of the lymphatics in the injured arm. Biopsy showed fibrous nodules with surrounding epithelioid cell granulomas that, on analysis, contained beryllium. Of even graver import are the radiologic findings of bilateral pulmonary mottling, evidence of impaired pulmonary function, and the presence of granulomas in a lung biopsy. It is probable that the recurring lymphatic lesions resulted from the original injury, but the chest lesions indicate an additional inhalation exposure.

Cutaneous and systemic findings of chronic beryllium disease are still seen, as evidenced by the recent report by Berlin and colleagues.[81] This patient had cutaneous lichenoid granulomas with a positive lymphocyte transformation test.

BERYLLIUM IN DENTAL AND MEDICAL DEVICES

Beryllium allergy has resurfaced after a scarcity of reports for many years. Haberman and colleagues[82] reported two cases of allergy induced by beryllium in a dental prosthesis. Both had positive patch tests only to beryllium (BeCl$_2$ 1% pet). In addition, a third patient had dermatitis localized to one arm in which he had an orthopedic implant for fracture stabilization. Again, the only reaction was to BeCl$_2$ but definite proof of beryllium in the implant could not be obtained. Vilaplana and colleagues[83] reported three cases of beryllium allergy, all with strongly positive patch tests to BeCl$_2$ (1% pet). One woman had oral stomatitis from beryllium in a denture, and a dental technician had hand dermatitis from working with beryllium. The third patient had dermatitis in the area of an orthopedic implant, but it was uncertain if the implant contained beryllium.

As is the case with other allergens that are not often used for testing, the true incidence of beryllium allergy is unknown, but it may be higher than is currently appreciated.

Brass and Bronze

Brass, which contains copper, zinc, tin, lead, and molybdenum, rarely causes allergic contact dermatitis. Lip trouble, among brass players, is usually due to irritant or pressure dermatitis. Some brass may contain traces of nickel. Bronze is an alloy of copper and tin. Traces of lead, phosphorous, nickel, and zinc may be present. Gun metal consists of bronze with zinc. The "gold leaf" that is claimed to be added to some eyeshadows is probably a fired bronze powder coated with stearic acid.

Cadmium Compound Reactions

In modern industry, cadmium is an important metal. It is used as a corrosion inhibitor, as a neutron brake in atomic reactors, as a stabilizer in plastics, in dry batteries, in dye production, in soldering and welding, and in photochemistry. The toxic effects of cadmium due to the inhalation of cadmium oxide (metal fume fever) are common. Such inhalation may produce respiratory tract inflammation, pulmonary edema, and decreased sense of smell. Renal toxicity may occur. Cadmium chloride does not appear to be a sensitizer in industry.[84,85]

CADMIUM RED (CADMIUM SELENIDE) IN DENTURES AND COOKING UTENSILS

A mixture of cadmium selenide and cadmium sulfide may be used as the pink pigment in acrylic resin. Pure Cadmium Selenide Red No. 1124 is used for the coloring of lucite dentures. Pure cadmium selenide reds are insoluble in perspiration, in natural water, and in dilute hydrochloride acids present in gastric juices. Cadmium red is soluble in muriatic acid. Cadmium reds are nonabsorptive through the skin. Although cadmium reds are classified as poisonous and cannot be used in food colors, they can be used as ingredients in the manufacture of dental rubber, enameled ware, and cooking utensils, or in the production of toys or tinware. In the manufacture of enameled ware, cadmium reds are not affected unless the enamel is destroyed by acids.

Kaaber and colleagues[86] stated that cadmium red is not a sensitizer.

A large German study found many questionable or positive patch tests to cadmium chloride (1% pet) in 719 patients.[87] There were 198 reactions, but only 6 were graded 2+ or 3+. The remainder were felt to be nonspecific irritant reactions, and in the authors' opinion, the stronger reactions were not relevant. The same authors later performed a dilution study and recommend testing with cadmium chloride 0.5% petrolatum, but only in those with a likely exposure to cadmium.[88]

Carbon Dermatoses

Carbon occurs in the pure state as the diamond and as graphite. It is used in electricity as the carbon arc through which the current is conducted and in carbon arc lighting and welding and in batteries.

Friedman[89] reported that the graphite in "lead" pencils produced an allergic dermatitis. Carbon black, consisting of finely divided amorphous forms of carbon, is used in pigments in rubber products and as filtering agents. Capusan and Mauksch[90] stated carbon black plant workers developed fissured hyperkeratoses of the palms and black tattoos of the hands and forearms.

Cerium

A patient treated a serious thermal burn with a topical containing cerium nitrate and silver sulfadiazine. Several years later, sarcoidal granulomas appeared. They contained cerium, demonstrated by electron probe X-ray microanalysis.[91]

Chromate

Chromium is ubiquitous; it is the fourth most common material in the earth's crust. Chromium is distributed widely in both the earth and the sea, and is more abundant than cobalt, copper, zinc, molybdenum, lead, nickel, and cadmium. Widespread exposure to chromium compounds is therefore not surprising. Chrome currently is the fifth most common metal allergen (see Table 32.5).

In contrast to other metals, allergy to chrome has been stable or declining in most reports.

The classic 3 major sources of chromate exposure are: 1) construction materials including concrete, cement, bricks, drywall, etc. 2) leather, and 3) chrome metal-working occupations. Many other occasional exposures to chromate, as noted below, can cause ACD.

CLINICAL FEATURES OF ALLERGIC ERUPTIONS CAUSED BY CHROMATES

Such eruptions tend to be insidious and persistent and are prone to relapse. Although the eruption may at times be acute and show oozing, it has a greater tendency to be dry, to fissure, and to lichenify. Chromate eruptions may mimic nummular eczema, atopic dermatitis, neurodermatitis, dry forms of dermatophytosis, and primary irritant reactions. Widespread chromate dermatitis may resemble ragweed dermatitis. Once chromate sensitivity has been established, the dermatitis tends to become more severe and more extensive and takes longer to clear with each exposure, even when there is prompt removal from contact with the chemical (Figures 32-2 and 32-3).[92,93]

CHRONICITY OF CHROMIUM DERMATITIS

Burry and Kirk,[94] writing in 1975, were quite pessimistic, labeling chromate-sensitized industrial workers "chrome cripples." In studies of contact dermatitis in southern

Table 32-5 Prevalence of Metal Allergy[a]

| | | Test Substances | | | | | | | | | | | |
| | | Nickel | | | | Chromate | | | | Cobalt | | | |
Study	Concentration (%)	Total tested	Total + (%)	M + (%)	F + (%)	Total tested	Total + (%)	M + (%)	F + (%)	Total tested	Total + (%)	M + (%)	F + (%)
NACDG, 2004	2.5	5129	18.7	NR	NR	5142	4.3	NR	NR	5141	8.4	NR	NR
UK 2002	5	4721	18.5	NR	NR	4721	3,4	NR	NR	4721	5.7	NR	NR
Israel 2000	5	943	17.4	5.7	25.5	943	10.6	8.8	11.8	943	7.5	3.9	10.1
NACDG, 1998	2.5	3,429	14.2	NR	NR	3,440	2.8	NR	NR	4,095	9.0	NR	NR
Hong Kong, 1987–1998	5	437	10.5	NR	NR	437	0.9	NR	NR	437	7.8	NR	NR
NACDG, 1996	2.5	3,108	14.3	NR	NR	3,106	2.0	NR	NR	3,087	8.0	NR	NR
NACDG, 1972	2.5	1,200	11%	NR	NR	1,200	7.6	NR	NR	NR	NR	NR	NR
Denmark, 1984 hand eczema	5	141	NR	6.5%	26.3%	141	NR	4.5%	7.7%	141	NR	8.7%	1.1%
Denmark, 1985–1986	5	2,166	15.6%	5.1%	20.7%	2,166	4.3%	5.0%	3.9%	2,166	4.6%	1.6%	6.1%
Eastern Europe, 1982	5	2,400	7.3%	2.1%	10.5%								
Netherlands 1984–1986	5	1,785	14.8%	3.2%	20.8%	1,785	4.6%	6.2%	3.8%	1,785	7.7%	4.7%	9.3%
Saskatoon 1983–1987	2.5	542	17.4%	8.5%	23.1%	542	6.1%	6.1%	6.1%	NR	NR	NR	NR
West Germany, 1977–1983	5	11,962	9.2%	2.6%	13.7%	11,962	4.3%	5.1%	3.7%	11,962	4.7%	3.0%	5.9%
Toronto, 1983–1987	2.5	447	11.9%	7.7%	16.9%	NR	NR	NR	NR	NR	NR	NR	NR
	5	629	10.5%	5.1%	16.7%	NR	NR	NR	NR	NR	NR	NR	NR

[a]NACDG, North American Contact Dermatitis Group; NR, not reported; M, male; F, female.
Note: All allergens tested in petrolatum potassium dichromate 0.5 (Europe & Canada) and 0.25% (NACDG), cobalt chloride 1% at all centers. From Reference 1.

Australia, they observed manual workers who had been sensitized by an obvious source of chromium or chromate salts and had been disabled by continuous or recurrent dermatitis, a few becoming virtually unemployable.

These investigators found that only minute quantities of chromium or chromate salts need be present in the environment to cause dermatitis in sensitized subjects. The contamination of factories and other workplaces by cement dust or chromate salts in solution (e.g., in diesel engine coolants) provides a constant source of allergen. The authors suggested that "[c]omplete responsibility for the dermatitis should always remain on the shoulders of the original employer's insurance company covering the [worker] at the time of sensitization. This would allow the disabled work[er] to experiment in a variety of tasks until he found one in which he was able to work free of dermatitis."

Burrows[95] found that only 8% of patients with chromate sensitivity from cement were free of dermatitis 10 to 13 years after the initial eruption. Breit and Turk[96] stated that a review of the available literature[93,97] showed that the prognosis for the dichromate-allergic patient was poor. They suggested that the only way to improve the situation was to prevent sensitization by strict avoidance of prolonged contact with dichromate-containing material.

Even with avoidance of chrome, however, many individuals develop chronic eczema. Since 1981, ferrous sulfate has been added to cement in Denmark.[98] Despite this, 12 of 17 workers with allergic hand eczema in 1981 suffered from chronic hand eczema in 1987. This occurred despite early retirement or change in occupation.[99]

PREVENTION OF CEMENT DERMATITIS

Fregert and colleagues[98] found that ferrous sulfate could be added to cement to reduce water-soluble hexavalent chromate to trivalent chromate, which is much less allergenic. Avnstorp[100] compared cement workers in 1981, before Denmark began adding ferrous sulfate to cement, to new workers in 1987. Significantly fewer workers (6/227) in 1987 had positive patch tests to chromate compared to 1981 workers (20/190). In contrast, in Australia, where iron sulfate is not added to cement, no change in the incidence of occupational chromate dermatitis was seen in 1989 compared to 1980.[101]

In a follow-up Danish study in 1996, of 4,511 consecutive patch test patients, 79 were allergic to chromate. Only 10 were related to cement contact, and 7 of these had been sensitized before 1981.[102] In contrast, in England, where ferrous sulfate is not used in cement, there

was no difference in positive patch test rates between 1983 and 1993.[103]

Unfortunately, for this technique to be effective, the iron sulfate must be added to fresh cement. In stored cement, the iron sulfate oxidizes to an inactive form. Also, this adds about 1% to the cost of the cement. Nonetheless, the benefits in reducing not only medical costs and work absenteeism but also the discomfort of chronic eczema would seem to suggest the benefit would outweigh the problems.

CHROME-TANNED LEATHER ARTICLES

After cement and related construction materials, leather is the next most common source of chromate allergy, except in certain occupational settings (Figure 32-4) (see Chapter 18.)

Chrome tanning is used particularly for light, flexible leathers, such as shoe uppers, and leather for other wearing apparel. The chromates are the principal cause of allergic dermatitis from leather articles.

Fisher's review of 20 patients with chromate sensitivity revealed that only 4 of them had shoe dermatitis. These four also suffered from hyperhidrosis.

Freeman[104] reported that in 55 patients with shoe allergy, 23.6% were caused by chromate. This was second only to rubber allergens as a whole (43.6%). There is a distinct international difference in causes of shoe allergy. In a report from India, 75% of cases were due to chromate, perhaps because of higher humidity and temperature there, resulting in more perspiration.[105]

Leather gloves must be avoided in workers with chromate sensitivity.

A report from Israel described 7 men who developed ACD to tefellin, and all were allergic to chromate. Tefellin is 2 leather boxes and a leather strap held closely against the skin for religious purposes.[106]

LESS COMMON SOURCES OF EXPOSURE TO CHROMATES

Chromium compounds have been long recognized for their primary irritant corrosive effects on the skin and for their potent skin-sensitizing properties and ability to produce allergic contact dermatitis. In occupational exposure, both effects are common, but in the general population, the allergic contact dermatitis is seen almost exclusively.

CHROMATES IN BLEACHING AGENTS

Javelle water (eau de javelle), a disinfecting and bleaching agent, is essentially a solution of sodium hypochlorite and sodium chloride. Sufficient potassium dichromate may be added (as a coloring and stabilizing agent) to cause dermatitis in dichromate-sensitive individuals.[107]

In contrast, of 20 household bleaches in common use in the United States, only 2 were found to contain detectable chromate.[108] In these two, the level was between 0.1 and 0.3 ppm, which is probably inadequate for allergy elicitation.

CHROMATES IN DETERGENTS

Phosphate-containing detergents have chromium salts, which may produce dermatitis in chrome-sensitive individuals.[109] Ingber and colleagues[11] found significant levels of chromium in some detergents on the Israeli market. Basketter et al found from 0.6 to 1.1 ppm chromate in various laundry and hand washing detergents in Europe.[110]

BRUSHLESS SHAVING CREAM

This is essentially a vanishing cream to which a lubricant has been added, forming an oil-in-water emulsion. Chromic acid or chromates may be added to prevent rusting of razor blades.

CHROMATED CATGUT

Tritsch and colleagues[111] reported an experiment with five chrome-sensitive individuals on whom implanted threads of chromic plain catgut produced a granulomatous inflammation with secondary involvement of the epidermis. Harp strings were shown to produce contact dermatitis in musicians.[112]

CHROME-PLATED MATERIALS

These metallic objects rarely cause allergic dermatitis, probably because of relative insolubility in sweat. This is in sharp contrast to nickel-plated objects, which are a common cause of allergic contact dermatitis.

Fregert[113] suggested that chromate-sensitive patients avoid the use of metal cigarette lighters, which may be chromium-plated. It has been Fisher's experience, however, that individuals with even a high degree of hypersensitivity to chromates can handle chrome-plated objects without difficulty.

CHROMATES IN MATCHES

Both in the United States and elsewhere, some matchheads contain chromates.[113] Perspiring fingers touching unlit matches may readily dissolve chromates from matchheads. In addition, the flame and fumes from a lit match may contain considerable amounts of the chemical. After the flame has been extinguished, the charred match-head still contains traces of chromates and, when placed in pockets, may contaminate pocket linings with chromates. Book matches may similarly contaminate pockets. Otitis externa may be caused by cleansing or scratching the ear canal with matches in sensitized individuals.

HIDE GLUES CONTAINING CHROME

Morris[114] cited several instances of ACD in chrome-sensitive individuals caused by contact with hide glues. Such glues are made by detanning chrome-tanned leather scraps in acids or in lime.

EPOXY RESIN ADHESIVE CONTAINING CHROME

A tile layer developed ACD to chromate.[115] The epoxy flooring adhesive was found to contain cement as a filler.

CHROME ALLOYS

Chromate dermatitis may occur in the manufacture of chrome alloys. Dermatitis that occurs from contact with the finished alloy, however, is usually due to metals other than chrome, particularly nickel.

"BLACKJACK DISEASE" CAUSED BY CHROMATES

Fregert and colleagues[116] reported an unusual occupational hazard of professional gamblers, roulette buffs, and card players—"blackjack disease," a dermatitis caused by exposure to chromium salts used for dyeing green felt or baize, which covers the gambling tables. These investigators stated that although the exact amount of chromates adhering to a player's hands after playing cards on a green felt tabletop is unknown, there is probably sufficient chromate to produce dermatitis in chromate-sensitive individuals.[117]

CHROMIUM IN FOOD AND DIETARY SUPPLEMENTS

Burrows[117] stated that minute quantities of chromium are also found in food: dairy products (mean 0.10 mg/g), meat and fish (mean 0.11 mg/g), vegetables (mean 0.03 mg/g), fruits (mean 0.02 mg/g), and grains (mean 0.04 mg/g). The highest concentrations in food occur in thyme (10.00 mg/g), black pepper (3.3 mg/g), and cloves (1.50 mg/g). Animal diets contain higher amounts (e.g., dog food pellets have 4.24 mg/g). Vegetation unlikely to be eaten, such as leaves of trees, contains higher quantities; for example, wild cherry leaves have 0.57 mg/g and pasture grass, 1.30 mg/g. Cigarettes contain 0.39 mg/g, and drinking water, 0 to 0.112 ppm. Total human body content is about 6 mg of chromium; there is a higher concentration in infants, and animals generally have very much higher concentrations.[118]

Burrows[117] stated that small quantities of potassium dichromate taken orally will produce an exacerbation of chromium dermatitis.[119] This is surprising, in view of the findings of Donaldson and Barreras,[118] who showed that most chromium is changed in the acid media of the stomach to trivalent chromium and not absorbed.

A severe exacerbation of dermatitis occurred in a bricklayer given a homeopathic drug that resulted in an intake of 60 mg of dichromate daily.[120]

Fowler[121] reported a man with scattered, generalized dermatitis of recent onset and patch tests positive only to chromate. The man reported that several weeks before the onset of the dermatitis, he began taking the dietary supplement chromium picolinate. The dermatitis resolved soon after he quit taking the supplement. Chromium picolinate is purported to be helpful in weight loss and control of blood sugar in diabetics, but adequate clinical trials are currently lacking. Fowler has seen several more cases in the last few years that are similar to this one.

ROLE OF CHROMATES IN INDUSTRIAL DERMATITIS

Table 32.6 lists the great variety of industrial exposures to chromates.[122] The following occupations are particularly well known for their risk to employees of chromium dermatitis: cement work, chromium plating, dyeing, printing, photography, work using antirust agents, and work with wood impregnated with chromium.[117]

Table 32-6 Occupational Exposures to Chromates

Aniline workers
Artificial flower makers
Automobile industry workers
Battery makers
Bleachers
Blueprint makers
Builders
Candle (colored) makers
Carbon printers (photography)
Cement makers
Ceramic workers
Chrome workers
Chromium platers
Color makers
Colorers (marble)
Compounders (rubber)
Crayon makers
Cutting oil makers
Dye makers
Dyers
Electroengravers
Electroplaters
Enamel makers

Table 32-6 (cont.) Occupational Exposures to Chromates

Enamelers
Etchers
Explosives (ammonia and pyroxylin) workers
Firefighters
Floor tile installers
Foundry workers
Frosters (glass and pottery)
Furniture polishers
Glass colorers
Glass polishers
Glaze workers (pottery)
Ink makers
Linoleum workers
Lithographers
Marble colorers
Match makers
Mixers (rubber)
Mordanters
Musicians (strings)
Paint makers
Painters
Paper hangers
Paper makers
Pencil (colored) makers
Photoengravers
Photographic workers
Photogravure workers
Pottery workers
Printers
Pulp makers
Railroad employees (diesel locomotives)
Rubber workers
Rustproofers
Stainless steel and other chrome alloy makers
Tannery workers
Television makers
Textile printers
Vulcanizers
Wallpaper printers
Waterproofers (paper and textiles)
Wax ornament workers
Welders
Woodworkers (handling wood impregnated with chromated zinc chloride)

In addition, chromium dermatitis has been reported from the following:[123–129] defatting solvent, food laboratories, oil from galvanized sheet metal, coolant oils, offset printing, milk testing, TV screens, magnetic tapes, detergents, bleaches, and boiler linings.

Automobile Industry

Primer paints containing zinc chromate have caused ACD among sensitized workers.[130] Hexavalent chromate used as a chromate dip to prevent corrosion of nuts and bolts used in automobile assembly has been reported as another cause.[131] Adequate rinsing of the nuts and bolts decreases the hazard. Chromium may be present in automobile antifreeze.

Ceramics Industry

Enamelers and decorators in the ceramics industry may occasionally react to chromates, although other metals, including nickel, cobalt, and red iron oxide, are more common allergens.[68]

Foundry Industry

In addition to cement, foundry sand may be contaminated with chromates by the addition of chromium magnesite bricks, which are used as refractory material in the steel furnace.

Pulp Industry

Fregert and colleagues[132] reported sensitization to chromium and cobalt in the processing of sulfate pulp.

Railroad Industry

Sodium dichromate is added to diesel locomotive radiator fluids as an antioxidant to prevent rusting of radiators and pipelines. Inasmuch as many workers acquired chromate dermatitis from this source in the past, various substitute antioxidants, such as borates and nitrates, have been tried, unsuccessfully.

Building Repair Industry

Spackle compounds, which are plaster-like mixtures used to repair defects in walls, contain chromates,[133] as do drywall (sheetrock), bricks, and mortar.

Chromates in Corundum

Corundum used in glass polishing may contain chromates.[134]

Chrome Plating

Lee and Goh[135] reported that 71% of chrome platers from 17 factories had chrome ulcers, dermatitis, or both or had scars from old ulcers. Mucosal irritation, mostly of the throat, was present in 57%. Workers in "hard" chrome plating, where the plating is thicker for industrial uses, were more likely to have mucosal irritation, whereas "bright" chrome (for decorative use) workers had a higher incidence of skin ulcers.

Welding Industry

Gases and fumes from welding, especially those from the welding of chromium steel alloys, may contain large amounts of not only chromium oxide but also hexavalent chromium.[136] Exposure may produce allergic contact dermatitis in individuals who are sensitized to chromates.

Shelley[137] reported a flare-up of a chrome dermatitis of the palms resulting from the inhalation of fumes from acetylene welding by a patient with a markedly positive patch test reaction to a 0.25% aqueous solution of potassium bichromate.

Zugerman[138] reported chromium dermatitis in arc welders. One of his patients was so sensitive to chromates that he was unable to work in any part of the plant without developing a cutaneous eruption.

Television Manufacturing Industry

Stevenson[139] studied patients with hand dermatitis who made color TV screens. Of 26 workers with hand dermatitis engaged in this process, 18 had chrome sensitivity.

Ammonium dichromate was used in making color television screens to produce cross-linking of light-sensitized polyvinyl alcohol. This enables fluorescent compounds (in turn red, green, and blue) incorporated in the polyvinyl alcohol to adhere to the screen. Although protective clothing and gloves were worn, examination of patients with a Wood's light showed persistence of the fluorescent compounds on the hands and nail folds even after repeated washing of the hands. Table 32.7 lists substances and industries that should be avoided by persons sensitive to chromates.

Table 32-7 Substances and Industries to be Avoided by Chromate-Sensitive Individuals

Chrome-plated metal—probably will not cause difficulty

Leather (most shoe, belt, and other chrome-tanned leather)

Construction industry (cement, mortar, plaster, drywall)

Bleaching agents (dichromate as coloring and stabilizing agent, javelle water)

Matchheads

Cosmetics with chromium oxide-green

Tattoos (chromium oxide and Casal's or Guignet's green)

Automotive industry:
    a. Primer paints (zinc chromate)
    b. Dips to prevent corrosion of nuts and bolts
    c. Welding with chrome alloys

Foundries (chromates are added to sand for bricks)

Antioxidants for radiators and pipelines for diesels

Building repair (spackle)

Rustproofing (protection of iron against corrosion and rusting; also used in coolants and grinding emulsions)

Some cutting oils

Catgut (chromated)

Paints and enamels (chromate pigments—especially green, orange, and yellow)

Detergents (phosphate-containing detergents usually have chromium)

Etching agent

Electroengraving of copper

PATCH TESTS WITH POTASSIUM DICHROMATE

Patch testing with potassium dichromate is generally carried out in the United States by using a concentration of 0.25% in petrolatum. In the past, 0.5% had been used, but this resulted in many irritant false-positive reactions. This also may have resulted in an erroneous diagnosis of chromate allergy if the investigator was unaware of the propensity for irritant reactions. European studies have shown that using a 0.375% concentration may be helpful but still results in false-positives.[140] Nonetheless, European researchers prefer to use the 0.5% concentration, then attempt to determine relevance on clinical grounds.

A study of 54 individuals found a linear correlation between reactivity and concentration in patients known to be allergic to chromate.[141] Using the T.R.U.E. test system, which provided for a high degree of control of allergen concentration, various dilutions of both chrome VI and chrome III were tested.

Forty-one percent reacted only to the 0.25% concentration, 41% reacted to 0.05%, and one reacted to 0.001%. This suggests that for screening purposes the 0.25% concentration, although occasionally giving a false-positive irritant reaction, is suitable. Testing at a lower level will miss many reactions, whereas more irritancy will occur at a higher concentration.

Kosann and colleagues[142] studied a 6-hour versus 48-hour patch test to chromate and found the shorter testing was unreliable.

Cement as it is ordinarily used is a primary irritant under a patch test. When it is diluted enough to avoid being a primary irritant, the chromium concentration may be so reduced that a positive patch test reaction will not be obtained, even if the patient has been sensitized to chromates.

CHROMIUM VALENCES AND CONTACT DERMATITIS

In lymphocyte stimulation tests, both trivalent and hexavalent chrome are capable of giving a strong positive response.[143] The reason that trivalent chrome is clinically less important is probably due to its very poor skin penetration compared to hexavalent chrome.

Hexavalent chromate is the most powerfully sensitizing chromate because of its solubility and capacity to penetrate the skin.

In the work by Nethercott and colleagues,[141] 54 patients allergic to hexavalent chromate were tested with higher levels of trivalent chromate with only a few reactions. The calculated minimum elicitation threshold (MET) for chrome VI was 90 ng/cm^2 and for chrome III was over 33,000ng/cm^2.

CHROME ULCERS

Chromates may have a corrosive, necrotizing effect on living tissue, forming ulcers, or "chromeholes."[144] Chrome ulcers on the skin and the perforation of the nasal septum are still common in workers exposed to strong chromate solutions in tanning, electroplating, and chrome production. Chrome ulcers generally occur on exposed areas of the body, chiefly on the hands, forearms, and feet, and they develop readily at the site of insect bites and other injuries. In the presence of chrome dust or vapors, ulceration of the nasal septum often occurs.

The typical chrome ulcer is a crusted, painless lesion. Removal of the adherent crust reveals a punched-out ulcer, 2 to 5 mm in diameter, with a thickened, indurated, undermined border and a base that is covered with exudate. Ulcers of the nasal septum may be painless, but with continued exposure or trauma, the lesions may extend to the underlying tissues and become painful. These lesions usually heal with an atrophic scar in several weeks if further chrome exposure is carefully avoided. No known therapy accelerates the process.[144]

Samitz[145] recommended that 10% ascorbic acid in an ointment be applied to the nasal septum for the prevention of chrome ulcers in exposed individuals. In addition, he stated that prompt washing of the exposed skin with an "antichrome solution," such as sodium pyrosulfite, or simply with water helps to diminish the degree of ulceration.

Burrows[117] stated that in Great Britain an ointment of lanolin and soft paraffin is used on exposed skin to prevent chrome ulcerations.

Hexavalent chrome is ulcerogenic, but trivalent chrome is not.[117] Apparently the oxidizing properties of hexavalent chromium compounds cause denaturation of the proteins of the skin. This process continues until all the hexavalent chromium is reduced to the trivalent state.

Cement Dermatitis and Burns

NATURE OF PORTLAND CEMENT

The original Portland cement is named for the Isle of Portland, Dorset, England.

Modern Portland cement is a type of hydraulic cement whose essential constituents are tricalcium silicate and dicalcium silicate, with varying amounts of alumina, tricalcium aluminate, and iron oxide. The pH is usually above 12, which is in the range of a strong alkali.

Table 32.8 shows the average composition of regular Portland cement, which contains large amounts of

Table 32-8 Average Composition of Regular Portland Cement	
Calcium oxide (CaO) 64%
Silicon dioxide (SiO$_2$) 21%
Aluminum oxide (Al$_2$O$_3$) 5.8%
Iron oxide (FeO$_3$) 2.9%
Magnesium oxide (MgO) 2.5%
Alkali oxides 1.4%
Sulfur oxide (SO$_3$) 1.7%

calcium oxide in combination with silicon dioxide (SiO$_2$) and aluminum oxide (Al$_2$O$_3$). Because excess calcium oxide, which is alkaline, can be formed during the processing of the raw materials in the manufacture of Portland cement, these cements can have varying degrees of alkalinity. Calcium oxide, known as lime, combines with water to form calcium hydroxide and, secondarily, sodium and potassium monoxide, which in the presence of water convert to sodium and potassium hydroxide. Severe burns and ulcerations can occur when this wet cement comes into close contact under pressure with the skin.

Cement can also produce an irritant dermatitis from its alkaline, hygroscopic, and abrasive properties. Allergic dermatitis can occur from the ubiquitous presence of hexavalent chromates in cement in patients who have become sensitized to this metallic salt. The chrome salt is an accidental contaminant of cement and is not an "additive" in the usual sense. Indeed, the earth's entire crust contains chromates in some amounts.

Fresh concrete contains about 15% cement. Mortar used for bricklaying and plaster often contains cement.

CEMENT DERMATITIS AND THE CHROMATES

Not only construction workers, but also artists and do-it-yourself home builders are exposed to cement and the hazards of cement dermatitis.

The main sensitizers in cement are the dichromates, but other metals, such as nickel and cobalt, may be present. Reports constantly appear from various countries indicating that cement continues to produce many cases of chromate dermatitis.[146,147] Soluble chromates have been identified in most of 25 samples of British cement.

Many workers may develop cement dermatitis, including masons, tile setters, and cement workers. Not infrequently, such dermatitis is persistent and tends to become widespread.

It is likely that the irritant effect and the alkaline content of cement interfere with the skin's defenses, permit-ting penetration and sensitization to the dichromates in cement to take place more readily. Not infrequently, individuals develop cement dermatitis after having worked with cement for many years without difficulty.

The incidence of cement dermatitis is highest among workers handling wet cement on small building jobs. In cement factories and on large-scale building jobs, the filling of cement and the mixing and placing of concrete are usually done mechanically, reducing contact with cement by the workers.

Some cement has been reported to contain, in addition to chromium, cobalt and nickel. Hypersensitivity to cobalt and nickel may produce cement eczema under such circumstances. Patch tests, therefore, should be performed not only with dichromate but also with nickel and cobalt in suspected cement dermatitis.

CEMENT BURNS RESULTING IN NECROTIC ULCERS DUE TO KNEELING ON WET CEMENT

Fisher[148] reported two cases of severe burns, with resulting ulceration and necrosis of the skin of the knees and legs caused by kneeling on premixed cement. In both instances, Portland premixed cement had been poured onto the ground to make patios. Neither patient was a professional in the handling of cement.

To smooth out the poured cement, which was uneven and lumpy, both patients had knelt down on their knees in order to facilitate the smoothing process with a board. The wet cement readily penetrated the patient's clothing and produced third-degree chemical burns of the knees and adjacent areas, necessitating hospitalization, debridement of the burn areas under anesthesia, and application of skin grafts.

In neither case had the patients been warned that wet cement should not be allowed to come in contact with the skin.

Hannuksela and colleagues[149] presented six patients who had been making a floor by leveling wet cement in a kneeling position. They all developed nearly identical curved ulcers on both sides of both patellae. The subjects were not aware of the irritating properties of fresh wet concrete. The features common to these six cases were a 2- to 6-hour exposure to calcium lye, insufficient protection that allowed the clothes to get wet, and pressure on the exposed areas. Immediately after stopping work, the patients noticed that the exposed skin was red; deep ulcers developed within 12 hours.

Warnings should be given by those who deliver or sell premixed cement to nonprofessional users that care should be taken not to allow the wet cement to make contact with skin.[150]

There appears to be fairly general agreement that direct skin contact, prolonged contact time, and pressure on exposed areas by kneeling or by persistent contact of cement against the skin by rubber boots, polythene sheeting, or rubber gloves are the conditions necessary for wet Portland cement to cause an acute ulcerative contact dermatitis.

Ready-mixed concrete as delivered to the site can be both more difficult to spread and marginally more alkaline than freshly mixed concrete. Wide fluctuations in alkalinity from batch to batch, however, are unlikely. Ready-mixed concrete is generally made in highly automated batching plants, where batching mistakes are very unlikely because they are specifically guarded against.[151] There are two main types of ready-mixed concrete: central mixed and transit mixed. With the first type, mixing is done at the plant and the drum on the truck merely agitates the mixture (2 to 6 rev/min). With the second type, batching only is done at the plant and mixing occurs on the truck (4 to 16 rev/min). Usually only 70 revolutions at mixing speed are required. Maximum haulage for central mixed concrete is usually 10 miles or half an hour, but distance and time can be increased by using transit mixing. None of the reports in the literature to date comment on which type of mixing was used in burn cases, but these details may be important to ascertain in future cases, if further light is to be shed on the etiology of cement burns.

BURNS FROM HARDENED CONCRETE

Stoermer and Wolz[152] reported that cement burns from contact with wet premixed cement is not uncommon. However, the available literature does not show reports of dermatitis caused by hardened concrete. They reported two patients who acquired "cement burns" by unloading concrete building stones from a truck. It was raining at the time, and their clothes were wet. In this case, particles of concrete stones were eluted with distilled water, and the pH value was 11.2. No additional chemicals were used in the cement.

CHROME CONTAMINATION OF THE ENVIRONMENT

Environmental chromium contamination has become a topic of interest in areas where chromite ore processing formerly occurred. Soil levels of up to 100 ppm chrome VI and 19,000 ppm chrome III have been reported in areas where slag has been used as landfill. The concern has been primarily because chrome VI may be an inhalation carcinogen. The risk of contact dermatitis and skin ulceration is also a potential problem, and cleanup standards based on the cutaneous risk have been proposed.

Based on threshold studies of levels of chrome needed to produce a positive patch test, along with presumed bioavailability of chrome in soil, it is likely that only a very few of the most highly sensitive individuals could develop ACD from environmental exposure.[141,153] A more recent unpublished study by Fowler and colleagues suggested that the lowest level of exposure at which 90% of allergic persons would react is between 100 and 400 ng/cm^2. This is significantly higher than the level proposed in the Nethercott study.

SPECIFIC TREATMENTS FOR CHROMATE DERMATITIS

In addition to the usual treatment of ACD, several options for prevention and treatment of chromate allergy have been proposed. Sodium dithionate (also known as sodium sulfoxylate or sodium hydrosulfite) has been used in the chrome industry to "neutralize" chrome splashes on the skin.[154] This is said to considerably diminish the incidence of chrome ulcers.

Romaguera and colleagues[155] devised a "barrier cream" for use in chromate allergy. The composition included tartaric acid, silicone, glycine, and other ingredients. Theoretically, the ingredients act as chelators and also reduce chrome VI to chrome III, which is less allergenic. The authors reported good results in a majority of chrome-allergic construction workers. Further studies with this compound may be warranted.

Miyachi and colleagues[156] reported that Dapsone (100 mg/day) improved hand eczema in five cement workers. Theoretically, the Dapsone reduced tissue superoxide radicals that may have led to clinical improvement. A controlled trial of this agent has not been performed as yet.

CHEMICAL TEST FOR CHROMATES

The object is placed in hot water to extract any chromium present. The solution is acidified with diluted hydrochloric acid. Then a 1% alcoholic solution of diphenyl carbazide is added. The development of a persistent red color is specific for hexavalent chromium salts. The test is sensitive to 10 ppm. Do not try this at home.

Cobalt Dermatitis

Cobalt is a shiny gray, magnetic, brittle metal, which is widely used in additives to produce blue color in porcelain, glass pottery, and enamels. In the earth it is often found with nickel and copper, with 44% coming from nickel ores. It is produced primarily in Australia,

Scandinavia, Russia, Canada, China, and Zambia.[157] It is commonly used as an alloy in steel for tools, aircraft engines, magnets, and orthopedic devices.

Cobalt may be detected (in the presence of 1,000 times as much nickel) by using a 1% aqueous solution of 2-nitroso-1-naphthol-4-sulfonic acid at pH 7 to 8, which produces a red coloration.

Allergic cobalt dermatitis was thought to be more common in Europe than in the United States, possibly because of the presence of cobalt in European detergents and of sufficient amounts in European cement to sensitize construction workers and those who work with clay and pottery.

This concept probably developed because for many years the (NACDG) did not routinely test with cobalt. However, current data show the rates of patch test reactions in North America to be similar to those in European studies.[2,158–160] (Table 32.5).

Another fallacy is that cobalt allergy almost always occurs in concert with nickel allergy. In fact, this is not true, even though metal objects that contain cobalt may also contain nickel. NACDG data indicated that 40% of patients positive to cobalt were negative to nickel (unpublished data). Edman[161] similarly found 23 of 73 (32%) cobalt-positive patients not allergic to nickel.

COBALT IN JEWELRY

Perryman and Fowler[162] tested 28 patients with known cobalt allergy to a new jewelry alloy containing platinum and cobalt.) The manufacturer felt the alloy would bind the cobalt tightly and thus be "hypoallergenic." In fact, only 5 (18%) reacted to a patch test with a disc of the alloy applied for 7 to 8 days continuously. This novel alloy is likely to be tolerated by most cobalt allergic patients.

Hindsen and colleagues[163] reported a case of cobalt dermatitis from jewelry and wonder if this will increase in Europe since the "nickel directive" has limited nickel content in jewelry.

VITAMIN B$_{12}$ AND COBALT DERMATITIS

Price and MacDonald[164] stated that allergy to vitamin B$_{12}$ (cyanocobalamin), a cobalt-containing compound, was recognized in two patients shown to be sensitive to cobalt on patch testing by Rostenberg and Perkins[165] and Fisher.[166] They reported a case of recurrent cheilitis in a patient who was found to be allergic to cobalt and who ingested vitamin B$_{12}$ tablets regularly. The patient developed an acute stomatitis of the hard palate when her dentist unwittingly fitted a denture containing a chrome cobalt alloy.

Fisher[166] reported one cobalt-allergic patient that was correlated with an allergic reaction to vitamin B$_{12}$ in injectable Berubigen (Upjohn). (One mL of Berubigen contains 43.4 mg of cobalt.) This cobalt-sensitive patient gave a positive patch reaction to 2% aqueous solution of cobalt chloride and to the vitamin B solutions in the strengths of 100 and 1,000 mg per mL. In addition, there were positive delayed scratch and intradermal reactions to the vitamin B$_{12}$ solutions. The patient noted that, following each injection of vitamin B$_{12}$, the injected area became red, tender, and pruritic, but not eczematous. Oral ingestion of vitamin B$_{12}$ produced similar flares in the sites of previous injections. The patient also had an intractable hand eczema.

In one reported case there was a delayed allergic reaction to intradermal injection, but not to subcutaneous and intramuscular injections, of vitamin B$_{12}$ (Cobione), a cobalt-containing compound.[167]

Kelensky and Schwank[168] described hypersensitivity to cobalt in a cream (Perilacin) used for hyperhidrosis. Patch tests were positive to cobalt, and in one patient, vitamin B$_{12}$ produced positive epicutaneous and intradermal test reactions.

COBALT DIET

Table 32.9 lists some foods thought to be high in cobalt.

OCCUPATIONAL COBALT DERMATITIS

Some of the described industrial exposures to cobalt include the following.

Industries Using Hard Metals

As reported in Skog,[169] cobalt is employed as a binding agent to make hard metal, which consists of metal carbides and a binding agent that are presented and sintered into plates. Wolfram carbide (a tungsten compound) and the carbides of titanium, nobilium, and tantalum are frequently used.

Hard metal is characterized by a high degree of wear resistance. Consequently, it is used for rock drills, cutting tools, drawing, pressing and stamping tools, and mechanical parts exposed to heavy strain.

Table 32-9 Foods High in Cobalt	
Apricots	Coffee
Beans	Liver
Beer	Nuts
Beets	Scallops
Cabbage	Tea
Cloves	Whole-grain flour
Cocoa and chocolate	

Hard metal dusts may produce primary irritant dermatitis with folliculitis or a chronic lichenified eczema. In addition, allergic eczematous contact dermatitis may develop, which is often due to the cobalt.

Fischer and Rystedt[170] reported that hard metal contains about 10% cobalt. Eight hundred fifty-three hard-metal workers were examined and patch tested with substances from their environment. Initial patch tests with 1% cobalt chloride showed 62 positive reactions. Allergic reactions to cobalt were reproduced in 9 men and 30 women by means of secondary serial dilution tests. Hand etching and hand grinding, which are traumatic to the hands, involved the greatest risk of cobalt sensitization. Twenty-four women, who had probably been sensitized by hard-metal work, had cobalt allergy and a simultaneous nickel allergy. They had probably been sensitized to nickel before their employment, then became sensitized to cobalt by hard-metal work, although cosensitization to jewelry or metalworking could occur.

Carbide Industry

McDermott[171] reported that cobalt is a common binding component in all grades of carbide. Pneumoconiosis and allergic sensitization from such cobalt-carbide compounds can occur.

Polyester Resin Industry

Cobalt naphthenate is commonly used in the manufacture of polyester resin. Several instances of allergic contact dermatitis were encountered in Great Britain that were attributed to workers handling cobalt naphthenate in polyester synthesis.[172]

Paint Industry

Cobalt siccatives or driers, which are present in certain paints, have been reported as producing allergic contact sensitivity in paint factory workers.[173] These are organic cobalt naphthenate or cobalt-resinate based on linseed oil.

Cement Industry

Although the cobalt content of cements may be low (less than 0.01%), cement workers may become sensitized to cobalt.

Two building workers in Cuba also had isolated cobalt allergy due to cement contact.[174]

Cobalt and chromate sensitivity may co-exist in the cement worker. Because these patients have positive patch test reactions to both chromate and cobalt, it is difficult to determine what role the cobalt hypersensitivity played in the production of the cement dermatitis.

In a 5-year study of 449 construction workers, cobalt was the second most common allergen (20.5%) after chromate (42.1%).[147]

Bricklaying

Camarasa[175] found that a high percentage of bricklayers in Barcelona showed hypersensitivity to both chromium and cobalt, but he noted that hypersensitivity to cobalt does not appear in patients allergic to chromium and working in other occupations. DeFonseca[176] concluded that cobalt has a higher sensitizing power than nickel and that sensitization to chromium augments sensitivity to cobalt.

Mueller and Breucker[177] found that in most of their 79 cobalt-sensitive patients, the most frequent cause of dermatitis was cement (29%), and that when these patients showed reactions to chromium and nickel, the sensitization was due to simultaneous exposure to the three metals and not to crossreactions.

Plastics Manufacturing

Cobalt-containing catalysts may be used in plastics manufacturing. Allergy to cobalt in workers has been reported.[178,179] Allergy to epoxy compounds in these workers is much more common, however. Cobalt naphthenate has been reported to cause ACD, with a negative patch test to cobalt chloride.[180]

Pottery Workers

Dermatitis from exposure to wet clay containing cobalt may occur.[181] Cobalt dermatitis from dry clay or finished wares is rare. Cobalt may be added to clay to neutralize the yellow color produced by impurities.

Cobalt is present in pigments used for amateur painting of pictures, china, and enameling. The dried paint or enamel is not an allergen. Cobalt is also used as a drying agent in linseed oil and printing inks.

Manufacture of Alloys Containing Cobalt

Alloys containing cobalt include alnico, duralumin, nobilium, permalloy, stellite, ticonium, and vitallium. Allergic dermatitis in workers making alloys of cobalt has been shown by patch tests to be due in some instances to the dust of metallic cobalt.[93] The dust also has been reported as causing asthma. It is believed that a dusty atmosphere containing metallic cobalt particles favors a sensitization to cobalt.

Miscellaneous Industries Using Cobalt

Currently, cobalt is used extensively in the carbide, glass, ceramic, enamel, electrical, and pigment industries. It may also be used in printing inks and in animal feeds. Cobalt in animal feeds has caused allergy in a Finnish pig farmer and an English animal feed worker.[182,183] Cobalt-2-ethylhexoate caused hand dermatitis in an offset printer.[184] Two of the ink driers he worked with contained this chemical. Inks, paints, and varnishes may contain cobalt and other heavy metal catalysts, which help speed the drying process.

UNUSUAL URTICARIAL REACTION TO COBALT

Nurnberger and Arnold[185] reported Quincke's edema as a manifestation of a cobalt allergy due to sensitization by cobaltous shell splinters in the arm. Injection of a cobalt-iron preparation was followed by a refractory bilateral periorbital edema. Patch testing showed a "monovalent" allergy to cobalt.

PHOTOSENSITIZATION DERMATITIS DUE TO COBALT

Camarasa and Alomar[186] reported a bricklayer with a chronic and severe eczema, combined with a chronic papular dermatosis in sun-exposed areas, associated with multiple sensitivities. Chromate, mercaptobenzothiazole, and parabens sensitized the patient in the usual way, but cobalt produced a reaction only after light exposure. This last fact justifies a new approach to those bricklayers suffering from dermatitis in areas exposed to sunlight and when their clinical course proves to be unsatisfactory or unexplained.

Romaguera and colleagues[187] found that four patients with chronic photocontact dermatitis were sensitive to cobalt salts. They presented as cases of contact dermatitis from cement or pig fodder with persistent lesions on exposed areas. Only two of them had standard patch test–positive reactions to chromate and cobalt, but all showed positive photo patch tests to cobalt. Photo-oxidation tests proved that cobalt salts are photosensitizing. The patients' chronic actinic dermatitis was due to exposure to cobalt salts.

PATCH AND INTRADERMAL TESTING WITH COBALT

A "reaction" peculiar to cobalt patch tests has been described by Storrs (FJ Storrs, M.D., personal communication). This consists of a "cayenne pepper" speckled appearance of the patch site without edema or uniform erythema, apparently due to a poral reaction. This is not an allergic reaction.

Allenby and Basketter[188] found that of six cobalt-allergic patients who reacted to cobalt chloride 1% aqueous, only one reacted to 0.1% aqueous. As long as the poral reaction is kept in mind, testing at 1% would seem reasonable.

In the past, intradermal testing with cobalt and other metal salts has been performed. Marcussen[189] outlined some of the difficulties with interpreting these tests, including impurity of the testing material and nonspecific immediate urticarial reactions. Currently, intradermal testing with metal salts is felt to be unnecessary, except in research protocols.

Copper Dermatitis

Copper, a common component of alloys and plating materials, may rarely be the offending agent in patients with metal dermatitis, particularly when patch testing excludes more commonly involved metals, such as nickel, chromium, mercury, cobalt, and gold.[190]

The rarity of allergic reactions to copper seems to be borne out, because in the 1970s and 1980s the Allergy Department of the New York Skin and Cancer Unit had been able to authenticate only three cases of allergic reactions to metallic copper or its salts. Researchers there studied a patient with a combined allergic reaction to gold and copper, agreeing with Epstein that multiple metal allergies in one individual are due to separate and simultaneously induced sensitivities by each offending metal. It must be remembered, however, that because routine testing with copper salts is not carried out, the true incidence of copper allergy may be underestimated, just as was done with gold in the past.

In the past, when copper salts were being used for iontophoresis for fungal infections on severely eczematized feet, no instances of dermatitis due to these salts were reported, proving how rarely sensitization to copper occurs.

Exposure to copper salts may take place from contact with insecticides, fungicides, food processing procedures, fertilizers, and mordants used in fur dyeing.[191]

D'Alibour's solution contains copper sulfate, zinc sulfate, and camphor water. Concentrated solutions of copper sulfate are caustic and produce primary irritation. Copper and copper alloy in silver metallic jewelry corrode readily on the skin, and, in the presence of adequate concentration of salt, a primary irritation is produced.

A report from India implicated copper allergy as a cause of orodynia and lichen planus in three dental patients. Unfortunately, patch test and clinical details were not given.[192]

Copper is ubiquitous in all US coinage except the zinc-coated steel pennies of 1943. In Saltzer's case[190] of copper sensitivity, a penny, a nickel, and a dime provoked erythema and vesiculation at the patch test site within 24 hours.

So-called copper itch, which is caused by a dust of copper precipitate, is probably due to the presence of arsenic in the mixture.[191] Cohen[193] reported toxic effects from copper dust, which include upper respiratory irritation, "metal fever," ulceration, and perforation of the nasal septum.

DERMATITIS DUE TO COPPER INTRAUTERINE DEVICES

One widely used contraceptive method is the copper intrauterine device (IUD). Copper metal in contact with biologic substrates is highly reactive. The copper ions thereby produced also have biologic effects. Thus, this device is a pharmacologic agent.

The biologic evidence, most clearly shown with laboratory animals, is that the copper IUD has its contraceptive effect by inhibiting implantations.[194] The copper-containing intrauterine device was developed to overcome such undesirable side effects as metrorrhagia, pain, and expulsion, common to previous appliances. The CU-7 brand of intrauterine copper contraceptive (Searle) has a plastic component composed of polypropylene homopolymer with barium sulfate added to render it radiopaque. Its shape approximates the number 7. Coiled around the vertical limb is pure virginal electrolytic copper wire. This wire provides a surface area of 200 mm^2.

Barranco[195] reported the first case of eczematous dermatitis due to a copper IUD, verified by patch testing.

Barkoff[196] stated that a 24-year-old woman developed an acute urticarial reaction secondary to a copper intrauterine contraceptive device. Allergy to copper was proven by scratch tests. The condition cleared with removal of the intrauterine device.

Dry and colleagues[197] tested for allergy to copper by patch tests in 69 women who were using copper IUDs and 50 young women who did not use any IUD. These 119 women also tested to nickel. Patch tests were performed with a 5% solution of copper sulfate and with a 10% glycerol solution of nickel sulfate. The tests were read immediately after removal of the patches after 48 hours of application.

The one positive test to copper was observed in a woman with known previous allergy to copper. She developed generalized dermatitis 8 days after placing the IUD. Replacement by Lippes loop (no copper involved) resulted in a rapid and definitive improvement.

Romaguera and Grimalt[198] also reported contact dermatitis from a copper-containing intrauterine contraceptive loop.

Karlberg and colleagues[199] noted that copper is a very rare sensitizer. After reviewing over 100 cases published before 1983, they accepted only four cases as true copper allergy, and 20 as probably relevant. The largest series

was that of Dhir and colleagues,[200] who found 10 workers allergic to copper sulfate in a furniture polish. However, they did not test for nickel or other allergy.

Van Joost and colleagues[201] pointed out that nickel and copper allergy may coexist, and both may be significant.

UNUSUAL REACTIONS TO COPPER

Pande and Gupta[202] reported a 17-year-old boy who developed thrombocytopenic purpura after ingesting 1% copper sulfate solution (2 mg/day) given for vitiligo. This probably represented an allergic rather than a toxic reaction. Reid[203] reported that within 2 hours of having a premolar tooth temporarily filled with black copper cement, a woman became almost completely covered with an itching urticarial rash. In this instance, the patient had already suggested that she might be allergic to certain dental cements. The rash subsided after a few hours, although mild skin irritation persisted for 2 or 3 days.

Green discoloration of seborrheic keratoses has been reportedly caused by excessive levels o copper in a therapeutic swimming pool.[204]

Gold

Before the late 1980s, there were scattered case reports of gold allergy, but most references, including early editions of this book, suggested that gold allergy was rare.[205–207] There are probably two reasons for this misconception. First, testing for gold allergy was rarely done and if done may have been inadequate because of poor allergens. Second, gold is metallurgically inert and therefore was thought to be immunologically inert.

Obviously, gold allergy is anything but rare, as has been established in numerous patch test centers in the last decade (Figure 32-5).[208] Prevalence of positive patch test reactions to gold has been as high as 9.5% in large series, and numerous papers have been published discussing various features of gold allergy. The NACDG from 1996 to 1998 tested over 4,000 patients and found that 9.5% were positive to gold sodium thiosulfate (0.5% pet).[2] Gold was the sixth most frequent allergen. Similarly, Bruze and colleagues,[209] from Sweden, reported prevalence of about 9% in consecutive patients. A number of other studies from Europe and Asia have reported rates anywhere from 1% to 23%.

In the early 1990s some investigators were concerned that many gold patch test reactions seemed to lack relevance. However, as more data accumulates, cases previously thought to be lacking in relevance have been shown to be caused by gold contact. For example, Fowler,[210] in 1988, reported two women with eyelid dermatitis and gold allergy. Since then, statistical analysis has confirmed the association in Sweden and North America.[209] The NACDG found that of 388 gold-allergic patients, 7.5% had eyelid dermatitis.[211] More recently, the NACDG showed that of 268 patients with eyelid dermatitis only, gold was the single most common allergen at 8.2% positive.[212]

Some patients have a definite positive allergic patch test to gold, but seem to be able to wear gold jewelry without incident, whereas others have eyelid or facial dermatitis that resolves upon discontinuation of gold use. Nedorost postulates that cosmetic powders, that contain microabrasives like titanium dioxide, may abrade jewelry and ac as carriers to the face.[213]

In addition to dermatitis, lichen planus, both oral and cutaneous, is not uncommonly associated with allergy to gold (or other metals) in dental work (see Chapter 33).[214] Scalf and colleagues[215] patch tested 10 metal allergens in 51 patients with oral lichen planus. Gold ranked second only to mercury with 20% positive.

The vast majority of gold-allergic patients are women, probably because of greater jewelry usage. Also, most have gold dental work (crowns or fillings), although most have no oral symptoms.[209,216] In a report from one center, 34% of patients with gold dental restorations had positive patch tests to gold, as compared to 11% of those without gold in the mouth (p<.001).[217]

PATCH TESTING FOR GOLD ALLERGY

Fowler[218] reviewed various published reports of gold allergy. Gold chloride, also called trichloride, is composed of gold in dilute hydrochloric acid. This acid compound may predispose to irritant reactions. The best agent for patch testing is gold sodium thiosulfate (GSTS) (0.5% pet), also known as sodium thiosulfatoaurate. Gold sodium thiomalate (injectable therapeutic gold) may also be used. Potassium dicyanoaurate is used in the electronics industry and may cause ACD and irritant contact dermatitis (ICD). It is not a reliable patch test allergen. Gold leaf is also not a reliable patch test allergen, because it is poorly soluble.

A German study confirmed that gold sodium thiosulfate at 0.5% petrolatum versus 0.25% pet was twice as likely to yield positive results.[219] Likewise a Swedish study showed the superiority of GSTS over the chloride.[220] This author appreciates their confirmatory findings (but could have saved them the trouble).

Persistence of positive gold patch tests is rather common. Fowler has noted that frequently the sites may be visible for up to 8 weeks, but are usually asymptomatic (personal observation). Colleagues from Denmark have quantified this, noting that 8 of 21 positive patch tests

(up to 2% aq) were present at 14 to 33 days after testing.[221] It must be noted that some concentrations used were much higher than those normally used.

EXPERIMENTAL GOLD ALLERGY STUDIES

Gold chloride was found to be a strong sensitizer in a human maximization test.[222] However, to date there have been no reports of successful sensitization to gold in animals, according to Bruze and Andersen.[223] This study demonstrates the frequent inadequacy of animal predictive tests in identifying human allergens.

Sometimes it may be difficult to separate irritant from allergic positive patch tests to gold. Christiansen and colleagues postulate that analysis of cytokines produced by lymphocytes from gold-allergic persons may be helpful at identifying true allergy.[224] They found interferon-gamma stimulation on lymphocyte stimulation tests to be about 82% sensitive and specific for true gold allergy.

NONECZEMATOUS PERSISTENT PAPULAR GOLD ERUPTIONS

Allergic gold dermatitis may be a "dermal" type of contact dermatitis characterized by minimal eczematous epidermal changes and by marked dermal involvement.[225]

Shelley and Epstein[226] emphasized that allergic gold dermatitis may manifest as a chronic papular eruption. Bowyer[227] reported that an allergic eczematous patch test to gold may become papular and that such a papular patch test will show a "dermal" infiltrate when examined histologically.

The so-called allergic "dermal" contact dermatitis produced by gold, neomycin, nickel, and ragweed is an allergic contact dermatitis in which the eczematous element is minimal or absent. The eruption remains edematous and erythematous throughout its course. Histologically, there is a normal epidermis or an epidermis with little spongiosis. There is usually edema and a dense perivascular small, round cell infiltrate in the dermis. "Dermal" contact dermatitis is combined occasionally with the usual papulovesicular eczematous variety, in which case, one can usually demonstrate both a positive patch and an intracutaneous reaction with the specific allergen.

Petros and Macmillan[228] reported that a contact sensitivity to gold developed in a patient 6 months after she had her ears pierced and started wearing gold earrings. The patient developed pruritus, soreness and swelling of the earlobes, as well as irritation and pruritus under her gold wedding band. A biopsy from one of the ear lesions showed a dense infiltration of the dermis with lymphocytes and plasma cells. There were no significant changes in the epidermis.

Suzuki[229] may have found one reason for the persistence of clinical findings in some cases of gold ACD. In this study, small microfragments of gold were found in the skin by X-ray microanalysis long after earrings were removed. In another study, five of eight patients developed persistent papules at intradermal gold test sites, which lasted up to 20 months.[230] X-ray microanalysis revealed gold in tissue macrophages.

In a letter published in the *Journal of the American Medical Association* in 1974, Fisher[231] pointed out:

"Even the use of pure gold earrings is not quite safe following ear piercing. While allergic gold sensitization from ear piercing is much rarer than nickel sensitization, it is, nevertheless, a definite hazard. Incidentally, gold dermatitis tends to be persistent, sometimes lasting for several months, even though there is no further contact with gold.

Sensitization to both nickel and gold can be avoided by piercing the ears with a stainless steel needle (18 to 20 gauge) and inserting stud earrings of stainless steel that give a negative reaction for a spot test for nickel."

There is speculation that the persistence of the dermatitis may be due to the persistent presence of gold in the dermis.

GOLD RING DERMATITIS

In some instances, dermatitis from a ring is due to a primary irritation from trauma, accumulated detergents, or the corrosive action of salts on the ring. Allergic gold ring dermatitis does occur commonly.

Comaish's case[232] of allergic gold ring dermatitis showed that both the dermatitis and the positive gold patch test reaction persisted for several months after exposure to the gold had ceased. Repeated patch tests with scraping from the ring (18 karat) and pure gold leaf were negative at 48 to 72 hours. Patch testing with gold chloride (chloroauric acid, 2%) showed a strongly positive eczematous response at 48 hours. Redness and infiltrated papules persisted at the site for more than 2 months but were fading at 3 months. Lack of reaction to ring scrapings and gold foil is typical and indicates that testing with gold salts in gold allergy is important.

Rytter and Schubert[233] showed a primary sensitization after wearing a gold ring for 18 months. A positive test was obtained with very low solutions of sodium gold thiosulfate, and a lymphocyte transformation gave a positive result.

NATURE OF WHITE GOLD

According to the US Treasury Department, white gold is a gold-base alloy with sufficient alloying constituents to give a white color. Palladium, to the extent of 10% in the alloy, gives an excellent white gold; a cheaper alloy contains 10% nickel and 5% zinc. As the gold content is lowered, other alloying constituents may be used; thus, in 14 and 18 karat alloys, nickel, copper, zinc, and silver are among the elements to be found.

The dimethylglyoxime test readily detects the presence of nickel in metallic gold. Whenever allergic dermatitis from a gold ring is suspected a dimethylglyoxime test and patch tests with gold sodium thiosulfate, copper sulfate, nickel sulfate and palladium chloride should be performed to determine which metal is the culprit.

So-called jeweler's gold is in reality "jeweler's metal" that contains copper, zinc, and tin.

SYSTEMIC GOLD REACTIONS

Systemic therapy with gold, for rheumatic and/or dermatologic diseases, is often complicated by cutaneous adverse effects. Lichenoid eruptions and dermatitis are both seen. British investigators, using lymphocyte transformation assays to gold and nickel, found that patients with lichenoid reactions often showed positive tests to gold but those with dermatitis often reacted to nickel. Nickel is a significant contaminant of the injectable gold tested (Myochrisin, Rhone-Poulenc).[234] Möller and colleagues[235] found positive gold patch tests in 7 of 20 candidates for gold therapy and therefore recommend testing all prospective patients before starting chrysotherapy. In another 10 gold-allergic patients given gold intramuscularly (IM), flares of previous test sites and transient fevers were noted.[236]

Chrysiasis

The deposition of gold in the skin, leading to blue-gray pigmentation, is termed chrysiasis. This occurs after the therapeutic administration of gold, usually for rheumatoid arthritis. It rarely occurs with cumulative doses under 50 mg/kg and is common with doses above 150 mg/kg.[237] Miller and colleagues[238] studied a case of chrysiasis and identified gold microparticles in the superficial dermis.

Gold Schnapps Syndrome

Russell and colleagues[239] reported three patients with lichenoid eruptions and gold allergy provoked by consuming schnapps that contained gold flecks. Each cleared after several months of avoiding the gold-containing liquor.

OCCUPATIONAL GOLD ALLERGY

Soluble gold salts can cause occupational dermatitis. Exposure to gold salts may take place in porcelain, gold plating, gilding glass, and photography.

Gold Dermatitis in the Gilding Industry

Nava and Briatico Vangoso[240] described six cases of allergy to gold salt. Four workers engaged in gilding presented dermatoses in acroexposed sites. An administrative employee showed urticaria, the origin of which must be attributed, besides the exposure to gold salts, to sensitivity to foods and other contact antigens. In the sixth patient, who had urticaria and past eczema at sites of gold objects (ring and watch), the dermatitis was attributed to gold, whereas the urticaria was due to food, fungi, and drugs.

Skin and Nail Lesions from Gold Potassium Cyanide

Budden and Wilkinson[241] reported a man whose work consisted of cleaning gold electrode contacts. These electrode contacts were placed in a basket containing a mixture of potassium cyanide and an oxidizing agent, metanitrobenzene sulfonic acid. The mixture resulted in the formation of gold potassium cyanide, $KAu(CN_2)$.

Four days before he was seen at the clinic, the patient developed some scattered pustules on the backs of the fingers of the right hand and erosions and crusting of the lower lip. The patient remained off work for 2 weeks, and both sets of lesions healed uneventfully. When he was seen at the end of that time, however, he had developed a purplish brown discoloration with some partial onycholysis of the free ends of most of his finger nails on the right hand. Four weeks later, his fingernails had also returned to normal. Potassium dicyanoaurate is available for patch testing from Chemotechnique diagnostics at a concentration of 0.1% aqueous.[242]

Indium

Indium is found in dental restoration alloys. Marcussen and colleagues[243] reported allergy to indium in individuals with suspected sensitivity to dental materials. In all, nine had at least a 2+ reaction to indium sulfide 10% aqueous, and one reacted to indium chloride 10% aqueous. Several concentrations of both indium sulfide and indium chloride were tested, with indium sulfide 10% aqueous the most likely to give a reaction. Unfortunately, no comment was made regarding possible irritant reactions or clinical relevance. Fowler has seen rare reactions to indium in dental patients.

Iridium

In the same study, five patients reacted to iridium chloride 1% aqueous. Ammonium hexachloroiridate was also used for testing, with poor results.[243] A report from Italy noted no positives to iridium chloride (1% aq) in 720 consecutive subjects.[391] Iridium is of the platinum group of metals. In industry it is often found in association with platinum, which is a fairly common airborne respiratory allergen. There is one report of contact urticaria and respiratory hypersensitivity to iridium in an electrochemical process worker.[244]

Iron

DISCOLORATION AND DERMATITIS DUE TO IRON SALTS

Hemmer and colleagues[245] tested 623 patients with suspected metal allergy to ferric chloride (2% aq) and ferrous sulfate (5% pet). They saw only five positive and two questionable reactions. On testing with a dilution series, only two reacted. Both were also allergic to nickel and cobalt. Relevance was doubtful.

Nater[246] reported an instance of epidermal hypersensitivity to iron, but the patch test reaction may have been the nonspecific pustular variety. Baer[247] cited a metalworker with an allergic reaction to iron who had a positive (eczematous) patch test reaction.

One patient has been reported to be allergic to yellow iron oxide in a mascara[248] (see Chapter 16.)

Seven of 190 Italian ceramics workers were positive to patch testing with red iron oxide (2% pet).[249] A number of other metal salts used for decorative coloring of pottery also gave positive patch tests. The only one more common, however, was nickel (15% vs 3.6%).

Allergic contact dermatitis due to iron is apparently rare.

FERROXYL TEST FOR IRON

The ferroxyl test may be used to show the presence of free iron in corroded metallic objects. The metallic article is immersed in a gel containing 1% sodium chloride and 0.2% ferricyanide. A positive reaction is indicated by a blue growth that resembles seaweed from the corroded metal.

PIGMENTATION AND TATTOOING FROM IRON

Monsel's solution (a ferric chloride solution) has long been used as a hemostyptic. The application of old or concentrated solutions, particularly to abraded skin sites, may produce a permanent red-brown pigmented iron tattoo. Monsel's solution should be fresh and well shaken before being used on cosmetically exposed areas such as the face, the breast, or the upper back.[250] Aluminum chloride may be used as an alternative styptic, which is free of complicating pigmentation.

EXOGENOUS SIDEROSIS— PIGMENTATION OF SKIN FROM IRON PARTICLES

Jirasek[251] reported a red-brown, tattoo-like eruption in welders doing spot welding, which he labeled "exogenous siderosis." Exogenous siderosis of the skin, also called "millers' disease," has occurred in the past in millers and in millstone cutters and was caused by penetration of minute fragments of steel flying from cutters during millstone shaping. Similar manifestations occurred in file makers. The same manifestations occurred in gasfitters in whom particles of soot, dust, and rust penetrated into the skin when scouring gas pipes with compressed air.

Exogenous siderosis took the form of a perifollicular, punctate, red-brown pigmentation of the forearm in a man whose work was dipping iron parts into hydrochloric acid. After an acute dermatitis had healed, permanent rusty hyperpigmentation persisted in the affected areas on the volar aspect of the wrist. Histologic examination confirmed the presence of an exogenous iron pigment in the upper layer of the corium.

Jirasek[251] stated that the occupational hyperpigmentation reported by him has undoubtedly the same features as the exogenous siderosis of the skin reported earlier in millers, file makers, gasfitters, and other workers. Such hyperpigmentation is not a disease but is an interesting occupational stigma, which, for the affected individuals, is only of cosmetic significance, although it is not negligible from the aesthetic aspect.

Kasteler and Fowler have seen a patient with extensive iron deposition in a surgical scar (JS Kasteler, M.D., Louisville, KY, personal communication, 2000). A young woman underwent placement of stabilizing rods in the back and shortly thereafter was given an intravenous iron preparation. She developed brownish speckled dots throughout the long vertical scars. Histologic examination confirmed the presence of iron.

Lead

The rarity of allergic reaction to lead is emphasized by Fregert,[252] who, reporting a "possible" case of lead allergy, asked, "Has anyone else seen patch-test reactions to lead salts?" Fregert's case was a truck driver who had, for several years, charged the accumulators used in trucks. He developed dermatitis on the distal part of the fingers, and he himself suspected that the dermatitis

was due to the lead electrodes and the hydrochloric acid. Patch testing in a standard series gave negative reactions. Two different samples of lead chloride (0.2% aq) and lead acetate (0.5% aq) gave positive reactions; lead metal gave a negative reaction. The dermatitis was possibly caused by lead dissolved in hydrochloric acid.

DERMATITIS ASSOCIATED WITH LEAD POISONING

Czarnecki and Fritsch[253] reported a case of contact sensitization to lead, which presented as an acute bullous contact dermatitis after application of an ointment containing lead oxide (unguentum diachylon Hebra). In patch testing, the patient reacted strongly to lead oxide and lead acetate. Further examination revealed chronic lead intoxication with neurologic and labyrinthine involvement. As a painter, the patient had had professional contact with lead paints up to 25 years previously for a period of 30 years. He had never noticed any contact allergies to his working materials.

Allen and colleagues[254] studied three patients who had blistering on exposed areas of the skin and who had biochemical evidence of lead poisoning. A causal relationship through abnormalities in porphyrin metabolism is suggested.

It should be noted that thousands of people have used a hair preparation called Grecian Formula containing lead salts to darken hair without any reports of allergic or toxic reactions. The preparation contains an aqueous solution of lead acetate and glycerin with a small quantity of suspended sulfur.

Manganese

Manganese is a gray-white, brittle metal, with the atomic number 25. Most use is in steel and iron production. It is a component of the pesticide maneb, which may cause ACD. It was used in American coinage in nickels from 1942 to 1945. Manganese dioxide (10% pet) gave a positive patch test reaction in 2 of 190 ceramics workers.[68] Manganese has been reported to cause oral symptoms from dental prostheses in very rare cases.[255,256] It has been reported to cause hand dermatitis in a metal worker, who worked with an aluminum alloy containing 2% manganese.[257] All other patch tests, including many metals were negative, while MgCl (5% pet) was strongly positive.

Metallic (Elementary) Mercury

Mercury is one of the oldest metals known. From a standpoint of exposure, allergy to mercury must be considered differently from other metals. With the other common metal allergens, exposure to the metal itself is by far the most common situation, whereas exposure to primary solutions or metal salts is unusual except in the occupational setting. Exposure to metallic mercury, however, rarely occurs except in dental materials, whereas exposure to organic mercurials such as thimerosal is fairly frequent. Allergy to organic mercurials is discussed in Chapter 17. For our purposes here, it is sufficient to note that a patch test reaction to thimerosal usually indicates mercury allergy but may also indicate allergy to the thiosalicylic acid portion of the molecule.[258]

An unusual cutaneous side effect caused by mercury led to the origin of patch testing. In 1895, Jadassohn[259] described a patient with acute eczematous dermatitis confined to the sites to which a gray mercurial ointment had been previously applied for treatment of pediculosis pubis. Subsequent application of the gray ointment to unaffected sites produced eczematous reactions. These observations were the first to show that contact sensitization can be induced by the simple application of a suspected substance to unaffected skin.

Boyd and colleagues from Tennessee have reviewed the recent literature on cutaneous disease caused by mercury exposure.[260] Their case had cutaneous granulomas from traumatic mercury inoculation.

REACTIONS TO MERCURY FROM BROKEN THERMOMETERS

Spilled mercury droplets from a broken thermometer can produce severe reactions in sensitized individuals, such as dermatitis, stomatitis, encephalitis, and even death.[261]

Spilled mercury droplets from a broken thermometer can be picked up with a clean, shiny piece of copper. A mixture of sulfur, calcium, and water or aerosol hair spray can also "fix" mercury droplets.

Swinyer[262] reported a patient with a 23-year history of recurrent eruptions after contact with mercury from a broken thermometer. The patient's initial sensitization occurred after a "romance" with mercury that started with several "backroom" experiments using the chemical from thermometers that he purposely broke. In one experiment, he "changed a penny to a dime" by spreading the copper-colored coin with the silver-colored mercury using his fingertips. Each subsequent exposure after sensitization produced a blistering rash, "like poison oak." Within 24 hours of mercury exposure, his eyes would swell shut. This reaction was followed by a rash that spread over his entire body. He joined a pipeline company, and his job necessitated limited exposure to a small pool of metallic mercury in a fuel flow measuring

device. This exposure resulted in repeated severe cutaneous eruptions.

Vermeiden and colleagues[263] described a patient who developed erythema multiforme from inhalation of metallic mercury vapor. The patient reported that before his rash, he had cleaned up broken thermometers for 7 hours a day for 7 days in a 10-day period. This task had been performed in a locked room, and he had not worn a mask. On later inspection, the mercury was still found in the seams of the wooden floor.

Gerstner and Huff[264] pointed out that elementary mercury, such as that present in a thermometer or barometer, evaporates at room temperature and can enter the body by inhalation. Irreversible damage to the central nervous system can arise, depending on the concentration in the air and the time of exposure. Drowsiness and general malaise can also follow exposure to mercury vapors. These symptoms were observed in their patient.

Nakayama and colleagues[265] studied patients with a generalized rash, mostly appearing 1 or 2 days after breaking a clinical thermometer or during dental treatment. Similar skin manifestations were revealed, suggestive at first glance of mercury exanthem (i.e., diffuse symmetrical erythema predominantly on major fluxural areas). An inverted triangular or V-shaped erythema on both upper anteromedial thighs was a common feature. Severe cases had miliary pustules or purpura on erythematous skin. Pruritus or burning sensation was relatively mild. Pyrexia or malaise was a complaint of more than half the patients. Most of the patients had a previous history of contact dermatitis to Mercurochrome, and by patch testing, these patients were found to have contact allergy to several mercurials, especially inorganic ones. Mercurochrome had been widely used as a topical disinfectant in Japan. This seems to be a possible cause of the high incidence of contact allergy to mercurials in Japan. Nakayama et al. believed that patients had developed systemic contact dermatitis due to inhalation of mercury vapor.

BABOON SYNDROME

A syndrome of striking, bright erythema of the buttocks combined with dermatitis in flexural areas has been termed the "baboon syndrome." Inhalation of mercury vapor causes this rare but distinctive eruption. As noted above, small pustules may appear in the red areas. Sometimes bullae may occur.[266,267] Broken thermometers are the usual source of exposure, but one case occurred from playing a commercial English game containing mercury.[268] Although mercury was causative in initial reports, the baboon syndrome may occur from systemic exposure to other contact allergens.

NUMMULAR DERMATITIS

A Japanese report noted 2 cases of nummular dermatitis whose disease cleared after removal of mercury containing fillings. Patch tests were strongly positive in both to ammoniated mercury 1% per and 0.05% aqueous.[269]

CUTANEOUS GRANULOMAS

These findings are often the result of intentional injection of mercury, traumatic injection, or repetitive topical application of mercury ointments.[270]

MERCURY AMALGAMS

Mercury, without being heated, unites with many metals to form combinations known as amalgams. Dermatitis from amalgams may be caused by metallic mercury or the other metals. Amalgams composed of silver (about 35%), zinc, tin (15%), copper, and mercury (25%) are used as fillings for teeth (see Chapter 32), and as dental cements. In addition, amalgams of mercury with gold, silver, or copper may be used.

Recently, mercury has been re-examined not only as an allergen but also as a cause of nonspecific symptoms, such as malaise, headache, and fatigue from exposure by dental fillings. Although the question of oral mercury toxicity is uncertain, allergic stomatitis and oral (and possibly systemic) lichen planus to mercury from dental exposure definitely occurs. This is discussed in depth in Chapter 32. To summarize, a number of studies have clearly documented that stomatitis, oral lichenoid lesions, or lichen planus, and sometimes orodynia, may be caused by allergy to dental metals. Mercury and gold have been most often implicated, but other metals may cause oral allergy as well.[271–275]

The most likely scenario where relevant mercury dental allergy may occur is when an oral lesion is directly adjacent to a mercury amalgam filling. In one study, 70% of 30 patients with this pattern were patch-test positive to mercury and of these 93% improved with removal of the amalgam.[276]

Dental workers are also at risk for sensitization and ACD to mercury.[277]

UNUSUAL SOURCES OF MERCURY EXPOSURE

Koch and Nickolaus[278] reported a 5-year-old boy with generalized dermatitis and positive patch tests to thimerosal (0.05% pet), amalgam (5% pet), mercury chloride (0.01% pet), and mercury ammonium chloride (1% pet). After common sources of mercury exposure were ruled out, chemical testing revealed the presence of mercury chloride in PVC boots. The authors stated that mercury may be used in both leather and plastic footwear and as an antimildew agent.

PATCH TESTING FOR MERCURY ALLERGY

Thimerosal is a component of most patch test screening series and is the usual allergen for detecting mercury allergy. Goncalo and colleagues[258] stated that most positive patch tests to thimerosal indicate mercury allergy, but some detect allergy to the thiosalicylic acid portion of the molecule. Elemental mercury, amalgam, and various inorganic mercury salts may also be used to detect mercury sensitivity. Both Nakada and colleagues[279] and Handley and colleagues[280] suggest using both ionized (ammoniated mercury or mercury chloride) and nonionized mercury (metallic mercury or amalgam) for completeness.

When testing with amalgam, a 5% concentration in petrolatum has been recommended.[281] Testing with individual components would also be advisable when indicated.

Molybdenum

In various stainless steel suture clips, molybdenum was present at about 1% concentration. Seven of 184 patients patch tested with ammonium heptamolybdate 1% had a 1+ reaction, and 4 had a 2+ or 3+ reaction. Correlation with delayed wound healing and local reactions was not well documented for molybdenum but was present in nickel allergy.[282] Molybdenum has been implicated in allergy to endovascular stents (See Chapter 19).

Nickel—Ubiquitous Contact Allergen

"The Romance of Nickel," a brochure distributed by the International Nickel Company,[283] will no doubt intrigue nickel-sensitive persons—particularly the statement that reads, "Nickel is with you and does things for you from the time you get up in the morning until you go to sleep at night." This almost continuous exposure is reflected in the increasing number of patients who are sensitized to nickel.[284] Throughout the world, nickel is reported to be one of the most common causes of allergic contact dermatitis, particularly in women.[1,2,285,286] Nickel produces more cases of ACD than all the other metals combined.

In men, nickel dermatitis has been deemed predominantly of occupational origin (Table 32.10). Now that more men are undergoing body piercing, the rates in

Table 32-10 Industrial Exposures to Nickel

Alkaline batteries
Blackening zinc and brass
Ceramics
Coating (electroplating)
Duplicating fluids and fluxes (brazing)
Dyes
Electrical wiring
Enamel (green: nickel oxides)
Fuel additives
Hardening of fats (acts as a catalyst)
Insecticides
Magnet cores
Mordant in dyeing and printing fabrics
Nickel alloys
Nickel plating
Paint for glass
Pigments for paint and wallpaper
Reagents and catalysts (plastics)

Note: Rubber gloves are not protective. Use heavy-duty vinyl gloves.

Table 32-11 Metal Allergy Demographics

Nickel
  Female > male
  Incidence increasing overall
  Younger > older
Association with hand eczema, systemic ACD
  Association with cobalt
  Association with ear piercing
  Association with palladium
Chromate
  Male > female
  Incidence decreasing or stable
  Older > younger
Cobalt
  Female > male
  Incidence increasing
  Younger > older
  Association with nickel

From Reference 1.

men are likely to increase and nonoccupational exposure may predominate. It should be noted that since industrial nickel solutions can pass through rubber gloves; heavy-duty vinyl gloves should be used instead. In women, the most common cause of nickel dermatitis is direct contact, primarily from jewelry, garments, and wristwatches, and secondarily from such occupations as metal industry, hair dressing, tailoring, and hotel and restaurant work.

Once an individual acquires nickel dermatitis, allergic sensitivity to nickel persists indefinitely. No portion of the skin from the scalp to the soles is invulnerable to nickel dermatitis. As an occupational disease in workers exposed to massive amounts of nickel salts, the eruption may be generalized and resemble scabies.

PATCH TESTING CURES "BASAL-CELL CARCINOMA"

One recent report showed that a lesion on the cheek that looked exactly like a basal-cell carcinoma was actually a chronic ulcer due to nickel allergy to the patient's eyeglass frame.[287]

EPIDEMIOLOGY OF NICKEL ALLERGY

Table 32.5 reviews a number of studies regarding prevalence of positive patch test reactions to metals. It can be seen that women are more commonly allergic than men by a factor of 2 to 6 times. There is general agreement that this is due to jewelry usage, specifically ear piercing. Christophersen and colleagues,[288] using multivariate analysis, examined various factors in nickel allergy. In addition to an increase in women, absence of atopy and presence of hand eczema independently correlated with nickel allergy (Table 32.11).

Uter and colleagues[289] performed a statistical analysis of nickel allergy in a multi-year, multi-center study from Germany and Austria. Out of almost 75,000 patients, nickel was positive in 15.5% (11,615). The strongest demographic correlation was in females versus males. Also, risk increased continuously with decreasing age. There was no association with atopy.

In Israel, 17.4% of 943 patients were positive to nickel, 25% of women and 6% of men. They also found more nickel–positive patients in the group under age 40.[290]

Schubert and colleagues[291] found that of 104 patients, 68 were free of nickel dermatitis 3 years after patch testing, and 13 had chronic hand eczema. Dietary nickel modification was not tried. Forty-two had changed jobs, 36 of whom had cleared.

Is environmental nickel pollution protective against ACD to nickel? Norwegian and Russian authors present the interesting hypothesis that high levels of nickel in the environment may protect from sensitization. They compared women from a Norwegian town with low levels of environmental nickel and two Russian towns with high levels. In the low-exposure group, 27.5% of women had nickel allergy, but only 7.2 % were allergic from the high exposure areas. Ear piercing rates were identical.[292]

NONINDUSTRIAL NICKEL DERMATITIS IN MEN

From Kuwait, Kanan[293] reported that the men are sensitized by the nickel-plated studs in their underwear.

Peltonen[294] stated that the most common sensitizers of men outside occupations dealing with metals seem to be wristwatches and watchstrap buckles. Like women, men are sensitized by the accessories on their clothing, particularly by buttons in jeans and belt buckles, but also by cheap jewelry. It was found that the participants of the study were not exposed to nickel in their occupations and that nickel sensitivity was found in men only in the young age group (which is more prone to wear jeans and jewelry). The incidence of nickel sensitization in men will increase as more men pierce their ears (or other body sites) to wear earrings. Men, however, may tend to wear fewer different earrings of higher quality, so they may not be as readily sensitized.

DIETARY COMPONENT OF NICKEL DERMATITIS

Even today, in the new millennium, the role of dietary nickel in causing and maintaining nickel dermatitis is vastly underappreciated. The simple fact, documented by a variety of studies, is that enough nickel in the diet of a sensitive individual can provoke dermatitis. The hands are the most common location for systemic nickel dermatitis (Figure 2-3), with manifestations including pompholyx or "regular" hand dermatitis. Other body areas may be affected as well. Evidence for the role of dietary nickel includes (a) flare of eczema and/or patch test sites upon oral nickel challenge; (b) improvement of dermatitis with a reduced nickel diet; (c) improvement of dermatitis by oral disulfiram, which chelates nickel and increases its excretion; and (d) preliminary suggestions that children with orthodontic devices (braces), who are therefore exposed to low continuous levels of ingested nickel, may have less subsequent nickel ACD.

NICKEL IN FOOD

The normal daily intake of nickel by American adults has been calculated at 0.3 to 0.6 mg (295). About 1% to 10% of nickel in food is absorbed in the gastrointestinal tract, and the remainder is excreted. The nickel content of foods is partially determined by the components of the soil in which it is grown, fungicides used on it, and the equipment used in handling the food.

Nickel in food may vary considerably from region to region. Certain foods are routinely high in nickel content. Legumes, nuts, grains, potatoes, chocolate, and fish are among the foods high in nickel.[296] (See Chapter 35 for a low-nickel diet.)

Horak and Sunderman[297] stated that fecal excretion is the major route for elimination of nickel from the human body. Hence, comprehensive evaluations of environmental or occupational exposures to nickel should include analyses of nickel in feces, as well as analyses of serum, urine, and hair.

It may be noted that appreciable losses of nickel also occur in the sweat. This observation may account for the diminished concentration of serum nickel in blast-furnace workers who were chronically exposed to extreme heat. The only other known route for the excretion of appreciable amounts of nickel is in a mother's milk.

The amount of nickel absorbed from food and water has been shown to vary considerably. Nielsen and colleagues[298] showed that peak serum nickel concentration was 13 times greater if nickel in water was given 30 minutes before a meal of scrambled eggs as compared to giving it simultaneously with the meal.

NICKEL IN TAP WATER

Fregert[299] stated that many nickel-sensitive patients with hand dermatitis suspect that tap water contains nickel and that their dermatitis is worsened by exposure to such water. In a previous study, Fregert had found no nickel, or only traces, when various samples of tap water that had been submitted by patients were analyzed. More recently, however, a nickel-sensitive woman with hand dermatitis reported that her condition was always worse when she was living in her own apartment but improved when she was in her parents' house. The first liters of running water obtained from the patient's home contained considerable amounts of nickel, especially from the hot tap (up to 0.13 mg/L), apparently due to corrosion of the tap and the linings of the boiler and tubes. Another factor may be the previous nickel-plating of chromium-plated metal; after long use, the nickel may reach the surface on water taps. On the basis of these findings, Fregert advised, "Nickel-sensitive persons should let the first liter of water run away in the morning."

On the basis of analyses of nickel concentrations in 969 water supplies in the United States during 1969 and 1970, Kopp and Kramer[300] found that the average concentration of nickel in water samples taken at the consumer's taps was 4.8 mg/L. With an estimated daily intake of 2 L of water, an adult would consume approximately 10 mg of nickel in drinking water each day. These investigators found the highest concentration of nickel in tap water from the Ohio River and Lake Erie river basins.

McNeely and colleagues[301] found that tap water from Sudbury, Ontario, the site of the largest open-pit nickel mines in North America, contained 200 mg/L of nickel—182 times greater than the concentration in tap water from Hartford, Connecticut, which contained 1.1 mg/L. In addition, the serum and urine concentrations of nickel in persons living in Sudbury were significantly higher than in those living in Hartford. These authors emphasized that there is no evidence that environmental exposures to nickel in Sudbury, Ontario, are associated with adverse effects in humans or animals or are deleterious in any way to the health of the inhabitants.

INGESTED NICKEL AS A CAUSE OF DERMATITIS

Fowler[1] reviewed the various studies of nickel intake in relation to flares of dermatitis. Various amounts of nickel, up to 5 or 6 mg, have been given in capsule form. Other studies have attempted dietary intervention to reduce nickel intake. With rare exceptions, ingestion of enough nickel can result in a flare of dermatitis, especially hand eczema of the "pompholyx" type. Kaaber and colleagues,[302] for example, found that 17 patients flared after ingestion of 2.5 mg of nickel. Nine of these improved after 6 weeks on a reduced-nickel diet. In another study, weekly nickel administration worsened dermatitis in 75% of 12 subjects, whereas only 25% on placebo worsened.[303] In Denmark, the estimated daily average nickel intake is about 0.3 mg, with a maximum of about 1 mg. A dose-response study there confirmed the ability of ingested nickel to cause dermatitis.[304] In 10 subjects fed 4.0 mg., 7 had a flare of dermatitis. Four of 10 given 1 mg and also 4 of 10 given 0.3 mg had dermatitis flares. Only 1 flared with placebo.

Veien[305] was enthusiastic about the benefits of a low-nickel diet, with at least some improvement being common, although total clearing may not occur. Further evidence for the role of systemic nickel in causing dermatitis is the finding that disulfiram, a nickel chelator, may result in improvement in nickel dermatitis and definitely increases nickel excretion.[303]

The Danish investigators performed a meta-analysis of 9 studies looking at dose-response issues in systemic nickel allergy.[306] They concluded that at least 1% of nickel-allergic persons will develop systemic ACD from daily exposure to "normal" amounts of dietary nickel, which they defined as 0.22 to 0.35 mg. Obviously more persons would be expected to react to higher intake.

The difficulty in predicting systemic nickel allergy is primarily due to our lack of knowledge regarding a person's dietary nickel intake at any given time. It can be stated without doubt that in most patients, a nickel intake above their "threshold level" will result in systemic dermatitis.

In a study of nine nickel-sensitive patients with various forms of hand eczema, Fowler[307] found that eight improved significantly after treatment with disulfiram 250 mg/day. None improved with placebo treatment. Side effects may include liver function abnormalities and drowsiness. Avoidance of alcohol during treatment must be absolute. An initial flare, caused by temporary mobilization of systemic nickel, may occur. Once improvement is achieved, intermittent treatment may maintain clearing.

ROLE OF COOKING UTENSILS IN NICKEL DERMATITIS

Katz and Samitz[308] found that sweat and household detergents were shown to have the capacity to release nickel from stainless steel. This finding substantiates the thesis that stainless-steel utensils can be sources of skin contact allergy with nickel.

Christensen and Möller[309] measured the release of nickel to boiling water from new and used saucepans of different materials. No nickel was released from aluminum, Teflon, and enamel. Certain amounts of nickel were released from stainless steel, but only at acid pH. When the pH was lowered, appreciable amounts of nickel were leached out into the boiling water from new as well as used saucepans. It was even shown that the amounts released were positively correlated with the acidity of the water. Patients with nickel allergy should thus avoid stainless-steel cooking utensils because some foodstuffs may provide an acid milieu during processing.

The amount of nickel released from cooking utensils in the present study was fairly small in comparison to the dose used in oral provocation, and therefore this is unlikely to be a major contributor to dietary intake.

In summary, then, ingested nickel from food, beverages, or cooking utensils can cause a flare of dermatitis in some individuals. Accordingly, well-motivated patients may see improvement if they can reduce their body burden of nickel through either dietary changes or disulfiram therapy.

POSSIBLE ROLE OF METALS IN DIET IN PATCH TEST–NEGATIVE PATIENTS

Veien and colleagues[310] claimed that the dermatitis of some patients with patch test–negative vesicular hand eczema flares after oral challenge with nickel, cobalt, or chromium salts.

In a controlled study, 202 patients (68 males and 134 females), with patch test–negative, symmetrical vesicular hand eczema, were challenged orally with 2.5 mg of nickel, 2.5 mg of chromium, and 1 mg of cobalt given as salts of the respective metals. A mixture of the three metal salts was given initially, and if this produced a flare of the eczema, the salts were administered individually at 1-week intervals.

Fifty-five patients reacted to the mixture of salts as well as to one or two of the individual salts. Three other patients were challenged openly with nickel alone. Male patients reacted primarily to chromate and cobalt, whereas female patients more commonly reacted to nickel and cobalt.

Fifty-six patients were instructed to follow diets planned to reduce the daily intake of the respective metals. The dermatitis of 36 patients cleared or improved markedly after 1 month of dieting. Responses to a questionnaire sent to these 36 patients indicated that 28 of them had followed the prescribed diet rigorously or intermittently for at least 1 year, because they experienced recurrence of the dermatitis if they stopped dieting. Six patients noted no long-term benefit, and two did not respond. The diet instructions for cobalt in this experiment are listed in Table 32.9.

Veien and colleagues[311] then challenged patients with various chronic dermatoses of obscure origin as follows: The 299 patients with chronic dermatitis of obscure origin were challenged orally in a controlled study, with 2.5 mg of nickel, 2.5 mg of chromium, and 1 mg of cobalt given as salts of the respective metals.

Flares of the dermatitis were seen in 12 of 61 patients with patch test–negative hyperkeratotic eczema, in 9 of 32 patients with patch test–negative perianal eczema, and in 7 of 143 patients with various other patch test–negative eczemas. In this latter group, flares were seen only among patients with nummular eczema or hand eczema. Among 34 patients with various positive patch tests not relevant to the current dermatitis, 3 patients with hand eczema experienced flares.

Patients who reacted to oral challenges with the metal salt to which they had a positive patch test included 3 of 9 with nickel allergy, 2 of 5 with cobalt allergy, and 6 of 15 with chromate allergy. These patients were tested openly.

Low metal diets were prescribed for 33 patients who had flares after oral challenge with specific metal salts. The dermatitis cleared or improved markedly for 23 of these patients after following the diet for at least 2 weeks. Responses to a questionnaire sent to the 23 patients indicated that 16 had followed the prescribed diet rigorously or intermittently for at least 1 year.

NICKEL IN URINE

Menné and colleagues,[312] commenting that the importance of internal exposure to nickel in patients with recurrent hand eczema and nickel allergy has become evident, undertook a study to investigate the value of urinary nickel determinations as an index of oral nickel intake. After administering 5.6 mg of nickel orally (as the sulfate), Menné and colleagues found increased nickel excretion over the next 2 to 3 days. Spruit and Bongaarts[313] also produced results showing increased urinary nickel levels for more than 24 hours after the adminis-

tration of 5 mg of nickel to two healthy volunteers. McNeely and colleagues[314] found that such diverse conditions as myocardial infarction, stroke, burns, hepatic cirrhosis, and uremia could produce abnormal concentrations of nickel in serum and, presumably, urine.

Spruit[315] found that the nickel (Ni) concentration in the urine of a rheumatic nonhypersensitive person that was usually about 1 mg Ni/L urine, increased to 9 mg Ni/L urine (range: 6 to 13 mg Ni/L) by the oral ingestion of 25 mg indomethacin per day over a period of 5 days. Prolonged ingestion of a medicine with food may thus increase the internal nickel absorption and possibly cause an exacerbation of nickel eczema in patients hypersensitive to that metal.

It is comforting for the clinician to learn that the nickel concentrations of blood plasma, urine, and scalp hair do not differ between patients who are hypersensitive and those who are nonsensitive to nickel. Even persons exposed occupationally to nickel, who may have 10 times more nickel in their plasma, urine, and hair than the normal "control" population, do not necessarily become allergic to nickel.[314]

NICKEL IN HAIR

Katz and colleagues[316] reported that the nickel content of human hair was found to be more dependent on the sex of the donor than on other parameters and that nickel sensitivity was not reflected in the nickel content of women's hair, although there is a significant difference between the nickel content of men's and women's hair.

NICKEL AND THE LAW

In response to the high rate of nickel allergy, the Danish Ministry of the Environment, on 27 June 1989, released Statutory Order No. 472.[317] The order essentially prohibits the sale of nickel-containing jewelry, eyeglass frames, or clothing accessories that give a positive dimethylglyoxime test. The European "Nickel Directive" essentially extended this prohibition throughout the EU. It came into force in July, 2001. The penalty for violation may be a fine or imprisonment. Enforcement today seems uncertain. A Swedish report 4 years later stated that 17% of ear-piercing posts and 8% of 786 consumer items and jewelry were above the legal limit.[318]

NICKEL SENSITIVITY AS A CAUSE OF INFUSION REACTIONS

Stoddart[319] reported that skin reactions developed in two patients who had had intravenous infusions and that in one of these there was also an alarming anaphylactoid reaction. It was suggested that sensitivity to the nickel in the infusion cannulas was the cause.

Smeenk and Teunissen[320] described seven patients with a contact allergy to nickel in whom cutaneous lesions, sometimes with fever, developed after administration of an intravenous infusion. The lesions consisted of vesiculobullous eruptions on the hands, more or less generalized exanthema, and occasional flares at the sites of earlier contact eczema due to nickel. It could be demonstrated experimentally that minute amounts of nickel, sufficient to cause the symptoms described, may be eluted from metallic needles by the infusion fluid. Their experiment consisted of a closed system in which 500 mL of physiologic saline was circulated four times during a 24-hour period through a stainless steel (8% nickel, 18% chrome) needle; 7 mg/L of nickel could be found in the solution. In a similar experiment lasting 48 hours (recirculated eight times), 80 mg/L of nickel was found.

TYPES OF NICKEL ERUPTIONS

Calnan[321] classified nickel dermatitis into two groups: (a) primary: areas in direct contact with metal (such eruptions are usually eczematous but are occasionally papular); and (b) secondary: selective symmetrical areas that are involved when the dermatitis spreads.

The secondary eruption behaves like an autosensitive hematogenous spread similar to an "id" phenomenon. It is usually symmetrical and is related to the activity of the primary site. The secondary site may be the elbow flexure, eyelids, sides of neck, and face. The eruption is sometimes said to become generalized.

The secondary or idlike eruption may be manifest occasionally as a noneczematous dermatitis, such as erythema multiforme, urticaria, or prurigo. It should be noted that this type of secondary symmetrical eruption is not often seen. Instead, a pompholyx type of eruption has been extensively described.

Both Calnan[321] and Epstein[322] remarked that nickel dermatitis is "peculiar," in that at times nickel dermatitis spreads without contact with nickel and at other times the dermatitis does not always appear at all sites of contact. In our opinion, however, the spread of nickel dermatitis to distant areas without contact with nickel may be more apparent than real. A careful history may reveal that in reality nickel did contact all the affected areas. Nickel-plated objects in wearing apparel may have a wide range of excursion on the skin. Bracelets and various other nickel-plated trinkets may move from the wrist to the elbows. Such bracelets may also contact the chest and abdomen if they are not removed when the patient undresses or bathes. Moreover, wandering, perspiring fingers may convey nickel in solution from metallic objects to distant sites.

The factor of perspiration has to be recognized in relationship to the production of nickel dermatitis. Because certain areas of skin may perspire more than others, it is to be expected that not all areas of the skin making contact with metallic nickel will necessarily dissolve out nickel salt in the same concentrations. Nickel-plated objects contacting relatively "dry" areas of skin may not produce dermatitis in nickel-sensitive individuals.

Some nickel-sensitive persons report that the dermatitis due to nickel is much worse in the summer. Fisher noted that several women stated that when they were perspiring freely, their costume jewelry would cause an itching, prickly sensation within 15 to 20 minutes and that an eruption would appear in about 45 to 60 minutes. These same persons can wear nickel-plated objects for several hours in the winter, or when they were not perspiring, without any symptoms of dermatitis. The chloride radical in sweat is apparently an important factor in dissolving the metallic nickel, permitting the soluble nickel salts to act.

The proof that the chloride in sweat can release nickel from a metallic object was demonstrated by placing a nickel-plated object in each of three jars. The first contained a solution resembling sweat (0.5% sodium chloride, 0.5% urea, and 0.17% lactic acid). The second jar contained alcohol. The third jar contained distilled water. The nickel coins were allowed to remain in the jars for 2 hours. A spot test with dimethylglyoxime was then done with the solutions remaining after the nickel objects were removed. Only the first jar gave a positive test result for nickel.[323] In addition, it should be noted that considerable amounts of nickel are excreted in sweat.

Other factors to be considered are friction and pressure. Adequate pressure is undoubtedly necessary to produce nickel dermatitis. Those areas in most intimate contact with nickel are the most likely to show nickel dermatitis. When pressure is avoided, dermatitis may not occur even in patients with marked hypersensitivity to nickel.

Talcum or other absorbent powder placed under a nickel-plated object may prevent dermatitis in nickel-sensitive persons for a short time. The powder acts both as a mechanical barrier, preventing contact of the nickel object with the skin, and as a sponge, absorbing perspiration that ordinarily would dissolve and remove soluble nickel salts from the metallic objects.

TYPES OF NICKEL HAND DERMATITIS

Hand dermatitis to nickel may be due to actual contact with nickel in sensitized individuals or to internal exposure.

Direct Contact

In men, nickel dermatitis of the hands is usually due to industrial exposure. In women, contact with inexpensive rings, knitting needles, or prolonged contact with nickel-plated objects will localize the dermatitis.

The prognosis is good in the industrial worker if the worker changes his or her job or if industrial hygiene improves.

Very low and short contact nickel exposure can flare hand dermatitis. Nielsen and colleagues[324] immersed one finger of 17 nickel-allergic volunteers for 10 minutes in a nickel solution of 10 ppm. This was done daily for one week, followed by 100 ppm daily for one week. Development of vesicles at day 14 was significantly higher ($p > .05$) in subjects compared to 18 controls.

Pompholyx or Dishydrosiform Dermatitis

Another type of hand dermatitis, which may be caused by external nickel sensitization, is pompholyx. This dermatitis is accompanied by recurring itching and vesicles in the palms and on the sides of the fingers. It should be noted that these types of hand dermatitis are not specific to nickel allergy.

Christensen[325] gave a follow-up report of 63 female patients with nickel allergy and hand eczema who were reinvestigated 6 years after the primary investigation. Christensen discovered that 30% of the patients were healed. Patients with the pompholyx eczema had the worst prognosis. The start of hand eczema was not correlated to any particular occupation. There was a strong correlation between a history of metal sensitivity and a positive patch test reaction. High frequencies of personal and family atopy were found, and atopy made the prognosis worse.

PATCH TESTS FOR NICKEL SENSITIVITY

Patch testing with nickel has been a common field of study. The following questions have been posed[326]: (a) What is the best vehicle for patch testing with nickel sulfate? (b) What is the optimum patch test concentration for nickel sulfate? (c) Are there any indications for intradermal patch testing with nickel? and (d) Are there patients with allergic hypersensitivity to nickel in whom patch test results to nickel are negative?

Vehicles for Testing with Nickel Sulfate

Most investigators use petrolatum as the diluent vehicle for nickel sulfate. In comparing patch test results of nickel sulfate in petrolatum with aqueous nickel sulfate, Fisher stated that 5% nickel sulfate in petrolatum gives an occasional negative reaction, whereas the aqueous solution in the same concentration gives a strongly positive patch test reaction.

In petrolatum, nickel and some other allergens may not always be evenly dispersed. Thus, there are nickel-poor or even nickel-free areas in these petrolatum patch test materials that could give rise to false-negative patch test reactions. In aqueous solutions of nickel sulfate, there is always an even distribution of the nickel salt.

Wahlberg[327] pointed out, in his experiments with both humans and guinea pigs, that distilled water was slightly more reliable than petrolatum as the suitable material for patch testing with metal compounds. He also pointed out, however, the following advantages of using petrolatum: (a) It possesses sealing capacity, (b) there is less risk of decomposition of the test substances in storage, and (c) petrolatum is somewhat better than water when using nonocclusive tapes.

Van Ketel[328] agreed that distilled water is more reliable than petrolatum as a suitable vehicle for metal compounds. He stated, however, that in certain patients with a definite nickel dermatitis, patch testing with nickel sulfate 2.5% to 5% in water did not give positive reactions. In these cases, the use of nickel sulfate 2.5% in dimethyl sulfoxide (DMSO) resulted in more positive patch test reactions than when dissolved in water. Originally, van Ketel tested with nickel sulfate 2.5% in 50% DMSO.

When Wall and Calnan[329] investigated an outbreak of occupational dermatitis in an electroforming plant in which there was a heavy exposure to nickel, they found that nickel chloride was a more reliable patch test allergen than nickel sulfate in petrolatum.

Nickel chloride, in a gel vehicle, such as the T.R.U.E. test, has been suggested to be somewhat more accurate than nickel sulfate in petrolatum because of better dispersion in the gel.[330]

Concentration of Nickel Sulfate for Patch Testing

Cronin[331] evaluated the efficacy of patch testing with 5% and 2.5% nickel sulfate in petrolatum by applying them concurrently to two series of routine patients, first in 1968 and again in 1973. In the first group, there were 75 nickel-sensitive patients, and in the second group there were 64. In both series, the weaker concentration (2.5%) failed to detect 20% of these sensitized persons. In the two groups, a few patients (8 of 139, or 6%) had positive test results to the 2.5% and negative results to the 5% concentration. This anomalous result was probably due to a fault in the technique, to greater pressure or occlusion of the weaker patch test, to irregularities in nickel dispersion, or to the "twinkling back" syndrome of Rietschel.

Cronin[331] concluded that the most suitable concentration for routine patch testing was 5% nickel sulfate in petrolatum and that because this concentration is a mild irritant in some patients, a purely poral or follicular reaction should be checked by repeating the 5% test, applying 2.5%, and checking the history.

Dooms-Goossens and colleagues[330] studied two women with histories of contact dermatitis to nickel-containing jewelry (dimethylglyoxime test positive) who failed to react to patch testing with 5% nickel sulfate in yellow petrolatum. Further patch testing was performed with nickel sulfate 2.5% and 5% in water and with 2.5% in DMSO 50%; no positive reactions were obtained. An intradermal test with 1:10,000 dilution in water also gave negative results.

Both patients were again patch tested with 10% nickel sulfate in yellow petrolatum, which resulted in positive reactions after 48 and 96 hours. These investigators point out that if both patients had not insisted and if the anamnesis had not been so clear, two diagnoses of nickel contact allergy would have been overlooked on the basis of the standard 5% concentration.

Occasionally, particularly in atopic individuals, pustular patch test reactions are obtained with nickel. These are nonspecific reactions of no clinical significance.

In Fisher's material,[326] a positive patch test reaction to 5% nickel sulfate solution was invariably strongly positive in individuals with proved allergic hypersensitivity to nickel. In a series of 50 individuals with nickel dermatitis, all showed a strongly positive patch test reaction, and 49 individuals showed positive intradermal reactions. In no instance did the intradermal test with nickel show any superiority over the patch test.

In Fisher's experience, every patient with proved nickel sensitivity also showed a positive patch test reaction to nickel coins. Moreover, a follow-up study revealed that more than 90% of the patients retained such strongly positive patch test reactions over a period of 2 to 17 years.

The NACDG has used nickel sulfate hexahydrate 2.5% in petrolatum for decades and finds it to be satisfactory.

Threshold Level of Nickel Reactivity

In a study by Emmett and colleagues,[332] 12 nickel-sensitive patients were tested with various dilutions of nickel sulfate in petrolatum or water. The lowest amount producing a reaction was 0.47 mg (0.01%) in petrolatum. The lowest amount to react in a significant number of patients was 1.5 mg (0.0316%). These low levels are easily attainable by sweat leaching of jewelry, for example. More recently Fischer and colleagues[333] reviewed the topic. They suggested that the 5% MET (the level at which 5% of nickel-sensitive persons would react) was

0.44 micrograms/cm^2 and that the 10% MET was 1.04 micrograms/cm^2.

In-vitro Testing for Nickel Allergy

Spiewak and colleagues[334] have extensively studied in-vitro lymphocyte testing to attempt to diagnose nickel allergy. They state that "[t]o date, no in vitro test is suitable for routine diagnosis of contact allergy." However, they present data that shows that T-lymphocytes from nickel-allergic patients, when treated with various cytokines, would produce significantly different levels of IL-5 and IL-13 than T-cells from normal control.

Other in-vitro testing methods have not, to our knowledge, been this carefully controlled and correlated with clinical manifestations of allergy.

Dimethylglyoxime Nickel Spot Test

The dimethylglyoxime (DMG) spot test for the detection of nickel has been modified and popularized by Fisher.[335] The spot test kit contains 1% dimethylglyoxime in alcohol solution (1 fl oz) and 10% ammonium hydroxide solution (1 fl oz). The directions are as follows: Add a few drops of each solution to the metallic object, solution, or skin to be tested. There is a positive reaction when a pink or red precipitate occurs, indicating the presence of available nickel in sufficient concentration (at least 1:10,000) to produce dermatitis in nickel-sensitive persons. Most metal alloys containing nickel give a positive reaction, except stainless steel, which is usually safe for use by those who are nickel-sensitive. The DMG spot test can detect the presence of nickel in "gold" and other jewelry when the patient and the jeweler are unaware of available nickel content.

Dr. Ronald Shore of the Hahnemann Medical College and Hospital of Philadelphia described a "modification" of the dimethylglyoxime test, as follows:

In our modification of this procedure, a few drops of dimethylglyoxime and ammonium hydroxide are successively placed on a cotton-tipped applicator, and the cotton tip is then rubbed against the test object. A positive result with this technique is the formation of a red precipitate on the applicator tip." This modification is the most commonly used DMGO test technique currently.

Previous editions of this text have given other more complicated chemical testing procedures for nickel, and the chemically inquisitive are directed to these editions if such information is desired.

Ear Piercing and Nickel Sensitivity

Many individuals become sensitized to nickel when their ears are pierced. Because injury to the skin from mechanical, physical, or chemical agents followed by intimate contact with nickel-plated earrings favors the development of allergic nickel dermatitis, piercing of earlobes followed by contact with jewelry containing nickel readily induces nickel sensitivity.

Ears should be pierced with stainless-steel instruments or needles, and only stainless-steel earrings should be worn for at least 3 weeks until the pierced opening is completely epithelialized. There are many so-called hypoallergenic earrings on the market, but no earrings should be recommended for nickel-allergic persons unless one obtains a negative result from a nickel dimethylglyoxime spot test.

The idea that the piercing of earlobes is important in developing nickel allergy is strongly supported by Rystedt and Fischer's investigations.[336] Among the nickel-allergic women, 95% had pierced earlobes. Piercing at an early age seems to increase the risk of incurring nickel sensitivity.

The piercing agent is probably not the main offender in nickel allergy. The nickel earrings used frequently after piercing are usually the cause of allergy. The environment of the hole in the earlobe is closed, and humid and irritant reactions often develop, especially after hair washing, when the rings are left in the earlobes. The shampoo that remains may cause an irritant contact dermatitis, which can induce nickel sensitivity.

Boss and Menné[337] agreed that the main cause of nickel sensitization in females is the piercing of ears. They stated that the manner of ear piercing today and the use of nickel-plated jewelry result in a nickel-sensitization rate of a minimum of 20% (11/53) among young females.

In a study of 700 Finnish teenagers, 31% with pierced ears were allergic to nickel, but only 2% without pierced ears were allergic.[338]

Nickel-sensitive individuals must wear stainless-steel earrings or more expensive precious metal earrings free of nickel. Some individuals coat "favorite" dermatitis-producing earrings with nail lacquer and can thus wear the earrings for a few hours without symptoms appearing.

JEAN NICKEL BUTTON DERMATITIS

Brandrup and Larsen[339] examined 79 nickel-sensitive patients (65 women and 14 men) with regard to a present or past eczema corresponding to contact with metallic buttons in jeans; 63% of the women and 64% of the men had or had had eczema of this kind. Among 40% of the women younger than 30 years of age, this was the primary site of manifestation. The seriousness of this sensitivity is illustrated by the fact that two-thirds of the nickel-sensitive patients with button dermatitis had

or had had eczema of the hands. The conclusion is that jean buttons should be made of a material that does not contain nickel, such as zinc alloys, which are used for some metallic buttons, or they should be designed in such a way that the button does not come into contact directly with the skin.[340] Brandrup and Larsen[339] stated that they had investigated the nickel release from 10 metallic buttons suspected of provoking contact dermatitis. The buttons represented identical types, although of various makes, and were used by 10 nickel-sensitive female patients whose nickel sensitivity was verified by positive patch tests.

The nickel release varied considerably. Two buttons had a particularly high release and were suspected of causing primary sensitization according to anamnestic information. Five buttons did not release more nickel than the blank synthetic sweat solution, but two of these buttons were dimethylglyoxime-positive. The dimethylglyoxime test seems to be better than the synthetic sweat/flameless atomic absorption model in predicting the risk of metallic alloys.

The jean nickel button dermatitis is usually most prominent in the navel area. The eruption may at times cover a large portion of the mid-abdomen. When the nickel-plated button is handled by someone with perspiring fingers, nickel dermatitis may occur in "ectopic" areas.

Brass or bone buttons may be substituted for the nickel-plated variety.

NICKEL IN EYESHADOW

Goh and colleagues[341] reported a nickel-allergic patient who reacted when wearing certain eyeshadow cosmetics. Patch test to the cosmetic was negative, but the sensitive eyelid skin reacted. The researchers found from 13 to 70 mg/g of nickel in some eyeshadows, well above the threshold for reactivity.

Eyeshadows, and possibly other cosmetics, should be considered as occult causes of dermatitis in nickel-allergic patients.

DERMO-JET NICKEL DERMATITIS

LaChapelle and Tennstedt[342] reported that 10 women allergic to nickel developed skin reactions at injection sites with a Dermo-Jet of 2% lidocaine solution and 0.9% saline solution. Ten women (age-matched), who were not allergic to nickel, were selected as controls and submitted to the same injections; they had no positive reactions. Nickel was leached out of the Dermo-Jet by tissue fluids producing the reaction. The dimethylglyoxime test showed that the internal rod of the reservoir as well as metallic internal parts of the nozzle leached appreciable amounts of nickel even before any clinical use.

De Corret and colleagues[343] reported that 20 blood donors developed a dermatitis at the site of venipuncture within a few hours of giving blood. A local anesthetic administered with a Dermo-Jet had been used before extracting blood. A used Dermo-Jet releases more nickel than a new Dermo-Jet.

OCCUPATIONAL NICKEL EXPOSURE

Shah and colleagues[344] evaluated 386 nickel-allergic patients for workplace exposure. In 84 (22.8%), nickel was felt to be a definite or possible occupational allergen. Hand dermatitis, as expected, was more common in the occupational group, and irritant dermatitis often coexisted. Commonly affected workers included hairdressers, retail clerks, food service workers, cleaners, and metal workers.

NICKEL DERMATITIS IN HAIRDRESSERS FROM PERMANENT-WAVE SOLUTIONS

Wahlberg[345] showed that hairdressers often develop nickel hypersensitivity through contact with utensils such as scissors and clips. Dahlquist and colleagues[346] demonstrated that hairdressers are in contact with permanent-wave liquids, which contain ammonium and glyceryl thioglycolate. Thioglycolic acid can form complexes with nickel ions.[346] Dahlquist et al. showed that commercial permanent-wave liquids readily release nickel from nickel-plated utensils used by hairdressers, but that similar objects, which are made of stainless steel, do not release any nickel.

UNUSUAL SOURCES OF NICKEL EXPOSURE

A worker making molded bricks developed ACD from nickel.[347]

In two reports, nickel in chalk apparently caused hand dermatitis in teachers.[348,349]

A metal strap to dissipate static electricity caused ACD in an electronics worker.[350]

Nickel allergy from a bedwetting alarm was confused with genital herpes in a 5-year-old girl.[351] In another case, a swallowed coin caused generalized dermatitis in a child.[352]

REACTIONS TO NICKEL-CONTAINING HEART VALVES

Lyell and colleagues[353] stated that life-threatening peri-prosthetic incompetence developed with two successive nickel-containing mitral-valve prostheses in a patient allergic to nickel. Neither prosthesis had been incorporated satisfactorily. The patient's present nickel-free prosthesis seemed to be satisfactory 22 months after insertion. Because allergy to nickel may have been involved in the failure of these prostheses, it is recommended that nickel-sensitive patients should be given nickel-free prostheses. (See Chapter 19.)

USE OF CHELATING AGENTS IN CHRONIC NICKEL DERMATITIS

Chelating agents such as disulfiram (Antabuse) have proved effective in nickel carbonyl poisoning. Menné and Kaaber[354] stated that the ingestion of nickel is important for the chronicity of hand eczema in nickel-sensitive patients. They tried the effect of chelating agents, because diethyldithiocarbamate (DDC) and tetra-ethylthiuram disulfide (TETD, Antabuse) have proved effective in the treatment of nickel carbonyl poisoning. A 66-year-old woman suffering from severe nickel dermatitis was treated in three periods: in the first period with DDC 100 mg four times daily (QID) for 20 days and later for two periods with TETD 100 mg three times daily (TID). An improvement was observed in all three experiments.

Christensen and Kristensen[355] and Kaaber and colleagues[356] conducted further studies with disulfiram (DSM). Using various dosages, these authors found that more often than not, DSM was helpful for nickel-sensitive hand eczema. However, hepatic toxicity may occasionally occur with DSM use. In one patient, a 49-year-old woman with no prior liver problems, elevated liver enzymes occurred after 8 weeks of taking DSM 200 mg/day.[357] The enzymes returned to normal after stopping the drug, then went up again on drug rechallenge.

Fowler[307] published a double-blind placebo-controlled crossover study showing that while on DSM 250 mg/day, eight of nine patients improved. In contrast, on placebo four patients had no change and five worsened. Side effects were minimal. Occasionally mild fatigue or lethargy may occur with the drug. Liver enzyme elevations have returned to normal when the drug is discontinued, but should be checked for.

Certainly, not all patients with cutaneous allergy to nickel are candidates for treatment with DSM. Some patients may not be willing to abstain from alcohol during treatment periods. Also, patients allergic to thiurams used in rubber processing may develop a systemic allergic reaction if given DSM, which is chemically related. Avoidance of the allergen, topical corticosteroids and emollients, systemic antihistamines, and occasional systemic steroid usage will control many patients with nickel contact dermatitis. However, despite these measures some patients have recurrent problems.

One other chelating agent, triethylenetetramine (Trientine), also chelates nickel, but is more effective at removing copper. Burrows and colleagues[358] found it to be ineffective in nickel hand eczema. It did not increase urinary nickel significantly, although copper excretion went up dramatically.

Topical chelation of nickel by L-histidine or ethylenediamine tetra-acetate acid (EDTA) in skin cleansers was effective in removing more nickel from the skin than control cleansers.[359] Perhaps incorporation of these agents in commercial skin cleansers would be useful in occupational nickel allergy.

UNUSUAL REACTIONS ASSOCIATED WITH NICKEL ALLERGY

Veien and colleagues[305] reported that the vesicular eruptions on palms and fingers, as well as urticaria and other noneczematous reactions following internal exposure to nickel, may be due to mechanisms other than delayed hypersensitivity. Precipitating antibodies against nickel sulfate bound to human albumin have been found in some patients with widespread erythema after oral challenge.

Chronic urticaria due to nickel has been reported by Warin.[360] McConnell and colleagues[361] reported asthma due to nickel sulfate in a metal-plate worker; a broncho-provocation challenge test with nickel sulfate duplicated the patient's symptoms, and circulating antibodies were found by hemagglutination tests. Block and Yeung[362] reported a second case study of asthma induced by nickel sulfate.

Espana and colleagues[363] carefully documented a case of chronic urticaria due to nickel in false teeth. In addition to a positive test, the patient had a positive response with severe urticaria and fever after ingesting a test dose of nickel sulfate. After removal of the dental prosthesis, she remained clear of skin lesions for 2 years. Oral lesions were not present.

In another case, localized urticaria of the upper lips was attributed to nickel in a dental implant. Removal was curative.[364]

Dr. Fisher reported that Estlander and colleagues of Helsinki, Finland, in a lecture entitled "Contact Allergy, Contact Urticaria, and Asthma Due to Nickel," described one patient, a 27-year-old woman, who had performed manual machine grinding of metal castings, which contain 9% nickel, for 2 years. She had used a respirator with a changeable filter at work. She had a long-standing cough and paroxysmal dyspnea followed by occasional urticaria on both arms after 2 months' employment. Both her cough and dyspnea grew worse during the second year of employment. Cheap metal objects had caused dermatitis since she

was 14 years old. Epicutaneous tests showed only a 2+ allergic reaction to 2.5% nickel sulfate (NiSO₄) in petrolatum. Skin prick tests showed no reactions to any common inhalant allergens. A scratch chamber test elicited a pseudopodial reaction to NiSO₄ at a concentration of 10 mg/mL. An open test on the volar aspect of the right arm with the same NiSO₄ solution elicited contact urticaria in 15 minutes. Bronchial and nasal provocation tests with the same NiSO₄ solution also were positive. The RAST was positive to nickel.

Cook[365] reported a patient with urticaria multiforme associated with nickel and cobalt dermatitis. Hjorth[366] found that nickel sensitivity could produce vasculitis.

"MECHANICAL" PREVENTION OF NICKEL DERMATITIS

Nickel-sensitive patients often use adhesive tapes or Band-Aids to cover nickel objects. Substitution of plastic for metallic knitting needles, buttons, pens, office supplies and bobby pins may be instrumental in clearing cases of nickel dermatitis. Plastic sleeves and plastic covers for eyeglass frames and nickel handles protected several patients from exposure to nickel.

Dr. Fisher noted that two patients found that talcum powder under metallic objects worn next to the skin protected them for several hours. Talcum powder as temporary prevention of nickel dermatitis may act in one of two ways: It may act as a mechanical barrier against the contact of nickel with the skin, and it may absorb perspiration, which dissolves some of the nickel from the metal object.

Some patients found that the avoidance of pressure prevented nickel objects from causing nickel dermatitis; that is, wearing nickel objects so that they touched the skin lightly often prevented the dermatitis. Some patients noted that they could tolerate nickel objects after losing weight.

Jewelry may be coated with nail polish or resin solutions. (Caution: The patient may become allergic to these solutions.) Also, a jeweler may apply rhodium or platinum plating to the inner surface of rings or other jewelry. Palladium should not be used, as crossreactions with nickel commonly occur.

Cooking utensils made of aluminum, Teflon, and enamel are safest for nickel-sensitive individuals.

Wall[367] demonstrated that nickel can penetrate rubber, but not vinyl gloves.

SUBSTITUTING ALTERNATIVES TO PREVENT NICKEL DERMATITIS

Table 32.12 lists suggested instructions for nickel-sensitive patients in order to prevent the recurrence and prolongation of nickel dermatitis.

Table 32-12 Instructions for Nickel-Sensitive Individuals

1. You are allergic to nickel and will probably remain so indefinitely.

2. You will be especially susceptible to a rash when the weather is hot and when you are perspiring.

3. Sweat can readily dissolve nickel out of metal, even through a layer of cloth, paint, nail polish, and adhesive tape.

4. Very small quantities of nickel can produce a rash where the nickel contacts the skin, and may even be conveyed by fingers to distant areas.

5. Many metals contain some nickel, including 14K yellow and white gold. Stainless steel contains nickel, but the nickel is so firmly bound in the steel that it does not leach out with ordinary contact, and so will not usually cause a rash.

6. Some earrings are marked "hypoallergenic" for nickel-sensitive individuals, but have proved to cause a rash because they are made of metals that release nickel.

7. You should learn how to do the chemical test for nickel called the dimethylglyoxime test. This will enable you to avoid buying jewelry that contains nickel-releasing metals and to test various metal objects to see whether they are safe for you to contact.

8. Be careful of the following wearing apparel: garter snaps, wire brassiere cup supports, zippers, hooks and snaps on undergarments, eyelets on shoes, metal arch supports, shoe and belt buckles, jewelry, medallions, ID tags, watch bands, metallic buttons on jeans. Substitute plastic snaps, buttons, and Velcro fasteners.

9. Coins can produce a rash if kept loose in a pocket for a prolonged period. Keep coins in a plastic bag.

10. Metal keys can cause a rash. You can substitute keys made of aluminum.

11. Be careful persistent skin contact with household items such as vacuum cleaners, sewing machines, needles, scissors, office equipment, paper clips, toy parts, and so forth.

12. Substitute wood for metal chairs and armrests, or put seat covers on and cover armrests with thick fabric. Many chrome-plated objects contain nickel.

13. Purchase all-plastic eyeglass frames. Some nickel-sensitive people continue to use metal eyeglass frames by buffing the metal with grade 0 steel wool, then coating with polyurethane varnish, then repeating the buffing and recoating. However, this is only a temporary measure.

14. A rash on your head and face including the eyelids may be caused by metallic items that touch the face or by contact from the hands with metal items, and then touching the face.

15. Nickel in the diet may cause skin problems, especially hand dermatitis. If you have dermatitis that doesn't resolve by avoiding contact with nickel, a low nickel diet may be helpful.

16. When you go for medical or dental treatment, tell your doctors that you are allergic to nickel. Short contact with nickel instruments will not be a problem, but prolonged skin contact for more than 30 minutes or so may produce a rash.

17. Should you require orthopedic surgery with the insertion of metal parts, your orthopedic surgeon may decide that you need special metals if you are nickel sensitive. The same holds true for a nickel-sensitive patient who may need other metallic medical devices.

18. If you contact nickel-containing liquids at work, remember that such liquids can penetrate rubber gloves. Heavy-duty vinyl gloves are more protective.

Niobium

Niobium, discovered in 1801, is a soft, grey metal used in steel alloys, primarily.[368] It is used especially where exceptional strength is needed such as in aerospace applications. It may be found in some jewelry, glassworking, and medical applications. Niobium compounds can be skin and eye irritants but allergy has not been reported.

Palladium

Palladium is a precious metal that may be used as a substitute for platinum. It may be found as a component of white gold and other jewelry alloys. It is becoming more commonly used in dental alloys. Exposure may also occur in the electronics and chemical industries. Some palladium salts are strong contact irritants, whereas others, such as palladium chloride, show minimum irritancy.[369]

Before the 1980s, only two reports of palladium allergy were found.[370,371] In 1991, however, a joint European study found 42 positive reactions in 1,521 patients (2.7%).[372] This suggests that the prevalence of allergy to palladium is either increasing or has been previously over-looked. Probably both of these conclusions are true. Palladium has been reported to cause a treatment-resistant granulomatous allergic contact dermatitis at ear piercing sites.[373] Perryman and Fowler[374] reported that 50 (9%) of 591 patients tested positive for palladium (1% pet). If only those with a strong (2+ or 3+) reaction were considered, still the rate was 4%. Only 70% were positive to nickel, indicating crossreactivity is not always found.

Aberer and colleagues[375] were alarmed at the frequency of positive reactions (8.3% of 1,382 consecutive patients). Only eight patients reacted to palladium alone, the rest being allergic to nickel. Six of these patients had oral complaints. These authors are concerned that increasing use of palladium in dental alloys may lead to a rise in stomatitis and other oral complaints. Filon and colleagues from Italy[376] tested over 4400 patients with PdCl 1% petrolatum. In all, 236 (5.3%) were positive, with an increasing incidence from the early to late 1990s. Only 7% were allergic to Pd alone. Virtually all the rest were allergic to nickel, and 33% were allergic to cobalt.

Both occupational and nonoccupational cases have been reported. Stomatitis and dermatitis are seen, depending on the exposure source.[375] Jewelry and dental materials constitute the most likely route of exposure in nonoccupational cases. The majority of reported patients have been women. Not surprisingly, patients allergic to palladium may not react to the pure metal, but only to the dissolved allergen.[377]

Palladium has been reported to cause a granulomatous reaction after ear-piercing.[378]

Most patients with palladium allergy are also allergic to nickel (Table 32.2). Many also react to cobalt. Because palladium and nickel are in the same group of metals (group VIII of the periodic table), it would seem that crossreactivity might occur. Wahlberg and Boman[379] executed a precisely designed study in guinea pigs to answer this question. Nickel, as a more common allergen, might be expected to be the primary sensitizer, with palladium as a secondary crossreactor. In fact, however, no animals sensitized to nickel reacted on challenge with palladium. In contrast, a number of animals sensitized only to palladium later reacted to nickel. This suggests that crossreactivity works in the direction of palladium to nickel only.

Similarly, in humans, Hindsen and friends gave oral nickel doses in a blinded fashion to patients who had previously been patch tested to nickel, palladium, and cobalt.[380] Flares at the patch test sites of both nickel and palladium occurred and in fact slightly more palladium sites flared than did nickel sites. They carefully excluded the presence of nickel from the palladium test material, and palladium from the oral nickel.

Clinically, palladium allergy may explain why some nickel-sensitive patients still react to "hypoallergenic" jewelry. Just as gold allergy has been overlooked, unsuspected palladium allergy may be occurring. Palladium should be suspected in jewelry allergy or allergic stomatitis.

Platinum

Fowler and family reported patch test results on 446 consecutive patients.[381] They tested 446 consecutive patients with ammonium tetrachloroplatinate 0.25% aqueous as part of diagnostic testing for presumed contact dermatitis. Only 2 female patients (0.4%) had a positive patch test. One was allergic to other metals including nickel, palladium, and gold. The other was not. Among this group, 99 were positive to nickel and 33 were positive to palladium. One of the positive patients routinely wore platinum jewelry and had facial dermatitis. Relevance was considered to be probable.

Santucci and colleagues tested 800 consecutive patients with hexachloroplatinic acid, potassium tetrachloroplatinate, and sodium hexachloroplatinate.[382]

No positives were seen, although they did report 4 reactions in another group of occupationally-exposed workers. Crossreactivity between platinum, palladium, iridium, and rhodium salts was demonstrated.

Metallic platinum, as used in jewelry, photography, dentistry, and the chemical and electrical industries, very rarely causes ACD, although dermatitis due to a platinum ring has been reported.[371] Rhodium is often used to plate white gold and platinum, and in this instance, the platinum dermatitis occurred when the rhodium plating wore off. Most jewelry made of platinum is either pure platinum or 90% platinum and 10% iridium.

In industry, soluble platinum salts, liquid platinum sprays, and splashes of platinum salts have been reported as causing dermatitis and asthma.[383] Platinosis is a disease caused not by metallic platinum but usually by its complex salts, primarily chloroplatinates, and affects mainly workers in platinum-refining workshops.[383] The cutaneous manifestations include pruritus, erythema, eczema, and urticaria, which are usually seen on the parts of the body exposed during work.

Roberts[384] coined the term "platinosis" for the symptom complex produced by platinum and its salts. His observations concurred exactly with other reports, and it was advised that sufferers from the effects of platinum salts should be transferred to other work. Roberts carried out scratch tests with aqueous solutions of sodium chloroplatinate on 60 platinum workers. He found that all subjects developed a 1+ reaction with a 1:10 dilution of the salt and that following the onset of symptoms, of either the cutaneous or the respiratory type, a reaction was always obtained with a 1:1,000 dilution. Roberts decided that initial scratch testing was an unreliable index of liability to develop future symptoms, and he claimed that a person with a strong personal or family history of atopic manifestations or of contact dermatitis was more likely to succumb to platinosis than others.

Baker and colleagues[385] reported that 15 of 107 platinum refinery workers had positive skin prick tests to platinum. Five of these had dermatitis. The researchers tested with disodium hexachloroplatinate and ammonium hexachloroplatinate at concentrations of 0.1% to 0.000001%. Thirty-nine controls were negative.

It is worth pointing out that scratch or intradermal testing can be hazardous to the point of being life-threatening in these patients. A single intradermal test using potassium hexachloroplatinate at a concentration of 1 mg/mL produced an anaphylactic reaction in the patient of Freedman and Krupey.[386] Successful hyposensitization was achieved in an analytical chemist who exhibited typical severe symptoms of hay fever, asthma, and contact urticaria when exposed to platinum complex salts in the course of his work.[387]

PATCH TESTING WITH PLATINUM SALTS

Complex salts of platinum are not readily soluble in distilled water, but solubility is improved if physiologic saline is used. These compounds dissolve in dilute hydrochloric acid, but such solutions are not suitable for patch testing. It is not even clear what is an appropriate concentration to be used for patch testing. Commercially available platinum patch tests include ammonium tetrachloroplatinate (0.25% aq) and ammonium hexachloroplatinate (0.1% aq).

In a study with mice, ACD was easily induced by repeat applications of sodium hexachloroplatinate (Na_2PtCl_6) 5% in acetone. This solution, however, caused a local irritant reaction on application. Sensitization was documented 6 days later with a 2% solution.[388]

This confirms the possibility of ACD to platinum, but does not help determine proper patch test materials for humans.

Rhodium

Rhodium has been reported to cause ACD in jewelers, specifically in goldsmiths.[389–391] In one case, patch test with rhodium sulfate (0.05% aq) was positive, although 40 controls were negative. Rhodium sulfate (2% pet) has also been used for testing. Currently, rhodium allergy from wearing jewelry has not been reported. Rhodium may be used to plate the inside of rings to attempt to block allergy to other metals.

Stingeni and colleagues[392] tested 720 patients consecutively with rhodium chloride (1%aq) with 2 positive reactions. Both also reacted to nickel and cobalt. Neither patient had known exposure to rhodium and the reactions were not considered relevant.

Rhodium, like other platinum group metals, can cause respiratory IgE-mediated reactions.[243]

Rubidium

Rubidium iodide (tested at 1% pet) was implicated as a cause of a facial dermatitis.[393] Eyedrops were the source of the rubidium. Testing in 20 controls was negative.

Silver (Ag) and its Salts

Metallic silver in jewelry or wire rarely causes dermatitis. Gaul[394] reported a patient with allergic reactions to silver coins, pure silver, and silver nitrate. A case report from England implicated silver allergy in a jeweler.[395] He was positive on patch testing to Ag nitrate (0.5% aq) but was also allergic to colophony.

SILVER NITRATE

Silver nitrate is kept in dark bottles because on exposure to air and light it decomposes, forming small amounts of nitric acid, silver nitrite, and colloidal silver, which liberate silver ions. Testing with old solutions of silver nitrate may, therefore, give irritant reactions.

ALLERGIC REACTIONS TO SILVER NITRATE

Marcussen[396] reported an allergic reaction to silver nitrate, as did Gaul and Underwood.[397] Gaul and Underwood's patient developed a vesicular reaction to the 10% silver nitrate used for marking patch tests. He recalled having applied in the past a solution of silver nitrate to an area of eczema on his heel and having to stop it after 2 weeks because the eczema suddenly worsened and spread. On patch testing, he reacted to 5% and 10% aged silver nitrate but not to 10% fresh silver nitrate. The ionized silver was thought to be the sensitizer in this patient and explained the discrepancy between the results of testing with old and with fresh solutions.

ARGYRIA FROM TOPICAL SILVER NITRATE AND OTHER SILVER SALTS

Marshall and Schneider[398] reported a case of systemic argyria secondary to the topical use of silver nitrate for bleeding gums caused by poorly fitting dentures.

Localized argyria may result from topical silver salts through either medicinal or occupational exposure. Buckley[399] reported a case of a duplicating-machine operator who developed localized argyria of her hands from daily immersion in photographic developing solutions. Handling of silver metal by silversmiths and the oral suctioning of silver nitrate solutions in the preparation of silver beads are other causes of reported occupational argyria.[400] The use of colloidal silver compounds such as mild silver protein (Argyrol) and strong silver protein (Protargol) for such varied indications as bladder irrigation, urethritis, nasal drops for cold prevention, mucosal ulcerations, cervicovaginitis, and conjunctivitis has been practiced. In the early twentieth century the use of silver arsphenamine for the treatment of syphilis was associated with a significant incidence of at least localized argyria. In 1935, Gaul and Staud[401] reported 70 cases of argyria secondary to oral, intranasal, or pharyngeal use of organic and colloidal silver compounds. It appears that Marcussen's series marked the end of widespread use of the silver colloid solutions, as no subsequent reports have rivaled his in number of cases or in frequency of detection. The current use of silver sulfadizine in the treatment of burns must be scrutinized carefully to avoid excessive systemic absorption of silver from the wounds.

"IMMEDIATE" REACTION TO ARGYROL

Criep[402] reported that argyrol, which is a colloidal solution of silver or silver oxide in alkaline proteins, produced immediate-type hypersensitivity after its use in the nose and as a pharyngeal spray. Scratch testing with 1% argyrol was positive and intradermal testing gave a severe local reaction and constitutional symptoms.

DERMATITIS FROM MISCELLANEOUS SILVER SALTS

Silver Coat

Heyl[403] stated that a patient acquired dermatitis from "silver coat." Silver coat is a powder consisting of silver cyanide with small amounts of sodium carbonate, sodium cyanide, and sodium nitrate. The patient's work involved the weighing of various precious metal salts for electroplating purposes, in powder form. Patch tests revealed a 3+ positive reaction to a 1% aqueous solution of "silver coat" but negative for gold potassium cyanide and silver metal.

Silver Fulminate

Although fulminates were widely used in the past as explosives, they are now little encountered. Fulminate itch is of historical interest. White and Rycroft[404] investigated a factory using silver fulminate in the manufacture of explosive snaps. Silver fulminate, known in the trade as "white salt," may produce stomatitis, particularly in women.

IONIC SILVER CHLORIDE COMPLEXED WITH THIOSULFATE

Marks[405] reported that a radiographer, who processed films by hand, developed a papular eczema under her watch strap. Patch tests were positive to 1% silver chloride complexed with sodium thiosulfate, to 1% silver nitrate, and to the fixing fluid. Although silver chloride is insoluble, it was suggested that it formed a soluble complex with sodium thiosulfate in the fixing tank and that this complex contaminated the patient's wristwatch strap. Ionic silver was postulated as the sensitizer.

Tellurium

tellurium is a brittle white metalloid with the atomic number 52, symbol Te. It is chemically related to selenium and sulfur.[406] It may be used in alloys of stainless steel, copper, and iron and may be found in ceramics, glasswork, and semiconductors. Systemic toxicity can occur and a characteristic odor of garlic, "tellurium breath" is noted. ACD has not been reported.

Tin

It is uncertain whether tin can cause ACD.

Menné and colleagues[407] described the first findings of positive patch tests to tin. They found 6 of 73 patients tested to tin-coated copper discs who gave 2 or 3+ reactions. All patients were nickel sensitive. The authors stated that no nickel contaminated the tin. They did not test patients to copper or other metals. The same authors later reported five positive reactions from 2,206 consecutive patients tested with tin chloride 1% petrolatum.[408] None were nickel positive. The total of doubtful or irritant reactions was 25. No relevance was found for the five positive reactions, so it is possible the reactions were irritant. The authors stated that biopsies from four of the patients, however, were believed to be allergic, histologically.

A probable case of true ACD to tin was recently reported.[409] A metalworker with heavy exposure to tin-containing metal dust developed airborne ACD on exposed surfaces. Patch testing was positive only to tin ($SnCl_2$), at 0.25%, 0.5%, and 1% in petrolatum. Lymphocyte testing was performed but did not yield positive results.

Tributyl tin oxide, a biocide in paint and a catalyst in the production of some rubber and plastic materials, is a well-known irritant.[410]

Titanium

Titanium is an inert metal used for some orthopedic devices and medical implants. Compared to other metals, titanium allergy is rarely reported.

There have been several reports of allergy to titanium in cardiac pacemakers. Granulomatous dermatitis in one case, with negative patch tests, was felt to be caused by titanium, because titanium was found on electron probe microanalysis in the granulomas.[411]

Two other cases of granuloma without positive patch tests have been reported.[412,413] In three other cases, positive patch tests confirmed titanium allergy.[414–416] Earlobe granulomas were attributed to a titanium alloy, but patch testing was not performed.[417] Titanium along with aluminum and vanadium were found in the granulomas. Excision was curative.

A frequent query to dermatologists from our patients and orthopedic colleagues involves concern over metallic orthopedic implants in metal-allergic individuals. Holgers and colleagues[418] studied 445 patients with titanium implants. In nine patients, a local skin reaction developed. None were allergic to titanium. In six cases, staphylococcal infection was causative, and in the others, allergy to other agents occurred.

Dujardin and colleagues[419] reviewed the literature in 1995 and found no cases of titanium allergy among 54 cases of dermatitis related to orthopedic implants. In a Japanese report, dermatitis following a stainless-steel implant resolved when a titanium implant was substituted.[420]

Perhaps the most extensively documented case of titanium allergy comes from Thomas and colleagues, in Germany.[421] A young man received pure titanium screws and a plate to repair a hand fracture. The fracture failed to heal and eczema in the affected area (spreading elsewhere eventually) developed after several weeks. Patch testing was totally negative, including TiO_2. However, a positive lymphocyte transformation test to TiO_2 was positive in the patient and negative in 40 controls. After removal of the titanium, the fracture healed and the eczema cleared.

Titanium salts are frequently used in sunscreens and other topical products. Basketter and colleagues[422] reported 3 positive reactions to ammonium titanium lactate (10%), used in a proposed deodorant. Patients were negative to titanium dioxide (10% pet).

Based on current reports, appropriate advice to our orthopedic colleagues would be:

1. Dermatitis from stainless-steel implants is unusual but may occur in metal-sensitive persons.
2. Titanium allergy is exceedingly rare, but has been documented to occur.
3. Titanium implants may be used in cases where metal allergy may be present clinically or if there are medicolegal concerns. Patch testing should be undertaken to document metal allergy where concern exists.
4. Unfortunately, the most appropriate allergen for patch testing for titanium allergy is unknown.

Vanadium

Vanadium pentoxide (10% pet) was positive in 1 of 190 ceramics workers. No irritant reactions were seen.[249] One report suggested a high rate of positive patch tests to vanadium in patients with dermatitis and loosening of hip prostheses. Clinical significance is uncertain at this time.[423]

Zinc Dermatitis and Discolorations

ZINC OXIDE AND ZINC POX

Although zinc oxide is completely inert allergenically, it is probably the most common cause of black dermographism produced by jewelry. Zinc oxide present in cosmetics, lotions, and dentifrices is much harder than most metals in jewelry and coins, leading to abrasion and deposition of minute metal particles. Zinc stearate is so soft that it cannot cause black dermographism. Zinc oxide ointment may be used in sunscreens, classically for protecting the nose and lips of lifeguards at the beach.

Calnan[424] described metal fume fever as an influenza-like illness due to inhalation of fumes of zinc oxide and other metals.

Zinc pox is an eruption from zinc oxide dust, especially localized to the moist intertriginous areas such as the axillae and the groin. A secondary infection may occur.[425]

ZINC CHLORIDE

Zinc chloride is a strong primary irritant and can produce ulcerations resembling those produced by chromic acid. Allergic reactions to this caustic zinc salt are rare. Sources of exposure are dental fillings, preservation and fireproofing of timber, solder flux, and Mohs' chemosurgery.

ZINC CHROMATE

This yellow pigment, made of zinc oxide and chromic acid, is widely used as an anticorrosion agent as an undercoat. Zinc chromate can cause chromate dermatitis in chromium-sensitive individuals.

ZINC METAL ALLERGY

Zinc was implicated as the cause of dermatitis localized at sites of acupuncture therapy.[426] Patch tests were positive only to zinc sulfate (2% pet), but no controls were tested.

ZINC PYRITHIONE

Zinc pyrithione has become a popular ingredient in many antiseborrheic shampoos. Zinc pyrithione sensitivity is rare.

Yates and Finn[427] reported that this antidandruff agent produced ACD. In addition, the patient had an actinic reticuloid syndrome.

Calnan[428] stated that scalp and facial dermatitis developed in a patient after the use of ZP11 shampoo, which contains zinc pyrithione. The patient also showed a positive patch test reaction to ethylenediamine hydrochloride. Calnan reported that zinc pyrithione also crossreacts with piperazine hydrochloride. There is a report that a patient with occupational piperazine dermatitis was also allergic to ethylenediamine.[429] A more recent case implicated zinc pyrithione in a combination of ACD and a flare of pustular psoriasis. Patch test to zinc pyrithione was positive.[430]

The dermatologist treating a patient sensitive to zinc pyrithione or ethylenediamine hydrochloride must be aware of the following: (a) Zinc pyrithione crossreacts with piperazine; (b) piperazine is a relative of ethylenediamine; (c) hydroxyzine hydrochloride (Atarax, Vistaril) is an ethylenediamine derivative; therefore, (d) zinc pyrithione, piperazine, Atarax, Vistaril, and ethylenediamine hydrochloride may crossreact.

Zinc acexamate, an oral medication used to treat gastric ulcers, caused a generalized dermatitis in a Spanish man. Patch test and oral challenge tests were positive.[431]

ZINC INSULIN ALLERGY

Feinglos and Jegasothy,[432] in an investigation of two unrelated patients who had local cutaneous hypersensitivity reactions after injection of any commercially available insulin preparation, have shown that the cause of the allergy was zinc. Zinc insulin- and zinc sulfate-induced proliferation of peripheral blood lymphocytes from these patients; they also induced the production of a specific leukocyte inhibitory factor. Intradermal skin tests for zinc were positive in both patients. Similar studies carried out in a patient whose cutaneous allergy to insulin was corrected by changing from mixed beef-pork to pure pork insulin were negative. Zinc-free insulin did not produce any allergy in the first patient. This previously unrecognized allergy should be considered in all patients whose insulin allergy does not respond to conventional therapy.

Zirconium Granulomas

These granulomas of the skin, originally seen following the use of zirconium sodium lactate as a deodorant, have also been seen following the use of zirconium oxide for the treatment of rhus plant dermatitis.[433,434] Soluble salts were used in the deodorants that produced granulomas. In the topical preparations for rhus dermatitis, mostly insoluble salts are used.

Palmer and Welton[433] reported a case of lupus miliaris disseminatus faciei in an individual who was exposed to a zirconium oven in a metal-alloy factory.

Zirconium, like beryllium, can produce sarcoid-like granuloma.[435]

CLINICAL APPEARANCE

The lesions usually appear 4 to 6 weeks after initial use of the zirconium preparation and are limited to the sites of contact. They appear as persistent, firm, shiny, erythematous, flesh- or apple-jelly-colored papules, which are solitary, grouped, or coalescent. Eczematous changes are also usually present. Pruritus is minimal or absent.[436]

HISTOLOGIC APPEARANCE

The epidermis is normal. In the dermis, large aggregates or tubercles of distinctive epithelioid and Langerhans cells are present. A minimal inflammatory reaction is occasionally present. Foreign body material is not detected by polarized light microscopy. Differentiation from sarcoidosis may not be possible histologically.[437]

MECHANISM OF PRODUCTION

Any defect in the protective layer of the skin enhances the development of hypersensitivity. The granulomas then develop in individuals who have acquired an allergic hypersensitivity to zirconium. In the axillae, minute abrasions from shaving, as well as excess friction and sweating, enhance the penetration of the zirconium salts of the deodorants. The preparations containing zirconium salts used for treatment of rhus dermatitis readily penetrate through the acutely inflamed skin and through denuded areas, vesicles, and bullae.

TESTS FOR ZIRCONIUM HYPERSENSITIVITY

Either patch or intracutaneous testing may be used to determine allergic hypersensitivity to zirconium salts. Regular patch test may be negative.

For "patch" testing, the zirconium preparation may be rubbed into a test site that has been prepared by multiple scratches or denuded by a dermal curet. The site is then covered with an occlusive dressing for 2 days. In sensitized individuals, a positive reaction consists of the development of reddish brown papules in about 4 weeks. Such papules show a sarcoidal granulomatous infiltrate histologically.

In intracutaneous testing, a small wheal is made by injecting a 1:10,000 dilution of sodium zirconium lactate. A positive reaction consists of a discrete papule, which appears in 8 to 14 days. In about a month, the papule clinically and histologically has the appearance of a sarcoid lesion. It may persist for 6 to 24 months.

Table 32-13 Industrial Exposure to Zirconium and its Salts

Zirconium metals
  Alloys
  Nuclear reactors
  Superconductors
  Surgical implants
  Vacuum tube parts
Zirconium acetate
  High-temperature electrical conductors
  Refactory applications
  Water repellents
  Zinc boride
  Zinc carbide
Zirconium hydroxide
  Pigments in glass
Zirconium naphthenate
  Ceramics
  Lubricants
  Paints
  Varnishes
Zirconium nitrate (as a preservative)
  Electronics
  Ceramic glazes
  Special glasses
Zirconium oxychloride
  Cosmetics
  Greases
  Textiles
Zirconium potassium fluoride in welding fluxes
Zirconium sulfate
  Chemicals
  Lubricants
  Reagent and catalysts
  Retannage
  Tanning of white leather
Zirconium tetrafluoride
  A component of molten salts for nuclear reactors

PROGNOSIS

Axillary granulomas produced by soluble zirconium lactate in deodorants usually disappear within a few months. Lesions produced by insoluble zirconium oxide preparations used for rhus plant therapy usually remain unchanged for several months to years and may be refractory to therapy. Temporary improvement is obtained by the use of corticosteroids either systemically or intralesionally.[438]

Table 32.13 lists the industrial exposures to zirconium and its salts.

Miscellaneous Compounds Sometimes Classified with Metals

The following compounds are sometimes included with metals, although strictly speaking, they are not typical metals.

PHOSPHORUS

A foundry worker with work-related hand dermatitis reacted to sodium hypophosphate (NaH_2PO_2) used in steel processing at both 1% and 5% aqueous. He also reacted to phosphorus sesquisulfide (P_4S_3).[439] Controls were not tested. No other explanation of the dermatitis could be found.

Phosphorus sesquisulfide has been previously reported to cause contact urticaria and dermatitis from safety matches.[440] Postinflammatory hypopigmentation has also been noted.

SELENIUM

Stedman's Medical Dictionary defines selenium as a metallic element chemically similar to sulfur. *Webster's Dictionary* and *Random House College Dictionary* define selenium as nonmetallic.

Selenium is often found together with tellurium. It is a semiconductor and acts as a rectifier and photoconductor. It is widely used in electronics, glass, and ceramics and occasionally as a rubber accelerator (selenium diethyldithiocarbamate), catalyst, dietary supplement, and trace element in animal feeds.

Selenium oxychloride (seleninyl chloride), a powerful solvent for metals and a chlorinating agent, is a strong vesicant that rapidly destroys the skin unless immediately removed by washing.

Some compounds of selenium are severe irritants and are readily absorbed through the lungs, gastrointestinal tract, and damaged skin. The most characteristic sign of absorption is the smell of garlic from the breath. Selenium dioxide, which is important in industry, is a light powder that dissolves in water or sweat to form noxious selenious acid. When selenium dioxide is inhaled, it causes pulmonary edema, conjunctivitis in the eyes, and burns or irritant dermatitis on the exposed skin. The nail beds become painful if it penetrates under the nails.[441]

In a selenium refinery plant, 11 employees developed dermatitis, conjunctivitis, and inflammation of the upper respiratory tract. Investigation showed no evidence of sensitization, and it was concluded that all of the effects were due to irritation.[442]

Senff and colleagues[443] report a well-documented case of selenium allergy. A laboratory technician developed hand eczema only when handling a selenite (Na_2SeO_3) containing culture medium. The only positive patch test was to selenite down to a dilution of 0.1% aqueous. Multiple control subjects were negative. Avoidance of the broth resulted in clearing.

Selenium sulfide is used in several topical agents, such as shampoos, for the treatment of seborrheic dermatitis and for the treatment of tinea versicolor. Allergic reactions to these preparations are rare.

SILICA AND SILICONE GRANULOMAS

Silicone implants have been implicated as causing a variety of systemic symptoms. This is beyond the scope of this text.

Shelley and Hurley[444] described silica granulomas as a nonallergic foreign body epithelioid reaction to silica in the colloidal form. Silicone powder can also produce granulomas.

Mason and Apisarnthanarax[445] reported a 38-year-old woman who had a migratory silicone granuloma of the left upper portion of the chest and left upper arm secondary to a ruptured breast implant. The initial diagnosis was factitial panniculitis. With the common use of silicone in cosmetic surgery, physicians should inquire into a possible history of silicone injections or implants before ascribing a factitial cause of foreign-body granulomas.

Silicone adhesives are used for bonding silicone elastomer (silastic medical adhesive) to itself or other implantable synthetics, such as Dacron, Teflon, and acrylic. A silicone adhesive has been implicated as a cause of dermatitis associated with an implanted cardiac pacemaker.[446]

Contact urticaria to silicone rubber in a military gas mask has been reported.[447]

TELLURIUM

Tellurium is used in the vulcanization of rubber, in alloys, as a color for glass, as a catalyst, and in the production of photoelectric devices and computer chips.

Blackadder and Manderson[448] reported poisoning in two research workers, both of whom had the characteristic smell of sour garlic in their breath, sweat, and urine. An unusual feature was a bluish black discoloration of the skin in streaks on the face and neck and in patches in the finger webs. This was thought to be due to the absorption of tellurium esters through the skin and the deposition of tellurium in the dermis and subcutaneous tissues. The patients recovered without treatment.

URANIUM

Thiers and colleagues[449] reported two men preparing uranium for an atomic energy plant who developed hand eczema. They were patch tested with 2% sodium and calcium salts of uranium, to which they reacted.

References

1. Fowler JF. Allergic contact dermatitis to metals. Am J Contact Dermat 1990;1:212.

2. Warshaw E, Belsito D, DeLeo V, et al. North American Contact Dermatitis Group patch test results, 2003–2004 study period. Contact Dermatitis 2007, accepted for publication.

3. Zug K, McGinley-Smith D, Belsito D, et al. Contact allergy in children: NACDG data 2001–2004. submitted for publication, 2007.

4. Larsson-Stymne B, Windstrom L. Ear piercing—a cause of nickel allergy in school-girls. *Contact Dermatitis* 1985;13:289.

5. Ehrlich A, Kucenic M, Belsito D. Role of body piercing in the induction of metal allergies. Am J Contact Dermat 2001;12:151.

6. Kanerva L, Jolanki R, Estlander T, et al. Incidence rates of occupational allergic contact dermatitis caused by metals Am J Contact Dermat 2000;11:155..

7. Ruff C, Belsito D. The impact of various patient factors on allergy to nickel, cobalt, and chromate. J Am Acad Dermatol 2006;55:32..

8. Wilkinson JV. Some metallurgical aspects of orthodontic stainless steel. Am J Orthod 1962;48:192.

9. Liden C, Menné T, Burrows D. Nickel containing alloys and platings and their ability to cause dermatitis. Br J Dermatol 1996;134:193.

10. Liden C, Rondell E, Skare L, et al. Nickel release from tools on the Swedish market. Contact Dermatitis 1998;39:127.

11. Ingber A, et al. Detergents and bleaches are sources of chromium contact dermatitis in Israel. Contact Dermatitis 1998;38:101.

12. Malten KE. Nickel sensitization and detergents. Acta Derm Venereol (Stockh) 1969;49:10.

13. Malten KE, Spruit D. The relative importance of various environmental exposures to nickel in causing contact hypersensitivity. Acta Derm Venereol (Stockh) 1969;49:14.

14. Quinones PA, Garcia Munox CM. Contact allergy due to nickel and chrome: presence of these compounds in detergents used in the household. Ann Derm Syph 1965;92:383.

15. Vilaplana J, et al. Cobalt content of household cleaning products. Contact Dermatitis 1987;16:139.

16. Basketter D, Angelini G, Ingber A, et al. Nickel, chromium, and cobalt in consumer products. Contact Dermatitis 2003;49:1.

17. Zugerman C. Contact dermatitis to yellow iron oxide. Contact Dermatitis 1985;13:107.

18. Levy J, Sewell M, Goldstein N. II. A short history of tattooing. J Derm Surg Oncol 1979;5:851.

19. Sulzberger MB, Tolmach JA. Allergic flare-up reactions in red tattooing: Observations on development and subsidence of mercurial sensitivity and on allergic granulomatous and sarcoid reactions. Hautarzt 1959;10:110.

20. Biro L, Klein WP. Unusual complications of mercurial (cinnabar) tattoo. Arch Dermatol 1967;96:2.

21. Lowenthal LJA. Reactions in green tattoos. Arch Dermatol 1960;82:237.

22. Bjoernber A. Allergic reaction to cobalt in light blue tattoo markings. Acta Derm Venereol (Stockh) 1961;41:259.

23. Bjoernber A. Reactions to light in yellow tattoos from cadmium sulfide. Arch Dermatol 1963;88:267.

24. Goldstein N. Mercury-cadmium sensitivity in tattoos: photoallergic reaction in red pigment. Ann Intern Med 1967;67:948.

25. Waldmann I, Vakilzadeh F. Allergische spatty preaktion auf roten azofarbdtoff in tatowiernngen. Hautarzt 1997;48:666.

26. Scutt R, Gotch C. The mystery of tattooing, skin deep. London: Peter Davies, 1974.

27. Nguyen LQ, Allen HB. Reactions to manganese and cadmium in tattoos. Cutis 1979;23:71.

28. Rubianes EI, Sánchez JL. Granulomatous dermatitis to iron oxide after permanent pigmentation of the eyebrows. J Derm Surg Oncol 1993;19:14.

29. Morales- Callaghan A, Aguilar-Bernier M, Martinez-Garcia G, et al. Sarcoid granuloma on a black tattoo. J Am Acad Dermatol 2006; 55:S71–3.

30. Flint GN. A metallurgical approach to metal contact dermatitis. Contact Dermatitis 1998;39:213.

31. Buckley WR, Lewis CE. The ruster in industry. J Occup Med 1960;2:25.

32. Burton JL, Pye RJ, Brooks DB. Metal corrosion by chloride in sweat. Br J Dermatol 1976;95:417.

33. Bang-Petersen N. Topical treatment of a "ruster." Br J Dermatol 1977;96:332.

34. Liden C, Carter S: Nickel release from coins. Contact Dermatitis 2001;44:160.

35. Bang Pedersen N, Fregert S, Brodeilius P, Gruvberger B. Release of nickel from silver coins. Acta Derm Venereol (Stockh) 1974;54:231.

36. Yeatman GW, van Dang V. Çao Gio (coin rubbing): Vietnamese attitudes toward health care. JAMA 1980;244:2748.

37. Gellis SS, Feingold M. Cao gio (pseudo-battering in Vietnamese children). Am J Dis Child 1976;130:857.

38. Yeatman GW, Shaw CS, Barlow MJ, et al. Pseudobattering in Vietnamese children. Pediatrics 1976;58:616.

39. Keller EL, Apthorp J. Folk remedies vs child battering. Am J Dis Child 1977;131:1173.

40. Tan A. Coin rubbing and related folk medicine. JAMA 1981;245:1819.

41. Kranke B, Aberer W. Multiple sensitivities to metals. Contact Dermatitis 1996;34:225.

42. Rystedt I. Relationship between nickel and cobalt sensitization in hard metal workers. Contact Dermatitis 1983;9:195.

43. Lammintausta K, et al. Inter-relationship of nickel and cobalt sensitization. Contact Dermatitis 1985;13:148.

44. Simonetti V, Manzini BM, Seidenari S. Patch testing with nickel sulfates comparison between 2 nickel sulfate preparations and 2 different test sites on the back. Contact Dermatitis 1998;39:187.

45. Seidenari S, Manzini BM, Belletti B. Pretreatment of the test area with 1-day occlusion improves the response rate to NiSO4 5% pet. patch tests in subjects with a positive history of nickel allergy. Contact Dermatitis 1995;33:152.

46. Seidenari S, Motolese A, Belletti B. Pre-treatment of nickel test areas with sodium lauryl sulfate detects nickel sensitivity in subjects reacting negatively to routine performed patch tests. Contact Dermatitis 1996;34:88.

47. Uter W, Fuchs T, Hausser M, et al. Patch test results with serial dilutions of nickel sulfate (with and without detergent), palladium chloride, and nickel and palladium metal plates. Contact Dermatitis 1995;32:135.

48. Meneghini C, Angelini G. Intradermal test in contact allergy to metals. Acta Derm Venereol (Stockh) 1979;59:123.

49. Marcussen PV. Comparison of intradermal test and patch test using nickel sulfate and formaldehyde. J Invest Dermatol 1963;40:263.

50. Möller H. Intradermal testing in doubtful cases of contact allergy to metals. Contact Dermatitis 1989;20:120.

51. Basketter D, Lea L, Cooeper K, et al. Identification of Metal Allergens in the Local Lymph Node assay. Am J Contact Dermat 1999;10:207.

52. Urbach E, Pillsbury DM. Black dermagraphism. JAMA 1943;121: 485.

53. Fisher AA. Black dermographism. A physical phenomenon. Cutis 1974;13:187.

54. Hurley HJ. Black dermographism (society transactions). Arch Dermatol 1960;81:329.

55. Fisher AA. What causes gold smudge? Jewelers' Circular-Keystone 1971;141:64.

56. Rapson WS. Skin contact with gold and gold alloys. Contact Dermatitis 1985;13:56.

57. Steinegeer S. Endemic skin lesions near an aluminum factory. Fluoride Quart Rept 1969;2:37.

58. Hemmer W, Wantke F, Focke M, et al. Evaluation of cutaneous hypersensitivity to aluminum by routine patch testing with AlCl3. Contact Dermatitis 1996;34:217.

59. Slater DN, et al. Aluminum hydroxide granulomas: light and electron microscopic studies and X-ray microanalysis. Br J Dermatol 1982;107:103.

60. Kaaber K, Nielsen AD, Veien, NK. Vaccination granulomas and aluminum allergy: course and prognostic factors. Contact Dermatitis 1992;26:304.

61. O'Driscoll J, et al. Contact Dermatitis to aluminum acetate eardrops. Contact Dermatitis 1991;24:156.

62. Kalveram K-J, Rapp-Frisk C, Sorck G. Misleading patch test results with aluminum Finn chambers® and mercury salts. Contact Dermatitis 1980;6:507.

63. Fischer T, Maibach H. Aluminum in Finn chambers® reacts with cobalt and nickel salts in patch test materials. Contact Dermatitis 1985;12:200.

64. Veien NK, Hattel T, Laurberg G. Systemically aggravated contact dermatitis caused by aluminum in toothpaste. Contact Dermatitis 1993;28:199.

65. Stevenson CJ. Antimony spots. Trans St Johns Hosp Derm Soc 1965;51:40.

66. White GP, Mathias CGT, Davin JS. Dermatitis in workers exposed in antimony in a melting process. J Occupational Med 1993;35:392.

67. Paschoud J. Occupational arsenic and antimony contact eczema. Dermatologica 1964;129:410.

68. Motolese A, Truzzi M, Giannini A, et al. Contact dermatitis and contact sensitization among enamellers and decorators in the ceramics industry. Contact Dermatitis 1993;28:59.

69. Birmingham D, Key MM. An outbreak of arsenical dermatitis in a mining community. Arch Dermatol 1965;91:457.

70. Holinquist R. Occupational arsenical dermatitis. Acta Derm Venereol (Stockh) 1951;31:26.

71. Barbaud A, Mougedelle J, Schnutz J. Contact hypersensitivity to arsenic in a crystal factory worker. Contact Dermatitis 1995;33:272.

72. Maier L: Beryllium health effects in the era of the beryllium lymphocyte transformation test. Appl Occup Environ Hyg 2001;16:514.

73. Bekris L, Viernes H, Farin F, et al,: Chronic Beryllium disease and glutathione biosynthesis genes. J Occup Environ Med 2006;48:599.

74. Day G, Stefanial A, Weston A, et al. Beryllium exposure: dermal and immunological consideration. Int Arch Occup Environ Health 2006;79:161.

75. Balkisson R, Newman L. Beryllium copper alloy (2%) causes chronic beryllium disease. J Occup Med 1999;41:304.

76. Stanton M, Henneberger P, Kent M, et al. Sensitization and chronic beryllium disease among workers in copper-beryllium distribution centers. J Occup Environ Med 2006;48:204.

77. Curtis CH. Cutaneous hypersensitivity to beryllium. Arch Dermatol 1951;64:470.

78. Nichol AD, Dominiquez R. Cutaneous granuloma from accidental contamination with beryllium phosphorus. JAMA 1949;140:855.

79. Dobson RL. General discussion on the treatment of chronic beryllium poisoning with ACTH and cortisone. AMA Arch Indus Hyg 1951;3:543.

80. Jones Williams W. Granulomatous diseases. Proc Roy Soc Med 1971;64:946.

81. Berlin J, Taylor J, Sigel J, et al, Beryllium Dermatitis, J Am Acad Dermatol 2003;49:939.

82. Haberman AL, Pratt M, Storrs FJ. Contact dermatitis from beryllium in dental alloys. Contact Dermatitis 1993;28:157.

83. Vilaplana J, Romaguera C, Grimalt F. Occupational and nonoccupational allergic contact dermatitis from beryllium. Contact Dermatitis 1992;26:295.

84. Raith L, Schubert H, Goring H-D. Contact dermatitis from cadmium chloride? Contact Dermatitis 1982;8:267.

85. Wahlberg JE. Routine patch testing with cadmium chloride. Contact Dermatitis 1977;3:293.

86. Kaaber S, Cramers M, Jepsen FL. The role of cadmium as a skin sensitizing agent in denture and non-denture wearers. Contact Dermatitis 1982;8:308.

87. Gebhardt M, Geier J. Evaluation of patch test results with denture materials series. Contact Dermatitis 1996;34:191.

88. Geier J, Vieluf D, Fuchs T. Patch testing with cadmium chloride. Contact Dermatitis 1996;34:73.

89. Friedman AA. Dermatitis of the breast from "lead" pencils. Arch Dermatol 1956;73:384.

90. Capusan I, Mauksch J. Occupational dermatoses of workers of a carbon black producing factory. Berufsdermatosen 1969;17:28.

91. Boye T, Terrier J, Coillot C, et al. Cerium induced granulomatous dermatitis (in French) Ann Dermatol Venereol 2006;133:50.

92. Nater JP. Possible causes of chromate eczema. Dermatologica 1963;126:160.

93. Fregert S. Occupational dermatitis in a 10 year material. Contact Dermatitis 1975;1:96.

94. Burry JN, Kirk J. Environmental dermatitis: chrome cripples. Med J Aust 1975;2:720.

95. Burrows D. Prognosis in industrial dermatitis. Br J Dermatol 1972;87:145.

96. Breit R, Turk RBM. The medical and social fate of the dichromate allergic patient. Br J Dermatol 1976;94:349.

97. Cronin D. Chromate dermatitis in men. Br J Dermatol 1971;85:95.

98. Fregert S, et al. Reduction of chromate in cement by iron sulfate. Contact Dermatitis 1979;5:39.

99. Avnstorp C. Follow-up of workers from the prefabricated concrete industry after the addition of ferrous sulphate to Danish cement. Contact Dermatitis 1989;20:365.

100. Avnstorp C. Risk factors for cement eczema. Contact Dermatitis 1991;25:81.

101. Halbert AR, Gebauer KA, Wall LM. Prognosis of occupational chromate dermatitis. Contact Dermatitis 1992;27:214.

102. Zachariae CO, Agner T, Menne T. Chromium allergy in consecutive patients in a country where ferrous sulfate has been added to cement since 1981. Contact Dermatitis 1996;35:83.

103. Olsavsky R, et al. Contact sensitivity to chromate: comparison at a London contact dermatitis clinic over a 10-year period. Contact Dermatitis 1998;38:329.

104. Freeman S. Shoe dermatitis. Contact Dermatitis 1997;36:247.

105. Bajaj A, Gupta S, Chatterjee A, Singh K. Shoe dermatitis in India. Contact Dermatitis 1991;24:149.

106. Trattner A, David M: Tefillin dermatitis. J Am Acad Dermatol 2005;52:831.

107. Nater JP. Possible causes of chromate eczema. Dermatologica 1963;126:160.

108. Hostynek J, Maibach H. Chromium in US household bleach. Contact Dermatitis 1988;18:206.

109. Feuerman EJ. Housewives' eczema and the role of chromates. Acta Derm Venereol (Stockh) 1969;39:288.

110. Basketter D, Angelini G, Ingber A, et al. Nickel, chromium, and cobalt in consumer products. Contact Dermatitis 2003;49:1.

111. Tritsch H, Orfanos C, Luckerath I. Experiments on the allergic skin reaction to chromated catgut. Hautarzt 1967;18:355.

112. Nethercott JR, Holness DL. Dermatologic problems of musicians. J Am Acad Dermatol 1991;25:870.

113. Fregert S. Otitis externa due to chromate of matches. Acta Derm Venereol (Stockh) 1962;42:473.

114. Morris GE. Chromate dermatitis from chrome glue and other aspects of the chrome problem. AMA Arch Industr Health 1955;11:368.

115. Lück H, Jentsch G. Chromium dermatitis caused by epoxy resin. Contact Dermatitis 1988;19:154.

116. Fregert S, Hjorth N, Gruyberger B. Chromate in bridge table felt. Contact Dermatitis Newsletter 1970;8:173.

117. Burrows D. Chromium and the skin. Br J Dermatol 1978;99:587.

118. Donaldson RM, Barreras RF. Intestinal absorption of trace elements of chromium. J Lab Clin Med 1966;68:484.

119. Veien NK, Kaaber K. Nickel, cobalt and chromium sensitivity in patients with pompholyx (dyshidrotic eczema). Contact Dermatitis 1979;5:371.

120. Van Ulsen J, Stolz E, Van Joost TH. Chromate dermatitis from a homeopathic drug. Contact Dermatitis 1987;16:53.

121. Fowler J. Systemic contact dermatitis caused by chromium picolinate. Cutis 2000;65:116.

122. Fisher AA. Chromates: prime causes of industrial allergic contact dermatitis. Cutis 1983;32:24.

123. Bang-Pedersen NB. Chromate in the food laboratory. Contact Dermatitis 1977;3:105.

124. Fregert S, Gruvberger B. Factors decreasing the content of water-soluble chromate in cement. Acta Derm Venereol (Stockh) 1973;53:267.

125. Einarsson O, Kylin B, Lindstedt G, Wahlberg JE. Chromium, cobalt and nickel in used cutting fluids. Contact Dermatitis 1975;1:182.

126. Malten KE. Cobalt and chromium in offset printing. Contact Dermatitis 1975;1:120.

127. Rudsky E, Czerwinska-Dihnz I. Sensitivity to dichromate milk testers: 6 cases of chromate allergy in milk testers. Contact Dermatitis 1977;3:107.

128. Krook G, Fregert S, Gruvberger B. Chromate and cobalt eczema due to magnetic tapes. Contact Dermatitis 1977;3:60.

129. Garcia-Perez A, Martin-Pascual A, Sanchez-Misiego A. Chrome content in bleaches and detergents: its relationship to hand dermatitis in women. Acta Derm Venereol (Stockh) 1973;53:353.

130. Engel HO, Calnan CD. Chromate dermatitis from paint. Br J Ind Med 1963;20:192.

131. Newhouse NL. A cause of chromate dermatitis among assemblers in an automobile factory. Br J Ind Med 1963;20:199.

132. Fregert S, Gruyberger B, Heijer A. Sensitization to chromium and cobalt in processing of sulphate pulp. Acta Derm Venereol (Stockh) 1972;52:221.

133. Samitz MH, Shrager J, Katz S. Studies on the prevention of injurious effects of chromates in industry. Industr Med Surg 1962;31:427.

134. Richter G, Heidelbach U. Chromate eczema after glass polishing with corundum. Berufsdermatosen 1969;17:8.

135. Lee HS, Goh CL. Occupational dermatoses among chrome platers. Contact Dermatitis 1988;18:89.

136. Fregert S. Chromate in welding fumes with special reference to contact dermatitis. Acta Derm Venereol (Stockh) 1963;43:119.

137. Shelley WG. Chromium in welding fumes as a cause of eczematous hand eruption. JAMA 1964;189:772.

138. Zugerman C. Chromium in welding fumes. Contact Dermatitis 1982;8:69.

139. Stevenson CJ. Fluorescence as a clue to contamination in TV workers. Contact Dermatitis 1975;1:242.

140. Burrows D, Andersen RE, Camarasa JS. Trial of 0.5% versus 0.375% potassium dichromate. Contact Dermatitis 1989;21:351.

141. Nethercott J, et al. A study of chromium-induced allergic contact dermatitis with 54 volunteers: implications for environmental risk assessment. Occup Environ Med 1994;51:371.

142. Kosann M, Brancaccio R, Shupack J, et al. Six-hour versus 48 hour patch testing with varying concentrations of potassium dichromate. Am J Contact Dermat 1998;9:92.

143. Siegenthaler U. Studies on contact sensitivity to chromium in the guinea pig. J Invest Derm 1983;80:44.

144. Samitz MH, Epstein E. Experimental cutaneous chromate ulcers in guinea pigs. Arch Environ Health 1962;5:463.

145. Samitz MH. Some dermatologic aspects of the chromate problem. Arch Industr Health 1955;11:361.

146. Goh CL, Gan SL. Change in cement manufacturing process, a cause for decline in chromate allergy? Contact Dermatitis 1996;34:51.

147. Conde-Salazar L, Guimaraens D, Villegas C, et al. Occupational allergic contact dermatitis in construction workers. Contact Dermatitis 1995;33:226.

148. Fisher AA. Cement burns resulting in necrotic ulcers due to kneeling in wet cement. Cutis 1979;23:272.

149. Hannuksela M, Suhonen R, Karvonen J. Caustic ulcers caused by cement. Br J Dermatol 1976;95:547.

150. Tosti A, Peluso AM, Varotti C. Skin burns due to transit-mixed Portland cement. Contact Dermatitis 1989;21:58.

151. Junger H, Witzani R. Cement ulcers. Dermatosen Beruf Umwelt 1978;26:121.

152. Stoermer D, Wolz G. Cement burns. Contact Dermatitis 1983;9:421.

153. Fowler J, Kauffman L, Marks J, et al. An environmental hazard assessment of low level dermal exposure to hexavalent chromium in solution among chromium sensitized volunteers. J Occup of Environ Med 1999;41:150.

154. Wall LM. Chromate dermatitis and sodium dithionite. Contact Dermatitis 1982;8:291.

155. Romaguera C, et al. Formulation of a barrier cream against chromate. Contact Dermatitis 1985;13:49.

156. Miyachi Y, et al. Auto-oxidative damage in cement dermatitis. Arch Dermatol Res 1985;277:288.

157. <www.thecdi.com/about-cobalt> accessed February 16, 2007.

158. Gollhausen R, et al. Trends in allergic contact sensitizations. Contact Dermatitis 1988;18:147.

159. Young E, Van Weelden H, Van Osch L. Age and sex distribution of contact sensitivity to standard allergens. Contact Dermatitis 1988;19:307.

160. Christophersen J, et al. Clinical patch test data evaluated by multivariate analysis. Contact Dermatitis 1989;21:291.

161. Edman B. Sites of contact dermatitis in relationship to particular allergens. Contact Dermatitis 1985;13:129.

162. Perryman J, Fowler J: A patch test study to evaluate the allergenicity of a metallic jewelry alloy in patients allergic to cobalt. CUTIS 2006;77:77.

163. Hindsen M, Persson L, Gruvberger B: Allergic contact dermatitis from cobalt in jewelry. Contact Dermatitis 2005;53:350.

164. Price ML, MacDonald DM. Cheilitis and cobalt allergy related to ingestion of vitamin B12. Contact Dermatitis 1981;7:352.

165. Rostenberg Jr A, Perkins AJ. Nickel and cobalt dermatitis. J Allergy 1951;22:467.

166. Fisher AA. Contact dermatitis at home and abroad. Cutis 1972;10:719.

167. Young WC, Ulrich CW, Fouts PJ. Sensitivity to vitamin B12 concentrate. JAMA 1950;143:893.

168. Kalensky J, Schwank R. Hypersensitivity to cobalt caused by an antihydrotic cream. Cesk Derm 1962;43:423.

169. Skog E. Skin affections caused by hard metal dust. Industr Med Surg 1963;32:266.

170. Fischer T, Rystedt I. Cobalt allergy in hard metal workers. Contact Dermatitis 1983;9:115.

171. McDermott FT. Dust in the cemented carbide industry. J Am Ind Hyg Assoc 1971;32:188.

172. Bourne LB, Milner FJM. Polyester resin hazards. Br J Industr Med 1963;200:100.

173. Pirila V. On occupational diseases of skin among paint factory workers, painters, polishers and varnishers in Finland: clinical and experimental study. Acta Derm Venereol (Stockh) 1947;27[Suppl 16]:1.

174. García J, Armisen A. Cement dermatitis with isolated cobalt sensitivity. Contact Dermatitis 1985;12:52.

175. Camarasa GJM. Cobalt contact dermatitis. Acta Derm Venereol (Stockh) 1967;47:287.

176. DeFonseca A. Joint sensitization with chromium, cobalt and nickel in cement eczema. Acta Derm Sifilgiogr 1970;61:151.

177. Mueller R, Breucker G. Cobalt as work-dependent eczematogen and as co-allergen with chromium and nickel. Derm Wochenschr 1968; 154:276.

178. Bhushan M, Craven NM, Beck MH. Contact allergy to methyl ethyl ketone peroxide and cobalt in the

manufacture of fibreglass-reinforced plastics. Contact Dermatitis 1998;39:203.

179. Jolanki R, Tarvainen K, Tatar T, et al. Occupational dermatoses from exposure to epoxy resin compounds in a ski factory. Contact Dermatitis 1996;34:390.

180. Schena D, Rosina P, Chieregato C, et al. Lymphomatoid-like contact dermatitis from cobalt naphthenate. Contact Dermatitis 1995;33: 197.

181. Pirila V. Sensitization to cobalt in pottery workers. Acta Derm Venereol (Stockh) 1953;33:193.

182. Tuomi ML, Rasanen L. Contact allergy to tylosin and cobalt in a pig farmer. Contact Dermatitis 1995;33:285.

183. Ratcliffe J, English JS. Allergic contact dermatitis from cobalt in animal feed. Contact Dermatitis 1998;39:201.

184. Kanerva L, Jolanki R, Estlander T. Offset printer's occupational allergic contact dermatitis caused by cobalt-2-ethylhexoate. Contact Dermatitis 1996;34:67.

185. Nurnberger F, Arnold W. Quincke's edema as a manifestation of a cobalt allergy due to a sensitization of cobaltous shell splinters. Berufsdermatosen 1969;17:21.

186. Camarasa JG, Alomar A. Photosensitization to cobalt in a bricklayer. Contact Dermatitis 1981;7:154.

187. Romaguera C, Lech M, Grimalt F, et al. Photocontact dermatitis to cobalt salts. Contact Dermatitis 1982;8:383.

188. Allenby CF, Basketter DA. Minimum eliciting patch test concentrations of cobalt. Contact Dermatitis 1989;20:185.

189. Marcussen PV. Intradermal test using cobalt chloride. Acta Derm Venereol (Stockh) 1963;43:472.

190. Saltzer EI. Allergic contact dermatitis due to copper. Arch Dermatol 1968;98:37.

191. Foussereau J, et al. Allergy to copper gas. Med France 1969;76:4489.

192. Santosh V, et al. Results of patch testing with dental materials. Contact Dermatitis 1999;40:50.

193. Cohen SR. A review of the health hazards from copper exposure. J Occup Med 1974;16:621.

194. Oster G, Salgo MP. The copper intrauterine device and its mode of action. N Engl J Med 1975;239:432.

195. Barranco VP. Eczematous dermatitis caused by internal exposure to copper. Arch Dermatol 1972;106:386.

196. Barkoff JR. Urticaria secondary to a copper intrauterine device. Int J Dermatol 1976;15:594.

197. Dry J, Leynadier F, Bennani A, et al. Intrauterine copper contraceptive devices and allergy to copper and nickel. Ann Allergy 1978;41:194.

198. Romaguera C, Grimalt F. Contact dermatitis from a copper-containing intrauterine contraceptive device. Contact Dermatitis 1981;7:163.

199. Karlberg A-T, Boman A, Wahlberg JE. Copper—a rare sensitizer. Contact Dermatitis 1983;9:134.

200. Dhir G, et al. Contact dermatitis caused by copper sulfate used as coloring material in commercial alcohol. Ann Allergy 1977;39:204.

201. Van Joost T, Habets JMW, Stolz I. The meaning of positive patch test to copper sulphate in nickel allergy. Contact Dermatitis 1988;8:101.

202. Pande RS, Gupta YN. Thrombocytopenic purpura following copper sulfate therapy. J Indian Med Assoc 1969;52:227.

203. Reid DJ. Allergic reaction to copper cement. Br Dent J 1968;124:92.

204. 204 Peterson J, Shook B, Wells, M: Cupric Keratoses. Cutis 2006;77:39.

205. Fregert S, Hjorth N. In: Rook AJ, et al., eds. Textbook of dermatology. Oxford: Blackwell Scientific Publications, 1968.

206. Malten KE, Mali J. Contact eczema due to gold. Allergic Asthma 1966;12:31.

207. Elgart ML, Higdon RS. Allergic contact dermatitis to gold. Arch Dermatol 1971;103:649.

208. Fowler J: Gold. Am J Contact Dermat 2001;12:1.

209. Bruze M, Edman B, Bjorkner B, et al. Clinical relevance of contact allergy to gold sodium thiosulfate. J Am Acad Dermatol 1994;31:579.

210. Fowler J. Allergic contact dermatitis to gold. Arch Dermatol 1988;124:181.

211. Fowler J, Taylor J, Storrs F, et al. Gold allergy in North America. Am J Contact Dermat 2001;12:3.

212. Warshaw E, Rietschel R, Belsito D, et al. Common Contact Allergens found in eyelid dermatitis. Contact Dermatitis 2007, accepted for publication.

213. Nedorost S, Wagman A. Positive patch test reactions to gold. Dermatitis 2006;16:67.

214. Koch P, Bahmer F. Oral lesions and symptoms relating to metals in dental restorations. J Am Acad Dermatol 1999;41:422.

215. Scalf L, Fowler J, Morgan K, Looney S. Dental metal allergy in patients with oral, cutaneous, and genital lichen planus. Am J Contact Dermat 2001;12:146.

216. Bjorkner B, Bruze M, Moller H. High frequency of contact allergy to gold sodium thiosulfate. Contact Dermatitis 1994;30:144.

217. Schaffran R, Storrs F, Schalock P. Prevalence of gold sensitivity in asymptomatic individuals with gold dental restorations. Am J Contact Dermat 1999;10:201.

218. Fowler JF. Selection of patch test materials for gold allergy. Contact Dermatitis 1987;3:280.

219. Koch P, Kiehn M, Frosch P. Epikutane Testung mit Goldsalzen. Zwei Multicenterstudien der Deutschen Kontaktallergiegruppe. Hautarzt 1997;48:812.

220. Moller H, Ahnlide I, Gruvberger B, Bruze M. Gold trichloride and gold sodium thiosulfate as markers of contact allergy to gold. Contact Dermatitis 2005;53:80.

221. Andersen K, Jensen C: Long lasting patch reactions to gold sodium thiosulfate occurs frequently in healthy volunteers. Contact Dermatitis 2007;56:214.

222. Kligman A. The identification of contact allergies by human assay. J Invest Dermatol 1966;47:393.

223. Bruze M, Andersen K. Gold—a controversial sensitizer. Contact Dermatitis 1999;40:295.

224. Christiansen J, Farm G, Eid-Foret R, et al. Interferon-gamma secreted from peripheral blood mononuclear cells as a possible marker for allergic dermatitis to gold. Contact Dermatitis 2006;55:101.

225. Fisher AA. Metallic gold: the cause of persistent allergic "dermal" contact dermatitis. Cutis 1974;14:177.

226. Shelley WB, Epstein E. Contact-sensitivity to gold as a chronic papular-eruption. Arch Dermatol 1963;87:388.

227. Bowyer A. Epidermal reactions and prolonged dermal reactions to patch testing with gold salts. Acta Derm Venereol (Stockh) 1967;47:9.

228. Petros H, Macmillan AJ. Allergic contact sensitivity to gold with unusual features. Br J Dermatol 1973;88:505.

229. Suzuki H. Nickel and gold in skin lesions of pierced ear-lobes with contact dermatitis. Arch Dermatol Res 1998;290:523.

230. Kalimo K, Rasanen L, Aho H, et al. Persistent cutaneous pseudo lymphoma after intradermal gold injection. J Cutan Pathol 1996;23:328.

231. Fisher AA. Ear piercing hazard of nickel-gold sensitization. [Letter]. JAMA 1974;228:1226.

232. Comaish S. A case of contact hypersensitivity to metallic gold. Arch Dermatol 1969;99:720.

233. Rytter M, Schubert H. Allergy due to a golden ring by primary epicutaneous sensitization. Dermatologica 1971;142:209.

234. Choy E, Gambling L, Best S, et al. Nickel contamination of gold salts: link with gold induced skin rash. Br J Rheumatol 1997;36:1054.

235. Möller H, Svensson A, Bjorkner B, et al. Contact allergy to gold and gold therapy in patients with rheumatoid arthritis. Acta Derm Venereol 1997;77:370.

236. Möller H, Bjorkner B, Bruze M. Clinical reactions to systemic provocation with gold sodium thiomalate in patients with contact allergy to gold. Br J Dermatol 1996;135:423.

237. Jeffrey D, Biggs D, Percy J, et al. Quantitation of gold in skin in chrysiasis. J Rheumatol 1975;2:28.

238. Miller M, Harford R, Yeager J, et al. A case of chrysiasis. Cutis 1997;59:256.

239. Russell M, Langley M, Truett A, et al. Lichenoid dermatitis after consumption of gold containing liquor. J Am Acad Dermatol 1997;36:841.

240. Nava C, Briatico Vangosa G. Allergy to gold salts. Med Lavoro (Milano) 1971;62:572.

241. Budden MG, Wilkinson DS. Skin and nail lesions from gold potassium cyanide. Contact Dermatitis 1978;4:172.

242. www.chemotechnique.se. accessed May 28, 2007.

243. Marcussen J, Cederbrant K, Heilborn J. Indium and iridium allergy in patients exposed to dental alloys. Contact Dermatitis 1998;38: 297.

244. Bergman A, Suedberg U, Nilsson E. Contact urticaria with anaphylactic reactions caused by occupational exposure to iridium salt. Contact Dermatitis 1995;32:14.

245. Hemmer W, Focke M, Wanke F, et al. Contact hypersensitivity to iron. Contact Dermatitis 1996;34:219.

246. Nater JP. Epidermal hypersensitivity to iron. Hautarzt 1960;11:223.

247. Baer R. Allergic contact sensitization to iron. J Allergy Clin Immunol 1973;51:35.

248. Zugerman C. Contact dermatitis to yellow iron oxide. Contact Dermatitis 1985;13:107.

249. Motolese A, et al. Contact dermatitis and contact sensitization among enamellers and decorators in the ceramics industry. Contact Dermatitis 1993;28:59.

250. Brehm G. Pigmentierung nach lokaler Anwendung von Eisenchloridlosung. Akt Dermatol 1976;3:117.

251. Jirasek L. Occupational exogenous siderosis of the skin. Contact Dermatitis 1979;5:334.

252. Fregert S. Allergic contact dermatitis from lead? Contact Dermatitis Newsletter 1973;13:352.

253. Czarnecki N, Fritsch P. Contact allergy to lead. Hautarzt 1978;29:445.

254. Allen BR, Hunter JAA, Beatties AD, Moore MR. Lead poisoning and blistering of the skin. Scot Med 1974;19:3.

255. Pardo J, Rodriguez-Serna M, DeLa Cuadra J, et al. Allergic contact stomatitis due to manganese in a dental prosthesis. Contact Dermatitis 2004; 50:41.

256. Ortiz-Ruiz A, Ramirez-Espinosa M, Lopez-Jornet P. Oral lichen planus and sensitization to manganese in a dental prosthesis. Contact Dermatitis 2006;54:214.

257. Dosil V, Martinez R, Fernandez R, etal. Allergic contact dermatitis due to manganese in an aluminum alloy. Contact Dermatitis 2006;54: 67–8.

258. Goncalo M, Figueiredo A, Goncalo S. Hypersensitivity to thimerosal: the sensitizing moiety. Contact Dermatitis 1996;34:201.

259. Sulzberger MB. Dermatologic allergy. Springfield, IL: Charles C Thomas Publisher, 1940.

260. Boyd A, Seger D, Vannucci S, et al. Mercury exposure and cutaneous disease. J Am Acad Dermatol 2000;43:81.

261. Frykholm KO, Wahlgren F. A fatal case of mercurial dermatitis with complication. Acta Derm Syph 1964;44:362.

262. Swinyer LJ. Allergic contact dermatitis from metallic mercury. Contact Dermatitis 1980;6:226.

263. Vermeiden I, Oranje AP, Vuzevski VD, Stolz E. Mercury exanthem as occupational dermatitis. Contact Dermatitis 1980;6:88.

264. Gerstner HB, Huff JE. Selected case histories and epidemiologic examples of human mercury poisoning. Clin Toxicol 1977;11:131.

265. Nakayama H, Niki F, Shono M, Hada S. Mercury exanthem. Contact Dermatitis 1983;9:411.

266. Zimmer J, Grange F, Straub P, et al. Mercury erythema after accidental exposure to mercury vapor. Ann Med Interne Paris 1997;148: 317.

267. Andersen K, Hjorth N, Menné T. The baboon syndrome: systemically induced allergic contact dermatitis. Contact Dermatitis 1984;10:97.

268. Le-Coz CJ, Boos V, Cribier BJ, et al. An unusual case of mercurial baboon syndrome. Contact Dermatitis 1996;35:112.

269. Adachi A, Horikawa T, Takashima T, et al. Mercury-induced nummular dermatitis. J Am Acad Dermatol. 2000;43:383.

270. Bradbery S, Feldman M, Brathwaite R, et al. Elemental mercury induced skin granulomas. Clin Toxicol 1996;34:209.

271. Veron C, Hildebrand HF, Martin P. Amalgames dentaires et allergie. J Biol Buccale 1986;14:83.

272. Laine J, et al. Resolution of oral lichenoid lesions after replacement of amalgam restorations in patients allergic to mercury compounds. Br J Dermatol 1992;126:10.

273. Laine J, Kalimo K, Happonen RP. Contact allergy to dental restorative materials in patients with oral lichenoid lesions. Contact Dermatitis 1997;36:141.

274. Camisa C, Taylor JS, Bernat Jr, et al. Contact hypersensitivity to mercury in amalgam restorations may mimic oral lichen planus. Cutis 1999;63:189.

275. Koch P, Bahmer FA. Oral lichenoid lesions, mercury hypersensitivity and combined hypersensitivity to mercury and other metals: histologically proven reproduction of the reaction by patch testing with metal salts. Contact Dermatitis 1995;33:323.

276. Thornhill M, Pemberton M, Simmons R, et al. Amalgam-contact hypersensitivity lesions and oral lichen planus. Oral Surg Oral Med Oral Pathol Oral Radiol Endod 2003;95:291.

277. Kanerva L, Lahtinen A, Toikkanen J, et al. Increase in occupational skin diseases of dental personnel. Contact Dermatitis 1999;40:104.

278. Koch P, Nickolaus G. Allergic contact dermatitis and mercury exanthem due to mercury chloride in plastic boots. Contact Dermatitis 1996;34:405.

279. Nakada T, Higo N, Iijima M, et al. Patch test materials for mercury allergic contact dermatitis. Contact Dermatitis 1997;36:237.

280. Handley J, et al. Mercury allergy in a contact dermatitis clinic in Northern Ireland. Contact Dermatitis 1993;29:258.

281. Von Mayenburg J, Rakoski J, Szliska C. Patch testing with amalgam at various concentrations. Contact Dermatitis 1991;24:266.

282. Lhotka C, Szekeres T, Fritzer-Szekeres M, et al. Are allergic reactions to skin clips associated with delayed wound healing? Am J of Surg 1998;176:320.

283. The romance of nickel. New York: International Nickel Co, 1960.

284. Fisher AA. Nickel—the ubiquitous contact allergen—possible significance of its presence in food, water, urine, hair and infusion fluids. Cutis 1978;22:544.

285. Hogan D, et al. Results of routine patch testing of 542 patients in Saskatoon, Canada. Contact Dermatitis 1988;19:120.

286. Lee T, Lam T. Patch testing of 490 patients in Hong Kong. Contact Dermatitis 1996;35:23.

287. Hague J, Ilchyshyn A: Nickel allergy mimicking basal cell carcinoma. Contact Dermatitis 2006;54:344.

288. Christophersen J, et al. Clinical patch test data evaluated by multivariate analysis. Contact Dermatitis 1989;21:291.

289. Uter W, Pfahlberg A, Gefeller O, et al. Risk factors for contact allergy to nickel. Contact Dermatitis 2003;48:33.

290. Freirich-Astman M, David M, Trattner A. Standard patch test results in patients with contact dermatitis in Israel. Contact dermatitis 2007;56:103.

291. Schubert H, et al. Epidemiology of nickel allergy: results of a follow-up analysis of patients with positive patch tests to nickel. Contact Dermatitis 1988;18:237.

292. Smith-Sivertsen T, Tchatchtchine V, Lund E: Environmental nickel pollution: does it protect against nickel allergy? J Am Acad Dermatol 2002;46:460.

293. Kanan MW. Contact dermatitis in Kuwait. J Kwt Med Assoc 1969;3: 129.

294. Peltonen L. Nickel sensitivity in the general population. Contact Dermatitis 1979;5:27.

295. Murphy G, Rhea K, Peeler JT. Levels of copper, nickel, rubidium and strontium in institutional total diets. Environ Sci Tech 1973;7:1.

296. Flyvholm M-A, Nielson GD, Andersen A. Nickel content of food and estimation of dietary intake. Z Lebensm Unters Forsch 1984;179:427.

297. Horak E, Sunderman Jr EW. Fecal nickel excretion by healthy adults. Clin Chem 1973;19:429.

298. Nielsen GD, Soderberg U, Jorgensen PJ, et al. Absorption and retention of nickel from drinking water in relation to food intake and nickel sensitivity. Toxicol Appl Pharmacol 1999;154:67.

299. Fregert S. Nickel in tap water. Contact Dermatitis Newsletter 1971;9:202.

300. Kopp JF, Kramer RC. Trace metals in waters in the United States. Cincinnati: US Department of the Interior, Division of Pollution Surveillance, 1967.

301. McNeely MD, Neckay MW, Sunderman Jr EW. Measurements of nickel in serum and urine as indices of environmental exposure to nickel. Clin Chem 1972;18:992.

302. Kaaber K, Veien NK, Tjell JC. Low nickel diet in the treatment of patients with chronic nickel dermatitis. Br J Dermatol 1978;98:197.

303. Sjovall P, Christensen OP, Möller H. Oral hyposensitization in nickel allergy. J Am Acad Dermatol 1987;17:774.

304. Jensen C, Menne T, Lisby S, et al. Experimental systemic contact dermatitis from nickel. Contact Dermatitis 2003;49:124.

305. Veien NK. Systemically induced eczema in adults. Acta Derm Venereol (Suppl) 1989;69:147.

306. Jensen C, Menne T, Johansen J. Systemic contact dermatitis after oral exposure to nickel. Contact Dermatitis 2006;54:79.

307. Fowler JF. Disulfiram is effective for nickel allergic hand eczema. Am J Contact Dermat 1992;3:175.

308. Katz SA, Samitz MH. Leaching of nickel from stainless steel consumer commodities. Acta Derm Venereol (Stockh) 1975;55:113.

309. Christensen, OB, Möller, H. Release of nickel from cooking utensils. Contact Dermatitis 1978;4:343.

310. Veien NK, Hattel T, Justesen O, Norholm A. Oral challenge with metal salts: 1. Vesicular patch-test-negative hand eczema. Contact Dermatitis 1983;9:402.

311. Veien NK, Hattel T, Justesen O, Norholm A. Oral challenge with metal salts: 2. Various types of eczema. Contact Dermatitis 1983;9:407.

312. Menné T, Mikkelsen HI, Solgaard P. Nickel excretion in urine after oral administration. Contact Dermatitis 1978;4:106.

313. Spruit JC, Bongaarts PFM. Nickel content of plasma, urine and hair in contact dermatitis. Dermatologica 1977;154:291.

314. McNeely MD, Sunderman Jr EW, Nechay MW, et al. Abnormal concentrations of nickel in serum in cases of myocardial infarction, stroke, burns, hepatic cirrhosis, and uremia. Clin Chem 1971;17:1123.

315. Spruit D. Increased nickel absorption following Indomethacin therapy. Contact Dermatitis 1979;5:62.

316. Katz SA, Bowen HJM, Comaish JS, et al. Tissue nickel levels and nickel dermatitis. Br J Dermatol 1975;92:187.

317. Menné T, Rasmussen K. Regulation of nickel exposure in Denmark. Contact Dermatitis 1990;23:57.

318. Liden C. Norberg K: Nickel on the Swedish market. Contact Dermatitis 2005;52:29.

319. Stoddart JC. Nickel sensitivity as a cause of infusion reactions. Lancet 1960;2:741.

320. Smeenk G, Teunissen PC. Allergic reactions to nickel from infusion equipment. Ned Tijdschr Geneeskd 1977;121:4.

321. Calnan CD. Nickel sensitivity in women. Arch Allerg Appl Immunol 1957;11:73.

322. Epstein S. Epidermal and dermal reactions in a case of sensitivity to nickel. J Invest Dermatol 1962;38:37, 1962.

323. Fisher AA. Nickel dermatitis. Cutis 1967;1:298.

324. Nielsen N, Menné T, Kristiansen J, et al. Effects of repeated skin exposure to low nickel concentrations: a model for allergic contact dermatitis to nickel in the hands. Br J of Derm 1999;141:676.

325. Christensen OB. Prognosis in nickel allergy and hand eczema. Contact Dermatitis 1982;8:7.

326. Fisher AA. Problems attending patch testing for nickel sensitivity. Cutis 1982;29:148.

327. Wahlberg JE. Petrolatum—a reliable vehicle for metal allergens? Contact Dermatitis 1980;6:134.

328. Van Ketel WG. Patch testing with nickel sulphate in DMSO. Contact Dermatitis 1978;4:167.

329. Wall LM, Calnan CD. Occupational nickel dermatitis in the electroforming industry. Contact Dermatitis 1980;6:414.

330. Dooms-Goossens A, Naert C, Chrispeels MI, et al. Is a 5 percent nickel sulphate patch test concentration adequate? Contact Dermatitis 1980;6:232.

331. Cronin E. Patch testing with nickel. Contact Dermatitis 1975;1:56.

332. Emmett EA, et al. Allergic contact dermatitis to nickel: bioavailability from consumer products and provocation threshold. J Am Acad Dermatol 1988;19:314.

333. Fischer L, Menne T, Johansen J: Experimental nickel elicitation thresholds. Contact Dermatitis 2005;52:57.

334. Spiewak R, Moed H, von Blomberg B, et al. Allergic contact dermatitis to nickel: modified in vitro test protocols for better detection of allergen-specific response. Contact Dermatitis 2007;56:63.

335. Fisher AA. The dimethylglyoxime test in the prevention and management of nickel dermatitis. Cutis 1990;46:467.

336. Rystedt I, Fischer T. Relationship between nickel and cobalt sensitization in hard metal workers. Contact Dermatitis 1983;9:195.

337. Boss A, Menné T. Nickel sensitization from ear piercing. Contact Dermatitis 1982;8:211.

338. Kerosuo H, Kullaa A, Kerosuo E, et al. Nickel allergy in adolescents in relation to orthodontic treatment and piercing of ears. Am J Orthod Dentofacial Orthop 1996;109:148.

339. Brandrup F, Larsen FS. Nickel dermatitis provoked by buttons in blue jeans. Contact Dermatitis 1979;5:148.

340. Larsen ES, Brandrup F. Nickel release from metallic buttons in blue jeans. Contact Dermatitis 1980;6:298.

341. Goh CL, Ng SK, Kwok SF. Allergic contact dermatitis from nickel in eyeshadow. Contact Dermatitis 1989;20:380.

342. LaChapelle JM, Tennstedt D. An anatomo-clinical study of delayed skin allergic reactions to nickel following intradermal injections of lidocaine with a Dermo-Jet. Contact Dermatitis 1982;8:193.

343. de Correst LF, Garrastazu MT, Soloeta R, Escayol P. Nickel contact dermatitis in a blood bank. Contact Dermatitis 1982;8:32.

344. Shah M, Lewis FM, Gawkrodger DJ. Nickel as an occupational allergen: a survey of 368 nickel sensitive subjects. Arch Dermatol 1998;134:1231.

345. Wahlberg JE. Nickel allergy and atopy in hairdressers. Contact Dermatitis 1975;1:161.

346. Dahlquist I, Fregert S, Gruvberger B. Release of nickel from plated utensils in permanent wave liquids. Contact Dermatitis 1979;5:52.

347. Hegyi E, Gasparík J. The nickel content of moulded bricks as building material. Contact Dermatitis 1989;21:63.

348. Raith L, Jaeger K. The nickel content of chalk-cause of dermatitis? Contact Dermatitis 1986;14:61.

349. Zanca A, et al. The release of nickel from blackboard chalk may cause contact dermatitis. Contact Dermatitis 1988;19:143.

350. Widström L, Bergström B, Wennerholm C. Nickel allergy and wrist strap to dissipate static electricity. Contact Dermatitis 1986;15:299.

351. Hanks JW, Venters WJ. Nickel allergy from a bed-wetting alarm confused with herpes genitalis and child abuse. Pediatrics 1992;90:458.

352. Lacroix J, Morin CL, Collin P-P. Nickel dermatitis from a foreign body in the stomach. J Pediatr 1979;95:428.

353. Lyell A, Bain WH, Thomson RM. Repeated failure of nickel-containing prosthetic heart valves in a patient allergic to nickel. Lancet 1978;2:658.

354. Menné T, Kaaber K. Treatment of pompholyx due to nickel allergy with chelating agents. Contact Dermatitis 1978;4:289.

355. Christensen OB, Kristensen M. Treatment with disulfiram in chronic hand nickel dermatitis. Contact Dermatitis 1979;4:221.

356. Kaaber K, Menné T, Hougaard P. Treatment of nickel dermatitis with Antabuse: double blind study. Contact Dermatitis 1983;9:297.

357. Kristensen ME. Toxic hepatitis induced by disulfiram in a non-alcoholic. Acta Med Scand 1981;209:335.

358. Burrows D, et al. Treatment of nickel dermatitis with Trientene. Contact Dermatitis 1986;15:55.

359. Healy J, Johnson S, Little MC, et al. An in vitro study of the use of chelating agents in cleaning nickel contaminated skin: an alternative approach to preventing nickel allergic contact dermatitis. Contact Dermatitis 1998;39:171.

360. Warin RP. Chronic urticaria. Contact Dermatitis 1982;8:117.

361. McConnell LH, Fink JN, Schlueter DP, et al. Asthma caused by nickel sensitivity. Ann Intern Med 1973;78:888.

362. Block GT, Yeung M. Asthma induced by nickel. JAMA 1982;247:1600.

363. Espana A, et al. Chronic urticaria after implantation of 2 nickel-containing dental prostheses in a nickel-allergic patient. Contact Dermatitis 1989;21:204.

364. Fernandez-Redondo V, Gomez-Centeno P, Toribio J. Chronic urticaria from a dental bridge. Contact Dermatitis 1998;38:178.

365. Cook LJ. Associated nickel and cobalt contact dermatitis presenting as erythema multiforme. Contact Dermatitis 1982;8:280.

366. Hjorth N. Nickel vasculitis. Contact Dermatitis 1976;2:356.

367. Wall LM. Nickel penetration through rubber gloves. Contact Dermatitis 1980;6:461.

368. http://en.wikipedia.org/wiki/niobium (accessed November 2006)

369. Campbell KI, et al. Dermal irritancy of metal compounds. Arch Environ Health 1975;30:168.

370. Munro-Ashman D, Munro DD, Hughes TH. Contact dermatitis from palladium. Trans St John Hosp Derm Soc 1969;55:196.

371. Sheard Jr C. Contact dermatitis from platinum and related metals: report of case. Arch Dermatol 1955;71:357.

372. Camarasa JG, et al. Palladium contact sensitivity. Contact Dermatitis 1991;24:370.

373. Goossens A, De Swerdt A, Connick K, et al. Allergic contact granuloma due to palladium following ear piercing. Contact Dermatitis 2006;55:338.

374. Fowler J, Hayden J. Palladium patch test reactivity. Exogenous Dermatol 2004;2:277.

375. Aberer W, et al. Palladium in dental alloys—the dermatologists' responsibility to warn? Contact Dermatitis 1993;28:163.

376. Filon F, Uderzo D, Bagnato E. Sensitization to palladium chloride: a 10 year evaluation, Dermatitis 2003;14:78.

377. Dodd DJ, Burrows D. Patch testing with pure palladium metal in patients with sensitivity to palladium chloride. Contact Dermatitis 1992;26:327.

378. Casper C, Groth W, Hunzelmann N. Sarcoidal type allergic contact granuloma. Am J Dermatopathol 2004;26:59.

379. Wahlberg JE, Boman A. Palladium chloride—a potent sensitizer in the guinea pig. Am J Contact Dermat 1990;1:112.

380. Hindsen M, Spiren A, Bruze M. Cross reactivity between nickel and palladium demonstrated by systemic administration of nickel. Contact Dermatitis 2005;53:2.

381. Fowler J, Perryman J, Quinlan B. Rarity of positive patch tests to platinum. Submitted for publication 2007.

382. Santucci B, Valenzano C, de Rocca M, et al. Platinum in the environment. Contact Dermatitis 2000;43:333–8.

383. Roberts AE. Platinosis. Arch Industr Hyg 1951;4:549.

384. Roberts AE. Platinosis. A five-year study of the effects of soluble platinum salts on employees in a platinum laboratory and refinery. AMA Arch Industr Hyg Occup Med 1951;4:549.

385. Baker DB, et al. Cross-sectional study of platinum salts sensitization among precious metals refinery workers. Am J Indus Med 1990;18:653.

386. Freedman SO, Krupey J. Respiratory allergy caused by platinum salts. J Allergy 1968;42:233.

387. Levene GM, Calnan CD. Platinum hypersensitivity: treatment by specific hyposensitization. Clin Allergy 1971;1:75.

388. Schuppe H, Kir G, Lerchenmuller C, et al. Contact hypersensitivity to disodium hexachloroplatinate in mice. Toxicol Lett 1997;93:125.

389. De la Cuadra J. Occupational contact dermatitis from rhodium and cobalt. Contact Dermatitis 1991;25:182.

390. Bodello P. Contact dermatitis to rhodium. Contact Dermatitis 1987;17:111.

391. Gomez dela Fuente E, Alvarez J, Vicente F, et al. Occupational contact dermatitis caused by rhodium. Dermatitis 2003;14:173.

392. Stingeni L, Brunelli L, Lisi P. Contact sensitivity to rhodium and iridium in consecutive patch tested subjects. Contact Dermatitis 2004;51:316.

393. Cameli N, et al. Contact dermatitis from rubidium iodide in eyedrops. Contact Dermatitis 1990;23:377.

394. Gaul LE. Incidence of sensitivity to chromium, nickel, gold, silver and copper compared to reactions to their aqueous salts including cobalt sulphate. Ann Allergy 1954;12:429.

395. Agarwal A, Gawkrodger D: Occupational allergic contact dermatitis to silver and colophonium in a jeweler. Dermatitis 2002;13:74.

396. Marcussen PV. Eczematous allergy to metals. Acta Allergolog 1962; 17:311.

397. Gaul LE, Underwood GB. The effects of aging a solution of silver nitrate on its cutaneous reaction. J Invest Dermatol 1948;11:7.

398. Marshall JP, Schneider RP. Systemic argyria secondary to topical silver nitrate. Arch Dermatol 1977;113:1077.

399. Buckley WR. Localized argyria. Arch Dermatol 1963;88:531.

400. Gettler AO, Rhoads CP, Weiss S. A contribution to the pathology of generalized argyria with a discussion of the fate of silver in the human body. Am J Pathol 1927;3:631.

401. Gaul LE, Staud AH. Clinical spectroscopy. JAMA 1935;104:1387.

402. Criep LH. Allergy to argyrol. JAMA 1943;121:421.

403. Heyl T. Contact dermatitis from silver coat. Contact Dermatitis 1979;5:197.

404. White IR, Rycroft RJG. Contact dermatitis from silver fulminate itch. Contact Dermatitis 1982;8:159.

405. Marks R. Contact dermatitis due to silver. Case report. Br J Dermatol 1966;78:606.

406. http://en.wikipedia.org/wiki/tellurium (accessed June , 2007).

407. Menné T, Andersen K, Kaaber K, et al. Tin: an overlooked sensitizer. Contact Dermatitis 1987;16:9.

408. De Fine-Olivarius F, et al. Skin reactivity to tin chloride and metallic tin. Contact Dermatitis 1993;29:110.

409. Nielsen N, Skov L. Occupational allergic contact dermatitis in a patient with a positive patch test to tin. Contact Dermatitis 1998;39:97.

410. Goh C. Irritant dermatitis from tri-n-butyl tin oxide in paint. Contact Dermatitis 1985;12:161.

411. Viraben R, Boulinguez S, Alba C. Granulomatous dermatitis after implantation of a titanium containing pacemaker. Contact Dermatitis 1995;33:437.

412. Verbov J. Pacemaker contact sensitivity. Contact Dermatitis 1985;12:173.

413. Brun R, Hunziker N. Pacemaker dermatitis. Contact Dermatitis 1980;6:212.

414. Abdallah HI, Balsara RK, O'Riordan AC. Pacemaker contact sensitivity: clinical recognition and management. Ann Thorac Surg 1994;57:1017.

415. Peters MS, Schroeter AL, van Hale HM, et al. Pacemaker contact sensitivity. Contact Dermatitis 1984;11:214.

416. Rueda M, Pons-Guirard AQ. Allergie au pacemaker. Nouv Dermatol 1994;13:183.

417. High W, Ayers R, Adams J, et al. Granulomatous reaction to titanium alloy. J Am Acad Dermatol 2006;55:716.

418. Holgers K, et al. Clinical, immunological, and bacteriological evaluation of adverse reactions to skin-penetrating titanium implants in the head and neck region. Contact Dermatitis 1992;27:1.

419. Dujardin F, Fevrier V, Lecorvaisier C, et al. Allergic dermatitis caused by metallic implants in orthopedic surgery. Rev Chir Orthop Reparatrice Appar Mot 1995;81:473.

420. Tan M, Suzuki H. Usefulness of titanium implants for systemic contact dermatitis due to orthopaedic prostheses. Contact Dermatitis 1995;33:202.

421. Thomas P, Bandl WD, Naier S, et al. Hypersensitivity to titanium osteosynthesis with impaired fracture healing, eczema, and T-cell hyperresponsiveness in vitro. Contact Dermatitis 2006;55:199.

422. Basketter D, Whitle E, Monk B. Possible allergy to complex titanium salt. Contact Dermatitis 2000;42:310.

423. Granchi D, Cenni E, Trisolino G, et al. Sensitivity to implant materials in patients undergoing total hip replacement. J Biomed Mater Res B Appl Biomater 2006; 77:257–64.

424. Calnan CD. Metal fume fever. Contact Dermatitis 1979;5:124.

425. Schwartz L, Tullipan L, Birmingham DS. Occupational diseases of the skin, 3rd ed. Philadelphia: Lea & Febiger, 1957.

426. Koizumi H, et al. Acupuncture needle dermatitis. Contact Dermatitis 1989;21:352.

427. Yates YM, Finn OA. Contact allergic sensitivity dermatitis and actinic reticuloid syndrome. Contact Dermatitis 1980;6:349.

428. Calnan CD. In: Fisher AA, ed. Highlights of the first international symposium on contact dermatitis. Cutis 1976;18:645.

429. Calnan CD. Occupational piperazine dermatitis. Contact Dermatitis 1975;1:126.

430. Nielsen N, Menné T. Allergic contact dermatitis caused by zinc pyrithione associated with pustular psoriasis. Am J Contact Dermat 1997;8:170.

431. Galindo P, Garrido J, Gomez E, et al. Zinc acexamate allergy. Contact Dermatitis 1998;38:301.

432. Feinglos MN, Jegasothy BV. Insulin allergy due to zinc. Lancet 1979;1:122.

433. Palmer L, Welton W. Lupus miliaris disseminatus faciei: zirconium hypersensitivity as possible cause. Cutis 1967;7:74.

434. Rublin L. Granulomas of axillae caused by deodorants. JAMA 1956;162:953.

435. Shelley WB, et al. Intradermal tests with metals and other inorganic elements in sarcoidosis and anthraco-silicosis. J Invest Dermatol 1958;31:301.

436. Epstein WL, Allen JR. Granulomatous hypersensitivity after use of zirconium-containing poison oak lotions. JAMA 1964;190:162.

437. Baler GR. Granulomas from topical zirconium in poison ivy dermatitis. Arch Dermatol 1965;91:145.

438. LoPresti PJ, Hambril GW. Zirconium granuloma following treatment of rhus dermatitis. Arch Dermatol 1965;92:188.

439. Costa C, Hunziker, N. Occupational dermatitis due to sodium hypophosphite. Contact Dermatitis 1988;19:313.

440. Payero M, et al. Contact urticaria and dermatitis from phosphorus sesquisulphide. Contact Dermatitis 1985;13:126.

441. Glover JR. Some medical problems concerning selenium in industry. Trans Assoc Industr Med Officers 1954;4:94.

442. Jirasek L, Kalensky J. Hypersensitivity to platinum, rhodium, gold, copper, antimony and other precious metals and occupational dermatitis caused by selenium. Cesk Dermatol 1975;50:361.

443. Senff H, et al. Allergic Contact dermatitis from selenite. Contact Dermatitis 1988;19:73.

444. Shelley WB, Hurley HJ. The pathogenesis of silica granulomas in man: a non-allergic colloidal phenomenon. J Invest Dermatol 1960;34:107.

445. Mason J, Apisarnthanarax P. Migratory silicone granuloma. Arch Dermatol 1981;117:366.

446. Raque C, Goldschmidt H. Dermatitis associated with an implanted cardiac pacemaker. Arch Dermatol 1970;102:647.

447. Elmer K, George R. Contact urticaria to the MCV-2A/P gas mask. Mil-Med 1996;164:377.

448. Blackadder ES, Manderson WG. Occupational absorption of tellurium: a report of two cases. Br J Industr Med 1975;32:59.

449. Thiers MM, Chanial G, Rivoire J, Muller F. Dermites professionnelles par sensibilisation aux urantes de sodium et de calcium. Arch Des Malades Professionelles Méd Travail Soc 1961;22:168.

CHAPTER 33

CONTACT STOMATITIS AND CHEILITIS

EXECUTIVE SUMMARY

Lesions and symptoms in the mouth and on the lips have a variety of causes. Included in the differential diagnosis of allergic or irritant contact stomatitis is a range of microbial (bacterial, fungal, and viral) infections, autoimmune and metabolic diseases, malignancy, and physical insults (trauma, thermal, and actinic damage). The lips are highly prone to development of allergic contact dermatitis (ACD) and irritant contact dermatitis (ICD). Lip "balms," cosmetics, sunscreens, and dentifrices are the most likely causes of allergic cheilitis. The mouth may be less likely to develop allergic reactions than the skin. Theories behind this include the concept that saliva washes away many allergens after only brief contact, and the concept that antigen-presenting cells are less available in the mouth. When allergic reactions do occur in the mouth, dental materials, including metals and acrylics in restorations (fillings), crowns, and dentures are often to blame. The most common positive reactions on patch testing include flavoring and fragrances, metals, especially gold and mercury, and acrylates. 2-hydroxyethylmethacrylate (1-HEMA) appears to be an excellent screening allergen for acrylic dental allergy. Dentifrices and foods are occasional causes of allergic stomatitis, and are perhaps more likely to cause irritant stomatitis. Oral lichen planus, while often idiopathic, may be caused by allergy to dental materials. One should have a high index of suspicion if the lesions are in direct proximity to fillings, crowns, or dentures. Patch testing in this instance should be done as part of an initial evaluation. Occasionally "burning mouth syndrome" may be caused by allergic contact, but patch testing should probably be deferred until other disorders have been ruled out.

The oral mucosa, like the skin, is subject to both primary irritation and allergic sensitization. In general, the mucosa is more resistant to primary irritants and is not as readily sensitized as is the skin, possibly because the keratin layer of the skin may contain proteins that more readily combine with simple chemicals to form allergens.[1]

The oral mucosa is constantly bathed in saliva, which washes food particles, debris, irritants, and sensitizers from the mucosal surface. Saliva also plays a considerable role in digestion through the action of enzymes, such as amylase and maltase. Saliva may solubilize allergens. In addition, saliva may contain yeasts, which can modify the clinical picture of the stomatitis.

Clinical Picture of Contact Stomatitis and Cheilitis

Often the subjective symptoms of contact stomatitis are more prominent than the physical signs. Patients may complain of loss of taste, numbness, a burning sensation, and pain in the involved area. Itching is not a usual symptom.

The appearance of the mucous membrane varies from a barely visible, mild erythema to a fiery red color with or without edema. Lingual papillae may disappear. In the presence of considerable edema, the mucosa takes on a smooth, waxy, glazed appearance. Vesiculation of the oral mucosa is rarely seen, because vesicles rupture quickly to form erosions. Erosions may be seen with allergy but also with primary immunobullous disease such as pemphigus, pemphigoid, lichen planus, lupus erythematosus and others. Vitamin deficiency and various infections are included in the differential diagnosis of stomatitis. Oral lichen planus may be idiopathic or allergic in nature.

In allergic reactions to denture material or restorations (fillings), there is often a relatively sharp demarcation between the red, inflamed mucosa covered by or adjacent to the dental material and the nearby uninvolved area.

The irritation of an ill-fitting plate may, however, give an appearance similar to that of allergic stomatitis. Similarly, allergic stomatitis from metal or acrylics used in dental implants or crowns often shows a sharp border just around the treated teeth. However, occasional cases of allergic stomatitis may not have localized lesions. Some cases of diffuse stomatitis or burning mouth syndrome (BMS) without lesions may be due to allergy.

Allergic stomatitis may be accompanied by cheilitis. The usual picture of allergic cheilitis, whether secondary to stomatitis or caused by contactants applied directly to the lips, is one of dryness, scaling or crusting, edema, fissuring, and angular cheilitis. Itching may be pronounced. It may be very difficult to tell from the clinical pattern, the difference between allergic cheilitis, irritant cheilitis, and actinic cheilitis. A riboflavin deficiency syndrome may be simulated.

In contrast to the distinct disease "perioral dermatitis," allergic cheilitis usually does not have a "grenz zone" of normal skin immediately adjacent to the vermilion border. Perioral dermatitis is more akin to acne than dermatitis, although it may have features of both.

PRIMARY IRRITATION OF THE ORAL MUCOSA BY HEAT AND CHEMICALS

Irritation Due to Heat

The oral mucosa can usually withstand excessively hot liquids and spicy foods with little or no evidence of irritation. The ingestion of hot liquids or hot foods, such as melted cheese in grilled cheese sandwiches and pizzas, however, may sometimes inflict severe, painful thermal burns with the formation of vesicles or bullae, particularly on the palate, tongue, and lips. The patient may treat such burns by sucking on ice chips or by applying ice-cold glycerin to the affected areas. If pain persists, a topical anesthetic such as lidocaine in an oral base may then be applied to painful sites.

Stomatitis Due to Chemical Injury

A previously common cause of chemical injury is repeated placement of aspirin tablets against a painful tooth. Chewing gum containing aspirin may also produce oral ulceration.[2,3] Although aspirin has no local anesthetic properties, it does have a strong caustic action on oral mucosa and can rapidly cause complete separation and sloughing of the epithelium. The prolonged use of undiluted perborate or hydrogen peroxide may also produce painful, superficial erosions of the oral mucosa.

The most severe injury from chemicals occurs in individuals who swallow caustics such as lye for suicidal purposes and in young children who accidentally ingest household caustics and acids. Such strong chemicals may cause severe necrosis and sloughing of the mucosa. In addition, caustic chemicals such as phenol, silver nitrate, and nitric acid may be accidentally placed against the mucosa during dental procedures.

Denture cleaners come in powder, pill, and cream form. Abramson[4] wrote that after having been soaked in a warm solution of a denture cleaner, "store teeth" should be rinsed thoroughly before being put back into the wearer's mouth. Cleaner and mouth were never intended to meet. Most active ingredients in the cleaners are acid, alkali, or oxygenating compounds, or a combination. Abramson[4] pointed out that studies indicate that alkalis are particularly destructive to esophageal tissue because they penetrate deep into tissue layers by liquefaction necrosis; acid burns are less destructive because they produce coagulation necrosis that blocks deeper penetration.

Necrotic and ulcerative lesions of the oral mucous membranes may be produced in patients receiving a solution of 9.8% sodium citrate and 14% citric acid (Shohl's solution) orally to alleviate metabolic acidosis. The lesions are due to a direct primary irritant effect of the solution. Shohl's solution should be diluted when used by patients who have difficulty swallowing or poor oral hygiene.

Stomatitis Nicotina

Prolonged smoking may produce distinct umbilicated papules on the palate.[5] The lesions arise from the ducts of the salivary glands and not from the glands themselves.

Reddy and colleagues[6] reported that 550 people with nicotine stomatitis and a control group of 2,850 were surveyed with respect to their smoking and other habits. The most important factor in the development of this type of stomatitis was reverse smoking of homemade *chuttas*. Other methods of smoking produced lesions less frequently and in a milder form. Women have more chance of developing stomatitis than men because many form a habit of smoking only the reverse way, whereas most men smoke either the ordinary way or the reverse way and so have less chance of developing lesions.

Cotton Roll Stomatitis

"Cotton roll stomatitis" is a complication of oral surgery. The saliva-absorbing cotton roll strips off tissue when it is removed, causing a superficial ulceration.

Ulcerative Stomatitis in Infants

Oral ulcerations in newborns and infants are commonly due to infectious diseases such as herpes simplex. Mennie and colleagues[7] reported a case of oral ulcers in a 17-day-old baby apparently due to direct irritation from contact with a solution of 18% sodium chloride with hypochlorous acid that the mother used to "disinfect" her breasts.

Allergic Contact Stomatitis

Allergic contact stomatitis occurs less frequently than allergic contact dermatitis, probably because of the following factors.

1. With the exception of dental materials, the period of contact of sensitizers with the buccal mucous membranes is brief.
2. Saliva dilutes and removes potential allergens and may buffer and neutralize chemicals.
3. The anatomical structure of the buccal mucosa, with its extensive vascularization, aids in rapid dispersion and absorption of the allergen, thereby preventing prolonged contact of the allergen with the mucosa.

When the skin is the original surface sensitized, the mucous membrane may or may not be involved on a clinical level. However, when the mucous membrane is first sensitized, the skin is usually involved. For example, sensitization to an ingredient in a dentifrice may produce allergic stomatitis, cheilitis, and circumoral dermatitis upon exposure to the allergen (Table 33.1).

Lowney[8] showed that a series of applications of dinitrochlorobenzene to the buccal mucosa induced a mild contact sensitivity in some subjects and not in others. Virtually all subjects then were refractory to subsequent attempts to induce sensitivity or raise the level of sensitivity previously induced. This finding, that partial tolerance to dinitrochlorobenzene can be induced by buccal administration of the compound, may become of importance if this technique works with other chemicals. It has been suggested that children who wear metallic orthodontic devices (braces) in the absence of nickel allergy may be less likely to become sensitized than children without braces.[9]

FLAVORINGS

Cinnamon flavorings, particularly cinnamic aldehyde, are probably the most frequent cause of allergic stoma-

Table 33-1 Some Causes of Allergic Stomatitis

Foods and flavors: *Myroxylon pereirae*, cinnamon and derivatives, menthol, peppermint, etc.

Preservatives and components of dentifrices: parabens, prolylene glycol, formocresol, etc.

Dental materials: metals, acrylics, other plastics and resins, eugenol, etc.

titis from dentifrices and foods. On patch testing, a positive result to *Myroxylon pereirae* (MP) or cinnamic aldehyde suggests that these flavorings should be avoided in the appropriate clinical setting (Figure 33-1).

Three patients developed an allergic cheilitis and stomatitis from the use of toothpaste containing cinnamic aldehyde. One patient experienced a flare-up of the condition after she added cinnamon to her coffee as a flavoring agent. Patch tests with 1% cinnamic aldehyde gave strongly positive reactions in the three patients (personal communication, Alexander Fisher, New York, NY, 2000).

Drake and Maibach[10] described a patient who had acute stomatitis and dermatitis from a popular toothpaste containing cinnamon oil flavor. Magnusson and Wilkinson[11] studied 16 patients for whom patch tests gave positive results who developed "oral" symptoms from a newly formulated "spicy" toothpaste containing cinnamic aldehyde. Kirton and Wilkinson[12] reported five additional cases of toothpaste cheilitis and stomatitis caused by cinnamic aldehyde. Tom's of Maine brand makes some toothpastes that are unflavored or fruit-flavored and should not affect the cinnamic-sensitive patient.

Another report linked cinnamon-containing or cinnamon-flavored oral preparations with red or white oral mucosal plaques and lichenoid oral lesions.[13] Histology revealed hyperkeratosis and a lichenoid infiltrate with many plasma cells.

A report from Korea indicates that a product called Eundan used as a breath freshener and smoking deterrent may cause allergic and/or irritant stomatitis. One herb, *Tinula helenium*, was shown to be a direct irritant. Another component, *Glycyrrhiza uralensis*, apparently acted as an allergen.[14]

ESSENTIAL OILS

In dentistry, essential oils are chiefly used as pharmaceutical aids, as mild antiseptics and anodynes, and as flavoring for dentifrices and mouthwashes. Several of these oils can produce allergic stomatitis and cheilitis.

The essential oils, particularly clove oil, eugenol, and cinnamon oil, may crossreact with balsam of Peru, which is used in dental cement liquids. In addition, these oils may crossreact with benzoin, rosin, vanilla, and the essential oils of orange peel.[15,16]

Anise oil is used as a flavoring agent, especially to disguise substances of disagreeable taste.

Cinnamon oil (cassia oil) is a very weak antiseptic. In dentistry, it is used primarily as a flavoring agent. Oil of cinnamon has further been identified as the cause of allergic cheilitis and stomatitis from toothpaste,[17] bubble gum, and lipstick. Ingestion of oil of cinnamon in dry vermouth may provoke a flare-up of pre-existing allergic contact dermatitis in sensitized individuals.[18] Cross-sensitization to MP may result from primary sensitivity to oil of cinnamon.

MENTHOL, USP

Menthol is used as a flavoring agent, as a component of zinc oxide-eugenol cements, and as a mint flavoring and cooling agent in toothpastes and mouthwashes, cough drops, candy, chewing gum, food, cigarettes, liqueurs, and mixed drinks.[19] Papa and Shelley[20] described dermatitis, cheilitis, and stomatitis from menthol.

Morton and colleagues[21] presented data on 12 patients with oral symptoms and allergy to menthol and/or peppermint. Five patients had burning mouth syndrome, four had oral ulcers, and three had oral lichen planus. Patch tests were positive to menthol (5% pet), peppermint oil (1% pet), or both. In six of nine that could be contacted later complete or significant clearing occurred with allergen avoidance. One other patient cleared with removal of a mercury filling.

EUGENOL

This is the main constituent of clove oil, oil of carnation, pimento oil, and oil of bay. In dentistry, eugenol is used in periodontal dressings, zinc oxide cement, and impression pastes.

Goransson and colleagues[22] observed three cases of eugenol hypersensitivity. In one, a eugenol impression paste produced allergic cheilitis and stomatitis. In the other two, an allergic eczematous reaction was produced from handling eugenol. Koch and colleagues[23] showed that eugenol is a potent sensitizer.

A case of a 10-year-old girl allergic to eugenol in chewing gum has been reported.[24] She had no oral lesions but only a circumoral dermatitis. Her chewing gum was shown to contain eugenol. In addition to eugenol, she was positive to isoeugenol, MP, and fragrance mix.

Eugenol may crossreact with MP, diethylstilbestrol, and benzoin.

ORAL LICHEN PLANUS AND LICHENOID REACTIONS CAUSED BY ALLERGIES

A wide variety of metals have been used by dentists and oral surgeons for fillings and prostheses, including aluminum, antimony, beryllium, chromium, cobalt, copper, gold, indium, iridium, mercury, nickel, osmium, palladium, platinum, rhodium, ruthenium, silicon, silver, tin, titanium, and tungsten. Of these metals used in dentistry, mercury and gold have most commonly been implicated as a producer of allergic reactions,[25] including lichen planus (LP), but most other metals have been reported occasionally as well.. All dental amalgams contain mercury and in addition may contain copper, silver, tin, and

other metals. According to the number of metals they contain, amalgams are classified as binary, tertiary, quaternary, and so forth.[26] Metal dentures containing chromium, nickel, and other metals may produce dermatitis, stomatitis, and LP, or lichenoid oral lesions.[27]

Oral lichen planus may be induced by metal allergy. Koch and Bahmer[28] presented a study with extensive patch testing of 19 patients with oral LP adjacent to fillings, 42 with oral LP not anatomically related to fillings, 28 with other oral diseases, 46 with burning mouth syndrome, and 59 controls with no oral symptoms or pathology. Fifteen of the 19 in the first group were positive to inorganic mercury, sometimes with positive reactions only developing after 10 to 17 days. Thirteen of these 15 had total or significant clearing after removal of the dental mercury. Mercury was positive in only 7 of the other 116 patients, suggesting that other oral lesions or symptoms are less likely to be related to dental metals. Gold allergy was found in 17 patients, and in 2 the gold was removed with lesional resolution. Palladium was positive in 19 patients and 8 controls with uncertain relevance. Biopsies from patch test reactions frequently showed lichenoid histology.

Scalf and colleagues[29] patch tested 51 patients with LP or "lichenoid reactions" to 12 metal allergens (Table 33.2). Twenty-five (49%) reacted to one or more mercury allergens and 38 (74.5%) reacted to at least one metal. Thirty-four patients had oral disease, with or without cutaneous or genital disease. All groupings, e.g., cutaneous disease only, cutaneous plus genital disease, oral plus genital, etc. gave positive patch-test rates of 75–80%. Nine of the patients with metal allergy decided to have the metals removed and all (100%) experienced complete clearing or significant improvement. In contrast, only

Table 33-2 Metal Patch Test Findings in 51 Patients with Oral Lichen Planus

Metal Allergen	Positive (Percent)	NACDG 1998 Positive	P-value
Mercury (thimerosal 0.1% pet, mercury 0.5% pet, or phenylmercuric acetate 0.05% pet	25 (49%)	10.9%	0.005
Gold sodium thiosulfate 0.5% pet	10 (19.6%)	9.5%	0.041
Palladium chloride 1% pet	9 (17.7%)	NT	
Nickel sulfate hexahydrate 2.5% pet	8 (15.7%)	14.2%	0.896
Cobalt chloride5% pet	8 (15.7%)	9.0%	0.169
Potassium dichromate 0.25% pet	5 (9.8%)	2.8%	0.028
Copper sulfate 2% pet	2 (3.9%)	NT	
Indium (III)sulfate 10.0% aq	2 (3.9%)	NT	
Iridium (III) chloride hydrate 1.0% aq	2 (3.9%)	NT	
Silver nitrate 1% aq	2 (3.9%)	NT	

From reference #29

62.5 % of those who did not replace dental metals showed improvement one year later.

Yiannias and colleagues[30] found that 25 of 46 patients (54%) with oral LP had positive patch tests. They tested with a variety of metals and other allergens (not including indium and iridium). Seventeen reacted to at least one metal, with gold the most common (14 patients). Only 3 reacted to mercury, 3 to silver and 4 to nickel.

These authors also noted one patient with allergy to acrylics in a dental retainer and 6 patients with relevant reactions to flavorings such as cinnamic aldehyde or MP.

Laeijendecker and colleagues[31] looked at 20 patients with oral LP adjacent to amalgam dental fillings, 20 with adjacent and spreading lesions, 20 with oral lesions elsewhere in the mouth, and 20 controls with ACD but not LP. Thirteen, 8, and 2 respectively reacted to one or more mercury allergens. None of the controls were positive. Sixteen of the twenty-one in the first two groups had complete healing with removal of the amalgam and the other 5 were improved. Of the two in the non-adjacent group one was improved and one unchanged.

From Israel, a report of 103 patients with various oral symptoms and or cheilitis found the following patch test positives: gold 17 (14%), nickel 13, mercury 11, palladium 7 and cobalt 6. Also 5 were allergic to hydroxyethyl methacrylate.[32]

Marcusson[33] tested 397 patients presenting to a patch test clinic with oral symptoms that were not specified in his report. The complaints, however, seemed to be temporally related to dental work. Twenty-three percent were positive to gold, a much higher rate than the 4% to 9% seen in most patch testing centers. Twenty-two percent were allergic to nickel, which is somewhat more than expected. Cobalt and chromate allergies were also slightly over-represented.

Mercury

Probably the most common contact with mercury in the general population occurs from mercury amalgam dental fillings. The possibility of toxicity from dental mercury has been a popular topic for debate. Essentially there are questions relating to putative mercury sensitivity: (a) Can dental mercury cause oral lesions, including lichenoid lesions? (b) Can dental mercury cause cutaneous urticaria, dermatitis, or LP in sensitive individuals? and (c) Can dental mercury cause nonspecific systemic complaints such as fatigue, malaise, and headache?

Generally, older reports suggested that mercury is unlikely to cause oral lesions, whereas virtually all recent literature, as noted above, implicates mercury (and other metals) as possible causes of stomatitis and LP.

Epstein[34] stated that the contact antigen formed with mercury is given specificity for the epidermis by protein conjugates characteristic of, or present only in, the epidermis, and that mercury sensitivity does not extend to the oral mucosa.

However, Fernstreom and colleagues[35] stated that patients who had previously been sensitized to mercury and had acquired a mercury dermatitis subsequently developed a stomatitis and a flare-up of the dermatitis when mercury amalgam fillings were used. These patients had a prompt remission when their mercury amalgam fillings were removed. Such flare-ups were attributed to mercury vapor, which is liberated by the amalgam fillings, both when the amalgam is being prepared and during insertion into the cavity. The authors consider the amount liberated from the filling after treatment to be negligible in comparison to the amount liberated while the filling is being inserted.

Cutaneous Reactions to Dental Mercury Gaul[36] reported on three patients with mercury dermatitis in whom epidermal sensitivity to mercury was demonstrated. In all three patients, however, silver amalgam dental fillings, containing approximately 50% metallic mercury, produced no irritation within the mouth.

Johnson and colleagues[37] found that the removal of mercury amalgam fillings cleared recalcitrant eczemas in mercury-sensitive individuals. Sidi and Casalis[38] described mercury-sensitive patients with chronic eczema that persisted until amalgam fillings were removed. Vickers[39] reported on a mercury-sensitive individual who developed a widespread, eczematous eruption, starting 24 to 48 hours after a mercury amalgam filling had been inserted. No oral lesions were described. Vickers speculated that the generalized dermatitis was due to mercury dropped on the mucosal surface of the mouth during the dental operation.

Spector[40] described a patient in whom there was a sudden appearance of extensive edema and urticaria involving the neck, face, and upper part of the back following installation of an amalgam filling. This reaction recurred on two occasions when the patient underwent dental treatment with silver amalgam. The eruption persisted for 7 to 10 days, then disappeared spontaneously without removal of the filling. Spector performed patch tests with the silver alloy alone, the mercury alone, and a combination of both. The patient had no reaction to the silver alloy alone. When the mercury alone or the combination was tested, the patient developed severe local erythema at the test site, with vesiculation, edema, and urticarial reactions on the elbows and neck. The author concluded that this was a rare instance of mercury sensitivity manifested by urticaria, edema, and a vesiculation.

Thomson and Russel[41] described a patient who, on several occasions after mercury amalgam dental restorations, developed first an urticarial and then an eczematous eruption on her face, trunk, and extremities. She had previously developed an eczematous eruption on the lower part of the abdomen and thighs and a vaginitis from the use of a contraceptive jelly containing a phenylmercuric salt. Patch tests were positive to 0.1% mercuric-chloride and silver amalgam. The dermatitis on each occasion lasted 10 to 14 days, then subsided, although the mercury amalgam fillings were not removed.

Frykholm[42] tried to determine whether exposure to mercury in amalgam restorations can be deleterious to health. First, he tried to measure the amount of mercury that escaped from the amalgam and the amount that was absorbed. Second, he endeavored to measure the quantity of mercury excreted in the urine and feces. He found that the average amount of mercury per millimeter of respired air in 30 minutes of treatment was 0.02 mg to 0.4 mg but that the upper values occurred only if copper amalgam was used. If the fillings were coated with saliva, the amount of vapor evolved was instantly reduced. His experiments on the solubility of mercury amalgam fillings in saliva and gastric juice showed that the freshly triturated amalgam was only slightly soluble. The amount of mercury reaching the circulation appeared to be insignificant. He concluded that amalgam restoration treatment exposes the patients to a small quantity of mercury mainly during insertion and that reports of reactions after amalgam restorations, even in mercury-sensitive persons, are uncommon, and the few cases reported usually involved a history of allergic contact to mercury.

In the cases discussed above, the usual time of onset of eczema or urticaria in mercury-sensitive patients is a few hours after an amalgam filling has been inserted. The eruption usually persists for 10 to 14 days, which fits well into Frykholm's work on mercury liberation after amalgam insertion.

The answers to the questions posed above would, at this time with current information, seem to be as follows. Mercury and other metal may produce oral lesions, including lichen planus–like lesions, at sites of mucosal contact. Generalized skin reactions and lesions elsewhere in the mouth are rarely related to dental metals but may occur.

Patch testing for mercury allergy Patch testing with mercury and its salts is somewhat tricky because irritant reactions may occur. Von Mayenburg and colleagues43 found that 13 of 27 patients with reactions to mercury salts also reacted to 20% amalgam in petrolatum. The amalgam contained 51% mercury, 34% silver, with the remainder being tin, zinc, and copper. Ten of the 13

reacted down to 5% amalgam in petrolatum. The authors suggested using a 5% or 10% concentration for testing. It should be remembered that mercury may react with aluminum in Finn chambers. Whether this is of clinical significance is unknown. If desired, plastic chambers may be used instead.

Patch testing with mercury of a patient with nonspecific symptoms without oral or cutaneous findings may be unreliable and lead to invalid conclusion due to the frequency of irritant and allergic reactions seen in healthy individuals. However, patch testing in patients with unexplained oral LP is definitely indicated.

Nickel

Foussereau and Laugier[44] cited a case of generalized eczema that occurred after a chromium-nickel denture had been fitted. Skin tests were strongly positive to nickel and chromium, and the dermatitis subsided after the denture was removed. No mention is made of oral reactions.

Van Loon and colleagues[45] showed that nickel in the mouth can produce allergic stomatitis in patients who exhibit positive nickel patch tests. Five such patients had a small nickel plate glued to a tooth for 7 days. All five patients developed stomatitis at the site, which showed histologic features of an allergic reaction on biopsy.

Allergic contact stomatitis and cheilitis can occur from nickel-plated instruments used in dental procedures.[46] Many nickel-sensitive individuals have acquired allergic stomatitis and cheilitis by holding between the lips nickel-plated objects, such as needles, pins, bobby pins, and metal lipstick holders.[47] Perlèche may be clearly simulated in nickel-sensitive individuals who hold nickel-plated coins, keys, and other objects at the corners of their mouths. One patient developed erosions of the gums resembling aphthous ulcers from holding metal bobby pins between the teeth.[48]

Gold

As noted above, gold allergy has been linked to oral LP fairly commonly. Gold is becoming recognized as a more common allergen than was previously appreciated.

Elgart and Higdon[49] described a case of allergic sensitivity to gold in which the gingival mucosa sloughed from contact with a gold crown and sites of previous gold contact dermatitis to jewelry flared. The cutaneous lesions subsided when the crown was removed.

Schaffran and colleagues[50] pointed out that individuals with gold dental work and no oral symptoms at all are often patch test positive to gold. Of those with gold in the mouth, 34% were positive, whereas only 11% without dental gold were positive.

Moller reviewed dental gold issues several years ago.[51] He correctly points out that the mere presence of a positive gold patch test does not guarantee that oral signs and symptoms are due to gold allergy. The mere fact of having gold dental work, seems to predispose to gold allergy even in the absence of clinical symptoms. Release of gold into saliva, however, has been demonstrated and blood levels are correlated with the amount of gold in the mouth.

Chrome-Cobalt Combination

Brendlinger and Tarsitano[52] described a woman with severe dermatitis and allergic reactions to several metals who recovered only after removal of a cast chrome-cobalt partial denture. Replacement with an all-acrylic resin partial denture was satisfactory.

Chrome-cobalt pins used to fasten porcelain teeth to acrylic dentures may produce stomatitis in individuals sensitized to cobalt. In a case observed by Fisher, such pins produced an extensive stomatitis and cheilitis in a cobalt-nickel-sensitized individual. The reaction occurred after the acrylic portion of the denture had worn away, exposing the pins. When the pins were covered with self-curing acrylic resin, the stomatitis cleared.

Ovrutsky and Ulyanov[53] and Moffa and colleagues[54] reported generalized and eczematous reactions from such chromium-containing dental casting alloys.

Platinum and Palladium

Sheard[55] stated that both metallic platinum and its salts are potent allergens and that reactions to dentists' platinum wiring may be allergic.

Palladium is becoming well recognized as an allergen usually in combination with nickel sensitivity.[56] It is used in dental alloys and therefore may be expected to cause stomatitis occasionally. However, three patients with a positive patch test to palladium chloride (2.5% aq) did not show any reactions to a palladium metal plate placed in the mouth for 7 days.[45] Perhaps a longer duration of exposure is needed for the palladium ions to be released.

A case of linear facial LP with a "peculiar sensation" in the mouth was caused by allergy to palladium. Patch tests were positive to both palladium and platinum. Removal of the palladium-containing dental work resulted in total resolution of symptoms.[57] A case of combined palladium and platinum allergy causing lichenoid stomatitis was reported from Germany.[58]

Beryllium

Beryllium has also been reported to cause two cases of allergic stomatitis.[59] The alloy rexillium was used in making dental prostheses.

Because of the high cost of gold, a number of base metal alloys may be substituted. Two major types of base metal alloys are available: a high nickel type (70% to 84% Ni) and a nickel-free type based in cobalt and chromium. Some of these alloys contain beryllium.

ALLERGIC AND IRRITANT STOMATITIS FROM OTHER MATERIALS

Corticosteroids

Allergy to topical corticosteroids is more common than has been previously appreciated. Tixocortol pivalate is a good patch test marker for hydrocortisone hypersensitivity. In a report from Switzerland, three women were allergic to tixocortol in a nasal spray, and one also had stomatitis from an oral lozenge containing the drug.[60]

Dental Impression Compounds

These preparations may contain stearin, stearic acid, paraffin wax, beeswax, and gutta-percha with synthetic or natural resins, such as shellac copak (kauri), coumarone-indene resins, and fillers. Of these ingredients, the resin is most likely to cause allergic stomatitis.

Some of the fluxes contain borax, boric acid, silica, and potassium fluoride. Most fluxes are strong irritants. Waxes such as paraffin, beeswax, carnauba, candelilla, and petrolatum are used by dentists. Several types of plaster containing mineral gypsum, potassium sulfate, potash alum, and alizarin S are used.

Van Groeningen and Nater[61] reported that of approximately 2,000 persons treated with Scutan, an epimine plastic for temporary crowns and bridges, and Impregum, a polyether impression material, a total of 10 patients complained of untoward reactions. Patch tests with the basic materials were performed on 4 of the 10 patients. Positive allergic reactions were obtained to patch tests with the catalyst methyl-*p*-toluene sulfonate 0.1% in dibenzyltoluol present in Scutan, and the catalyst methyldichlorobenzene sulfonate 0.1% in dibenzyltoluol present in Impregum. Four control subjects did not react to these concentrations.

Scutan, the temporary dental splint material, contains no monomers and is not an acrylic derivative. Impregum is an impression rubber material used for the construction of inlays, crowns, and bridges. It is usually in contact with the oral mucosa for only a short period.

Resinous Substances Used in Dentistry

ACD and urticaria from dental resin-based products are considered rare.[62] However, it is often difficult to assess which materials are present in a patient's mouth. Very little is known about how components released from dental restorations act as sensitizers or cause dermatologic sequelae in presensitized individuals.

MP, a balsamic resin of plant origin, is a component of some cement liquids. Copal is another resin of plant origin and is a constituent of some cavity varnishes. This resin should not be confused with Copalite, which is a synthetic resin. Mastic is composed principally of masticinic acid and used in some cavity varnishes. Also called colophony, rosin is an ingredient of many mixtures used for sealing pulp canals. Rosin in chloroform solution has been used as a varnish for pulp protection in deep cavities. It has been added to zinc oxide or to eugenol as an ingredient of pulp capping preparations, surgical packs, impression pastes, and other preparations.[63]

Resins: Epoxy and Acrylate Hensten-Pettersen[64] reported in 1981 that, over the previous 15 years, more than 100 similar new brands of resin-based cold-curing materials had been introduced. Methyl methacrylate and other acrylic resin-based composite materials, pit and fissure sealants, orthodontic adhesives, glazes, veneers and repair kits for porcelain-fused-to-metal restorations, root canal sealers, and temporary crowns are now commonly used in dentistry and occasionally cause allergy.

Depending on the composition, the polymerization is induced by chemical agents or ultraviolet or visible light sources. The materials are based on monomers of different types: methacrylate monomers and urethane-based-dimethacrylates, epoxybisphenо resins, and ethylene-amino derivatives.

In addition, the chemicals involved in the polymerization processes are present: benzoyl peroxide, hydroquinone, camphoroquinone, phthalates, tertiary aromatic and aliphatic amines, benzoin ethers, ultraviolet stabilizers, and antioxidants and their derivatives.[65] Even though the materials set to a hard state in the oral environment, the amount of residual unreacted endgroups of dimethyl acrylates may vary from 15% to 50%, leading to a slow release of degradation products such as formaldehyde.[66]

One case of oral lichen planus documented by biopsy was thought to be caused by resin that was exposed to the mucosa from a broken denture.[63] Removal of the material cleared the eruption.

In the United States, an epoxy-acrylate resin system is generally used for most bonding. "Bis" stands for the epoxy resin bisphenol A, which reacts with glycidyl methacrylate. Thompson and colleagues[67] studied the unpolymerized material extracted from cured orthodontic bonding resin, which was analyzed by ultraviolet spectrophotometry. Under certain conditions, substantial amounts of the material (approximately 14%) were leached from bracketed teeth. Significant amounts of unpolymerized material remaining in cured orthodontic bonding resins can be readily leached out by various aqueous solutions, such as saliva, water, soda water, and ethanol solutions.

Acrylic Denture Materials

Most dentures today are processed from acrylic resins that are heat cured. Self-curing acrylics that harden without heat are available for repairing and relining. Heat-cured acrylic dentures cause occasional allergic reactions.[68]

The acrylic monomer usually contains an inhibitor or stabilizer, such as hydroquinone, and the polymer, an initiator or catalyst, such as benzoyl peroxide or dimethyl-*p*-toluidine (or a tertiary amine). When the monomer and polymer are mixed in the cold, the benzoyl peroxide initiates the reaction and a hard, solid, high-molecular-weight polymer is produced. The mixture can also be heat cured, when no initiator is required. In the heat process the reaction is essentially complete, but after cold cure it is likely that very small amounts of the monomer will be left unpolymerized. This residual monomer is capable of inducing stomatitis and angular cheilitis in sensitized individuals.

Certain additives in acrylic denture material may also be sensitizers. Thus, hydroquinone, the inhibitor in the monomer, may be the sensitizer rather than the acrylic monomer itself. Benzoxyl peroxide may account for some instances of methacrylate sensitivity.

Crissey[69] cited four instances in which allergic stomatitis resulted from heat-cured acrylic dentures. The onset of symptoms followed fitting of the acrylic dentures by periods varying from 1 week to 4 years. These cases had the following features in common: (a) the clinical picture of stomatitis, including angular stomatitis; (b) relief of symptoms when the dentures were removed, and subsequent flare-up on reinsertion; (c) positive patch test reactions (cheek) to filings from the heat-cured acrylic prostheses and the acrylic monomer; and (d) negative patch test reactions to polystyrene denture material.

Both dental personnel and their patients are at risk for ACD due to acrylates in dentures. Thirty patients and 18 dental workers reacted to acrylates in one report.[70] all but one reacted to 2-hydroxyethyl methacrylate (2% pet). The other reacted to bis-GMA (2% pet). A variety of other acrylates were positive as well, but these two alone would have screened for 100% of identified allergy in these patients.

In a report from India, two patients with oral lesions reacted to triethyleneglycol dimethacrylate.[71]

Acrylic dentures may also contain plasticizers (dibutyl or dimethyl phthalate), pigments (mercuric sulfate, ferric oxide, carbon black, and selenium compounds), and cross-linking agents (glycol dimethyl acrylate and divinyl benzene) to prevent crazing, and an inhibitor, such as hydroquinone.

Tosti and colleagues[72] reported one case of contact stomatitis in a 62-year-old woman traced to *N,N*-dimethyl-para-toluidine used as an accelerator for the acrylic reaction.

Hydroquinone, used to stabilize acrylic monomer, caused cheilitis and stomatitis in one patient who was also allergic to several metals.[73] Van Joost and colleagues[74] reported four denture reactors. One person reacted to methyl methacrylate, one to bisphenol A, and two to a product called Lurene, in which the allergen was not identified.

Patients may complain of a burning sensation for several hours after first use of an acrylic denture that has been relined or repaired. Such complaints may be related to the presence of solvents such as ethyl or amyl acetate, diethyl carbonate, and glycerol triacetate.

NONALLERGIC CAUSES OF DENTURE STOMATITIS

Inflammation of the mucous membrane beneath artificial dentures is often referred to as "denture-sore mouth." The oral mucosa of the palate and the maxillary edentulous alveolar ridges are the most common sites of involvement. The tissue beneath the denture may appear bright red and edematous, and the patient may complain of soreness, rawness, dryness, and burning sensations in the area in contact with the denture. Occasionally perlèche may be the only sign of denture stomatitis. Usually these reactions are irritant in nature due to poor-fitting dentures or trapped food particles.[75]

Wakkers-Garritsen and colleagues[76] stated that it is remarkable that the denture-sore mouth (DSM) syndrome appears to occur mainly in women patients. In their group of 24 persons, 19 were women. The DSM complaints generally started between ages 40 and 60 years; the mean age was 49 years. In most cases, complaints commenced with the first prosthesis. Using other prostheses from different materials made no appreciable difference; in one case, seven successive dentures were made of different compounds without any real improvement.

These data, combined with the fact that in 12 of 24 cases complaints started within 1 hour of mucosal contact, suggest a nonallergic cause of the complaints. This is supported by the negative results of the patch test reactions. Mechanical factors are difficult to assess. In many cases, however, patients stated that the fitting of their dentures was correct, a fact that was confirmed by functional analysis. Evidence of heat accumulation beneath the dental plates in patients complaining of DSM could not be detected. Finally, the investigators could not confirm the suggested causal role of *Candida albicans* or related yeasts. These investigators had an impression that all patients included in this investigation were very tense and nervous. Further studies to elicit these psychologic factors are necessary.

Traumatic Suction Effect of Ill-Fitting Dentures

Nonallergic denture-sore mouth caused by trauma is quite common. Traumatic denture-sore mouth produces an erythematous, "cluster of grapes" appearance owing to a suction effect produced by the rocking back and forth of ill-fitting dentures. When a denture is constructed, a depression is created in this area to prevent "denture rock." This depression causes a suction effect.

Dry Mouth Syndrome

Klein[77] stated that "dry mouth syndrome" is one of the most prevalent complaints after age 65. This is one of the factors contributing to the increase in dental caries, inability to wear dentures, burning sensation in the mouth, and decreased sensitivity of the taste buds of many individuals in this age group. The source of this problem is diminution of salivary flow caused by acinar destruction and hyalinization, adhesions and obstructions with atrophy of salivary ducts, and infection or disease within the stoma of the glands themselves. Not every individual develops this condition, and many aged patients have adequate salivary flow well into the 80s or even beyond. Sjögren's syndrome, tumors of the salivary glands, and diabetes may also cause dry mouth syndrome.

Role of Candidiasis in Denture Stomatitis

Denture stomatitis may be caused by oral candidiasis and, like acute atrophic candidiasis, is a red rather than a white lesion. It occurs as a uniform or patchy atrophic erythematous lesion, almost exclusively limited to the palate of denture wearers. It is usually, but not always, seen under dentures that are worn 24 hours a day. It is generally described as sore or burning rather than painful and occurs more commonly in women than men. Two predisposing factors stand out; the space between denture and palate can be regarded as an ideal culture chamber and the denture acts in the manner of an occlusive dressing, keeping any organisms on its surface in close contact with the mucosa.

Taaffe and Rigott[78] found that *Candida* occurred more commonly in the oral mucosa of denture-wearing patients than in the control subjects. There was no evidence of increased prevalence of *Candida* at other mucocutaneous sites, and the amount of *Candida* recovered from the stools did not suggest involvement at other sites in the alimentary system.

A large proportion of patients with this condition also have angular cheilitis (perlèche), similarly infected with

C. albicans. The dentures are often implicated in that their shape and dimensions allow deep creasing or folding at the angles of the mouth. These creases are continually moist with saliva because they form a capillary channel between the inside of the mouth and the facial skin. In patients without dentures, similar changes may occur with aging and subsequent overlap of the upper lip.

Treatment involves soaking the dentures in an antiseptic solution at night, and perhaps construction of new dentures. Oral mycostatin suspensions or troches containing clotrimazole are also helpful. Systemic agents such as fluconazole may be useful as well.

ANTISEPTICS AND PRESERVATIVES IN ORAL MEDICATIONS AND FOODS

Certain antiseptics that are added to dentifrices, mouthwashes, and topical oral medications and anesthetics to retard or prevent microbial growth have been shown to be sensitizers. Such chemicals include parahydroxybenzoic acid (parabens), dichlorophene (G-4), hexachlorophene (G-11), phenylmercuric nitrate, Merthiolate, ethylenediamine hydrochloride, the quaternary ammonium compounds, benzoic gum, and benzyl benzoate.

Parabens

Parabens are bacteriostatic, fungistatic, and antioxidant in their action and are widely employed as preservatives (see Chapter 16).

The US Food and Drug Administration requires that the labels on foods and topical prescription drugs indicate the presence of parabens. This requirement does not apply to oral preparations and dentifrices. Sensitive patients may therefore find it difficult to avoid contact with these agents. Parabens in dentifrices may produce cheilitis and circumoral dermatitis. Fortunately, even paraben-sensitive individuals usually tolerate paraben-containing oral medications, provided the mucosa is intact.

Dichlorophene (G-4) and Hexachlorophene (G-11)

According to Fisher in previous editions of this text, dichlorophene in dentifrices has caused allergic cheilitis. Patients have become sensitized to this preservative and have developed stomatitis with a cherry-red tongue and loss of taste and numbness. The lips become dry and scaly, and fissuring at the corners of the mouth suggests vitamin B deficiency. Hexachlorophene, in contrast, has almost never produced allergic sensitivity.

Formaldehyde

This chemical, present in Thermodent dentifrice and in desensitizing agents and used in root canal therapy as formocresol, may produce allergic stomatitis. Fowler has seen a case of hand eczema in a dental office worker due to formocresol (J. Fowler, Louisville, KY, 1998).

Sodium Perborate

This oxidizing agent is an occasional sensitizer. In the United States, sodium perborate sensitivity is rare. Sodium perborate is present in Kleenite, a denture cleansing preparation.

Quaternary Ammonium Compounds

The members of this chemical family, which includes benzalkonium chloride (Zephiran) and benzethonium chloride (Phemerol), are rare sensitizers, but not uncommonly produce irritant reactions.

Merthiolate and Phenylmercuric Nitrate

Merthiolate contains not only a mercurial component but also thiosalicylic acid. Allergic stomatitis and cheilitis may occur in sensitized individuals. Mercury in dental fillings is more often a cause of stomatitis.

Gallates

The gallates (octyl, propyl, and lauryl or dodecyl) are used as preservatives in foods and cosmetics, especially ones containing fats or oils. Cheilitis and stomatitis occasionally have been reported to these agents.[79] In one case, a 6-year-old boy had recurrent lip swelling for 1 year due to lauryl gallate in margarine.[80]

BHA

Butylated hydroxyanisole (BHA) caused lip swelling in a woman.[81] Food challenge test was positive.

ETHYLENEDIAMINE HYDROCHLORIDE

This stabilizer, present in Mycolog cream, has produced many instances of allergic cheilitis and circumoral dermatitis. Flare-ups of the cheilitis may be produced by the administration of aminophyllin, which contains ethylene diamine hydrochloride as one of its ingredients. In addition, flare-ups may be produced by the administration of such antihistamines as Pyribenzamine and hydroxyzine, which are ethylenediamine derivatives (see Chapter 16).

ANTISEPTICS USED IN DENTAL SURGERY

Maurice and colleagues[81] reported severe allergic contact stomatitis and dermatitis around the mouth from iodoform in a ribbon gauze known as BIPP used in packing a dental socket. Systemic iodine toxicity has occurred using this gauze in large cavities.

The sensitizing and irritant phenolic compounds used in root canal work and periapical infections include creosote and the parachlorophenols. Thymol and hexyl-resorcinol may produce crossreactions with resorcin.

Merk and colleagues[82] reported allergic contact stomatitis from hexetidine in a gargle.

Penicillin

Contact sensitivity has been widely reported after use of topical oral penicillin preparations, such as troches. Severe anaphylactoid reactions have occurred in penicillin-sensitive individuals after the endodontic use of a paste containing penicillin, bacitracin, dihydrostreptomycin, and sodium caprylate.[83]

Tetracyclines

Undesirable oral mucosal reactions have been noted from the use of lozenges containing tetracycline, and patients being treated systemically and topically with this antibiotic may develop a transitory yellowish brown discoloration of the tongue, which is not allergic in nature.

Allergic mucosal reaction to antibiotic-containing lozenges may be due to the antibiotic or coloring or flavoring agents.

Eczematous eruptions of the fixed type do occasionally result from systemic administration of tetracyclines.[84] Furthermore, cross-fixed drug reactions from systemic use of Aureomycin, Achromycin, and Terramycin have been described.[85] Such reactions may produce erosions of the mouth and lips.

REACTIONS TO LOZENGES AND TROCHES

These preparations may contain antibiotics, quaternary ammonium compounds, local anesthetics (particularly benzocaine), hexylresorcinol, iodine compounds, flavoring agents, or tyrothricin. Allergic reactions to antibiotic-containing lozenges may be due to the antibiotic or to the coloring or flavoring agents.

When an oral topical medication is suspected of producing allergic contact stomatitis, testing must be performed with all the individual ingredients in the preparation, regardless of whether they are active or inert. Inert flavoring and coloring agents and preservatives are just as important causes of allergic contact stomatitis and cheilitis as are the active antiseptic or anesthetic chemicals present in the lozenges and troches.

TOPICAL ANESTHETICS AS MUCOSAL SENSITIZERS WITH SPECIAL REFERENCE TO BENZOCAINE

Benzocaine, a common sensitizer, continues to be used in many topical anesthetic compounds.

Such preparations are often used as mouthwash or gargle in the treatment of aphthous stomatitis, "teething pains," herpes simplex, denture irritation, trench mouth, cheilosis, avitaminosis, thrush, gingivitis, and throat irritations.

The topical administration of anesthetic aerosol sprays can produce in benzocaine-sensitive individuals a shock-like syndrome. Lidocaine (Xylocaine), mepivacaine (Carbocaine), or dyclonine hydrochloride (Dyclone) usually can be safely substituted in benzocaine-sensitive patients when surface anesthesia is required, although allergy to these agents occurs occasionally as well.

Benzocaine-sensitive patients may show crossreactions with the ester group of local anesthetics that are derived from para-aminobenzoic acid: procaine (Novocain), butethamine (Monocaine), tetracaine (Pontocaine), and propoxycaine (Ravocaine). Metabutethamine (Unacaine), which is based on meta-aminobenzoic acid, meprylcaine (Oracaine), and isobucaine (Kincaine), which is based on benzoic acid, may also cause cross-reactions with benzocaine.

The injection of these local anesthetics into benzocaine-sensitive individuals may lead to localized swelling of the oral mucosa at the site of injection. On rare occasions, generalized urticaria or anaphylaxis will result from the injection of procaine into benzocaine-sensitive patients.

The following injectable local anesthetics rarely crossreact with benzocaine and, because they are based on an "amide" structure, are usually safely used in benzocaine-sensitive patients: lidocaine (Xylocaine), mepivacaine (Carbocaine), prilocaine (Citanest), and pyrrocaine (Dynacaine). Patch testing with the individual allergens should be performed, however, even though crossreactivity is rare.

It should be emphasized that patch tests with local anesthetics may not reveal the immediate, urticarial, or anaphylactic type of reaction. Scratch or intradermal testing may be helpful in this regard.

INGREDIENTS OF DENTIFRICES AND MOUTHWASHES

In 1995, Sainio and Kanerva[86] published a list of 48 toothpastes then on the Finnish market, many of which are also available in the United States. About 50% contained one or more allergens, such as peppermint oil, parabens, other flavors, and other preservatives.

Most powder and paste dentifrices contain flavoring, coloring agents (certified dyes), abrasives, and soaps or synthetic detergents, particularly "foaming" alkyl sulfates or sarcosinates. In addition, toothpastes may contain glycerine, propylene glycol, sorbital solution, alcohol, and thickeners, such as tragacanth, alginate, carrageen (Irish moss), and cellulose derivatives. Some dentifrices include antiseptics, preservatives, fluorides, and ammonium compounds. Saccharin and the cyclamates may be added.[87,88]

Mouthwashes are medicated liquids used for cleansing the mouth for therapeutic or cosmetic purposes and, like dentifrices, may contain alcohol, flavorings, antiseptics, and preservatives The alkyl sulfates, sarcosinates, and sulfonates are synthetic "foaming" detergents. So-called antienzyme dentifrices may contain these surfactants, which are claimed to prevent transformation of sugar to acid in the oral cavity. These surface-active agents very rarely produce allergic reactions.

Sims[89] claimed that antienzyme dentifrices may produce ulcerative lesions of the oral mucosa and sore tongue in patients with allergic sensitivity to the antienzyme. Sodium lauryl sarcosinate, a foaming, surface-active agent in some dentifrices, has been claimed to act as an antienzyme. Allergic reactions to this agent have not been proved.

The abrasives in dentifrices (e.g., chalk, calcium carbonate, bentonite, pumice, hydrated aluminum, calcium phosphate, zinc oxide, sodium chloride, sodium bicarbonate, and the magnesium salts) are very rare sensitizers. The quaternary ammonium compounds are very rare sensitizers. The preservatives, essential oils, formalin, flavorings, antiseptics, antibiotic agents, and alcohol are more common sensitizers. Rarely do coloring agents cause allergy.

If not properly diluted, many mouthwashes may produce an irritant stomatitis from the presence of such antiseptics and astringents as sodium perborate, zinc chloride, borax, menthol, thymol, phenol, iodine, methyl salicylate, alcohol, boric acid, creosols, surfactants, and flavors.

The fluorides are very rare sensitizers[90,91] but frequently produce nonspecific nonallergenic pustular patch test reactions.[92] Virtually all mass-marketed toothpastes produced in the United States now contain fluoride.

Saunders[93] claimed that fluoride toothpastes can produce circumoral dermatitis.

There is one report of a possible urticarial reaction to a fluoride dental treatment solution in an atopic child.[94]

ULCERS CAUSED BY CONTACT ALLERGENS

On rare occasions, contact of the sensitized patient's oral mucosa with the specific allergen may produce erosions or ulcers rather than a diffuse stomatitis. Such lesions may be indistinguishable from aphthous ulcers or erosive lichen planus.[95]

Sugarman[96] cited a case of hypersensitivity to a mint chewing gum in which the lesions were characterized by an aphthous-appearing ulcer.

Cancellieri[97] listed contact sensitivity to dentifrices, teeth whiteners, mouth purifiers, chewing gum, drugs, food, acrylic resin liquid, and monomers in dentures as capable of producing chronic aphthous ulcers. Fisher[25] observed nickel-sensitive women with ulcers of the lips and oral mucosa caused by the holding of nickel-plated objects, such as bobby pins or hair clips, in their mouths. Fregert and colleagues[98] studied a patient with allergic hypersensitivity to alcohol, as shown by positive patch test reactions, who developed a burning sensation, erythema, and aphthae of the oral mucosa whenever she ingested alcoholic beverages.

DENTAL BRACES AND NICKEL ALLERGY

A large, population-based Danish study showed that the prevalence of nickel allergy was significantly reduced in adolescents who had received dental braces prior to body piercing.[9] This suggests that a low level of systemic nickel intake, from the braces, acted to tolerize the children and protect against subsequent sensitization. However, the reverse is not true, so that an already sensitized person may sometimes develop oral or lip or even systemic symptoms after applicati0on of nickel braces. Other Danish investigators have shown that stainless steel braces release measurable nickel into artificial saliva.[99]

Cheilitis and Perlèche

The vermilion border of the lips has a modified epithelium, which is more likely to develop allergic contact sensitivity reactions than is the oral mucosa. Allergens in contact with both the oral mucosa and the lips may produce only cheilitis.

An angular cheilitis may be the only manifestation of allergic hypersensitivity to denture materials and dental fillings,. Allergic cheilitis may first manifest itself merely with dryness and fissuring. Edema and crusting may supervene from contact with strong allergens over a prolonged period. Allergic contact cheilitis may result from contact with allergens in dental preparations and oral care products; topical agents directly applied to the lips, such as antichap agents, lipsticks, and sunscreens; foods and flavorings; and allergens transported by touching the lips, such as nail polish, metals in jewelry, or other contactants. Because the hands are relatively resistant, cheilitis or facial dermatitis may occur in the absence of hand dermatitis.

Freeman and Stevens[100] retrospectively analyzed 75 cases of cheilitis seen in a contact dermatitis clinic. Irritant cheilitis was diagnosed in 36%, mostly attributed to

Table 33-3 NACDG Clinically Relevant Patch Test Results for Cheilitis

Allergen	% of Patients with ACC
Fragrance mix 8% pet	30.0
Myroxylon pereirae (balsam of Peru) 25% pet	23.3
Nickel sulfate 2.5% pet	21.7
Sodium gold thiosulfate 0.5% pet	13.3
Neomycin sulfate 20% pet	11.7
Cobalt chloride 1% pet	10.0
Propylene glycol 30% aq	8.3
Lanolin alcohol 30% pet	6.7
Cinnamic aldehyde 1% pet	6.7
Bacitracin 20% pet	5.0
Benzophenone-3 3% pet	5.0
Methyldibromoglutaronitrile/phenoxyethanol 2% pet	5.0%
Tea tree oil, oxidized 5% pet	5.0%
Budesonide 0.01% pet	5.0%
Mercaptobenzothiazole 1% pet	3.3%
Formaldehyde 1% aq	3.3%
Potassium dichromate 0.25% pet	3.3%
Tosylamide formaldehyde resin 10% pet	3.3

chronic lip licking. Allergy was found in 25%. Common allergens included fragrances and flavorings, preservatives, lanolin, oxybenzone, and colophony. Sunscreens, lipsticks, toothpastes, medicaments, and cosmetics were causative, along with one case of nickel allergy in a flutist. Atopic dermatitis was found in 9%. Women accounted for two-thirds of the cases, and the ages ranged from 9 to 79 years.

Similarly, Zug and colleagues presented data from the NACDG on cheilitis.[101] In a 4-year period, 196 patients (out of 10,061 total) who were patch tested had a diagnosis of lip dermatitis, without involvement elsewhere. Women accounted for 84%. Allergic contact was the final diagnosis in 75 (38%). Fragrance and flavoring allergens and nickel were the most common relevant allergens, followed by gold and neomycin (Table 33.3). Almost one-third of the patients had positive patch tests to allergens not on the NACDG screening series. Lipsticks accounted for 26% of these cases that were not identified by standard screening allergens. Other cosmetic and toiletry products, including sunscreens, accounted for most of the remaining cases.

SELECTED CAUSES OF ALLERGIC CHEILITIS AND PERLÈCHE

Cheilitis from Dentifrices

Bactericidal agents, essential oils, and preservatives in toothpastes and mouthwashes may produce allergic cheilitis.[102] Examples of these allergens are listed above.

Lipstick Cheilitis

A number of additives in lipsticks may produce allergic cheilitis. The most common are flavoring agents, sunscreens, vehicle components like lanolin and propylene glycol, and preservatives. Dyes and other components are rare allergens (see Chapter 16).

Propolis

Propolis, also known as bee glue, is a brownish resin collected by bees and used to seal their hives. Warshaw and colleagues[103] have published an extensive review. Since lip salves fairly common contain propolis, cheilitis from allergy to this material is not rare. Crossreactivity may commonly be seen with MP and the cinnamates.[104] Ingestion of propolis from lozenges, dentifrices, etc. may cause cheilitis, stomatitis and systemic ACD.[105]

Cheilitis Caused by Nail Polish and Nail Hardeners

Patients allergic to nail polish who bite their nails may develop cheilitis and perlèche. The usual sensitizer in nail polish is tosylamide-formaldehyde resin. So-called hypoallergenic nail polish contains an alkyd resin. Acrylates in artificial nails may cause cheilitis and facial dermatitis.

Huldin[106] observed three cases of hemorrhage of the lips in nail-biting patients who used nail hardeners, which contain formaldehyde. This phenomenon disappeared with discontinuation of the nail hardener and recurred when it was reused. Examination of the lips revealed many small (1 mm to 3 mm) hemorrhages in the midportion of the lips, which blended out toward the angle of the mouth. Most of these changes were noted on the vermilion border of the lower lip.

Cheilitis Caused by Foods

Klauder[107] described a patient with sensitivity to carrots who developed a cheilitis and perioral dermatitis when she ate this vegetable raw or cooked.

Patients who are sensitized to poison ivy may acquire an allergic cheilitis from eating mango, which contains a catechol related to poison ivy oleoresin.

Individuals who remove orange peels with their teeth may develop an allergic cheilitis from orange peel. The specific sensitizer is limonene, an essential oil. Mitchell and Rook[108] reported a case of cheilitis caused by the volatile oil of oranges. The volatile orange oils may produce not only cheilitis but also circumoral dermatitis and hyperpigmentation.

Lupton[109] described a persistent cheilitis caused by coffee. In this instance, the coffee also produced a positive patch test reaction on the skin.

Perlèche Caused by Nickel

Nickel-sensitive individuals who habitually place between the lips nickel-plated objects such as hairpins, bobby pins, pens, pencils, and metal lipstick holders readily develop "allergic" nickel perlèche. In several instances of "nickel" perlèche, there was sufficient nickel present in the labial commissures to give a positive reaction to dimethylglyoxime.[110]

Perlèche Caused by Rubber

Rubber-sensitive individuals who chew on rubber pencil erasers, rubber bands, and the rubber tips of toothbrushes have acquired this type of perlèche. In one instance, a rubber dam used in a dental procedure produced "allergic" perlèche. In five of six instances of "rubber" perlèche, the actual sensitizer proved to be mercaptobenzothiazole, a rubber accelerator.

Other Causes of Cheilitis or Perlèche

Allergic cheilitis has resulted from application of triamcinolone acetonide (Mycolog cream) for angular cheilitis presumably caused by monilia. In these instances, the actual sensitizer was the ethylenediamine stabilizer in the cream.[111]

The erythrosin in disclosing tablets (Xpose and Red Cote), which are used to identify dental plaque, is a photosensitizer. If the disclosing solution made with this dye contaminates the lips and is not removed, exposure to sunlight may produce a photosensitizing cheilitis. Other disclosing solutions and tablets may contain iodine or Mercurochrome.

IRRITANT PERLÈCHE AND CHEILITIS

Role of Saliva in Production of "Irritant" Perlèche

"Perlèche" (from the French word, perlècher, meaning "to lick thoroughly") is used to describe inflammatory processes occurring at the angles of the mouth.

Perlèche caused by contact irritants or sensitizers may exactly mimic the angular cheilitis resulting from monilia, riboflavin deficiency, and the split papules of secondary syphilis. Saliva plays a major role in the production of perlèche, particularly the irritant variety.[110]

The salivary enzymes such as amylase and maltase, which play a role in the digestion of food, probably are irritating when they are in contact with the skin. Other enzymes present in saliva, such as acid and alkaline phosphatase, cholinesterase, lipase, sulfatase, galactosidase, lysozyme, hyaluronidase, catalase, glycogenase, hexokinase, carbonic anhydrase, and mucinase, are no doubt also irritants when in intimate, prolonged contact with the skin.

Any process that increases the flow of saliva, which, in turn, becomes trapped at the angles of the mouth, will produce perlèche. Chewing tobacco and gum, which increases the flow of saliva, can produce an angular cheilitis. Probably the most exotic variety of "chewer's perlèche" is observed in eastern India, where betel chewing is a common practice among both men and women. The betel leaf is coated with a paste of lime and various astringents, placed in the mouth, and chewed. The constant chewing keeps the mouth full of saliva, which trickles to the labial commissures. The continuous friction and rubbing of the moist opposing surfaces at the angles of the mouth produces perlèche with maceration, erosion, and fissures.[112]

Excess salivation with drooling and moisture at the corners of the lips favors irritation and secondary infection. Those "lickers" who habitually place the tongue moistened with saliva at the corners of their mouth soon acquire perlèche.

"Pickers" who excoriate the labial fissures with their nails or other objects develop a "mechanical" form of perlèche. Irritant metabolic products formed in saliva are capable of producing irritation at the corners of the mouth. Thus, the first sign of uremic stomatitis may be an angular cheilitis that gradually extends to the entire buccal mucosa. This type of stomatitis is due to ammonia produced by the action of bacterial urease on the increased salivary urea.[113]

Saliva also plays an important role in the formation of angular cheilitis in which faulty dentition is a factor. In edentulous individuals, in those wearing ill-fitting dentures, or in elderly individuals with marked attrition of the teeth, there is a closing of the vertical dimension so that the jaws approximate one another more closely, resulting in a folding of the skin and mucosa at the angles of the lips. These folds trap saliva and moisture. The saliva accumulating in the retaining folds irritates and macerates the labial fissures, producing perlèche.

Male patients with chronic angular cheilosis often keep the lips firmly approximated when shaving because of the discomfort after cutting over the inflamed tissues. They thus maintain abrasive areas of "stubble" in the contiguous portions of skin of the upper and lower lips. Consequently, an intact epidermis cannot develop. Such patients should be instructed to shave over the infected areas with the mouth stretched wide open.

Differential Diagnosis

A careful history and proper patch tests may help clinch a diagnosis of allergic contact angular cheilitis and aid in the differential diagnosis of the following types of perlèche.

Angular stomatitis (angular cheilitis, cheilosis) is the most common and characteristic oral manifestation of riboflavin deficiency. The lesion may be unilateral or bilateral. The first visible alteration is a whitening or pallor of the mucosa of the labial commissures. As the lesions progress, there is fissuring or cracking with ulceration. Candidal perlèche is most common in diabetics, debilitated individuals, those taking antibiotics for long periods, and HIV patients. Occasionally moniliasis will complicate perlèche caused by contact allergy or some dental problems. Staphylococcal or streptococcal infections occur particularly in sick or ill-nourished children and may occur in epidemic form. Atopic and seborrheic dermatitis involving the face may be associated with angular cheilitis. Patients taking isotretinoin (Accutane and others) for acne often develop dry skin of the face with inflammation of the angles of the mouth and scaling of the lips. Thomas and colleagues[114] warned that factitious cheilitis must be distinguished from contact and actinic cheilitis on the basis of history and laboratory examination. Actinic cheilitis usually occurs with a background of obvious facial actinic damage in fair-skinned individuals. Goldman[115] cited trauma from the use of dental floss as a factor in the development of perlèche on the right side of the mouth. The patients called attention to this problem. Unwaxed dental floss applied to the bicuspids and molars rubbed against the commissure area of the lips, especially when the mouth was wide open.

Management of Perlèche

Schoenfeld and Schoenfeld[116] emphasized the following factors in the management of perlèche.

The dermatologist should take a close look at the palate. If inflammation is present, either a new denture or a relining of the old denture is probably indicated.

Drooling, nocturnal or otherwise, contributes a great deal to angular cheilitis. Indeed, without the macerating action of saliva (along with its function as a vehicle for *Candida albicans*), many cases would not occur. Anything that promotes drooling, such as sucking on a pipe, pencil, or thumb in the corner of the mouth, predisposes the patient to this condition.

Orthodontic appliances cause a temporary change in lip contour and promote salivation that together can cause drooling and subsequent cheilitis. A teenager wearing braces and taking antibiotics for acne is obviously a good candidate for the condition. Luckily, both treatments are relatively temporary, and the eventual prognosis is excellent.

Persistent mouth breathing caused by any one or combination of factors, such as malocclusion, persistent rhinitis, or enlarged adenoids, allows saliva to collect in the angles of the mouth with subsequent cheilitis.

Therapy for angular cheilitis consists of two parts. The main approach should be first, to correct the underlying causes, then to treat with antimicrobial and/or anti-inflammatory preparations locally, which will accomplish permanent clearing of the lesions. Frequent application is required, because the area is constantly bathed by saliva. Usually simple elimination of the focus of irritation will clear the condition. Intralesional injection of diluted triamcinolone may reduce inflammation. Combining a low-strength topical corticosteroid or calcineurin inhibitor with the antifungal agent may be helpful. Lip balms should be used cautiously because they often contain sensitizers. Petrolatum may be used safely if desired.

Although palliative treatment of angular cheilitis is simple and effective, recurrences will continue to plague the patient unless all the etiologic factors are treated.

Patch Testing in Stomatitis, Cheilitis, and Perlèche

Screening patch test trays contain a number of allergens that may cause stomatitis, cheilitis, and perlèche. These include metals, rubber allergens, preservatives, flavorings (MP and the fragrance mix), and topical medications. Supplemental allergens, such as acrylates, other metals, dental resins, cosmetic ingredients, sunscreens, and other items listed in this chapter, may be useful for complete diagnostic accuracy. Cosmetic products such as lipsticks and salves can usually be tested "as is." However, testing with dental materials and dentifrices themselves requires caution (Table 33.4).

PRECAUTIONS FOR PATCH TESTING WITH DENTIFRICES AND MOUTHWASHES

Soaps or synthetic detergents in a dentifrice may produce primary irritant reactions under a closed patch test, so these materials should be diluted by at least a factor of 10 for testing. Positive reactions to patch tests with a dentifrice or mouthwash should always be checked by testing at least five controls. If they also show positive reactions, the product is a primary irritant as tested.[117] Mouthwashes often contain alcohol and other ingredients that may partially evaporate and cause irritation under a closed patch test. These products should generally first be tested uncovered on the back or forearm, and only tested with a closed patch under dilution. Alternatively, a repeated open application test (ROAT) may be helpful in testing these agents. Apply the product to the antecubital space twice daily for 7 days. A positive test implies allergy, if controls are negative. A negative test, however, may be falsely negative due to inadequate concentration of an allergen in the product.

Table 33-4 Ingredients of Dentifrices and Mouthwashes—Concentrations and Vehicles for Patch Testing

Contactant	Concentration and vehicle	Comment
Abietic acid	2% pet	In denture adhesive powders
Acetic acid	3% aq	Astringent in mouthwash
Acetone (dimethyl ketone)	As is (open)	Solvent for celluloid-like material in dentifrices
Alcohol, USP 70%	As is (open)	Solvent and astringent in mouthwashes
Aluminum acetate	10% aq	Astringent
Aluminum chlorhydroxide	10% aq	Astringent
Aluminum chloride	2% aq	Astringent
Aluminum sulfate	2% aq	Astringent
Aluminum sulfocarbolate	2% aq	Astringent
Ammonium fluoride	2% aq	May produce nonspecific pustular patch test reaction
Ammonium persulfate	2% aq	Ammoniated dentifrices
Ammonium phosphate	2% aq	Ammoniated dentifrices
Anise oil	25% co	Flavoring agent
Benzalkonium chloride, USP	0.1% aq	Present in mouthwashes
Benzocaine	5% pet	Topical anesthetic
Benzoic acid	5% petA	Antibacterial agent in mouthwashes
Benzothonium chloride	0.1% aq	Antimicrobial agent
Benzoyl peroxide	10% pet	Used in acrylic resins
Benzyl alcohol	5% pet	Present in flavoring agents
Betadine solution (povidone-iodine)	As is	Mouthwash and gargle
Betanaphthol	10% oo	Antibacterial agent in mouthwash
Boric acid	Powder as is	Antiseptic in mouthwash
Camphor oil	10% pet	Flavoring agent; antimicrobial
Caraway seed oil	25% co	Flavoring agent
Carnation oil	10% aq	Flavoring agent
Cassia flavor	5% oo	Chinese cinnamon flavoring agent
Cetylpyridinium chloride	0.1% aq	Quaternary ammonium antimicrobial
Chlorophyllin, sodium copper	5% aq	Antimicrobial
Chlorothymol	2% aq	Antiseptic in mouthwash
Cinnamic acid	5% pet	Flavoring agent
Cinnamic aldehyde	2% pet	Flavoring agent (Lavoris)
Cinnamon oil	5% oo	Flavoring agent
Citric acid	1% aq	Astringent in mouthwash
Clove oil	25% co	Eugenol is chief constituent
Coriander oil	10% co	Flavoring agent
Coumarin	5% pet	A cinnamic acid flavor
Dequalinium	0.1% aq	Quaternary ammonium compound
Dichlorophene	2% aq	Preservative in toothpaste
Domiphen bromide	0.1% aq	Quaternary ammonium compound
Essential oils	1% alc	Flavoring, antiseptic, and anodyne agents
Ethylenediamine	10% pet	Stabilizing agent
Ethylenediamine tetra-acetic acid	10% aq	Stabilizing agent
Eucalyptus oil	1% alc	Flavoring agent
Eugenol	5% pet	Flavoring agent (derived from clove oil)
Formaldehyde	1% aq	Preservative
Geraniol	10% pet	Flavoring agent
Ginger oil	25% co	Flavoring agent
Glycerine	As is	Humectant and sweetener
Glyoxide	As is (open)	Contains urea peroxide
Gum arabic (acacia)	As is	Binder in denture adhesive powders
Hexachlorophene	2% aq	Antimicrobial agent
Hexetidine	1% aq	Antibacterial agent
Hexylresorcinol	As is	Antiseptic in mouthwash

Table 33-4 (cont.) Ingredients of Dentifrices and Mouthwashes—Concentrations and Vehicles for Patch Testing

Contactant	Concentration and vehicle	Comment
Irish moss (carrageen)	As is	Binder in toothpastes
Isodine	As is	Mouthwash with povidone-iodine
Javelle water (potassium hypochlorite)	10% aq	Antiseptic mouthwash
Karaya gum (sterculia gum)	As is	Denture adhesive powders
Krameria, tincture (tinctura rhatanhiae)	5% alc	Astringent in mouthwash
Lactic acid	3% aq	Astringent in mouthwash
Laurel oil	25% co	Flavoring agent
Lavender oil	1% alc	Flavoring agent
Limonene, oil of	1% alc	Flavoring agent
Linalool	10% pet	Flavoring agent
Mace, oil of (nutmeg)	10% alc	Flavoring agent
Menthol	1% pet	Flavoring agent
Methylbenzathonium chloride	0.1% aq	Quaternary ammonium disinfectant
Methyl cellulose	As is	Binder in dentifrices
Methyl salicylate	2% oo	Flavor in Listerine and Reef
Myroxylon Pereirae	10% pet	Present in denture cement liquids, may crossreact with cinnamates, essential oil flavors, and eugenol
Myrrh, tincture	10% alc	Disinfectant—Astringosol
Nitrobenzene	10% oo	Flavoring agent
Nitrofurazone	1% pet	Antibacterial agent in mouthwash
Nutmeg oil (mace)	10% alc	Flavoring agent
Oleyl alcohol	20% pet	Solvent for essential oils
Orange oil	1% alc	Flavoring agent
Orris root	as is	Flavoring agent
Oxychlorosene	1% aq	Antimicrobial
Pancreatin	As is	Mixture of enzymes
Peppermint oil	25% co	Flavoring agent
Phenol	1% aq	Antimicrobial, astringent
Phenolic compounds	1% aq A	myl, heptyl, and octyl phenols
Pimiento	10% co	Flavoring agent
Polyethylene glycol	10% aq	Humectant and solvent
Polyethylene sorbitan monooleate	5% aq	Emulsifying agent in mouthwashes
Polysorbate 80, USP	10% pet	Emulsifier and dispersing agent in dentifrices
Potassium chlorate	10% aq	Antiseptic oxidizing agent in mouthwash
Propylene glycol	30% aq	Humectant and binder
Sassafras	2% oo	Flavoring agent
Sodium alginate (Algin)	As is	Emulsifier in dentifrices
Sodium alkyl sulfate	2% aq	"Foaming" surfactant
Sodium fluoride	0.5% aq	May give nonspecific pustular patch test reaction
Sodium hypochlorite	10% aq	Antiseptic
Sodium monofluorophosphate	0.5% aq	Fluoride compound
Sodium monoglyceride sulfonate	2% aq	"Foaming" surfactant in Gleem
Sodium laurel sulfate	2% aq	"Foaming" agent in dentifrice
Sodium-N-alkyl sarcosinate	2% aq	"Foaming" agent
Sodium perborate	as is	Oxidizing agent
Sorbisol	10% aq	Humectant in dentifrices
Spearmint, oil of	1% alc	Flavoring agent
Stannus fluoride	0.5% aq	Fluoride agent
Strontium chloride	2% aq	
Tannic acid	1% aq	Astringent mouthwash
Thyme, oil of	25% co	Flavoring agent
Thymol (isopropyl metacresol)	1% pet	Antibacterial agent
Tragacanth	1% aq	Emulsifier and binder in dentifrices

Table 33-4 (Cont.) Ingredients of Dentifrices and Mouthwashes—Concentrations and Vehicles for Patch Testing		
Contactant	Concentration and vehicle	Comment
Tyrothricin	As is	Present in Tyrolaris mouthwash
Urea (carbamide)	10% aq	Ammoniated toothpastes
Wintergreen, oil of (gaultheria oil)	1% alc	Flavoring agent
Zinc chloride	2% aq	Astringent in Lavoris, Astringosol
Zinc oxide	As is	Combined with eugenol in many dental preparations
Zinc peroxide	As is	Astringent, antiseptic
Zinc sulfate	5% aq	Astringent
Zinc sulfocarbolate	5% aq	Astringent

alc, alcohol; aq, aqueous; as is, full strength; co, castor oil; oo, olive oil; open, uncovered; pet, petrolatum; sat, saturated

In the event that an allergic patch test reaction is obtained with a dentifrice or mouthwash, an effort should be made to ascertain the specific sensitizing ingredient. Furthermore, aimed testing may be possible with the cooperation of the product manufacturer.

DIRECT TESTING OF ORAL MUCOSA

In the past, testing of the oral mucosa has been occasionally performed. In past editions of this text, Fisher has suggested the following:

The suspected ingredient is incorporated into Orabase, which is an adhering paste composed of pectin, gelatin, sodium carboxymethylcellulose, and plasticized hydrocarbon gel. The mixture is applied to the inner side of the dried lip and left in place for 24 hours. Positive reactions marked by erythema of the mucosa may occur the next day, with the reaction reaching its peak at 48 hours after the allergen has been applied.

Another method of direct testing of the mucosa is to place the allergen inside a rubber or plastic cup that is then tied to the surface of the teeth in such a fashion that the allergen, held in the cup with collodion, is in contact with the buccal fold.

Dentures may be used to keep suspected allergens against the mucosa in those who use such appliances.

It must be strongly emphasized that using any of these nonstandard testing methods can produce false-positive irritant reactions as well as false-negative reactions, so clinical correlation is essential.

TESTING FOR ALLERGIC SENSITIVITY TO ACRYLIC DENTURES

Patch testing by strapping the denture to the forearm may lead to diagnostic errors, because redness, papulation, vesiculation, and even bullae may result from nonspecific pressure effects. This practice is not recommended. Patch testing with heat-cured dentures or with denture grindings also may give false reactions from friction and pressure. Testing with the monomer and other separate ingredients avoids false-positive reaction from the hardness of the denture or the sharpness of filings (Table 33.5).

The identification of specific allergens in denture materials can be difficult, because many combinations of chemicals and additives may be used. Crossreactivity between acrylates is common, but not definite.

Kaaber and colleagues[118] studied the significance of sensitizing compounds in the denture base for the etiology of the burning mouth syndrome (BMS) in 53 denture-wearing persons, 7 males and 46 females. Patch tests were performed with standard concentrations of benzoyl peroxide, dibutylphthalate, dimethyl-*p*-toluidine, formaldehyde, hydroquinone, methylmethyl acrylate, and *p*-phenylenediamine, as well as cadmium sulfate, potassium dichromate, cobalt chloride, and nickel sulfate. Furthermore, patch testing was performed with filings from the denture mixed with the patients' own saliva. Positive skin reactions to dimethyl-*p*-toluidine, hydroquinone, formaldehyde, methylmethyl acrylate, *p*-phenylenediamine, potassium dichromate, cobalt chloride, and nickel sulfate were observed in 15 persons, including 3 patients with reactions to filings from their dentures.

In 12 cases a causal connection could be traced between the oral symptoms and the denture base, indicating that contact sensitivity to base materials of the denture plate plays a greater role in the pathogenesis of BMS in edentulous persons than was previously suggested.

In our experience, patch testing with dentures or with filings of dentures often produces false-positive reactions from nonspecific pressure of hard particulate matter. Patch tests should be performed with commercially available allergens if at all possible. The liquid monomer or the other basic denture materials in solution or in

Table 33-5 Suggested Screening Tray for Patch Testing for Stomatitis, Cheilitis, and Perlèche

Metals
  Nickel sulfate
  Cobalt chloride
  Gold sodium thiosulfate
  Potassium dichromate
  Metallic mercury
  Thimerosal (mercury)
  Palladium chloride
  Platinum
  Copper sulfate
  Beryllium sulfate
  Indium sulfate
  Iridium chloride
Acrylates and plastics
  Bis-GMA
  Epoxy resin
  2-hydroxyethyl methacrylate
  Methyl methacrylate
  Rosin
Flavorings
  Benzyl alcohol
  Cinnamic aldehyde
  Clove oil
  Eugenol
  Fragrance mix
  Menthol
  Myroxylon pereirae
Disinfectants, vehicles, and preservatives
  Benzalkonium chloride
  Domiphen
  Cetylpyridinium chloride
  Sodium benzoate
  Benzethonium chloride
  Dichlorophene
  Hexylresorcinol
  Lanolin
  Paraben mix
  Propylene glycol

petrolatum may be tested, but must be highly diluted to avoid irritant reactions and active sensitization.

Fowler[119] has seen a case of a dental worker allergic to acrylates wherein positive reactions were seen 4 weeks after testing, performed on two separate occasions.

Therapy of Allergic and Irritant Cheilitis and Stomatitis

In mild cases, prompt removal of the specific contact allergen or irritant is all that is necessary to effect a cure.

For swelling of the lips with an intact epithelium, the application of petrolatum with or without cold compresses is helpful. When the swelling of the lips is accompanied by fissuring and crusting, a nonsensitizing topical antibiotic ointment such as mupirocin may be used, along with a topical steroid or calcineurin inhibitor such as desonide ointment, tacrolimus ointment, or pimecrolimus cream. Ointments may be preferable because they generally contain less sensitizers. Yeast cheilitis may have a clinical appearance identical to allergy, so a fungal culture should be performed in recalcitrant cases. An antifungal topical and/or oral fluconazole is useful in such cases. Commercial lip balms should be avoided since they usually contain many potential allergens.

When there is edema of the oral mucosa, sucking on ice chips is indicated. Painful erosions or ulcers may be covered with triamcinolone acetonide (Kenalog in Orabase) or other topical steroids. An effective way to apply the topical steroid is to place the gel or ointment on a gauze pad, then place the pad against the affected area for 15 to 30 minutes. It may be held in place by the teeth or tongue. Topical calcineurin inhibitors may be useful as well. For painful lesions, lidocaine (Xylocaine Viscous) or other local anesthetics may be applied. Ulcer-Ease Mouth Rinse (Med-Derm Co., Kingsport, TN) and other over-the-counter mouth rinses with antiseptic and analgesic properties may be useful to help control discomfort.

Diphenhydramine hydrochloride (Benadryl, and others) has local anesthetic properties and may help with relief of symptoms. Some dermatologists make a mixture of this agent plus nystatin and tetracycline as a "shotgun" approach to alleviating oral symptoms.

References

1. Fisher A. Contact stomatitis, glossitis, and cheilitis. Otolaryngol Clin North Am 1974;7:827.

2. Claman HN. Mouth ulcers associated with prolonged chewing of gum containing aspirin. JAMA 1967;202:651.

3. Cohen L. Ulcerative lesions of the oral cavity. Int J Dermatol 1980;19:62.

4. Abramson A. Causes of stomatitis. Medical World News, 28 June 1974, p. 19.

5. Forsey RR, Sullivan TJ. Stomatitis nicotina. Arch Dermatol 1961;83:112.

6. Reddy C R, Ramulu C, Raju MVS, Reddy PG. Relation of reverse smoking and other habits to the development of stomatitis nicotina. Indian J Cancer 1972;91:223.

7. Mennie S, Piccinno R, Pistritto MG. Ulcerative stomatitis in a neonate due to a chlorine antiseptic. Contact Dermatitis 1988;18:320.

8. Lowney E D. Unresponsiveness to a contact sensitizer in man. J Invest Dermatol 1968;51:411.

9. Mortz C, Lauritsen J, Bindsley-Jensen C, et al. Nickel sensitization in adolescents and association with ear piercing, use of dental braces, and hand eczema. Acta Derm Venereol 2003;83:359.

10. Drake T E, Maibach H I. Allergic contact dermatitis and stomatitis caused by a cinnamic-aldehyde flavored toothpaste. Arch Dermatol 1976;112:202.

11. Magnusson B, Wilkinson DS. Cinnamic aldehyde in toothpaste: 1. clinical aspects and patch tests. Contact Dermatitis 1975;1:70.

12. Kirton V, Wilkinson W. Sensitivity to cinnamic aldehyde in a toothpaste: 2. further studies. Contact Dermatitis 1975;1:77.

13. Miller RL, Gould AR, Bernstein ML. Cinnamon-induced stomatitis venata. Oral Surg Oral Med Oral Pathol 1992;73:708.

14. Kim SC, Hong KT, Kim DH. Contact stomatitis from a breath refresher (Eundan). Contact Dermatitis 1988;19:309.

15. Hjorth N. Eczematous allergy to balsams. Copenhagen: Munksgaard, 1961.

16. Calap Calatayud J. Allergy to balsam of Peru. Med Esp 1969;61:119.

17. Fisher AA. Allergic contact stomatitis. Cutis 1975;15:149.

18. Kern AN. Contact dermatitis from cinnamon. Arch Dermatol 1960;81:599.

19. Camarasa G, Alomar A. Menthol dermatitis from cigarettes. Contact Dermatitis 1978;4:169.

20. Papa CM, Shelley WB. Menthol hypersensitivity. JAMA 1964;189:546.

21. Morton CA, Garioch J, Todd P, et al. Contact sensitivity to menthol and peppermint in patients with intra-oral symptoms. Contact Dermatitis 1995;32:281.

22. Goransson J, et al. Some cases of eugenol sensitivity. Svensk Tandlak T 1967;60:545.

23. Koch G, Magnusson B, Nyquist G. Contact allergy to medicaments and materials used in dentistry: II. Sensitivity to eugenol and colophony. Odont Rev 1971;22:275.

24. Beswick S, Ramsay H, Tan B. Contact dermatitis from flavourings in chewing gum. Contact Dermatitis 1999;40:49.

25. Fisher AA. Allergic reactions due to metals used in dentistry. Cutis 1974;14:797.

26. Foussereau J, Laugier P. Allergic eczema from metallic foreign bodies (tooth fillings and denture alloys). Clin Dermatol 1966;52:221.

27. Frykholm KO, Frithiof A, Fernstrom AI, et al. Allergy to copper derived from dental alloys as a possible cause of oral lesions of lichen planus. Acta Derm Venereol 1969;49:268.

28. Koch P, Bahmer F. Oral lesions and symptoms related to metals used in dental restoration: a clinical, allergological, and histologic study. J Am Acad Dermatol 1999;41:422.

29. Scalf L, Fowler J, Morgan K, Looney S. Dental metal allergy in patients with oral, cutaneous, and genital lichenoid reactions. Am J Contact Dermat 2001;12:146.

30. Yiannias J, el-Azhary R, Hand J, et al. Relevant contact sensitivities in patients with the diagnosis of oral lichen planus. J Am Acad Dermatol 2000;42:177.

31. Laeijendecker R, Dekker S, Burger P, et al. Oral lichen planus and allergy to dental amalgam restorations. Arch Dermatol 2004;140:1434.

32. Khamaysi Z, Bergman R, Weltfriend S. Positive patch test reactions to allergens of the dental series and the relation to the clinical presentation. Contact Dermatitis 2006;55:216.

33. Marcusson JA. Contact allergies to nickel sulfate, gold sodium thiosulfate and palladium chloride in patients claiming side-effects from dental alloy components. Contact Dermatitis 1996;34:320.

34. Epstein S. The antigen-antibody reaction in contact dermatitis. Ann Allergy 1952;10:633.

35. Fernstreom A, et al. Mercury allergy with eczematous dermatitis due to silver amalgam fillings. Br Dent J 1962;113:206.

36. Gaul L. Immunity of the oral mucosa in epidermal sensitization to mercury. Arch Dermatol 1966;93:45.

37. Johnson H, Schonberg I, Bach N. Chronic atopic dermatitis, with pronounced mercury sensitivity: partial clearing after extraction of teeth containing mercury amalgam fillings. Arch Derm Syph 1951;63:279.

38. Sidi E, Casalis J. Les intolerances de la muqueuse buccale. Presse Med 1951;59:730.

39. Vickers CF. Mercury sensitivity. Contact Dermatol Newsletter 1961;2.

40. Spector LS. Allergic manifestations to mercury. JAMA 1951;42:320.

41. Thomson J, Russell JA. Dermatitis due to mercury following amalgam dental restoration. Br J Dermatol 1970;82:292.

42. Frykholm KO. On mercury from dental amalgam: its toxic and allergic effects and some comments on occupational hygiene. Acta Odontol Scand 1957;22[Suppl 15]:230.

43. Von Mayenburg J, Rakoski J, Szliska C. Patch testing with amalgam at various concentrations. Contact Dermatitis 1991;24:266.

44. Foussereau J, Laugier P. Allergic eczema from metallic foreign bodies (tooth fillings and denture alloys). Clin Dermatol 1966;52:221.

45. van Loon LAJ, et al. Contact stomatitis and dermatitis to nickel and palladium. Contact Dermatitis 1984;11:294.

46. Fisher AA, Shapiro A. Allergic eczematous contact dermatitis due to metallic nickel. JAMA 1956;161:717.

47. Wilson H_T. Nickel dermatitis. Br J Dermatol 1955;67:291.

48. Calnan C_D. Nickel sensitivity in women. Int Arch Allergy 1957;1:73.

49. Elgart M, Higdon R. Allergic contact dermatitis to gold. Arch Dermatol 1971;103:649.

50. Schaffran R, Storrs F, Schalock P. Prevalence of gold sensitivity in asymptomatic individuals with gold dental restorations. Am J Contact Dermat 1999;10:201.

51. Moller H. Dental gold alloys and contact allergy. Contact Dermatitis 2002;47:63.

52. Brendlinger DL, Tarsitano JJ. Generalized dermatitis due to sensitivity to a chrome-cobalt removable partial denture. J Am Dent Assoc 1970;81:395.

53. Ovrutsky GD, Ulyanov AD. Allergy to chromium using steel dental prosthesis. Stomatologia 1976;55:660.

54. Moffa JP, Beck WD, Hoke AW. Allergic response to nickel-containing dental alloys. J Dent Res 1977;56[Special Issue B]:107.

55. Sheard Jr C. Contact dermatitis from platinum and related metals. Arch Dermatol 1955;71:357.

56. Fowler JF. Allergic contact dermatitis to metals. Am J Contact Dermat 1990;1:212.

57. Mizoguchi S, Setoyama M, Kanzaki T. Linear lichen planus in the region of the mandibular nerve caused by an allergy to palladium in dental metals. Dermatology 1998;196:268.

58. Koch P, Baum HP. Contact stomatitis due to palladium and platinum in dental alloys. Contact Dermatitis 1996;34:253.

59. Haberman AL, Pratt M, Storrs FJ. Contact dermatitis from beryllium in dental alloys. Contact Dermatitis 1993;28:157.

60. Bircher AJ, Pelloni F, Langauer-Messmer S, Muller D. Delayed hypersensitivity reactions to corticosteroids applied to mucous membranes. Br J Dermatol 1996;135:310.

61. Van Groeningen G, Nater JP. Reactions to dental impression materials. Contact Dermatitis 1975;1:373.

62. Tinkelman DG, Tinkelman CL. An unusual etiology of urticaria. Pediatrics 1979;63:339.

63. Garcia-Bravo B, Pons A, Rodriguez-Richardo A. Oral lichen planus from colophony. Contact Dermatitis 1992;26:279.

64. Hensten-Pettersen C. Dermatitis and dental materials. Contact Dermatitis 1981;7:174.

65. Bowen RL. Compatibility of various materials with oral tissues: 1. the components in composite restorations. J Dent Res 1979;58:1493.

66. Ruyter IF, Svendsen SA. Remaining methacrylate groups in composite restorative materials. Acta Odontol Scand 1978;36:75.

67. Thompson LR, Miller EG, Bowles WH. Leaching of unpolymerized materials from orthodontic bonding resin. J Dent Res 1982;61:989.

68. Fisher AA. Allergic sensitization of the skin and oral mucosa to acrylic denture materials. JAMA 1954;156:238.

69. Crissey JT. Stomatitis, dermatitis and denture materials. Arch Dermatol 1965;92:45.

70. Goon A, Isaksson M, Zimerson E, et al. Contact allergy to (meth)acrylates in the dental series in Southern Sweden. Contact Dermatitis 2006;55:219.

71. Santosh, et al. Results of patch testing with dental materials. Contact Dermatitis 1999;40:50.

72. Tosti A, et al. Contact stomatitis due to N_1N-dimethyl-para-toluidine. Contact Dermatitis 1990;22:113.

73. Torres V, et al. Allergic contact cheilitis and stomatitis from hydroquinone in an acrylic dental prosthesis. Contact Dermatitis 1993;19:102.

74. van Joost TH, van Ulsen J, Van Loon J. Contact allergy to denture materials in the burning mouth syndrome. Contact Dermatitis 1988;18:97.

75. Fisher A. Allergic sensitization of the skin and oral mucosa to acrylic resin denture materials. J Prosthet Dent 1956;6:600.

76. Wakkers-Garritsen BG, Timmer LH, Nater JP. Etiological factors in the denture sore mouth syndrome: an investigation of 24 patients. Contact Dermatitis 1975;1:337.

77. Klein DR. Oral soft tissue changes in geriatric patients. Bull NY Acad Med 1980;56:721.

78. Taaffe A, Riggott JM. Aetiological factors in denture stomatitis. Br J Dermatol 1982;107:38.

79. Pemberton M, et al. Allergy to octyl gallate causing stomatitis. Br Dent J 1993;175:106.

80. Lewis FM, Shah M, Gawkrodger DJ. Contact sensitivity to food additives can cause oral and perioral symptoms. Contact Dermatitis 1995;33:429.

81. Maurice PDL, et al. Allergic contact stomatitis and cheilitis from iodoform used in a dental dressing. Contact Dermatitis 1988;18:114.

82. Merk H, Ebert L, Goerz G. Allergic contact dermatitis due to the fungicide hexetidine. Contact Dermatitis 1982;8:216.

83. Epstein S. Dermal contact dermatitis from neomycin. Ann Allergy 1958;16:268.

84. Welsh L. The fixed drug eruption. Arch Dermatol 1961;84:1012.

85. Welsh L. Cross-fixed drug eruption from three antibiotics. Arch Dermatol 1955;71:521.

86. Sainio EL, Kanerva L. Contact allergens in toothpastes and a review of their hypersensitivity. Contact Dermatitis 1995;33100.

87. Kierland R. What's new. Int J Dermatol 1971;10:208.

88. Accepted dental therapeutics, 33rd ed. Chicago: American Dental Association, 1968.

89. Sims W. Oral lesions caused by antienzyme dentifrices. US Armed Forces J 1955;6:995.

90. Shea J, Gillespie S, Waldbott G. Allergy to fluoride. Ann Allergy 1967;25:388.

91. Douglas T. Fluoride dentifrice and stomatitis. Northwest Med 1957;56:1037.

92. Fisher A, et al. Pustular patch test reactions. Arch Dermatol 1959;80:742.

93. Saunders M. Fluoride toothpastes: a cause of acne-like eruptions. Arch Dermatol 1975;111:793.

94. Camarasa J, et al. Contact urticaria from sodium fluoride. Contact Dermatitis 1993;28:294.

95. Pay DK, Shelley WB. Necrotic ulcerations secondary to oral neomycin troches. Arch Dermatol 1965;91:136.

96. Sugarman MM. Contact allergy due to mint chewing gum. Oral Surg 1950;3:1145.

97. Cancellieri CP. Chronic aphthous ulcers (canker sores) due to inhalant allergen sensitivity. J Allergy 1958;29:503.

98. Fregert S, et al. Alcohol dermatitis. Acta Derm Venereol 1969;49:493.

99. Jensen C, Lisby S, Baadsgaard O, et al. Release of nickel ions from stainless steel alloys used in dental braces. Contact Dermatitis 2003;48:300.

100. Freeman S, Stephens R. Cheilitis: analysis of 75 cases referred to a contact dermatitis clinic. Am J Contact Dermat 1999;10:198.

101. Zug K, Kornik R, Belsito D, et al. Patch testing patients with lip dermatitis: data from the NACDG 2001–2004. Submitted for publication, 2007.

102. Dooms-Goossens A, Degreef H, Verhoeve L. Hidden contact allergens in ORL—pharmaceutical preparations. Acta Otorhinolaryngol Belg 1979;33:474.

103. 103.Walgrave S, Warshaw E, Glesne L: Allergic contact dermatitis from propolis. Dermatitis 2005;16:209.

104. Hausen B, Evers P, Stuwe H, et al. Propolis allergy IV. Contact Dermatitis 1992;26:34.

105. Fernandez S, Luaces L, Madoz S, et al. Allergic contact stomatitis due to therapeutic propolis. Contact Dermatitis 2004;50:321.

106. Huldin DH. Hemorrhages of the lips secondary to nail hardeners. Cutis 1968;4:709.

107. Klauder JV. Sensitization to carrots. Arch Dermatol 1956;74:149.

108. Mitchell J, Rook JC. Botanical dermatology—plants and plants injurious to the skin. Philadelphia: Lea & Febiger, 1979.

109. Lupton ES. Cheilitis due to coffee. Arch Dermatol 1961;84:798.

110. Fisher AA. Perleche (angular cheilitis) due to contactants. Cutis 1974;14:499.

111. Epstein E, Maibach H. Ethylenediamine allergic contact dermatitis. Arch Dermatol 1968;98:476.

112. Singh G. Betel chewer's perlèche. Br J Dermatol 1973;89:98.

113. Gruskin S, Tolman D, Wagoner R. Oral manifestations of uremia. Minn Med 1970;53:495.

114. Thomas III J, Greene S, Dicken C. Factitious cheilitis. J Am Acad Dermatol 1983;8:368.

115. Goldman L. Dental floss as a factor in the development of perleche. Arch Dermatol 1979;115:108.

116. Schoenfeld R, Schoenfeld F. Angular cheilitis. Cutis 1977;19:213.

117. Fisher A. Patch tests for allergic reactions to dentifrices and mouthwashes. Cutis 1970;6:554.

118. Kaaber S, Thulin H, Nielsen E. Skin sensitivity to denture base materials in the burning mouth syndrome. Contact Dermatitis 1979;5:90.

119. Fowler J. Late patch test reactions to acrylates in a dental worker. Am J Contact Dermat 1999;10:224.

CHAPTER **34**

TREATMENT OF CONTACT DERMATITIS

EXECUTIVE SUMMARY

While topical and systemic corticosteroids are the most widely used treatment for contact dermatitis, other programs of care come into play in specific circumstances. A low-nickel diet for vesicular hand dermatitis can be helpful in select nickel-sensitive cases. Disulfiram has also been used. Oral desensitization to *Toxicodendron* and *Parthenium* can be tried. Azathioprine has been successful in some Parthenium cases. Acitretin and psoralen plus ultraviolet A (PUVA) have been used in hand dermatitis. Grenz-ray therapy is highly effective but not widely available. Oral cyclosporine A has been proven effective. Itraconazole suppressed elicitation of contact dermatitis to strong allergens in an animal model. Fexofenadine can suppress the pruritus that accompanies contact dermatitis. Topical tacrolimus and pimecrolimus have activity against contact dermatitis, but pimecrolimus was not effective against *Toxicodendron*.

Intentional induction of contact dermatitis has been used as a treatment for inflammatory skin disorders, particularly alopecia areata, but side effects ranging from dyspigmentation to urticaria and erythema multiforme have occurred.

Irritant contact dermatitis is sometimes managed without corticosteroids with Burow's solution, anhydrous lanolin, Lassar's paste, zinc oxide, and Mastisol for fissures.

Acute Contact Dermatitis

Acute poison ivy dermatitis is the most common example of an acute allergic contact dermatitis. Systemic corticosteroid therapy is of great benefit and should be considered in all but mild cases of acute allergic contact dermatitis. For adults, 40 to 60 mg of prednisone per day, in two or three divided doses, is the treatment of choice. Generally, this dosage should be tapered gradually, resulting in a total treatment time of 10 to 14 days. An easily remembered dosage schedule for prednisone is 10 mg four times daily for 3 days, three times daily for 3 days, two times daily for 3 days, then once daily for 3 days. Further tapering is not necessary, and steroid side effects, although possible, are very rare with this length of treatment. Tapering the treatment too soon often results in a rebound of the initial dermatitis.

In cases of localized acute contact dermatitis, or in patients in whom even a short course of systemic steroids is contraindicated, a potent topical corticosteroid cream can be used. Fluorinated steroids such as these, however, should not be used on the face or intertriginous areas except for periods of less than 1 to 2 weeks. Cream bases, which may provide some drying effect, are preferable to ointments, which may trap moisture.

To further enhance the drying of acute, weepy lesions, moist compresses that have a soothing effect and remove crust and debris are helpful. Moisten a clean, absorbent cloth with an astringent, such as aluminum sulfate and calcium acetate (Domeboro), or even plain tap water, and apply for 20 to 30 minutes several times a day. Alternatively, bathing in oatmeal baths (Aveeno) is useful when large body areas are involved.

Itching is often severe in acute contact dermatitis and is usually best treated by steroids rather than antihistamines. However, antihistamines initially may have an added effect and also may induce drowsiness, which may be beneficial to the patient. Hydroxyzine, 10 to 25 mg, or diphenhydramine, 25 to 50 mg two to four times daily as needed and tolerated, may be useful. Other sedating antihistamines may be used, but sometimes nonsedating antihistamines such as cetirizine may be helpful.

722

Chronic Contact Dermatitis

In contrast to their use in the treatment of acute contact dermatitis, systemic steroids should be used cautiously in the treatment of chronic contact dermatitis because the condition may require months or even years of therapy. The first line of treatment beyond prevention and avoidance is the use of emollients to decrease itching and reduce dryness and scaling. Lotions containing alpha-hydroxy acids, such as glycolic acid or lactic acid, are available over the counter and are especially useful for thick, scaly plaques. Low- to medium-strength topical steroids, such as hydrocortisone valerate, alclometasone, or desonide, are useful. Some ointments, however, are greasy; the patient's acceptance of them must be considered when prescribing these products.

Intralesional injection of triamcinolone acetonide (Kenalog), 4 to 10 mg per mL, is useful in occasional thick plaques, but caution must be exercised because of the potential for atrophy. Antihistamines are of some benefit in minimizing itching, but intolerance may develop, thus limiting their effectiveness. In selected cases, Kenalog 40 mg to 60 mg intramuscularly, which has a beneficial effect of 3 to 6 weeks' duration, may be used without serious risk of adverse effects.

Treatment of Dermatitis in Special Circumstances

NICKEL DERMATITIS

Systemic nickel dermatitis may sometimes occur in the form of dyshidrosiform hand eczema or may occur in other areas of the body. A low-nickel diet, as discussed elsewhere in this text, may be helpful. If both external and internal allergen avoidance is not successful, disulfiram 250 mg four times daily may be tried. This agent binds nickel and allows it to be excreted in the urine and stool. Absolute avoidance of alcohol is essential in taking this drug because alcohol intake will result in nausea and vomiting. In addition, liver function test results should be monitored before and during treatment. Readers should check the references and review the studies on this agent before prescribing it.

PARTHENIUM DERMATITIS

Oral hyposensitization to plant allergens has been helpful in some patients, but with *Toxicodendron* a side effect of pruritus ani was common. *Parthenium hysterophorus* has caused dermatitis in India by direct contact and by airborne exposure. At times this allergen has produced epidemic levels of dermatitis. Oral hyposensitization

was found useful in 66% of a series of 24 patients, but about 30% worsened and had to drop out of the study. There was no pruritus ani in this series.[1] For patients with chronic parthenium dermatitis, an alternative to the phototherapy approach outlined in the previous section is the use of azathioprine. In a study of 15 Parthenium-sensitive patients with extensive contact dermatitis who had contraindications to corticosteroids, oral azathioprine (100–150 mg per day) was used. This produced a slow improvement. No significant side effects occurred in this study, but it took between 6 and 12 months to obtain substantial benefit. By the end of the year of treatment, near-total clearing had occurred.[2] A novel treatment program using 300 mg of azathioprine once-weekly for 6 months was studied in 12 patients (10 males and 2 females) who had experienced airborne contact dermatitis for 3 to 19 years. An excellent response (defined as 80–100% clearing) was seen in 7 of the 12 patients, and 60% clearance was found in an additional 5. This weekly dosing schedule reduced costs by 60% and the authors reported no significant side effects.[3]

GARLIC DERMATITIS

Hubbard and Goldsmith report a curry chef with garlic-induced dermatitis of the non-dominant hand, who was successfully treated with acitretin 25mg/day and another such chef who responded to topical psoralen-ultraviolet A after a period of 12 weeks.[4]

METALS

Prevention of patch test reactions to nickel, cobalt, and copper but not to palladium were achieved by application of a 10% diethylenetriaminepentaacetic acid (DTPA) cream. The cream was evaluated in a double-blind manner.[5]

SKIN-PROTECTIVE PRODUCTS

Generally, skin protectants or "barrier creams" have proven unsatisfactory in the care of patients with contact dermatitis. However, a number of new products that may prove to be of some use have been introduced to the marketplace as of this writing. Also, in occasional cases some of the older barrier creams used in industry may have some benefit. It must be kept in mind, however, that barrier creams may trap allergens, actually worsening dermatitis. Furthermore, individuals may be allergic to some components of barrier creams.

The one barrier product that has been proven of definite use is IvyBlock Lotion for the prevention of dermatitis from poison ivy, oak, and sumac. The protective nature of this product has been well documented. It should be applied to all exposed areas before possible contact with the offending plants. Protection is expected for at least 4 hours but may last as long as 8 hours. The mechanism of action is uncertain, but perhaps the active ingredient in IvyBlock (quaternium-18 bentonite) may bind the urushiol allergen and prevent its penetration. Accordingly, after exposure any exposed areas should be washed with soap and water. It is uncertain at this time whether IvyBlock Lotion provides protection from other allergens. Fowler (personal observation) has noted some success in using this product in individuals with airborne Compositae dermatitis.

Noncorticosteroid Management Options for Contact Dermatitis

GRENZ-RAY TREATMENT

Grenz rays are useful in the management of chronic dermatitis, including chronic contact dermatitis. The equipment to perform this treatment is not as commonly available as it once was due to concerns about the hazards of ionizing radiation. Grenz rays are softer than superficial X rays. In a study of chronic symmetrical hand eczema, significant benefit was demonstrated using 3 Gy (300 rad) weekly for 6 weeks.[6] In a study of six patients who were nickel sensitive, a dilution series of nickel patch tests were placed on both sides of the back, and one side was treated with 3 Gy weekly for 3 weeks. Almost nothing was seen at the sites treated with grenz rays, and monoclonal antibody staining of skin biopsy specimens showed severe depletion of Langerhans cells at the treated sites.[7] A similar study of irritant reactions found a slight but not significant difference between sodium lauryl sulfate patch tests applied to skin pretreated with grenz rays.[8] Chronic vesicular hand dermatitis was treated with 1,200 cGy in 8 fractions in a group of 9 patients. Six MV of photons were employed. During a follow-up period of 1 to 45 months, complete resolution was seen in 7 of 15 treated sites (47%) and reduced severity or frequency of flare-ups were seen in the remaining sites.[9]

PHOTOTHERAPY

A comparison of ultraviolet B (UVB) light versus bath psoralen plus ultraviolet A (PUVA) phototherapy for the management of hand dermatitis in 13 patients treated for 6 weeks found no significant difference.[10]

PUVA has been successfully used to manage photosensitive Compositae-sensitive patients, however. The dose of methoxsalen used was 0.3 mg/kg. The patients were started on 60mg of prednisone at the same time that they started PUVA at 1 joule less than the minimal phototoxic dose (MPD). Treatments were administered on a Monday-Wednesday-Friday schedule, 1.5 hours after ingestion of methoxsalen. Treatments were increased 1 J if the MPD was greater than 6 J, or increased by 0.5 J if the MPD was 6 J or less. The prednisone dose was decreased to 40 mg at week 2, further tapered to 20 mg at week 3, and then discontinued. The maximum UVA exposure was 10 J per treatment. The frequency of phototherapy was tapered after 6 weeks to twice a week and then once a week. This schedule was successful.[11]

CYCLOSPORINE

Oral cyclosporine at a dose of 3 mg/kg per day for 6 weeks was used to treat 27 patients with hand dermatitis. The mean decrease in disease activity was 54%,[12] which is somewhat disappointing. Topical use of cyclosporine has also been disappointing.[13] A comparison between cyclosporine and betamethasone-17,21-diproprionate in 41 patients found that 50% improved with cyclosporine and 30% improved with betamethasone.[14]

ITRACONAZOLE

A study done in mice found that itraconazole could suppress the elicitation of contact dermatitis to the strong allergens dinitrofluorobenzene and oxazolone. Itraconazole had no effect on the induction phase of contact sensitization nor did it effect irritant reactions. Only the elicitation of contact dermatitis in sensitized animals was suppressed. The mechanism seems to be an inhibition of IFN-gamma.[15]

FEXOFENADINE

Pruritus created by diphenylcyclopropenone used to treat alopecia areata was studied to see if the H1-receptor antagonist fexofenadine could benefit patients by symptom relief. No corticosteroids were used by patients undergoing this treatment. Itching peaked 6–12 hours after application of diphenylcyclopropenone and fexofenadine partially but rapidly reduced the severity of itching for 72 hours.[16]

TACROLIMUS AND PIMECROLIMUS

Topical tacrolimus has been shown to inhibit both irritant and allergic contact dermatitis in the guinea pig.[17] In rats, its inhibitory action was stronger than alclometasone dipropionate, and it is thought to inhibit the activation of sensitized T-lymphocytes.[18] The benefits of tacrolimus ointment in atopic dermatitis make it a potentially useful drug for the management of some cases of contact dermatitis.[19] A study of experimentally induced chronic nickel contact dermatitis in humans found tacrolimus ointment 0.1% significantly more effective and placebo.[20] Similarly, tacrolimus ointment 0.1% was found to significantly reduce erythema, oozing, scaling and itching in a nickel sulphate-induced steroid-resistant allergic contact dermatitis compared to placebo.[21]

A comparison of tacrolimus 0.1% ointment (Protopic) to mometasone furoate 0.1% ointment found the two compounds to be statistically equal in their ability to suppress induced nickel dermatitis when both agents were applied under occlusion. In the study, both tacrolimus and mometasone furoate were significantly better than petrolatum.[22]

Treatment of experimentally induced Toxicodendron dermatitis with pimecrolimus used twice a day found no significant difference in time for resolution of itch or rash compared to placebo and the average dermatitis score was equivalent. The authors concluded that pimecrolimus 1% cream is ineffective in the treatment of this dermatitis.[23] The difference in mechanism of action of pimecrolimus, tacrolimus, and cyclosporine A was studied in a mouse model. Pimecrolimus did not impair sensitization at the highest dose tested (120 mg/kg); both cyclosporine A and tacrolimus did. The conclusion was that pimecrolimus has a more selective immunomodulatory effect that inhibits the elicitation phase but not the sensitization phase of contact dermatitis.[24] In a human study of experimentally induced nickel contact dermatitis that compared pimecrolimus 1% cream, tacrolimus 0.1% ointment, clobetasol propionate 0.05% ointment, and triamcinolone acetonide 0.1% ointment, the four agents were found equal in their ability to suppress the dermatitis.[25]

Allergic Contact Dermatitis as Treatment

The use of squaric acid dibutylester (SADBE) to treat alopecia areata and warts provides an opportunity to observe the natural history of contact allergy. Of 40 patients who had been treated with SADBE and required retreatment 1 to 7 years later, 23 (57.5%) were found to have lost their allergy. Reinstitution of topical immunotherapy required 10 to 10,000 times more SADBE to re-establish the sensitized state, suggesting a degree of tolerance developed in such individuals.[26] Complications of the use of contact dermatitis as a treatment for alopecia areata include vitiligo, persistent hypo/hyperpigmentation, erythema multiforme-like eruption, psoriasis, contact urticaria, and generalized urticaria. Diphenylcyclopropenone (DCP) was reported to cause a dose-dependent diffuse urticaria that could be managed by reducing the cutaneous exposures to 0.00001% or less.[27] A study done in mice attempted to identify a mechanism

by which contact dermatitis intentionally induced to treat alopecia areata might work. The study found that the chemokine milieu created by allergen treatment severely hampered dendritic cell migration from the skin to the draining lymph nodes. This produced less T cell activation, which allowed hair follicle recovery.[28] An alternative theory suggests that inflammation depletes intracellular glutathione shifting Th1 cells into Th2 activity. Furthermore, inflammatory cytokines induce COX-2, which produces PGE2, which in turn increases cAMP intracellularly, suppresses macrophage functions, and increases IL-4, which is a Th-2 cytokine.[29] It is unclear which of these possible mechanisms is the actual mechanism.

Treatment of Irritant Contact Dermatitis

In the acute phase of irritant contact dermatitis of the feet, the use of foot baths with cool Burow's solution (1 part to 20 parts water for 20 minutes twice daily) reduces inflammation and edema. In the presence of secondary infection, appropriate antibiotics should be prescribed. After the foot baths, zinc oxide ointment or plain Lassar's paste may be applied. If the dermatitis is oozing, an absorbent paste composed of the following substances can be applied:

- Burow's solution 10 mL
- Anhydrous lanolin 20 g
- Plain Lassar's paste up to 60 g

In the presence of fissuring, the following ointment may be used:

- Mastisol (Ferndale Laboratories) 2 mL
- Zinc oxide ointment up to 20 g

Often, the dermatitis produced by saliva and food juices does not respond to creams and ointments. Adherent protective pastes, such as plain Lassar's paste, give better results. When an infant's skin is bathed constantly by saliva or irritating fluids, the application of an absorbent and protective paste composed of the following substances is useful:

- Burow's solution 5 mL
- Anhydrous lanolin 10 g
- Talc USP 10 g
- Zinc oxide ointment up to 6 g

Management of Chronic Otitis

Patients who have chronic or infectious eczematoid dermatitis of the ear should have patch tests performed.

Table 34-1 Otic Preparations Free of Propylene Glycol
Americaine Otic[a]
Auralgan Otic Solution[a]
Coly-Mycin S Otic with Neomycin and Hydrocortisone[b]
Debrox Drops
Decadron Phosphate Sterile Ophthalmic Solution[c]
Metreton Ophthalmic Solution Sterile[c]
Otic Domeboro Solution
Otobiotic Otic Suspension
Otocort Ear Drops[b]

[a]Not recommended because of benzocaine content.
[b]Not recommended because of neomycin content.
[c]Advocated for both ophthalmic and otic use.

VoSol HC is an otic solution containing 1% hydrocortisone in an acid-nonaqueous propylene glycol solution that, although free of antibiotics, is antibacterial, antifungal, and anti-inflammatory. This is an effective solution except for individuals who are sensitive to propylene glycol.

When everything else fails in the treatment of dermatitis and itching of the external ear canal, carbol-fuchsin paint is effective. The deep red color of the solution, however, is a disadvantage.

Cerumenex eardrops to soften wax may produce an acute otitis externa with spreading dermatitis to the face, neck, and back. The actual sensitizer in Cerumenex was a polypeptide in several reported cases.[30–32] Propylene glycol in Cerumenex may also be a sensitizer. Table 34.1 lists propylene glycol–free otic preparations.

Instructions for Prevention of Irritant Dermatitis in Individuals Who Have Atopic Dermatitis

- *Clothing:* Clothes worn close to the skin should be smooth and loose. Rough and starched cuffs and collars are irritating. Avoid contact with wool. Linen, cotton, poplin, gabardine, suede, chamois, and synthetic fibers, such as orlon and nylon, are usually well tolerated. Wash all new clothing before use, and be sure that all soaps and detergents are removed after each washing. Wear sandals or perforated shoes whenever possible. Avoid prolonged use of tennis shoes.
- *Furniture and room furnishings:* Keep rooms, especially the bedroom, as uncluttered as possible. Avoid dust-gathering draperies and carpets. Small cotton scatter rugs are permitted. Avoid use of upholstered furniture. Plain wooden furniture is preferable.

- *Toys:* Avoid fuzzy or woolen toys, such as teddy bears. Toys made of wood, rubber, paper, or plastics are permitted.
- *Pets:* It is best not to allow dogs, cats, or birds in the house. If the presence of such pets is necessary, they must be excluded from the bedroom. Turtles and fish are permitted anywhere in the house.
- *Dust and molds:* Exposure to all kinds of dust must be avoided as much as possible. Dust on the skin is irritating, and the inhalation of dust may also cause increased itching. Moldy objects should also be avoided for the same reasons.
- *Overheating and excessive perspiration:* Patients should indulge in activities that involve minimal sweating. Swimming, particularly in salt water, seems to agree with most patients who have atopic dermatitis.
- *Tension:* Nervous excitement and tension may cause itching and scratching. If trying situations, such as school examinations or difficult business or social situations, are anticipated, taking prescribed medication beforehand may be helpful.
- *Scratching:* Scratched skin quickly becomes inflamed and damaged, with resultant retardation in healing. Patting or rubbing may be less harmful than scratching. Keep fingernails short. The application of ice or ice-cold water on cotton cloths to localized areas may stop the itching.
- *Soaps and cleaning agents:* Strong detergents, cleansers, and solvents, such as turpentine and benzene, are particularly harmful to atopic skin. Mild soaps may be tolerated. Because one cannot predict the soap substitute that will work for a particular individual, several, such as Soydome, Lowila, Dermolate, or Aveeno Bar, may have to be tried.

Adults who have atopic dermatitis of the hands present special problems. Frequently, atopic dermatitis clears with the exception of the hands, where the eruption may remain for prolonged periods. The use of rubber or cotton-lined gloves is unsuccessful because atopic skin does not tolerate the occlusion and the resulting sweat retention and maceration. People who have atopic dermatitis of the hands should use long-handled brushes for dishwashing, cleaning, and doing most other household chores.

Treatment of Contact Dermatitis Superimposed on Atopic Dermatitis

In general, treatment of contact dermatitis complicating an atopic eczema is the same as that of contact dermatitis on nonatopic skin, with the exceptions noted in this section.

WET DRESSINGS

Potassium permanganate or silver nitrate dressings should be avoided because they are often irritating to atopic skin. Burow's solution (1 part to 20 parts water) or wet dressings of a 1% boric acid solution are better tolerated. Occasionally, even these dressings are too drying. If the inflamed skin is dry, hot, and edematous, the application of a thin layer of plain petrolatum and a superimposed ice bag or ice-cold water compresses may be more soothing.

TUB BATHS

In generalized acute cases, tub baths may be indicated. An ointment-based moisturizer or corticosteroid should be used after bathing to prevent overdrying.

TOPICAL CORTICOSTEROID THERAPY

In uncomplicated atopic dermatitis, topical corticosteroid creams and ointments are often efficacious. Occlusive dressings with Saran Wrap generally are tolerated in air-conditioned circumstances or cool climates but not in ambient surroundings that lead to sweating. Even in a cool setting, occlusion will be tolerated only for 1 to 2 hours. If intense pruritus occurs, treatment will be counterproductive and should be abandoned.

SYSTEMIC CORTICOSTEROID THERAPY

In general, the use of systemic corticosteroid therapy is avoided in atopic dermatitis because of the chronicity of the disease and because the patient may become dependent on this mode of therapy. In the presence of severe or generalized contact dermatitis in the atopic individual, however, systemic corticosteroid therapy should be used in the absence of contraindications. Such systemic therapy is indicated particularly when the contact dermatitis is of an allergic nature and the contactant has been discovered. In such instances, systemic therapy does not need to be prolonged for more than 2 or 3 weeks.

An efficient, economical method of systemic corticosteroid therapy in such cases is the administration of 60 g of prednisone daily for 2 days, 40 mg daily for 3 days, 30 mg daily for 2 days, 20 mg daily during the second week, and finally 10 mg daily during the third week. A gradual tapering of the steroid over 2 to 3 weeks tends to prevent a severe rebound dermatitis. Children may receive 20 mg of prednisone for 3 days and then a gradually decreasing dose for 3 weeks.

Management of Epoxy-Resin Dermatitis

Most problems encountered with handling epoxy-resin or curing-agent systems can be prevented by following good personal hygiene and safety practices that include protection for the skin and eyes; good ventilation, including exhaust hood facilities; avoidance of inhalation of vapors; and use of fire prevention safeguards.

Pegum[33] has shown that epoxy resins penetrate rubber gloves. Better protection is obtained with heavy-duty vinyl gloves.

Epoxy resin can be removed by acetone, alcohol, or methyl ethyl ketone followed by acid-type cleansers and a conditioning cream; however, overuse of these solvents can provoke an irritant dermatitis.

Instructions for Patients Who Have Household Eczema ("Dishpan Hands")

1. Use long-handled brushes for dishwashing and for cleaning and scouring pots, stoves, and dishwashing machines.[34]
2. Heating and sweating inside a rubber glove may be as bad for the hands as the irritation from soaps and cleansers. White cotton gloves must be worn inside the rubber gloves. Loose-fitting gloves may be more comfortable and less irritating than gloves that fit snugly. Try not to wear rubber gloves for more than 30 minutes at a time. Do not put hands into very hot water when wearing rubber gloves, because the heat may penetrate the gloves and irritate the hands. Many patients have found that rubber gloves sometimes make their hands worse because they have become allergic to the rubber. If this occurs, switch to light-weight or heavy-duty vinyl gloves. Soak dishes in hot, soapy water for 30 minutes and let the water cool before washing so that the hands are not overheated by the hot water.
3. Bathe babies with one's bare hands, because soaps used for this purpose are mild and do not usually irritate the skin. If the hand dermatitis is acute and rubber gloves are worn, however, put a pair of cotton gloves over the rubber gloves so that the baby can be handled without danger of slipping through the wet rubber gloves.
4. Handling diapers, which contain much ammonia, may irritate the hands. Pick up such diapers with forceps or tongs, place them into a basin containing 1 teaspoon of boric acid powder to 1 quart of water, and allow them to remain in this solution for about 1 hour to neutralize the ammonia.
5. Wear cotton gloves to prevent the hands from getting excessively soiled while doing dry, dusty, and dirty housework. This makes the need for excessive cleaning of the hands unnecessary. If the fingertips are free of dermatitis, cut off the tips of the gloves to allow air to circulate about the hands and thereby prevent excessive sweating.

6. Contact of the hands with fruit juices, fruits, vegetables, and raw meats may irritate the skin. Use canned or frozen products until the hands are better. Avoid direct contact of the inflamed skin with the irritating juices of onions and garlic.

7. Wool causes itching and irritation in many individuals; contact with it should be minimized.

8. Avoid exposure of the hands to hair tonics and lotions. Use a brush or cotton-tipped swab to apply such preparations to the scalp.

9. When pouring or measuring detergents or bleaches, be careful that they do not splash onto the hands and forearms. Patients who have hand eczema should use bleaches in powder form or those that are premeasured and packaged in plastic containers.

10. Cleansing of the skin in hand dermatitis:

A. Do not use household cleansers on the hands. These products are made to remove dirt from dishes, clothes, walls, and floors and are too harsh for use on the skin. Also avoid the use of solvents such as turpentine or benzene. These chemicals are harsh because they defat the skin and cause marked dryness and cracking. Do not use deodorant soaps or antibacterial soaps, because they have chemicals that can irritate or cause allergic reactions. Use plain, unscented soaps. If the hands are dry, use a superfatted soap.

B. Avoid prolonged or too frequent washing of the skin. Gently pat the skin dry with a soft cloth or tissues. Avoid vigorous rubbing. Remember that some people seem to tolerate unlimited washings of the hands with soap and water, whereas others get dry and irritated skin even with minimal washing. Do not use soaps that sting and are excessively drying.

C. Even the mildest soap must be rinsed off the hands gently and thoroughly.

D. In the acute stage, when the hands are swollen and red, avoid cleansing the skin with soap. Bathe the hands in Burow's solution (1 part to 20 parts water). If the skin feels dry after this procedure, gently swab it with olive oil and apply the prescribed medication. Remove rings from fingers when washing the hands.

PRINCIPLES OF TREATMENT OF HAND DERMATITIS

The following directions are general guidelines only; they may need to be modified to suit individual cases.

1. Use an unscented soap or hand cleanser free of color, antiseptics, deodorants, vitamins, and tar.

2. Wash hands with lukewarm water and use the soap sparingly. Rinse hands thoroughly. Dry gently with a clean towel and do not forget to dry between the fingers. Wash the hands as infrequently as possible, preferably no more than two or three times daily.

3. Take off rings when washing hands. Soap caught under a ring may produce a flare-up of hand dermatitis.

4. Avoid hobbies or household chores that involve direct contact with solvents, turpentine, waxes, adhesives, and epoxy resins unless protective gloves can be worn.

5. Do not use strong corticosteroid topical medications over prolonged periods. These may produce skin atrophy.

6. If the skin is dry, a corticosteroid ointment gives better results than a cream. If an ointment is considered too messy, use a cream in the daytime and an ointment at night.

7. Wear thin polyethylene gloves at night for several hours to enhance the effect of the ointment and to prevent spread of the ointment to the bedclothes.

8. Avoid use of creams that contain anything you are shown to be allergic to on patch testing. Use a fragrance-free moisturizing cream liberally, as recommended by your physician.

9. Guidelines regarding gloves:

A. Plastic (vinyl) gloves are better protection against some chemicals than latex rubber gloves, to which some people become allergic. Try to limit the wearing of gloves to approximately 30 minutes or less at a time. Wear thin cotton gloves underneath vinyl gloves to absorb perspiration.

B. While doing dry, dusty, and dirty work, wear cotton gloves to prevent the hands from getting excessively soiled. Wash your gloves, not your hands.

C. Woolen gloves cause irritation of many people's hands.

D. Neither vinyl nor rubber gloves stop penetration of some chemicals, such as hair perming chemicals and many solvents. A plastic polymer glove, such as the 4-H Glove, is usually more protective against these chemicals.

10. Avoid handling the following items with bare hands:

A. Fruit juices and the inside of the skin of fruits; raw meats, fish, and vegetables, especially raw onions and garlic

B. Detergents, turpentine, and kerosene

C. Hair tonics (use a cotton-tipped swab or a brush.)

D. Shampoos (use vinyl gloves.)

GENERAL MEASURES IN MANAGEMENT OF HAND DERMATITIS

In addition to the special measures and instructions already suggested in this chapter, most patients who have contact dermatitis of the hands require antieczematous and antibacterial therapy and may benefit from the following suggestions.

- *Wet dressings:* In the acute phase, when itching, edema, and oozing are features, compresses with cold water to which crushed ice has been added are valuable, except in the presence of vascular disease of the hands, particularly Raynaud's syndrome. In the presence of infection, the addition of Burow's solution (1 tablespoon to a pint of cold water) is indicated. In most instances, it is inadvisable to use wet potassium permanganate dressings on the hands because it produces uncomfortable drying and crusting and discoloration of the nails, which may be embarrassing to the ambulatory patient. Another water additive used to make a wet dressing is Prophyllin Powder (Dystan), a copper-chlorophyll product that produces a soothing compress solution.
- *Proper cleansing:* Avoid excessive hand washing. The skin of the hands does not have to be cleansed completely before each application of a topical remedy. Only those scales, crusts, and debris that come away easily with gentle cleansing should be removed.
- *Topical medication:* Following the use of the wet dressings, topical corticosteroid medications may be applied to the hands. For ambulatory patients, creams may be used in the daytime, whereas ointments are applied overnight. Often, ointments are more effective than creams on the palms. Such ointments may be kept in place and their effect enhanced with plastic gloves, which are used for several hours at a time.
- Dermatitis of the hands readily becomes secondarily infected. Practically all fissured, crusted hand eczemas are infected and can benefit from antibiotic treatment. Fisher recommends a corticosteroid cream for daytime use and erythromycin ointment (Ilotycin) for nighttime use. Oral erythromycin or another antibiotics active against staphylococcal and streptococcal infections may be helpful.
- *Systemic treatment:* Systemic corticosteroid therapy may be indicated when the dermatitis of the hands is severe and spreading and does not respond quickly to topical remedies. In the absence of the usual contraindications to such therapy, 40 to 60 mg of prednisone or its equivalent may be given for several days. The dosage should be decreased by 10 to 15 mg every few days over a 10- to 14-day period. Such gradual tapering of steroid therapy prevents the rebound of the contact dermatitis that may take place when corticosteroid therapy is stopped too abruptly. Alternatively, 40 to 60 mg intramuscularly of triamcinolone acetonide (Kenalog and others) may be useful for its prolonged duration of action. The offending contac-

tant should be searched for and eliminated in order to prevent recurrences.

- *Treatment of fissures:* Fissures can be carefully coated with a cyanoacrylate glue such as Krazy Glue or Super Glue. Care must be taken that the fingers are not glued together.
- *Occlusive dressings:* In the chronic phase of a hand dermatitis, the use of corticosteroid ointments covered with an occlusive dressing such as Saran Wrap may expedite healing. This form of therapy should be avoided in individuals who have atopic backgrounds and who have hyperhidrosis.
- *Protective bandages:* The patient should avoid the use of Band-Aids and other adhesives directly on the skin. Light, white cotton gloves are useful to protect the hands and to keep topical remedies in place. Even an ordinary gauze bandage may irritate the skin of the hands. Soft, closely woven cotton or linen dressings are preferred.
- *Sedation:* For the tense, pruritic, sleepless patient, cyproheptadine hydrochloride (Periactin) 4 mg twice a day or hydroxyzine hydrochloride (Atarax) 10 mg three times daily may be prescribed for their antipruritic and sedative effects. Other antihistamines may be similarly used.
- *Scale reduction:* In thick, keratotic hand eczema, the following mixture may be useful: salicylic acid (2%), liquor carbonis detergens (LCD) (2%), hydrocortisone (2.5% cream) or triamcinolone (0.1% cream 60 g), and Velvachol (as much as suffices, up to 240 g).
- *Other treatments:* Hand PUVA or grenz ray therapy may be useful in stubborn chronic cases of hand eczema. Care must be taken with topical psoralen products because burning is more likely than with systemic psoralen administration.

References

1. Handa S, Bijaylaxmi S, Sharma VK. Oral hyposensitization in patients with contact dermatitis from *Parthenium hysterophorus*. Contact Dermatitis 2001;44:279.

2. Sharma VK, Chakrabarti A, Mahajan V. Azathioprine in the treatment of Parthenium dermatitis. Int J Dermatol 1998;37:299.

3. Verma KK, Bansal A, Sethuraman G. Partenium dermatitis treated with azathioprine weekly pulse doses. Indian J Dermatol Venereol Leprol 2006;72:24.

4. Hubbard VG, Goldsmith P. Garlic-fingered chefs. Contact Dermatitis 2005;52:165.

5. Wohrl S, Kriechbaumer N, Hemmer W, et al. A cream containing the chelator DTPA (diethylenetriaminepenta-acetic acid) can prevent contact allergic reactions to metals. Contact Dermatitis 2001;44:224.

6. Lindelof B, Wrangsjo K, Liden S. A double-blind study of grenz ray therapy in chronic eczema of the hands. Br J Dermatol 1987;117:77.

7. Lindelof B, Liden S, Lagerholm B. The effect of grenz rays on the expression of allergic contact dermatitis in man. Scand J Immunol 1985;21:463.

8. Lindelof B, Lindberg M. The effect of grenz rays on irritant skin reactions in man. Acta Derm Venereol 1987;67:128.

9. Duff M, Cruchfield III CE, Moore J, et al. Radiation therapy for chronic vesicular hand dermatitis. Dermatitis 2006;17:128.

10. Simons JR, Bohnen IJ, van der Valk PG. A left-right comparison of UVB phototherapy and topical photochemotherapy in bilateral chronic hand dermatitis after 6 weeks' treatment. Clin Exp Derm 1997;22:7.

11. Burke DA, Corey G, Storrs FJ. Psoralen plus UVA protocol for Compositae photosensitivity. Am J Contact Dermat 1996;7:171.

12. Granlund H, Erkko P, Reitamo S. Long-term follow-up of eczema patients treated with cyclosporine. Acta Derm Venereol 1998;78:40.

13. De Rie MA, Meinardi MM, Bos JD. Lack of efficacy of topical cyclosporin A in atopic dermatitis and allergic contact dermatitis. Acta Derm Venereol 1991;71:452.

14. Granlund H, Erkko P, Eriksson E, Reitamo S. Comparison of cyclosporine and topical betamethasone-17,21-dipropionate in the treatment of severe chronic hand eczema. Acta Derm Venereol 1996; 76:371.

15. Ausaneya U, Kawada A, Aragane Y. Itraconazole suppresses an elicitation phase of a contact hypersensitivity reaction. J Invest Dermatol 2006;126:1028.

16. Katagiri K, Arakawa S, Hatano Y, et al. Fexofenadine, an H1-receptor antagonist, partially but rapidly inhibits the itch of contact dermatitis induced by diphenylcyclopropenone in patients with alopecia areata. J Dermatol 2006;33:75.

17. Lauerma AI, Stein BD, Homey B, et al. Topical FK 506: suppression of allergic and irritant contact dermatitis in the guinea pig. Arch Dermatol Res 1994;286: 337.

18. Sengoku T, Moritak, Sakuma S, et al. Possible inhibitory mechanism of FK 506 (tacrolimus hydrate) ointment for atopic dermatitis based on animal models. Eur J Pharmacol 1999;379:183.

19. Fleischer AB Jr. Treatment of atopic dermatitis: role of tacrolimus ointment as a topical noncorticosteroidal therapy. J Allergy Clin Immunol 1999;104(3 pt 2):S126.

20. Belsito DV, Wilson DC, Warshaw E, et al. A prospective randomized clinical trail of 0.1% tacrolimus ointment in a model of chronic allergic contact dermatitis. J Am Acad Dermatol 2006;55:40.

21. Pacor ML, Di Lorenzo G, Martinelli N, et al. Tacrolimus ointment in nickel sulphate-induced steroid-resistant allergic contact dermatitis. Allergy Asthma Proc 2006;27:527.

22. Alomar A, Puig L, Gallardo CM, et al. Topical tacrolimus 0.1% ointment (Protopic ®) reverses nickel contact dermatitis elicited by allergen challenge to a similar degree to mometasone furoate 0.1% with greater suppression of late erythema. Contact Dermatitis 2004;49:185.

23. Amrol D, Keitel D, Hagaman D, et al. Topical pimecrolimus in the treatment of human allergic contact dermatitis. Ann Allergy Asthma Immunol 2003;91:563.

24. Meingassner JG, Fahrngruber H, Bavandi A. Pimecrolimus inhibits the elicitation phase but does not suppress the sensitization phase in murine contact hypersensitivity, in contrast to tacrolimus and cyclosporine A. J Invest Dermatol 2003;121:77.

25. Bhardwaj SS, Jaimes JP, Liu A, et al. A double-blind randomized placebo-controlled pilot study comparing topical immunomodulating agents and corticosteroids for treatment of experimentally induced nickel contact dermatitis. Dermatitis 2007;18:26.

26. Mastrolonardo M, Lopalco PL, Diaferio A. Topical immunotherapy with contact sensitizers: a model to study the natural history of delayed hypersensitivity. Contact Dermatitis 2002;47:216.

27. Francomano M, Seidenari S. Urticaria after topical immunotherapy with diphenylcyclopropenone. Contact Dermatitis 2002;47:310.

28. Gupta P, Freyschmidt-Paul P, Vitacolonna M, et al. A chronic contact eczema impedes migration of antigen-presenting cells in alopecia areata. J Invest Dermatol 2006;126:1559.

29. Namazi MR. Two novel molecular mechanisms to account for the therapeutic efficacy of contact dermatitis against alopecia areata. Int Immunopharmacol 2006;6:862.

30. Kroon S. Contact dermatitis from oleyl polypeptide in Ceruminex ear drops. Contact Dermatitis 1981;7:271.

31. Boxley JD, Dawber RP. Contact dermatitis to one ingredient of Xeruminex ear drops. Contact Dermatitis 1976;2:233.

32. Grice K, Johnstone CI. Contact dermatitis from Xerumenex. Br Med J 1972;1:508.

33. Pegum JS. Penetration of protective gloves by epoxy resin. Contact Dermatitis 1979;5:281.

34. Grimalt F, Romaguera C. Dry and fissured skin limited to the index finger of the right hand as a unique manifestation of housewife's dermatitis. Contact Dermatitis 1977;3:54.

CHAPTER 35

SPECIFIC INSTRUCTIONS FOR PATIENTS WITH COMMON CONTACT ALLERGENS

General Instructions for a Positive Patch Test

1. A positive test indicates that an adverse reaction may occur if your skin comes in contact with the identified substance. Usually this will be a rash that itches and persists for several days or even several weeks.

2. It is important to avoid direct skin contact with the allergen as no method like "allergy shots" to desensitize to this type of allergen is presently available.

3. When an allergen is avoided, improvement in skin rashes starts slowly, and in most cases the full benefit of the avoidance will occur within 3–6 weeks. However, with severe or prolonged dermatitis the full benefits may not be seen for up to 3 months.

4. Being in the same room or area with an allergen that has been identified by patch testing is generally not a problem unless the substance can be blown into the air or is extremely volatile. It must touch your skin for the dermatitis to occur.

5. The parts of the skin that come in greatest contact with the allergen will usually have the greatest amount of rash. Areas protected from direct exposure to the allergen will usually show less rash.

6. If avoidance of skin contact with materials thought to contain your allergen fails to result in improvement of your dermatitis within 3–6 weeks, then there must be other factors involved in causing your rash. There may be an additional allergen to worry about, or allergy may not be your only problem. Some people do not clear as quickly as others because they have "sensitive skin" that is more easily irritated by everyday, normally harmless exposures. Discuss this with your doctor.

Neomycin

You are allergic to neomycin. This antibiotic is a common ingredient in over-the-counter triple antibiotic ointments. Examples would be Neosporin, Neopolycin, and Mycitracin. It will be listed on the ingredient label. Betadine ointment is a chemically unrelated antibiotic that you could substitute for neomycin. Also, two prescription ointments (called mupirocin and retapulmin) are safe for you. Let all your doctors know that you are allergic to neomycin and related antibiotics. These include gentamicin and tobramycin and are called aminoglycosides. You should avoid these as well.

Benzocaine

You are allergic to benzocaine. This is an anesthetic and is used to numb the skin or make the nerve endings in the skin less sensitive. It is commonly found in skin care products for burns, cuts, sores, and rashes. Benzocaine is a common ingredient found in medication for teething babies, hemorrhoidal preparations, and some cough and sore throat medications. Many other anesthetics that end in "caine" may also cause your skin to break out, but one that is safe for use is lidocaine (Xylocaine). You should let your doctor know you are allergic to benzocaine so that no such materials are used on your skin, mouth, or gums at the dentist's or doctor's office or in any of your prescriptions. Always check labels for this, as it will be noted if it is present.

Thimerosal

You are allergic to thimerosal. This is also known as Merthiolate. Some immunizations contain thimerosal that can lead to local reactions (such as soreness at the injection site), but serious systemic reactions almost never occur. Most products with thimerosal are used on moist areas of the body, such as around the eyes, ears, nose, and genital areas. Contact lens solutions and other eye, ear, and nasal medications may be sources of thimerosal.

Imidazolidinyl Urea

The substance to which you are allergic is one that will normally be found on labels. If you are purchasing anything for use on your skin, first inspect the package for the ingredient list. If you have products at home that do not have a label or the container does not list the ingredients, it would be best to go to the store where the product was purchased and inspect the original package. In the United States, products that are sold for consumer use on the skin as a cosmetic or toiletry item must be labeled with the ingredients listed in decreasing order of concentration. The first item listed is present in the greatest concentration, and the last listed is at the lowest concentration. Many of the allergenic materials are present in very low concentrations and are listed near the end of the ingredient list. Products sold as medical devices at present only have to reveal the "active" ingredients.

Sometimes a product will contain so little of a material that you are allergic to that skin contact may be harmless. However, you cannot count on this and should try to avoid all the products that have the potential to cause trouble.

You are allergic to imidazolidinyl urea. This is a preservative commonly used in skin care products. By reading labels, you should be very successful at avoiding this allergen. A similar preservative called diazolidinyl urea should probably also be avoided, because many, but not all, people who are allergic to one may react to both.

Quaternium-15

The substance to which you are allergic is one that will normally be found on labels. If you are purchasing anything for use on your skin, first inspect the package for the ingredient list. If you have products at home that do not have a label or the container does not list the ingredients, it would be best to go to the store where the product was purchased and inspect the original package. In the United States, products that are sold for consumer use on the skin as a cosmetic or toiletry item must be labeled with the ingredients listed in decreasing order of concentration. The first item listed is present in the greatest concentration, and the last listed is at the lowest concentration.

Many of the allergenic materials are present in very low concentrations and are listed near the end of the ingredient list. Products sold as medical devices at present only have to reveal the "active" ingredients.

Sometimes a product will contain so little of a material that you are allergic to that skin contact may be harmless. However, you cannot count on this and should try to avoid all the products that have the potential to cause trouble.

You are allergic to quaternium-15, which is a preservative. It is also used to purify some water-soluble coolants in industrial settings. In industry, it is known as Dowicil 200. Quaternium compounds with other numbers are usually totally different and generally not of concern. It may be present in products frequently recommended by dermatologists, but you should avoid these if quaternium-15 is on the label.

Lanolin

The substance to which you are allergic is one that will normally be found on labels. If you are purchasing anything for use on your skin, first inspect the package for the ingredient list. If you have products at home that do not have a label or the container does not list the ingredients, it would be best to go to the store where the product was purchased and inspect the original package. In the United States, products that are sold for consumer use on the skin as a cosmetic or toiletry item must be labeled with the ingredients listed in decreasing order of concentration. The first item listed is present in the greatest concentration, and the last listed is at the lowest concentration. Many of the allergenic materials are present in very low concentrations and are listed near the end of the ingredient list. Products sold as medical devices at present only have to reveal the "active" ingredients.

Sometimes a product will contain so little of a material of which you are allergic that skin contact may be harmless. However, you cannot count on this and should try to avoid all the products that have the potential to cause trouble.

You are allergic to lanolin, which is also known as wool alcohol or wool wax alcohol. Another very similar chemical that you should avoid is called Amerchol. Prudence would dictate avoidance of all lanolin products, especially on areas where the skin is already irritated.

Rubber Allergens

You have been found to be allergic to a rubber chemical. Although some forms of rubber are familiar, others are not. Elastic materials are generally rubber based and may contain your allergen. Rubber cements are used to hold together many items where flexibility is required, such as shoes. Adhesives and tapes may contain these materials, as may hoses and belts.

Some rubber allergens are found in agricultural products, such as fungicides, although others may be found in pet care products. Some polyurethane foam rubber products have been found to contain these allergens. Cloth-covered foam materials and clothing that contains spandex are other possible sources.

Specific rubber allergen groups are listed below.

MERCAPTOBENZOTHIAZOLE AND MERCAPTO MIX

In addition to the above, pay attention to pesticides, animal repellents, and veterinarian products.

THIURAM MIX

May be found in Playtex rubber gloves. Cotton liners do not protect against this allergen. May also be found in fungicides and the prescription drug Antabuse.

CARBA MIX

Also found in the same items noted for thiuram mix. Both have been found in polyurethane foam rubber. Might cross-react with iodopropynyl butylcarbamate, a preservative in skin care products.

BLACK RUBBER MIX

This is more common in industrial black rubber and automobile tires. Sometimes other colors of rubber contain these chemicals. These allergens have been found in some undergarment elastic. Some persons allergic to this mix have problems from dyes used on synthetic fabrics, such as rayon, polyester, and acrylics.

If you are having a problem with gloves, vinyl gloves do not contain rubber chemicals and should be safe for you.

Cinnamic Alcohol and Aldehyde

You are allergic to a form of cinnamon (either cinnamic alcohol or cinnamic aldehyde). This is both a flavor and a fragrance. Use of unscented or fragrance-free products is necessary to minimize skin contact with cinnamon. Sometimes cinnamon is part of a mixture of flavor chemicals and not readily apparent by taste or smell.

Ingestion of cinnamon-flavored items may cause some, but not all, cinnamon-sensitive people to have a rash or itching. If you feel this is a possible cause for your symptoms, you should avoid obvious cinnamon-flavored

food and beverage items, as well as colas, sweet vermouth, bitters, and chocolate.

Cassia oil is another name for these allergens.

Epoxy Resin

You are allergic to epoxy resin. This is generally found in two-part glue and paints or other coatings that have to be mixed shortly before use. Dentists use epoxies; therefore, you should inform your dentist of your allergy. Sometimes epoxy resin may remain in some plastics. If you are concerned about a plastic item, it must come in contact with your skin and the rash should occur at this site. Heated epoxy resins may become fumes that lead to rashes on sensitive exposed skin, such as the eyelids.

Paratertiary Butylphenol Formaldehyde Resin

You are allergic to paratertiary butylphenol formaldehyde resin. This is found in glues, such as those used in shoes and other adhesives. Rubber items may contain this substance. It has also been found in duplicating paper, printing inks, and some plastics. Some handles on cookware are made of plastic containing this allergen. Some plywood is glued together with it. Commercial deodorants and commercial germicidal detergents may contain it. It is also often found in adhesives used for leather goods, such as wallets, wristwatch straps, and handbags.

Colophony

You are allergic to colophony or rosin. This is obtained from the sap of pine trees. It is frequently used to make things sticky, such as glues and adhesives. Adhesive tape is one example. Polish for furniture, floors, and cars may contain colophony. Solder used in electronics often contains rosin, as does some welding flux. Paper products contain colophony, as does printer's ink. Some putty and wood doughs are sources of this allergen. The rosin bag on the pitcher's mound and rosin for violin bows are familiar sources of this allergen. Occasionally, cosmetics may contain colophony, especially eye cosmetics.

Paraphenylenediamine

You are allergic to paraphenylenediamine. This is a dark dye usually found in hair dyes. The most common problem with this allergen is in dying hair. It can similarly cause problems if it gets on your skin while you are dying other objects, such as furs or cloth. Photographic chemicals may contain paraphenylenediamine. Some clothing dyes may cause reactions, but for this to explain your rash, the skin that has the rash would have to be the skin contacted by the suspect clothing. Similarly, some rubber goods may have chemical contents that will cause your skin to develop a rash. Some industrial chemicals that are found in rubber may be chemical cousins to this allergen and cause rashes when in contact with skin.

The labels on hair dyes may have names that are somewhat different from paraphenylenediamine, but cause just as much of a problem. Avoid the following:

p-toluenediamine
1,4-benzenediamine
p-aminodiphenylamine
1,4-phenylenediamine
2,4-diaminoanisole
p-ami noaniline
o-aminophenol

Some people with this allergy also have trouble with sulfa drugs and sunscreens based on PABA (para-aminobenzoic acid). Others may have trouble with anesthetics such as benzocaine. Your doctor should tell you if these are concerns in your case.

Henna is a safe hair coloring, but some henna products, especially temporary tattoos, contain PPDA. Also, most people allergic to this chemical can tolerate semi-permanent hair coloring rinses.

Formaldehyde

You are allergic to formaldehyde. Skin contact with formaldehyde is required for this to cause a rash. Avoid contact with items that list formaldehyde as an ingredient on the label. Some formaldehyde-sensitive persons cannot tolerate even the tiniest amount of skin contact with formaldehyde, but most are not this severely sensitive. There are five commonly used topical preservatives that are in the formaldehyde family: quaternium-15, imidazolidinyl urea, diazolidinyl urea, bronopol, and DMDM hydantoin. Most formaldehyde-allergic people need to avoid all of these, but occasionally you may tolerate a product with a low level of one of these.

If your occupation brings you in contact with some of the following circumstances, you may be getting formaldehyde on your skin and causing rashes: embalming fluid; photographic chemicals; industrial disinfectants and fumigations; automotive fluids; medical dialysis fluids; paints; leather processing; some printing processes such as etching. The manufacturing process of plastics and plywood is often a source of formaldehyde exposure to workers.

Fumes of formaldehyde will not usually cause difficulty because the concentration is so low. If your rash is in skin exposed to air and the most sensitive areas of that exposed skin are a prominent part of your problem, then fumes of formaldehyde may be of concern. Smoke from fires or cigarettes will contain formaldehyde.

Clothing that is "permanent press" is treated with formaldehyde-related materials. You should generally avoid wearing any permanent-press treated clothing. You may tolerate wearing loose, cool permanent press clothes for a short period occasionally.

Ethylenediamine

You are allergic to ethylenediamine. This chemical is an ingredient in the original formula of Mycolog Cream. The company that makes Mycolog no longer makes a formula that contains your allergen. Mycolog II is safe for use from an allergen standpoint. However, the generic forms of Mycolog are made with the original formula, which should be avoided.

If you have asthma, your doctor may wish to give you an intravenous medication that is known as aminophylline. It breaks down into your allergen and should be avoided. You should let your doctor know about your allergy.

Some medicines used for itching may cause you to have a rash. They are chemically almost identical with ethylenediamine and may be mistaken as the same chemical by your body. It may be wise to avoid these closely related materials, which are in the antihistamine category:

hydroxyzine (Atarax, Visteril)
tripelennamine (Pyribenzamine)
meclizine (Bonine, Antivert)
chlorcyclizine (Mantadil)
cyclizine (Marezine)
buclizine (Bucladin-S)

There are industrial exposures that may apply to your case if you work with electroplating, film developing chemicals, some dying processes, and some other solvents. Epoxy hardeners often contain chemicals related to ethylenediamine. If you work with epoxy glues, coatings, paints, or plastics you may come into contact with ethylenediamine.

Myroxylon Pereirae (formerly called Balsam of Peru)

You are allergic to *Myroxylon pereirae* (Balsam of Peru). This is a sweet-smelling natural substance from pine or fir trees. Allergy to balsam of Peru most frequently means that you are allergic to a fragrance chemical or perfume. However, because this is a natural product and contains many different substances, it is difficult to be exact as to which fragrance chemical is at fault. The prudent person would avoid scented products and favor fragrance-free or unscented ones instead.

Some medical products will contain balsam of Peru, and it may be listed on the ingredient label in some cases. Check products that may be used in the diaper area and for hemorrhoid treatment. There are closely related chemicals that enjoy a medical use, such as benzoin and benzyl alcohol, and if these appear on the label of a skin care product, it would be best to avoid them.

Naturally occurring ingredients in foods may contain substances so closely related or identical to substances present in balsam of Peru that when ingested they may cause your rash. If avoiding external sources of balsam of Peru has not resulted in clearing of your problem, then a period of dietary avoidance of the substances listed below may be worthwhile. (Dietary restrictions may take 3 to 4 weeks to show benefit. If you improve, you should add back one food per week to see if avoidance really makes any difference. Frequently, only one or two foods are truly found to be at fault, but it is still necessary to eliminate all the other possible causes for the diet restrictions to be properly evaluated.)

Avoid citrus peel and related flavors in any food, such as candy, gum, baked goods, spiced teas, tobaccos, ice cream, cola, and citrus soft drinks. Avoid spices, such as cinnamon, cloves, vanilla, curry, tomato ketchup, chili sauce, chutney, pickled herring, pickled vegetables, paté, vermouth, and bitters.

Potassium Dichromate

You are allergic to chromates. This allergen is found in a variety of substances. The powdered form of cement and some wet cement contain chromates that cause problems mainly for members of the construction trades. If the powdered form of cement is blown by wind onto your skin, a rash may develop on the exposed areas; otherwise, direct skin contact with the material is required for a rash to develop. Other construction materials including brick, mortar, and drywall may contain chromates. Leather goods are treated with chromates and may cause you to have a rash. This is usually a problem when the leather becomes wet by sweat or moisture from other sources. Some chromate-allergic people have no trouble with leather shoes as long as they wear socks and their shoes do not get wet.

Coatings used to prevent rust generally are chromates and must be kept off your skin. These are used in industry to galvanize sheet metal and protect metals in general, and they are also found in home-use rust preventatives. Yellow and green paints are also a potential source of chromates. Other items may be of concern, such as some textiles, cosmetics, and the green felt on pool tables, and nongreen items such as blueprints, lithography fluids, match heads, and wood preservatives.

Kathon (Methylchloroisothiazolinone/Methylisothiazolinone)

This preservative is in common use in many shampoos, cleansers, and especially in cosmetic and skin care products. Usually the name Kathon is not listed on the label, but the longer name noted above (methylchloroisothiazolinone/methylisothiazolinone) is what you will see on the label. You need to read very carefully to be sure you do not use any products that contain this chemical. This chemical is used in industry in water-cooling plants and metalworking fluids.

Nickel

You are allergic to nickel. This metal allergen accounts for most, but not all, costume jewelry reactions. Nickel objects often are shiny and appear chrome plated. Not all metal will contain nickel. Direct skin contact with the metal object containing nickel will cause a rash at that specific site. For example, metal eyelash curlers may cause eyelid rashes. Cleaning your ears with a metal bobby pin may cause ear canal rashes. Metal pins and snaps in clothing may cause spots of itchy, reddened skin at such sites, such as around the belly button.

Stainless steel contains nickel, but it is so tightly bound to the metal that it takes much longer contact to cause problems. In general, it takes about 3 minutes of skin contact with a common metal object to start to move the nickel from the metal into your skin. Wet contact with metal will shorten the length of time for the transfer to occur and start a rash.

A test kit is available called the dimethylglyoxime test (DMGO). This kit will allow you to test metal items for the presence of nickel at home or work. Keep in mind that nickel will go through rubber gloves with or without cotton liners. Avoidance of skin contact is the key to getting better.

DIET INSTRUCTIONS FOR NICKEL-SENSITIVE PEOPLE

Sometimes after avoiding all skin contact with an allergen, such as nickel or chromate, the rash may persist. In some cases, the same amounts of these allergens that occur naturally in foods will be responsible for the rash continuing. When this is the case, it is necessary to avoid the foods listed below for 3 to 4 weeks to rid the body of a continued stimulation that could be causing the rash. If your skin improves with the diet, you may add back one food per week to see if your rash returns or flares. This will confirm the importance of continuing to avoid the food in question. It will also ensure that you are not needlessly giving up a food you enjoy. Frequently, only one or two food items will be critical to your getting better. It is necessary to begin with strict avoidance of all the possibilities in order to determine the role of diet in your care.

Various food items and drinks can aggravate nickel eczema even though the nickel content of these foods may be low. Such food items include beer, wine (in particular, red wine), herring, mackerel, tuna, tomato, onion, carrot, and certain fruits, in particular, apples and citrus fruits (juice). The vegetables mentioned can usually be tolerated when cooked.

The first liter (quart) of water taken from the tap in the morning should not be used in food preparation, as nickel may be released from the tap during the night.

These foods are OK	Avoid these foods	These foods are OK	Avoid these foods
Meat, fish, etc.		Cornflakes	products
Eggs	Shellfish, such as shrimp,	Cornmeal	Multigrain breads
Fish	mussels, and crawfish	Cornstarch	Oatmeal
Meat (all kinds)		Macaroni	Rice (unpolished)
Poultry		Popcorn	Rye bran
Dairy products		Rice (polished, white rice	Sesame seeds
Butter	Chocolate milk	in moderation)	Sunflower seeds
Cheese		Spaghetti	Wheat bran and other bran
Milk in all forms		Wheat flour	and fiber products,
Yogurt (unflavored)		Whole grain rye and wheat	including cereals, bran
Vegetables		bread (in moderation)	biscuits, and fiber tablets
Asparagus	Beans (green, brown, white)		Whole grain breads and biscuits
Beets, red		*Fruit, berries, etc.*	
Broccoli	Kale		
Brussels sprouts	Leeks	Bananas (in moderation)	Dates
Cabbage, white	Lentils	Berries (all except	Figs
Cauliflower	Lettuce	raspberries)	Pineapple
Chinese cabbage	Peas (green and split)	Peaches	Prunes
Corn	Soy protein powder (used	Pears	Raspberries
Cucumber	in sausages, sandwich	Raisins	
Dill	meat, products made	Rhubarb	
Eggplant	from minced meat,	*Drinks*	
Garlic (in moderation)	bread, soup	Alcoholic beverages (distilled products	Chocolate and cocoa drinks
		and drinks made from these)	Tea from drink dispensers
Mushrooms	concentrates,	Carbonated beverages	
Onions (in moderation)	bouillon, etc.)	Coffee and tea (not too strong	
		and in moderation)	
Parsley	Spinach	*Miscellaneous*	
Peppers, green, red	Sprouts made from beans	Margarine	Almonds
Potatoes	and alfalfa	Yeast	Baking powder (in large amounts)
Grains and grain products			Hazel nuts and other nuts
Breakfast foods made of rice	Bran		Linseed, linseed oil
Cakes and biscuits not	Buckwheat		Peanuts
containing almonds or	Millet		Sweets containing chocolate,
			marzipan, nuts, and strong licorice
other nuts, cocoa, or	Muesli and other similar		Vitamins containing nickel
chocolate	breakfast cereal		

Nickel-plated kitchen utensils, such as eggbeaters and tea balls, should be replaced.

Acid foods, such as stewed fruits and rhubarb, cooked in stainless-steel utensils should be avoided. The acids in the foods can cause nickel to be released from the utensils. Tinned foods should be eaten only in moderation.

Provided by: Niels K. Veien, MD, PhD, The Dermatology Clinic, Vesterbro 99, DK-9000 Alborg, Denmark.

Cobalt

This is a metal found in some costume jewelry and other everyday inexpensive metal objects. More often it is found in "hard metal" objects such as industrial drills, cutting tools, etc. In addition, it may be found in construction materials such as concrete, drywall, brick, and mortar. Occasionally, it is found in cosmetics as a coloring agent and may be found in wet, uncured pottery.

Many individuals allergic to cobalt are also allergic to nickel and chromate. These metals also are often found in jewelry and construction materials, as noted above. Cobalt is occasionally used in industry in the manufacture of plastic and rubber materials, but this should only be a problem for workers in these industries, not for consumers handling plastic or rubber.

Cocamidopropyl Betaine

This is a substance found in many skin care products, especially soaps, shampoos, and hair conditioners, but also other products, including skin lotions, makeup removers, and even contact lens cleaners. This chemical is called a surfactant, which means it is used to help dissolve oils and to let other substances mix together. It should be fairly easy to avoid this substance because it should be listed on labeling by this name.

It may also be found in some household cleaning products.

Fragrances

Fragrance allergy may be difficult to deal with because there are literally several hundred individual chemicals, both natural and synthetic, that are used in fragrances. A person who is allergic to fragrances on patch testing may have problems with perfumes and colognes but also with the fragrances in other skin and hair care products, laundry products, and so on. Therefore, individuals with a fragrance allergy should use fragrance-free products as much as possible. If an individual wishes to use a fragrance-containing product, the product should be site tested by applying a small amount of the product to the inside of one elbow twice a day in the same spot for 7 days. If no redness or itching develops at that site, then that particular fragrance-containing product is probably safe for use.

It is generally not advised that individuals with a fragrance allergy apply fragrance materials to their clothing. Some individuals with a fragrance allergy may develop dermatitis when eating certain foods and spices in the family of balsams. Your doctor can discuss this more fully with you if this is suspected.

Glutaraldehyde

This chemical is also called glutaral. This is a sterilizing solution and preservative that is commonly found in medical and dental offices. It is occasionally used in dental products and shampoos. It is commonly found in industrial hand cleaners as a disinfectant. It is also present in embalming fluid and is used as a tanning agent for some leather products. Many people have problems from exposure to medical and dental instruments that have been cleaned with this chemical. It is also used as an agent in some photographic processes.

Glyceryl Thioglycolate

This is a chemical that is the main ingredient in most currently used hair permanent solutions that are known as acid perms or heat perms. There is an older permanent solution that contains another chemical called ammonium thioglycolate. Most people who are allergic to the glyceryl thioglycolate can tolerate ammonium thioglycolate. Unfortunately, glyceryl thioglycolate is a chemical that penetrates normal rubber gloves; therefore, these do not protect individuals from this chemical. 4-H gloves provide a good barrier and will not allow the chemical to penetrate. These can be obtained from commercial glove suppliers.

Gold

Gold allergy is much more common than previously believed. Obviously, some people will react at sites where their skin comes in contact with gold jewelry, such as the ears, fingers, and neck. However, some people do not react on the hands because the skin there is relatively strong and does not break out as easily. Some individuals will develop dermatitis on the face, eyelids, or other sensitive areas of the body just by touching and wearing gold jewelry. Because these areas are more sensitive, occasional contact of jewelry on the skin can cause problems. It is recommended that people who are allergic to gold should avoid wearing gold jewelry as much as possible. Use on special occasions for short times is probably acceptable. Platinum or sterling silver can be worn safely, but white gold should be avoided as well. For special jewelry items an individual may wish to wear, a jeweler can usually plate the back of the jewelry with rhodium or platinum, which helps to block the contact of gold with the skin. Many individuals with gold allergy have gold dental work. It is unlikely that gold dental work will cause problems on the skin. However, if an individual has mouth sores in areas of contact with gold dental work, then this problem may be helped by changing to a dental filling to which the patient is not allergic. In addition, there are some cases of lichen planus that have been shown to be related to gold allergy in dental work.

Parabens

These are chemicals that are commonly used as preservatives to kill microorganisms in skin and hair care products. You will often see a prefix before the word "paraben" on label ingredients, such as "butyl" or "propyl." Any of the parabens must be avoided. Occasionally, these chemicals may be used as preservatives in medications taken internally. If there is any question about this, your pharmacist should be consulted, and he or she should be able to determine if parabens are present in a medication you are taking. Sometimes individuals can tolerate using a preparation that contains these chemicals on normal skin, but if the same preparation is used on skin that is already irritated, then an allergic reaction may develop. Also, sensitive areas such as the face are more likely to react than other skin surfaces.

Propylene Glycol

This is a thick, liquid substance that is used in many skin care products and cosmetics as a thickener and to give an antibacterial effect. It should be in the ingredient list on products. It is also found in many prescription and over-the-counter cortisone-type creams. In addition, propylene glycol may be used as a swimming pool or mobile home antifreeze. It is also used in some food products, especially condiments, salad dressings, and prepared baked goods. However, it is sometimes found in other unexpected food products, such as some cake mixes. It should be included in food ingredient labeling. In most cases, individuals allergic to propylene glycol do not need to avoid other glycols, including butylene glycol, hexylene glycol, and polyethylene glycol. As with other allergens, sometimes you may tolerate skin contact

with products that contain only a low level of this chemical- but it is safest to avoid it entirely if possible.

Diazolidinyl Urea

The substance to which you are allergic is one that will normally be found on labels. If you are purchasing anything for use on your skin, first inspect the package for the ingredient list. If you have products at home that do not have a label or the container does not list the ingredients, it would be best to go to the store where the product was purchased and inspect the original package. In the United States, products that are sold for consumer use on the skin as a cosmetic or toiletry must be labeled with the ingredients listed in decreasing order of concentration. The first item listed is present in the greatest concentration, and the last listed is at the lowest concentration. Many of the allergenic materials are present in very low concentrations and are listed near the end of the ingredient list. Products sold as medical devices at present only have to reveal the "active" ingredients.

Sometimes a product will contain so little of a material to which you are allergic that skin contact may be harmless. However, you cannot count on this and should try to avoid all the products that have the potential to cause trouble.

You are allergic to diazolidinyl urea. This is a preservative commonly used in skin care products. By reading labels, you should be very successful at avoiding this allergen.

Bacitracin

You are allergic to bacitracin. This antibiotic is a common ingredient in over-the-counter triple antibiotic ointments. Examples are be Neosporin, Neo-Polycin, and Mycitracin. Bacitracin is also available by itself. It will be listed on the ingredient label. Povidone-iodine ointment is a chemically unrelated antibiotic that you could substitute for bacitracin. Two prescription antibiotic ointments, mupirocin and retapulmin can be used instead of bacitracin.

Budesonide

You are allergic to budesonide, a type of corticosteroid or cortisone that is a marker for allergy to a wide range of cortisone products. It would be best to avoid the following corticosteroids, even though some of them may be safe for use on your skin surface. Avoid triamcinolone, amcinonide, fluocinolone acetonide, halcinonide, flucinonide, desonide, and any others that end with the letters "...ide". There may be corticosteroids that you can safely take. Cortisone allergy is not as rare as once believed, and many doctors are unfamiliar with cortisone allergy. Internal cortisones that you may be able to safely take include dexamethasone, hydrocortisone, prednisone. Check with your doctor for others.

Tixocortol-21-Pivalate

You are allergic to a corticosteroid known as tixocortol-21-pivalate. The cortisone is representative of a class of cortisone that you should avoid. The more common members of this class are hydrocortisone, prednisone, prednisolone, and methylprednisolone. There may be other cortisones that you can safely take, but these are best avoided. Cortisone allergy is something with which many doctors are unfamiliar. It is not as rare as once believed. High doses of cortisones like prednisone may appear to give benefit because of their pharmacological properties, but as the dose is reduced, the immunologic reaction (allergy) becomes apparent. Potentially safer internal corticosteroids include dexamethasone and betamethasone, but you should check with your doctor about this.

Mixed Dialkyl Thioureas

Diethyl thiourea and dibutyl thiourea are included in the allergen referred to as mixed dialkyl thioureas. These are chemicals added to neoprene rubber products. Common sources of exposure to these chemicals are rubber weather stripping, wet suits for diving, some polyvinyl chloride adhesives, neoprene rubber gloves, orthopedic knee and elbow sleeves, and the insoles of athletic shoes. Industrial anticorrosive compounds may contain these thioureas, as may some industrial detergents. Diazo copy paper, which is used for industrial textile patterns and architectural plans, also contains these agents. They may be found in other types of rubber in addition to neoprene.

Tosylamide Formaldehyde Resin

You are allergic to a chemical found in nail polish. This material imparts durability to the polish and is not associated with any specific color. It is even found in clear nail polish. You should choose a nail polish that does not contain this material, such as Clinique and Almay nail polishes. You may also check the labels of nail polish of other companies to determine if they will be safe for your use. Older bottles of nail polish may list this ingredient under the name toluene-sulfonamide formaldehyde resin. The new name is tosylamide formaldehyde resin, but the ingredient is the same.

Ethyleneurea Melamine Formaldehyde Resin

You are allergic to a chemical used to make fabric wrinkle resistant or permanent press. This allergen will not appear on the label of the garments you buy. Several very closely related chemicals are also used to make fabrics wrinkle resistant, and because they are all very similar chemically, you should avoid all permanent press clothing. These chemicals are related to formaldehyde, to which you may also be sensitive.

Some types of fabric are more likely to be treated with your allergen. These include cotton-polyester blends, 100% cotton wrinkle-resistant fabrics, wrinkle-resistant linen, shrink-proof woolens, rayon, corduroy, and any blends of cotton, rayon, wool, or other synthetic or natural fibers. It is important to remember that 100% cotton is not a guarantee of safety, as cotton can be treated with these chemicals. If a garment wrinkles and requires ironing, it is likely to be safe.

Fabrics that are unlikely to be treated with these chemicals include 100% cotton denim, 100% linen, 100% silk, 100% polyester, 100% nylon, and 100% ultrasuede.

Chloroxylenol

The substance to which you are allergic is one that will normally be found on labels. If you are purchasing anything for use on your skin, first inspect the package for the ingredient list. If you have products at home that do not have a label or the container does not list the ingredients, it would be best to go to the store where the product was purchased and inspect the original package. In the United States, products that are sold for consumer use on the skin as a cosmetic or toiletry must be labeled with the ingredients listed in decreasing order of concentration. The first item listed is present in the greatest concentration, and the last listed is at the lowest concentration. Many of the allergenic materials are present in very low concentrations and are listed near the end of the ingredient list. Products sold as medical devices at present only have to reveal the "active" ingredients.

Sometimes a product will contain so little of a material to which you are allergic that skin contact may be harmless. However, you cannot count on this and should try to avoid all the products that have the potential to cause trouble.

You are allergic to chloroxylenol. This is a preservative commonly used in skin care products. By reading labels, you should be very successful at avoiding this allergen. It may be found in products such as burn remedies, hair dressings, Absorbine Jr., carbolated Vaseline, feminine hygiene products, and in some prescription topical corticosteroids. It is found in powders such as ZeaSORB, Desitin, and Aveeno. It is also known as PCMX, p-chloro-meta-xylenol, and 4-chloro-3,4-xylenol.

Iodopropynyl Butylcarbamate

The substance to which you are allergic is one that will normally be found on labels. If you are purchasing anything for use on your skin, first inspect the package for the ingredient list. If you have products at home that do not have a label or the container does not list the ingredients, it would be best to go to the store where the product was purchased and inspect the original package. In the United States, products that are sold for consumer use on the skin as a cosmetic or toiletry must be labeled with the ingredients listed in decreasing order of concentration. The first item listed is present in the greatest concentration, and the last listed is at the lowest connection. Many of the allergenic materials are present in very low concentrations and are listed near the end of the ingredient list. Products sold as medical devices at present only have to reveal the "active" ingredients.

Sometimes a product will contain so little of a material to which you are allergic that skin contact may be harmless. However, you cannot count on this and should try to avoid all the products that have the potential to cause trouble.

You are allergic to iodopropynyl butylcarbamate. This is a preservative commonly used in skin care products. By reading labels, you should be very successful at avoiding this allergen.

2-Bromo-2-Nitropropane-1,3-Diol

The substance to which you are allergic is one that will normally be found on labels. If you are purchasing anything for use on your skin, first inspect the package for the ingredient list. If you have products at home that do not have a label or the container does not list the ingredients, it would be best to go to the store where the product was purchased and inspect the original package. In the United States, products that are sold for consumer use on the skin as a cosmetic or toiletry must be labeled with the ingredients listed in decreasing order of concentration. The first item listed is present in the greatest concentration, and the last listed is at the lowest concentration. Many of the allergenic materials are present in very low concentrations and are listed near the end of the ingredient list.

Products sold as medical devices at present only have to reveal the "active" ingredients.

Sometimes a product will contain so little of a material to which you are allergic that skin contact may be harmless. However, you cannot count on this and should try to avoid all the products that have the potential to cause trouble.

You are allergic to 2-bromo-2-nitropropane-1,3-diol. This is a biocide and preservative. It can be found in skin care products and is used in industry to prevent the growth of microorganisms in water-based fluids such as coolants used by machinists. By reading labels, you should be very successful at avoiding this allergen in consumer products. The material safety data sheet on water-soluble coolants should be consulted for the presence of this material in industry. Industrially, it may be referred to as Bronopol.

Methyldibromoglutaronitrile

The substance to which you are allergic is one that will normally be found on labels. If you are purchasing anything for use on your skin, first inspect the package for the ingredient list. If you have products at home that do not have a label or the container does not list the ingredients, it would be best to go to the store where the product was purchased and inspect the original package. In the United States, products that are sold for consumer use on the skin as a cosmetic or toiletry must be labeled with the ingredients listed in decreasing order of concentration. The first item listed is present in the greatest concentration, and the last listed is at the lowest concentration. Many of the allergenic materials are present in very low concentrations and are listed near the end of the ingredient list. Products sold as medical devices at present only have to reveal the "active" ingredients.

Sometimes a product will contain so little of a material to which you are allergic that skin contact may be harmless. However, you cannot count on this and should try to avoid all the products that have the potential to cause trouble.

You are allergic to methyldibromoglutaronitrile. This is a preservative commonly used in skin care products. By reading labels, you should be very successful at avoiding this allergen. You may find this listed on labels as methyldibromoglutaronitrile/phenoxyethanol. This is another form of your allergen, and you should avoid this too. Some Lubriderm products contain this material, as may other skin care products. In some countries this compound is called dibromodicyanobutane+phenoxyethanol. Another name for this chemical is Euxyl K 400.

DMDM Hydantoin

The substance to which you are allergic is one that will normally be found on labels. If you are purchasing anything for use on your skin, first inspect the package for the ingredient list. If you have products at home that do not have a label or the container does not list the ingredients, it would be best to go to the store where the product was purchased and inspect the original package. In the United States, products that are sold for consumer use on the skin as a cosmetic or toiletry must be labeled with the ingredients listed in decreasing order of concentration. The first item listed is present in the greatest concentration, and the last listed is at the lowest concentration. Many of the allergenic materials are present in very low concentrations and are listed near the end of the ingredient list. Products sold as medical devices at present only have to reveal the "active" ingredients.

Sometimes a product will contain so little of a material to which you are allergic that skin contact may be harmless. However, you cannot count on this and should try to avoid all the products that have the potential to cause trouble.

You are allergic to DMDM hydantoin. This is a preservative commonly used in skin care products. By reading labels, you should be very successful at avoiding this allergen.

PLATE 1

Figure 2-1: Example of an irritant reaction to a non-standard patch test chemical. Note the turbid, pustular quality of the bulla.

Figure 2-2: A remarkably strong 3+ reaction to gold sodium thiosulfate in a renal transplant patient who was taking oral tacrolimus, mycophenolate mofetil, and prednisone to prevent transplant rejection.

Figure 2-3: Dishydrosiform hand dermatitis in a patient allergic to nickel.

Figure 2-4A: Metal cardiology stent, in this case used for patch testing. **B**: Reaction to the metal stent seen in A. The traumatic purpura is an artifact caused by pressure.

Figure 2-5: Multiple positive patch test results. In this case all were found to have present or past relevance.

Figure 2-6: Reaction to colophony (center), surrounded by a tape reaction. The tape (which contains no colophony) was present on all four quadrants of the back, but no reaction to the tape occurred in the other three quadrants. This is an example of spillover.

PLATE 2

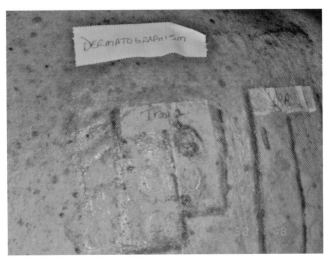

Figure 2-7: Strong dermatographic response to pressure from tape. Not an allergic reaction.

Figure 2-8: Plantar dermatitis due to rubber allergy (mercaptobenzothiazole).

Figure 2-9A: Correct application of Finn chamber patch tests, from the bottom up.

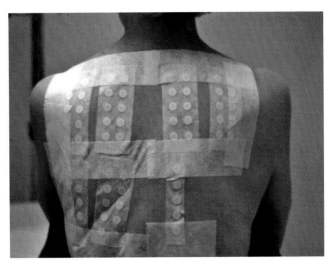

Figure 2-9B: Use of additional Scanpor tape to reinforce the patches.

Figure 2-9C: Small strips of tape bearing the numbers of the patches are left in place upon patch test.

PLATE 3

Figure 2-10: Patch test reactions

Figure 2-10A: Borderline or inconclusive.

Figure 2-10B: 1+.

Figure 2-10C: 2+.

Figure 2-10C: 3+.

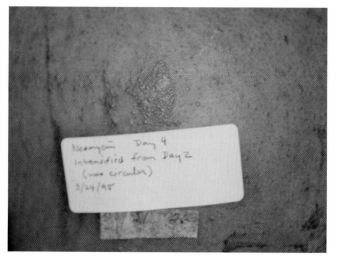

Figure 2-11: Patch test intensification. The affected area was round at the day 2 reading but was enlarged and irregularly shaped at the day 4 reading, seen here.

Figure 5-1: Atopic dermatitis in a child.

PLATE 4

Figure 6-1: Eyelid dermatitis due to cocamido-propyl betaine in shampoo.

Figure 6-2: Eyelid dermatitis from thiuram contained in foam sponges used to apply eye make-up.

Figure 6-3: Contact dermatitis due to an otic preparation. The reaction has spread beyond the area of intentional use.

Figure 6-4: Dermatitis of the earlobe due to earring allergy. Hyperpigmentation is common in more darkly pigmented individuals.

Figure 7-1A: The sole of this patient's foot has turned red and mildly edematous, but is non-vesicular. Her foot was normal 2 days prior to this photograph and had been normal for about 1 year.

Figure 7-1B: The application of two alkyl thiourea patch tests caused not only strong 2+ reactions on her back but also induced this change on her feet, where she had originally experienced dermatitis.

Figure 7-2A: Consort dermatitis. Sunscreen rubbed off the skin of the patient's boyfriend onto hers, with no direct application. The allergen proved to be homosalate found in Coppertone lotion.

Figure 7-2B: Here, the material was applied directly to the leg, causing follicular dermatitis from homosalate in Coppertone lotion.

PLATE 5

Figure 7-3: Waxy, corrugated, non-vesicular change resulting from exposure to a solvent used to remove labels from clothing. This is an irritant reaction.

Figure 7-4: Purpuric contact dermatitis of the feet due to allergy to footwear.

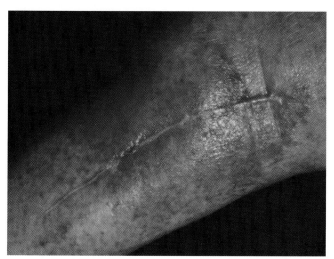

Figure 7-5: Purpuric changes resulting from use of cocoa butter in an effort to improve scar formation. Patch tests to cocoa butter were negative. The rubbing of firm blocks of cocoa butter caused the purpuric change.

Figure 9-1A,B: Reactions to clonidine transdermal patches.

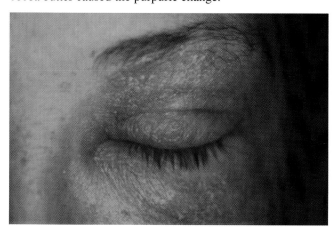

Figure 12-1: Allergic contact dermatitis of the eyelid from neomycin.

Figure 12-2: Allergic contact dermatitis overlying a tattoo. The patient was instructed to apply triple antibiotic ointment but proved allergic to neomycin and bacitracin.

PLATE 6

Figure 15-1: Facial and neck dermatitis due to allergy to hydrocortisone cream.

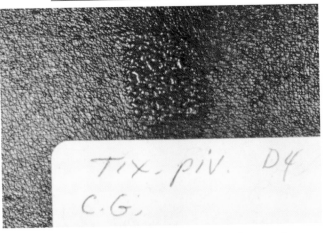

Figure 15-2: Vesicular patch test reaction to tixocortol pivalate, which screens for allergy to hydrocortisone.

Figure 15-3: Reaction to tixocortol pivalate, seen in the largest reaction area on the left lower back.

Figure 15-4: A rim reaction. This reaction is considered a true positive reaction when the test substance is a corticosteroid.

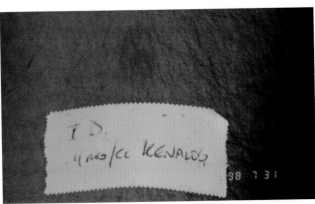

Figure 15-6: Positive intradermal test to triamcinolone acetonide (4 mg/mL).

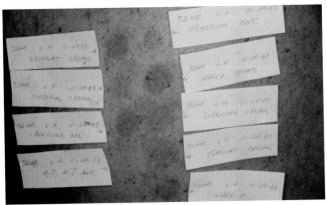

Figure 15-5: Multiple reactions to commercial topical corticosteroid products. All the reactions are from Class B and Class D corticosteroids, which can crossreact. The negative patch test result on the lower left is to 20% hydrocortisone in petrolatum; this is a member of Class A, which does not usually crossreact with Classes B and D.

PLATE 7

Figure 16-1: Allergic contact dermatitis to quaternum-15 in a moisturizer.

Figure 16-2: Allergic contact dermatitis to thimerosal.

Figure 16-3: Rare case of allergic contact dermatitis from polyvinylpyrrolidone (PVP)/hexadecene copolymer in a bath product.

Figure 16-4A,B,C: Allergy to cocamidopropyl betaine (CAPB). Results of a controlled use test with a shampoo and shower gel containing CAPB.

PLATE 8

Figure 17-1A,B: Nail changes and hyperpigmentation in a housekeeper at a nursing home. She was allergic to thiuram, nickel, and chromium. The palms and fingers show particularly pronounced hyperpigmentation.

Figure 17-2A,B: Hand dermatitis due to nickel in a metalworker.

PLATE 9

Figure 18-1A,B,C: Allergic contact dermatitis from formaldehyde in permanent-press clothing.

Figure 18-2: Allergic contact dermatitis to elastic in clothing.

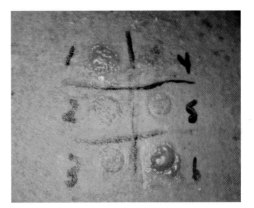

Figure 18-3: Strongly positive patch test results to disperse textile dyes.

Figure 18-4: Shoe dermatitis corresponding to a specific component of the shoe (not covering the entire foot).

Figure 18-5: Shoe dermatitis involving most of the foot, due to athletic footwear. The box toe of the shoe is a different material and the toes were spared.

Figure 18-6: Plantar allergic contact dermatitis from rubber in shoes.

PLATE 10

Figure 19-1: Dermatitis of the leg in a patient with a recent knee implant. Patch test was positive to acrylates.

Figure 19-2: Dermatitis from rubber lining of wrist support.

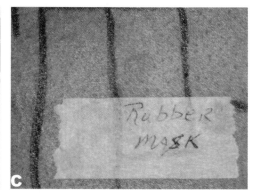

Figure 19-3A,B,C: Facial allergic contact dermatitis from rubber respirator mask, with patch test positive to mask (also mercaptobenzothiazoles [MBT]).

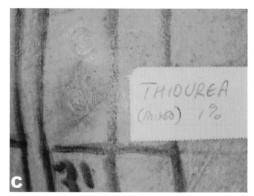

Figure 19-3A,B,C: Allergy to thiourea.
A,B: Two cases of allergy to thiourea in neoprene knee sleeves.
C: Positive patch test to thiurea.

PLATE 11

Figure 20-1: Fragrance allergy.

Figure 21-1: Poison ivy (light green "leaves of three") growing among regular ivy.

Figure 21-2A,B: Allergic contact dermatitis to Toxicodendron. **A:** The less-known early edematous stage, preceding the development of the characteristic blisters by a day or two. **B:** The more recognized, vesicular stage of Toxicodendron dermatitis.

Figure 21-3: Diagnosis of Toxicodendron dermatitis. The black dot is not an artifact but is highly concentrated urushiol, a clue to this diagnosis.

PLATE 12

Figure 24-1: Allergic contact dermatitis of the hand due to thiuram allergy in latex gloves worn by this health care worker.

Figure 24-2: Positive prick tests to latex protein extracted from two different samples of gloves. A positive reaction must be at least half the size of the histamine control.

Figure 24-3A,B: Severe allergic contact dermatitis in a metalworker due to Bioban P-1847.

Figure 27-1: Dermatitis from epoxy resin in an electronics worker.

Figure 27-2: Acrylate allergy in a dental worker.

Figure 28-1: Contact urticaria to sorbic acid, found in foods and cosmetics. A 1% aqueous solution was applied to create this reaction, which developed in 5 minutes.

PLATE 13

Figure 28-2: Reaction to a dye used for tattooing permanent eye make-up.

Figure 29-1: Contact urticaria to latex in a patient with spina bifida.

Figure 31-1: Dermatographism.

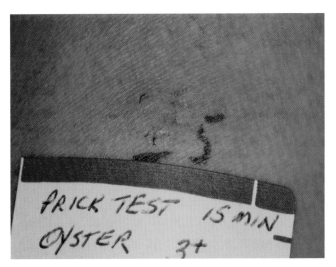

Figure 31-2: Contact urticaria to oyster in a fish-restaurant worker, with positive prick test.

Figure 31-3: Contact urticaria to acrylic acid.

PLATE 14

Figure 32-1: Nickel allergy from eyeglass frames.

Figure 32-2: Chronic, severe hand eczema in a cement worker with chromate allergy.

Figure 32-3: Acute irritant dermatitis from kneeling in wet cement.

Figure 32-4: Allergic contact dermatitis due to chromate in leather wallet.

PLATE 15

Figure 32-5A: Allergic contact dermatitis to gold.

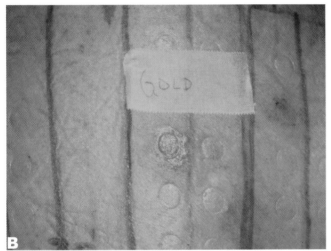

Figure 32-5B: Allergic contact dermatitis to gold.

Figure 32-5C: Allergic contact dermatitis to gold.

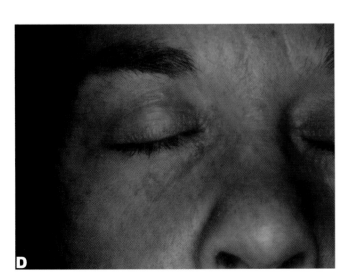

Figure 32-5D: Allergic contact dermatitis to gold.

Figure 32-5E: Allergic contact dermatitis to gold.

PLATE 16

Figure 33-1A,B: Two cases of allergic cheilitis due to cinnamic aldehyde.

Figure References

Figures 2–9A; 9–1A,B; 21–2A,B; and 21–3 from Rietschel RR, Conde-Salazar L, Goossens A, et al. Atlas of Contact Dermatitis. London: Martin Dunitz, 1999. Reproduced with permission.

APPENDIX

This appendix is intended as a quick reference for selected allergens. Please see the text for a more complete discussion of uses and patch-test concentrations for specific allergens.

Explanation of Terms used in the Appendix

1. *Primary sensitizer.* Testing with this substance may sensitize the patient. The patch test re-action usually is delayed for at least 5 days.
2. *Photosensitizer.* This substance should be tested both covered and with exposure to sun-light or ultraviolet radiation.
3. *Controls.* The substance may be a primary irritant. The patch test reaction should be checked with at least three normal controls.
4. *Para-amino.* This refers to chemicals that have an amino group in the para position, including paraphenylenediamine, paraaminobenzoic acid, and aminosalicylic acid. Cross-reactions occur with certain local anesthetics, sulfonamides, sunscreens and azo, and aniline dyes.
5. *Sensitizes to alcohol.* Exposure to this chemical combined with the ingestion of alcohol produces an aldehyde syndrome consisting of flushing of the skin, nausea, and vomiting.

Key to Abbreviations used in the Appendix

ACD:	allergic contact dermatitis
acet.:	acetone
alc.:	alcohol 70%
aq.:	aqueous
as is:	undiluted
chlor.:	chloroform
c.o.:	castor oil
con.:	concentration
MEK.:	methylethylketone
o.o.:	olive oil
pdr.:	powder
pet.:	petrolatum
sat.:	saturated
sol.:	solution
veh.:	vehicle

Contactant	Concentration and Vehicle	Exposure	Crossreactions	Comment
Abietic acid	2% pet.	Rosins, colophony, adhesives, balsams, typewriting paper, denture adhesive powder, pine resin	Hydroabietalcohols	Forms about 80% of American rosin
Abieto-formo-phenolic resin	2% pet.	Printing ink	Rosin	
Abitol (dihydroabietyl alcohol)	1% pet.	Cosmetics, plastics, adhesives	Rosin	
Acacia (gum arabic)	50% aq.	Ink, matches, lithography, mucilage, pharmaceutical vehicle, offset sprays in printing, adhesives, stiffeners for rayon, pastry, denture adhesive powder		May contain alcohol
Aceclofenac	10% pet.			Metabolized to diclofenac Photoallergic contact dermatitis
Acetanilide	5% pet.	Analgesics, antipyretics, dye manufacture, cellulose ester varnishes		
2-Acetexycyclonhexahone oxime	1% pet.	In the synthesis of lysine		
Acetic acid	3% aq.	Vinegar, flavoring agent, wart remedy, astringent mouthwash		Causes aphthous ulcer?
Acetone	10% o.o.	Industrial solvent, nail polish remover, diabetic urine, solvent for celluloid material in dentifrices		Anti-irritant
1-Acetyl-2-phenylhydrazine	1% pet.	Anaerobic sealant		A dimethacrylate
N-acetylcysteine	10% aq.			Eye drops, mucolytic
Achromycin Ointment (Lederle)	As is	Topical medication	Tetracyclines	
Acid fuchsin	1% pet.	Azo dyes	Para-amino compounds	
Acridine	1% pet.	Yellow dyes, acriflavine, tar		Photosensitizer
Acriflavine	1% pet.			An acridine dye photo-sensitizer
Acrylic monomer (methylmethacrylate)	10% o.o.	Synthetic resins, dentures, artificial nails, adhesives, paints, plastic, glass, sealer of screws in automobile industry, orthopedic prostheses		Can penetrate rubber gloves. May contain hydroquinone benzoylperoxide, tertiary amines, can cause contact urticaria
Acrylonitrile	0.1% pet.	Used in Plexidur plastic splints		
Acyclovir	1% pet.	Topical and systemic		

Contactant	Concentration and Vehicle	Exposure	Crossreactions	Comment
Adhesive tape (acrylate)	As is	Dermicel (J & J), Steri-strip Brand SkinClosures, Micropore Brand SurgicalTape (3M)		Some brands colophony
Adhesive tape (rubber)	As is			May contain rubber additives, rosin, turpentine, and lanolin
Aerosol OT (dioctylester of sodium sulfosuccinic acid)	1% aq.	Surfactant, anionic synthetic detergents, bubble baths		Controls
Akrinol Cream (acrisorcin; Schering)	As is		Hexylresorcinol	
Alantolactone	0.1% pet.	Sensitizer in Compositae plants		Known as Helenin in Denmark
Alcohol (industrial denatured)	As is			Contains methyl alcohol and acetone
Alcohol (ethyl)	70—95%		Amyl, butyl, methyl, isopropyl alc	Test reaction may occur very rapidly; may cause contact urticaria
Alcohol (isopropyl, "rubbing")	As is	Cosmetics, medicinal preparations		Denaturing agents include tartar emetic, quinine, salicylic acid, colchicine, alkaloids and azo dyes
Alcohol (methyl, methanol, wood)	As is	Chemical synthesis, antifreeze, solvent in shellac, varnish, paint remover, denaturant in denatured alcohol		*Synonyms:* methyl hydrate, methyl hydroxide, acetone, alcohol, wood spirits, wood naphtha, Columbian spirits, carrinol
Alizarin dyes: Alizarin red Alizarin 778 Alizarin sulfate	As is 1% alc. 10% aq.	Synthetic dyes, red paints, hair dyes, chemical indicators		
Alkyldiaminoethylglycine hydrochloride	0.01%aq.	Tego®		
Alkyl ethoxy sulfate	1% pet.	Liquid dishwashing products		
Alkyl phenoxyl polyethoxyethanols	2% aq.	Wetting agent and emulsifier		
Allantoin	0.5% aq.	Topical medications, "healing agent," cosmetics, vaginal creams, shampoos		Uric acid derivative
Allyl glycidyl ether	0.25% MEK[a]	Reactive epoxy diluent		
Allyl phenoxyacetate	1% pet.	Carpet shampoo		
Almond oil	As is	Brilliantines, hair dressings, spices, flavoring agents		

Contactant	Concentration and Vehicle	Exposure	Crossreactions	Comment
Aloe arborescens	As is	Plant and laxative		
Aloe vera	10% pet.	Anthraquinone compound	Benzoin and Balsam of Peru (topical medicinal)	
Alpha-chlorobenzaldehyde-phenylhydrazone	0.1% aq.	To prepare optical fluorescing compound as an optical whitener		
Alpha-phenyl-indol in PVC	2% pet.	Stabilizer in polyvinyl chloride		
Alpha-terthienyl	1% pet.	Thiophene compound present in Chrysanthemum family of plants		
Alprenolol	2% aq.	Beta-adrenergic blocking agent		
Alrosol C (fatty acid amidecondensate)	1% aq.	Surfactant, nonionic synthetic detergents		Controls irritant
Alstroemeria	As is	South American plant		
Alum (aluminum and potassium sulfate)	10% aq.	Styptic agents, purification of water, baking powders, mouthwashes, astringents		
Aluminum acetate	10% aq.	Mordants, siccatives, astringents, deodorants, fur dyeing, fabric finishing, waterproofing, dye compounds, disinfectants		Rare sensitizer. May produce nonspecific follicular reaction
Aluminum chlorhydroxide	10% aq.	Deodorants, antiperspirants, astringents		
Aluminum chloride	2% aq.	Astringents, antiseptics, antiperspirants		Rare sensitizer. Irritation from pore closure
Aluminum metal	As is	Finn-Chambers		
Aluminum powder	As is in pet.	Astringents, instruments		Rare sensitizer
Aluminum sulfate	2% aq.	Astringents, antiseptics, antiperspirants		Rare sensitizer. Irritation from pore closure
Aluminum sulfocarbolate	2% aq.	Astringents, antiseptics, antiperspirants		Rare sensitizer. Irritation from pore closure
Amaranth pink	5% pet.	Color elixir phenobarbital, foods, alcohol		
Amerchol L-101	1% pet.	Lanolin alcohol	Lanolin	
Amino-azobenzene	0.25% pet.	Leather dyes, textiles	Para-amino compounds	
Amino-azotoluene hydrochloride	1% pet.	Leather dyes	Para-amino compounds	

Contactant	Concentration and Vehicle	Exposure	Crossreactions	Comment
Amino-azotoluene	1% pet.	Scarlet red topical medications	Para-amino compounds	
3-Amino-1,2,4-triazole	5% pet.	Herbicide		
Aminoethylethanolamine	1% aq.	Aluminum cables		Used to solder aluminum electric wires
Aminoguanidine hydrochloride	5% pet.	Herbicide		
o-Aminophenol	10% pet.	Fur and hair dye		Paraphenylenediamine
Aminophylline	1% aq.	Pharmaceutical industry, rectal suppositories (Rectalad, Aminet, Heogen)	Phenergan, pyribenzamine	Composed of ethylenediamine and theophylline
Ammoniated mercury	2% pet.	Topical medications	Organic and inorganic mercurials, mercury amalgam	Incompatible with sulfur and iodine pigment changes
Ammonium fluoride	2% aq.	Glass industry, insecticides, rust removers, dentistry, Aluminum Brite (Copper Brite Co.)		Patch tests may produce large nonspecific pustules. Keep in dark wax-coated bottle
Ammonium persulfate	2% aq.	Flour and hair bleaches, disinfectants, deodorants, ammoniated dentifrices	Potassium-sodium persulfate	May produce urticaria, shock by contact
Ammonium phosphate	2% aq.	Ammoniated dentifrices		
Ammonium rhodanate	1% pet.	Photography		
Ammonium thioglycolate	5% aq. test open			
Ammonyx lo	5% aq.	Surfactant and antiseptic for surgical scrubs Present in chlorhexidine		
Ampholyt G	1% aq.	Disinfectant, present in Tego		
Ampicillin sodium	5% aq.	Use fresh preparation		Occupational hazard in nursing personnel
Amyl acetate (banana oil) Amyl cinnamic alcohol Amyl cinnamic aldehyde	10% o.o. 5% terpene 5% terpene	Solvents, nail polish removers, waterproofing, sheet metal, enamelware, woodworking		
Amyl dimethylaminobenzoate	1% pet.	Ultraviolet cured ink		
Amyltricresol	1% aq.	A phenol mercury compound in Pentacresol Mouthwash		
Anethole	5% pet.	Toothpaste flavoring		Found in oils of anise, star anise, and fennel
Anileridine	As is	Injectable narcotic		Occurs in pharmacists and those who inject narcotics

Contactant	Concentration and Vehicle	Exposure	Crossreactions	Comment
Aniline	10% o.o.	Dyes, drugs, cloth marking inks, paints, paint removers	Para-amino compounds	A colorless aminobenzene. May containn aphthylamine
Aniline black	10% o.o.	Fur dyes	Para-amino compounds	
Aniline blue	2% pet.	Cosmetics, carbons, fur dyeing, hairdyes, nail polish, rubber, photographics, inks, colored pencils, crayons	Para-amino compounds	
Aniline dyes	5% pet.	Crayons, diaper markings, shoe polishes	Para-amino compounds	Toxic to infants when used for diaper markings
Anise oil	25% c.o.	Flavoring agents in dentistry, liqueurs (anisette), confectioneries, perfumes, soaps		Derived from seeds of carrot family
Anisyl alcohol	5% pet.			
Anthracene	Pure	Tar		Photosensitizer
Anthralin ointment (Cignolin)	0.05% pet.	Anthra-Derm Ointment (Dermik), Anthryl (Reed & Carnrick)		Irritant when covered. Controls
Anthraquinone	2% pet.	Yellow vat dyes, makes seeds distasteful to birds, laxatives		From anthracine, a coal tar derivative
Antimony chloride Antimony oxide	2% aq. Pure	Alloys, type metals, batteries, foils, ceramics, safety matches, ant pastes, textiles, tartar emetic, Fuadin, base for paints, vitreous enamels, fireproofing plastics		Irritant and toxic
Antimony sulfide	2% aq.	Matches, putty		
Antipyrine (phenazone)	5% pet.	Auralgan Ear Drops (Ayerst), Tympagesic Ear Drops (Warren-Teed)		Auralgan also contains benzocaine and hydroquinoline. May cause erythema multiforme
Antisapstain	1% pet.	Antifungal agent for timber		Can cause irritant and allergic reactions
Antistine (antazoline)	0.5% aq. sol or 1% pet.	Eye and nose drops	Pyribenzamine, Neoantergan, Diatrin, Neohetramine, Trimeton, Benadryl, aminophylline	Derivative of ethylenediamine
Antivy (CIBA)	As is (patch-scratch)			Contains zirconium oxide. Allergic granuloma
Apomorphine	1% aq. scratch test	For the treatment of alcoholism. Exposure nurses, pharmacists who dispense the drug.		

Contactant	Concentration and Vehicle	Exposure	Crossreactions	Comment
Apraclonidine	10% aq.	Brimonidine, clonidine		
Aquaphor (Duke Lab.)	As is		Lanolin	Cholesterolated Vaselineand lanolin alcohol. Cholesterolated absorbent ointment base
Aracel C (Sorbitansesquioleate)	5% o.o.	Pharmaceuticals		In Polysorb Hydrate
Araldite 502	0.1% acet.	Low molecular weight epoxy resins		
Araldite 6060	10% acet.	High molecular weight epoxy resins		
Arctic Syntex M (sodiummonoglyceride sulfide)	5% aq.	Surfactant, synthetic detergents		Controls
Argyrol	10% aq. (open)	Antiseptics		
Arlacel	10% aq.	Emulsifier in soaks and detergents		
Arlacel A (mannidemonooleate)	5% aq.	Surfactant, nonionic synthetic detergents; pharmaceuticals		Controls
Arnica, tincture of	20% alc.	Rubefacients	Chrysanthemum	Arnica and chrysanthemum, belonging to the aster family or Compositae
Arning's Tincture	As is (open)		Balsam of Peru	Contains anthrarobin, tumenol ammonium, ether, tincture of benzoin
Arsenate (potassium)	1% aq.	Fowler's solution		
Arsenate (sodium	10% pet.	Insecticides, ant poisons, weed killers, wallpaper paints, glass, ceramics	Other arsenicals	Frequent pustular patch test reaction
Arsenic trioxide (white arsenic)	5% in starch pdr.	Insecticides, soaps, hair tonics, depilatories, caustics, weed killers, poisonbaits, fungicides, glasses, enamels, alloys	Sodium arsenate	Frequent pustular patch test reaction
Artemesia	As is	Compositae plant test		Ingested as folk remedy, may cause systemic contact dermatitis
Artichoke	Patch test with stem as is or alcohol extract of stem	Food handlers and gardeners	Crossreacts with Compositae	
Arylalcanoic acids	1% pet.	Rubifacient used in Europe		Present in Motrin
Asterol (diamthazole)	5% pet.	Antifungal agents		
Atranorin	0.1% pet.	Lichen substance present in oak moss		

Contactant	Concentration and Vehicle	Exposure	Crossreactions	Comment
Atronin	1% pet.	May be photosensitizer. Present in lichens and perfumes		
Aureomycin Ointment, Powder (Lederle)	As is		Tetracyclines	
Azidamphenicol	5% pet.	Antibiotic closely related to chloramphenicol		
Azo dyes	2% pet.	Foods, drugs, cosmetics, clothes, ballpoint pens, ink	Para-amino compounds	
Azodicarbonamide	1% pet.	Used in the manufacture of polyvinylchloride Polyolefin plastics		
Bacitracin	20% pet.	Wybiotic Troches, Tyrotrace, Baciguent, Baci-Wax, Mycitracin, Epimycin A, Bacimycin, Cortisporin, Polysporin, Neo-polycin, Neosporin, Tetrazets	Polymyxin B colistine	May coreact with neomycin. Can cause contact urticaria
Balsam of Peru: see *Myroxolon pereirae*				
Balsam of tolu	1% alc.	Cough mixtures, throat lozenges, benzoin tincture, tolu varnish, coating for pills, perfumes	Benzoin tincture, balsam of Peru	
Barium sulfide	2% aq.	Depilatories	Freshly prepared	
Bay rum	As is	Hair tonics	Eugenol, clove oil, cinnamon oil	Combination of Jamaica rum and oil of bay
Bee glue (propolis)	As is			May contain raw beeswax
Beeswax (cera alba [bleached],cera flava [unbleached])	30% pet.	Adhesives, plasters, textile waterproofing agent, ointments, cosmetics, polishes, cosmetic stiffeners	Balsam of Peru	May be contaminated with bee glue
Beeswax-turpentine mixture	5% pet.	Eyeglass frames		To produce smooth gloss on plastics
Befunolol	1% aq.	Carteolol		Beta blocker
Benadryl (diphenhydramine hydrochloride; Parke, Davis)	2% pet.	Caladryl Ointment (Parke, Davis)	Dramamine	
Benomyl (benlate)	1% pet.	Insecticide		
Benoquin (monobenzone; Elder)	As is	Depigmenting agent	Hydroquinone	Contains monobenzyl-ether of hydroquinone
Benzaldehyde	5% pet.	Oil of bitter almond, preservatives, biologicals	Vanilla, balsam of Peru	Contact urticaria

Contactant	Concentration and Vehicle	Exposure	Crossreactions	Comment
Benzalkonium chloride	1:1000 aq.sol. = 0.1%	Antiseptic detergents, mouthwashes, preservative in ophthalmic solutions, Zephiran solution, medicated paper tissues (Zephiran towelettes)		May be irritant
Benzene (benzol)	5% o.o.	Coal tar distillates, motor fuels, commercial solvents		Synonyms: phenylhydride, coal tar naphtha
Benzene hexachloride	5% pet.	Insecticide Kwell (Reed & Carnrick)		May cause chloracne, porphyria
Benzethonium chloride (Phemerol)	1:1000 aq. sol. = 0.1%	Antiseptic detergents		Present in Colgate mouthwash, feminine hygiene sprays
Benzidine (para-diamino-diphenyl)	3% alc.	Tests for blood, derivatives are optical bleaches		
Benzine	50% o.o.	Petroleum solvents		Synonyms: petroleum benzine, petroleum ether
Benzisothiazoline	1% pet.	Preservative in gum arabic, industrial preservative, Biocide in pottery industry		
Benzocaine	5% pet.	Numerous topical anesthetic compounds (see text)	Para-amino compounds	Synonyms: anethesin, ethyl aminobenzoate, Anesthone, parathesin. May cause contact urticaria. Rare photo-sensitizer
Benzoic acid	5% pet.	Balsam of Peru, Whitfield's ointment, essential oils, mouthwashes, preservatives for fruit, pharmaceuticals		Extremely rare sensitizer
Benzoin	10% alc.	Tincture of benzoin, compound tincture of benzoin, Arning's tincture, benzoinated lard (adeps benzoatus), antioxidant in creams, perfumes, expectorants, throat lozenges, raw beeswax, bee glue, preservative in adhesives, gums of myrrh, locust, golbam	Balsam of Peru, benzyl cinnamate, benzyl alcohol, eugenol, vanilla, alpha-pinene, Storax	
Benzophenone	5% pet.	Sunscreens (Solbar, Sunguard, Uval), textiles, plastics, rubber products, paints, varnishes, cosmetics		May produce urticarial and contact sensitivity. Synonyms: SpectraSorb UV 284
Benzoquinone	1% pet.	Present in plants and wood		
Benzotriazole	0.5% pet.			

Contactant	Concentration and Vehicle	Exposure	Crossreactions	Comment
Benzoxonium chloride	0.1% aq.	Benzalkonium chloride, domiphen bromide		
Benzoyl peroxide	1% pet.	Polyester and acrylic resins, Quinolor Ointment (Squibb), burn dusting powder, flour improver, benzoyl peroxide ointment. Acne medications: Persadox, Benoxyl, Loroxide,Vanoxide, Oxy 5, Oxy 5 HC, etc.	Benzoic acid derivatives, cinnamon, cocaine, Surfacaine, Metacaine	Not stable Irritant Discolors textiles
Benzyl alcohol	5% pet.	Essential oils, balsam of Peru, food flavorings, perfumes, antiseptic and local anesthetics	Balsam of Peru Perfumes	Preservative in allergy extracts and injectables
Benzyl benzoate	2% pet.	Balsam of Peru, balsam of tolu, perfumes, nail polish plasticizer, Topocide (Lilly)	Diethylstilbestrol	
Benzyl salicylate	2% pet.	Perfumes, detergents, sunscreens (methoxsalen), psoralens	Essential oil	May enhance photosensitization
Bergamot, oil of	2% pet.	Eau de Cologne Shalimar, hair tonics, toilet water, china painting, ceramics		A photosensitizer. Test open and closed
Beryllium chloride	0.5% pet.	Cathode tube and fluorescent lights, alloys, electrical equipment, ceramics, fluorophors		May produce granulomas, as can beryllium SO$_4$
17-β-estradiol	0.1% eth.			
Beta-cyclocostunolide	0.1% pet.			Can be detected with sesquiterpene lactone mix
Betadine (povidone-iodine; Purdue Frederick)	As is (open)			Iodine in polyvinyl pyrrolidine Irritant
Betanal	2% aq.	Herbicide (phenmedipham)		
Betanaphthol	10% o.o.	Glues, adhesive solvent, book binding, mouthwashes, hair tonics		
Bimatoprost	0.003% aq			Lumigan
Bioban P-1487	0.5% pet.	Cutting oils		
Biocide (Tektamer 38)	1% pet.	In paste glue		Formaldehyde releaser?
Bis-(4-chlorophenol) methylchloride	1% chlor.	Insecticide-related DDT		

Contactant	Concentration and Vehicle	Exposure	Crossreactions	Comment
Bis(diethyl and dibutyldithio-carbamato) zinc	1% pet.	Rubber	Thiuram Comp.	
Bismarck brown	5% pet.	Dyeing silks, wools, leathers	Para-amino compounds	
Bismuth oxide	0.5% pet.			
Bisphenol A	1% acet.	Epoxy resin converter, antioxidant, component of oil-soluble phenolicresins	Diethylstilbestrol, organic silicone compounds, monobenzylether of hydroquinone	
Bithionol	1% pet.	Antiseptic no longer used in US	Chlorinated salicylanilides	Photosensitizer
Bitrex	2% pet.	Disinfectant		
Bitter almond, oil of	10% o.o.		Benzoin, balsam of Peru	A benzaldehyde poison
Borax (sodium borate)	Sat. aq.	Refrigerant, antiseptics, soaps, detergents, abrasives, bath salts, cosmetics, flux		
Boric acid	3% aq.	Antiseptics, detergents, cosmetics		
Boron trifluoride-ethylamine	1% pet.	Epoxy resin hardener (formaldehyde-releasing agent)		
Brilliant green	2% aq.	Dyes		
British antilewisite (BAL; 2–3,dithiopropanol; dimercaprol)	5% pet.	Chelating agents		
1-Bromo-3-chloro-5,5-dimethylhydantoin	2% aq.			Hot tub bromine
9-Bromofluorene	**Do not test**	Chemistry laboratory		Erythema multiforme reaction
Bronopol	0.25% pet.	Preservative in cosmetics		
Brucine	1% pet.	Denatured alcohol		A strychnine compound
BTC (lauryl dimethyl benzyl-ammonium chloride)	0.1% aq.	Surfactant, cationic synthetic detergents, bubble baths		Irritants
Budesonide	0.1% pet.	Topical corticosteroids	Grp. B corticosteroids	
Bufexamac	1% pet.	Topical analgesic in Italy and Belgium		
Burow's solution (liquor aluminum acetatis)	10% aq.	Astringents, antiseptics		Very rarely sensitizes
Butacaine	5% pet.	Topical anesthetic	Para-amino-compound	Based on para-aminobenzoic acid
Butethamine (Monocaine)	5% pet.	Local anesthetic	Para-amino compound	Based on para-aminobenzoic acid

Contactant	Concentration and Vehicle	Exposure	Crossreactions	Comment
Butyl acetate	25% o.o.	Solvents, nail polish removers		
Butyl acrylate	0.1% pet.	Plastics, spectacle frames		
Butyl aminobenzoate	As is	Local anesthetic	Procaine, benzocaine	Butesin picrate Proprietary name
Butyl glycidyl ether	1% o.o.	Reactive epoxy resin diluent		
p-tert-Butylcatechol	0.1% acet.	Oil antioxidant		May cause depigmentation
Butylhydroxyanisol	1% pet.	Antioxidant		
Butylhydroxytoluene	1% pet.	Antioxidant		
p-tert-Butylphenol formaldehyde resin	10% pet.	Adhesive—contains little or no formaldehyde		
Butyrolactone (Antara)	As is	Organic solvent		Useful solvent for patch testing of resins
Cadmium sulfide (Capsebon)	1% aq.	Tattoos, photo-conducting material, forms pink pigment in acrylic dentures with cadmium selenide		Photoallergic
Calcium chloride	0.5% pet.	EEG Electrode Paste, dehydrating agents, antimildew		A primary irritant
Calcium cyanamide	1% aq.	Fertilizer and pesticide anthelmintic		Found in Carbodiimide—irritant—does not produce cyanide effects
Calcium lignosulfonate	10% aq.	Animal food	Paper pulp	Paper and wood
Calcium oxide (quicklime)	Do not patchtest	Unslaked lime, caustic lime, burnt lime		Not a sensitizer. Burns skin when moistened. See also lime, slaked
Calcium thioglycolate	5% aq.	Depilatories		
Camomile, oil of	25% o.o.	Cosmetics, mirror manufacturing, vegetable hair dyes		Compositae
Camphor oil Camphor powder Camphor crystals	10% pet.	Used in dentistry as camphorated chlorophenol, preservatives, plasticizer, nail polish, lacquers, varnishes, moth repellents, embalming fluids, explosives, pharmaceuticals		Some camphors contain oil of laurel

Contactant	Concentration and Vehicle	Exposure	Crossreactions	Comment
Canada balsam	25% pet.	Cement for lenses, fine lacquers, mounting slides	Turpentine, balsam of Peru	
Capsicum, tincture of	1% alc.	Hair tonics, rubefacient, tear gas (OnGuard)		
Captan	0.25% pet.	Pesticide, antifungal	Phaltan	A dicarboximide
Captopril	10% aq.		Other ACE inhibitors usually negative	
Caraway seed oil	25% c.o.	Spices in baking, liqueurs, soaps, flavor in dentifrices		May cause contact urticaria
Carbamide (urea)	10% aq.	Therapeutic agent, Ammident, Colgate and Dr. Lyons toothpaste		
Carbitol (diethylene glycol)	10% aq.	Solvents, stabilizer of emulsions		
Carbocaine Hydrochloride (mepivacaine; Winthrop)	2% aq.	Local anesthetics	Lidocaine	Not based on para-amino-benzoic acid
Carbolfuchsin paint (Castellani's paint)	As is (open)			Contains resorcin. Keep in dark bottle
Carbon disulfide	10% o.o.	Industrial solvents, laboratories, rayon industry		
Carbon paper	As is	Typing, lithography, blue printing, photocopying		Reported sensitizers: Triphenyl phosphate, oleyl alcohol, nigrosine
Carbon tetrachloride	10% o.o.	Solvents, floor waxes, cleansers, fire extinguisher fluids, insecticide sprays, antiseborrheic lotion		Synonyms: carbon tet, tetrachloromethane and perchloromethane
Carbowax	As is	Cosmetics, pharmaceutical vehicles		Solid polyethyleneglycols
Carboxylase (cocarboxylase, coenzyme B)	10% aq.	Manufacture of thiamine	Thiamine chloride	
Carboxyphenyl	As is	Manufacturer of photo processing		
Carbromal (bromodiethyl-acetylurea)	1% in propylene glycol	Carbrital (Parke, Davis), Tabor0ea (Table Rock)	Barbiturates	Purpuric patch test
Carbyne	1% aq.	Herbicide		
Cardamom	50% aq.	Confectionery spice	Terpenes	
Carmine dye	5% pet.	Rouge, lip pomade, ink, stains, food		Contains cochineal, a dried insect
Carnation oil	5% pet.	Eugenol, "Flubber" putty, flavoring agent, perfume		

Contactant	Concentration and Vehicle	Exposure	Crossreactions	Comment
Carnauba wax	50% mineral oil	Orange skin protective, old phonograph records, furniture, shoe andfloor waxes, candles, electrical insulation, cosmetics, lipsticks, cologne sticks		Obtained from South American palm trees. A solid that becomes fluid when rubbed with a circular motion
Casalic green	2% aq.	Chromium oxide powder, green tattoos, Guinget Cream		
Cashew nut shell oil	3% alc.	Voodoo dolls, swizzle sticks, mucilage, printer's ink, varnishes, brake pads	Rhus and other Anacardiaceae	
Cassia flavor	5% o.o.	Chinese cinnamon		
Castor oil	As is	Cosmetic emollient		
Catechol	3% o.o.	Plastic industry, rubber	Resorcin, hydroquinone	
Cauliflower	As is	Cruciferae plant	Cabbage, brussels sprout, grape seed	
CD-2 (amino diethylamino monohydrochloride; diethyl paraphenylenediamine)	1% aq.	Color film developers		Lichen planus type of eruption
CD-3 (color developer)(amino-4-N-ethyl-N-(methane-sulfon-aminoethyl)-m-toluidine)	1% pet.			
Cedarwood oil	10% o.o.	Essential perfume oil		A photosensitizer
Celecoxib	5% pet.			
Cellulose	As is	Sodium carbomethyl cellulose used in Japanese cake mix Surgical is oxidized regenerated cellulose		
Cement (clay and limestone)	As is (open)	Construction industry irritant		May contain cobalt, nickel and chromates
Cephalosporin	As is or scratch test 0.5% aq.	Handling or taking drug	Penicillin	Positive patch test in adverse drug reaction
Ceramol	30% pet.			Blend of cetyl and stearyl alcohol with sodium lauryl sulfate
Ceresin (ozokerite)	30% pet.	Cosmetic stiffeners		
Cerium oxide	As is	Polishing eyeglass lenses		
Cetirizine	2.5% pet.	Ethylenediamine, Piperazine		May cause depigmentation

Contactant	Concentration and Vehicle	Exposure	Crossreactions	Comment
Cetyl alcohol	30% pet.	Fatty alcohol present in lanolin, Chloromycetin Cream, Vioform HC Lotion, Neo-Cord-Dome Lotion, Pragmatar	Stearyl alcohol	Synonyms: hexadecyl or palmityl alcohol. Can cause contact urticaria
Cetyl pyridinium bromide	1:1000 aq.sol.			Used in Hungarian contraceptives
Cetyl pyridinium chloride(Ceepryn)	1:1000 aq.sol.	Cepacol, Micrin, Reef, Scope		A quaternary ammonium compound
Chalk dyes	1% pet.	Colored chalk dyes Pigment red, pigment yellow		
Chamomile tea	5% aq.	Artemesia and mugwort		May cause severe bullous eruption
Chicory	Leaf or juice as is	Handling of plants		Used as coffee substitute
Chloracetopenone (CN)	0.1% alc.	Tear gas		Test open. A severe irritant and primary sensitizer
Chloral hydrate	10% aq.	Hair tonics, suppositories, Calmitol Ointment, veterinary anesthetics	Chlorobutanol	
Chloramine	2% aq.	Water disinfectants	Sod. hypochlorite	
Chloramphenicol	2% pet.	Antibiotic		
Chloramphenicol (Chloromycetin [Parke,Davis])	5% pet.	Antibiotic cream, Genetris Pessaries	DNCB	
Chlordane	5% acet.	Insecticides		
Chlordantoin	1% pet.	Antifungal agent found in Clocandil vaginal cream		
Chlorhexidene	1% aq.	Antiseptic		May be irritant
Chlorhexidine digluconate	0.5% aq.	Antiseptic		
Chlorinated alkalis	0.5% aq.	Javelle water, Labarraque's solution, Carrel-Dakin's solution, Clorox, chlorinated lime, chloramine	Sodium hypochlorite	
Chlorinated naphthalene	As is	Electric wires, motors, electrical equipment, transformers		Produces acneiform eruptions
Chloroacetamide	0.2% aq.	Preservative in cosmetics, pharmaceuticals, coolant oils, pesticides		
Chlorobenzene	5% o.o.	Insecticides		Produces acneiform eruptions

Contactant	Concentration and Vehicle	Exposure	Crossreactions	Comment
Chlorobenzylidene malonitrile(CS)	1% alc. (open)	Tear gas		Test open. A severe irritant and primary sensitizer
Chlorobutanol crystals	5% o.o.	Dentalone (Parke, Davis), sedative dressing (Krutchen), local anesthetics, preservative for parenteral solutions and pharmaceuticals, biologic fluids	Chloral hydrate	
Chlorocresol	2% pet.	Valisone Cream, topical medications, pesticides	Chloroxylenol	
Chloroform	40% o.o.	Solvent for gutta percha, gum copal, acrylic dentures, UltraBrite and McLean's Toothpaste, anesthetics, liniments		
Chloro-meta-cresol	1% pet.	Preservative		p-Chloro-meta-cresol
Chloromethylisothiazolinone	0.5% pet.	Antibacterial preservative in cosmetics and shampoos		Present in Kathon
p-Chloro-o-cresol	0.1% alc.	Preservative		Phenolic compound
Chloro-2-phenylphenol (Dowicide 32)	1% pet.(open and closed)	Liquid soap, disinfectants, fungicides		Photosensitizer
Chlorphenesin	1% pet.	Plant growth inhibitor found in fungicides		
Chlorophyll	1% pet.	Deodorizers		
Chlorophyllins	5% aq.	Deodorizers, cosmetics, suntan preparations, Green Mint Mouthwash		
Chloroquin	5% pet.	Pharmaceuticals	Atabrine	
Chlorosalicylamide	1% white pet.	Antimycotic agent (Jadit)		Photosensitizer
Chlorothalonil	0.0001% aq.	Paint, wood preservative, floriculture		Vapors at 0.4 ppm cause airborne dermatitis
Chlorothion	1% alc.(open)	Insecticides		
Chlorothymol	2% alc. or 0.1% aq.	N.F. Antiseptic Solution. *Antiseptic solutions:* Gray Cross, C.S.I. *Foot powders:* Upjohn Medicated, Dr. Solvey, Ward's Foot Balm, K4. *Douches:* Lanteen, Verazeptol. Liniments: Neurabalm, Balsam of Myrrh, Rex Rub. Key Nose Drops. Formula DC Vaginal Jelly. *With benzocaine:* Idol, Lanocaine		

Contactant	Concentration and Vehicle	Exposure	Crossreactions	Comment
Chloroxylenol	1% pet	Chloroxylenol Solution B.P., Absorbine, Jr., Redux EGG Paste, NulloFoot Cream, Rezamid Cream Lotion,Acne Aid, Cenathesin, First aid petroleum jelly. *Sprays:* Feminine hygiene "My Own" (EMKO), Unburn, Unguentine, Top Brass, Stopette Deodorant. *Powders: ZeaSORB*, Desitin, Aveeno	Chlorocresol	Synonyms: p-chloro-meta-xylenol; 4chloro-3,5-xylenol; Ottasept; PCMX; Bezytol
Chlorpromazine chloride (Thorazine)	1% pet.	Medical, nursing and chemistry personnel	Phenothiazines	Photoallergic and phototoxic
Chromium sulfate	2% aq.	Textile inks, paints, varnishes, leather processing, lithographing, fur dyeing, electroplating, blueprinting		Trivalent chromium
Chromium trichloride	0.5% aq.	See Chromium sulfate		Use 1/100 for intradermal testing
Chrysarobin	0.03% pet.	Topical medications		Obtained from goa powder (Indian tree)
Chrysoidine brown	5% pet.	Leather dyes	Para-amino compounds	
Cidex	1% aq.	Cold sterilizing solution	To be freshly prepared	Is 2% buffered glutaraldehyde
Cinchona, tincture of	1% alc.	Hair tonics, rubefacients		
Cinnabar (red mercuric sulfide)	1% pet.	Red tattoos, topical medications		Only mercurial compatible with sulfur May cause lichenoid and granulomatous allergic reactions
Cinnamates (2-ethoxyethyl-p-methoxy)	1% pet.	Sunscreens		Photosensitizer
Cinnamic acid	5% pet.	Styrax, balsam of Peru, menthyl and benzyl cinnamates in sunscreens: RVPaque (Elder), SunDare Lotion (Texas Pharmacal), Sun Bath (Revlon), Sun Tan Gelee (Rexall)		Contact urticaria
Cinnamic aldehyde	1% pet.	Cinnamon oil, cassia oil, cinnamon powder, patchouli oil, flavoring agents, toilet soaps, perfumes	Balsam of Peru, benzoin	Depigmentation Contact urticaria
Cinnamon oil	2% pet.	Cassia bark, flavoring agents, vermouths, gum, toothpastes, confections, cola beverages, tobacco, bubble gum, lipsticks	Balsam of Peru, cinnamic aldehyde, bay leaf, marjoram	Contact urticaria
Citric acid (citron oil)	1% aq.	Transfusions, nicotine stain remover, astringent mouthwash		Cause of aphthous ulcers?
Citronella oil (lemon grass oil)	1% pet.	Perfumes, insect repellents		

Contactant	Concentration and Vehicle	Exposure	Crossreactions	Comment
Citrus Red 2	2% acet.	Dye for Florida orange peel		An azo dye
Clindamycin	1% aq.	Antibiotic		
Clorox	1% aq.	Detergents, chlorinated alkalines		
Clove oil	1% pet.	Eugenol, antiseptics, local anesthetics, mucilage, perfumes, condiments, chewing gum	Balsam of Peru, diethylstilbestrol, benzoin	
Coal tar	5%, pet.	Adhesives, creosotes, insecticides, phenols, wood working, preservation of wood		Photosensitizing
Cobalt chloride	2% aq. or 1% pet.	Tattoos, pottery, clays, cements, hematinics, alloys, anodes, glass enamels, adhesives, fly paper, hair dyes, carbides, pigments	Vitamin B$_{12}$	Vitamin B$_{12}$ (Cobione) isa cobalt compound
Cobalt naphthenate	2% pet.	Polyester resins, rubber industry	Other cobalt salts	
Cobalt sulfate	2% aq.	Alloys, dyeing, lacquers, glass, paints, oilcloth colors, enamels, permanent ink for porcelain		
Cobaltous aluminate (azure orcobalt blue)	2% aq.	Blue tattoo pigment		
Cocaine hydrochloride	1% aq.			Based on benzoic acid
Cocaine liquid	1% aq.	Topical anesthetics, mydriatic		Based on benzoic acid
Cocamidopropyl betaine	1% aq.	Hair and bath products		Non-ionic surfactant
Coconut oil	Pure	Soaps, oleomargarine, cooking fat, baking ingredients, confections		
Coconut soap (sodium salt)	2% aq.	Surfactant, synthetic detergents, bubble baths		Control
Cocobolo wood	As is	Musical instruments, kitchen utensil handles, woodworking industry		
Coins, U.S.A.	As is	Penny Nickel Dime Quarter Half dollar		95% copper, 5% zinc 75% copper, 25% nickel 90% copper, 8% nickel 90% copper, 8% nickel 60% copper, 40% nickel (All U.S. coins except the penny give a positive dimethylglyoxime testreaction)

Contactant	Concentration and Vehicle	Exposure	Crossreactions	Comment
Collodion	As is			Contains ether, absolute ethyl alcohol and pyroxylin
Collodion, flexible	As is			Contains colophony (rosin) and castor oil
Colocynth extract	1% alc.	Denaturing agent in alcohol		
Colophony	See Rosin			
Congo red	2% pet.	Azo dye		Diagnostic aid in amyloidosis, indicator of free HCl in gastric contents
Coniferyl benzoate	1% pet.	Benzoin	Benzyl cinnamate, benzyl alcohol, eugenol, benzoin, vanilla	
Copper sulfate	2% pet.	Insecticides, fungicides, food processing, fertilizers, mordant in fur dyeing, coin alloys, D'Alibour solution		A rare sensitizer
Coriander, oil of	10% c.o.	Flavoring agents		
Costus root oil	0.1% pet	Plants		
Cottonseed oil	As is	Cosmetics, margarine, vegetable shortening		
Coumarin	10% o.o.	Flavorings (including vanilla), perfumes, cosmetics, optical bleaches		A cinnamic acid derivative Photosensitizer
Creosote (creosote oil)	10% o.o.	Expectorants, preserving wood, waterproofing, lumber industry		A photosensitizer
Cresol	1% aq.	Antiseptics		
Crotamiton	5% pet.	Scabies treatment		
Crystal violet	1% aq.	Gentian violet		
Curcumin	1% pet.			
Cutting oil	As is (open) or 50% o.o.			Controls. May contain additives
Cyclaine (hexylcaine hydrochloride; Merck Sharp & Dohme)	1% aq.	Local anesthetics	Procaine p-Amino-compounds	
Cyclohexamide (actidione)	1% pet.	Culture media, garden spray	Neomycin	
Cyclohexanol peroxide	0.5% pet.	Polyester resin hardener		

Contactant	Concentration and Vehicle	Exposure	Crossreactions	Comment
n-Cyclohexyl benzothiazyl sulfenamide	1% pet.	Rubber	Mercapto derivatives	
Dammar resin	20% pet.	Plasters, varnishes, lacquers		Resin from East Indies plant
Dangard	0.25% pet.	Q.E.D. Shampoo sold by barbers		
DDT (dichlorodiphenyl-trichloroethane)	1% pet.	Insecticides, chlorobenzene derivatives		May produce chloracne and possibly porphyria
Decyl alcohol	5% pet.	Lanolin		An aliphatic alcohol
Depilatories	As is (open)			Controls
Dequalinium chloride	0.1% aq.	Micrin Mouthwash, antiseptics		A quaternary ammonium compound
Desenex (WTS-Pharmacraft)	As is	Antifungal agents		Rare sensitizer
Detergent 1011 (secondary amide of lauric acid)	1% aq.	Surfactant, nonionic synthetic detergents		Controls
Detergent, enzyme	0.25% aq.			Test the pure subtilisms 0.1% aq.
Dexketoprofen	2% pet.			Topical NSAID
Diallyl phthalate	0.1% acet.	Polyester resin industry		A strong irritant
Diaminodiphenylmethane	0.5% pet.	Rubber antioxidant, epoxy resin curingagent, intermediate in germicides, surface active agents, pharmaceuticals, corrosion inhibitors, phosphateinsecticides	Amino compounds Polyurethane resins	Photosensitizer
Diazolidinyl Urea (Germall II)	1% aq.	Preservative in cosmetics		
Diazonium	1% alc. (open).	Phosphate inseticides		
Diazonium compounds	10% aq.	Ozalid photocopy paper		Contains 4-nn'-diethyl-amino benzene diazonium chloride
Dibenzothiazyl disulfide	1% pet.	Rubber	Mercapto derivatives	
Di-beta-naphthyl para-phenylenediamine	1% pet.	Rubber	Paraphenylene derivatives	
Dibromsalan (dibromosalicylanilide)	1% pet.	Deodorant soaps, White Lifebuoy		Photoallergic
Dibutyl phthalate	5% pet.	Plasticizer for synthetic resins, nail lacquer		
Dibutyl tin maleate	1% pet.	Plasticizer in plastic (Elastiglass)		
Dichlorobenzene	5% chloroform	Mothballs		A primary sensitizer

Contactant	Concentration and Vehicle	Exposure	Crossreactions	Comment
Dichlorodiphenyl (methylcarbinol)	5% acet. (open)	Organic insecticides		
1,2,4-Dichloronitrobenz ene (dinitrochlorobenzine) (DNCB)	0.1% acet.	Algicide in air conditioner NALCO-205		A primary sensitizer
Dichlorophene (G4)	1% aq.	Fungicides, antimildew agents, preservative in creams, dentifrices	Hexachlorophene	
Dichloropropane	1% pet.	Used in production of plastic products		
Diclofenac	2.5–5.0% pet.			
N-(2-(diethylamino)ethyl)-acrylamide	1% pet.			
Diethylene glycol monobutyl ether	1% aq.			
Diethylenetriamine	0.1% aq.	Epoxy resin amine	Ethylenediamine HCL	
Diethylethanolamine	0.1% aq.	Amine polyurethane catalyst		
Diethyl-meta-toluamide (DEET)	5% alc. (open)	Black Flag, Off, 7—11, RVPellent (Elder)		May produce bullous eruption
Diethylparaphenylenediamine (CD₂)	1% pet.	Color film developers	Para-amino compound	Lichen planus reaction
Diethylstilbestrol	0.1% in ethyl alc.	Aquarant "E" (Webster), Furestrol Suppositories (Eaton), diethylstilbestrol suppositories (Lilly)	Dienestrol, hexestrol,bisphenol A, monobenzyl-ether of hydroquinone, eugenol, stilbene benzophenone benzylbenzoate	Contact urticaria
Diethylthiourea	1% pet.			Sensitizer in diver's wetsuit
Difluorodiphenyl-trichloroethane	5% acet.	Insecticides		
Difolantan	1:1000 aq.	Fungicide for farm crops		Derivative of dicarboximide
Digalloyltrioleate	3% pet.	A-Fil, Neo-A-Fil (Texas Pharmacal), Sunprotectol (Lamond)		Sunscreens may be photosensitive
Dihydrostreptomycin sulfate	20% pet.	Pharmaceutical and nursing personnel	Neomycin, kanamycin, streptomycin	
Dihydroxyacetone	10% aq.	Man Tan, Magictan, Positan, Tan-O-Rama, Tansation, Tanfastic		Rare sensitizer
Dihydroxyphenyl	0.1% pet.	Rubber		
Diisocyanatohexane	1% aq.	Textile finish		
Diisopropyl fluorophosphate	1% alc.(open)	Insecticides		Usually occupational
Dilan	5% acet.(open)	Insecticides		

Contactant	Concentration and Vehicle	Exposure	Crossreactions	Comment
Dimethoxane	1% pet.	Preservative in water systems and emulsions		
Dimethylamino propylamine	1% pet.	Epoxy resin hardener		Irritant
Dimethylaniline	1% pet	Polyester resin accelerator		
Dimethylglyoxime	10% in Carbowax	Chemical test for nickel		
Dimethyl paratoluidine	2% pet.	Accelerators, acrylic resins		
Dimethyl phthalate	20% pet.	Plasticizer for synthetic resins, insect repellents		761
Dimethyl sulfate	Do not test			Forms sulfuric acid
Dimethyl sulfoxide (DMSO)	90% aq.	Industrial solvents, topical medicaments		Primary urticariogenic agent
Dimethylol dihydroxy ethylene urea (Fixapret CPN)	4.5% aq.	Permanent press clothing	Other textile resins	
Dimethylol urea formaldehyde	10% pet.	Crease resistant, drip-dry clothing		Releases formaldehyde
Dimite dichlorodiphenyl-ethanol	5% acet.(open)	Insecticides		
Di-β-naphthyl-p-phenylenediamine	1% pet.	Rubber antioxidant	IPPD	
Dinitrochlorobenzene (DNCB)	0.1 % acet.	Investigative sensitizer, algicide in water cooling systems	Chloromycetin (chloramphenicol)?	A primary sensitizer
Dinobuton	1% pet.	Insecticide in Acrex		
Dioctyl phthalate	1% pet.	Plastics and rubber		
Dioctyl sodium sulfosuccinate	1% aq.	Wetting compounds, anionic surfactant		
Diodoquin (diiodohydroxyquin; Searle)	5% pet .	Amebicides	Vioform, Quinolor,Sterosan	
Dioxane	1% aq.	Degreasing solvent		
Dipentamethylene thiuramdisulfide	1% pet.	Rubber	Other thiuram compounds	
Diphenyl	2% pet.	Dielectrics	Fungicide for oranges	
Diphenylcyclopropenone	0.1% acet.	Chemistry experiments		
Diphenylguanidine	1% pet .	Rubber accelerator		
Dipivefrin chloride	1% aq.	Epinephrine (sometimes)		
Diphenylparaphenylenediamine	1% pet.	Rubber accelerator (black rubber)	PPDA derivative	

Contactant	Concentration and Vehicle	Exposure	Crossreactions	Comment
Dipropylenetriamine	1% pet.	Epoxy resin hardener		
Dithiomorpholine	1 % pet.	Rubber vulcanizer		
Dithionone	1% pet.	Pesticide		Merck product
Divinyl benzene (styrene)	1% o.o.	See Styrene		
dl-chlorpheniramine maleate	1% pet.			
DMDM Hydantoin	1% aq.	Preservative		Other names: Bis-(hy-droxymethyl) dimeth-ylimidazolidinedione, Dimethylol-Dimethyl Hydantoin Glydant, Imidazolidinedione-Bis(hydroxymethyl) Dimethyl
Domiphen bromide	0.1% aq.	Quaternary compound in Scope Mouthwash		A "Quat" compound
Dorzolamide hydrochloride	5% pet			Trusopt eyedrops
Dowicide(s)	1% pet.	Germicides, fungicides, antiseptics, disinfectants		A series of phenolic substances
Dowicide A (sodium-o-phenylphenate)	1% pet.	Dowicide A, B, and G used in paper money		Not absorbed through skin. An oil solution (5%) is well tolerated on human skin, but aqueous solutions of the sodium salt are irritating in concentrations exceeding 0.5%.
Dowicide B (sodium 2,3,5-trichlorophenate)	1% pet.	Water-soluble fungicide		
Dowicide C (sodium chloro-o-phenyl phenate)	1% pet.	Water-soluble antiseptic		
Dowicide D (2-chloro-4-phenyl-phenol sodium)	1% pet.	Germicide		
Dowicide E (2-bromo-4-phenyl-phenol sodium)	1% pet.	Fungicide		
Dowicide F (sodium tetrachlorophenate)	1% pet.	Used as germicide, antiseptic, fungicide		
Dowicide G (sodium pentachlorophenate)	1% pet.	Industrial antiseptic		
Dowicide H (sodium tetrachlorophenoxide)	1% pet.	Industrial antiseptic		
Dowicide 1 (o-phenyl phenol)	1% pet.	Germicide, antiseptic, fungicide		
Dowicide 3 (chlorophenylphenol)	1% pet.	Germicide, antiseptic, fungicide		

Contactant	Concentration and Vehicle	Exposure	Crossreactions	Comment
Dowicide 4 (2-chloro-4-phenylphenol)	1% pet.	High-efficiency germicide		
Dowicide 6 (tetrachlorophenol)	1% pet.	Germicide, antiseptic, fungicide		
Dowicide 7 (pentachlorophenol)	1% pet.	Oil-soluble antiseptic, germicide, fungicide		
Dowicil 200	1% pet.	Bactericide		Release formaldehyde
Duponol WA (sodium lauryl sulfate)	1% aq.	Surfactant, anionic synthetic detergents		Controls
Duraspan (International Latex)	As is	Polyurethane elastomer (Spandex)		
Dyclone (dyclonine hydrochloride; Dow Chemical)	1% aq.	Local anesthetics		Not based on para-aminobenzoic acid
Dyes Certified Disperse Orange 3 Blue Disperse Yellow 3 Red1	2% pet. 1% pet.	Foods, drugs, cosmetics Nylon dyes	Para-amino compounds	
Ecogaine	2% aq.	Local anesthetics	Procaine, benzocaine P-amino compound	Based on para-aminobenzoic acid
Edathamil (calcium EDTA versenate)	1% aq.	Chelating agent		
Eldoquin (Elder)	See Hydroquinone			
Emulsifying wax	30% pet.			Contains alkyl stearyl alcohol
Eosin	50% pet.	Fluorescent dyes, pharmaceuticals		A photosensitizer
Ephedrine	1% pet.	Nose drops		
Epichlorhydrin	0.1% alc.	Epoxy resin	Propene oxide	
Epon 828	1% acet.	Epoxy resins		
Epon 1001	1% acet.	Epoxy resins		
Epoxy acrylate	0.5% pet.	UV inks and varnishes	Other acrylates	
Epoxy glue hardener	0.5% pet.	One part of 2 tube preparation, house-hold glue, collages, sculptures		May contain triethylene-tetramine or diamino-diphenylmethane
Epoxy glue resin	1% acet.			Has caused contact urticaria
Epoxy glycidyl ether	0.1% acet.			Epoxy resin diluent
Erythromycin stearate	1% pet.	Antibiotic		

Contactant	Concentration and Vehicle	Exposure	Crossreactions	Comment
Erythrosin	2% pet.	Fluorescent dyes		A photosensitizer
Esoterica (Mitchum)	As is	Skin-lightening cream		Contains ammoniated mercury
Essential oils	1% alc. Or 2%pet.	Flavor in dentifrices, mouthwashes, medicinal elixirs, perfumes		May be photosensitizer
Ether	60% o.o.	Anesthetics, solvents		May be irritant
Ethoxyethyl-p-methoxycinna-mate	5% pet.	Sunscreen		Photosensitivity
Ethoxyquin	1% o.o.	Apple packing, animal feed additive		A quinoline
Ethyl acetate	5% mek.	Solvent for varnishes, lacquers and nitrocellulose plastics, component of nail-polish removers		Trace amounts in foods and alcoholic beverages
Ethyl acrylate	0.1% pet.	Crosslink agent in rubber		
Ethyl butyl thiourea	1% pet.	Neoprene adhesive		
Ethyl cetab (cetylethyldimethyl-ammoniumbromide)	0.1% aq.	Surfactant, cationic synthetic detergents		Controls"Quat" compound
Ethyl hexyl acrylate	0.5% pet.			
Ethyl parahydroxybenzoate	5% pet.	Preservative in pharmaceuticals, cosmetics, foods, cleansers	Other parabens	May cause systemic contact dermatitis
Ethylene dichloride	50% o.o.	Solvents, plastics, rubber, insecticides, hobby crafts		
Ethylene glycol	5% alc.	Antifreeze solvent	Propylene glycol	
Ethylene glycol monomethylether acetate (Egmea)	1% mek.	Used to cement nose pads to eyeglass frames		May contain traces of ethyl acetate
Ethylene oxide	0.01% aq.	Sterilizing gas for surgical instruments, towels, sheets, gloves, anesthesia masks, chemical reactor		Powerful vesicant
Ethylene urea, melamine formaldehyde resin (Fixapret AC)	5% pet.	Permanent press clothing	Other textile resins	
Ethylenediamine hydrochloride	1% pet.	Mycolog Cream, parent substance of certain antihistamines and aminophylline; dyes, rubber, fungicides,waxes, resins, insecticides, asphalt; present in Tincture Merthiolate (Lilly)	Aminophylline, Pyribenzamine, Antistine, Diethyltetramine Piperaine citrate Piperazine	Can cause systemic contact dermatitis

Contactant	Concentration and Vehicle	Exposure	Crossreactions	Comment
Ethylenediamine tetraacetate (Versene)	1% aq.	Stabilizing agent in many ophthalmic solutions, chelating agent		
Etofenamate	0.5% pet.			Contact and photocontact Topical NSAID
1,3-Ethylhexanediol	5% o.o.	Insect repellent		Irritant
Eucalyptus oil	1% alc.	Gutta percha for root canal fillings	Balsam of Peru, benzoin, vanilla, oil of orange peel	
Eugenol	25% pet.	Oil of carnation (hyacinth), oil of bay, pimento oil (allspice), clove oil, flower oils, cinnamon oil, foodspices, perfumes, zinc oxide dental cement, flavoring agent, dental impression agent	Iso-Eugenol Balsam of Peru Benzoin Propanoid	Derived from clove oil Has caused contact urticaria
Eurax Cream and Lotion (10%n-ethyl-o-crotonotoluide;Geigy)	As is	Scabicide		
Euxyl K400	0.5% pet.	Cosmetics, skin care products	Mix of phenoxyethanol and methyldibromoglutaronitrile	
Evafanol AS-1	1% aq.	Fabric finish		Anti-"pilling" agent
Evans Blue Dye	1% aq.	Azo dye		Used in lymphangiography
Eyeglass frames, plastic	Shavings (controls)			Possible allergens: cellulose acetate, cellulose propionate, resorcinol monobenzoate, anthraquinone p-tertiarybutyl phenol, azodyes, beeswax-turpentine mixture, ethyleneglycol, ethylene oxideand ethyl acetate
Eyeglass nose pad				Ethylene glycol mono-methyl ether acetate (welds nose pad to eyeglass frames)
Fentichlor	1% pet. (open and closed)	Antiseptic and fungicide, cosmetics, pharmaceuticals		A photosensitizer
Fepradinol	2% eth.			NSAID, causes eczema and photodermatitis
Ferric chloride	2% aq.	Monsel's solution, styptic		Very rare sensitizer
Flit	25% o.o.	Insecticide		
Fluorescein	10% pet.	Dyes, eyeglass cleaner		Photosensitizer
Fluorouracil	5% pet.	Cytotoxic drug		Phototoxic?

Contactant	Concentration and Vehicle	Exposure	Crossreactions	Comment
Formaldehyde resins	10% pet.	Plastics, textile finishes		
Urea formaldehyde	10% pet.	Glues, plastics, textile finishes		
Melamine formaldehyde	1% pet. or 1% isopropyl alcohol			
Others				
Formalin (40% sol. of formaldehyde gas)	1 or 2% aq.sol.	*Cosmetics:* shampoos, antiperspirants, Sub-Rosa Cream Deodorant, nail hardener, nail polish, resins, Thermodent Toothpaste, soaps, permanent wave lotions. *Medical:* root canal preparation (Forno-Cresol) disinfectant, wart remedies, fungicides, insecticides, tissue fixative, embalming fluid, denatured alcohol, orthopedic casts, renal dialysis unit, vaccines. *Industrial:* tanning white leather, tex-tile finish (antiwrinkle), synthetic gums and adhesives, synthetic resins and rubber, paper, photography, antimildew in leather, glues, wet strength paper	Glutaraldehyde?	Hexamethylenetetra-mine (methenamine) liberates formaldehyde in the presence of acids. Formaldehyde-releasing agents. May cause contact urticaria
Formic acid spirits	1% aq.	Hair tonics		
Fowler's solution (potassium arsenite solution)	As is			Equivalent to 1% arsenic trioxide
Fuchsin	1% pet.	Basic fuchsin, rosaniline, therapeutic dye, fuchsin silver nitrate. Marking patch test sites—irritant		
Fumaronitrile	**Do not test**	Plasticizer for vinyl resin herbicide, soil fumigant		A potent irritant and vesicant. May also be allergen
Furacin (nitrofurazone; Eaton)	As is	Topical bacterial agent	Contains Carbowax	Water-soluble Furacin preparations have a base of polyethylene glycols
Gallium oxide	1% pet.	Semiconductor industry		
Garamycin (Gentamycin)	20% pet.	Antiseptic topical medication	Neomycin, kanamycin	Contact urticaria
Garlic	5% aq. extract		Balsam of Peru, tars, onion	Controls
Gasoline	50% o.o.			
Gentian violet (methylrosaniline chloride)	1% aq.	Stain, indicator, antiseptics, vaginal creams, tablets, aerosols	Rivanol	Intradermal test with 0.05 mL of a 1:5000 dilution
Geraniol	5% pet.	Flavoring agent, perfume, geranium oil		

Contactant	Concentration and Vehicle	Exposure	Crossreactions	Comment
Ginger oil	25% c.o.	Condiments, candy gastric medications, rubefacient		
Ginkgo fruit pulp	1:10 acet.		Rhus, cashew	Ginkgo tree is a member of Anacardium genus
Glospan (Globe Manufacturing Co.)	As is	Polyurethane elastomer (spandex)		Lycra spandex is free of mercaptobenzothiazole
Glue	As is open or 10% acet.	Furniture, shoes, books, toys, waterproofing		Rubber, epoxies, chromates, formaldehyde, polyvinyl acetateresins
Glutaraldehyde	1% aq. freshly prepared	Tissue fixative, antiperspirants, antiseptics, tanning agent for soft leather, embalming fluids, shampoo preservative, dentifrices	Formaldehyde?	Tans and dries skin May discolor skin
Glycerin	10% aq.	Emollient, pharmaceutical vehicle, mounting medium in microscopy		Very rare sensitizer
Glyceryl monooleate	30% pet.	Emulsifier, soaps, cosmetics		
Glyceryl monostearate	30% pet.	Emulsifier, cosmetics, food products, medicinals		
Glyceryl monothioglycolate	2.5% pet.	Permanent waves		
Glycol dimethyl acrylate	5% o.o.	Synthetic resins		Prevents crazing, cracking of resins
Gly-Oxide	As is	Mouthwash providing hydrogen peroxide		Contains urea peroxide
Gold chloride	1% aq.	Photographers		Pustular patch test reaction
Gold leaf	As is	Gilding, topical ulcer medication		
Gold sodium thiosulfate	0.5% pet.	Jewelry, dental		Persistent positive
Gold trichloride	1% aq.	Jewelry		
Gramicidin	5% pet.	Antibacterial topical agent, mouthwashes		
Graphite (black lead)	As is	Lead pencils, crucibles, rubber surfaces, lubricants		
Grotan BK	2% pet.			
Grotan HD-2	0.15% pet.			
Grotan K	1% pet.			
Guaiacol	5% pet			

Contactant	Concentration and Vehicle	Exposure	Crossreactions	Comment
Guaiazulene	1% pet.	Used in Italian lipsticks, dentifrices; anti-inflammatory agent		
Guanine (2-amino-6-hydroxypurine)	5% pet.	Pearly nail lacquer		Obtained from fish scales
Guignet's green (chromium oxide)	2% aq.	Green tattoo pigment		
Gum(s)	50% aq.	Resinous plant exudates		Contains carbohydrates forming mucilaginous substances with water
Gum arabic (acacia)	50% aq.	See Acacia		
Gutta percha	As is aqueous suspension brittle when exposed to air	Resins, rosins, root canal mixtures		Latex of Malaysian trees contains more resin than does rubber
Hair lotions, tonics, and sprays	As is (open)			May contain: *rubefacient*—chloral hydrate, formic acid spirits, quinine salts, tincture capsicum or cinchona, cantharidin; phenolic compounds—chlorthymol, resorcinol, betanaphthol; *other antiseptics*—salicylic acid, formaldehyde, mercurybichloride; *tars*—coal tar derivatives, oil of cade; *vehicle*—alcohol and volatile solvents, perfumes
Haloprogin	1% pet.	Antifungal, antibacterial		
Henna	10 mg powder in 100 mL water or ether	Vegetable dye, synthetic henna (Lawsonia, hydroxynaphthoquinone—the coloring matter of henna leaves)		Rarely sensitizes May cause contact urticaria
Heroin	3% pet.			
Hexachlorophene (G-11)	1% pet.	Soaps, detergents, creams, oils, pharmaceuticals	Bithionol, chlorinated salicylanilides Dichlorophene	Now restricted by FDA primarily to prescription items, photosensitizer
Hexahydrophthalic anhydride	1% pet.			
Hexamethylenetetramine (methenamine)	1% pet.	Many proprietary urinary antiseptics often combined with mandelic acid. Also a rubber accelerator	Formaldehyde	Liberates formaldehyde in the presence of acids
Hexanedioldiacrylate	0.1% pet.	Ultraviolet cured inks		Photosensitizer
Hexetidine	alc.	Antibacterial agent in Sterisol mouthwash, douches		Synonyms: ethylhexyl, hexahydro, methylimidaso, imidasolel

Contactant	Concentration and Vehicle	Exposure	Crossreactions	Comment
Hexylresorcinol	1% pet.	Contraceptives, Sucrettes, Tetrazets, ST37, Crystoids, Caprikol (Merck), Akrinol Cream, Listerine, Lanteen Jelly (Esta), Nymore		
Holocaine (phenacaine) Hcl.	1% aq.	Local anesthetics	Benzocaine, procaine, p-amino compounds	
Homatropine	1% aq.	Eye drops		
Hyamine 1622 (p-diisobutylphenoxyethoxyethyldimethyl benzyl-ammonium chloride)	0.1% aq.	Surfactant, cationic synthetic detergents, bubble baths, Clesk Lotion (Dara), Quinette Inserts (Arnar-Stone)		"Quat"
Hydralizine hydrochloride, bromide or sulfate	1% aq. or 1% pet.	Wide industrial exposure, metal, plastics, rubber products, rocket fuel, photography, insecticides, fungicides, preservatives. Parent substance for drugs listed in adjacent column	Apresoline, isonicotinicacid, hydrazide, phenylhydrazine, Nardil (derived from hydrazinehydrobromide)	
Hydroabietyl alcohol (abitol)	10% pet.	Film former in mascara and adhesive		Abietic acid
Hydrochloric acid	1% aq.	Chemical industry, Acidulin (Lilly), Convertin (Ascher), Muripsin (Norgine), Normacid (Stuart)		Rarely sensitizes Irritant
Hydrocortisone acetate or free alcohol	2.5% alc.			Test with tixocortol pivalate 1%
Hydrogen peroxide solution	3% aq.	Bleaches, oxidizing agents, antiseptics		
Hydrogen sulfide	2% aq.	Petroleum refineries, tunnels, mines, rayon plants		Irritant
Hydrophilic ointment U.S.P.	As is			Contains sodium laurylsulfate, propylene glycol, stearyl alcohol, methyl paraben, propyl paraben, white petrolatum, distilled water
Modified				Modified hydrophilic ointment contains glycerin instead of propylene glycol
Hydrophilic petrolatum(U.S.P.)	As is			Contains stearyl alcohol, cholesterol, white wax, white petrolatum
Hydroquinone	1% pet.	Rubber inhilbitor polyester, acrylic, photography, Eldoquin and Eldopaque (Elder), Artra (White), Dermablanch (Brayten)	Resorcin, pyrocatechol, monobenzylether of hydroquinone	Depigmenting agent May be irritant

Contactant	Concentration and Vehicle	Exposure	Crossreactions	Comment
Hydroquinone, monobenzylether of	See Monobenzylether of hydroquinone			
Hydroxycitronell	1% pet.	Perfume		Causes hyperpigmentation
Hydroxyethyl methacrylate	5% pet.	Anaerobic metal sealant		
2-hydroxyethyl salicylate	5% aq.			Anti-inflammatory gels
8-Hydroxyquinoline	5% pet.	Antibacterial		Bioform, Diodoquin
Hypochloride	2% aq.	Kasenol Mouthwash, Oxychlorosene		
Ibuprofen	10% pet.			
Ichthyol (ichthammol; sulfonated bitumen)	10% pet.	Topical medications, Derma Medicone (Medicone), Ichthymall (Mallinckrodt)		Rarely sensitizes
Idoxuridine	1% pet.	Antiviral agent	Other pyrimidine drugs	
Igepal (nonylphenoxypolyethylene oxyethanol)	1% aq.	Surfactant, synthetic detergents, bubble baths		Controls
Igepon T.H.C. (sodium oleyllaurate)	1% aq.	Surfactant, synthetic detergents, bubble baths		Controls
Imidazolidinyl urea (Germall115)	2% pet.	Antibacterial, antifungal		
Indalone	As is (open)	Insect repellents		
Indane	5% acet. (open)	Insecticides: chlordane, heptachlor, aldrin, dieldrin, endrin, diendrin		
Indigo	5% pet.	Tattoos, stains, blue dye		
Indium chloride	1% pet.			
Ink(s)	As is (open)			Acid and basic dyes, ironsalts, tannic acid, gallates, phenol, silver nitrate, alkalies, castor oil
Ink eradicator	As is (open)			Active agents are tinchloride, sodium bisulfite, sodium hypochlorite, sodium chloride
Iodine crystals	0.5% alc.	Betadine	Iodoform, radiopaque iodine, iodized medications, thymol iodide	Old iodine solutions exposed to light are irritants. Incompatible with sulfur and mercury

Contactant	Concentration and Vehicle	Exposure	Crossreactions	Comment
Iodine, tincture of	As is (open)		Same as Iodine crystals	Is an irritant when covered
Iodixanol	5% aq.			Visipaque
Iodochlorhydroxyquin	3% pet.	Vioform, Sterosan, Chinoform, Clioquinol	Chloroquinadol Hydroxyquinoline	Topical agents may produce irritant & allergic reaction
Iodoform (formyl triiodide)	5% pet.	Local anesthetics, antiseptics	Iodine, formaldehyde	
Ioprep	As is (open)			Irritant when occluded
Irgasan GF3 (Cloflucarban[Geigyl)	0.5% pet.	Safeguard soap; used abroad as bacteriostat in vinyl gloves; shampoos		A carbanilide
Irgasan DP 300 (Triclosan[Geigyl; 2,4,4-trichloro-2-hydroxydiphenyl ether)	0.5% aq.	Surgical scrub soaps; Dial, ColgateP300, Palmolive and Calgan antiseptic soaps; Right Guard, Calm and Dial underarm deodorants and antiperspirants; commercial laundry products, disposable paper products, paper lining for rodent cages, industrial fabric softener, fabric bacteriostat		Widely used bacteriostat
Iridium chloride	1% pet.			
Irish moss (carrageen)	As is	Cosmetics, wave sets, dentifrices, mucilage		Trade names: Sea Kem, Viscarin, Chondrus extract
Iron chloride	2% aq.			
Isobutyl-p-aminobenzoate	5% pet.	Sunscreen	p-amino compounds	
Isocyanate monomer	1.1% acet.	Polyurethane resins	Diaminodiphenylmethane	
Isodine	As is	Mouthwash		Like Betadine, is iodine in PVP
Iso-eugenol	5% pet.	Balsam of Peru—Eugenol		
Isophorone diamine	0.1% o.o.	Epoxy resin hardener		
Isopropyl alcohol	10% aq.	Antiseptic, solvent		
Isopropyl myristate	10% alc. or 2% pet.	Cosmetics, pharmaceuticals, Decaspray, aerosol sprays		Alcohol ester of fatty acid
Isopropyl-n-phenyl para-phenylene-diamine (IPPD)	0.1% pet	Rubber antioxidant (black rubber)	Hair dye, paraphenylenediamine derivatives	May cause lichenoid orpurpuric eruptions. Trade names: Cysone, Eastone, Fleezwax, Flexaone, Santoflex, Nonox-2A

Contactant	Concentration and Vehicle	Exposure	Crossreactions	Comment
Isothane (laurylisoquinolinium bromide)	0.1% aq.	Surfactant, cationic synthetic detergents, bubble baths		Controls "Quat" Compounds
Isothiouronium (PBA-1)	0.1% aq.	Persulfate bleach accelerator		
Jaborandi leaves, tincture of	As is (open)	Hair tonics		
Jasmin absolute	10% pet.	Perfume		
Jasmin, oil	10% pet.	Fragrance		Causes pigmented cosmetic dermatitis
Jasmine synthetic	10% pet.	Perfume		
Javelle water (potassiumhypochlorite)	10% aq.	Disinfecting and bleaching agents	Chloramine	European preparations may contain dichromates
Jojoba oil	20% o.o.	Cosmetics		Replacement for spermacetic OTC treatment wrinkles, dry skin
Juniper tar (oil of cade)	25% c.o.	Alma-Tar (Schieffelin)		
Kanamycin	20% pet.	Antibiotic		Neomycin
Karaya gum (Sterculia gum)	As is10% aq.	Hair-waving lotions, denture adhesivepowders, cement for ileostomy appliances, furniture polishes		Obtained from sterculia ureus
Kathon	0.5% pet.	Antibacterial preservative in cosmetics, shampoos	Contains methylchloroisothiazolinone and methylisothiazolinone	
Kerosene	60% o.o.	Solvents, curing tobacco, heating, cooking, lighting, waterless handcleansers		Irritant
Ketone	10% o.o.	Organic solvents, acetone		
Ketoprofen	1% pet.	Etoprofen, loxoprofen		Topical NSAID
Krameria, tincture of (tincturarhatanhiae)	5% alc.	Poultices for hemorrhoids, oral and mucosal astringents, combined withtincture of myrrh		Primary sensitizer
Kwell (Reed & Carnrick)	As is	Pediculosis remedy		Contains benzene hexachloride
Lactic acid	3% aq.	Astringent mouthwash, pharmaceutical creams		
Lamotrigine	10% pet.			Stevens-Johnson syndrome
Lanoconazole	1% pet.			Antifungal

Contactant	Concentration and Vehicle	Exposure	Crossreactions	Comment
Lanolin	As is	Wool fat, wool wax, adhesives, cosmetics, pharmaceuticals	Eucerin Wool alcohols	Wool alcohols may be the specific sensitizers
Lansoprazole	10% pet.			
Lantrol (dewaxed lanolin)	As is			
Latex	As is	Rubber, gutta percha, chicle, balata, fig		Fig tree latex is a sensitizer and photosensitizer
Laurel oil	2% pet.	Flavoring agent, felt hats, camphor laurel, plastics, perfumes, pharmaceuticals		
Lauryl alcohol	20% pet.	Lanolin		An aliphatic alcohol
Lauryl gallate	0.1% pet.	Antioxidant in margarine and cosmetics		
Lavender oil	1% alc. Or pet.	Colognes, cosmetics, soaps, china, ceramics and paintings	Balsam of Peru, rosin, wood tar, essential oils	A photosensitizer, pigmentation, essential oil
Lead acetate	0.5% aq.			
Lead arsenate	20% pet.	Fungicides, insecticides		
Lead chloride	0.2% aq.	Fur processing, felt processing, mordants, printing, solder, and flux		
Lead oxide (red lead)	2% alc.	Matches, glazes for ceramics, paints		
Lemon grass oil	2% pet.	Perfume		
Lemon oil	2% pet.	Perfume		
Lidocaine (Xylocaine)	1% pet.	Anesthetic		Amide
Lime, slaked (calcium hydroxide)	As is	Hydrated lime		Controls. See also Calcium oxide (quicklime)
Limonene, oil of (Pipentene)	2% pet.	Orange, lemon peel, perfumes, lemonwood	Turpentine, celery, bergamot, dill	Main sensitizer of orange and lemon peel
Linalool, oil of	10% pet.	Flavoring in dentifrices		
Lindane	1% pet.	Pesticide		Hexachlorocyclohexane,gammahexane Has caused urticaria
Linseed oil	As is	Paints, varnishes, sculpturing, furniture polishes, refinishing waxes, car ron oil, putty, folk medicine		
Lipstick	As is			Indelible variety may photosensitize

Contactant	Concentration and Vehicle	Exposure	Crossreactions	Comment
Lycra (Du Pont)	As is	Polyurethane elastomer (spandex)		
Lysol (compound cresol solution)	1% aq.	Disinfectant		
Mace, oil of (nutmeg)	1% alc.	Flavoring agent		
Mafenide acetate	8% pet.	Burn remedy (Sulfamylon Cream)		
Magnesium peroxide	10% pet.	Oxidizing agent—McLean's Toothpaste		
Malachite green	2% aq.	Dye		
Malathion	1% alc.(open) 0.5% pet.	Insecticides		A primary sensitizer
Maleic anhydride	1% aq.	Epoxy resin		
Maneb	1% pet.	Present in fungicides, pesticides, known as manganese ethylene bis-dithiocarbamate		
Manganese chloride	5% pet.	Pigment in rubber goods, alloy in iron and steel, dry batteries, brick, pottery, dyeing industry, drying paint sand varnishes, glass making, printing, dyeing textiles		
Mastic	As is (open)	Varnishes, styptic, astringent, cements, microscopy, dentistry		Resin of European mastic tree
Matches and match boxes(striking surfaces)	As is			Principal ingredients are potassium chlorate, red phosphorus, phosphorus sesquisulfide (phosphorus trisulfide), antimony sulfide, chromates, red lead, glue, cornstarch, coloring agents, rosin, paraffin May cause airborne dermatitis and contact urticaria
Melamine formaldehyde	10% pet.	Clothing finishes, epoxy resins, synthetic resins		
Menthol	1% pet.	Flavoring agents, rubefacients, dusting powders, douches, foods, cigarettes, liqueurs, mixed drinks, Listerine, Reef, Chloraseptic, face cream, toothpaste, mint candies, coughdrops, aerosol room spray	Contact urticaria	
Mercaptans	10% aq.	Depilatories, glue	Thioglycolic acid, BAL (dimercaprol)	
Mercaptobenimidazole	1% pet.			
Mercaptobenzothiazole	1% pet.	Rubber accelerator	Mercapto derivatives	

Contactant	Concentration and Vehicle	Exposure	Crossreactions	Comment
Mercolized cream (Dearborn)	As is	Skin lightener cream		Contains ammoniated mercury Irritant
Mercresin Tincture (Upjohn)	As is (open)		Organic and inorganic mercurials	Irritant when covered. Contains organic mercury and cresol
Mercurochrome Solution (merbromin; Hynson, Westcott & Dunning)	As is	Organic mercurial antiseptic	Organic and inorganic mercurials Metallic mercury	
Mercurous chloride (calomel)	0.5% pet.	Topical and systemic medicaments	Organic and inorganic mercurials Metallic mercury	May produce eczematous "contact-type" dermatitis medicamentosa
Mercury (metallic)	0.5% pet.	Dentistry, thermometer		
Mercury bichloride	0.05% aq.	Disinfectants, processing artificial silk, bronzing, dental laboratories, electric wiring, electroplating, electric equipment, paints, electric storage batteries, reagents, embalming fluid, fur processing, felt curing, engraving, printing, thermometers, metal work, mirror finishing, lamp bulbs, photography, photogravure, insecticides, skin lighteners	Organic and inorganic mercurials Metallic mercury	May cause nonspecific pustular patch test reactions Irritant
Mercury-salicylic ointment	As is (open)	Topical medications		May irritate glabrous skin
Merthiolate (thimerosal)	0.1% pet.	Preservative in cosmetics, topical medications, dentifrices, germicides Contact lens solutions		Contains an organicmercurial and thiosalicylic acid. Tincture of Merthiolate contains ethylenediamine
Mesna	1% aq.			Mistabron
Metacide	1% alc. (open)	Insecticides		
Metaphen (nitromersol; Abbott)	0.5% pet.	Germicides	Inorganic mercurials	
Metaphenylenediamine	0.1% aq.	Epoxy hardeners		
Methoxychlor	5% acet.	Insecticides		
8-Methoxypsoralen	0.001% alc.	Plants of Umbelliferae family, perfume oils (oil of bergamot), Trisoralen (Elder)		A photosensitizer
Methyl acetate	10% o.o.	Organic solvents		
Methyl acrylate	0.1% pet.	Textiles, leather		Susceptible to cold and water

Contactant	Concentration and Vehicle	Exposure	Crossreactions	Comment
Methyl alcohol (methanol)	Pure as is	Solvents, thinners, artificial leather manufacture, dry cleaning, antifreeze, rubber cement, celluloid,gums, resins, chemical processing		*Synonyms:* methyl hydrate, methyl hydroxide, acetone, alcohol, wood spirits, wood naphtha, carbinol, Columbian spirits, colonial spirits
Methyl bromide	**Do not test**	Fire extinguisher fluid, refrigerants, fumigants		Severe irritant
Methyl cellulose	2% aq.	Binder in dentifrices		
6-Methyl coumarin	10% alc.	Perfume		Photosensitizer
Methyl dichlorobenzene sulfonate	0.1% acet.	Dental impression material		
Methyl diisocyanate (MDI)	1% pet.			
Methyl ethyl ketone	As is (open)	Solvents		
Methyl ethyl ketone peroxide	0.5% acet.	Polyester resin catalyst		
MEK peroxide (methyl ethylketone peroxide)	1% pet.			
Methyl heptene carbonate	0.1% alc.	Perfumes, blend fixatives in lipsticks, soaps		
Methyl methacrylate	2% pet.	Resin used in dentistry, bone cement, adhesive artificial nails		
Methyl morpholine	0.1% aq.	Polyurethane catalyst		
Methyl orange	2% pet.	Indicator		
Methyl parahydroxybenzoate	5% pet.	Preservatives, pharmaceuticals, cosmetics, food, cleansers	"Parabens"	May cause systemic contact dermatitis
Methyl salicylate	2% o.o.	Flavoring in dentifrices, Listerine, Reef, oil of wintergreen, rubefacients	Sodium salicylate aspirin	A primary sensitizer May cause systemic contact dermatitis
Methylbenzethonium chloride	0.1% aq.	Germicides, disinfectants, Diaparene (Breon)		Quaternary ammonium disinfectant
Methylchloroisothiazoli-none/ methylisothiazolone (MCI/MI or Kathon CG)	100 ppm	Cosmetics, skin and hair care products Industrial water systems, cutting oils		
Methylene blue	2% pet.	Dyes, platinum bleach	Phenothiazines	A photosensitizer
Methylisothiazolinone	0.5% pet.	Antibacterial preservative in cosmetics, shampoos		Present in Kathon

Contactant	Concentration and Vehicle	Exposure	Crossreactions	Comment
n-Methylol-chloracetamide	5% pet.	Preservative, coolant oils, and cosmetics found in Danish Product Parmetol		
n-Methylolacrylamide	0.1% pet.	Combined with vinyl acetate coatings, adhesives, varnishes		
Metol	1% pet.	Photography	p-amino compound	p-Methylaminophenolsulfate
Metycaine (piperocaine; Lilly) HCL	1% aq.	Local anesthetics, suppositories, ophthalmic ointment		Based on benzoic acid, not on para-amino-benzoic acid
Miconazole nitrate	2% pet.	Antifungal agents		
Miconazole nitrate	2% pet.	Antimycotic agent		
Miranol HM (Lauroyl imidazoline)	2% aq.	Surfactant, synthetic detergents, bubble baths		Controls
Miranol SM (capryl imidazoline derivative)	1% aq.	Surfactant, synthetic detergents, bubble baths		Controls
Mirbane oil	10% o.o.			
Mirbane oil (nitrobenzene)	25% c.o.	Substitute for oil of bitter almonds, manufacturing aniline dyes		
Mitomycin C	0.1% pet.	Bladder instillation		Acral eruption
Monobenzylether of hydroquinone (agerite alba; monobenzone)	1% pet.	Rubber antioxidant, depigmenting agent, Benoquin (Elder)	Hydroquinone	Sensitizer and producer of leukoderma
Monoglycerol para-amino benzoate	5% pet.	Sunscreening agents	Para-amino compounds	A photosensitizer
Monosulph (sulfated castor oil)	2% aq.	Surfactant, synthetic detergents, bubble baths		Controls
Monsel's solution	As is (open)	Styptic		Contains approximately 20% iron
Morphine	1% aq.		Apomorphine	Primarily urticariogenic on scratch or intracutaneous testing
Morpholine	1% pet.	Present in Sulfasan—vulcanizing agent		
Morpholinylmercaptobenzo-thiazole	1% pet.	Rubber accelerator	Other mercapto derivatives	
Mucilage	As is			Plant substances forming adhesive liquids with water
Musk ambrette	5% alc.	Aftershave lotion, perfume		Photosensitizer

Contactant	Concentration and Vehicle	Exposure	Crossreactions	Comment
Musk ambrette	5% pet.	Perfume		Photosensitizer
Mustard oil	0.1% pet.	Flavoring in food products, soaps, drugs, folk medicine		Contains allyl thiocyanate
Myristyl alcohol	5% pet.	Lanolin Pharmaceuticals		
Myroxylon pereirae	25% pet.	Topical medications, cements, (Warner-Chilcott), Rectocaine Suppositories (Moore Kirk), Endacaine Compound Suppositories, Granulex, Rectal Medicone Suppositories and Ointment, Wyanoids HC, Calmol 4, Melynor Ointment (Davies RoseHoyt), cosmetics, hair tonics, per-fumes, flavoring industry, china painting, oil painting	Benzoin, rosin, benzoic acid, benzyl alcohol, cinnamic acid, essential oils, orange peel,eugenol, cinnamon, clove, Tolu balsam, storax, benzyl benzoate, wood tars	An important sensitizer A perfume allergy indicator May cause contact urticaria Systemic ACD
Myrrh, tincture	10% alc.	Astringosol and Odora Lorvic Disinfectants		
Nacconol NRSF (alkylaryl sulfonate)	1% aq.	Surfactant, anionic synthetic detergents, bubble baths		Controls
Nail polish	As is			Sulfonamide resin most common sensitizer. Dye may be photosensitizer
Naphtha	50% o.o.	Solvents, dry cleaning agents, varnishes, fuel		
Naphthalene	2% alc.	Mothballs, moth flakes, deodorant cakes, synthetic intermediate		
Naphthol A-S	1% pet.	Textiles		Dye coupler
Neomycin	20% pet.	Topical medications, cosmetics, soaps, deodorants	Other aminoglycosides, antibiotics	If reaction to patch test is negative, check with 1/100 intradermal testing
Neoprene	20% in equal parts of toluene and ethylacetate	Rubber industry, thiourea		
Neroli, oil of	2% pet.	Essential perfume oil, liqueurs		A photosensitizer
Nesacaine (chloroprocaine hydrochloride; Strasenburgh)	2% aq.	Local anesthetics	Para-amino compounds	
Neticonazole	1% pet.			Antifungal
Neutral red	0.1% aq.	Dye added to quaternary ammonium salts to control pH		Neutral red is red at pH6.8 and yellow at 8.0 Photosensitizer

Contactant	Concentration and Vehicle	Exposure	Crossreactions	Comment
Neutronyx 600 (aromaticpolyglycol ether condensate)	1% aq.	Surfactant, nonionic synthetic detergents, bubble baths		Controls
Nickel sulfate	2.5% pet. (USA), 5% pet. (EU)	Hairpins, curlers, bobby pins, eyelash curlers, earrings, eyeglass frames, nickel coins, dental instruments, metal lipstick holders, clasps of necklaces, zippers, medallions, metal identification tags, wire support of brassiere cups, garter clasps, metal chairs, handles of doors, handbags, carriages, umbrellas, thimbles, needles, scissors, pens, watchbands, metallic eyelets ofshoes, metal arch supports, safety pins on sanitary napkins, hair dyes and bleaches, electric wiring, telephone wiring, silver work, mordantin dyes, insecticides, fungicides, nickel plating, nickel-containing alloys		Pustular patch test reactions
Nicotine (base)	10% aq.	Transdermal patches		
Nicotine sulfate	5% aq.	Agricultural sprays, insecticides, "black leaf"		Do not test with nicotine base
Nigrosine	2% pet.	Dye, varnish leather, platinum blond hair bleach		
Nigrosine base (Solvent black7)	1% pet. or 1% mek.	Carbon paper, shoe polish, crayons, typewriter ribbon, inks, leather finish		
Nimesulide	5% pet.			Topical NSAID
Ninol 2012 (fatty acid alkanolamine condensate)	1% aq.	Surfactant, non-ionic synthetic detergents, bubble baths		Controls
Nitric acid	Do not test	Explosives, dyes, celluloid manufacture, artificial pearls, precious stones		Powerful irritant
Nitrobenzene (oil of mirbane;artificial oil of bitter almonds)	10% o.o.	Shoe dyes, flavoring in foods, soaps, perfumes		Odor like that of oil of bitter almonds
Nitrofurazone	1% pet.	Antibacterial agent, mouthwashes, Furacin (Eaton)		
Nitrogen mustard	As is	Topical agent for mycosis fungoides		May produce urticariaand anaphylaxis
Nitroglycerin	0.2 mg/mL in water	Angina treatment		Ointment, disc

Contactant	Concentration and Vehicle	Exposure	Crossreactions	Comment
Nitrose dimethyl aniline	1% alc.	Dye		Primary sensitizer
Nonic 218	2% aq.	Surfactant, non-ionic synthetic detergents, bubble baths		Control
Nonoxynol-6	0.5% aq.	Industrial waterless hand cleanser		
Nonoxynol-9	0.5% aq.	Spermicidal in emulsifying agent; birth control sponges		
Nordihydroguaiaretic acid	2% pet.	Fat antioxidant		
Norethisterone acetate	0.1% eth.			
Novocain (procaine; Winthrop)	5% pet.		Para-aminobenzoic acidesters	Does not crossreact with Xylocaine. Based on para-aminobenzoic acid
Nupercaine (Cinchocaine hydrochloride)	1% pet.	Anesthetic		
Nutmeg oil (mace)	1% alc.	Condiments, flavoring agent		
Nylon dyes	1% pet.			Disperse Orange 3 andYellow 3
Nystatin	3% alc.	Mycolog Cream, Nystaform-HC, Mycostatin, Nilstat, Nysta-Dome, Achrostatin, Declostatin, Florotic, Myconef, O-V Statin, Tetrex-F		Rare sensitizer
Oak moss, absolute	2.0% pet.	Perfume	Atranorin	
Oak moss, synthetic	5% pet.	Perfume		
Octyl alcohol	20% pet.	Lanolin		
2-Octyl dodecanol	30% pet.	Lanolin		
Oleyl alcohol	30% pet.	Lanolin, hair lotions, brilliantines, cosmetics, superfatting agent, solvent for essential oils	Stearyl alcohol	
Omite	1% pet.	Plant Parasiticide (Japanese)		Irritant
Optical bleaches	1% aq.	"Whiter-than-white" detergent, blan-cophores, stilbene derivative, Solium methyl umbelliferones		Photosensitizers
Orange peel	As is	May be covered with carnauba wax, colored with azo dye (Citrus Red 2), sprayed with arsenic	o-Phenyl phenol	Controls. Orange peel may be irritant under patch

Contactant	Concentration and Vehicle	Exposure	Crossreactions	Comment
Orange peel, oil of	1% alc.	Colognes, perfumes, baking, candies, beverages	Turpentine, celery, bergamot, caraway, dill, balsam of Peru	Contains terpenes, oil oflimonene, carotene
Orcinol (dihydroxytoluene)	2% alc.	Antiseptic	Resorcinol	5-Methyl resorcinol
Orris root	Pdr. pure	Dentifrices, perfumes, teething rings, adhesives, back plasters		
Orthodichlorbenzene	5% alc.	Leather dyes		
Orthoform	25% pet.	Topical anesthetics	Paraamino compounds	Based on para-aminobenzoic acid, primary sensitizer
Orthophenyl phenol	1% pet.	Cosmetic preservative Preservative in paper linings of lids of cosmetic jars Same as Dowicide 1		May cause depigmentation
Orvus WA (sodium lauryl sulfate)	1% aq.	Surfactant, anionic synthetic detergents, bubble baths		Controls
Ovotran	5% acet.	Insecticides		
Oxaine (oxethazine; Wyeth) HC1.	2% aq.	Gastrointestinal topical anesthetics		
Oxalic acid	0.1% aq.	Bleaches, stain removers, rust removers, metal cleansers		Irritant
Oxybenzone (Benzophenone-3) (Eusolex 4360)	2.0% pet.	Sunscreens, cosmetics		Regular and photo ACD
Oxychlorosene	1% aq.	Hypochlorite in Kasdenol Mouthwash		Prepare fresh for testing
Oxyquinoline sulfate	1% pet.	Contraceptive, antiseptic		
Ozokerite (ceresin)	30% pet.	Cosmetics, candles, waxes		
Paints	As is (open) or 10% pet.			
Palladium chloride	1% pet.	Jewelry, dental	Nickel	
Pancreatin	5% pet.	Enzyme mixture, Pycopay Toothpaste	Trypsine, chemotrypsine	
Panthenol (pantothenol)	30% pet.	Vitamin B₅, Aquasol A, Panthoderm		Alcohol of pantothenic acid
d-Panthenyl Ethyl Ether	1% pet.	Present in hair lotion and cosmetics, part vitamin B complex		

Contactant	Concentration and Vehicle	Exposure	Crossreactions	Comment
Paper money	As is		U.S. paper bills may contain formaldehyde and Dowicides (chlorinated phenols) to prevent mildew	
Para-aminobenzene	1% pet.	Organic dye		Para-amino compounds
Para-aminobenzoic acid (aminobenzoic acid)	10% pet.	Pabafilm sunscreening agent, Solar Cream (Doak), synthesis of local anesthetics, vitamin B complex, brewer's yeast	Paraphenylenediamine, procaine, sulfonamides, azo dyes, benzocaine P-amino compounds	The acid is less soluble and less sensitizing than are its salts Photosensitizer
Para-aminophenol	2% pet.	Analgesics, fur dyes	Paraphenylenediamine	
Paraben mixture	15% pet.	Preservative in topical agents, cosmetics, foods, cleansers		3% each of ethyl, methyl, propyl, butyl and propyl parahydroxybenzoic acid
Para-chloro-meta-xylenol	1% pet.	Cosmetic and topical medication	May crossreact with chloro-metacresol	
Parachlorophenol	1% aq.			
Paradichlorobenzene	1% alc.	Mothproofing, toilet bowls, deodorants		May produce purpura
Paraffin	Equal parts soft paraffin	Petrolatum (soft yellow paraffin)		
Parahydroxybenzoic acid (methyl and ethyl propylparabens)	5% pet.	Parabens as preservatives in pharmaceuticals, cosmetics, foods		Sensitizer in topical creams
Para-oxon	1% alc. (open)	Insecticides		
Paraphenylenediamine(PPDA)	2% pet. in adark bottle	Hair dyes, fur dyes, leather processing, rubber vulcanizing, printer's ink, photographic work, x-ray fluids, lithographing	Azo and aniline dyes, procaine, benzocaine, para-aminobenzoic acid, HydroDIURIL, carbutamide sulfonamides, para-aminosalicylic acid	Many weakly positive patch test reactions are not significant Has caused "tightness"of the chest
o-nitro-Paraphenylenediamine	1% pet.			
Pararosaniline	Sat. sol.	Dye		
Para-tertiary butyl phenol	1% pet.	Adhesive, resins, duplicating paper, rubber industry, leather industry		May cause leukoderma Antioxidant
Para-tertiary butyl phenolformaldehyde resin (PTBFR)	1% pet.	Adhesives shoes/leather	PTBP	
Parathion	1% alc. (open)	Insecticides		

Contactant	Concentration and Vehicle	Exposure	Crossreactions	Comment
Paratoluenediamine sulfate	1% pet.	Chemistry laboratories		
Paris green (Schweinfurt or emerald green)	2% acet.	Paint pigment, wood preservative, insecticide sprays	P-amino compound	Copper acetoarsenite compound
Parsnip, parsley (wild)	As is (moist)			Photosensitizer
Parsol 1789 (4-tert-butyl-4'-methoxydibenzoyl-methane)	2% pet.	Sunscreen		Photo ACD UVA absorber
Patchouli, oil of	1% pet.	Cosmetics, perfume	Essential oils	
Pearl essence Natural	As is	Frosted nail polish		A suspension of guanine crystals (from fish scales) in amyl acetate or acetone
Synthetic	As is	Lacquers, plastics		Metal stearates, lead, barium hypophosphites, bismuth oxychloride, metallic silver, zinc ammonium phosphate and hydrolysis of products of titanium chloride on protein films
Pencil colors				Lead (graphite) is not a sensitizer. Indelible pencils—methyl or crystal violet—are not sensitizers. Green and yellow colored pencils may contain lead chromate
d-Penicillamine	1% aq.	Ophthalmic or systemic	Penicillin	
Penicillin (powder or ointment)	10,000 IU/gram pet.	Topical use, pharmaceuticals, nursing and medical professions, cheese processers, fruit handlers		Contact allergy may be accompanied by anaphylactic variety
Pentachloronitrobenzene (PCNB)	0.5% pet.	Agricultural fungicide		
Pentachlorophenol	1% alc.	Weed killers, insecticides, wood preservatives, adhesives		
3-Pentadecylcatechol	0.1% pet.	Anacardiaceae: rhus, mango, cashew, India nut marking tree		A primary sensitizer
Pentaerythritol triacrylate (PETA)	0.1% pet.	UVR cured ink		Phototoxic
Pentoxol	As is	Organic solvents		
Peppermint oil	1% pet.	Flavoring agent, perfumes	Balsam of Peru, rosin, wood	An essential oil
Perchlorethylene (tetra-chloroethylene)	25% o.o.	Dry cleaning		Sensitizes to alcohol

Contactant	Concentration and Vehicle	Exposure	Crossreactions	Comment
Perfumes	As is (open and closed)		Balsam of Peru, benzylsalicylate, phenylac-etaldehyde	May produce berloque dermatitis
Permanent wave solutions	2% aq.	Glyceryl, ammonium thioglycolates		
Permanganate, potassium	1% aq.	Oxidizing agents, neutralizer of alka-loids, disinfectants		
Peroxide catalysts Acetyl Benzoyl peroxide Cumene hydroperoxide Cyclohexanone Lauroyl Methyl ethyl ketone	0.5% acet. Or 1% pet.	Polyester resins Acrylate resins		
Petitgrain Oil	5% pet.	Perfume oil		A photosensitizer
Petrolatum	As is	Vaseline, soft yellow paraffin or white		Best vehicle for most patch test substances, rarely sensitizing
Petroleum	20% o.o.	Insecticides, rodenticides, gasoline, solvents		
Phenanthrene	1% pet.	Tar		A photosensitizer
Phenergan Cream (Wyeth)	As is		Promethazine, phenothiazine (Thorazine, Thephorin)	A photosensitizer
Phenol (carbolic acid)	1% aq.	Dermal Chemabrasive (Budkon), Carbolated Vaseline, carbolfuchsin, Chloraseptic Lozenges and Mouthwash (Eaton), P&S Liquid and Ointment, Panscol Ointment (Baker)	Resorcin, cresols, hydroquinone	Irritant
Phenolformaldehyde	5% pet. or 1% alc.	Clothing, finishes, epoxy resins		
Phenolic compounds	1% aq.	Mouthwashes		Amyl, heptyl and actylphenols in mouthwashes
Phenolphthalein	0.5% alc.	Indicator, laxative		Test at site of fixed drug eruption
Phenothiazine	1% aq. (photosensitizer— 1 % pet. test open and closed)	Veterinarian anthelmintic, fly control, methylene blue Chloropromazine Phenothiazine HCl.Tripenelamine	Phenergan	Present in Sparine, Thorazine, Compazine, Stelazine, Temaril, Largon, Tindal, Dartal, Mellaril, Vesprin, Prolixin, Repoise, Dermitil
Phenyl indole	2% pet.	Found in polyvinylchloride fabrics		
Phenoxybenzamine	0.1% pet.	Chemical laboratory		Irritant

Contactant	Concentration and Vehicle	Exposure	Crossreactions	Comment
Phenoxyethenol	1% pet.	Preservative in cosmetics Antimicrobial		Rare sensitizer
2- phenoxy ethylacrylate	0.01% pet.			Insulin pumps
Phenylacetaldehyde	2% pet. or 0.5% alc.	Perfumes, flavoring agents		
Phenylbetanaphthylamine	1% pet.	Rubber antioxidant		
Phenylcycloparaphenylenediamine	1% pet.	Rubber, Black Rubber		
Phenylephrine	1% pet.	Eye drops—Mydriatic eye drops		
Phenylglycidyl ether	1% o.o.	Epoxy resin		
Phenylglycidyl ether	0.25% acet.	Epoxy resin		
Phenylisopropyl para-phenylenediamine (IPPD)	0.1% pet.	Rubber (black)		Can cause lichenoid or purpuric eruptions
Phenylmercuric acetate and borate	0.1% pet.	Fungicides, germicides, preservatives in cosmetics, contraceptives, Nylmerate (Holland-Rantos)	Organic and inorganic mercurials	May be a primary irritant in 0.1% aq.
Phenylmercuric nitrate	0.05% pet.	Preservatives, vaginal cream, contraceptives, Pher-Mer-Nite, Merpecto-gel		
Phenyl salicylate (salol)	1% pet.	Plastics, lacquers, adhesives, waxes, polishes, suntan oils, plasticizers		
Phosphorus trisulfide (phosphorus sesquisulfide)	As is	Safety matchboxes, matches, ignition paper, diesel motors, high-pressure lubricants, asphalt		Airborne allergen May cause contact urticaria
Phthalic anhydride	1% alc.	Epoxy resins		A primary sensitizer
Phytomenadione	10% pet.	Vitamin K, parenteral		
Picric acid (trinitrophenol)	5% aq.	Dye industry, explosives, artificial flowers, antiseptics		
Picryl chloride	1% acet.			A primary sensitizer
Piketoprofen	1% pet.			Topical NSAID
Pimaric acid	10% pet.			
Pimento	10% c.o.	Flavoring agent, all spice		
Pine oil	5% pet.	Disinfectants, deodorants, liquid scrub soaps		Controls Irritant

Contactant	Concentration and Vehicle	Exposure	Crossreactions	Comment
Pine tar	25% pet.			
Pinene	15% o.o.			
Piperazine	1% aq.	Vermifuges, Antepar, Pipizan, Multifuge, Perin, Ascarey	Ethylenediamine HC1.	May flare from ingestion of Atarax (hydroxyzine hydrochloride)
Pitch	As is (open)	Various tars		A photosensitizer
Plants	As is—leaf, flower, pollenbulb			Risk of false positive reaction
Plaster of Paris (gypsum; calcium sulfate)	As is	Cast, moldings		Some reinforced with formaldehyde resin
Plastibase (Squibb)	As is	Quinolor Ointment		Contains 5% polyethylene plastic resin
Plastic(s)Monomer Polymer	0.1—1% acet. or pet. As is			
Plastic cement	As is (open)	Industrial, toys, models, glue sniffers		Contains volatile hydrocarbons and solvents, formaldehyde, formaldehyde resins, nitrocellulose
Platinum bleaches for hair	As is	Methyl violet, methylene blue, nigrosine		Applied after peroxide bleach
Platinum-amm. tetrachloroplatinate or hexachloroplatinate	0.25% aq. and 0.1% aq., respectively			May cause a pustular reaction
Plexoderm (Crookes-Barnes)	As is		Balsam of Peru	
Poison ivy extract or oleoresin	0.1% acet.	Identical to poison sumac and poison oak	Oleoresin of Japanese lacquer tree, cashew nut, mango fruit, India inktree, ginkgo tree	A primary sensitizer
Polyester (unsaturated)	1% acet.			
Polyester monomer	10% acet.	Polyester resin		
Polyethylene glycol	As is	Polyethylene glycol ointment (U.S.P.), Furacin (Eaton), Plastibase (Squibb), Carbowax, hair dressings		Nos. 200 to 700 are liquids. Nos. 1000 to 6000 are solids (Carbowax) Rare sensitizer
Polymethyl methacrylate (acrylic polymer powder)	As is	Dentistry, synthetic resins		Acrylic monomer may sensitize; the polymer very rarely does so
Polymyxin B sulfate	3% pet	Numerous topical medications		Rare sensitizer
Polysorb-80 U.S.P. Polysorbate-80	5% aq.	Emulsifier and dispersing agent, surfactant		Tween 80
Polysorb Hydrate (Fougera)	5% o.o.			Sorbitan sesquioleate in wax-petrolatum

Contactant	Concentration and Vehicle	Exposure	Crossreactions	Comment
Polysulfide liquid polymer	1% acet.	Epoxy resin plasticizer		
Polyvinyl pyrrolidone	As is	Hair lacquers, cosmetics, pharmaceuticals, Betadine, Isodine		
Pontamine black powder	2% pet.	Fur dyes		
Pontocaine (tetracaine hydrochloride; Winthrop)	2% aq.	Local anesthetics	P-amino compounds	
Potassium carbonate	1% aq.	Soaps, cleaning agents, lye, Drano, Pronto		
Potassium chlorate	1% aq.	Matches, oxidizer in mouthwashes		
Potassium dichromate	0.25% pet. (USA), 0.5 pet. (EU)	*General:* leather, bleaches, matches, yellow paints, spackle compounds, detergents. *Industrial:* fur industry, photography, photo engraving lithography, electroplating, tanning agents, mordants in dyeing, yellow and orange paints, ink manufacture, stainless steel, chrome plating, match making, polishing steel, diesel engine radiator fluid, welding, acetylene workers, cement, rubber, glass, linoleum, wood impregnated with chromated zinc chloride, alloys, containing chrome, antirust compounds	Trivalent chromium compounds	Sensitizer, also irritant and producer of chrome ulcers. False positive reactions common in patients with acute dermatitis or irritable skin and in atopics
Potassium hydroxide	**Do not test**	Soaps, cleaning agents, cuticle remover		Irritant
Potassium iodide	30% pet.	Photographic emulsions, animal and poultry feed, table salt, medications		Halogens often produce pustular patch test reactions. Control test in Duhring's disease with potassium bromide
Potassium peroxymonosulfate	5% pet.			Hot tub "shock"
Potassium persulfate	2.5% aq.	Bleaches, germicides	Ammonium persulfate	
Potassium and sodium dicyanoaurate	0.001% ethanol			
Potosan	1% alc. (open)	Insecticides		
Pramoxine hydrochloride (4-n-butoxyphenyl gamma-morpholino-propyl ether hydrochloride)	1% aq.	Topical anesthetics: Anugesic Ointment and Suppositories (Warner-Chilcott), Aural Acute (Saron), Drotic Ear Drops (Ascher), Phorm Ointment (Ascher), Tronothane Hydrochloride (Abbott), Vio Hydro-cortisone Cream (North American Pharmacal), Pramasone Lotion (Ferndale), Prax Cream (Ferndale)		Does not crossreact with benzocaine or xylocaine

Contactant	Concentration and Vehicle	Exposure	Crossreactions	Comment
Primin (6-methoxy-2n-pentyl-p-benzoquinone)	0.0025%ethyl ether	Allergen in primula plant		
Primrose (Primula obconica) Expressed Leaf	25% aq. / As is	Main English plant sensitizer / Main English plant sensitizer	Daisy family / Daisy family	Primary sensitizer / Primary sensitizer
Procaine hydrochloride (Novocain)	2% aq.	Other local anesthetics based on p-amino compound (benzocaine)	Benzocaine, para-aminobenzoic acid, para-aminosalicylic acid, paraphenylenediamine	Does not crossreact with Xylocaine
Proflavine dihydrochloride	1% pet.	Topical fluorescent dye		Advocated for herpes simplex. Caution: a sensitizer
Promethazine HCL	2% pet.		Phenothiazines	Photosensitizer; has caused contact urticaria
Propantheline bromide	1% aq.	Pro-Banthine (Searle) when incorporated in topical agents as an antiperspirant		Treatment of axillary hyperhidrosis
Propolis	As is	Cosmetics, medicaments		"Bee glue"
Propylene glycol	30% aq.	Vehicle for 5-fluorouracil, humectant, cosmetics, Synalar Solution, Lidosporin		
Propylene oxide	1% alc.	Chemical intermediate in preparing polyurethanes; also used in solvent, fumigant; present in Danish product Medi-Swab		
Propyl gallate	1% pet.	Cosmetics, lipsticks	Other gallates?	Antioxidant
Propyl parahydroxybenzoate (propyl paraben)	5% pet.	Preservative in topical agents, cosmetics, foods, cleansers	Other parabens	
Pyrethrum powder	2% pet.	Insecticides, mothproofing	Chrysanthemum, turpentine, ragweed	Contains pyrethrins and cinerins
Pyribenzamine hydrochloride (tripelennamine)	2% pet.	Antihistamine	Sulfapyradine, Antistine	An ethylenediamine derivative
Pyridine	30% o.o.	Tar		A photosensitizer
Pyrocatechol	2% in 95% alc.		Hydroquinone, resorcin	
Pyrogallol	1% pet. or3% aq.	Hair dyes, tars	Resorcin	
Pyrrolinitrin	1% pet.	European antimycotic medication		
Quassin (extract of Jamaica bitter wood)	2% acet.	Lacquers, paper, waterproofing, denatured alcohol		Contains sucrose octa-acetate

Contactant	Concentration and Vehicle	Exposure	Crossreactions	Comment
Quaternary ammonium compounds	0.1% aq.	Cetrimide, antiseptic detergents such as Phemerol, Zephiran, Ceepryn, Diaprene		Rare sensitizers, may cause ulceration of genitalia in concentrated solutions
Quaternium-15 (Dowicil 200)	2% pet.	Preservative		Formaldehyde-releasing agent
Quicklime (unslaked lime; calcium oxide)	Caustic; **do not test**	Mortar, cement, fertilizers, soap, glass, metals, depilatories, manufacture of calcium cyanide, calcium carbide		See Lime, slaked and Calcium oxide
Quillaja	1% alc.	Emulsifying agent, solution of coal tar, cosmetics		Derived from South American rosaceous tree bark
Quince seed	As is	Hair straighteners, mucilage, gums, cosmetics		
Quinidine sulfate	1% aq.	Pharmaceutical industry, contraceptives		Eczematous or purpuric patch test reaction
Quinine sulfate or hydrochloride	1% aq.	Contraceptives, sunscreens, hair tonics, quinine tablets, vermouth, gin, vodka, denatured alcohol		Photosensitizer
Quinolor Compound Ointment (Squibb)	Half strength with pet.		Vioform, Sterosan, Diodoquin	Contains chlorhydroxyquinoline, benzoylperoxide, methyl salicylate, menthol and eugenol in Plastibase vehicle. Some preparations contain eucalyptol, white thyme oil
Quinoxaline dioxide	5% pet.	Growth promoter animal foodstuffs		Photosensitizer
Quotane Ointment and Lotion (dimethisoquin hydrochloride; Smith, Kline & French)	As is	Topical anesthetic		Not related to para-aminobenzoic acid
Ragweed	1:1000 acet.		Chrysanthemum, pyrethrum, turpentine	Plant leaves and pollen may also be used for testing
Ranitidine hydrochloride (Zantac)	1% pet.	H$_2$ antagonist		
Rapeseed oil (Factice)	As is	Adhesives, lubricant		
Red mercuric oxide	3% pet.	Antiseptics, bleaching agents	Organic and inorganic mercurials	
Resorcin	5% pet.	Acne remedies, hair tonics, suppositories, eye drops, tanning, explosives, resins, dyes, cosmetics, frecklecream, dyeing and printing	Euresol, phenol, hexylresorcinol, orcinol, hydroquinone, pyrocatechol, pyrogallol, hydroxyquinone	Deteriorates when exposed to light. Dispense in dark bottle. May be irritant
Resorcin green	2% pet.	Azo dye	Para-amino compounds	

Contactant	Concentration and Vehicle	Exposure	Crossreactions	Comment
Resorcinol monoacetate (Euresol [knoll])	5% aq.	Clantis (Dara), Resulin Resorcitate (Schieffelin), Sulforcin (Texas Pharmacal), RMS Lotion (Ar-Ex), Acne-Dome (Dome)	Resorcin	
Resorcinol monobenzoate	1% pet.	Colored eyeglass frames	Balsam of Peru	Ultraviolet inhibitor
Retinoic acid	0.1% pet.	Acne therapy		Irritant
Rezifilm (Squibb)	As is			Contains tetramethylthiuram disulfide
Rhodamine	5% pet.	Red lipstick dye		A photosensitizer
Rhodium sulfate	2% pet.	Jewelry making		
Rhulicream, Rhulispray, Rhulitol (Lederle)	As is (patchscratch)	Topical agent for plant dermatitis		Allergic granuloma fromzirconium
Riasol (Shield)	As is	Proprietary preparation for psoriasis		Mercury as coconut oilsoap
Rigithane 112	1% alc.	Polyurethane resins		
Rigithane catalyst	10% aq.	Polyurethane resins		
Roccal (alkyldimethyl-benzyl-ammonium chloride)	0.1% aq.	Surfactants, cationic synthetic detergents, bubble baths, benzalkonium chloride		Controls "Quat"
Rodannitrobenzene	1% pet.	Pesticides	Paraphenylenediamine	
Rosaniline (basic fuchsin)	2% aq.	Therapeutic dye		
Rose bengal	2.5% pet.	Dyes		Photosensitizing
Rose, oil of	1% alc./1% pet	Perfume, unguentum aquae rosae		
Rosin (colophony): gum rosin (from turpentine), wood rosin (from pine stump)	10% pet.	Yellow bar soap, adhesive tape, insulating tape, Scotch Tape, glossy paper, flypaper, polish, paints, inks, epilating wax, rosin bags for ball players, rosin for violin bows	Balsam of Peru, turpentine (gum rosin) Wood tars Methyl abieate	Contains abietic acid and 1-pinearic acid
Rotenone powder (Derris root)	5% in talcum	Insecticide		From roots of rotenone-bearing plants (Derris and Lonchocarpus)
Rubber accelerators	1% pet.	Mercaptobenzothiazole, tetramethylthiuram monosulfide, diphenyl-guanidine		Of the rubber accelerators, these are the most common sensitizers
Rubber antioxidants	1% pet.	Monobenzylether of hydroquinone, phenyl-beta-naphthylamine, isopropyl paraphenylenediamine		Of the rubber antioxidants, these are the most common sensitizers

Contactant	Concentration and Vehicle	Exposure	Crossreactions	Comment
Rubber, finished products	As is	Rubber box toes of shoes, rubber cements, dress shields, elastic in hairnets, panties, dental plates, edge ofeyelash curler, kneeling pads, rubber support pessary and diaphragms, dental sheeting, head rests, condoms, rubberbands, finger guards, art gum erasers, stethoscopes, rubber handgrip of vibrators, aprons, mammary prostheses, goggles, adhesive tape, "Flubber" (a putty-like toy), tire treads, tubes, wire insulation, drug sundries, calendered stocks		Rubber accelerators and antioxidants are the most common cause of rubber dermatitis
Rubber peptizer	1% pet.	Thio-beta-naphthol		Keeps rubber soft
Rubidium iodide	1% pet.	Topical medications		
Rust removers	**Do not test** (see cornment)			Contains irritants such as naphtha, ammonium sulfide, oxalicacid, hydrofluoric acid, concentrated solution of phosphoric acid, inorganic heavy metal salts. For testing, see individual chemicals or begin with 1% solutions and use controls
Ruthenium	0.15 powder	Electronics		
Salicylates	2% o.o.		Aminosalicylic acid	Amyl, benzyl, glyceryl, menthyl, ethylhexyl phenyl and propylene salicylates may be used as sunscreens
Salicylic acid	1% pet.	Many topical agents, including Whit-field's ointment		Rare sensitizer. Salicylic acid and mercury combinations may be irritants when covered
Saligenin (salicyl alcohol)	2% aq.	Topical local anesthetics		Rarely sensitizes
Sandalwood oil	1% pet.			Photosensitizer
Sassafras oil	1% pet.	Flavoring agents		
Sawdust	As is			Test dry and moist
Scarlet red (aminoazotoluene)	As is 2.5% pet.	Dye, therapeutic agent for burns and ulcers	Para-amino compounds	
Sedormid	Sat. sol. in propylene glycol	This drug is not being made at present		Purpuric patch test reaction
Selenium sodium oxide	0.1% aq.	Electronics		

Contactant	Concentration and Vehicle	Exposure	Crossreactions	Comment
Selenium sulfide	3% pet.	Selsun (Abbott), glass, photoelectric cells, coloring of acrylic dentures		May be irritant
Selsun (Abbott)	As is (open)	Therapeutic shampoo		Contains selenium sulfide
Sesame oil	50% o.o.	Vehicle for intramuscular medications, synergist for pyrethrins, cosmetics, pharmaceuticals		
Shampoos	5% aq. sol (open) 2% aq. (closed)			Controls
Shellac	As is	Paint, varnish, hair dressings, waxes		May have methyl alcohol and arsenic trisulfide Controls
Shoe polish	5% pet.			
Silicone fluids (dimethylpolysiloxanes)	As is	Cosmetics, greases, antifog agent, eyeglasses, glass		May cause blepharitis, lacrimation
Silver bromide	2% aq.	Photography, mirror finishing		
Silver nitrate	1% aq.	Caustic pencils and hair dyes		Pustular patch test reaction
Simazine	1% pet.			
Siroil (Siroil)	As is	Proprietary psoriasis remedy		Contains mercury, irritant
Soaps	1% aq.			Controls
Sodium alginate (algin)	As is	Emulsifiers, mucilage, ice cream, wave sets		
Sodium alkyl sulfate	0.5% aq.	Foaming surfactant in detergents, Ultrabrite, Gleem, McLeans, Pepsodent, pharmaceuticals, cosmetic creams		May contain formaldehyde
Sodium amidotrizoate	10% aq.	A radiopaque substance in angiography and renography		
Sodium arsenate	10% aq.	Arsenical soaps, insecticides, hair tonics		
Sodium bisulfite	10% aq.	Antioxidant in food		May cause anaphylaxis in asthmatic patients
Sodium carbonate	10% aq.	Soap additives		Irritant
Sodium diethyldithiocarbamate	10% in Carbowax	Treatment of nickel carbonyl poisoning		
Sodium fluoride	0.5% aq.	Glass etchings, dentifrices		Pustular patch test reaction common

Contactant	Concentration and Vehicle	Exposure	Crossreactions	Comment
Sodium fusidate	2% pet.	Fucidin Ointment		
Sodium hydroxide	**Do not test**	Soaps, cleaning agents, lye—Drano, Pronto		Powerful irritant
Sodium hypochlorite	0.5% aq.	Bleaching solutions, cleansing agents Antiseptic	Chloramine	Controls, irritant
Sodium hyposulfite	0.5% aq.	Antiseptic		
Sodium lauryl sulfate(Duponal C)	1% aq.	Emulsifying agent in cosmetics, pharmaceuticals, "foaming" dentifrices		Fatty alcohol sulfate Primary irritant Controls
Sodium metabisulfite	2% pet.	Antioxidant in pharmaceuticals, printing, and photography		
Sodium monofluorophosphate	0.5% aq.	Surfactant (Colgate Toothpaste)		Pustular patch test reactions
Sodium monoglyceride sulfonate	1% aq.	Surfactant (Gleem Toothpaste)		Controls
Sodium n-lauroyl sarcosinate	1% aq.	Antienzyme, dentifrices, emulsifiers, surfactant in cosmetics, pharmaceuticals		Controls
Sodium perborate	10% pet.	Dentures, household cleansers, cold hair-waving neutralizers, mouthwashes, Vince, Amosan		
Sodium pyrithione	0.3% aq.	Metalworking fluids, water-based printer's ink, antidandruff shampoo		Also known as sodiumomadine
Sodium stearate	1% aq.	Cosmetics		Controls
Sodium stearoyl lactylate	2% pet.			Emulsifier
Sodium sulfide	2% aq.	Bleaching agent for cotton, paper, stainremover for tetryl and potassium permanganate, preservative for dyes and foods, Wandex (Research Supplies)		Controls Has caused contact urticaria Unstable in solution
Sodium sulfide	2% aq.	Sulfur dyes, hides, insecticides, depilatories		
Sodium thiosulfate	5% aq.	Fungicides, stain removers, hair dye developers, Tinver, Komed Lotion, Microsyn		
Solithane 113	1% alc.	Polyurethane prepolymer		
Solithane catalysts C-113–300 C-113–328	1% alc. 2% aq.	Polyurethane catalyst Polyurethane catalyst		

Contactant	Concentration and Vehicle	Exposure	Crossreactions	Comment
Sorbic acid	2% pet.	Preservative, Hytone Cream (Dermik), Aristocort Cream (Lederle), Fluorone Cr. (Upjohn), Maxiflor (Herbert), Kenalog Cr. (Squibb), Pramasone Cr. (Ferndale)		Present in many fruits, especially strawberries. Urticariogenic agent
Sorbitol	10% aq.	Humectants, cosmetics, pharmaceuticals		
Sorsis Cream (Ar-Ex)	As is	Topical agent for psoriasis		Contains ammoniated mercury
Span 20 (sorbitan monolaurate)	5% o.o.	Surfactant, nonionic synthetic detergents, bubble baths	Other Spans	Controls
Span 80 (sorbitan monooleate)	5% o.o.	Surfactant, nonionic synthetic detergents, bubble baths	Other Spans	Controls
Spandelle (Firestone)	As is	Polyurethane elastomer (spandex)		Not a sensitizer
Sparklers				*Green sparklers* contain barium nitrate, potassium perchlorate and aluminum powder; *red sparklers* contain strontium carbonate, nitrate, potassium perchlorate and aluminum powder
Spearmint oil	2% pet.	Flavoring agents		
Spermaceti	As is	Cosmetics, pharmaceuticals, candles		
Spice, oil of	5% pet.			
Spiramycin	1% pet.	Veterinary antibiotic		
Stannous fluoride	0.5% aq.	Dentifrices, including Crest, Cue, Fact, Superstripe, Dr. Lyons Fluoride, McKesson Fluoride		Pustular patch test reaction
Stearamidoethyl Diethylamine Phosphate	0.5% pet.	Cosmetic emulsifier		
Stearic acid	5% pet.	Cosmetics, soaps		Pustular patch test reaction common
Stearyl alcohol	30% pet.	Lanolin, aliphatic alcohol in lanolin, cosmetics, textile finishes, antifoam agent, lubricant	Oleyl alcohol Cetyl alcohol	May cause contact urticaria
Sterosan Cream (Geigy) (chlorquinaldol)	As is	Bacteriostatic and fungistatic cream and ointment	Vioform, Diodoquin, Quinolor	Free of iodine
Stilbene triazine	0.5% aq.	Optical bleaches, brightening agents, soaps, detergents, cosmetics, textiles		Photosensitizer

Contactant	Concentration and Vehicle	Exposure	Crossreactions	Comment
Stoddard Solvent (high flashpoint petroleum distillate)	25% o.o.	Dry cleaning, paint thinner		
Streptomycin	2.5% aq. 1% pet.	Medical, nursing and pharmaceutical personnel	Dihydrostreptomycin, kanamycin, neomycin	Has caused systemic contact dermatitis
Strontium chloride	2% aq.	Sensodyne dentifrice		
Strontium sulfide	2% aq.	Depilatories		
Styrax USO (storax)	2% pet.	Plexoderm, perfumes, contains topical medication	Benzoin styrene, balsam of Peru	A balsam with cinnamic acid
Styrene (vinyl benzene)	1% o.o.	Synthetic rubber, alkyd, acrylic and polyester resins, extractive of storax balsam, compound tincture of benzoin, soaps, wines, berries	Benzoin compounds	
Styrene oxide	1% o.o.	Reactive epoxy diluent		
Subtilins	0.1% aq.	Detergent enzymes		
Sulfacetamide, topical	5% pet.	Sultrin (Ortho), many ophthalmic and acne topical medications		Rarely sensitizes
Sulfanilamide, topical	5% pet.	AVC, Otomide, Vagitrol, Sufamil	Para-amino compounds	A photosensitizer
Sulfobromophthalein	5% aq.	Diagnostic dyes		Anaphylactic or immediate rather than delayed allergens
Sulfonamide	5% pet.	Blexcon (Madland), Gantrisin (Roche), Vagitrol (Syntex)	Para-amino compounds	Sulfonamide diuretics may be photosensitizers
Sulfonamide-formaldehyde resin	10% pet.	Main sensitizer in nail lacquer		
Sulfonated imidazole	0.5% aq.	Optical bleaches, brightening agents, soaps, detergents, cosmetics, textiles		Photosensitizer
Sulfur	5% pet.	Topical medications, gunpowder, matches, bleaches, insecticides, fungicides		*Precipitated sulfur* contains calcium sulfide; *sublimed* sulfur is a pure yellow sulfurpowder. Incompatible with iodine and mercury
Sulfuric acid	Do not test			Strong irritant
Sulisobenzone (2-hydroxy-4-methoxy-benzophenone-5-sulfonic acid)	10% pet.	Sungard, Uval, Spectra Sorb UV 284, Uvinulms-40		Sunscreen
Surfacaine (cyclomethycaine; Lilly)	1% pet.	Topical anesthetic, Surfacaine Cornpound, Surfadil		Not based on para-aminobenzoic acid

Contactant	Concentration and Vehicle	Exposure	Crossreactions	Comment
Synthetic detergents	2% aq.			Controls
Tagamet (Cimetidine)	1% pet.	Pharmacist		
Talc (talcum) U.S.P.	As is	Cosmetics, pharmaceuticals		May produce granulomas in wounds
Tannic acid	0.25% aq.	Mordant in dyes, sizing paper and silk, polished fabrics, tortoise shellframes, rubber manufacture, tanning leather, photography, sunscreens and medicines for burns, Dalidyne (Dalin), Astringent lotion, Onycho-Phytex (Unimed), artificial nail preparation, tannic jelly		Rare sensitizer
Tantalum	1% powder	Electronics		·
Tar				
Coal	5% pet.	Alphosyl, Balnetar, Carbo-Cort, Daxalan, Ionil T, Polytar, Pragmatar, Sebical Tar Shampoo, Sebutone, Supertah, Tarbonis, Tar Distillate, Tarpaste, Topigel, Tropsor Lotion, Unguentum Bossi, Ze-Tar-Quin, Zetar Shampoo and Emulsion		Photosensitizer
	As is	Liquor carbonis detergens, Epidol, Tridentar (Spirt), Hydro-Tar (Schieffelin), Pentarcort (Dalin), Methatar (Borden), Ulcortar (Ulmer), Cor-Tar Quin Cream and Lotion (Dome)		Photosensitizers. Contains coal tar, Quillaja bark, alcohol
Wood	12% (3% each of pine, beech, juniper and birch)	Almay-Tar (Schieffelin), oil of cade (juniper tar)		Not photosensitizers
Tartar emetic	3% aq.	Dye mordant, counterirritant, denaturing agent in rubbing alcohol		
Tashan Cream (Hoffman-La Roche)	As is			The vitamin E in this preparation reported to be a sensitizer. See Vitamin E
Tattoo pigments		Blue—Cobalt Blue—Cobalt Chloride 2% pet.Green—Chromium—Potassium Dichromate 0.5% pet. Red—Mercury sulfide—Mercury 0.5% pet. Yellow—Cadmium Sulfide—1% aq. Purple—Manganese—Manganese oxide Pure		*Black:* carbon, iron oxide, logwood (may contain potassium dichromate). *Blue:* cobaltous aluminate. *Brown:* ferric sulfate. *Flesh:* iron oxide. *Green:* Chromium oxide, chromium sesquioxide (casalis green), hydrous chromium oxide (Guignet's green), copper salts mixed with azo dyes. *Red:* cadmium selenide, cinnabar, sienna. *Violet:* manganese violet. *White:* Zinc oxide. *Yellow:* cadmium sulfide

Contactant	Concentration and Vehicle	Exposure	Crossreactions	Comment
TEACoco a/k/a Potassium pyrosulfite	5% aq.	Pharmaceutical antioxidant. Printing, photography. Shampoos, cosmetics		
TEGON	0.1 % aq.	European antiseptic detergent		Dodecylic aminoethylglycine hydrochloride
Terpineol	5% pet.	Thyme, pharmaceutical		
Terraclor	0.5% pet.			
Tertiary butyl catechol	1% acet.	Polyester resin inhibitor, antioxidant, lubricating oils, paint, rubber, plastics		May produce leukoderma
Tertiary butyl phenol	1% acet.	Detergents, synthetic oils, disinfectants		May produce leukoderma
p-Tertiary butyl phenolformaldehyde, resin	1% pet.	Resins, glues		
Tetrabromofluorescein + eosin	50% pet.	Dye in lipsticks, pharmaceuticals		Photosensitizer
Tetracaine (Pontocaine[Winthrop]) Amethocaine	1% pet.	Local anesthetics, PNS suppositories (Winthrop), Vertussin Loz tablets (Warren-Teed), Rectodyne Ointment (Semed)	Procaine, benzocaine P-amino compounds	Based on para-amino-benzoic acid
Tetrachlorodiphenylethane (TDE)	5% acet.	Insecticides		
Tetrachloroisophthalonitrile (TCPN)	0.01% acet.	Agricultural fungicide		
Tetrachlorosalicylanilide (TCSA, Impregon)	0.5% pet.	Antiseptic used in soaps	Tribromosalicylanilide, bithionol, hexachlorophene	A photosensitizer
Tetraethylthiuram disulfide (disulfiram, Antabuse)	1% pet.	Rubber industry, medications	Thiram compound Carbamates	Sensitizes to alcohol
Tetrahydracurcumin	1% pet.			
Tetrahydroxy benzophenone	1% pet.			
Tetralin (tetrahydronaphthalene)	25% o.o.	Plumbing, steam fitting	Thiram compounds	
Tetramethylthiuram disulfide (thiram, febram, fermate)	1% pet.	Rubber industry, insecticides, fungicides, germicides, Rezifilm (Squibb)	Disulfiram, Antabuse, Carbamates, Thiram	Sensitizes to alcohol
Tetramethylthiuram monosulfide	1% pet.	Rubber accelerator	Tetrathiuram disulfides, carbamates	Sensitizes to alcohol
Tetryl	Sat. sol. in ether	Munitions		Produces yellow stain; often causes folliculitis
Thallium sulfate	1% aq.	Rodenticides, insecticides, depilatories		Toxic hair loss

Contactant	Concentration and Vehicle	Exposure	Crossreactions	Comment
Thephorin (phenindamine tar trate; Hoffman-La Roche)	2.5% pet.			Potential topical sensitizer
Thermometer fluids (Metallic mercury)	0.5% pet.			*Clinical:* mercury. *Indoor and outdoor:* triethyl phosphate, toluene, xylene, alcohol
Thiamine chloride (vitamin B₁)	50% aq.	Pharmaceuticals	Cocarboxylase (coenzyme B)	
Thimerosal	See Merthiolate			
Thio-beta-naphthol	1% pet.	Rubber peptizer		
Thiocolchicoside	1% pet.			Topical muscle relaxant
Thioglycolic acid	5% aq.	Depilatories		
Thiokol polysulfide polymers	1% acet.	Epoxy resin systems		
Thiophene compound	1% pet.	Phototoxic Compositae plants		
Thiophenol	0.1% alc.	Merthiolate (Lilly)		
Thiosalicylic acid	0.1% alc.	Merthiolate (Lilly)		Sensitizer in thiosalicylic acid
Thiourea, dialkyl esters	0.1% pet.	Rubber Diazo paper	Thiuram?	
Thorazine (Smith Kline & French)	1% pet.	Medical, nursing, pharmaceutical personnel handling and injecting the drug. Excreted in urine (contaminated linen)	Phenothiazine drugs, Phenergan, Theruhistin, Pyrrolazote	Photosensitizer
Thyme, oil of	1% alc.	Waterproofing, flavoring agent, Quinolor Compound (Squibb)	Niaouli Oil	
Thymol (isopropyl metacresol)	1% pet.	Dentifrices, mouthwashes, antiseptics, antimildew, Listerine, Chloraseptic, douches		
Thymol iodide	25% pet.	Antiseptics		
Tiger Balm	As is	Chinese proprietary ointment	Balsam of Peru	Contains balsams
Tin (stannic chloride)	0.5% pet.	Metal, plating		
Tinactin (Schering)	As is	Fungicide		Contains tolnaftate 1%, butylated hydroxytoluene polyethylene glycol
Tinuvin-P (hydroxy-5-methyl-phenyl benzotriazole)	1% pet.	UV absorber, plastics, dyes, dental, cosmetics, spandex, ostomy bags, plastic watch straps		

Contactant	Concentration and Vehicle	Exposure	Crossreactions	Comment
Titanium dioxide	10% pet.	Sunscreens		
Titanium oxalate	1% aq.	Electronics, metal implants		
Tixocortol pivalate	1% pet.	Corticosteroid allergy marker	Hydrocortisone	
Tobacco	As is			
dl-alpha-Tocopherol	10% pet.	Vitamin E		
Toilet water	As is			Photosensitizer
Tolnaftate	1% pet.	Tinactin Solution Antifungal medication		Iso-z-naphthyl-m-n-di-methylthiocarbanilate
Toluene	50% o.o.	Solvents, rubber, adhesives, dyes, perfumes, thermometer fluids, nonclinical thermometer fluids		
Toluene diisocyanate (TDI)	1% pet.	Isocyanate compounds—pulmonarytoxin		
Toluene sulfonamide resin	2% pet.			
p-Toluenesulfonyl chloride	0.5% alc.	Furan plastics, dye manufacture, synthetic tanning		
Toluidine Red	10% o.o.	Aniline dye		Photosensitizer
Toothpastes and powders Soapless With soap or detergent	As is (open) 2% aq.			Controls
Topocide (Lilly)	As is	Miticide, insecticide		Benzyl benzoate, benzocaine, and DDT
Trafuril Ointment (European)	5% pet.	Primary urticariogenic agent		
Tragacanth	1% aq.	Powders, cosmetics, candy manufacture, calico printing, drying agent, drug filler, sizing paper, printing, wave-setting fluids		Vegetable gum
Trenimon (2,3,5-triethylene-imino-1,4-benzoquinone)	0.05% pet.	Chemotherapeutic agent		
Tretinoin	0.005% alc.			Retin A, retinoic acid
Triacetin (glyceryl triacetate)	As is	Cigarette filters, Enzactin (Ayerst), antifungal agent		
Triazine	0.5% aq.	Film hardener		
Tribenoside	1% pet.			Anti-hemorrhoidal, excreted as benzoic acid

Contactant	Concentration and Vehicle	Exposure	Crossreactions	Comment
Tribromosalicylanilide (TBS)	1% pet.	Antiseptic in soaps—Green Lifebuoy, Praise, Safeguard	Tetrachlorosalicylanilide, bithionol, hexachlorophene	A photosensitizer
Trichloroacetic acid	**Do not test**			Primary irritant
Trichloroethylene (ethylenetrichloride, acetylene trichloride)	5% o.o.	Metal degreasing, solvent for oils, greases, paints, varnishes, dye; leather manufacturing, dry cleaning, refrigerant, anesthetics, insecticides, perfumes		Sensitizes to alcohol
Triclosan (Irgasan DP 300)	2% pet.	Antiseptic		
Tricresyl ethyl phthalate	5% pet.	Plasticizer in nail adhesive		
Tricresylphosphate (tritolyl phosphate)	5% pet.	*Plasticizer:* vinyl films, resins,polyester, cellulose, nail lacquer. *Lead scavenger:* in gasoline, fire retardant. *Carbon paper*	Triphenylphosphate	
Triethanolamine	5% pet.	Cosmetics, pharmaceuticals, epoxy hardener		
Triethanolamine	1% pet.	Cosmetic surfactant		
Triethylenediamine	0.1% aq. 0.5% pet.	Polyurethane resin catalyst, epoxy hardener		
Triethylenetetramine	0.1% aq. 0.5% pet.	Epoxy resin		
Trimethylolpropane triacrylate (TMPTA)	0.1% pet.	UVR Cured ink		
Trimeton Ointment (prophen-pyridamine; Schering)	As is	Tripoton, Inhiston	Antistine	
Trinitrobenzene	1% acet.			Primary sensitizer
Trinitrotoluene	20% pet.	Explosives		Causes yellow discoloration
Tri-ortho-cresyl-phosphate	**Do not test** (very toxic)	Plastic coatings, fireproofers, lubricants, gasoline		In Morocco, vegetable oil adulterated with this compound produced paralysis in thousands
Triphenylmethane	1% pet.	Dyes		
Triphenyl phosphate	5% pet.	Cellulose acetate carbon paper		
Trisodium phosphate	2% aq.	A "builder" added to detergents and soaps		
Triton 25 (para-octyl phenolethylene oxide)	0.1% aq.	Wetting agent in cosmetic and pharmaceutical preparations, textiles, metal cleaning, dry cleaning solvent, solvent in ballpoint inks		
Triton X-100 (alkylated arylpolyether alcohol)	1% aq.	Surfactant, nonionic synthetic detergents, bubble baths		Controls

Contactant	Concentration and Vehicle	Exposure	Crossreactions	Comment
Triton X-200 (sodium salt ofalkylated aryl polyether sul-fonate)	1% aq.	Surfactant, anionic synthetic detergents, bubble baths		Controls
Triton X-400 (stearyldimethyl-benzylammonium chloride)	0.1% aq.	Surfactant, cationic synthetic detergents, bubble baths		Controls" Quat"
Tromantadine	0.5% pet.	Antiviral drug		
Trometamol	0.5% aq.			A tris-buffer
Turkey Red Oil	1% o.o.	Surfactant, agricultural textile industry		
Turpentine	10% o.o. or (turpentine peroxides) 0.3% pet.	Synthetic resins, pine oleoresins, furniture and stove polish, varnish, wax solvent, cleaning fluid, paint thinner, adhesives, insecticides. *Liniments*: Sloans, Minards, Johnson's Anodyne, Mentholatum, Penetromide	Chrysanthemum, ragweed, pyrethrum,colophony (rosin), balsams (pine and spruce)	Sensitizer is alpha-carene or alpha-pinene Irritant
Turpentine peroxide	0.3% pet.	Present in Sloan's Liniment and Secaderm Cream		
Tween 20 (sorbitan monolauratepolyoxyethylene derivative)	5% aq.	Surfactant, nonionic synthetic detergents, bubble baths		Controls
Tween 80 (sorbitan monooleatepolyoxyethylene derivative)	5% aq.	Surfactant, nonionic synthetic detergents, bubble baths		Controls
Tylosin (Tylan)	5% pet.	Animal feed	Spiramycin?	Antibiotic
Tyrothricin	20% pet.	Tyrolaris Mouthwash, Creams and Ointments, Isodettes, Otalgine Drops (Purdue Frederick)		
Ultrawet K (sodium aralkyl sulfonate)	1% aq.	Surfactant, synthetic detergents, bubble baths		Controls
Umbelliferone (7-hydroxy-coumarin)	2% pet.	Sunscreening agents, optical bleaches	Furocoumarin	A cinnamic acid derivative. Photosensitizer
Undecylenic acid	4% pet.	Sweat, topical antifungal medications		Rare sensitizer
Unguentum Bossi (Doak)	As is	Psoriasis remedy		Contains ammoniated mercury, tar and sulfosalicylic acid

Contactant	Concentration and Vehicle	Exposure	Crossreactions	Comment
Urea (carbamide)	10% aq.	Amino Cery (Milex), Carbamine (Key Pharmaceuticals), Carmol Cream (Ingram), Debrox (International Pharmaceutical), Gly-Oxide (International Pharmaceutical), Kerid Drops (Blair), Otomide (Schering), Panafil Ointment (Rystan), Panafil-White Ointment (Rystan), Ureaphil (Abbott), Stilbamidine, deodorants, dentifrices, hand creams (Aquacare), formaldehyde resins		Rare sensitizer. Urea frost (urea particles of face in uremia). Cause of ammoniacal dermatitis and stomatitis.Tsyrkunol, L: Occupational Skin Diseases in Workers Engaged in Production of Nitrogen-Mineral Fertilizers, P. Westndner.-Vener., 6,31, 1963. Synthetic urea is an irritant
Urea formaldehyde	10% pet.	Plastics, finishes		
Urea peroxide (Gly-Oxide)	As is			
Uric acid	1% aq.	Allantoin (a derivative of uric acid)		Rarely sensitizes
Usnic acid	1% pet.	Lichens, lichen mosses, clothing dyes, litmus paper	Furocoumarins	
Vanadium pentoxide	10% pet.	Electronics		
Vanilla (alcoholic extract)	10% acet.	Flavoring agent in foods, tobacco, beverages, perfumes	Balsam of Peru, benzoin, oil of cloves Coumarin	Vanilla lichen—a dermatitis due to mites infesting vanilla pods
Vanillin	10% pet.	Aromatic crystalline principle ofvanilla	Balsam of Peru, benzoin, oil of cloves, eugenol Coumarin	Vanillism—allergic dermatitis, rhinitis and asthma from vanilla
Vegetable gums	1% pet.			Karaya, gum arabic (acacia) and tragacanth are the most sensitizing gums
Vermouth	As is (open)	Handlers and imbibers		Some vermouths contain oil of cinnamon and quinine
Vinegar	As is	Condiments, preservative, fermenting beer, cider, malt, wine, lead subacetate		Acetic acid content causes aphthous ulcers?
Vinyl benzene (styrene)	1% o.o.	See Styrene		
Vinyl films	As is			Sensitizers in vinyl films may be *plasticizers*, such as tricresylphosphate, dioctyl-phthalate, ester of adipic acid, and epoxy resins, or *stabilizers*, such as dibutyl tin maleate

Contactant	Concentration and Vehicle	Exposure	Crossreactions	Comment
Vioform Ointment, Cream, Lotion (iodochlorohydroxyquin; CIBA)	As is	*Related compounds:* Entero-Vioform (CIBA), HEB-Cort V Cream and Lotion (Barnes-Hind), Hysone (Mallard), Lidaform-HC Creme and Lotion (Dome), Nystaform Ointment (Dome), Nystaform-HC Ointment and Lotion (Dome), Pentarcort (Dalin), Racetico Cream (Lemmon), Vioform Inserts (CIBA), Vioform Hydrocortisone (CIBA), Vio-Hydrosone Cream (North American Pharmacal), Quinoform, 1-Quinn Dermaform, Domeform, Torofor (Torch), HEB-Cort, Hyquin Cream, Topigel	Diodoquin, Sterosan, Quinolor Ointment Broxyquinolene	Iodine containing hydroxyquinoline
Virginamycin	2.5% pet.	Pristinamycin		Antibiotic
Vitamin A	0.1% pet.	Hand and cosmetic creams, vitamin A and D ointment		May be tested as Retinol acid "pure"
Vitamin A acid (Tretinoin)	0.1% pet.	Topical acne medications		An irritant. Rare sensitizer.
Vitamin B$_1$ (thiamine chloride, Betabion Hydrochloride, Aneurin Hydrochloride)	10% pet.	Pharmaceutical industry	Cocarboxylase, coenzyme B (diphosphothiamin)	Sensitized workers flare and acquire "systemic" contact dermatitis after ingestion or injection of thiamine chloride
Vitamin B$_6$ (pyridoxine; 2- methyl-3-nitro-4-meth- oxyly-methyl-5-cyano-6-chlopyridine)	10% pet.	Pharmaceutical industry	Pyridine derivatives in production of castor oil	Berufdermatosen, 13, 28, 1965. Allergic contact dermatitis in production of B, and of castor oil, another pyridine derivative
Vitamin B$_{12}$ (cyanocobalamine, Betalin 12, Berubigen, Cobione)	10% pet.	Pharmaceuticals Animal feed additive	Cobalt	0.4% of B$_{12}$ molecule iscobalt. See text for cobalt patient whose dermatitis flared from injection of B$_{12}$. Positive patch test reactions obtained with injectable B$_{12}$ preparations
Vitamin E (alpha-tocopherol)	As is in pet.	Tashan Cream, Vitamin E Deodorant Spray (Mennen), Vitamin LE Soap (Altabra from Italy)		Brodkin, R.H., et al.: Sensitivity to Topically Applied Vitamin E (in Tashan Cream). ArchDerm 90, 76, 1965
Vitamin E Deodorant Spray (Mennen)	As is			Contains propellant, Alcohol SD-40, vitamin E, silicone fluid and perfume. (The sensitizer in many cases proved to be vitamin E in this spray)
Vitamin K (Menadiol sodium diphosphate [Kappadione, Synkayvite]; menadione sodium bisulfite [Hykinonel])	0.1% aq.	Production of vitamin K		Jirasek, L.: Hypersensitivity to Vitamin K. Cesk. Derm., 40, 17, 1965
White henna (magnesium carbonate)	As is in pet.	Hair bleaches		

Contactant	Concentration and Vehicle	Exposure	Crossreactions	Comment
White spirits	25% o.o.	Solvent, thinner, turpentine substitute		
Wintergreen, oil of (gaultheria oil)	1% alc.	Flavoring agent, rubefacient, antiseptic, Banalg Liniment (Cole), Ger-O-Foam (Geriatric), Panalgesic (Poythress)	Salicylates	Rich in methyl salicylate
Witch hazel (Hamamelis)	As is	Topical medications, rubefacient, Tucks Pads, Cream, Ointment (Fuller); Hazel-Balm (Arnar-Stone)		Contains tannins and 70–80% alcohol
Wood (sawdust)	As is			Risk of false positive reaction. Controls
Wood tars		See Tar, wood		
Wool alcohols	30% pet.	Lanolin, eucerin, lanolin derivatives		Main sensitizer in lanolin
Xylene (Sylol)	50% o.o.	Solvents, paint removers, lacquers, degreasing cleansers, insecticides, pesticides		
Xylocaine (lidocaine; diethylaminoacet-2,6-xylidide hydrochloride)	2% aq.	Local anesthetic, solution, ointment, jelly, suppositories		Does not crossreact with benzocaine
Ylang-ylang oil	5% pet.	Cosmetics		Cause pigmentation
Zephiran chloride (benzalkonium; Winthrop)	1:1000 aq.sol.	Cationic antiseptic detergent, antirust powder and tablets		
Zinc bisdiethyldithiocarbamate	1% pet.	Rubber antioxidant		
Zinc chloride	1% aq.	Astringents, plumbing, welding, wood preservative		
Zinc ethylenebisdithiocarbamate	1% pet.	Rubber antioxidant		
Zinc oxide	10% pet.	Adhesives, paints, galvanizing, zinc plating, drying agents, dental cements, automobile tires, white ointments and powders, cosmetics		Rare sensitizer. May cause black dermographism
Zinc peroxide	10% pet.	Oxidizing medications, bleaches, healing agents, deodorants, astringents		
Zinc phenosulfonate	1% alc.	Astringents, cosmetics, deodorants (Secret, Top Brass, Arrid, Hi & Dry, Manpower)		
Zinc pyrithione	1% alc.	Dandruff therapy		Photosensitivity
Zinc stearate	10% pet.			May cause irritant granulomas

Contactant	Concentration and Vehicle	Exposure	Crossreactions	Comment
Zinc sulfate	2% pet.	Astringent, styptic pencil		
Zineb	1% pet.	Pesticide	Carbamates	Ethylene-bis(dithiocarbamate) zinc
Ziradyl (Parke, Davis)	As is (patch-scratch)	Topical agent for plant dermatitis		Zirconium oxide, Benadryl. Allergic granuloma
Ziram	1% pet.	Pesticide		
Zircobarb Lotion (Vogel)	As is (patch-scratch)	Topical agent for plant dermatitis		Hydrous zirconium.Allergic granuloma
Zirconium lactate, sodium	0.1% aq. (1:10,000 intracutaneous)	Antiperspirants		Allergic granuloma
Zirconium oxide	0.1% pet.	Ziradyl, Zirium, Zirnox, Rhulihist, Rhulicream, Rhulitol, Ivarest, Allergesic, Zotox		Allergic granuloma
Zirconium silicate	As is (patch-scratch)	Pepsodent Toothpaste		
Zirconyl hydrochloride	10% pet.	Secret Roll-on Deodorant		"Safe" zirconium?
Zirium (Ulmer)	As is (patch-scratch)	Topical agent for poison ivy dermatitis		Zirconium oxide and thenylpyramine. Allergic granuloma
Zirnox (Bristol)	As is (patch-scratch)	Topical agent for plant dermatitis		Allergic granuloma

SUBJECT INDEX

A

Abietic acid, 385, 611
    relationship to colophony, 419
Abitol, 419
Abrasive agents, 332
Absorbent gelling material (AGM), 39
Acacia (gum arabic), 183
    added to foods, 328
Acaricides, 500t
Accroides (yacca), 607t
ACD. *See* Acute contact dermatitis;
        Allergic contact dermatitis
        (ACD)
Aceclofenac, 248–249
Acetaminophen (propacetamol), 246
Acetarsone, 221
Acetate, 193–194
Acetone, 530
Acetylated lanolin (Modulan), 143,
        294
Acetylcysteine, 147
Acetylsalicylic acid (aspirin), 246
    causing systemic contact
        dermatitis, 116
Acetylsulfanilamide, 220t
Achromycin
    mucosal reactions to, 710
Acid dyes, 351
Acitretin
    for garlic dermatitis, 723
Acne
    in black skin from petrolatum, 132
    occupational, 96–97, 524
        cause of, 96t, 525t
    preparations
        containing mercury
            compounds, 195t
        containing resorcinol, 130, 130t
        topical, 201
Acneiform eruptions
    and contactants, 96
    resulting from cosmetics, 300–301

Acne venenata, 97
    with black skin, 52–53
Acral dermatitis, chronic
    with high IgE, 331
Acral lentiginous melanoma, 81
Acrex, 499
Acridine dyes, 204
Acriflavine (acridine) dyes, 204
Acroangiodermatitis
    Kaposi sarcoma-like, 99
Acrokeratoderma
    transient reactive
        papulotranslucent, 75
Acrylamide, 162, 162t
Acrylate
    causing allergic and irritant
        stomatitis, 707
    in inks, 553t
    orthopedic surgery, 372
    in paints, 494t
    in printing plates, 552
    in sculptured nails, 81
Acrylate-resin-based adhesive tapes,
    386
Acrylic(s), 342–343
    patch testing, 554
    possible exposures to, 549t
Acrylic acid
    causing ICU, 627
Acrylic bone cement
    causing ACD, 334
    causing allergic reactions in
        artificial joint rejection, 552
    causing paresthesia, 334
    used in orthopedic prostheses, 552
Acrylic dentures
    causing allergic and irritant
        stomatitis, 707
    patch testing, 717–718
Acrylic monomer, 157–158
    patch testing, 157–158
Acrylic nails, 550
Acrylic plastics, 549

Acrylic resins
    general uses of, 549
    system components, 554
Acrylic socks, 354
Acrylonitrile, 343
    causing paresthesia, 472
ACTAMAR, 200, 458–459
    cross-reaction, 459
ACTH. *See* Adrenocorticotrophic
        hormone (ACTH)
Actifed syrup, 236
Actinic cheilitis, 714
Actinic dermatitis, chronic, 463
Actinic reticuloid syndrome, 94
Acupuncture needle
    dermatitis, 382
    materials, 382t
Acute contact dermatitis, 433, 722
    prednisone, 722
Acute generalized exanthematous
        pustulosis (AGEP), 104, 115, 149
    corticosteroids, 259
    prednisone, 259
Acute onycholysis
    from chemicals, 80
Acyclovir (Zovirax), 225
    causing systemic contact
        dermatitis, 115
Additives
    animal feed, 160, 161t
    chewing gum, 44t
    food, 326–327, 327t, 566, 567t,
        569, 573t
    rubber, 583t, 587, 589
    topical products, 285–286
    in topical products, 285–286
Adhesive(s)
    aids in patch testing, 25–26
    anaerobic, 551–552
    bandages, 385
    Cyanoacrylate
        first-aid treatment for skin
            bonded with, 550

809